Mass Spectrometry

Jürgen H. Gross

Mass Spectrometry

A Textbook

Third Edition

Springer

Jürgen H. Gross
Institute of Organic Chemistry
Heidelberg University
Heidelberg, Germany

DOI 10.1007/978-3-319-54398-7

Printed on acid-free paper

This Springer imprint is published by Springer Nature
The registered company is Springer International Publishing AG
The registered company address is: Gewerbestrasse 11, 6330 Cham, Switzerland

Preface

When non-mass spectrometrists are talking about mass spectrometry, it rather often sounds as if they were telling a story out of Poe's *Tales of Mystery and Imagination*. Indeed, mass spectrometry appears to be regarded as a mysterious method, just good enough to supply some molecular weight information. Unfortunately, this rumor about the dark side of analytical methods may reach students way before their first contact with mass spectrometry. Possibly, some of this may have been bred by some mass spectrometrists who used to celebrate each mass spectrum they obtained from the very first gigantic machines of the early days. Of course, there were also those who enthusiastically started in the 1950s toward developing mass spectrometry out of the domain of physics to become a new analytical tool for chemistry. Within the more than a hundred years since J. J. Thomson's seminal work, there has been a lot that has happened and a lot now to be known and learned about mass spectrometry.

How All This Began

Back in the late 1980s, J. J. Veith's mass spectrometry laboratory at the Technical University of Darmstadt was bright and clean, had no noxious odors, and thus presented a nice contrast to a preparative organic chemistry laboratory. Numerous stainless steel flanges and electronics cabinets were tempting to be explored and – whoops – infected me with CMSD (chronic mass spectrometry disease). Staying with Veith's group slowly transformed me into a mass spectrometrist. Inspiring books such as *Fundamental Aspects of Organic Mass Spectrometry* or *Metastable Ions*, out of stock even in those days, did help me very much during my metamorphosis. Having completed my doctoral thesis on fragmentation pathways of isolated immonium ions in the gas phase, I assumed my current position. Since 1994, I have been head of the mass spectrometry laboratory at the Chemistry Department of Heidelberg University where I teach introductory courses and seminars on mass spectrometry.

When students then asked what books to read on mass spectrometry, there were various excellent monographs, but the ideal textbook still seemed to be missing – at least in my opinion. Finally, 2 years of writing began.

A Third Edition

Now, *Mass Spectrometry – A Textbook* is here in its third edition. For me, the author, preparing the third edition meant an obligation to update and further improve the content of this book. The extent of overall coverage and global organization has not changed as much for this edition as in the transition from the first to the second edition – nonetheless, many new sections have been added to adequately present the recent innovations in this ever-developing field of mass spectrometry. No chapter has remained untouched. Each of the 15 chapters has carefully been reworked and augmented with hundreds of additions, changes, and corrections.

What's New?

Since the second edition, new techniques have gained importance, and some instrumentation has received notable attention and attained considerable commercial success. To keep pace with recent developments, Chap. 4 now includes TOF instruments with folded flight paths, the dynamically harmonized FT-ICR cell, more on hybrid instruments, and ion mobility spectrometry–mass spectrometry. The increasing relevance of high-resolution and accurate mass measurements is even strongly reflected in Chap. 3. The five chapters dedicated to soft ionization methods (CI, APCI, APPI, FAB, LSIMS, FI, FD, LIFDI, ESI, LDI, MALDI) as well as those on ambient desorption/ionization (DESI, DART, REIMS, etc.) and on tandem mass spectrometry have been substantially updated and upgraded. There is also much more on chromatographic techniques (GC, LC) and their coupling to mass spectrometry in Chap. 14.

The way we are using books and literature in general has dramatically changed during the last decade. Back in 2001, when I started preparing the first edition of this book, regular visits to the libraries of several institutions in the area were on my schedule to collect some vast amount of literature. Today, almost all journal articles are electronically available within seconds, and even textbooks are now being extensively used in their e-book versions. This had also some impact on the layout and production process of this book.

In the light of an ever-growing abundance of methods, instruments, tools, and rules in mass spectrometry, the ease of how a complex field of analytical science can be grasped mentally certainly deserves attention. Therefore, the emphasis of my work was on refinement in terms of presentation, convenience of use, and ease of learning. Obviously, a textbook ranging around 900 pages may deter the novice, and thus, my focus was on a didactic and educational approach. Although the actual number of pages has notably increased once again, you will find the textbook easier to read, and you will benefit when transferring theory in actual practice such as spectral interpretation and method selection.

Overall, the third edition of *Mass Spectrometry – A Textbook* comes with lots of didactical improvements:

- Numerous passages have been rewritten and improved while remaining short and concise. Care has been taken not only to explain *how* but also *why* things are done a particular way.
- The number of figures has been notably increased, and about one third of them are now in full color. More photographs and schematics mean easier comprehension of contents, often providing valuable insight into the practical aspects of instrumentation and according procedures.
- Flowcharts have been introduced to describe procedures and approaches to mass spectral interpretation or aid in decision making.
- Bulleted enumerations have been introduced wherever a larger number of features, arguments, assumptions, or properties regarding a subject warrant a clear presentation.
- More examples, especially of methods and applications, are given and some *how-to-style* paragraphs provide practical guidance.
- Examples and notes now come with a short subheading that immediately tells what the particular section is all about.
- All chapters conclude with a concise summary that is subdivided into compact sections highlighting the basic concepts of the subject area, its figures of merit, typical applications, and its role in current MS. Chapter 4 ("Instrumentation") provides summaries of all types of mass analyzers.
- Digital object identifiers (DOIs) are included in the lists of references to facilitate the retrieval of references for e-book users. For those of you who, like me, still prefer a hardbound book, the DOIs offer an additional level of comfort. So, I am pretty convinced that the tedious work of collecting DOIs was very much worth the effort.
- The book's website has been updated providing new exercises and supplementary material (www.ms-textbook.com).

Deepest Gratitude

To all readers of the previous editions of *Mass Spectrometry – A Textbook*, I would like to express my deepest gratitude. Without their interest in wanting to learn more about mass spectrometry by the use of this book, all the efforts in writing it would have been a mere waste of time, and moreover, without their demand for updates, there would be no next edition. I also would like to thank the instructors all over the world who adopted and recommended this book for their own mass spectrometry courses.

Being an author of a textbook means to retrieve, collect, compile, sort, and balance knowledge, findings, and inventions of others. Most of what is written here relies on the intelligence, skill, integrity, and devotion of hundreds of researchers who have contributed to mass spectrometry each in their own way.

Many kind people have supported me in the process of compiling this and the previous editions. I appreciate the detailed knowledge and great thoroughness allocated by Kenzo Hiraoka, Yasuhide Naito, Takemichi Nakamura, and Hiroaki Sato to the translation of the first edition into Japanese. The valuable and welcome comments from readers from all over the world and, in particular, from book reviewers and colleagues have revealed some shortcomings, which now could be adequately addressed.

For the second edition, several competent and renowned colleagues had contributed by carefully checking the according contents in their fields of expertise. I want to express my special thanks to Jürgen Grotemeyer, University of Kiel, for checking Chap. 2 ("Principles of Ionization and Ion Dissociation"); Alexander Makarov, Thermo Fisher Scientific, Bremen (Chap. 4, "Instrumentation"); Christoph A. Schalley, Freie Universität Berlin (Chap. 9, "Tandem Mass Spectrometry"); Belá Paizs, German Cancer Research Center, Heidelberg (Chap. 11, "Matrix-Assisted Laser Desorption/Ionization"); Zoltán Takáts, Universität Gießen (Chap. 13, "Ambient Mass Spectrometry"); and Detlef Günther, ETH Zürich (Chap. 15, "Inorganic Mass Spectrometry").

For the first edition, I want to thank P. Enders, Springer-Verlag Heidelberg ("Introduction"); J. Grotemeyer, University of Kiel ("Gas Phase Ion Chemistry"); S. Giesa, Bayer Industry Services, Leverkusen ("Isotopes"); J. Franzen, Bruker Daltonik, Bremen ("Instrumentation"); J. O. Metzger, University of Oldenburg ("Electron Ionization and Fragmentation of Organic Ions and Interpretation of EI Mass Spectra"); J. R. Wesener, Bayer Industry Services, Leverkusen ("Chemical Ionization"); J. J. Veith, Technical University of Darmstadt ("Field Desorption"); R. M. Caprioli, Vanderbilt University, Nashville ("Fast Atom Bombardment"); M. Karas, University of Frankfurt ("Matrix-Assisted Laser Desorption/Ionization"); M. Wilm, European Molecular Biology Laboratory, Heidelberg ("Electrospray Ionization"); and M. W. Linscheid, Humboldt University, Berlin ("Hyphenated Methods").

Again, many manufacturers of mass spectrometers and mass spectrometry supply are gratefully acknowledged for generously providing schemes and photographs. The author wishes to express his thanks to those scientists, many of them from Heidelberg University, who allowed to use material from their research as examples and to those publishers, who granted the numerous copyrights for the use of figures from their publications. The generous permission of the National Institute of Standards and Technology (S. Stein, G. Mallard, J. Sauerwein) to use a large set of electron ionization mass spectra from the NIST/EPA/NIH Mass Spectral Library is also gratefully acknowledged.

Permission to prepare this third edition alongside my official professional duties, granted by Oliver Trapp, former director of OCI, and Heinfried Schöler, former dean of the Faculty of Chemistry and Earth Sciences, is sincerely acknowledged. Many thanks to my team Doris Lang, Iris Mitsch, and Norbert Nieth for smoothly running the routine analyses in our MS facility. Once more, Theodor C. H. Cole accomplished a great job in polishing up my English. Finally, I am again grateful to my family for their patience and solidarity in times when I had to come home late or needed to vanish on Saturdays during the writing of this book.

Have a good time studying, learning, and enjoying the world of mass spectrometry!

Jürgen H. Gross

Institute of Organic Chemistry (OCI)
Heidelberg University
Im Neuenheimer Feld 270
69120 Heidelberg, Germany
email: author@ms-textbook.com

Contents

Introduction

1

Learning Objectives

- The relevance of mass spectrometry
- Mass spectrometry – Basic concepts
- How mass spectra are displayed and communicated
- The performance features of mass spectrometry
- Basic terminology and conventions in data presentation
- Aims and scope and general organization of this textbook

1.1 Mass Spectrometry: Versatile and Indispensable

Mass spectrometry (MS) is an indispensable analytical tool in chemistry, biochemistry, pharmacy, medicine, and many related fields of science. No student, researcher or practitioner in these disciplines can really get by without a substantial knowledge of mass spectrometry.

Structure elucidation of unknown substances, environmental and forensic analytes, quality control of drugs, foods, and polymers – all rely to a great extent on mass spectrometry [1–7]. Mass spectrometry is employed to analyze combinatorial libraries [8], sequence biomolecules [9], and to explore metabolism in single cells [10, 11]. Today, "mass spectrometry is interwoven with biology to an extent that basic considerations of proteomics research are dealt with in a MS journal" [12]. Crude oils, derived products, and other highly complex mixtures, like dissolved organic matter (DOM), are analyzed by ultrahigh-resolution mass spectrometry [13–15]. Miniaturized mass spectrometers [16] contribute to our safety or can be employed in space missions [17, 18]. There are even some potential uses of mass spectrometry in homes and gardening [19].

J.H. Gross, *Mass Spectrometry*, DOI 10.1007/978-3-319-54398-7_1

Table 1.1 Fields of application of mass spectrometry

Key application and field of application	Explanation
Elemental and isotopic analysis Physics Radiochemistry Geochemistry	Elemental identification and isotopic abundance measurement of both short-lived and stable species in physics and radiochemistry (nuclear waste), in geochemistry and more recently in the life sciences.
Organic and bio-organic analysis Organic chemistry Polymer chemistry Biochemistry and medicine	Identification and structural characterization of molecules from small to very large as provided either by chemistry, physiological processes, or polymer chemistry.
Structure elucidation Organic chemistry Polymer chemistry Biochemistry and medicine	Mass spectrometric experiments can be arranged consecutively to study mass-selected ions in tandem mass spectrometry (MS/MS or MS^2). Eventually products are subjected to a third level (MS^3) and so forth (MS^n).
Characterization of ionic species and chemical reactions Physical chemistry Thermochemistry	Tandem MS provides an elegant means for the study of unimolecular or bimolecular reactions of gas phase ions and for the determination of ion energetics.
Coupling to separation techniques Quality control Environmental analysis Complex mixture analysis Forensics Petroleum chemistry Food chemistry	MS can be coupled to separation methods such as gas chromatography (GC) and liquid chromatography (LC). In 'hyphenation', i.e., as GC-MS or LC-MS, MS delivers high selectivity and low detection limits for the analysis of trace compounds in complicated matrices or the deconvolution of complex mixtures.
Mass spectral imaging Biomedical studies Pharmaceutical developments Material sciences	Mass spectra can be obtained from micrometer-sized areas on surfaces, translating the lateral distribution of compounds on surfaces (microelectronics, slices of tissue) into images, which in turn can be correlated to optical images.
Miniaturization Field portable MS Space missions Military applications	Mass spectrometers can be very small. Portable instruments allow for environmental on-site analysis, detection systems for explosives and warfare chemicals, and last but not least for many space missions.

Whatever the analytical interest may be: mass spectrometry aims to identify a compound from the molecular or atomic mass(es) of its constituents. The information delivered by mass alone can be sufficient for the identification of elements and the determination of the molecular formula of an analyte. The relative abundance of isotopologs helps to decide which elements contribute to such a formula and to estimate the number of atoms of a contributing element. Under the conditions of certain mass spectrometric experiments, fragmentation of ions can deliver information on ionic structure. Thus, MS elucidates the connectivity of atoms within smaller molecules, identifies functional groups, determines the (average) number and eventually the sequence of constituents of macromolecules, and in some cases even yields their three-dimensional structure (Table 1.1).

1.2 Historical Sketch

1.2.1 The First Mass Spectra

The first instrument to separate ions by mass-to-charge ratio was constructed by Joseph John Thomson (Nobel Prize in physics in 1906 for the discovery of the electron) in his attempt to understand electric discharges in gases and to analyze the charged gas phase species involved. His work [20–23] led to the discovery of atoms, isotopes, and thus to his recognition as the father of mass spectrometry (Fig. 1.1). While Thomson's original book from 1913 is hard to come by, there is a reprint by the *American Society for Mass Spectrometry* (ASMS) that is readily available.

Particularly due to Francis William Aston's work in the following decade, the new revolutionary technique soon provided means for the atomic characterization of numerous elements [24–28] for which Aston was awarded the Nobel Prize in chemistry in 1922 [29, 30]. Further Nobel Prizes related to MS are tabulated in the Appendix.

1.2.2 Thomson's Parabola Spectrograph

Thomson's apparatus, the parabola spectrograph, employs parallel magnetic and electric fields to achieve a deflection of ionic species depending on charge sign, charge, and mass. Ions exiting the ion source are passed through a collimator to create a roughly parallel beam that is then sent into the analyzer (Fig. 1.2) [23, 31]. The electric field of a planar capacitor deflects ions vertically either upward (cations in this illustration) or downward (anions) depending on their

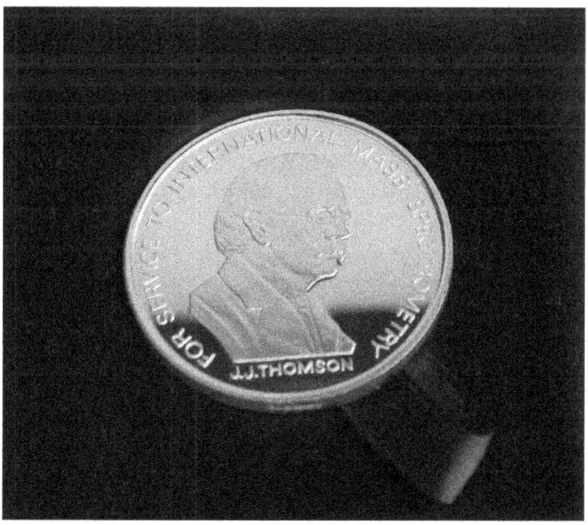

Fig. 1.1 The Thomson Medal in honor of Joseph John Thomson, generally regarded as the father of mass spectrometry, is awarded by the *International Mass Spectrometry Foundation* (IMSS) to outstanding scientists in the field of mass spectrometry

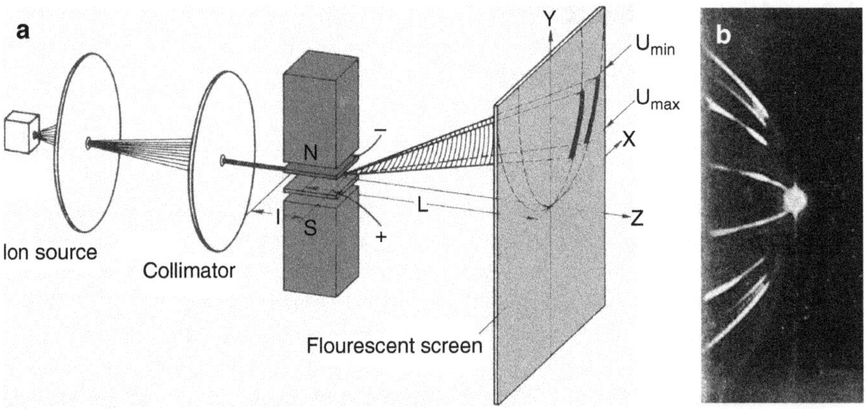

Fig. 1.2 Parabola spectrograph as constructed by J. J. Thomson. (**a**) Schematic, (**b**) photograph of the light emission from the fluorescent screen as obtained with this instrument (shown rotated by 90° with respect to the schematic) (Adapted from Ref. [31] with kind permission of Curt Brunnée)

charge sign. As fast ions will be deflected by a smaller angle than slower ones, the angle of y-deflection is a measure of ion kinetic energy. The magnetic field bends the beam horizontally in a way that depends on the mass-to-charge ratio and, again, charge sign. Heavier ions stay closer to the axis while lighter ones are pushed further out. Overall, this results in light emission on the fluorescent screen along parabolic branches, one branch per ion species that allow reading the ion momentum from the x-axis and kinetic energy from the y-axis. Thus, this apparently simple device simultaneously delivers a wealth of information. (Details on how magnetic and electric fields effect ion separation will be dealt with in Sect. 4.3.)

1.2.3 Milestones

Thomson and Aston only marked the beginnings of what expanded into more than a century of exciting developments in mass spectrometry, the major milestones of which were recently compiled [32]. From the 1950s to the present, mass spectrometry has made major strides and innovations are still being made at an enormous pace [29, 30, 33, 34].

The pioneering mass spectrometrist worked with home-built rather than commercial instruments. These machines, typically magnetic sector instruments using electron ionization, delivered a few mass spectra per day, providing that the device was delicately handled. Intimate knowledge of such an instrument and interpretation skills of the according EI spectra would provide the mass spectrometrist with a previously unknown wealth of insight into structural details [35–40]. The life sciences, in particular, have provided a great impetus for new developments that expand the mass range to higher molecular weights and increasingly fragile molecules. Environmental and pharmaceutical research has been a driving force in reaching even lower limits of detection. Current research is aimed at methods of ion sampling, ion generation, and subsequent ion transfer into mass analyzers for superior performance.

Nowadays, the output of mass spectra has reached an unprecedented level. Highly automated systems produce thousands of spectra per day when running a routine application where samples of the very same type are to be treated by an analytical protocol that has been carefully elaborated by an expert beforehand. A large number of ionization methods and types of mass analyzers has been developed and combined in various ways. Thus, people sometimes feel overwhelmed by the mere task of selecting one out of about a dozen of promising techniques available for their particular sample. It is precisely this diversity that makes a basic understanding of the concepts and tools of mass spectrometry more important than ever. On the other extreme, there are mass spectrometry laboratories specialized on employing only one particular method – preferably matrix-assisted laser desorption/ionization (MALDI) or electrospray ionization (ESI). In contrast to some 50 years ago, the instrumentation is now concealed in a sort of "black box", more appealingly designed to resemble an espresso machine. So let us take a look inside!

1.3 Aims and Scope of This Textbook

This book is tailored to be your guide to mass spectrometry – from the first steps to your daily work in research. Starting from the very principles of gas phase ion chemistry and isotopic properties, it leads you through the design of mass analyzers, mass spectral interpretation, and applied ionization methods. The book closes with chapters on chromatography-mass spectrometry coupling and one on inorganic mass spectrometry. In total, it comprises fifteen chapters that can be read independently from each other. However, for the novice it is recommended to work through from start to finish, occasionally skipping over more advanced sections (Table 1.2). Now in its 3rd edition, "Mass Spectrometry – A Textbook" continues to be your companion from undergraduate to graduate studies in chemistry, biochemistry, and other natural sciences, and aims to hold its value when serving as a hands-on reference in the course of professional life.

Step by step, you will understand how mass spectrometry works and what it can do as a powerful tool in your hands – equally well for analytical applications as for basic research. An improved layout and additional high-quality figures, about one third of them now in color, will make is easier and quicker to acquire the new knowledge. Many tables and flow charts have been added, compiling facts and comparing topics. Interrelationships are pointed to where appropriate. The correctness of scientific content has been examined by leading experts. Each chapter begins with a set of Learning Objectives and now also closes with a brief Summary followed by an elaborate list of references, emphasizing tutorial and review articles, book chapters, and monographs in the respective fields. Titles are included with all citations to help with the evaluation of useful further reading [41] and *digital object*

Table 1.2 Chapters of this book: overview for orientation

No.	Chapter title	Comment
1	Introduction	Getting ready, getting started
2	Principles of Ionization and Ion Dissociation	Tools of the trade. Basics needed for the understanding of any of the subsequent chapters
3	Isotopic Composition and Accurate Mass	
4	Instrumentation	
5	Practical Aspects of Electron Ionization	Electron ionization: the classical key to organic MS and indispensable part of every introductory course
6	Fragmentation of Organic Ions and Interpretation of EI Mass Spectra	
7	Chemical Ionization	Traditional, nonetheless still highly relevant soft ionization methods
8	Field Ionization and Field Desorption	
9	Tandem Mass Spectrometry	Fully controlled dissociation of mass-selected ions for many interesting purposes
10	Fast Atom Bombardment	More soft ionization methods. The latter two represent today's most relevant techniques in MS
11	Matrix-Assisted Laser Desorption/ Ionization	
12	Electrospray Ionization	
13	Ambient Desorption/Ionization	Exciting rather new field based on advances in atmospheric pressure ionization methods
14	Hyphenated Methods	Coupling of separation techniques to MS
15	Inorganic Mass Spectrometry	There is even more: a glimpse beyond the horizon of organic and biomedical MS

identifiers (DOIs) have been added to facilitate retrieval of the articles. References for general further reading on mass spectrometry are compiled at the end of this Introduction.

The coverage of this book is basically restricted to what is called "organic mass spectrometry" in a broad sense. It includes the ionization methods and mass analyzers currently in use, and in addition to classical organic compounds it covers applications to bio-organic samples such as peptides and oligonucleotides. Of course, transition metal complexes, synthetic polymers, and fullerenes are discussed as well as environmental or forensic applications. Elemental analysis, the classical field of inorganic mass spectrometry has been added to get a taste of mass spectrometry beyond molecular species.

Exercises

Many elaborate examples are included in this textbook, while conventional "problems and solutions" sections are omitted. Exercises complementing each chapter are available for free on the textbook's dedicated website at http://www.ms-textbook.com.

1.3.1 Facets of Mass Spectrometry

There is no single "golden rule" in approaching the wide field of mass spectrometry. In any case, it is necessary to learn about the ways of sample introduction, generation of ions, their mass analysis, and their detection as well as about data recording and presentation of mass spectra – and what's more is the art of interpreting mass spectra. All these aspects are correlated to each other in many ways and in their entirety contribute to what is referred to as mass spectrometry (Fig. 1.3). In other words, mass spectrometry is multi-facet rather than to be viewed from a single perspective. Like a view onto a globe does not reveal the complete surface of our planet, but roughly just one continent at a time, mass spectrometry needs to be explored from various vantage points [42].

1.4 What Is Mass Spectrometry?

Now, what is mass spectrometry? Well in any case, mass spectrometry is special in many ways. Up front, most *mass spectrometrists* do not fathom to be addressed as *mass spectroscopists*.

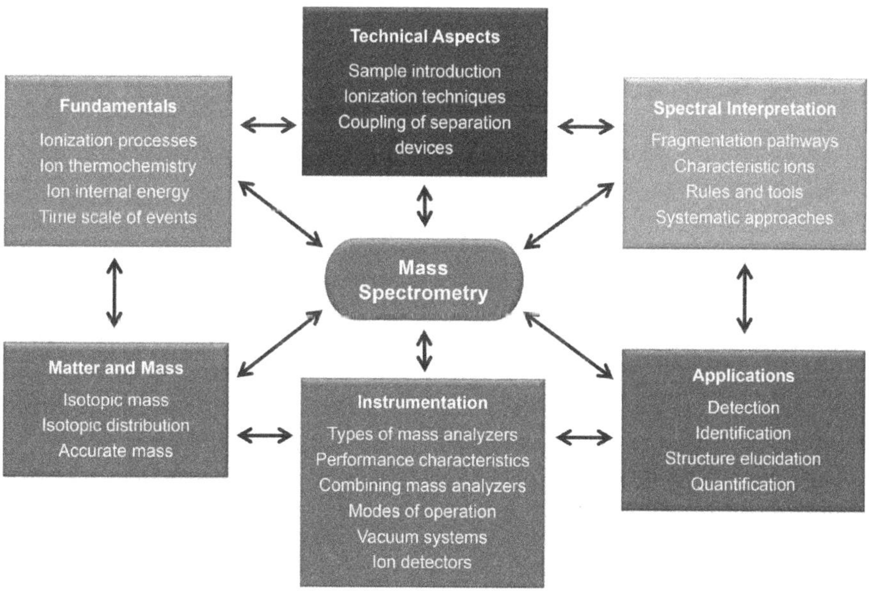

Fig. 1.3 The many facets of mass spectrometry. Each aspect is closely related to the others in various ways. Their assemblage yields an impression of the dimensions of MS

Zeroth law of mass spectrometry

"First of all, never make the mistake of calling it 'mass spectroscopy'. Spectroscopy involves the absorption of electromagnetic radiation, and mass spectrometry is different, as we will see. The mass spectrometrists sometimes get upset if you confuse this issue" [43].

Indeed, there is almost no book using the term *mass spectroscopy* and all scientific journals in the field bear *mass spectrometry* in their titles. You will find such highlighted rules, hints, notes, and definitions throughout the book. This more amusing one – we might call it the "zeroth law of mass spectrometry" – has been taken from a standard organic chemistry textbook. The same author completes his chapter on mass spectrometry with the conclusion that "despite occasional mysteries, mass spectrometry is still highly useful" [43].

Historical remark

Another explanation for this terminology originates from the historical development of our instrumentation [29]. The device employed by Thomson for the first mass-separating experiments was a type of *spectroscope* showing blurred signals on a fluorescent screen [44]. Dempster constructed an instrument with a deflecting magnetic field angled at 180°. In order to detect different masses, it could either be equipped with a photographic plate – a so-called *mass spectrograph* – or it could have a variable magnetic field to detect different masses by focusing them successively onto an electric point detector [45]. Later, the term *mass spectrometer* was coined for the latter type of instruments using a *scanning* magnetic field [46].

1.4.1 Basic Principle of Mass Spectrometry

"The basic principle of *mass spectrometry* (MS) is to generate ions from either inorganic or organic compounds by any suitable method, to separate these ions by their *mass-to-charge ratio* (m/z) and to detect them qualitatively and quantitatively by their respective m/z and abundance. The analyte may be ionized thermally, by electric fields or by impacting energetic electrons, ions or photons. The ... ions can be single ionized atoms, clusters, molecules or their fragments or associates. Ion separation is effected by static or dynamic electric or magnetic fields." Although this definition of mass spectrometry dates back to 1968 when organic mass spectrometry was in its infancy [47], it is still valid. However, some additions should be made. First, ionization of a sample can be effected not only by electrons, but also by (atomic) ions or photons, energetic neutral atoms, electronically excited atoms, massive cluster ions, and even electrostatically charged microdroplets can also be used to effect. Second, as demonstrated with great success by the time-of-flight

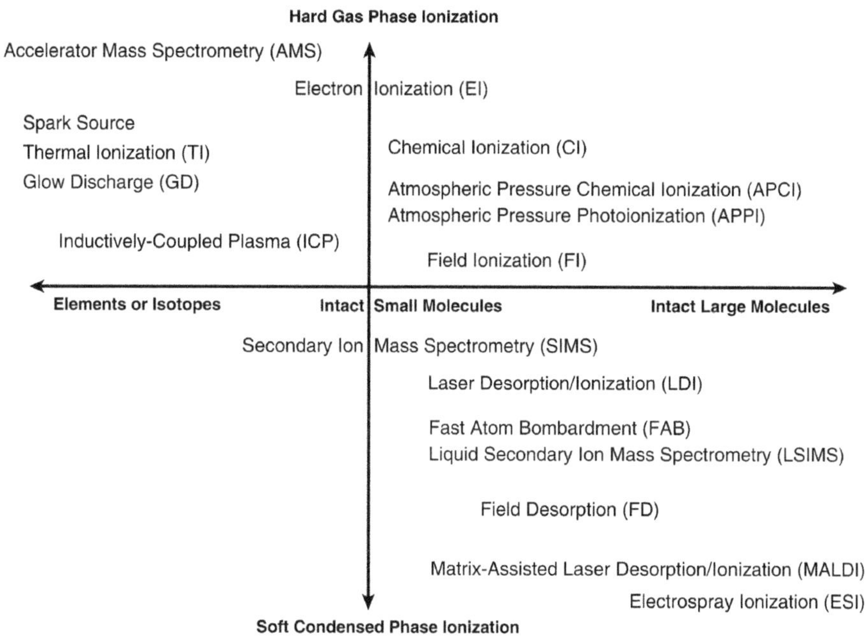

Fig. 1.4 Mass spectrometric techniques for different needs arranged by main fields of application and estimated relative hardness or softness (Reproduced from Ref. [42] by permission. © Wiley-VCH, Weinheim, 2009)

analyzer, ion separation by *m/z* can also be effected in field-free regions, provided the ions possess a well-defined kinetic energy at the entrance of the flight path.

The large variety of ionization techniques and their key applications can be roughly classified by their relative hardness or softness and (molecular) mass of suitable analytes (Fig. 1.4).

1.4.2 Mass Spectrometer

Obviously, almost any technique to achieve the goals of ionization, separation and detection of ions in the gas phase can be applied – and actually has been applied – in mass spectrometry. Fortunately, there is a simple basic scheme that all mass spectrometers follow. A mass spectrometer consists of an *ion source*, a *mass analyzer*, and a *detector* which are operated under high vacuum conditions. A closer look at the front end of such a device might separate the steps of *sample introduction*, *evaporation*, and successive *ionization* or *desorption/ionization*, respectively, but it is not always trivial to identify each of these steps as clearly separated from each other. Since the 1990s, mass spectrometers are operated under total data system control. The latter is also highly important for data acquisition, customization of spectral plots, and in-depth data analysis (Fig. 1.5).

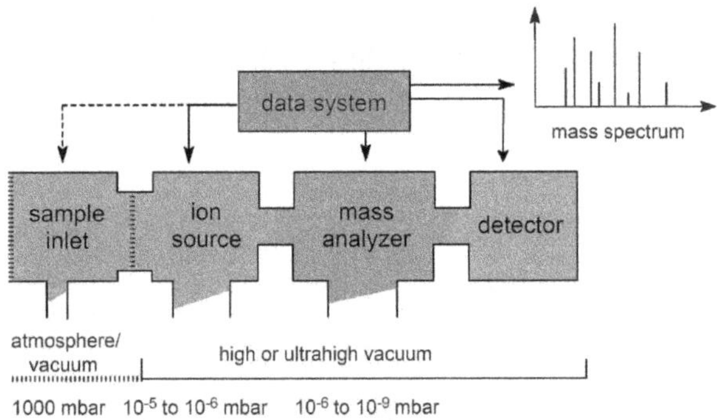

Fig. 1.5 General layout of mass spectrometers. Several types of sample inlets can be attached to the ion source housing. Transfer of the sample from atmospheric pressure into the high vacuum of the ion source and mass analyzer is accomplished by use of a vacuum lock (Sect. 5.2) or other types of interfaces (Sect. 12.2)

The *consumption of analyte* by its examination in the mass spectrometer is an aspect deserving our attention: Whereas other spectroscopic methods such as nuclear magnetic resonance (NMR), infrared (IR) or Raman spectroscopy do allow for sample recovery, mass spectrometry is destructive, i.e., it consumes the analyte. This is apparent from the process of ionization and translational motion through the mass analyzer to the detector during analysis. Although some sample is consumed, it may still be regarded as practically nondestructive, however, because the amount of analyte needed is in the low microgram range or even by several orders of magnitude below. In turn, the extremely low sample consumption of mass spectrometry makes it the method of choice when most other analytical techniques fail because they are not able to yield analytical information from nanogram amounts of sample.

1.4.3 Mass Scale

Plotting mass spectra on a physical scale of mass per electric charge (kg C^{-1}) would be very inconvenient to use. Thus, mass spectrometrists have adopted the use of a scale of atomic mass per number of elementary charges and termed it *mass-to-charge ratio*, *m*/*z*, (read "m over z" and write *m*/*z*) [48]. There is only one correct writing convention: the location of a peak on the abscissa is to be reported as "at *m*/*z x*".

Unfortunately, *m*/*z* is a rather artificial construct, as it has not received the status of a physical unit. Instead, *m*/*z* is dimensionless by definition. It may be understood as the ratio of the numerical value of ionic mass on the atomic mass scale and the number of elementary charges of the respective ion. The number of elementary charges is often, but by far not necessarily, equal to one. As long as only singly charged ions are observed ($z = 1$) the *m*/*z* scale directly reflects the atomic mass scale. However, there can be conditions where doubly, triply, or even highly charged ions are being created from the analyte depending on the ionization method employed.

Thomson versus *m/z*
Some mass spectrometrists use the unit *thomson* [Th] (to honor J. J. Thomson) instead of the dimensionless quantity *m/z*. Although the thomson is accepted (or tolerated), it is not an SI unit. The Thomson is equivalent to *m/z* in that there is no conversion factor between these units.

The distance between peaks on that axis has the meaning of a neutral loss from the ion at higher *m/z* to produce the fragment ion at lower *m/z*. Therefore, the amount of this neutral loss is given as "*x* u", where the symbol u stands for *unified atomic mass*. It is important to notice that the mass of the neutral is only reflected by the difference between the corresponding *m/z* values, i.e., $\Delta(m/z)$. This is because the mass spectrometer detects only charged species, i.e., the charge-retaining group of a fragmenting ion. Since 1961 the *unified atomic mass* [u] has been defined as $^1/_{12}$ of the mass of one single atom of the nuclide ^{12}C, which, by convention, has been set to precisely 12 u (Sect. 3.1).

Dalton versus u
Mass spectrometrists working in the biomedical field tend to use the *dalton* [Da] (to honor J. Dalton) instead of the *unified atomic mass* [u]. The dalton also is not an SI unit. The dalton is equivalent to unified atomic mass in that there is no conversion factor between these units.

1.4.4 Mass Spectrum

A *mass spectrum* is the two-dimensional representation of signal intensity (ordinate) versus *m/z* (abscissa). The position of a *peak*, as signals are usually called, reflects the *m/z* of an ion that has been created from the analyte within the ion source. The *intensity* of this peak correlates to the *abundance* of that ion.

Sometimes but not necessarily, the peak at highest *m/z* results from the detection of the intact ionized molecule, the *molecular ion*, $M^{+\bullet}$. The *molecular ion peak* is usually accompanied by several peaks at lower *m/z* caused by fragmentation of the molecular ion to yield *fragment ions*. Consequently, the respective peaks in the mass spectrum may be referred to as *fragment ion peaks*.

The most intense peak of a mass spectrum is called *base peak*. In most representations of mass spectral data the intensity of the base peak is normalized to 100% *relative intensity*. This largely helps to make mass spectra more easily comparable. The normalization can be done because the relative intensities are basically independent from the absolute ion abundances registered by the detector.

Our first mass spectrum In the electron ionization mass spectrum of a particular hydrocarbon, the molecular ion peak and the base peak of the spectrum happen to correspond to the same ionic species at *m*/*z* 16 (Fig. 1.6). The fragment ion peaks at *m*/*z* 12–15 are spaced at $\Delta(m/z) = 1$. Obviously, the molecular ion, $M^{+\bullet}$, fragments by loss of $H^\bullet$ which is the only possibility to explain the peak at *m*/*z* 15 by loss of a neutral of 1 u mass. Accordingly, the peaks at lower *m*/*z* might arise from loss of an H_2 molecule (2 u) and so forth. It is rather obvious that this spectrum corresponds to methane, CH_4, showing its molecular ion peak at *m*/*z* 16 because the atomic mass of carbon is 12 u and that of hydrogen is 1 u, and therefore 12 u + 4 × 1 u = 16 u. Removal of one electron from a 16 u neutral yields a singly-charged radical ion that is detected at *m*/*z* 16 by the mass spectrometer. Of course, most mass spectra are not that simple, but this is how it works.

1.4.5 Statistical Nature of Mass Spectra

It is important to be aware that a single molecule can only yield one ion of one *m*/*z* value. This ion may either reflect the intact molecule or any of its fragment ions. Statistics on thousands of ion formations and dissociations are needed to generate a useful mass spectrum exhibiting signals at different *m*/*z* where each of them can be assigned a relevant relative intensity. To understand this, simply imagine a single methane molecule that gets ionized and detected as a molecular ion: this would lead to a spectrum showing a single line at *m*/*z* 16, the intensity of which would have no meaning beyond 'yes' and 'no' (Fig. 1.7a). Alternatively, the molecular ion might fragment to yield a single CH_3^+ ion at *m*/*z* 15; again, the spectrum would show only one line. In fact, such a spectrum could not tell us whether the peak is caused by a molecular or a fragment ion. Eight ions might lead to a spectrum where each ion corresponds to 33.3% relative intensity (as in Fig. 1.7c) even though other distributions would be possible. Eleven ions could scale the intensity in 20%

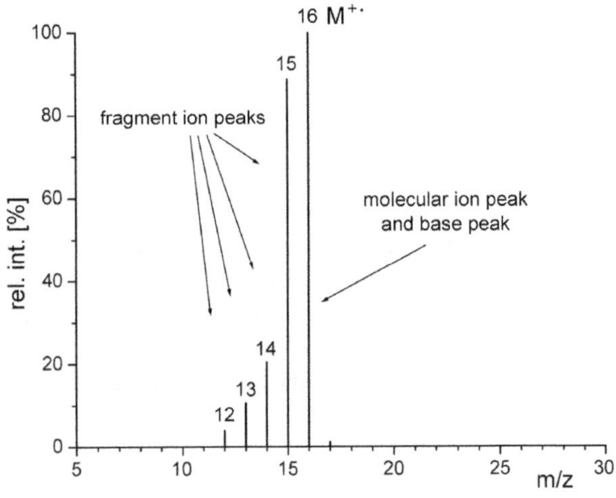

Fig. 1.6 Electron ionization mass spectrum of a low-mass hydrocarbon (Adapted with permission. © National Institute of Standards and Technology, NIST, 2002)

steps, while 23 ions could lead to a spectrum with 10% steps. It is evident that a spectrum with intensity levels as accurate as 0.1% has to be based on thousands of ions (Fig. 1.7f).

Attomole sensitivity? Sometimes, instruments are advertised to offer attomol sensitivity. Is this possible at all? The amount of 1 amol = 10^{-18} mol still corresponds to $6.022 \times 10^{23} \times 10^{-18} = 6.022 \times 10^{5}$ molecules. Assuming 10% of the sample could be ionized and 10% of this fraction would be detected, the resulting spectrum would still be based on 1% of the sample molecules, i.e., 6000 ions. Obviously, attomole sensitivity touches on the limit of what is required to deliver a useful spectrum.

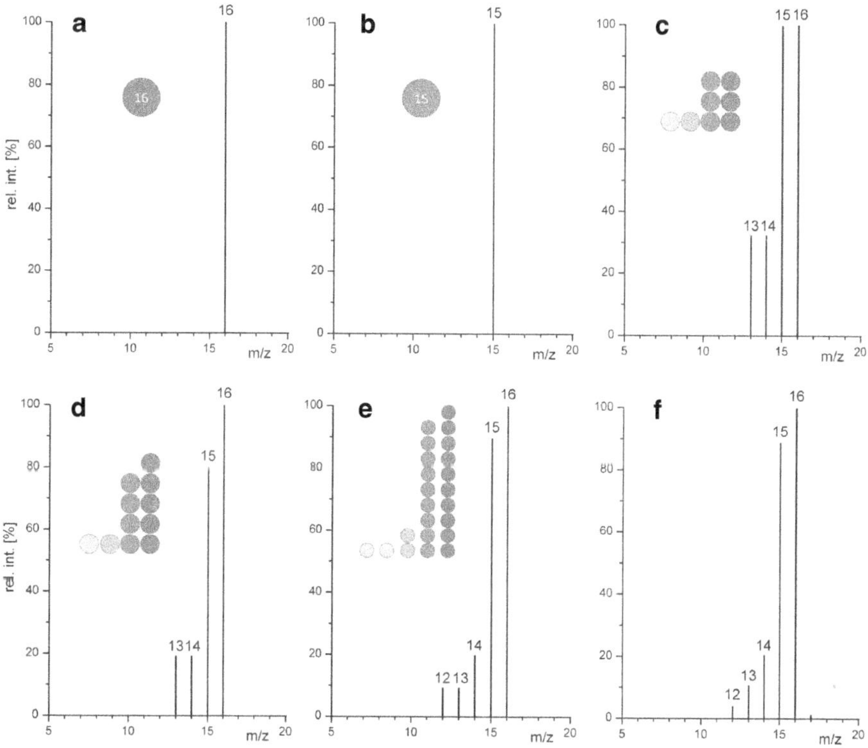

Fig. 1.7 Statistical nature of mass spectra and the appearance of methane spectra based on very low numbers of ions. (**a**) and (**b**) by one ion, (**c**) by eight ions, (**d**) by eleven ions, (**e**) by 23 ions, and (**f**) by thousands. The isotope peak of 1.1% relative intensity at *m/z* 17 is only visible and meaningful in the case of (**f**)

Avoid overload
There is also an upper limit for the number of ions and neutrals per volume inside the ion source from the point of which the appearance of spectra will significantly change due to ion–molecule reactions (Sect. 7.2).

1.4.6 Bars, Profiles, and Lists

The above spectra are represented as a *bar graph* or *histogram*. Such *data reduction* is common in mass spectrometry and useful as long as peaks are well resolved. The intensities of the peaks can be obtained either from measured peak heights or more correctly from peak areas. The position, i.e., the *m/z* ratio, of the signal is determined from its centroid. Noise below some user-defined cut level is usually subtracted from the bar graph spectrum. If peak shape and peak width become important, e.g., in case of high-mass analytes or high-resolution measurements, spectra should be represented as *profile data* as initially acquired by the mass spectrometer. *Tabular listings* of mass spectra are used to report mass and intensity data more accurately (Fig. 1.8).

Accurate intensity data is important for the analysis of isotope patterns. Also, accurate mass data can be used to derive the elemental composition of ions (Sect. 3.5).

1.5 Ion Chromatograms

Gas chromatography (GC) and liquid chromatography (LC) result in the separation and subsequent elution of the components of a mixture from the chromatographic column at individual *retention times*. When a mass spectrometer is employed as the

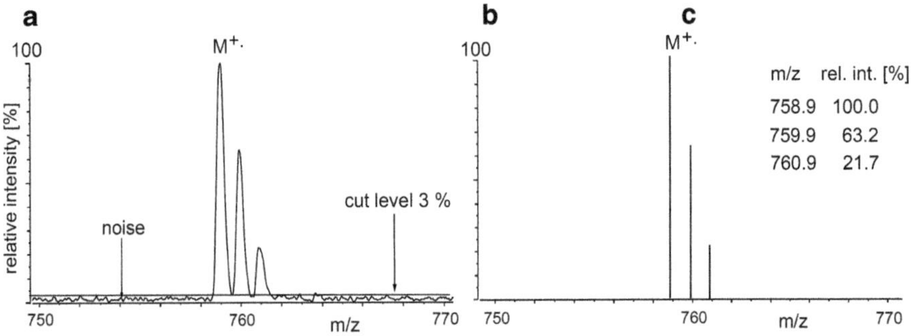

Fig. 1.8 Tetrapentacontane, $C_{54}H_{110}$: Three representations of the molecular ion signal in the field desorption mass spectrum (Sect. 8.6) (**a**) profile spectrum, (**b**) bar graph representation, and (**c**) tabular listing

chromatographic detector (GC-MS and LC-MS, Sects. 5.4 and 5.5; Chap. 14) its output must somehow represent the chromatogram that would otherwise have been obtained with "classic" chromatographic detectors (FID, TCD, UV). The chromatogram as produced by the mass spectrometer is composed of a large *set of consecutively acquired mass spectra*, each providing mass spectral data of the eluting species. Thus, the components can be identified one after the other by their individual mass spectra. Because mass spectral chromatograms represent ionic abundances as a function of retention time, these are termed *ion chromatograms.*

The *total ion current* (TIC) can either be measured by a *hardware TIC monitor* before mass analysis (nA to μA range), or its equivalent can be *reconstructed* or *extracted* after mass analysis [49]. Both adjectives, reconstructed and extracted, serve to illustrate that the chromatogram has been obtained post-acquisition from a set of spectra by a computational process that selects user-defined signals to build the trace.

True TIC
Modern instruments do not anymore support hardware TIC measurements, but until the 1970s, there used to be a hardware TIC monitor on the electronics panel. The TIC was obtained by measuring the ion current caused by those ions hitting the ion source exit plate instead of passing through its slit.

Thus, the TIC represents a measure of the overall intensity of ion production or of mass spectral output as a function of time, respectively. The TIC obtained by means of *data reduction* [50], i.e., by summation of peak intensities of each mass spectrum as successively acquired during analysis, is termed *total ion chromatogram* (TIC). For this purpose, the sums of all ion intensities belonging to each of the spectra is plotted as a function of time or scan number, respectively.

The term *total ion current chromatogram* (TICC) refers to a chromatogram obtained by plotting the total ion current detected in each of a series of mass spectra recorded as a function of retention times of the chromatographically separated components of a mixture (which essentially is implicated by: TIC). Sometimes we find combinations such as *reconstructed total ion current* (RTIC) or *reconstructed total ion current chromatogram* (RTICC, Table 1.3).

The term *reconstructed ion chromatogram* (RIC) was and still is used by many to describe the intensity of a given *m*/*z* or *m*/*z* range plotted as a function of time or scan number. Recently, the term *extracted ion chromatogram* (EIC) has been used to describe a chromatogram created by plotting the intensity of the signal observed at a chosen *m*/*z* value or set of values in a series of mass spectra recorded as a function of retention time. Plotting RICs or EICs is especially useful to identify a target compound of known *m*/*z* from complex GC-MS or LC-MS data. In other words, the RIC allows to retrieve the retention time of the target compound. RICs can also be used to uncover the relationship of certain *m*/*z* values to different mass spectra obtained from the measurement of a single (impure) sample. Thus, RICs

Table 1.3 Ion chromatograms

Acronym	Full name	Explanation
TIC	Total ion chromatogram	Sum of all signal intensities per spectrum vs. retention time. TIC is recommended.
TICC	Total ion current chromatogram	
RTIC	Reconstructed total ion chromatogram	
RTICC	Reconstructed total ion current chromatogram	
RIC	Reconstructed ion chromatogram	Signal intensity at selected *m/z* vs. retention time. Both are in use.
EIC	Extracted ion chromatogram	
BPC	Base peak chromatogram	Base peak intensity of each spectrum plotted vs. retention time.

(EICs) often reveal valuable information on impurities accompanying the main product, e.g., remaining solvents, plasticizers, vacuum grease, or synthetic by-products (Sect. 5.2 and Appendix A.9).

Finally, the *base peak chromatogram* (BPC) is a chromatogram obtained by plotting the intensity of the base peak detected in each of a series of mass spectra recorded as a function of retention time. BPCs can be useful to enhance the visibility of compound peaks in a complex chromatogram, especially when soft ionization methods are employed that cause most of the ion current to occur in one ionic species.

Ion chromatograms Polycyclic and nitro musks are frequently used as fragrances in cosmetic products. A GC-MC procedure for their identification and quantitation employs the characteristic RICs (EICs) of tonalide (AHTN), $C_{18}H_{26}O^{+\bullet}$, *m/z* 258, and xylene musk (MX), $C_{12}H_{15}N_3O_6^{+\bullet}$, *m/z* 297 [51]. Although eluting simultaneously (peak **3** in Fig. 1.9), EICs allow to separate both components by choosing characteristic *m/z* values, e.g., of the respective molecular ions or abundant fragment ions. The concentration of the solution injected was in the order of 1 μg ml^{-1} per component.

A certain degree of fractionation is also observed during evaporation of mixtures from a *direct insertion probe* (DIP), although the separation by far cannot be compared to that of chromatographic systems. Nonetheless, plotting the TIC or a RIC yields an overview of the temporal distribution of component spectra across a measurement using a DIP (Sect. 5.2).

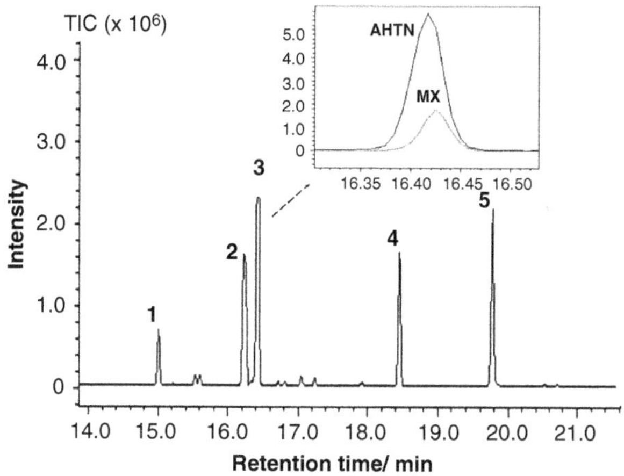

Fig. 1.9 Typical GC-MS chromatogram, i.e., TIC (TICC) in full scan mode for synthetic musks and some standards. However, the elution of two components occurs almost simultaneously and leads to superimposed peaks. The inset shows the characteristic RICs (EICs) of tonalide (AHTN), $C_{18}H_{26}O^{+\bullet}$, *m/z* 258, and xylene musk (MX), $C_{12}H_{15}N_3O_6^{+\bullet}$, *m/z* 297 (Reproduced from Ref. [51] with permission. © The Japan Society for Analytical Chemistry, 2009)

1.6 Performance of Mass Spectrometers

1.6.1 Sensitivity

The term *sensitivity* specifies the overall response of any analytical system for a certain analyte when operated under well-defined conditions. The *sensitivity* is defined as the slope of a plot of analyte amount vs. signal strength. In mass spectrometry, sensitivity is reported as electric charge of a specified ion species reaching the detector per mass of analyte used. The sensitivity is given in units of C μg^{-1} for solids [49]; for gaseous analytes, it can be specified as the ratio of ion current to analyte partial pressure in units of A Pa^{-1} [50].

According to the above definition, sensitivity does not only depend on the ionization efficiency of EI or any other ionization method. Also relevant are the extraction of ions from the ion source, the mass range acquired during the experiment, and the transmission of the mass analyzer. Therefore, the complete experimental conditions have to be stated with sensitivity data.

Calculating sensitivity Magnetic sector instruments are specified to have a sensitivity of about 4×10^{-7} C μg^{-1} for the molecular ion of methylstearate, *m/z* 298, at $R = 1000$ in 70 eV EI mode. One microgram of methylstearate is equivalent to 3.4×10^{-9} mol or 2.0×10^{15} molecules. The charge of 4×10^{-7} C corresponds to 2.5×10^{12} electron charges of 1.6×10^{-19} C each. Vice versa, in dividing the number of molecules per microgram by the number of charges at the detector we may conclude that only one out of 800 molecules is finally detected.

1.6.2 Limit of Detection

The *limit of detection* (LOD), also termed *detection limit*, is almost self-explanatory, yet it is often confused with sensitivity. The limit of detection defines the smallest flow or the lowest amount of analyte necessary to obtain a signal that can be discerned from the background noise. The detection limit is valid for one well-specified analyte upon treatment according to a particular analytical protocol [49, 50, 52].

Of course, the sensitivity of an instrumental setup is of key importance to low detection limits; nevertheless, the detection limit is a clearly different quantity. The detection limit may either be stated as a relative measure in trace analysis, e.g., 1 ppb of dioxin in waste oil samples (equivalent to 1 $\mu g\ kg^{-1}$ of sample), or as an absolute measure, e.g., 1 femtomol of substance P in MALDI-MS.

1.6.3 Signal-to-Noise Ratio

The *signal-to-noise ratio* (S/N) describes the uncertainty of an intensity measurement and provides a quantitative measure of a signal's quality by quantifying the ratio of the intensity of a signal relative to noise.

Noise results from the electronics of an instrument, and thus noise is not only present *between* the signals but also *on* the signals. Consequently, intensity measurements are influenced by noise. Real and very numerous background signals of various origin, e.g., matrix compounds as employed in fast atom bombardment (FAB) or matrix-assisted laser desorption/ionization (MALDI), column bleed in gas chromatography (GC), and other impurities can appear to be electronic noise, so-called "chemical" noise. In the strict sense, this should be distinct from electronic noise and should be reported as *signal-to-background ratio* (S/B) [52]. In practice, this can be difficult to do.

Electronic noise is statistical in nature, and therefore can be reduced by elongated data acquisition and subsequent summing or averaging of the spectra, respectively. Accordingly, an intensive peak has a better S/N than a low-intensity peak within the same spectrum.

The reduction of noise is proportional to the square root of acquisition time or number of single spectra that are averaged [53], e.g., the noise is reduced by a factor of 3.16 by averaging 10 spectra or by a factor of 10 by averaging 100 spectra, respectively.

How much noise? Signals are regarded to be clearly visible at $S/N \geq 10$, a value often stated in the context of detection limits. A mass spectrometer in good condition yields $S/N > 10^4$, which means in turn that even isotopic peaks of low

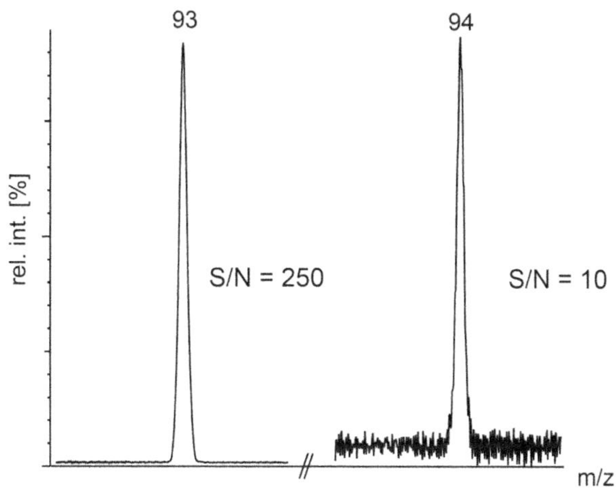

Fig. 1.10 Signal-to-noise ratio. Among the signals due to the toluene molecular ion, the first isotopic peak at *m/z* 93 has S/N = 250, while the second isotopic peak at *m/z* 94 has S/N = 10

relative intensity can be reliably measured, provided there is no interference with background signals. Among the signals from the toluene molecular ion in the below figure, the first isotopic peak resulting from $[^{13}C^{12}C_6H_8]^{+\bullet}$ at *m/z* 93, still had S/N = 250 while the second isotopic peak resulting from $[^{13}C_2{}^{12}C_5H_8]^{+\bullet}$ at *m/z* 94 just had S/N = 10 (Fig. 1.10). The theoretical ratio of intensities of the peaks at *m/z* 92 : 93 : 94 is given by 100 : 7.7 : 0.3, i.e., the ratio of intensities directly reflects the S/N ratio. Pursuing this consideration, we may expect the peak at *m/z* 92 that corresponds to $[^{12}C_7H_8]^{+\bullet}$ to have had S/N = 3250. In practice, S/N $\geq$ 1000 means that noise is essentially invisible in the spectral plot.

1.7 Terminology – General Aspects

General consensus regarding terms, acronyms, and symbols is of paramount importance for adequate communication in mass spectrometry. The currently accepted terminology is chiefly governed by the following publications:

- 1991: Compilation by Price under the guidance of the *American Society for Mass Spectrometry* (ASMS) [54].
- 1995: Compilation by Todd representing the official recommendations of the *International Union of Pure and Applied Chemistry* (IUPAC) [55].
- 2006: Terminology reference book by Sparkman [52].
- 2013: Update of terms and definitions by IUPAC [56]; a project that started in 2005 [57] and went through several stages of comments and suggestions [58–60].

Still, terminology in MS is not perfectly uniform. IUPAC in its 1995 version, for example, stays in opposition to the vast majority of practitioners, journals, and books when talking about *mass spectroscopy*, while both, Price and Sparkman are using *mass spectrometry*. IUPAC accepts terms such as *daughter ion* and *parent ion* as equivalent to *product ion* and *precursor ion*, respectively. Sparkman discourages the use of *daughter ion* and *parent ion* as these are archaic and gender-specific terms. None of these collections is fully comprehensive. Nevertheless, there is about 95% agreement between these guidelines to terminology in mass spectrometry and their overall coverage can be regarded as highly sufficient, making the application of any of these beneficial to oral and written communication.

Unfortunately, misleading and redundant terms are used throughout the literature, and thus, we need at least to understand their intention even if we are not going to use them actively. Terminology in this book avoids outdated or vague terms and special notes are given for clarification where ambiguities might arise.

Acronyms galore
Mass spectrometrists like to communicate their work using countless acronyms [61, 62], and thus there is no sense in trying to avoid them here. All acronyms are explained at first use in a chapter and are included in the subject index. For convenience, one hundred common MS acronyms are provided in the Appendix.

1.7.1 Basic Terminology in Describing Mass Spectra

One should be aware of some basic, but often misunderstood, terminology when describing mass spectra.

1. We may refer to a whatever-*type* (*mass*) *spectrum*, e.g., an *EI mass spectrum*. But, as MS means *mass spectrometry* as a method, the term *MS spectrum* is clearly incorrect.
2. Multi-stage MS (MS/MS equal to MS^2) refers to *tandem mass spectrometry*. Analogous to 1, it is correct to say *tandem mass spectra*, not *MS/MS spectra*.
3. Ions are detected *at* a certain *m*/*z* value. Correct phrasings are "the molecular ion at *m*/*z* 16" or "$M^{+\bullet}$, *m*/*z* 16" or "$CH_4^{+\bullet}$, *m*/*z* 16", for example.
4. Ranges in spectra or ranges set in operating a mass spectrometer are to be referred to in the form of "*m*/*z* 10–100" or "*m*/*z* 10 to *m*/*z* 100".
5. Mass spectrometers separate ions by mass-to-charge ratio, *m*/*z*. The abscissa of a mass spectrum is to be labelled only as "*m*/*z*". Any other labels like "mass", "*m*/*z* [Da]", or even worse "*m*/*z* [a.m.u]", are wrong.
6. Ions are correlated with peaks in a spectrum, not neutrals. Assigning an ion to a peak is already an act of interpretation.
7. Neutral losses (rarely called dark matter [52]) are exclusively recognized from the distance between peaks expressed in terms of the difference $\Delta(m/z)$. The mass of the corresponding neutral is then given in units of u.
8. A signal or peak is only the graphical representation of the mass spectrometer's detector output. It can just be observed, but not act by itself in any way.

Table 1.4 Symbols

Symbol	Meaning
•	Unpaired electron in radicals
+	Positive even-electron ions
–	Negative even-electron ions
+•	Positive radical ions
–•	Negative radical ions
	Arrow for transfer of an electron pair
	Single-barbed arrow for transfer of a single electron
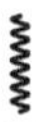	Indicates the position of a cleaved bond
⟶	Fragmentation or reaction
—o→	Occasionally for rearrangement fragmentation

9. Ions can act. Typically they fragment, dissociate, rearrange, react, isomerize.
10. It is advisable to use the common symbols compiled in Table 1.4, in particular, charge should precede the radical, as in +• or –•.

1.8 Units, Physical Quantities, and Physical Constants

The consistent use of units for physical quantities is a prerequisite in science, because it simplifies the comparison of physical quantities, e.g., temperature, pressure, or physical dimensions. Therefore, the *International System of Units* (SI) is used throughout the book. This system is based on seven units that can be combined to form any other unit needed. Nevertheless, mass spectrometers often have long lifetimes and 20-year-old instruments being scaled in inches and having pressure readings in Torr or psi may still be in use. In the Appendix of this book you will find tables that provide collections of SI units together with frequently needed conversion factors and a collection of physical constants and quantities.

1.9 Further Reading

This book provides extensive reference lists at the end of each chapter. Nonetheless, it may be useful to have the most relevant MS books compiled in one list.

First of all, there are some classical mass spectrometry books deserving our grateful attention [31, 63–73]. Then, some other introductory mass spectrometry books are to be mentioned [74–78]. Finally, various monographs covering MS in dedicated chapters are available; these are listed here in chronological order [30, 79–136].

1.10 Quintessence

Basic Principle
Mass spectrometry (MS) separates isolated ions in the gas phase by their mass-to-charge ratio. This is accomplished by means of electric and magnetic fields or combinations thereof. The fields may be constant in time, variable, or alternating, depending on the type of mass analyzer. Any sample needs thus to be transformed into the state of isolated gas-phase ions. There is a large variety of ionization techniques to perform this transition for almost any sample. The fact that the instrument's response relies on the detection of gaseous ions provides the basis for the outstanding low sample consumption of MS, generally in the nanogram to microgram range per sample. As sample consumption in MS is minimal, its potential applications are diverse and manifold.

Historical Development
Mass spectrometry was developed about a century ago. Initially applied to the characterization of elements and their isotopic composition, MS left the realms of physics in the 1940s to be applied for hydrocarbon analysis. From there, MS became a tool for compound characterization in organic chemistry and then expanded into biomedical and countless other natural sciences.

Applications of Mass Spectrometry
Mass spectrometry (MS) can be applied for the analysis of all classes of chemical compounds either elemental or molecular, pure or in complex mixtures. MS is thus widely applied not only in chemistry and the life science in the widest sense but also plays a significant role in pharmacology, geology, physics, and other sciences. MS is clearly interdisciplinary in itself and in regard to its different fields of application. It is the particular strength of MS to deliver analytical information from the tiniest amounts of a sample.

Important Terms and Concepts
The method is termed mass spectrometry (MS), the entire instrument is called a mass spectrometer. It consists of sample introduction system, ion source, mass analyzer, detector, and data system. A mass spectrum represents the output of a mass spectrometer. Mass spectra are plotted as (relative) signal intensity versus dimensionless mass-to-charge ratio, *m/z*. Alternatively, mass spectral data can be supplied in tabular form.

References

1. He F, Hendrickson CL, Marshall AG (2001) Baseline Mass Resolution of Peptide Isobars: A Record for Molecular Mass Resolution. Anal Chem 73:647–650. doi:10.1021/ac000973h
2. Cooper HJ, Marshall AG (2001) Electrospray Ionization Fourier Transform Mass Spectrometric Analysis of Wine. J Agric Food Chem 49:5710–5718. doi:10.1021/jf0108516

3. Hughey CA, Rodgers RP, Marshall AG (2002) Resolution of 11,000 Compositionally Distinct Components in a Single Electrospray Ionization FT-ICR Mass Spectrum of Crude Oil. Anal Chem 74:4145–4149. doi:10.1021/ac020146b
4. Mühlberger F, Wieser J, Ulrich A, Zimmermann R (2002) Single Photon Ionization (SPI) via Incoherent VUV-Excimer Light: Robust and Compact Time-of-Flight Mass Spectrometer for On-Line, Real-Time Process Gas Analysis. Anal Chem 74:3790–3801. doi:10.1021/ac0200825
5. Glish GL, Vachet RW (2003) The Basics of Mass Spectrometry in the Twenty-First Century. Nat Rev Drug Discovery 2:140–150. doi:10.1038/nrd1011
6. Zuccato E, Chiabrando C, Castiglioni S, Calamari D, Bagnati R, Schiarea S, Fanelli R (2005) Cocaine in Surface Waters: A New Evidence-Based Tool to Monitor Community Drug Abuse. Environ Health 4: online journal. doi: 10.1186/1476-069X-4-14
7. Harris WA, Reilly PTA, Whitten WB (2007) Detection of Chemical Warfare-Related Species on Complex Aerosol Particles Deposited on Surfaces Using an Ion Trap-Based Aerosol Mass Spectrometer. Anal Chem 79:2354–2358. doi:10.1021/ac0620664
8. Enjalbal C, Maux D, Combarieu R, Martinez J, Aubagnac J-L (2003) Imaging Combinatorial Libraries by Mass Spectrometry: From Peptide to Organic-Supported Syntheses. J Comb Chem 5:102–109. doi:10.1021/cc0200484
9. Maux D, Enjalbal C, Martinez J, Aubagnac J-L, Combarieu R (2001) Static Secondary Ion Mass Spectrometry to Monitor Solid-Phase Peptide Synthesis. J Am Soc Mass Spectrom 12:1099–1105. doi:10.1016/S1044-0305(01)00296-3
10. Amantonico A, Urban PL, Zenobi R (2010) Analytical Techniques for Single-Cell Metabolomics: State of the Art and Trends. Anal Bioanal Chem 398:2493–2504. doi:10.1007/s00216-010-3850-1
11. Zhang L, Vertes A (2015) Energy Charge, Redox State, and Metabolite Turnover in Single Human Hepatocytes Revealed by Capillary Microsampling Mass Spectrometry. Anal Chem 87:10397–10405. doi:10.1021/acs.analchem.5b02502
12. Aebersold R (2003) A Mass Spectrometric Journey into Protein and Proteome Research. J Am Soc Mass Spectrom 14:685–695. doi:10.1016/S1044-0305(03)00289-7
13. Koch BP, Witt M, Engbrodt R, Dittmar T, Kattner G (2005) Molecular Formulae of Marine and Terrigenous Dissolved Organic Matter Detected by Electrospray Ionization Fourier Transform Ion Cyclotron Resonance Mass Spectrometry. Geochim Cosmochim Acta 69:3299–3308. doi:10.1016/j.gca.2005.02.027
14. Klitzke CF, Corilo YE, Siek K, Binkley J, Patrick J, Eberlin MN (2012) Petroleomics by Ultrahigh-Resolution Time-of-Flight Mass Spectrometry. Energy & Fuels 26:5787–5794. doi:10.1021/ef300961c
15. Marshall AG, Chen T (2015) 40 Years of Fourier Transform Ion Cyclotron Resonance Mass Spectrometry. Int J Mass Spectrom 377:410–420. doi:10.1016/j.ijms.2014.06.034
16. Snyder DT, Pulliam CJ, Ouyang Z, Cooks RG (2015) Miniature and Fieldable Mass Spectrometers: Recent Advances. Anal Chem 88:2–29. doi:10.1021/acs.analchem.5b03070
17. Fenselau C, Caprioli R (2003) Mass Spectrometry in the Exploration of Mars. J Mass Spectrom 38:1–10. doi:10.1002/jms.396
18. Goesmann F, Rosenbauer H, Bredehoeft JH, Cabane M, Ehrenfreund P, Gautier T, Giri C, Krueger H, Le Roy L, MacDermott AJ, McKenna-Lawlor S, Meierhenrich UJ, Caro GMM, Raulin F, Roll R, Steele A, Steininger H, Sternberg R, Szopa C, Thiemann W, Ulamec S (2015) Organic Compounds on Comet 67P/Churyumov-Gerasimenko Revealed by COSAC Mass Spectrometry. Science 349:497–499. doi:10.1126/science.aab0689
19. Pulliam CJ, Bain RM, Wiley JS, Ouyang Z, Cooks RG (2015) Mass Spectrometry in the Home and Garden. J Am Soc Mass Spectrom 26:224–230. doi:10.1007/s13361-014-1056-z
20. Thomson JJ (1909) Positive Rays. Phil Mag 16:657–691. doi:10.1080/14786441008636543
21. Thomson JJ (1911) Rays of Positive Electricity. Phil Mag 20:752–767. doi:10.1080/14786441008636962

22. Thomson JJ (1912) Further Experiments on Positive Rays. Phil Mag 24:209–253. doi:10.1080/14786440808637325
23. Thomson JJ (1913) Rays of Positive Electricity and Their Application to Chemical Analysis. Longmans, Green and Co., London
24. Aston FW (1919) The Constitution of the Elements. Nature 104:393. doi:10.1038/104393b0
25. Aston FW (1919) A Positive-Ray Spectrograph. Phil Mag 38:707–715. doi:10.1080/14786441208636004
26. Aston FW (1919) Neon Nature 104:334. doi:10.1038/104334d0
27. Aston FW (1920) The Mass-Spectra of Chemical Elements. Phil Mag 39:611–625. doi:10.1080/14786440508636074
28. Aston FW (1922) List of Elements and Their Isotopes. Proc Phys Soc 34:197
29. Grayson MA (ed) (2002) Measuring Mass – From Positive Rays to Proteins. ASMS and CHF, Santa Fe and Philadelphia
30. Jennings KR (ed) (2012) A History of European Mass Spectrometry. IM Publications, Charlton Mill
31. Brunnée C, Voshage H (1964) Massenspektrometrie. Karl Thiemig Verlag KG, München
32. Doerr A, Finkelstein J, Jarchum I, Goodman C, Dekker B (2015) Nature Milestones: Mass Spectrometry. Nature Meth 12:1–21. doi: www.nature.com/milestones/mass-spec
33. Busch KL (2000) Synergistic Developments in Mass Spectrometry. A 50-Year Journey From "Art" to Science. Spectroscopy 15:30–39
34. Muenzenberg G (2013) Development of Mass Spectrometers from Thomson and Aston to Present. Int J Mass Spectrom 349–350:9–18
35. Meyerson S (1986) Reminiscences of the Early Days of Mass Spectrometry in the Petroleum Industry. Org Mass Spectrom 21:197–208. doi:10.1002/oms.1210210406
36. Quayle A (1987) Recollections of Mass Spectrometry of the Fifties in a UK Petroleum Laboratory. Org Mass Spectrom 22:569–585. doi:10.1002/oms.1210220902
37. Maccoll A (1993) Organic Mass Spectrometry – the Origins. Org Mass Spectrom 28:1371–1372. doi:10.1002/oms.1210281203
38. Meyerson S (1993) Mass Spectrometry in the News, 1949. Org Mass Spectrom 28:1373–1374. doi:10.1002/oms.1210281204
39. Meyerson S (1994) From Black Magic to Chemistry. The Metamorphosis of Organic Mass Spectrometry. Anal Chem 66:960A–964A. doi:10.1021/ac00091a001
40. Nibbering NMM (2006) Four Decades of Joy in Mass Spectrometry. Mas Spectrom Rev 25:962–1017. doi:10.1002/mas.20099
41. Gross ML, Sparkman OD (1998) The Importance of Titles in References. J Am Soc Mass Spectrom 9:451. doi:10.1016/S1044-0305(98)00002-6
42. Gross JH (2009) Mass Spectrometry. In: Andrews DL (ed) Encyclopedia of Applied Spectroscopy. Wiley-VCH, Weinheim
43. Jones M Jr (2000) Mass Spectrometry. In: Organic Chemistry. W. W. Norton & Company, New York
44. Griffiths IW (1997) J. J. Thomson – the Centenary of His Discovery of the Electron and of His Invention of Mass Spectrometry. Rapid Commun Mass Spectrom 11:2–16. doi:10.1002/(SICI)1097-0231(19970115)11:1<2::AID-RCM768>3.0.CO;2-V
45. Dempster AJ (1918) A New Method of Positive Ray Analysis. Phys Rev 11:316–325. doi:10.1103/PhysRev.11.316
46. Nier AO (1990) Some Reflections on the Early Days of Mass Spectrometry at the University of Minnesota. Int J Mass Spectrom Ion Proc 100:1–13. doi:10.1016/0168-1176(90)85063-8
47. Kienitz H (1968) Einführung. In: Kienitz H (ed) Massenspektrometrie. Weinheim, Verlag Chemie
48. Busch KL (2001) Units in Mass Spectrometry. Spectroscopy 16:28–31
49. Price P (1991) Standard Definitions of Terms Relating to Mass Spectrometry. A Report From the Committee on Measurements and Standards of the Amercian Society for Mass Spectrometry. J Am Soc Mass Spectrom 2:336–348. doi:10.1016/1044-0305(91)80025-3

50. Todd JFJ (1995) Recommendations for Nomenclature and Symbolism for Mass Spectroscopy Including an Appendix of Terms Used in Vacuum Technology. Int J Mass Spectrom Ion Proc 142:211–240
51. Lv Y, Yuan T, Hu J, Wang W (2009) Simultaneous Determination of Trace Polycyclic and Nitro Musks in Water Samples Using Optimized Solid-Phase Extraction by Gas Chromatography and Mass Spectrometry. Anal Sci 25:1125–1130. doi:10.2116/analsci.25.1125
52. Sparkman OD (2006) Mass Spectrometry Desk Reference. Global View Publishing, Pittsburgh
53. Kilburn KD, Lewis PH, Underwood JG, Evans S, Holmes J, Dean M (1979) Quality of Mass and Intensity Measurements from a High Performance Mass Spectrometer. Anal Chem 51:1420–1425. doi:10.1021/ac50045a017
54. Price P (1991) Standard Definitions of Terms Relating to Mass Spectrometry. A Report From the Committee on Measurements and Standards of the Amercian Society for Mass Spectrometry. J Am Soc Mass Spectrom 2:336–348. doi:10.1016/1044-0305(91)80025-3
55. Todd JFJ (1995) Recommendations for Nomenclature and Symbolism for Mass Spectroscopy Including an Appendix of Terms Used in Vacuum Technology. Int J Mass Spectrom Ion Proc 142:211–240. doi:10.1016/0168-1176(95)93811-F
56. Murray KK, Boyd RK, Eberlin MN, Langley GJ, Li L, Naito Y (2013) Definitions of Terms Relating to Mass Spectrometry (IUPAC Recommendations 2013). Pure Appl Chem 85:1515–1609. doi:10.1351/PAC-REC-06-04-06
57. Murray KK, Boyd RK, Eberlin MN, Langley GJ, Li L, Naito Y, Tabet JC (2005) IUPAC Standard Definitions of Terms Relating to Mass Spectrometry. Abstracts of Papers, 229th ACS National Meeting, San Diego, CA, United States, March 13–17, 2005, ANYL-212
58. Murray KK (2007) Web Glossaries the Wiki Way. Chem Int 29:23–25
59. Naito Y (2007) Commentary on Terms and Definitions Relating to Mass Spectrometry. J Mass Spectrom Soc Jpn 55:149–156. doi:10.5702/massspec.55.149
60. Murray KK, Boyd RK, Eberlin MN, Langley GJ, Li L, Naito Y (2009) Standard Definitions of Terms Relating to Mass Spectrometry (IUPAC Recommendations). Pure Appl Chem provisional recommendations in state of review
61. Busch KL (2002) SAMS: Speaking with Acronyms in Mass Spectrometry. Spectroscopy 17:54–62
62. Busch KL (2002) A Glossary for Mass Spectrometry. Spectroscopy 17:S26–S34
63. Field FH, Franklin JL (1957) Electron Impact Phenomena and the Properties of Gaseous Ions. Academic Press, New York
64. Beynon JH (1960) Mass Spectrometry and its Applications to Organic Chemistry. Elsevier, Amsterdam
65. Biemann K (1962) Mass Spectrometry. McGraw-Hill, New York
66. Biemann K (1962) Mass Spectrometry – Organic Chemical Applications. McGraw-Hill, New York
67. Biemann K, Dibeler VH, Grubb HM, Harrison AG, Hood A, Knewstubb PF, Krauss M, McLafferty FW, Melton CE, Meyerson S, Reed RI, Rosenstock HM, Ryhage R, Saunders RA, Stenhagen E, Williams AE, McLafferty FW (eds) (1963) Mass Spectrometry of Organic Ions. Academic Press, London
68. Kiser RW (1965) Introduction to Mass Spectrometry and its Applications. Prentice-Hall, Englewood Cliffs
69. Budzikiewicz H, Djerassi C, Williams DH (1967) Mass Spectrometry of Organic Compounds. Holden-Day, San Francisco
70. Aulinger F, Kienitz H, Franke G, Habfast K, Spiteller G, Kienitz H (eds) (1968) Massenspektrometrie. Weinheim, Verlag Chemie
71. Cooks RG, Beynon JH, Caprioli RM (1973) Metastable Ions. Elsevier, Amsterdam
72. Levsen K (1978) Fundamental Aspects of Organic Mass Spectrometry. Weinheim, Verlag Chemie

73. Howe I, Williams DH, Bowen RD (1981) Mass Spectrometry: Principles and Applications. McGraw-Hill, New York
74. Chapman JR (1993) Practical Organic Mass Spectrometry: A Guide for Chemical and Biochemical Analysis. Wiley, Chichester
75. McLafferty FW, Turecek F (1993) Interpretation of Mass Spectra. University Science Books, Mill Valley
76. De Hoffmann E, Stroobant V (2007) Mass Spectrometry – Principles and Applications. Wiley, Chichester
77. Watson JT, Sparkman OD (2007) Introduction to Mass Spectrometry. Wiley, Chichester
78. Ekman R, Silberring J, Westman-Brinkmalm AM, Kraj A (2009) Mass Spectrometry: Instrumentation, Interpretation, and Applications. Wiley, Hoboken
79. Porter QN, Baldas J (1971) Mass Spectrometry of Heterocyclic Compounds. Wiley Interscience, New York
80. Dawson PH (1976) Quadrupole Mass Spectrometry and Its Applications. Elsevier, New York
81. Beckey HD (1977) Principles of Field Desorption and Field Ionization Mass Spectrometry. Pergamon Press, Oxford
82. McLafferty FW (ed) (1983) Tandem Mass Spectrometry. Wiley, New York
83. Castleman AW Jr, Futrell JH, Lindinger W, Märk TD, Morrison JD, Shirts RB, Smith DL, Wahrhaftig AL, Futrell JH (eds) (1986) Gaseous Ion Chemistry and Mass Spectrometry. Wiley, New York
84. Benninghoven A, Werner HW, Rudenauer FG, Benninghoven A (eds) (1987) Secondary Ion Mass Spectrometry: Basic Concepts, Instrumental Aspects, Applications and Trends. Wiley Interscience, New York
85. Busch KL, Glish GL, McLuckey SA (1988) Mass Spectrometry/Mass Spectrometry. Wiley VCH, New York
86. Briggs D, Brown A, Vickerman JC (1989) Handbook of Static Secondary Ion Mass Spectrometry. Wiley, Chichester
87. March RE, Hughes RJ (1989) Quadrupole Storage Mass Spectrometry. Wiley, Chichester
88. Wilson RG, Stevie FA, Magee CW (1989) Secondary Ion Mass Spectrometry: A Practical Handbook for Depth Profiling and Bulk Impurity Analysis. Wiley, Chichester
89. Caprioli RM (ed) (1990) Continuous-Flow Fast Atom Bombardment Mass Spectrometry. Wiley, Chichester
90. Prókai L (1990) Field Desorption Mass Spectrometry. Marcel Dekker, New York
91. Assamoto B (ed) (1991) Analytical Applications of Fourier Transform Ion Cyclotron Resonance Mass Spectrometry. Weinheim, VCH
92. Harrison AG (1992) Chemical Ionization Mass Spectrometry. CRC Press, Boca Raton
93. Splitter JS, Turecek F (eds) (1994) Applications of Mass Spectrometry to Organic Stereochemistry. Weinheim, Verlag Chemie
94. Yinon J (ed) (1994) Forensic Applications of Mass Spectrometry. CRC Press, Boca Raton
95. Schlag EW (ed) (1994) Time of Flight Mass Spectrometry and its Applications. Elsevier, Amsterdam
96. Lehmann WD (1996) Massenspektrometrie in Der Biochemie. Spektrum Akademischer Verlag, Heidelberg
97. Dole RB (ed) (1997) Electrospray Ionization Mass Spectrometry – Fundamentals, Instrumentation and Applications. Wiley, Chichester
98. Cotter RJ (1997) Time-of-Flight Mass Spectrometry: Instrumentation and Applications in Biological Research. American Chemical Society, Washington, DC
99. Platzner IT, Habfast K, Walder AJ, Goetz A, Platzner IT (eds) (1997) Modern Isotope Ratio Mass Spectrometry. Wiley, Chichester
100. Niessen WMA, Voyksner RD (eds) (1998) Current Practice of Liquid Chromatography-Mass Spectrometry. Elsevier, Amsterdam
101. Tuniz C, Bird JR, Fink D, Herzog GF (1998) Accelerator Mass Spectrometry – Ultrasensitive Analysis for Global Science. CRC Press, Boca Raton

102. Roboz J (1999) Mass Spectrometry in Cancer Research. CRC Press, Boca Raton
103. Chapman JR (ed) (2000) Mass Spectrometry of Proteins and Peptides. Humana Press, Totowa
104. Kinter M, Sherman NE (2000) Protein Sequencing and Identification Using Tandem Mass Spectrometry. Wiley, Chichester
105. Snyder AP (2000) Interpreting Protein Mass Spectra. Oxford University Press, New York
106. Taylor HE (2000) Inductively Coupled Plasma Mass Spectroscopy. Academic Press, London
107. Montaudo G, Lattimer RP (eds) (2001) Mass Spectrometry of Polymers. CRC Press, Boca Raton
108. Budde WL (2001) Analytical Mass Spectrometry. ACS and Oxford University Press, Washington, DC and Oxford
109. de Laeter JR (2001) Applications of Inorganic Mass Spectrometry. Wiley, New York
110. Rossi DT, Sinz MW (eds) (2002) Mass Spectrometry in Drug Discovery. Marcel Dekker, New York
111. Pramanik BN, Ganguly AK, Gross ML (eds) (2002) Applied Electrospray Mass Spectrometry. Marcel Dekker, New York
112. Ardrey RE (2003) Liquid Chromatography-Mass Spectrometry – An Introduction. Wiley, Chichester
113. Pasch H, Schrepp W (2003) MALDI-TOF Mass Spectrometry of Synthetic Polymers. Springer, Heidelberg
114. Henderson W, McIndoe SJ (2005) Mass Spectrometry of Inorganic and Organometallic Compounds. Wiley, Chichester
115. Kaltashov IA, Eyles SJ (2005) Mass Spectrometry in Biophysics: Conformation and Dynamics of Biomolecules. Wiley, Hoboken
116. March RE, Todd JFJ (2005) Quadrupole Ion Trap Mass Spectrometry. Wiley, Hoboken
117. Siuzdak G (2006) The Expanding Role of Mass Spectrometry in Biotechnology. MCC Press, San Diego
118. Becker JS (2008) Inorganic Mass Spectrometry: Principles and Applications. Wiley, Chichester
119. Boyd RK, Basic C, Bethem RA (2008) Trace Quantitative Analysis by Mass Spectrometry. Wiley, Chichester
120. Le Gac S, van den Berg A (eds) (2009) Miniaturization and Mass Spectrometry. The Royal Society of Chemistry, Cambridge
121. Ramanathan R (ed) (2009) Mass Spectrometry in Drug Metabolism and Pharmacokinetics. Wiley, Hoboken
122. Schalley CA, Springer A (2009) Mass Spectrometry and Gas-Phase Chemistry of Non-Covalent Complexes. Wiley, Hoboken
123. Santos LS (ed) (2009) Reactive Intermediates: MS Investigations in Solution. Wiley-VCH, Weinheim
124. Cole RB (ed) (2010) Electrospray and MALDI Mass Spectrometry: Fundamentals, Instrumentation, Practicalities, and Biological Applications. Wiley, Hoboken
125. Li L (ed) (2010) MALDI Mass Spectrometry for Synthetic Polymer Analysis. Wiley, Hoboken
126. Lehmann WD (2010) Protein Phosphorylation Analysis by Electrospray Mass Spectrometry: A Guide to Concepts and Practice. Royal Society of Chemistry, Cambridge
127. Barner-Kowollik C, Gruendling T, Falkenhagen J, Weidner S (eds) (2012) Mass Spectrometry in Polymer Chemistry. Wiley-VCH, Weinheim
128. Hiraoka K (ed) (2013) Fundamentals of Mass Spectrometry. Springer, New York
129. Hillenkamp F, Peter-Katalinic J (eds) (2013) MALDI MS: A Practical Guide to Instrumentation, Methods and Applications. Wiley-VCH, Weinheim
130. Eiceman GA, Karpas Z, Hill HH Jr (2014) Ion Mobility Spectrometry. CRC Press, Boca Raton
131. Ellis AM, Mayhew CA (2014) Proton Transfer Reaction Mass Spectrometry: Principles and Applications. Wiley-Blackwell, Chichester

132. Prohaska T, Irrgeher J, Zitek A, Jakubowski N (eds) (2015) Sector Field Mass Spectrometry for Elemental and Isotopic Analysis. Royal Society of Chemistry, Cambridge, UK
133. Fujii T (ed) (2015) Ion/Molecule Attachment Reactions: Mass Spectrometry. Springer, New York. doi:10.1007/978-1-4899-7588-1
134. Domin M, Cody R (eds) (2015) Ambient Ionization Mass Spectrometry. Royal Society of Chemistry, Cambridge, UK
135. Hübschmann HJ (2015) Handbook of GC-MS – Fundamentals and Applications. Wiley-VCH, Weinheim
136. Cramer R (ed) (2016) Advances in MALDI and Laser-Induced Soft Ionization Mass Spectrometry. Springer, Cham. doi:10.1007/978-3-319-04819-2

Principles of Ionization and Ion Dissociation

2

Learning Objectives

- Electron ionization process and ionization energy
- Internal energy of ions and internal energy distribution
- Energetic considerations governing the fragmentation of excited ions
- Quasi-equilibrium theory and rates of unimolecular dissociations
- Time scale of mass spectrometry
- Selected tools of gas phase ion chemistry
- Ion–molecule reactions

The mass spectrometer can be regarded as a kind of chemical laboratory, especially designed to study ions in the gas phase [1, 2]. In addition to the task it is commonly used for – creation of mass spectra for a generally analytical purpose – it allows for the examination of fragmentation pathways of selected ions, for the study of ion–neutral reactions and more. Understanding these fundamentals is prerequisite for the proper application of mass spectrometry with all technical facets available, and for the successful interpretation of mass spectra because "analytical chemistry is the application of physical chemistry to the real world" [3].

In the first place, this chapter deals with the fundamentals of gas phase ion chemistry, i.e., with ionization, excitation, ion thermochemistry, ion lifetimes, and reaction rates of ion dissociation. The advanced sections are devoted to more practical aspects of gas phase ion chemistry such as the determination of ionization and appearance energies or of gas phase basicities and proton affinities. Finally, ion–molecule reactions are briefly discussed [4].

A basic coverage of some topics of this chapter may also be found in physical chemistry textbooks; however, much better introductions are given in the specialized literature [4–12]. Detailed compound-specific fragmentation mechanisms, ion–molecule complexes, and more are dealt with later (Chap. 6).

J.H. Gross, *Mass Spectrometry*, DOI 10.1007/978-3-319-54398-7_2

2.1 Gas Phase Ionization by Energetic Electrons

Mass spectrometers are designed to create ions from neutrals in order to be able to accelerate and to force them into direction-controlled motion with the aim to ultimately achieve *m/z* analysis of these ions. The mass analyzer of any mass spectrometer handles only charged species, i.e., ions that have been created from atoms or molecules, occasionally also from radicals, zwitterions, or clusters. It is the task of the ion source to perform this crucial step and there is a wide range of ionization methods in use to achieve this goal for the whole variety of analytes. Neutrals cannot be investigated – their translational motions are neither affected by electric nor by magnetic fields. Nevertheless, some neutrals by chance may hit the detector thereby contributing to noise on the signal.

The classical procedure of ionization involves shooting energetic electrons on a gaseous neutral. This is called *electron ionization* (EI). Electron ionization has formerly been termed *electron impact ionization* or simply *electron impact* (EI). For EI, the neutral previously must have been transferred into the highly diluted gas phase, which is done by means of any sample inlet system suitable for the evaporation of the respective compound. In practice, the gas phase may be regarded highly diluted when the mean free path for the particles becomes long enough to make bimolecular interactions almost impossible within the lifetime of the particles concerned. This is easily achieved at pressures in the range of 10^{-4} Pa usually realized in electron ionization ion sources. Here, the description of EI is restricted to what is essential for an understanding of the ionization process as such [13, 14] and the consequences for the fate of the freshly created ions.

2.1.1 Formation of Ions

When a neutral is hit by an energetic electron carrying several tens of electronvolts (eV) of kinetic energy, some of the energy of the electron is transferred to the neutral. If the electron, in terms of energy transfer, collides very effectively with the neutral, the energy transferred can exceed the *ionization energy* (*IE*) of the neutral. Then – from the mass spectrometric point of view – the most desirable process can occur: ionization by ejection of one electron generating a *molecular ion*, a positive *radical ion*:

$$M + e^- \rightarrow M^{+\bullet} + 2e^- \tag{2.1}$$

Depending on the analyte and on the energy of the primary electrons, doubly charged and even triply charged ions may be observed:

$$M + e^- \rightarrow M^{2+} + 3e^- \tag{2.2}$$

$$M + e^- \rightarrow M^{3+\bullet} + 4e^- \tag{2.3}$$

While the doubly charged ion, M^{2+}, is an *even-electron ion*, the triply charged ion, $M^{3+\bullet}$, again is an *odd-electron ion*. In addition, there are several other events possible from the electron–neutral interaction, e.g., a less effective interaction will bring the neutral into an electronically excited state without ionizing it.

Ionization of a molecule EI predominantly creates singly charged ions from the precursor neutral. If the neutral was a molecule as in most cases, it started as having an even number of electrons, i.e., it was an *even-electron (closed-shell) molecule*. The molecular ion formed must then be a radical cation or an *odd-electron (open-shell) ion* as these species are termed. For methane we obtain:

$$CH_4 + e^- \rightarrow CH_4^{+\bullet} + 2e^- \tag{2.4}$$

Ionization of a radical In the rare case the neutral was a radical, the ion created by electron ionization would be even-electron, e.g., for nitric oxide:

$$NO^\bullet + e^- \rightarrow NO^+ + 2e^- \tag{2.5}$$

Ionization of a polycyclic aromatic hydrocarbon The EI mass spectrum of a phenanthroperylene derivative shows a series of comparatively intensive doubly-charged ions, the one at m/z 178 being the doubly-charged molecular ion, the others representing doubly-charged fragment ions (Fig. 2.1) [15]. The occurrence of doubly-charged ions of moderate abundance is quite common in the mass spectra of polycyclic aromatic hydrocarbons (PAHs). For another example of multiply-charged ions in EI spectra cf. Sect. 3.8, for the LDI spectrum of this compound cf. Sect. 11.5.

2.1.2 Processes Accompanying Electron Ionization

In addition to the desired generation of molecular ions, several other events can result from electron–neutral interactions (Fig. 2.2). A "soft" collision of a neutral molecule with an electron is less effective. Such an interaction merely transforms the neutral into an electronically excited state without ionizing it. As the energy of the primary electrons increases, the abundance and variety of the ionized species will also increase, i.e., electron ionization may occur via different channels, each of which gives rise to characteristic ionized and neutral products. This includes the production of the following type of ions: molecular ions, fragment ions, multiply charged ions, metastable ions, rearrangement ions, and ion pairs [13].

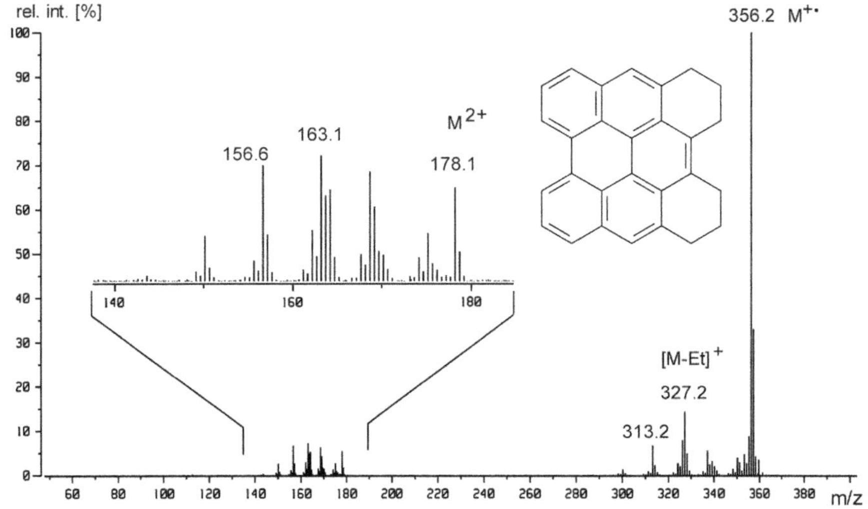

Fig. 2.1 EI mass spectrum of 1,2,3,4,5,6-hexahydrophenanthro[1,10,9,8-*opqra*]perylene. All signals in the expanded inset correspond to doubly-charged ions (Adapted from Ref. [15] with permission. © Elsevier Science, 2002)

In principle, the electron may also be captured by the neutral to form a negative radical ion. However, *electron capture* (EC) is rather unlikely to occur with electrons of 70 eV since EC is a resonance process because no electron is produced to carry away the excess energy [16]. Thus, EC only proceeds effectively with electrons of very low energy, preferably with thermal electrons (Sect. 7.6). Nonetheless, molecules containing strongly electronegative elements may form negative ions: the ionization efficiency of this process is very low, however.

Exceptions

The generation of negative ions from tungsten hexafluoride, WF_6, has been studied under conventional EI conditions. At higher electron energies, $WF_6^{-\bullet}$, WF_5^-, and F^- ions have been detected [17]. Highly fluorinated organic analytes such as perfluorokerosene, C_nF_{n+2}, also yield negative ions, but sensitivity is lower by some orders of magnitude than for positive-ion EI.

2.1.3 Ions Generated by Penning Ionization

Non-ionizing electron–neutral interactions create electronically excited neutrals. The ionization reactions occurring when electronically excited neutrals like noble gas atoms, A*, collide with a ground state molecule, M, can be divided into two classes [19]. The first process is *Penning ionization* (Eq. 2.6) [20], the second is *associative ionization*, also known as the Hornbeck-Molnar process (Eq. 2.7) [21]:

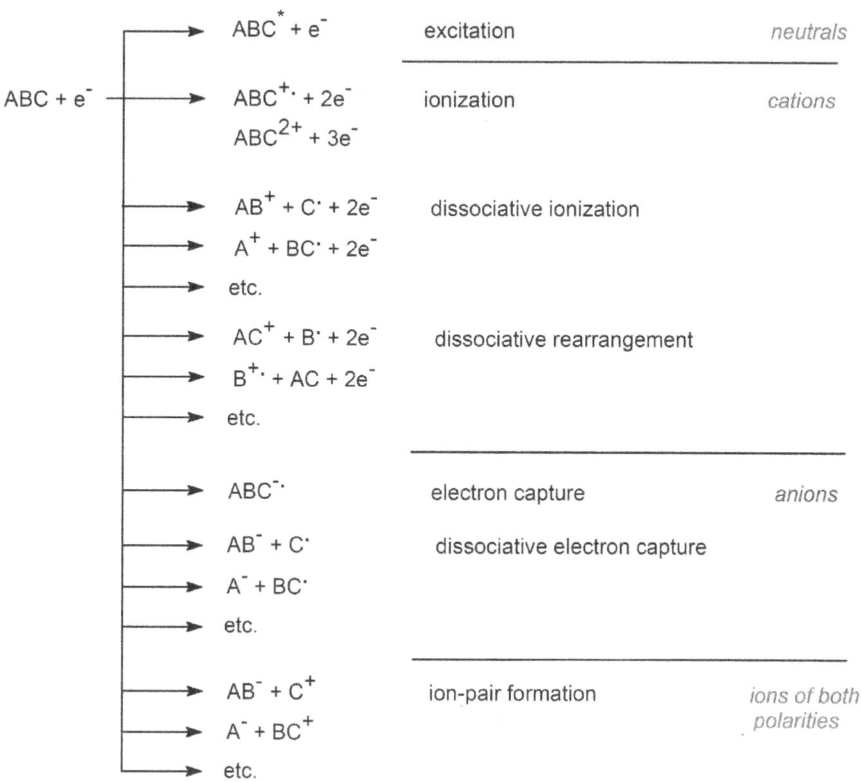

Fig. 2.2 Processes under electron ionization conditions. Under certain conditions, Penning ionization can also play a role (Adapted from Ref. [18] with permission. © Springer-Verlag Heidelberg, 1991)

$$A^* + M \rightarrow A + M^{+\bullet} + e^- \tag{2.6}$$

$$A^* + M \rightarrow AM^{+\bullet} + e^- \tag{2.7}$$

Penning ionization occurs with the (trace) gas M having an ionization energy lower than the energy of the metastable state of the excited (noble gas) atoms A*. The above ionization processes have also been employed to construct ion sources [19, 22], but until the advent of *direct analysis in real time* (DART, Sect. 13.8) and *glow discharge mass spectrometry* (GD-MS, Sect. 15.4), Penning ionization sources were not widely used in analytical MS.

2.1.4 Ionization Energy

It is obvious that ionization of the neutral can only occur when the energy deposited by the electron–neutral collision is equal to or greater than the *ionization energy* (*IE*) of the corresponding neutral. Formerly, ionization energy has erroneously been termed *ionization potential* (*IP*), as derived from the technique for its experimental determination (Sect. 2.10).

Definition
The *ionization energy* (*IE*) is defined as the minimum amount of energy that needs to be absorbed by an atom or molecule in its electronic and vibrational ground states in order to form an ion that is also in its ground states by ejection of an electron.

Lone pairs provide a good source from which electrons can be ejected. For that reason the *IE*s of ethanol and dimethylether, for example, are lower than those of ethane. It has been shown that the *IE* of a polysubstituted alkane is in principle equal to the *IE* of a structurally otherwise identical monosubstituted alkane bearing the sort of heteroatom which is energetically least demanding for electron loss [23]. The other substituent, provided it is separated by at least two carbon atoms, exerts a very small effect upon the *IE*. For example, the *IE* of dimethylsulfide, CH_3SCH_3, 8.7 eV, almost equals that of the larger methionine, $CH_3SCH_2CH_2CH(NH_2)COOH$. Introduction of an oxygen decreases the *IE* to a lesser extent than nitrogen, sulfur, or even selenium, since these elements have lower electronegativities, and thus, are energetically favorable sources to eject an electron. The bottom line of *IE*s is reached when π-systems and heteroatoms are combined in the same molecule (Table 2.1).

Range of *IEs*
Ionization energies of most molecules are in the range of 7–15 eV.

2.1.5 Ionization Energy and Charge-Localization

Removal of an electron from a molecule can formally be considered to occur at a σ-bond, a π-bond, or at a lone electron pair with the σ-bond being the least favored and the lone electron pair being the most favored position for *charge-localization* within the molecule, an assumption directly reflected in the *IE*s (Table 2.1). Noble gases do exist as atoms having closed electron shells and therefore, they exhibit the highest *IE*s. They are followed by diatomic molecules with fluorine, nitrogen, and hydrogen at the upper limit. The *IE* of methane is lower than that of molecular hydrogen but still higher than that of ethane and so forth until the *IE* of long-chain

Table 2.1 Ionization energies of selected compounds[a]

Compound	*IE*[b] [eV]	Compound	*IE*[b] [eV]
Hydrogen, H_2	15.4	Helium, He	24.6
Methane, CH_4	12.6	Neon, Ne	21.6
Ethane, C_2H_6	11.5	Argon, Ar	15.8
Propane, n-C_3H_8	10.9	Krypton, Kr	14.0
Butane, n-C_4H_{10}	10.5	Xenon, Xe	12.1
Pentane, n-C_5H_{12}	10.3		
Hexane, n-C_6H_{14}	10.1	Nitrogen, N_2	15.6
Decane, n-$C_{10}H_{22}$	9.7	Oxygen, O_2	12.1
		Carbon monoxide, CO	14.0
Ethene, C_2H_4	10.5	Carbon dioxide, CO_2	13.8
Propene, C_3H_6	9.7		
(*E*)-2-Butene, C_4H_8	9.1	Fluorine, F_2	15.7
		Chlorine, Cl_2	11.5
Benzene, C_6H_6	9.2	Bromine, Br_2	10.5
Toluene, C_7H_8	8.8	Iodine, I_2	9.3
Xylene, o-C_8H_{10}	8.6		
Indene, C_9H_8	8.6	Water, H_2O	12.6
Naphthalene, $C_{10}H_8$	8.1	Ethanol, C_2H_6O	10.5
Biphenyl, $C_{12}H_{10}$	8.2	Dimethylether, C_2H_6O	10.0
Anthracene, $C_{14}H_{10}$	7.4	Ethanethiol, C_2H_6S	9.3
Coronene, $C_{24}H_{12}$	7.3	Dimethylsulfide, C_2H_6S	8.7
		Ammonia, NH_3	10.1
Aniline, C_6H_7N	7.7	Dimethylamine, C_2H_7N	8.2
Triphenylamine, $C_{18}H_{15}N$	6.8	Triethylamine, $C_6H_{15}N$	7.5

[a]*IE* data taken from Ref. [25] with permission. © NIST 2016
[b]All values have been rounded to the first digit

alkanes approaches a lower limit [24]. The more atoms are contained within a molecule the easier it finds a way for stabilization of the charge, e.g., by delocalization or hyperconjugation. Molecules with π-bonds have lower *IE*s than those without, causing the *IE* of ethene to be lower than that of ethane. Again the *IE* is reduced further with increasing size of the alkene. Aromatic hydrocarbons can stabilize a single charge even better and expanding π-systems also help making ionization easier.

Once the molecular ion is formed, the electron charge is never really localized in a single orbital, although assuming so is often a good working hypothesis for mass spectral interpretation [26, 27]. Nonetheless, the concept of charge localization is contradictory to electronegativity that dictates the positive center of an ion should not reside on the more electronegative atom [28]. In case of the molecular ion of pyrrole only 5% of the positive charge reside on the nitrogen, while the adjacent two carbons take about 20% each, and the five hydrogens compensate for the remainder by almost equally contributing ~10% each [28]. Whatever species, it

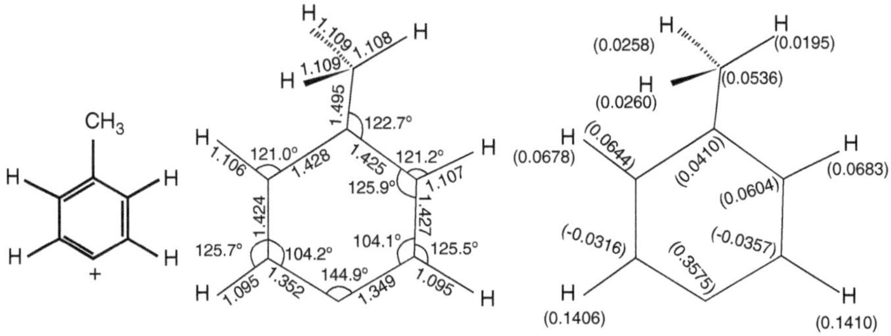

Fig. 2.3 *para*-Tolyl ion, $[C_7H_7]^+$: structural formula (*left*), calculated geometries (*center*) and calculated distributions of formal charge (*right*) (Reproduced from Ref. [32] with permission. © American Chemical Society, 1977)

turns out that the charge is delocalized over the whole molecular ion in a way that every atom of the molecule gets involved to some extent [29–31].

Charge delocalization For the *para*-tolyl ion only ~36% of the electron charge rests at the *para*-carbon atom (Fig. 2.3) [32]. In addition, the ionic geometry loses the symmetry of the corresponding neutral molecule.

2.2 Vertical Transitions

Electron ionization occurs extremely fast. The time needed for an electron of 70 eV to travel 1 nm through a molecule, a distance roughly corresponding to half a dozen bond lengths, is only about 2×10^{-16} s, and even larger molecules can be traversed in the low femtosecond range. The molecule being hit by the electron can be considered to be at rest because the thermal velocity of a few 100 m s^{-1} is negligible compared to the speed of the electron rushing through. Vibrational motions are slower by at least two orders of magnitude, e.g., even the fast C–H stretching vibration takes 1.1×10^{-14} s per cycle as can be calculated from its IR absorbance at around 3000 cm^{-1}.

According to the *Born-Oppenheimer approximation*, electronic motions and nuclear motions can be separated due to the large mass difference between nuclei and electrons [33–35]. Furthermore, the *Franck-Condon principle* states that electronic transitions will occur on a much faster timescale than it takes the nuclei to move to their new equilibrium positions [35–37]. Applied to the interaction of an energetic electron with a gaseous molecule this means that the positions of the atoms and thus bond lengths remain unaltered during ionization. In diagrams where energy is plotted on the ordinate and bond length on the abscissa, such transitions are represented as *vertical transitions* (Fig. 2.4).

The probability of a particular transition from the ground state neutral to a certain vibrational level of the ion is expressed by its *Franck-Condon factor*. The

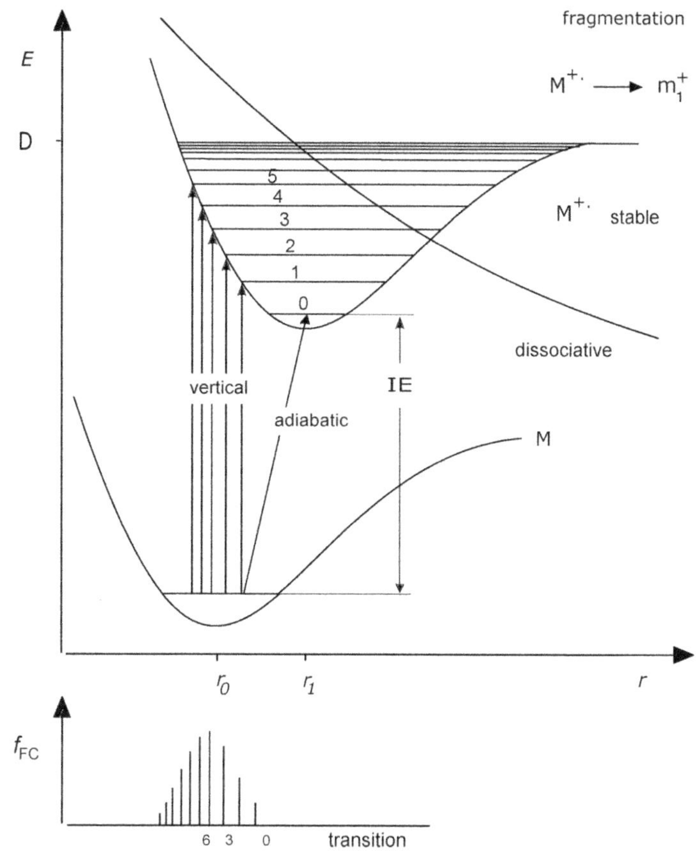

Fig. 2.4 Illustration of the transitions from the neutral to the ionic state for a diatomic molecule. Electron ionization can be represented by a vertical line in this diagram. Thus, ions are formed in a vibrationally excited state if the internuclear distance of the ionic state, r_1, is longer than in the ground state, r_0. Ions having internal energies below the dissociation energy D remain stable, whereas fragmentation will occur above. In few cases, ions are unstable, i.e., there is no minimum on their potential energy curve. The lower part schematically shows the distribution of Franck-Condon factors, f_{FC}, for various transitions

Franck-Condon factors originate from the fact that the probability for a transition is highest where the electronic wave functions of both ground state and excited state have maximum overlap. While for the ground state this is at equilibrium position, the wave functions of higher vibrational states have their maxima at the turning points of the motion.

No matter where the electron has formally been taken from, ionization tends to cause weakening of the bonding within the ion as compared to the precursor neutral. Weaker bonding means longer bond lengths on the average and this goes with a higher tendency toward dissociation of a bond.

In terms of potential energy surfaces, the situation can easiest be visualized by focusing on just one bond within the molecule or simply by discussing a diatomic molecule. A diatomic molecule has only one vibrational motion – bond stretching vibration – and therefore its potential energy can be represented by a potential energy curve rather than potential energy surface. The minimum of the potential energy curve of the neutral, which is assumed to be in its vibrational ground state, is located at shorter bond length, r_0, than the minimum of the radical ion in its ground state, r_1 (Fig. 2.4). Consequently, ionization is accompanied by vibrational excitation because the transitions are vertical, i.e., because the positions of the atoms are actually fixed during this short period.

The distribution of Franck-Condon factors, f_{FC}, describes the distribution of vibrational states for an excited ion [38]. The larger r_1 is, as compared to r_0, the more probable will be the generation of ions excited even well above the dissociation energy. Photoelectron spectroscopy allows for both the determination of adiabatic ionization energies and of Franck-Condon factors (Sect. 2.10.4).

The counterpart of the vertical ionization is a process where ionization of the neutral in its vibrational ground state would yield the radical ion also in its vibrational ground state, i.e., the $(0 \leftarrow 0)$ transition. This is termed *adiabatic ionization* and should be represented by a diagonal line in the diagram. The difference $IE_{vert} - IE_{ad}$ can lead to errors in ionization energies in the order of 0.1 – 0.7 eV [8].

The further fate of the ion depends on the shape of its potential energy surface. In case there is a minimum and the level of excitation is below the energy barrier for dissociation, D, the ion can exist for a very long time. Ions having an *internal energy* above the dissociation energy level will dissociate at some point leading to causing fragment ions within a mass spectrum. In some unfavorable cases, ions bear no minimum on their energy surface at all. These will suffer spontaneous dissociation and consequently, there is no chance to observe a molecular ion.

Metaphorically speaking

To understand the situation of the molecule imagine an apple through which a bullet is being shot: the impacting bullet passes through the apple, transfers an amount of energy, tears some of the fruit out and has long left it when the perforated apple finally drops or breaks into pieces.

2.3 Ionization Efficiency and Ionization Cross Section

The ionization energy represents the absolute minimum energy required for ionization of the neutral concerned. This means in turn that in order to effect ionization, the impacting electrons need to carry at least this amount of energy. If this energy were then to be quantitatively transferred during the collision, ionization would take place. Obviously, such an event is of rather low probability and therefore, the

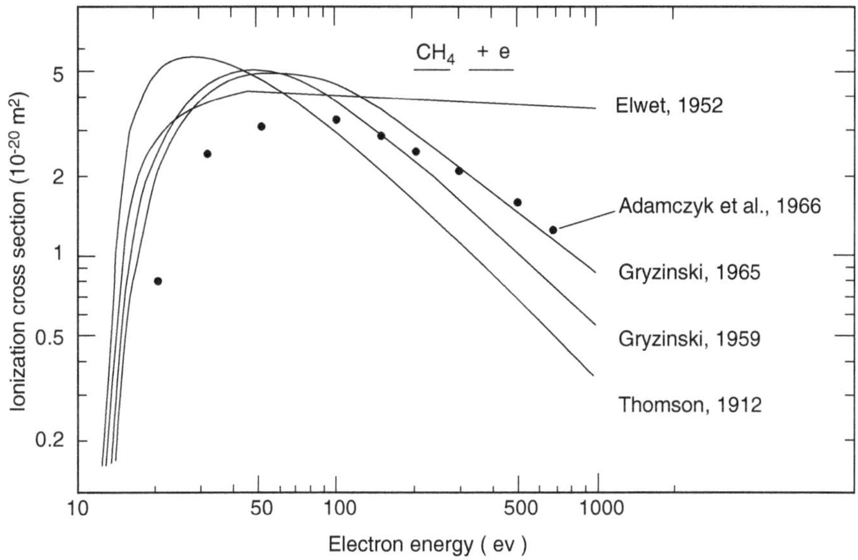

Fig. 2.5 Ionization cross sections for CH_4 upon electron ionization as obtained by several research groups (Reproduced from Ref. [13] with permission. © Elsevier Science, 1982)

ionization efficiency is close to zero with electrons carrying just the *IE* of the pertinent neutral. However, a slight increase in electron energy brings about a steady increase in ionization efficiency.

Strictly speaking, every molecular species has an ionization efficiency curve of its own depending on the *ionization cross section* of the specific molecule. In the case of methane, this issue has been studied repeatedly (Fig. 2.5) [13]. The ionization cross section describes an area through which the electron must travel in order to effectively interact with the neutral and consequently, the ionization cross section is given in units of square-meters.

Fortunately, the curves of ionization cross section vs. electron energy are all of the same type, exhibiting a maximum at electron energies around 70 eV (Fig. 2.5). This explains why EI spectra are almost always acquired at 70 eV.

Reasons for measuring EI spectra at 70 eV

- All atoms or molecules can be ionized at 70 eV, whereas at 15 eV such gases as He, Ne, Ar, H_2, and N_2 are not.
- The plateau of the ionization efficiency curve at ~70 eV implies small that variations in electron energy are negligible; actually EI at 60–80 eV work just as well.
- Therefore: better reproducibility of spectra, allowing comparison of spectra obtained from different mass spectrometers or from mass spectral databases (Sect. 5.9).

2.4 Internal Energy and the Further Fate of Ions

When an analyte is transferred into the ion source by means of any kind of sample introduction system it is in thermal equilibrium with this inlet device. As a result, the energy of the incoming molecules is represented by their thermal energy. This is the last opportunity to control the temperature, being a macroscopic property. After that, gas phase dilution would preclude any further collisions from taking place, and accordingly, any intermolecular energy transfer that would provide the basis for reaching thermal equilibrium and the validity of the Boltzmann distribution governing condensed phases and normal pressure gas phases. Thus, ionization changes the situation dramatically, as comparatively large amounts of energy need to be "handled" internally by the freshly formed ion. Even though part of this energy will contribute to translational or rotational energy of the molecule as a whole, the major fraction has to be stored in internal modes. Among the internal modes rotational excitation cannot store significant amounts of energy, whereas vibration and especially electronic excitation are capable of an uptake of several electronvolts each [39, 40].

2.4.1 Degrees of Freedom

Any atom or molecule in the gas phase has *external degrees of freedom*, because atoms and molecules as a whole can move along all three dimensions in space (along x, y, and z directions). This yields three *translational degrees of freedom*. From the kinetic gas theory the average translational energy can easily be estimated as $^3/_2kT$ delivering 0.04 eV at 300 K and 0.13 eV at 1000 K.

In case of diatomic and other linear molecules there are two rotations (around the x and y axes) and for all other molecules three rotations (around the x, y, and z axes). Thus, we have two or three more degrees of freedom contributing another kT or $^3/_2kT$ of energy, respectively, for the latter summing up to 0.08 eV at room temperature and 0.26 eV at 1000 K. This does not change independently of the number of atoms of the molecule or of their atomic masses.

In contrast to the external degrees of freedom, the number of *internal degrees of freedom*, notably *vibrational degrees of freedom*, s, increases with the number of atoms within the molecule, N. These internal degrees of freedom represent the number of vibrational modes a molecule can access. In other words, each of N atoms can move along three coordinates in space yielding $3N$ degrees of freedom in total, but as explained in the preceding paragraph, three of them have to be subtracted for the motion of the molecule as a whole and an additional two (linear) or three (nonlinear) have to be subtracted for rotational motion as a whole. Thus, we obtain for the number of vibrational modes

$$s = 3N - 5 \text{ in case of diatomic or linear molecules} \quad (2.8)$$

$$s = 3N - 6 \text{ in case of nonlinear molecules.} \quad (2.9)$$

It is obvious that even relatively small molecules possess a considerable number of vibrational modes.

Thermal energy of a molecule The thermal energy distribution curves for 1,2-diphenylethane, $C_{14}H_{14}$, $s = 3 \times 28 - 6 = 78$, have been calculated at 75 and 200 °C [41]. Their maxima were obtained at ~0.3 eV and ~0.6 eV, respectively, with almost no molecules exceeding twice that energy of maximum probability. At 200 °C, the most probable energy roughly corresponds to 0.008 eV per vibrational degree of freedom, which is a very small as compared to binding energies.

This indicates that excited vibrational states are almost fully unoccupied at room temperature and only the energetically much lower-lying internal rotations are effective under these conditions. Upon electron ionization, the situation changes quite dramatically as can be concluded from the Franck-Condon principle and therefore, energy storage in highly excited vibrational modes becomes of key importance for the further fate of ions in a mass spectrometer. In case of an indene molecule having 45 vibrational modes, the storage of 10 eV would mean roughly 0.2 eV per vibration, i.e., roughly a 20-fold value of thermal energy, provided the energy is perfectly randomized among the bonds.

2.4.2 Appearance Energy

As explained by the Franck-Condon diagram, hardly any molecular ions will be generated in their vibrational ground state. Instead, the majority of the ions created by EI is vibrationally excited and many of them are well above the dissociation energy level, the source of this energy being the 70 eV electrons. Dissociation of $M^{+\bullet}$, or fragmentation as it is usually referred to in mass spectrometry, leads to the formation of a fragment ion, m_1^+, and a neutral. These two processes can be written in generalized form as:

$$M^{+\bullet} \rightarrow m_1^+ + n^\bullet \quad (2.10)$$

$$M^{+\bullet} \rightarrow m_1^{+\bullet} + n \quad (2.11)$$

Reaction (2.10) describes the loss of a radical, whereas Reaction (2.11) corresponds to the loss of a molecule, thereby conserving the radical cation

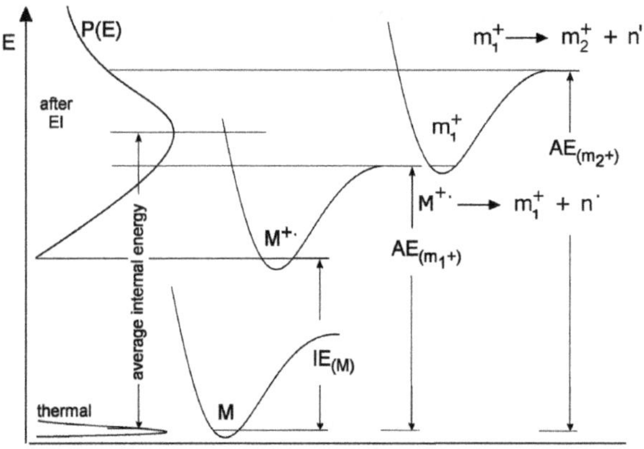

Fig. 2.6 Definition of the appearance energy and visualization of changes in internal energy distributions, $P_{(E)}$, of relevant species upon electron ionization and subsequent fragmentation (energy scale compressed for the ions)

property of the molecular ion in the fragment ion. Bond breaking is a endothermal process and thus the potential energy of the fragment ion is usually located at a higher energy level (Fig. 2.6).

Definition

The amount of energy needed to be transferred to the neutral M to allow for the detection of the fragment ion m_1^+ is called the *appearance energy* (*AE*) of that fragment ion. The old, and also incorrect, term *appearance potential* (*AP*) is still found in the literature.

In fact, the ions are not generated by one specific internal energy applying for all ions, but via a broad energy distribution $P_{(E)}$. One should keep in mind, however, that such a distribution is only valid for a large set of ions as each individual one bears a defined internal energy, ranging from just above *IE* to well beyond 10 eV for certain ones. Fragmentation of those highly excited ions from the tail of the $P_{(E)}$ curve yields fragment ions having still enough energy for a second dissociation step, $m_1^+ \rightarrow m_2^+ + n'$ or even a third one. Each of the subsequent steps can in principle also be characterized by an appearance energy value.

2.4.3 Bond Dissociation Energies and Heats of Formation

Great efforts have been made to generate accurate and reliable ion thermochemistry data. Once such data is available, it can be employed to elucidate fragmentation mechanisms and in addition, it is useful for obtaining some background on the energetic dimensions in mass spectrometry.

Heats of formation of neutral molecules, $\Delta H_{f(RH)}$, can be obtained from combustion data with high accuracy. Bond dissociation energies can either be derived for *homolytic bond dissociation*

$$R - H \rightarrow R^{\bullet} + H^{\bullet}, \Delta H_{Dhom} \tag{2.12}$$

or *heterolytic bond dissociation*

$$R - H \rightarrow R^{+} + H^{-}, \Delta H_{Dhet} \tag{2.13}$$

The homolytic bond dissociation enthalpies give the energy needed to cleave a bond of the neutral molecule which, in the gas phase is in its vibrational and electronic ground states, to obtain a pair of radicals which also are not in excited modes. Homolytic bond dissociation enthalpies are in the range of 3–5 eV (Table 2.2). The heterolytic bond dissociation energies apply for the case of creating a cation and an anion in their ground states from the neutral precursor which means that these values include the amount of energy needed for charge separation; they are in the order of 10–13 eV (Table 2.3). Due to the significantly altered bonding situation, breaking of a bond is clearly less demanding in molecular ions than in neutral molecules.

Energetics of $H^{\bullet}$ loss from $CH4^{+\bullet}$ The minimum energy needed to form a CH_3^+ ion and a hydrogen radical from the methane molecular ion can be estimated from the heat of reaction, ΔH_r, of this process. According to Fig. 2.6, $\Delta H_r = AE_{(CH3+)} - IE_{(CH4)}$. In order to calculate the missing $AE_{(CH3+)}$ we use the tabulated values of $\Delta H_{f(H\bullet)} = 218.0$ kJ mol^{-1}, $\Delta H_{f(CH3+)} = 1093$ kJ mol^{-1}, $\Delta H_{f(CH4)} = -74.9$ kJ mol^{-1},

Table 2.2 Homolytic R–H bond dissociation enthalpies, ΔH_{Dhom}, and heats of formation, $\Delta H_{f(X\bullet)}$, of some selected bonds and radicals [kJ mol^{-1}] [a]

	Radical $X^{\bullet}$	$H^{\bullet}$	$CH_3^{\bullet}$	$Cl^{\bullet}$	$OH^{\bullet}$	$NH_2^{\bullet}$
	$\Delta H_{f(X\bullet)}$	218.0	143.9	121.3	37.7	197.5
$R^{\bullet}$	$\Delta H_{f(R\bullet)}$					
$H^{\bullet}$	218.0	436.0	435.1	431.4	497.9	460.2
$CH_3^{\bullet}$	143.9	435.1	373.2	349.8	381.2	362.8
$C_2H_5^{\bullet}$	107.5	410.0	354.8	338.1	380.3	352.7
i-$C_3H_7^{\bullet}$	74.5	397.5	352.3	336.4	384.5	355.6
t-$C_4H_9^{\bullet}$	31.4	384.9	342.3	335.6	381.6	349.8
$C_6H_5^{\bullet}$	325.1	460.1	417.1	395.4	459.0	435.6
$C_6H_5CH_2^{\bullet}$	187.9	355.6	300.4	290.4	325.9	300.8
$C_6H_5CO^{\bullet}$	109.2	363.5	338.1	336.8	440.2	396.6

[a] Values from Ref. [42]

Table 2.3 Heterolytic R–H bond dissociation enthalpies, ΔH_{Dhet}, and heats of formation of some molecules and ions [kJ mol^{-1}] [a]

Ion	ΔH_{Dhet}	$\Delta H_{\text{f(R+)}}$	$\Delta H_{\text{f(RH)}}$
Proton, H^+	1674	1528	0.0
Methyl, CH_3^+	1309	1093	–74.9
Ethyl, $C_2H_5^+$	1129	903	–84.5
n-Propyl, $CH_3CH_2CH_2^+$	1117	866	–103.8
i-Propyl, $CH_3CH^+CH_3$	1050	802	–103.8
n-Butyl, $CH_3CH_2CH_2CH_2^+$	1109	837	–127.2
sec-Butyl, $CH_3CH_2CH^+CH_3$	1038	766	–127.2
i-Butyl, $(CH_3)_2CHCH_2^+$	1109	828	–135.6
t-Butyl, $(CH_3)_3C^+$	975	699	–135.6
Phenyl, $C_6H_5^+$	1201	1138	82.8

[a]Values from Refs. [9, 43–45]

and $IE_{(\text{CH4})} = 12.6\text{ eV} = 1216\text{ kJ mol}^{-1}$. First, the heat of formation of the methane molecular ion is determined based on the experimental value of $IE_{(\text{CH4})}$:

$$\Delta H_{\text{f(CH4+}\bullet)} = \Delta H_{\text{f(CH4)}} + IE_{(\text{CH4})} \tag{2.14}$$

$$\Delta H_{\text{f(CH4+}\bullet)} = -74.9\,\text{kJ mol}^{-1} + 1216\,\text{kJ mol}^{-1} = 1141.1\,\text{kJ mol}^{-1}$$

Then, the heat of formation of the products is calculated from:

$$\Delta H_{\text{f(prod)}} = \Delta H_{\text{f(CH3+)}} + \Delta H_{\text{f(H}\bullet)} \tag{2.15}$$

$$\Delta H_{\text{f(prod)}} = 1093\,\text{kJ mol}^{-1} + 218\,\text{kJ mol}^{-1} = 1311\,\text{kJ mol}^{-1}$$

Now, the heat of reaction is obtained from the difference

$$\Delta H_{\text{r}} = \Delta H_{\text{f(prod)}} - \Delta H_{\text{f(CH4+}\bullet)} \tag{2.16}$$

$$\Delta H_{\text{r}} = 1311\,\text{kJ mol}^{-1} - 1141.1\,\text{kJ mol}^{-1} = 169.9\,\text{kJ mol}^{-1}$$

The value of 169.9 kJ mol^{-1} (1.75 eV) corresponds to $AE_{(\text{CH3+})} = 14.35$ eV, which is in good agreement with published values of about 14.3 eV (Fig. 2.7) [25, 46]. It should be noted that the value of 169.9 kJ mol^{-1} is only 40% of the homolytic C–H bond dissociation enthalpy of the neutral methane molecule, thereby indicating the weaker bonding in the molecular ion. Based on mass spectrometric techniques alone, one would have measured $IE_{(\text{CH4})}$ and $AE_{(\text{CH3+})}$ to determine $\Delta H_{\text{f(CH4+}\bullet)}$ and $\Delta H_{\text{f(CH3+ H}\bullet)}$, respectively.

The heat of formation of organic radicals and positive ions decreases with their size and even more importantly with their degree of branching at the radical or ionic site. A lower heat of formation is equivalent to a higher thermodynamic stability of the respective ion or radical. The corresponding trends are clearly expressed by the values given in Tables 2.2 and 2.3. This causes the fragmentation pathways of

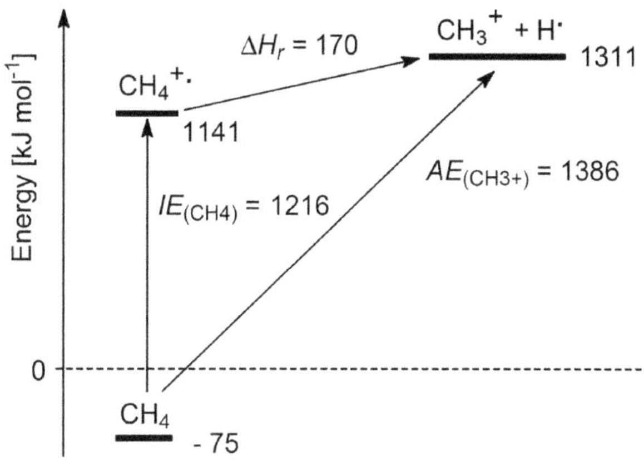

Fig. 2.7 Diagram showing the relative energy levels of species involved in ionization of methane and loss of an H$^\bullet$ from the molecular ion. Values are given in kJ mol^{-1} and rounded to integer numbers

molecular ions proceeding by formation of secondary or tertiary radicals and/or ions to become dominant over those leading to smaller and/or primary radical and ionic fragments, respectively (Sect. 6.2).

Isomeric $C_4H_9^+$ ions An impressive case showing the effects of isomerization upon thermal stability is that of butyl ions, $C_4H_9^+$. This carbenium ion can exist in four isomers with heats of formation that range from 837 kJ mol^{-1} in the case of *n*-butyl over 828 kJ mol^{-1} for *iso*-butyl (also primary) to 766 kJ mol^{-1} for *sec*-butyl to 699 kJ mol^{-1} in the case of *t*-butyl, meaning an overall increase in thermodynamic stability by 138 kJ mol^{-1} (Sect. 6.6) [43].

2.4.4 Randomization of Energy

The best evidence for randomization of internal energy over all vibrational modes of a molecular ion prior to any fragmentation is delivered by EI mass spectra themselves. If there was no randomization, fragmentation would occur directly at any bond that immediately suffers from the withdrawal of an electron. As a result, mass spectra would show an almost statistical bond breaking throughout the molecular ion. Instead, mass spectra reveal a great deal of selectivity of the molecular ion when choosing fragmentation pathways. This means the molecular ion explores many pathways up to its respective transition states and prefers the thermodynamically (and as we will see, also kinetically) more favorable ones. The same is true for fragment ions.

From a purely thermodynamic point of view the situation can be elucidated by considering a hypothetical molecular ion having some internal energy and being “faced to the selection” of a fragmentation pathway (Fig. 2.8).

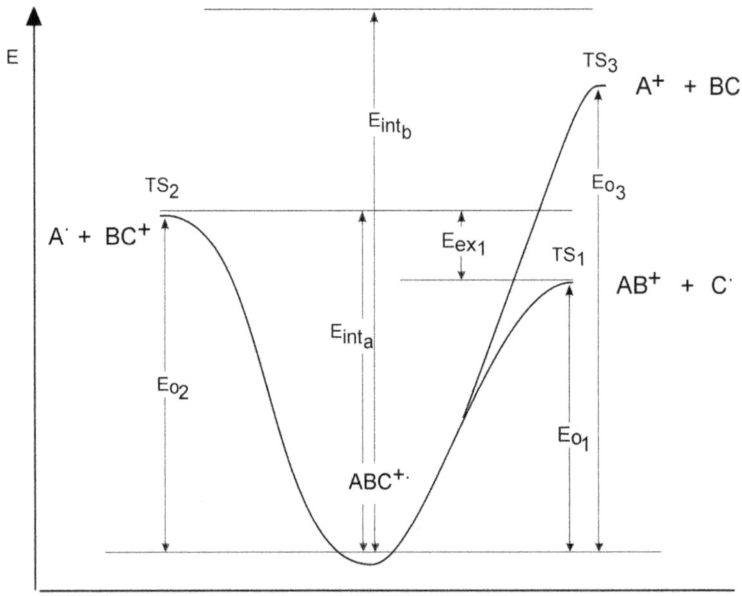

Fig. 2.8 Competition of fragmentation pathways strongly depends on the internal energy of the fragmenting ion and on the activation energies, E_0, of the transition states, i.e., the "energy barriers" of the respective reactions

Ions aren't individuals, are they?
Sometimes we refer to ions as if they were able to decisively act as individuals. However, we have to keep in mind that ion fragmentations result from a statistical distribution of internal energy among the internal degrees of freedom available. As from the perspective of the final result, it may nonetheless appear as if the ion had "chosen" to dissociate via a particular pathway.

(a) The molecular ion $ABC^{+\bullet}$ has an internal energy E_{inta} being slightly above the activation energy, E_{02}, required to cross the transition state TS_2 leading to the formation of $A^\bullet$ and BC^+, but definitely more than needed to dissociate into AB^+ and $C^\bullet$. The difference between the energy content E_{inta} and E_{01} is termed *excess energy*, $E_{\text{ex}} = E_{\text{int}} - E_0$, of the transition state TS_1. In this case either ionic product would be observed, but the third pathway could not be accessed.

(b) The molecular ion $ABC^{+\bullet}$ has an internal energy E_{intb} being clearly higher than any of the three activation energies. Here, formation of all possible products should occur.

A simple comparison of activation energies does not allow, however, to predict the relative intensities of the ions AB^+ and BC^+ or of AB^+, BC^+, and A^+, respectively. In fact, from this model one would expect similar or even equal abundances of all accessible fragment ions. Actual mass spectra show greatly differing intensities of signals resulting from competing decomposition pathways. This reveals the oversimplification of the preceding passage.

Not just energy alone

Thermodynamic data such as heats of formation and activation energies alone are not sufficient to adequately describe the unimolecular fragmentations of excited ions.

2.5 Quasi-Equilibrium Theory

The *quasi-equilibrium theory* (QET) of mass spectra is a theoretical approach for describing the unimolecular decompositions of ions and hence their mass spectra [47–49]. QET is an extention of the Rice-Ramsperger-Marcus-Kassel (RRKM) theory with the aim of accommodating the conditions of mass spectrometry and represents a landmark in the theory of mass spectra [12]. Within the mass spectrometer almost all processes occur under high vacuum, i.e., in the highly diluted gas phase – one needs to be aware of how this contrasts to chemical reactions in the condensed phase as usually carried out in the laboratory [50, 51]. In essence, bimolecular reactions rarely occur in the vacuum of a mass spectrometer. As long as ions are formed and reacting under these conditions we are dealing with the chemistry of *isolated ions in the gas phase*. Isolated ions are not in thermal equilibrium with their surroundings as assumed by the RRKM theory. In fact, being isolated in the gas phase means for an ion that it may only internally redistribute energy and that it may only undergo unimolecular reactions such as isomerization or dissociation. This is why the theory of unimolecular reactions is of paramount importance in mass spectrometry.

QET is not the sole theory in the field; indeed, there are several apparently competitive statistical theories for describing rate constants of unimolecular reactions [11, 49]. However, none of these theories has been able to quantitatively describe all reactions of a given ion. QET, however, is well established and even in its simplified form allows sufficient insight into the behavior of isolated ions. Thus, we start from the basic assumptions of QET. Along this scheme we will be led from the neutral molecule to ions, and from transition states and reaction rates to fragmentation products and thus, through the basic concepts and definitions of gas phase ion chemistry.

2.5.1 QET's Basic Premises

According to QET the rate constant, k, of a unimolecular reaction is basically a function of excess energy, E_{ex}, of the reactants in the transition state and thus $k_{(E)}$ strongly depends on the internal energy distribution of any particular ion. QET is thus based on the following essential premises [47, 52]:

1. The initial ionization is "vertical", i.e., there is no change of position or kinetic energy of the nuclei while it is taking place. With the usual electron energy any valence shell electron may be removed.
2. The molecular ion will be of low symmetry and have an odd electron. It will have as many low-lying excited electronic states as necessary to form essentially a continuum. Radiationless transitions then will result in transfer of electronic energy into vibrational energy on a time scale comparable to the periods of nuclear vibrations.
3. These low-lying excited electronic states will in general not be repulsive; hence, the molecular ions will not dissociate immediately, but rather remain together for a time sufficient for the excess electronic energy to become randomly distributed as vibrational energy over the ion.
4. The rates of dissociation of the molecular ion are determined by the probabilities of the energy randomly distributed over the ion becoming concentrated in the particular fashions required to give several activated complex configurations yielding the dissociations.
5. Rearrangements of the ions can occur in a similar fashion.
6. If the initial molecular ion has sufficient energy, the fragment ion will in turn have enough energy to undergo further decomposition.

The characteristics of the ionization process as described in Sect. 2.2 justify the first assumption of QET. Further, it is obvious that electronic excitation occurs together with vibrational excitation and thus, the second assumption of QET is met.

2.5.2 Basic QET

QET focuses on the dynamic aspects of ion fragmentation. It describes the *rate constants* for the dissociation of isolated ions as a function of internal energy, E_{int}, and activation energy of the reaction, E_0. By doing so, it compensates for the shortcomings of the merely thermodynamic treatment above.

QET delivers the following expression for the unimolecular rate constant:

$$k_{(E)} = \int_{0}^{E-E_0} \frac{1}{h} \times \frac{\rho^*(E_{int}, E_0, E_t)}{\rho_{(E)}} dE_t \tag{2.17}$$

In this equation, $\rho_{(E)}$ is the density of energy levels for the system with total energy E_{int}, and $\rho^*_{(E,E0,Et)}$ is the density of energy levels in the activated complex, i.e., transition state, with activation energy E_0 and translational energy E_t in the reaction coordinate. The reaction coordinate represents the bond which is actually being broken. The expression is slightly simplified by approximating the system by as many harmonic oscillators as there are vibrational degrees of freedom:

$$k_{(E)} = \left(\frac{E_{int} - E_0}{E_{int}}\right)^{s-1} \frac{\prod_{j=1}^{s} \nu_j}{\prod_{i=1}^{s-1} \nu_i *} \tag{2.18}$$

Then, the exponent is given by the number of degrees of freedom, s, minus 1 for the bond actually being broken. For a strict treatment of fragmenting ions by QET one would need to know the activation energies of all accessible reactions and the probability functions describing the density of energy levels.

In the most simplified form, the rate constant $k_{(E)}$ can be expressed as:

$$k_{(E)} = \nu \times \left(\frac{E_{int} - E_0}{E_{int}}\right)^{s-1} \tag{2.19}$$

where ν is a frequency factor which is determined by the number and density of vibrational states. The frequency factor thereby replaces the complex expression of probability functions. Now, it becomes clear that a reaction rate considerably increases with growing E_{ex}.

$$k_{(E)} = \nu \times \left(\frac{E_{ex}}{E_{int}}\right)^{s-1} \tag{2.20}$$

Unfortunately, as with all oversimplified theories, there are limitations for the application of the latter equation to ions close to the dissociation threshold. In these cases, the number of degrees of freedom has to be replaced by an effective number of oscillators which is obtained by use of an arbitrary correction factor [8]. However, as long as we are dealing with ions having internal energies considerably above the dissociation threshold, i.e., where $(E - E_0)/E \approx 1$, the relationship is valid and can even be simplified to give the quasi-exponential expression

$$k_{(E)} = \nu \times e^{-(s-1)^{E_0}/_E} \tag{2.21}$$

Calculating $k_{(E)}$ For $\nu = 10^{15}$ s^{-1}, $s = 15$, $E_{int} = 2$ eV, and $E_0 = 1.9$ eV the rate constant is calculated as 3.0×10^{-5} s^{-1}. For the same parameters but $E_{int} = 4$ eV we obtain $k = 6.3 \times 10^{10}$ s^{-1} being a 2.1×10^5-fold increase. This means that a reaction is extremely slow at small excess energies but becomes very fast as soon as there is some substantial excess energy available.

2.5.3 Rate Constants and Their Meaning

The rate constants of unimolecular reactions have the dimension *per second* (s^{-1}). This means the process can happen x times per second, e.g., $k = 6.3 \times 10^{10}\ s^{-1}$ being equivalent to 1.6×10^{-11} s *per fragmentation on the average*. Note the emphasis "on the average", because rate constants are macroscopic and statistical in nature as they get their meaning only from considering a very large number of reacting particles. A single ion will have a lifetime of 1.6×10^{-11} s *on the average* in this case; however, a specific one in consideration might also decay much sooner or later, with the actual decay occurring at the speed of vibrational motions. The dimension s^{-1} also means there is no dependence on concentration as it is the case with second- or higher order reactions. This is because the ions are isolated in the gas phase, alone for their entire lifetime, and the only chance for change is by means of unimolecular reaction.

2.5.4 $k_{(E)}$ Functions – Typical Examples

Although the general shape of any $k_{(E)}$ function resembles the ionization efficiency curve to the left of the maximum, these must not be confused. At an excess energy close to zero, the rate constant is also close to zero but it rises sharply upon slight increase of the excess energy. However, there is an upper limit for the rate of a dissociation that is defined by the vibrational frequency of the bond to be cleaved. The fragments are not able to fly apart at a higher velocity than determined by their vibrational motion (Fig. 2.9).

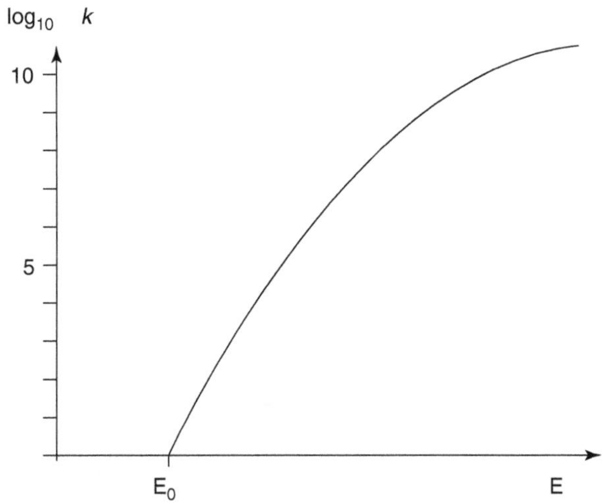

Fig. 2.9 General shape of a log k vs. E plot as determined by the simplified QET. At $E = E_0$ the reaction is extremely slow. A slight increase in energy causes k to rise sharply

2.5.5 Reacting Ions Described by $k_{(E)}$ Functions

According to our knowledge of rate constants, Fig. 2.8 now calls for a different interpretation. At an internal energy E_{inta} the molecular ion $ABC^{+\bullet}$ can easily cross the transition state TS_1 to form AB^+ and $C^\bullet$. The products of the second reaction can in principle be formed, even though the excess energy at TS_2 is so small that the product ion BC^+ will almost be negligible. The third pathway is still not accessible. At an internal energy E_{intb} the excess energy is assuredly high enough to allow for any of the three pathways with realistic rates to observe the products. Nevertheless, due to the strong dependence of the rate constant on E_{ex}, the reaction over TS_3 will be by far the least important.

2.5.6 Direct Cleavages and Rearrangement Fragmentations

The reactions of excited ions are not always as straightforward as expected. Of course, the existence of multiple fragmentation pathways for an ion consisting of several tens of atoms brings about different types of reactions all of which certainly will not lead to the same $k_{(E)}$ function [53].

The $k_{(E)}$ functions of two reactions of the same type, appear to be "parallel" in comparison, starting out at different activation energies (Fig. 2.10a), whereas different types of reactions will show a crossover of their $k_{(E)}$ functions at intermediate excess energy (Fig. 2.10b).

For example, case (**a**) depicts two competing homolytic bond cleavages. Homolytic bond cleavages are simple fragmentations of molecular ions creating an even-electron ion and a radical. One cleavage might require a somewhat higher activation energy than the other ($E_{02} > E_{01}$) because of the difference between the bonds to be cleaved, but once having enough excess energy their rates will rise sharply. The

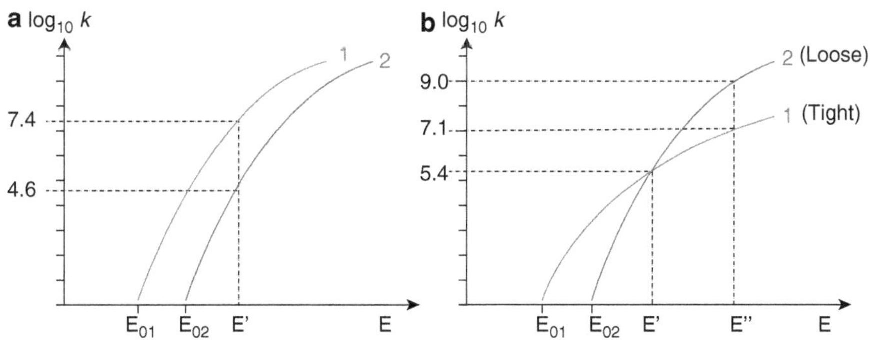

Fig. 2.10 Comparison of different types of reactions by their $k_{(E)}$ functions. Reactions of the same type show $k_{(E)}$ functions that are "parallel" (**a**), whereas $k_{(E)}$ functions of different types tend to cross over at intermediate excess energy (**b**). In **a**, reaction **1** would proceed $10^{2.8}$ (630) times faster at an internal energy E' than would reaction **2**. In **b**, both reactions have the same rate constant, $k = 10^{5.4}\ s^{-1}$, at an internal energy E', whereas reaction **2** becomes $10^{1.9}$ (80) times faster at E''

more energy is pushed into the ion, the faster the bond rupture can occur. A further increase of excess energy will become ineffective only when the rate approaches the upper limit as defined by the vibrational frequency of the bond to be cleaved.

Case (**b**) compares a *rearrangement fragmentation* (reaction 1) with a *homolytic bond cleavage* (reaction 2). During a rearrangement fragmentation the precursor ion expels a neutral fragment which is an intact molecule after having rearranged in an energetically favorable manner. Rearrangements commence at low excess energy, but then the rate approaches the limit relatively soon, while cleavage starts out later, then overrunning the other at higher excess energy. The differences can be explained by the different transition states of both types of reactions. The cleavage has a *loose transition state* [41], i.e., there is no need for certain parts of the molecule to assume a specific position while the cleavage proceeds. The dissociation merely requires enough energy in the respective bond so that the binding forces can be overcome. Once the bond is stretched too far, the fragments drift apart. The rearrangement demands less excess energy to proceed, because the energy for a bond rupture on one side is compensated for by the energy received when a new bond is formed by the accepting position. Compared to the simple cleavage, such a transition state is usually termed *tight transition state* (Sect. 6.12). Then, the neutral is expelled in a second step. Such a reaction obviously depends on the suitable conformation for rearrangement at the same time when sufficient energy is put into the bond to be cleaved. Furthermore, the second step has to follow in order to yield the products. Overall, there is no use in having more than enough energy until the ion reaches the conformation needed. Thus, after considering either basic type of fragmentation, the fifth assumption of QET is justified, because there is no reason why rearrangements should not be treated by QET.

2.6 Time Scale of Events

We have just learned that ionization occurs on the low femtosecond timescale, direct bond cleavages require between some picoseconds to several tens of nanoseconds, and rearrangement fragmentations usually proceed in much less than a microsecond (Fig. 2.11). All those chemical reactions are strictly unimolecular, because the reacting ions are created in the highly diluted gas phase – circumstances that prevent bimolecular reactions of the ions during their residence time within the ion source. This dwell time is determined by the extraction voltages applied to accelerate and focus ions to form a beam and by the dimensions of that ion source. In standard EI sources the ions spend about 1 μs before they are ejected by action of the accelerating potential [54].

Therefore, a reaction needs to proceed within that certain period of time to make the products detectable in the mass spectrum, and for this purpose there is a need for some excess energy in the transition state.

Finally, some fragment ions may even be formed after the excited species has left the ion source, so to speak in the “afterglow”, giving rise to metastable ion dissociation. As the ions then travel at speeds of some 10^4 m s^{-1} they pass the mass

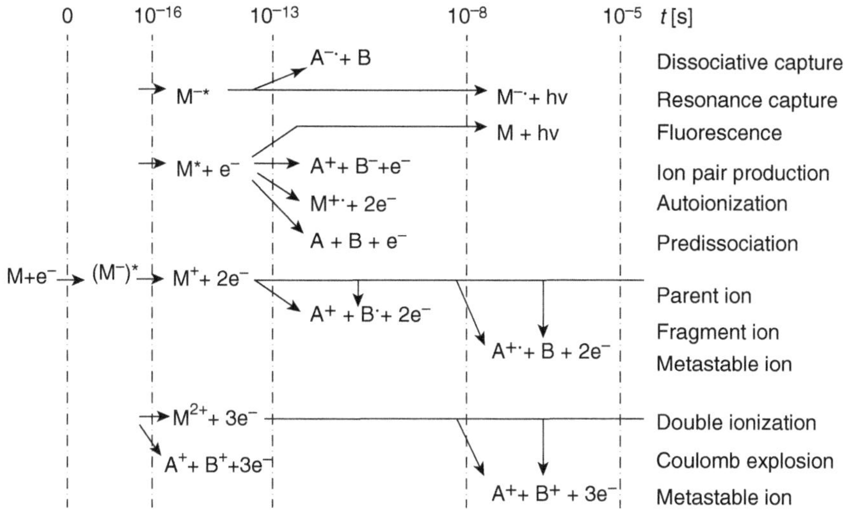

Fig. 2.11 Schematic time chart of possible electron ionization processes (Adapted from Ref. [40] with permission. © Wiley & Sons, 1986)

analyzer in the order of 10–50 µs (Fig. 2.12) [10]. Even though this particular case has been adapted for a double-focusing magnetic sector mass spectrometer, an ion of *m/z* 100, and an acceleration voltage of 8 kV, the effective time scales for other types of beam instruments (quadrupole, time-of-flight) are very similar under their typical conditions of operation (Table 2.4).

2.6.1 Stable, Metastable, and Unstable Ions

The terminology for ions has been coined as a direct consequence of the classical mass spectrometric time scale. Nondecomposing molecular ions and molecular ions decomposing at rates below about 10^5 s^{-1} will reach the detector without fragmentation and are therefore termed *stable ions*. Consequently, ions dissociating at rates above 10^6 s^{-1} cannot reach the detector. Instead, their fragments will be detected and thus they are called *unstable ions*. A small percentage, however, decomposing at rates of 10^5–10^6 s^{-1} will just fragment on transit through the mass analyzer – those are termed *metastable ions* (Figs. 2.11, 2.12, and 2.13) [5, 6, 10].

Definition

stable ions, $k < 10^5$ s^{-1}

metastable ions, 10^5 s$^{-1} < k < 10^6$ s^{-1}

unstable ions, $k > 10^6$ s^{-1}

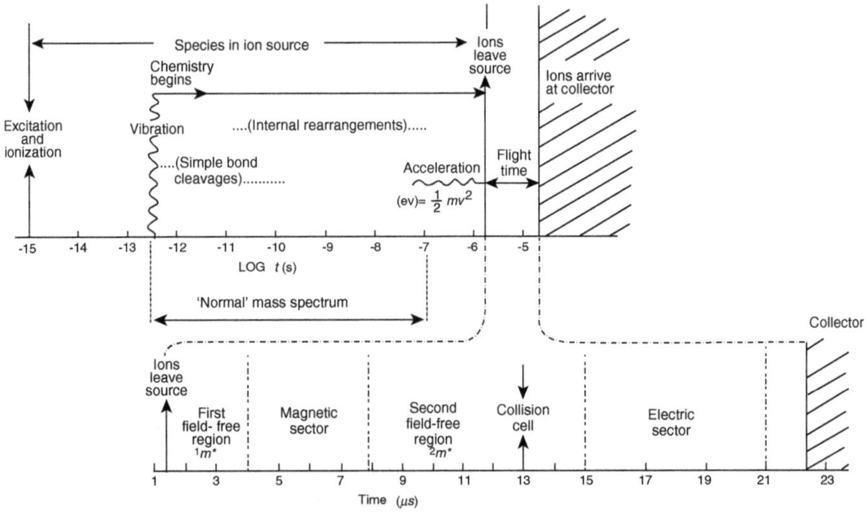

Fig. 2.12 The mass spectrometric time scale and its correlation to the classical instrumental framework. Note the logarithmic time scale for the ion source that spans nine orders of magnitude (Reproduced from Ref. [10] with permission. © John Wiley & Sons, Ltd., 1985)

Table 2.4 Typical ion flight times in different types of mass spectrometers

Mass analyzer	Flight path [m]	Acceleration voltage [V]	Typical *m/z*	Flight time [μs]
Quadrupole	0.2	10	500	57
Magnetic sector	2.0	5000	500	45
Time-of-flight	2.0	20,000	2000	45

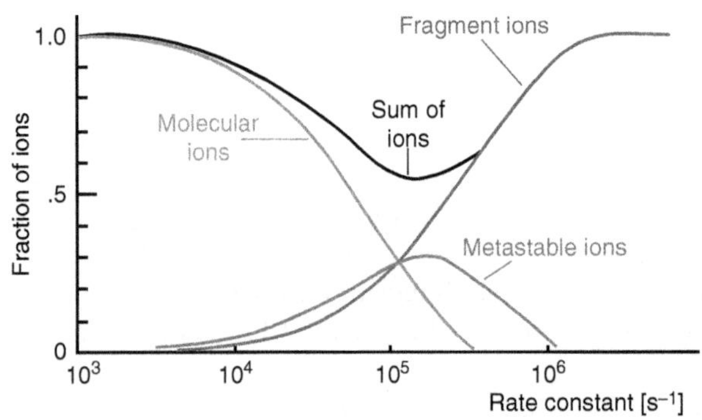

Fig. 2.13 Correlation between rate constants of ion dissociations and terminology referring to ion stability as employed in mass spectrometry (Adapted from Ref. [55] with permission. © The American Institute of Physics, 1959)

There is no justification for such a classification of ion stabilities outside the mass spectrometer because almost all ions created under the conditions inside a mass spectrometer would spontaneously react in the atmosphere or in solvents. Nevertheless, this classification is useful as far as ions isolated in the gas phase are concerned and is valid independently of the type of mass analyzer or ionization method employed.

2.6.2 Time Scale of Ion Storage Devices

Many modern instruments make use of ion storage in some way. Linear radiofrequency multipoles can be axially segmented or equipped with trapping plates to their ends to raise switchable potential walls that allow to accumulate, store, and eject ion packages as required. The most prominent of those devices is the *linear* (*quadrupole*) *ion trap* (LIT). The other type, the so-called three-dimensional *quadrupole ion trap* (QIT) stores ion clouds to have them ready for mass analysis by bringing them successively from stable to unstable ion trajectories that end up with ejection from the trap onto a detector. Fourier transform ion cyclotron resonance (FT-ICR) relies on storage of ions on circular paths to detect the angular frequencies of coherent ion packages as they repeatedly pass a pair of detection plates. The recent *Orbitrap* mass analyzer employs a different operational concept but shares the time frame with FT-ICR. Even during their transport from the ion source to the mass analyzer of the above instruments, ions are often repeatedly being accumulated, stored and passed to another section of the instrument before they finally enter the compartment for *m*/*z* analysis. (For details of mass analyzers refer to Chap. 4.)

The time span of ion accumulation can easily extend from milliseconds to seconds, the passage between functional units of the instrument may take tens of microseconds to milliseconds, and the *m*/*z* analysis requires storage times from milliseconds (QIT, LIT) to seconds (FT-ICR, Orbitrap).

This way, modern mass spectrometry instrumentation has gone beyond the classical mass spectrometric time scale. Especially the time frame after leaving the ion source has drastically been extended. It is still important, however, to understand the considerations of the classical mass spectrometric time scale as it governs the processes in many types of ion sources (electron ionization, chemical ionization, field ionization and field desorption, laser desorption) and as it is still basically valid for a wide range of mass analyzers. One should be aware though of the 10^3–10^6-fold expansion of the time scale for cases where ion storage is involved. Furthermore, the handling of ions on the extended time scale is only possible if they are stable, i.e., non-decomposing, and this is in accordance with our previous definition of ion stability in terms of being just below threshold for dissociation during their dwell time in the instrument. Without the use of extremely soft ionization techniques (such as electrospray ionization), those ion-storing instruments would not have any ions to store nor to be analyzed.

2.7 Internal Energy – Practical Implications

Even comparatively small molecular ions can exhibit a substantial array of first-, second-, and higher-generation fragmentation pathways due their internal energy in the order of several electronvolts [53]. Typically, ion dissociations are endothermic, and thus each fragmentation step consumes some of the ions' internal energy. Highly excited ions may carry enough internal energy to allow for several consecutive cleavages, whereas others may just undergo one or even none (Sect. 2.4.2). The latter reach the detector as still intact molecular ions. The fragmentation pathways of the same generation compete with each other, their products being potential precursors for the next generation of fragmentation processes.

Branching pathways Imagine the hypothetical molecular ion $ABYZ^{+\bullet}$ undergoing three competing first-generation fragmentations, two of them rearrangements, one a homolytic bond cleavage (Fig. 2.14). Next, three first-generation fragment ions have several choices each, and thus the second-generation fragment ions $Y^{+\bullet}$ and YZ^{+} are both formed on two different pathways. The formation of the same higher-generation fragment ion via two or more different pathways is even more common. There are, for example, two pathways leading to an ion of composition Y. A closer look reveals that one of the composition Y ions occurs as $Y^{+\bullet}$ and another as Y^{+}. It is important to understand that $Y^{+\bullet}$ and Y^{+} are different species despite having identical empirical formulas, because $Y^{+\bullet}$ is an odd-electron ion while Y^{+} is an even-electron ion. Nevertheless, they would both contribute to one common peak at the same nominal *m*/*z* in a mass spectrum of ABYZ (Sect. 3.1.4).

In an EI mass spectrum of ABYZ, all ionic species would be detected which are formed as a result of numerous competing and consecutive reactions, but there is no simple rule which of them should give rise to intensive peaks and which of them would be hardly noticed.

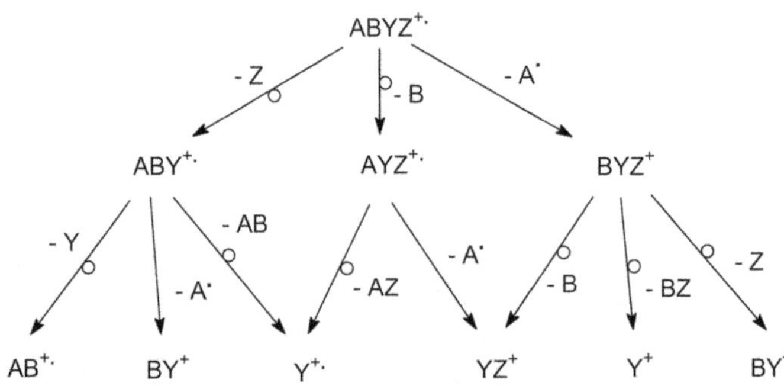

Fig. 2.14 Possible fragmentation pathways for hypothetical molecular ions $ABYZ^{+\bullet}$ having internal energies typical for EI. Simple bond cleavages cause radical losses, while rearrangement fragmentations (*circled arrows*) typically lead to losses of intact neutral molecules. Loss of a molecule preserves electronic state and charge state of the ion

Obviously, the first-generation fragment ions should be more closely related to the initial structure of ABYZ than those of the second or even third generation. Fortunately, such higher generation (and therefore low-mass) fragment ions can also reveal relevant information on the constitution of the analyte. In particular, they yield reliable information on the presence of functional groups (Chap. 6).

Fragmentation trees similar to that shown here can be constructed from any EI mass spectrum, providing ten thousands of examples for the sixth assumption of QET, that fragment ions may again be subject to dissociation, provided their internal energy suffices.

QET is realistic
The assumptions of QET have turned into basic statements governing the behavior of isolated ions in the gas phase and thus, in mass spectrometry in general.

2.8 Reverse Reactions – Activation Energy and Kinetic Energy Release

2.8.1 Activation Energy of the Reverse Reaction

By merely considering thermodynamic and kinetic models we may be able to understand how ions are formed and what parameters are effective to determine their further fate in the mass spectrometer. However, the potential energy surfaces considered in this context only reached up to the transition state (Fig. 2.6). Without explicitly mentioning it, we assumed the curves to stay on the same energetic level between transition state and the products of ion dissociation, i.e., the sum of heats of formation of the products would be equal to the energy of the transition state. This assumption is almost correct for homolytic bond cleavages in molecular ions because the recombination of an ion with a radical proceeds with almost negligible activation energy [5, 6]. In other words, the *activation energy of the reverse reaction*, E_{0r} (or often simply called *reverse activation energy*) is then close to zero. This explains why the result of our simple estimation of the activation energy for hydrogen radical loss from the molecular ion of methane could be realistic (Sect. 2.4.3).

In case of rearrangement fragmentations the situation is quite different, because one of the products is an intact neutral molecule of comparatively high thermodynamic stability, i.e., having negative or at least low values of ΔH_f (Table 2.5). Once the transition state is passed, the reaction proceeds by formation of products energetically much lower than the transition state. In case of the reverse reaction, this would require some or even substantial activation energy transfer to the fragments to allow their recombination, and thus $E_{0r} > 0$ (Fig. 2.15).

Table 2.5 Gas phase heats of formation, ΔH_f, of some frequently eliminated molecules[a]

Molecule	ΔH_f [kJ mol^{-1}][b]	Molecule	ΔH_f [kJ mol^{-1}][b]
CO_2	−393.5	HCl	−92.3
HF	−272.5	NH_3	−45.9
H_2O	−241.8	HBr	−36.4
CH_3OH	−201.1	C_3H_6 (propene)	20.4
H_2CO	−115.9	C_2H_4	52.5
CO	−110.5	HCN	135.1

[a]*IE* data extracted from Ref. [25] with permission. © NIST 2002
[b]All values have been rounded to one digit

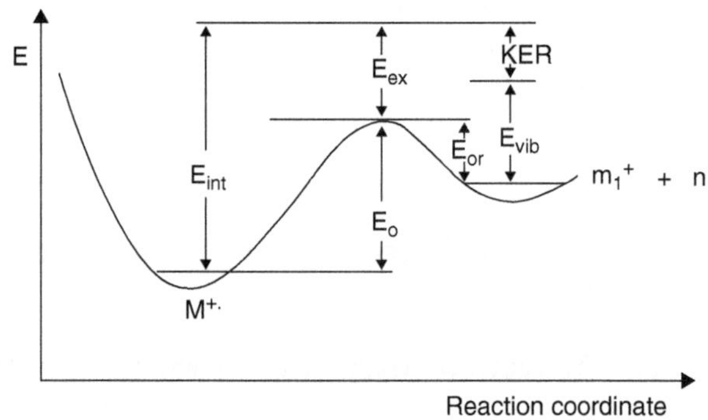

Fig. 2.15 Definition of E_{0r} and origin of KER. The excess energy of the decomposing ion in the transition state relative to the sum of the heats of formation of the ionic and neutral product is partitioned into vibrational excitation of the products plus KER

2.8.2 Kinetic Energy Release

The total excess energy, E_{extot}, of the precursor ion relative to the heats of formation of the products in their ground state, comprises the excess energy in the transition state, E_{ex}, plus the activation energy of the reverse reaction, E_{0r}:

$$E_{extot} = E_{ex} + E_{0r} \tag{2.22}$$

Although most ion fragmentations are endothermic, there is still a significant amount of energy to be redistributed among the reaction products. Much of E_{extot} is redistributed as vibrational energy, E_{vib}, among the internal modes, thereby supplying the energy for consecutive fragmentation of the fragment ion. Nonetheless, some of the energy is converted into translational motion of the fragments relative to their center of gravity. This portion of E_{extot} is released in the direction of the bond that is being cleaved, in other words, into separation from each other. This is termed *kinetic energy release*, KER (Fig. 2.14) [5, 6, 10, 56, 57].

The larger the sum of E_{ex} + E_{0r} the larger is the expected KER. Large reverse activation energy, especially when combined with repulsive electronic states in the transition state, will cause significant KER that has been observed up to 1.64 eV [58–61]. Significant KER also has been measured in the rare case of exothermic fragmentations [62]. On the other hand, homolytic cleavages and ion–neutral

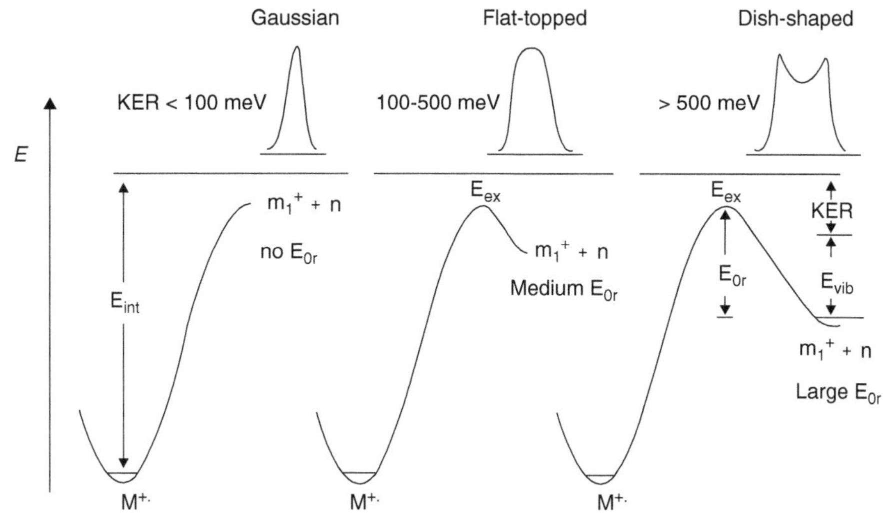

Fig. 2.16 Influence of the reverse activation energy on KER and, thus, on peak shapes in metastable ion decompositions (suitable experimental setup being a prerequisite). *From left*: no or small reverse barrier causes Gaussian peak shape, whereas medium E_{0r} yields flat-topped peaks and large E_{0r} causes dish-shaped peaks

complex-mediated reactions tend to proceed with very small KER in the range of 1–50 meV (Fig. 2.16).

KER allows us to look beyond

The importance of KER measurements results from the fact that the potential energy surface between transition state and products of a reaction can be reconstructed [56]. Thus, KER and *AE* data are complementary in determining the energy of the transition state.

2.8.3 Energy Partitioning

The observed KER consists of two components, one from E_{ex} and one from E_{0r}. This splitting becomes obvious from the fact that even if there is no E_{0r}, a small KER is always observed, thus demonstrating partitioning of E_{ex} between E_{vib} and E_{trans*} (KER):

$$E_{ex} = E_{vib} + E_{trans*} \tag{2.23}$$

Diatomic molecular ion dissociations represent the only case with clear energy partitioning, as all excess energy of the decomposition has to be converted to translational energy of the products ($E_{ex} = E_{trans*}$). For polyatomic ions the partitioning of excess energy can be described by a simple empirical relationship between E_{ex} and the number of degrees of freedom, s [7, 63]:

$$E_{trans*} = \frac{E_{ex}}{\alpha \times s} \tag{2.24}$$

with the empirical correction factor $\alpha = 0.44$ [63]. According to Eq. 2.24 the ratio E_{trans*}/E_{ex} decreases as the size of the fragmenting ion increases. This influence has been termed *degrees of freedom effect* (DOF) [64–66].

Consequently, E_{trans*} becomes rather small for substantial values of s, e.g., 0.3 eV/(0.44 × 30) = 0.023 eV. Therefore, any observed KER in excess of E_{trans*} must originate from E_{0r} being the only alternative source [62]. The analogous partitioning of E_{0r} is described by:

$$E_{trans} = \beta E_{or} \tag{2.25}$$

with $\beta = 0.2$–0.4 and $^1/_3$ being a good approximation in many cases.

Partitioning factor

In practice, most of the observed KERs (except at <50 meV), can be attributed to E_{trans} from E_{0r} [62], and as a rule of thumb, the ratio $E_{trans} \approx 0.33\ E_{or}$ may be assumed as the partitioning factor.

2.9 Isotope Effects

Most elements are composed of more than one naturally occurring *isotope*, i.e., having nuclei of the same *atomic number* but different *mass numbers* due to different numbers of neutrons [67]. The mass number of an isotope is given as a superscript preceding the element symbol, e.g., ^{1}H and ^{2}H (D) or ^{12}C and ^{13}C (Sect. 3.1).

Obviously, mass spectrometry is ideally suited for distinguishing between isotopic species, and isotopic labeling is used for mechanistic as well as analytical applications (Sect. 3.3). However, isotopic substitution not only affects ionic mass, but rather "isotopic substitution can have several simultaneous effects, and this complication sometimes produces results which are at first sight curious" [68].

Any effect exerted by the introduction of isotopes are termed *isotope effects*. Isotope effects can be *intermolecular*, e.g., upon $D^\bullet$ loss from $CD_4^{+\bullet}$ vs. $H^\bullet$ loss from $CH_4^{+\bullet}$, or *intramolecular*, e.g., upon $H^\bullet$ loss versus $D^\bullet$ loss from $CH_2D_2^{+\bullet}$.

2.9.1 Primary Kinetic Isotope Effects

Kinetic isotope effects represent one particular type of isotope effect. They are best rationalized when considering the potential energy diagram of both $H^\bullet$ and $D^\bullet$ loss from equivalent positions in the same isotopically labeled (e.g., deuterated) molecular ion (Fig. 2.17) [5, 6, 69]. The diagram is essentially symmetric, with the only differences arising from the zero-point energy (ZPE) terms. Since H$^•$ and D$^•$ are being lost from the same molecular ion, the single ZPE to start from is defined by this species. The transition states leading up to H$^•$ and D$^•$ loss possess ZPE terms associated with all the degrees of freedom of the dissociating ion except the one involved in that particular reaction. The transition state corresponding to H$^•$ loss must therefore have a lower ZPE because it contains a C–D bond that is not involved in the actual cleavage. This corresponds to a lower ZPE than is provided by the C–H bond-retaining transition state that leads to D$^•$ loss. Therefore, an ion with an internal energy E_{int} has a larger excess energy E_{exH} when it is about to eliminate H$^•$ than if it cleaved off a D$^•$. The activation energy for H$^•$ loss is thereby lowered making it proceed faster than D$^•$ loss ($k_H/k_D > 1$).

The reason for the lower ZPE of the deuterium-retaining species is found in its lower vibrational frequencies due to the double mass of D as compared to H at almost identical binding forces. According to classical mechanics the vibrational frequency ν_D should therefore be lower by the inverse ratio of the square roots of their masses, i.e., $\nu_D/\nu_H \approx 1/1.41 \approx 0.71$ [70].

The term *primary kinetic isotope effect* applies if the effect is exerted on a bond where the isotope itself is involved during the reaction. It seems clear that there is no single well-defined value of the kinetic isotope effect of a reaction (Fig. 2.17) and that it strongly depends on the internal energy of the decomposing ions. In the rare case when E_{int} is just above the activation energy for H$^•$ loss but still below that for D$^•$ loss, the isotope effect would be infinite. As ions in a mass spectrometer usually exhibit comparatively wide distributions of E_{int}, the probability for such a case is extremely low. However, kinetic isotope effects can be large in case of

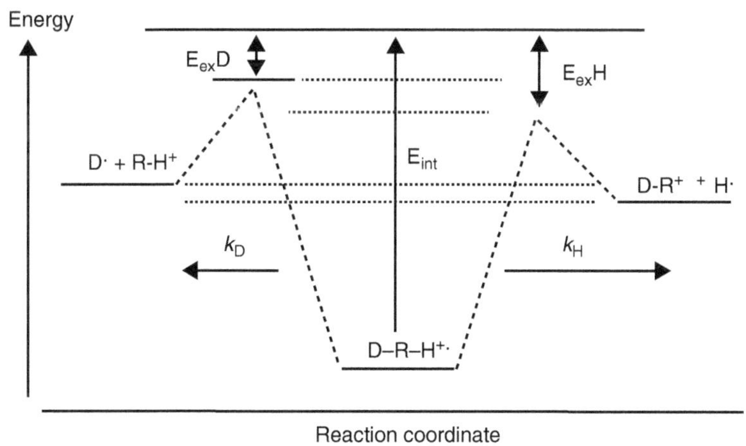

Fig. 2.17 Origin of kinetic isotope effects [5, 6, 69]. The change in vibrational frequencies, and thus in density of states causes somewhat higher activation energy and consequently smaller excess energy for the reaction of the deuterated bond, and thus reduces k_D

decomposing metastable ions ($k_H/k_D \approx 2$–4) because these ions possess only small excess energies. Such circumstances make them sensitive to the difference between E_{exD} and E_{exH}. On the other hand, ions that decompose in the ion source usually have high internal energies, and thus smaller isotope effects are observed ($k_H/k_D \approx$ 1–1.5).

While the mass of H remarkably differs from that of D (2 u/1 u = 2), the relative increase in mass is much lower for heavier elements such as carbon (13 u/12 u ≈ 1.08) [71] or nitrogen (15 u/14 u ≈ 1.07). In consequence, kinetic isotope effects of those elements are particularly small and special attention has to be devoted for their proper determination.

Revealing the rate-determining step Isotopic labeling does not only reveal the original position of a rearranging atom, but can also reveal the rate-determining step of multi-step reactions by its marked influence on reaction rates. Thus, the examination of H/D and $^{12}C/^{13}C$ isotope effects led to the conclusion that the McLafferty rearrangement of aliphatic ketones (Sect. 6.8) rather proceeds stepwise than concerted [71].

Facts about isotope effects

- Isotope effects dealt with in mass spectrometry are usually *kinetic isotope effects* resulting from different rate constants of bond breaking and bond formation without (k_H) or with (k_D) a heavier isotope involved, respectively.
- Unimolecular reactions involve *intramolecular kinetic isotope effects*, i.e., there are two competing fragmentations only differing in the isotopic composition of the products exhibit different rate constants k_H and k_D [72].
- Kinetic isotope effects are called *normal* if $k_H/k_D > 1$ and *inverse* if $k_H/k_D < 1$. Inverse kinetic isotope effects are rarely observed.
- Isotope effects can also be observed on KER [61, 73], e.g., the KER accompanying H_2 loss from methylene immonium ion varies between 0.61 and 0.80 eV upon D labeling at various positions [61].

2.9.2 Measurement of Isotope Effects

Mass spectrometry measures the abundance of ions vs. their *m/z* ratio, and it is common practice to use the ratio $I_{mH}/I_{mD} = k_H/k_D$ as a direct measure of the isotope effect. The typical procedure for determining isotope effects from intensity ratios is to solve a set of simultaneous equations [74–77].

Isotope effect on propene loss The transfer of a D compared to the transfer of an H during propene loss from partially labeled phenylpropylethers is accompanied by an isotope effect, the approximate magnitude of which was estimated as follows [77]:

$$[1,1-D_2]:\frac{[C_6H_6O]^+}{[C_6H_5OD]^+}=\frac{\alpha i}{1-\alpha} \tag{2.26}$$

$$[2,2,3,3,3-D_5]:\frac{[C_6H_6O]^+}{[C_6H_5OD]^+}=\frac{(1-\alpha)i}{\alpha} \tag{2.27}$$

where α is the total fraction of H transferred from positions 2 and 3 and i is the isotope effect favoring H over D transfer. Unfortunately, the situation is more complicated if more than just one complementary pair is being studied, and an exact solution will no longer be feasible. Then, a numerical approach is required to approximate the i value [77, 78].

Also, a rigorous treatment of isotope effects within the framework of QET reveals that the assumption $I_{mH}/I_{mD} = k_H/k_D$ represents a simplification [72]. It is only valid for when the studied species populate a small internal energy distribution, e.g., as metastable ions do, whereas wide internal energy distributions, e.g., those of ions fragmenting in the ion source after 70 eV electron ionization, may cause erroneous results. This is because the $k_{(E)}$ functions of isotopic reactions are not truly parallel [79], but they do fulfill this requirement over a small range of internal energies (Figs. 2.17 and 2.18).

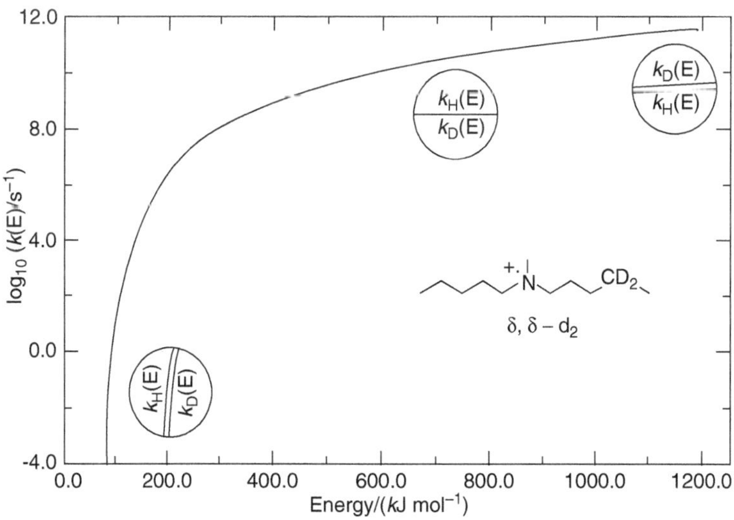

Fig. 2.18 Calculated $k_{H(E)}$ and $k_{D(E)}$ curves for the α-cleavage of deuterated amine molecular ions. The curves can be regarded as parallel over a small range of internal energies, but they are not in the strict sense. They may even cross to cause inverse isotope effects in the domain of highly excited ions (Reproduced from Ref. [79] with permission. © Wiley & Sons, 1991)

2.9.3 Secondary Kinetic Isotope Effects

Secondary kinetic isotope effects are observed if an isotopic label is located adjacent to or remote from the bond that is being broken or formed during the reaction. Again, these depend on the internal energy of the decomposing ions. Secondary kinetic isotope effects, i_{sec}, are generally much smaller than their primary analogs.

Isotope effects depend on internal energy The ratio $[M–CH_3]^+/[M–CD_3]^+$ from isopropylbenzene molecular ions decomposing by benzylic cleavage (Sect. 6.4) vary from 1.02 when fragmenting within the ion source (70 eV EI) over 1.28 for metastable ions in the 1st FFR to 1.56 in the 2nd FFR. This clearly demonstrates the dependence of the secondary kinetic isotope effect on ion internal energy [80].

It is convenient to specify the value normalized *per heavier isotope present*, $i_{secnorm}$, because of the possible presence of a number of heavier isotopes, n_D [69, 79]:

$$i_{\text{sec norm}} = \sqrt[n_D]{i_{\text{sec}}} \tag{2.28}$$

Competing α-cleavages Secondary kinetic isotope effects on the α-cleavage of tertiary amine molecular ions occur with deuterium labels either adjacent to or remote from the cleaved bond (Sect. 6.2). The label reduces the fragmentation rate relative to the non-labeled chain by factors of 1.08–1.30 per D in case of metastable ion decompositions (Fig. 2.19), but the isotope effect vanished for ion source processes [81]. The reversal of these kinetic isotope effects for short-lived ions (10^{-11}–10^{-10} s) could be demonstrated by field ionization kinetic measurements, i.e., then the deuterated species decomposed slightly faster than their non-labeled isotopologs [69, 79].

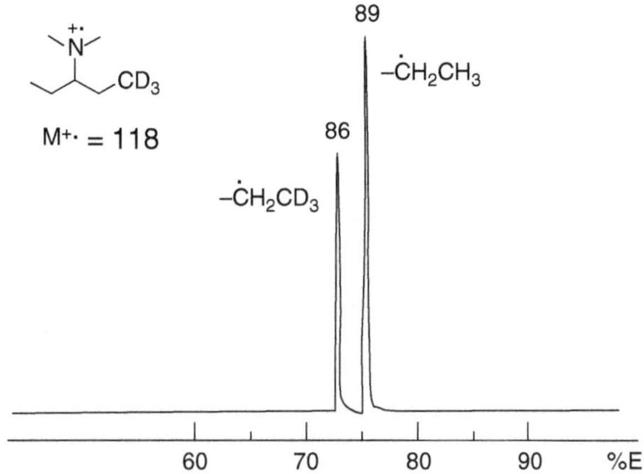

Fig. 2.19 Observation of secondary H/D isotope effects on the α-cleavage of tertiary amine molecular ions. For convenience, *m/z* labels have been added to the original energy scale of the MIKE spectrum (Adapted from Ref. [81] with permission. © American Chemical Society, 1988)

2.10 Determination of Ionization Energies

2.10.1 Conventional Determination of Ionization Energies

Ionization energies [82] can comparatively easily be determined – one simply needs to read out the lower limit of the electron energy at a vanishing molecular ion signal. Unfortunately, doing so yields only coarse approximations of the real ionization energy of a molecule. The accuracy of *IE* data obtained by this simple procedure will be about ± 1 eV. One of the associated problems is measuring the electron energy itself. The electrons are thermally emitted from a hot metal filament (1600–2000 °C), and therefore, their total kinetic energy is not only defined by the potential applied to accelerate them, but also by their thermal energy distribution [24]. In addition, electron ionization preferably creates vibrationally excited ions (Sect. 2.1), because ionization is a threshold process, i.e., it will take place not just when the energy needed to accomplish the process is reached, but also for all higher energies [83]. This causes a systematic error in that vertical *IE*s are obtained being higher than the adiabatic *IE*s one would like to measure. Further drawbacks are:

- Due to inhomogeneous electric fields within the ionization volume, the actual electron energy also depends on the location where ionization takes place.
- The fact that the low electron acceleration voltages of 7 – 15 V have to be superimposed on the ion acceleration voltage of several kilovolts causes low precision of the voltage settings in commercial magnetic sector instruments.
- There is additional thermal energy of the neutrals roughly defined by the temperature of the inlet system and the ion source.

2.10.2 Improved *IE* Accuracy from Data Post-processing

The slightly diffuse energy of the electrons effects that the ionization efficiency curves do not approach zero in a straight line; they rather bend close to the ionization threshold and exponentially approximate zero. Even if the electron energy scale of the instrument is properly calibrated against *IE*s of established standards, the accuracy of the *IE* data obtained from direct readout is only ±0.3 eV (Fig. 2.20a).

To overcome the unpredictability of the actual onset of ionization, the *critical slope method* has been developed [24, 84], among several other methods [85]. It makes use of the fact that, according to theory, realistic values of *IE* are expected at the position of the ionization efficiency curve where the slope of a semilog plot of the curve is

$$\frac{d}{dV}(\ln N_i) = \frac{n}{n+1}\frac{1}{kT} \tag{2.29}$$

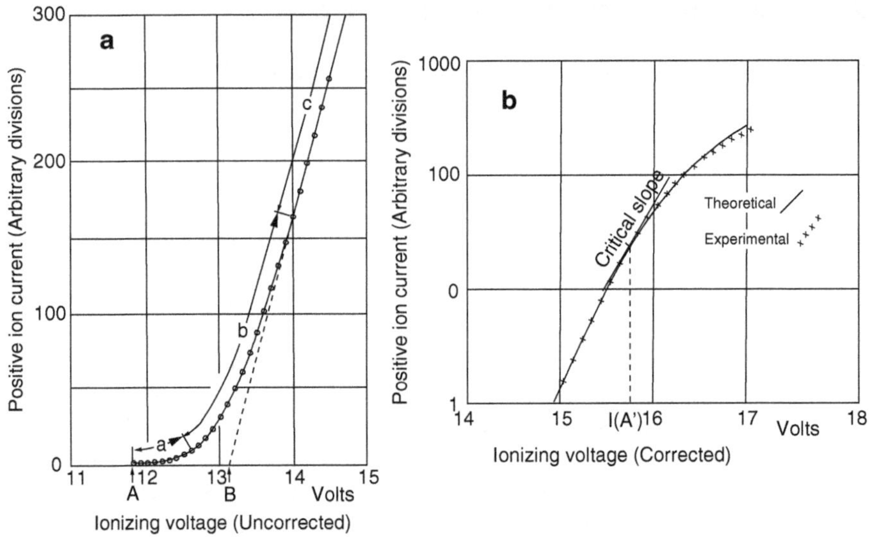

Fig. 2.20 Ionization efficiency curve of argon plotted on a linear scale (**a**) and as semilog plot (**b**). Extrapolation of the linear portion of (**a**) gives erroneous *IE*s, whereas the x-position of the tangent of an empirical critical slope to the semilog plot yields accuracies of $\pm$ 0.05 eV (Reproduced from Ref. [24] by permission. © American Chemical Society, 1948)

with N_i being the total number of ions produced at an electron acceleration voltage V, and with an empirical value of $n = 2$ (Fig. 2.20b).

2.10.3 *IE* Accuracy – Experimental Improvements

If reliable thermochemical data [25, 86] is required, the above disturbing effects have to be substantially reduced [82]. One way is to use an *electron monochromator* (accuracy up to ±0.1 eV) [87, 88]. An electron monochromator is a device for selecting nearly monoenergetic electrons from an electron beam [89]. Alternatively, *photoionization* (PI) may be employed instead of EI. Photoionization yields even more accurate results (±0.05 eV) than the electron monochromator [90]. In any case, the half width of the electron or photon energy distribution becomes small enough to detect detailed structural features of the ionization efficiency curves such as electronic transitions. Both techniques have been widely employed to obtain *IE* data (Table 2.1).

2.10.4 Photoionization Processes

The absorption of UV light by a neutral can result in electronically excited states that undergo relaxation either by emission of light or by emission of an electron.

Thus, the photon in *photoionization* (PI) serves the same purpose as the energetic electron in EI:

$$M + h\nu \rightarrow M^{*} \rightarrow M^{+\bullet} + e^{-} \quad (2.30)$$

Of course, the energy absorbed must lead into in a continuum state, i.e., at least provide the ionization energy of the neutral. Typical photon sources for PI are frequency-quadrupled Nd:Yag lasers delivering photons at 266 nm wavelength (4.6 eV) and ArF excimer lasers at 193 nm (6.3 eV). Both light sources clearly deliver photons well below the *IE* of most molecules. Fortunately, the absorption of energy has not to be a one-photon process. Instead, stepwise accumulation of energy from less energetic photons is also feasible. Thus, the normal procedure to achieve PI is *multiphoton ionization* (MUPI) [91].

The next stepping-stone to photoionization is finding the electronic levels of the neutral, because nonresonant ionization has rather low cross-sections that translate into poor ionization efficiencies along with high photon flux requirements. Resonant absorption of photons is more effective by several orders of magnitude [92]. Ideally, resonant absorption of the first photon leads to an intermediate state from where absorption of a second photon can forward the molecule into a continuum. This technique is known as 1 + 1 *resonance-enhanced multiphoton ionization* (REMPI). From a practical point of view, the second photon should be, but not necessarily has to be, of the same wavelength (Fig. 2.21) [93]. Proper selection of the laser wavelengths provides compound-selective analysis at extremely low detection limits [91, 92, 94, 95].

Ultrashort laser pulses in the picosecond rather than the conventional nanosecond regime prevent the molecules from unwanted relaxation or fragmentation prior to molecular ion formation. The REMPI mass spectra of diphenylmercury, for example, only exhibit a molecular ion peak when sub-picosecond laser ionization is employed [96].

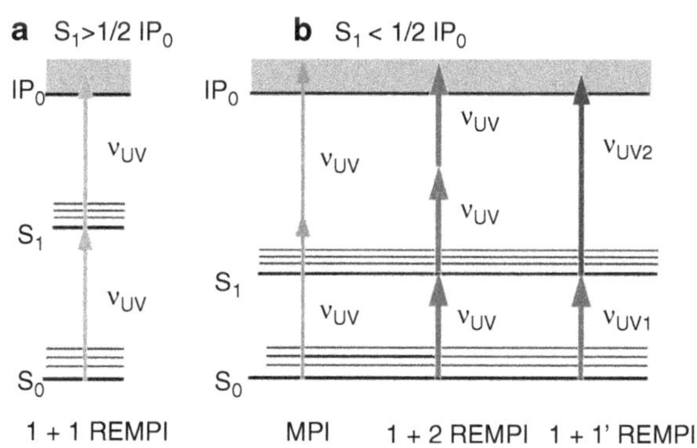

Fig. 2.21 Photoionization schemes. (**a**) Resonant 1 + 1 REMPI, (**b**) nonresonant MPI, resonant 1 + 2 REMPI, and resonant 1 + 1' REMPI with two different wavelengths (Adapted from Ref. [93] with permission. © The Vacuum Society of Japan, 2007)

2.10.5 Photoelectron Spectroscopy and Derived Methods

Photoelectron spectroscopy (PES, a non-mass spectral technique) [97] has proven to be very useful in providing *IE*s, but also to reveal the electronic and vibrational structure of atoms and molecules. Energy resolutions reported from PES are in the order of 10–15 meV. The low resolution of PES still prevents the observation of rotational transitions [83], and to overcome these limitations, PES has been further improved. In brief, the principle of *zero kinetic energy photoelectron spectroscopy* (ZEKE-PES or just ZEKE, also a non-mass spectral technique) [98–100] is based on distinguishing excited ions from ground state ions.

First, imagine a neutral interfering with a photon carrying some meV more than its *IE*. The neutral is going to expel a kinetic electron moving away due to this slight excess energy, E_{kinel}, defined by:

$$E_{\mathrm{kinel}} = h\nu - IE \tag{2.31}$$

Next, consider the situation for $h\nu = IE$. Here, the electron can merely be released, but it cannot move away from the freshly formed ion. After a short moment (1 μs) it is possible to separate *zero kinetic energy electrons* from others in space. Applying an extraction voltage along a given drift direction will then add a different amount of kinetic energy to the kinetic electrons (as these have traveled further) than to those ejected at threshold, i.e., they differ in speed. A time-of-flight measurement of the electrons therefore produces one signal for each group of electrons. (For another application of this concept cf. Sect. 4.2.5).

Photoelectron spectroscopy of O_2 The electronic and vibrational states of the oxygen molecular ion has been perfectly resolved by PES (Fig. 2.22), thus allowing to directly read out the Franck-Condon factors and to identify the $(0 \leftarrow 0)$ transitions corresponding to adiabatic ionization [101].

2.10.6 Mass-Analyzed Threshold Ionization

The main disadvantage of PES and ZEKE experiments lies in the detection of electrons making the measurements sensitive to impurities, because the electrons could arise from these instead of the intended sample. This can be avoided by detecting the produced ions instead – the corresponding technique is known as *mass-analyzed threshold ionization* (MATI) [102]. In MATI experiments, the neutrals are excited in a field-free environment by means of a tunable light source (usually a multi-photon laser process) very close to the ionization threshold. Often, a two-photon scheme is employed where the first photon is used to arrive at an electronically excited state of the neutral (Fig. 2.20) by adjusting the wavelength appropriately. Keeping the wavelength of the first photon constant, the wavelength of the second photon is then scanned as to just ionize this excited species (the spectra shown in Fig 2.23 only refer to the second photon's wavelength).

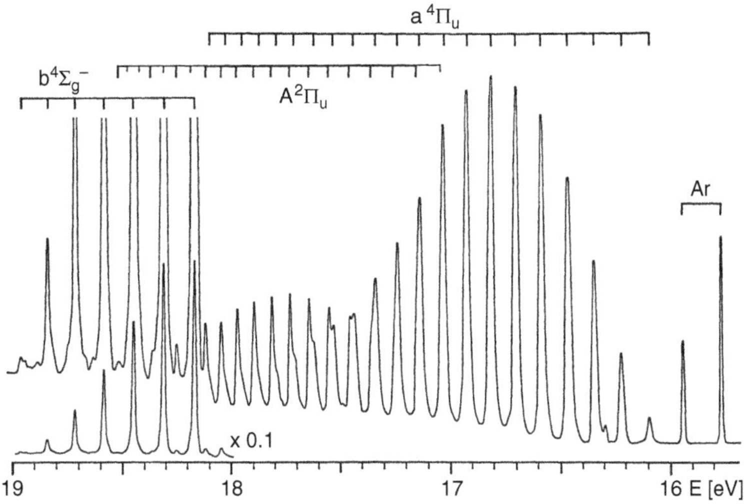

Fig. 2.22 High-resolution photoelectron spectrum of O_2, showing overlapping vibrational progressions from transitions to different electronic states of the ion. The range of *IE* is not shown. The two peaks on the *right* are from argon used for calibration of the energy scale (Reproduced from Ref. [101] with permission. © Royal Swedish Academy of Sciences, 1970)

Possible prompt ions are removed after about 0.1 μs by a weak positive electric field. Then, the near-threshold Rydberg species are ionized by applying a negative electric field pulse. The purpose of the external electric field is to create a potential gradient that affects the weekly bound electron at an energy level very close to the ionization threshold in a way that this electron is stripped of the excited molecule to effect its ionization (cf. field ionization process, Sect. 8.2). In addition, the electric field accelerates those ions towards a time-of-flight mass analyzer [102–104]. Thus, we are finally back to a real mass spectral technique. In contrast to ZEKE, the mass selectivity of MATI allows not only for the study of molecules [102, 104], but permits consideration of dissociating complexes and clusters [83, 105, 106].

Comparison of PI, MATI and ZEKE-PES The ionization spectra at the first ionization threshold of pyrazine, $C_4H_4N_2$, as obtained by PI, MATI, and ZEKE-PES look clearly different (Fig. 2.23) [102]. The PI spectrum is a plot of ion current versus wavelength of the probe laser. PI spectra show a simple rise of the curve at *IE*, while MATI and ZEKE yield a sharp peak at ionization threshold plus additional signals from lower vibrational ionization thresholds.

Using the relationship $\Delta E = h\nu$ and substituting $\nu = c/\lambda$ allows to calculate the energy of the absorbed second photon. In case of pyrazine the wavelength for ionization of the electronically excited $0_0^{\ 0}$ state is $\lambda = 227$ nm. Thus, using $h = 4.14 \times 10^{-15}$ eVs ($= 6.63 \times 10^{-34}$ Js) yields for the second step $\Delta E = 4.14 \times 10^{-15}$ eVs $\times$ (2.99×10^8 m s^{-1}/2.27×10^{-7} m) $= 5.45$ eV. The

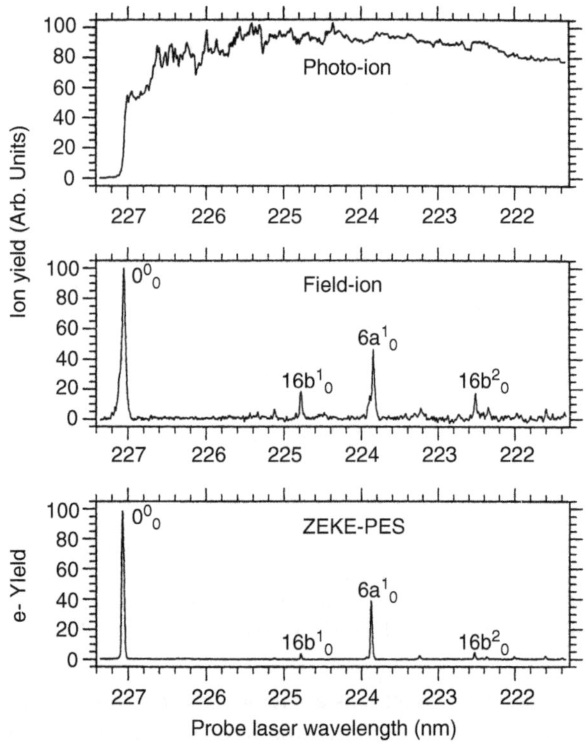

Fig. 2.23 Comparison of PI (*top*), MATI (*middle*) and ZEKE (*bottom*) spectra of pyrazine (Reproduced from Ref. [102] with permission. © American Institute of Physics, 1991)

adiabatic ionization energy of pyrazine can be obtained by adding the energy of the first photon. Overall, this delivers $IE_{\mathrm{py}} = 9.29$ eV [107].

2.11 Determining the Appearance Energies

The techniques used for the determination of appearance energies are essentially identical to those described above for *IE*s. However, even when using the most accurately defined electron or photon energies, great care has to be taken when determining *AE*s because of the risk of overestimation due to kinetic shift. Provided that there is no reverse activation energy for the particular reaction, the *AE* value also delivers the sum of heats of formation of the dissociation products. If substantial KER is observed, the *AE* may still be used to determine the activation energy of the process.

2.11.1 Kinetic Shift

Fragment ion abundances observed by means of any mass spectrometer strongly depend on ion lifetimes within the ion source and on ion internal energy

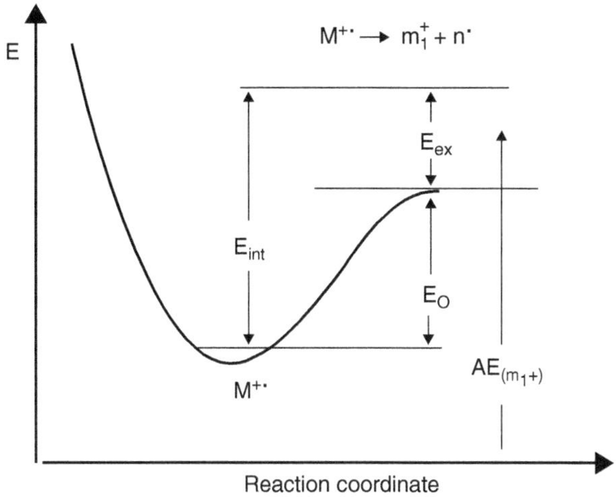

Fig. 2.24 Kinetic shift. The excess energy in the transition state affects *AE* measurements such that it always causes experimental values to be overestimated due to the need for some excess energy in the transition state

distributions, i.e., kinetic aspects play an important role for a mass spectrum's appearance. As explained by QET the rate constant of an ion dissociation is a function of excess energy in the transition state of the respective reaction, and there is a need of substantial excess energy to make the rate constant exceed the critical $10^6\ s^{-1}$ needed to dissociate during the residence times within the ion source. Therefore, appearance and activation energies are always in excess of the true values by the above amount. This phenomenon is known as *kinetic shift* (Fig. 2.24) [41, 55]. Often, kinetic shifts are almost negligible (0.01–0.1 eV), but they can be as large as 2 eV [41], e.g., an activation energy of 2.07 eV for $C_3H_6^{+\bullet} \rightarrow C_3H_5^+ + H^\bullet$ is accompanied by a kinetic shift of 0.19 eV [82]. As $k_{(E)}$ functions greatly differ between reactions and especially between homogeneous bond cleavages and rearrangement fragmentations, it is not an easy task to correct the experimental *AE*s by subtraction of E_{ex}. The influence of the kinetic shift can be minimized by increasing the ion source residence time and/or by increasing the detection sensitivity of the instrument.

Kinetic shift

The *kinetic shift* denotes the overestimation of *AE*s due to the contribution of excess energy in the transition state necessary to yield rate constants larger than $10^6\ s^{-1}$. The determination of *IE*s is not negatively affected by kinetic shift as kinetics is not involved in electron or photon ionization.

2.11.2 Breakdown Graphs

Employing the above techniques, one can examine the fragmentations of a molecular ion as a function of internal energy by constructing a so-called *breakdown graph*.

This involves plotting the ion intensities of interest, i.e., those of a certain *m/z*, vs. electron energy or vs. ion internal energy if the *IE* has been subtracted before [108]. Typically, a molecular ion can access a considerable number of fragmentation pathways as soon as there are some 1–3 eV of internal energy available. Breakdown graphs can be used to compare the energetic demands of those different fragmentation pathways. In addition, breakdown graphs help to correlate ion internal energy distributions derived from other methods such as photoelectron spectroscopy [109] with mass spectral data.

Breakdown graph of 4-methyl-1-pentene For 4-methyl-1-pentene, the breakdown graph, the internal energy distribution from the photoelectron spectrum, and the 70-eV EI mass spectrum are compared (Fig. 2.25) [110]. From the fragmentation threshold to about 2 eV of internal energy the breakdown graph is dominated by the $[C_4H_8]^{+\bullet}$ ion, *m/z* 56. In the range 2–4.5 eV the $[C_3H_7]^+$ ion, *m/z* 43, becomes most prominent. However, $[C_4H_8]^{+\bullet}$ only has 60% of the intensity of $[C_3H_7]^+$. It is obvious from the graphs that the 0.5–1 eV internal energy region, where $[C_4H_8]^{+\bullet}$ is the

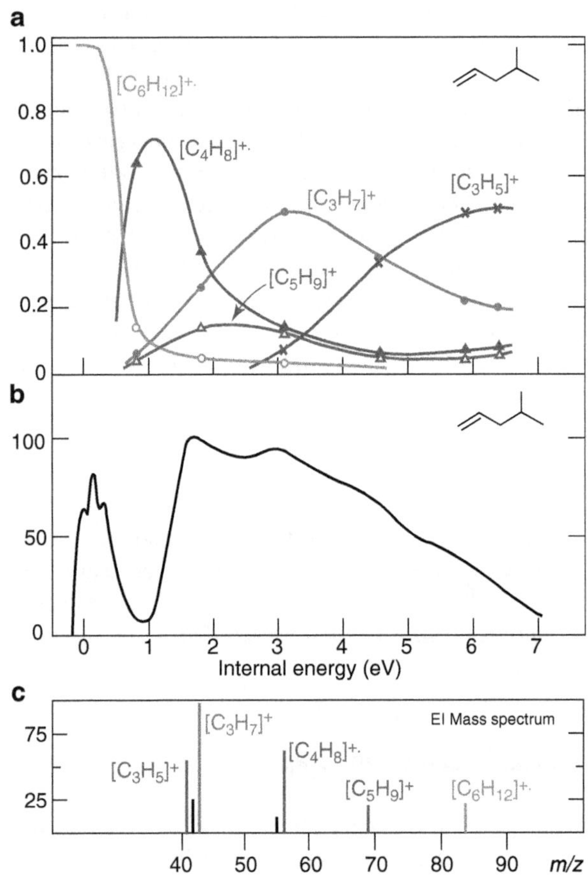

Fig. 2.25 4-Methyl-1-pentene: relationship of breakdown graph (**a**), internal energy distribution from PES (**b**), and mass spectrum (**c**) (Adapted from Ref. [110] by permission. © Wiley & Sons, 1982)

predominating fragment ion, corresponds to a region of the internal energy distribution having a low ion population. This explains why $[C_3H_7]^+$ constitutes the base peak of the spectrum. Beyond 5 eV of internal energy, the $[C_3H_5]^+$ ion, *m/z* 41, becomes the most prominent fragment ion.

2.12 Gas Phase Basicity and Proton Affinity

Not all ionization methods rely on unimolecular conditions as strictly as EI does. Chemical ionization (CI, Chap. 7), for example, makes use of reactive collisions between ions generated from a reactant gas and the neutral analyte to achieve its ionization by some bimolecular process such as proton transfer. The question which reactant ion can protonate a given analyte can be answered from *gas phase basicity* (*GB*) or *proton affinity* (*PA*) data. Proton transfer, and thus the relative proton affinities of the reactants, also play an important role in many ion–neutral complex-mediated reactions (Sect. 6.13). In the last decade, *proton transfer reaction* (PTR) MS has emerged as a tool for analyzing *volatile organic compounds* (VOCs) in air (Sect. 7.3) [111, 112]. Therefore, PTR-MS is in the focus of interest for analytical work concerning environmental issues and in occupational health and safety.

Here, we deal with *proton affinity* and gas *phase basicity* as thermodynamic quantities. Consider the following gas phase reaction of a (basic) molecule, B:

$$B_g + H_g{}^+ \rightarrow [BH]_g{}^+ \tag{2.32}$$

The tendency of B to accept a proton is then quantitatively described by

$$-\Delta G_r{}^0 = GB_{(B)} \quad \text{and} \quad -\Delta H_r{}^0 = PA_{(B)}, \tag{2.33}$$

i.e., the gas phase basicity $GB_{(B)}$ is defined as the negative free energy change for the proton transfer, $-\Delta G_r{}^0$, whereas the proton affinity $PA_{(B)}$ is the negative enthalpy change, $-\Delta H_r{}^0$, for the same reaction [113, 114]. From the relation

$$\Delta G^0 = \Delta H^0 - T\Delta S^0 \tag{2.34}$$

we obtain the expression

$$PA_{(B)} = GB_{(B)} - T\Delta S^0 \tag{2.35}$$

with the entropy term $T\Delta S^0$ usually being relatively small (25–40 kJ mol^{-1}). Furthermore, in case of an equilibrium

$$[AH]^+ + B \rightleftharpoons A + [BH]^+ \tag{2.36}$$

with the equilibrium constant K_{eq} for which we have

Table 2.6 Selected proton affinities and gas phase basicities [25, 113, 117]

Molecule	$PA_{(B)}$ [kJ mol^{-1}]	$GB_{(B)}$ [kJ mol^{-1}]
H_2	424	396
CH_4	552	527
C_2H_6	601	558
H_2O	697	665
$H_2C{=}O$	718	685
$CH_3CH{=}CH_2$	751	718
C_6H_6 (benzene)	758	731
$(CH_3)_2C{=}CH_2$	820	784
$(CH_3)_2C{=}O$	823	790
$C_{14}H_{10}$ (phenanthrene)	831	802
C_4H_8O (tetrahydrofurane)	831	801
$C_2H_5OC_2H_5$	838	805
NH_3	854	818
CH_3NH_2	896	861
C_5H_5N (pyridine)	924	892
$(CH_3)_3N$	942	909

$$K_{eq} = [BH^+]/[AH^+] \times [A]/[B] \tag{2.37}$$

the gas phase basicity is related to K_{eq} by [115, 116]

$$GB_{(B)} = -\Delta G^0 = RT \ln K_{eq} \tag{2.38}$$

For the experimental determination of *GB*s and *PA*s refer to Sect. 9.17. Some representative values are compiled in Table 2.6.

2.13 Ion–Molecule Reactions

Most of what we have dealt with in gas phase ion chemistry so far has been referring to properties and *unimolecular reactions* of isolated ions. While these conditions are typical for ions formed by electron ionization and for ions during their transit through mass analyzers in general, *intermolecular reactions* may nonetheless occur within an ion source or some other (dedicated) part of a mass spectrometer. Intermolecular reactions require multiple soft collisions to occur between the reactants – such conditions are normally enabled as the vacuum is reduced to 0.01–1 mbar. Coulombic repulsion prevents an ion from reacting with an ion of equal charge sign; nevertheless, an ion may react with a neutral molecule. In the most simple case, the neutrals just belong to the same molecular species that is currently being introduced for ionization. Molecular ions may thus react with their corresponding neutral molecules, e.g.:

$$CH_4^{+\bullet} + CH_4 \rightarrow CH_5^{+} + CH_3^{\bullet} \quad (2.39)$$

$$H_2O^{+\bullet} + H_2O \rightarrow H_3O^{+} + OH^{\bullet} \quad (2.40)$$

In fact, both reactions shown here are of high relevance. The reaction of methane (Eq. 2.39) was discovered early by mass spectrometry [118] and led to the development of chemical ionization mass spectrometry (CI, Chap. 7) [119]. The analogous reaction with water (Eq. 2.40) presents a crucial step towards protonation of analyte molecules in atmospheric pressure chemical ionization (APCI) and direct analysis in real time (DART, Sect. 13.8).

2.13.1 Reaction Order

Isolated ions only undergo unimolecular reactions like isomerization (Eq. 2.41) or ion dissociation (Eq. 2.42):

$$ABC^{+} \rightarrow CAB^{+} \quad (2.41)$$

$$ABC^{+} \rightarrow AB^{+} + C \quad (2.42)$$

This type of reaction is referred to as *first-order reaction*. The rate of a first-order reaction, i.e., the change of the concentration of the precursor ion $[ABC^+]$ as a function of time, is solely determined by the concentration of this precursor ion, $[ABC^+]$, and its internal energy. This is why the rate constant, k, of a reaction of first order has the dimension of s^{-1} (or Hz, like a frequency). Thus we have the relationship:

$$-d[ABC^{+}]/dt = k[ABC^{+}] \quad (2.43)$$

The rates of the reactions of methane and water molecular ions with their corresponding neutrals as described in the preceding paragraph (Eqs. 2.39 and 2.40) depend on both the concentration of the respective molecular ions and that of the neutrals. In a generalized form, a *bimolecular reaction* can be written as:

$$AB^{+} + C \rightarrow ABC^{+} \quad (2.44)$$

Accordingly, its rate is now determined by:

$$-d[AB^{+}]/dt = k[AB^{+}]\,[C] \quad (2.45)$$

The last type of reaction that may occur in the gas phase requires a third body, N, as inert collision partner. The role of N is to carry away some of the reaction enthalpy, and thus, to stabilize the product by cooling it down a bit. A *termolecular reaction* (or *trimolecular reaction*) is represented as:

$$AB^+ + C + N \rightarrow ABC^+ + N^* \quad (2.46)$$

Now, the rate is affected by the concentration of three partners:

$$-d[AB^+]/dt = k[AB^+]\,[C]\,[N] \quad (2.47)$$

An example of a termolecular reaction is given by the dimerization of nitrogen molecular ions in an excess of nitrogen gas to form the short-lived $N_4^{+\bullet}$ ion:

$$N_2^{+\bullet} + N_2 + N_2 \rightarrow N_4^{+\bullet} + N_2^* \quad (2.48)$$

In this special case, nitrogen molecules serve as both reactant and inert collision partner. Thus, the reaction rate can be represented as follows:

$$-d[N_2^{+\bullet}]/dt = k[N_2^{+\bullet}]\,[N_2]^2 \quad (2.49)$$

Again, this reaction is key to analyte ion formation in atmospheric pressure chemical ionization (APCI, Sect. 7.8) and direct analysis in real time (DART, Sect. 13.8). Actually, it is the step before $H_2O^{+\bullet}$ formation via charge transfer to neutral water.

2.13.2 Solution Phase Versus Gas Phase Reactions

The thermochemistry of gas phase *ion–molecule reactions* greatly differs from what is common in solution phase [2, 51, 67], Sect. 3.3 in [120] and Chap. 7 in [4]. In solution phase, ions are surrounded by solvent molecules which, in polar solvents, align towards the ion as to compensate some of its charge by solvation. In order to interact with a substrate molecule, the ion needs to overcome the energy barrier of solvation, which in turn necessitates some activation energy.

From hydrated to isolated OH^- The nucleophilic displacement reaction between OH^- and CH_3Br to yield CH_3OH and Br^- has been studied at various degrees of hydration of the OH^- ion. $[(H_2O)_nOH]^-$ ions, $n = 0, 1, 2, 3, n$, were generated in a H_2O/H_2 flowing plasma and allowed to react with CH_3Br [50]. The rate constant of the S_N2 reaction decreased by four orders of magnitude upon transition from nonsolvated to triply solvated OH^- ions. Semiquantitative reaction coordinate profiles reveal the typical transition from a solution phase reaction with substantial activation energy of 96 kJ mol^{-1} (23 kcal mol^{-1}) to a double minimum profile for the gas phase reaction of isolated ions that exhibits an exothermal formation of the encounter complex $[OH^- \cdots CH_3Br]$ (Fig. 2.26).

Obviously, isolated gas phase ions have no desolvation barrier to be overcome. Any approaching neutral is attracted by *ion–dipole interactions*. In other words, the initially isolated ion tends to build up some sort of solvation sphere in the gas phase. Provided the ion collides gently with the molecule, i.e., at or slightly above thermal

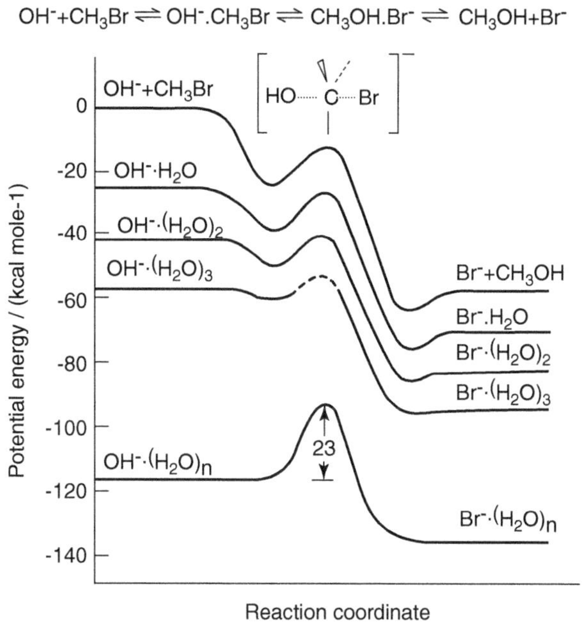

Fig. 2.26 Possible semiquantitative reaction coordinate profiles for the nucleophilic displacement reaction between OH^- and CH_3Br at various degrees of hydration of the OH^- ion. The activation energy in case of the hydrated hydroxide (*bottom*) is drastically diminished as the solvation is removed and finally turns into exothermal formation of the encounter complex (*top*) (Adapted from Ref. [50] with permission. © American Chemical Society, 1981)

energy (0.1–2 eV), the attractive forces trap the reactants into an *ion–neutral complex* (the term *ion–molecule complex* is also used). The ion–neutral complex may either persist as such or it may present the encounter complex of the reactants undergoing an ion–molecule reaction. Formation of this first intermediate is exothermal (Fig. 2.27) [2, 51, 67], Sect. 3.3 in [120] and Chap. 7 in [4]. If the activation energy towards some products is lower than the energy required for the reverse reaction, i.e., dissociation back into the substrates, the product complex can be formed. The excess energy of the product complex will then result in dissociation of this second ion–molecule complex to liberate the product ion and product neutral [51]. Overall, this kind of process is exothermal and very fast.

Wealth of information

Isolated gas phase ions and their reactions are free from obscuring factors like counterions, aggregates, and solvent effects. With mass spectrometry one can thus examine reaction pathways and steering factors of reactions, to reveal basic aspects of acidity and basicity, and moreover, to compare an established condensed phase reaction to its counterpart in the gas phase, thereby revealing the role of solvent effects on the process. Therefore, the intrinsic properties of "naked" ions and reactions are revealed by the toolbox of mass spectrometry [2].

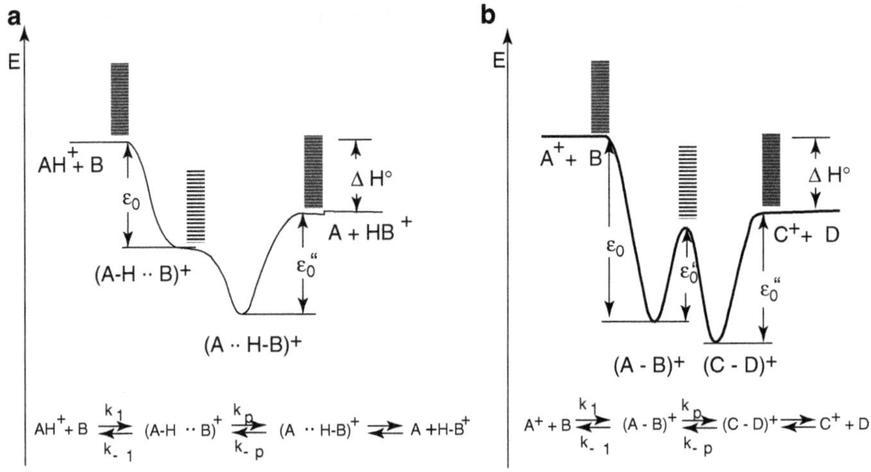

Fig. 2.27 Potential energy versus reaction coordinates of typical gas phase ion–molecule reactions. (**a**) Proton transfer reaction, (**b**) electrophilic displacement via S_N2 reaction. Note that both reactions can proceed without activation of the substrate and that both are exothermal (Reproduced from Ref. [51] with permission. © Elsevier Science, 1991)

2.14 Summary of Gas Phase Ion Chemistry

Line of Thoughts

This chapter started from basic considerations on how ionization of atoms and molecules is brought about and on why this partly determines the further fate of the incipient ionic species. Based on electron ionization, we learned about such key topics as ionization energy, ionization cross section, ion internal energy and its dissipation within the ion as well as appearance energy of fragmentation reactions. The quasi-equilibrium theory explains how these energetic parameters translate into competing ion dissociation pathways. From there, we went to the mass spectrometric time scale and the concept of stable, metastable, and unstable ions and moved from the classical instrumentation to some recent types of ion-trapping mass analyzers. Then, some dedicated topics were focused on, such as kinetic isotope effects, the estimation of the activation energy of reverse reactions from kinetic energy release, and the determination of ionization energies by several advanced techniques. Finally, we moved from the realm of isolated ions and their unimolecular reactions and further expanded on topics of gas phase proton affinity, basicity, and ion–molecule reactions.

Relevance

From a merely analytical point of view, the importance of gas phase ion chemistry studies may not immediately become evident. Nonetheless, we have to keep in mind that all the established fragmentation pathways used in structure elucidation were discovered and characterized by using the gas phase ion chemistry toolbox of mass spectrometry. Additionally, these techniques have revealed intrinsic properties of ions and reactions and have provided new insights in processes of industrial relevance. Furthermore, gas phase ion chemistry elucidates ion formation processes and crucial factors influencing ion yield not only for the manifold established ionization techniques but it may eventually also lead to the development of new capable methods.

References

1. Porter CJ, Beynon JH, Ast T (1981) The Modern Mass Spectrometer. A Complete Chemical Laboratory. Org Mass Spectrom 16:101–114. doi:10.1002/oms.1210160302
2. Schwarz H (1991) The Chemistry of Naked Molecules or the Mass Spectrometer as a Laboratory. Chem Unserer Zeit 25:268–278. doi:10.1002/ciuz.19910250507
3. Kazakevich Y (1996) Citation used by permission. hplc.chem.shu.edu; Seton Hall University, South Orange, NJ
4. Hiraoka K (ed) (2013) Fundamentals of Mass Spectrometry. Springer, New York
5. Cooks RG, Beynon JH, Caprioli RM (1973) Metastable Ions. Elsevier, Amsterdam
6. Levsen K (1978) Fundamental Aspects of Organic Mass Spectrometry. Weinheim, Verlag Chemie
7. Franklin JL (1979) Energy distributions in the unimolecular decomposition of ions. In: Bowers MT (ed) Gas Phase Ion Chemistry. Academic Press, New York
8. Beynon JH, Gilbert JR (1979) Energetics and mechanisms of unimolecular reactions of positive ions: mass spectrometric methods. In: Bowers MT (ed) Gas Phase Ion Chemistry. Academic Press, New York
9. Vogel P (1985) The study of carbocations in the gas phase. In: Carbocation Chemistry. Elsevier, Amsterdam
10. Holmes JL (1985) Assigning Structures to Ions in the Gas Phase. Org Mass Spectrom 20:169–183. doi:10.1002/oms.1210200302
11. Lorquet JC (1981) Basic Questions in Mass Spectrometry. Org Mass Spectrom 16:469–481. doi:10.1002/oms.1210161102
12. Lorquet JC (2000) Landmarks in the Theory of Mass Spectra. Int J Mass Spectrom 200:43–56. doi:10.1016/S1387-3806(00)00303-1
13. Märk TD (1982) Fundamental Aspects of Electron Impact Ionization. Int J Mass Spectrom Ion Phys 45:125–145. doi:10.1016/0020-7381(82)85046-8
14. Märk TD (1986) Electron impact ionization. In: Futrell JH (ed) Gaseous Ion Chemistry and Mass Spectrometry. Wiley, New York
15. Wolkenstein K, Gross JH, Oeser T, Schöler HF (2002) Spectroscopic Characterization and Crystal Structure of the 1,2,3,4,5,6-Hexahydrophenanthro[1,10,9,8-*opqra*]Perylene. Tetrahedron Lett 43:1653–1655. doi:10.1016/S0040-4039(02)00085-0
16. Harrison AG (1992) Fundamentals of gas phase ion chemistry. In: Chemical Ionization Mass Spectrometry. CRC Press, Boca Raton
17. De Wall R, Neuert H (1977) The Formation of Negative Ions from Electron Impact with Tungsten Hexafluoride. Z Naturforsch A 32:968–971. doi:10.1515/zna-1977-0910
18. Schröder E (1991) Massenspektrometrie – Begriffe und Definitionen. Springer, Heidelberg
19. Jones EG, Harrison AG (1970) Study of Penning Ionization Reactions Using a Single-Source Mass Spectrometer. Int J Mass Spectrom Ion Phys 5:137–156. doi:10.1016/0020-7381(70)87012-7
20. Penning FM (1927) Über Ionisation durch metastabile Atome. Naturwissenschaften 15:818. doi:10.1007/BF01505431

21. Hornbeck JA, Molnar JP (1951) Mass-Spectrometric Studies of Molecular Ions in the Noble Gases. Phys Rev 84:621–625. doi:10.1103/PhysRev.84.621
22. Faubert D, Paul GJC, Giroux J, Betrand MJ (1993) Selective Fragmentation and Ionization of Organic Compounds Using an Energy-Tunable Rare-Gas Metastable Beam Source. Int J Mass Spectrom Ion Proc 124:69–77. doi:10.1016/0168-1176(93)85021-5
23. Svec HJ, Junk GA (1967) Electron-Impact Studies of Substituted Alkanes. J Am Chem Soc 89:790–796. doi:10.1021/ja00980a010
24. Honig RE (1948) Ionization Potentials of Some Hydrocarbon Series. J Chem Phys 16:105–112. doi:10.1063/1.1746786
25. http://webbook.nist.gov/
26. Baldwin M, Kirkien-Konasiewicz A, Loudon AG, Maccoll A, Smith D (1966) Localized or Delocalized Charges in Molecule-Ions? Chem Commun:574. doi:10.1039/C19660000574
27. McLafferty FW (1966) Generalized Mechanism for Mass Spectral Reactions. Chem Commun:78–80. doi:10.1039/C19660000078
28. Wellington CA, Khowaiter SH (1978) Charge Distributions in Molecules and Ions: MINDO 3 Calculations. An Alternative of the Charge Localization Concept in Mass Spectrometry. Tetrahedron 34:2183–2190. doi:10.1016/0040-4020(78)89024-3
29. Baldwin MA, Welham KJ (1987) Charge Localization by Molecular Orbital Calculations. I. Urea and Thiourea. Rapid Commun Mass Spectrom 1:13–15. doi:10.1002/rcm.1290010110
30. Baldwin MA, Welham KJ (1988) Charge Localization by Molecular Orbital Calculations. II. Formamide, Thioformamide and *N*-Methylated Analogs. Org Mass Spectrom 23:425–428. doi:10.1002/oms.1210230522
31. Weinkauf R, Lehrer F, Schlag EW, Metsala A (2000) Investigation of Charge Localization and Charge Delocalization in Model Molecules by Multiphoton Ionization Photoelectron Spectroscopy and DFT Calculations. Faraday Discuss 115:363–381. doi:10.1039/B001092H
32. Cone C, Dewar MJS, Landman D (1977) Gaseous Ions. 1. MINDO/3 Study of the Rearrangement of Benzyl Cation to Tropylium. J Am Chem Soc 99:372–376. doi:10.1021/ja00444a011
33. Born M, Oppenheimer JR (1927) Zur Quantentheorie der Molekeln. Ann Phys 84:457–484. doi:10.1002/andp.19273892002
34. Seiler R (1969) A Remark on the Born-Oppenheimer Approximation. Int J Quantum Chem 3:25–32. doi:10.1002/qua.560030106
35. Lipson RH (2009) Ultraviolet and Visible Absorption Spectroscopy. In: Andrews DL (ed) Encyclopedia of Applied Spectroscopy. Wiley-VCH, Weinheim
36. Franck J (1925) Elementary Processes of Photochemical Reactions. Trans Faraday Soc 21:536–542. doi:10.1039/TF9262100536
37. Condon EU (1926) Theory of Intensity Distribution in Band Systems. Phys Rev 28:1182–1201. doi:10.1103/PhysRev.28.1182
38. Dunn GH (1966) Franck-Condon Factors for the Ionization of H_2 and D_2. J Chem Phys 44:2592–2594. doi:10.1063/1.1727097
39. Märk TD (1982) Fundamental Aspects of Electron Impact Ionization. Int J Mass Spectrom Ion Phys 45:125–145. doi:10.1016/0020-7381(82)80103-4
40. Märk TD (1986) Electron impact ionization. In: Futrell JH (ed) Gaseous Ion Chemistry and Mass Spectrometry. John Wiley and Sons, New York
41. McLafferty FW, Wachs T, Lifshitz C, Innorta G, Irving P (1970) Substituent Effects in Unimolecular Ion Decompositions. XV. Mechanistic Interpretations and the Quasi-Equilibrium Theory. J Am Chem Soc 92:6867–6880. doi:10.1021/ja00726a025
42. Egger KW, Cocks AT (1973) Homopolar- and Heteropolar Bond Dissociation Energies and Heats of Formation of Radicals and Ions in the Gas Phase. I. Data on Organic Molecules. Helv Chim Acta 56:1516–1536. doi:10.1002/hlca.19730560509
43. Lossing FP, Semeluk GP (1970) Free Radicals by Mass Spectrometry. XLII. Ionization Potentials and Ionic Heats of Formation for C_1–C_4 Alkyl Radicals. Can J Chem 48:955–965. doi:10.1139/v70-157

44. Lossing FP, Holmes JL (1984) Stabilization Energy and Ion Size in Carbocations in the Gas Phase. J Am Chem Soc 106:6917–6920. doi:10.1021/ja00335a008
45. Cox JD, Pilcher G (1970) Thermochemistry of Organic and Organometallic Compounds. Academic Press, London
46. Chatham H, Hils D, Robertson R, Gallagher A (1984) Total and Partial Electron Collisional Ionization Cross Sections for Methane, Ethane, Silane, and Disilane. J Chem Phys 81:1770–1777. doi:10.1063/1.447848
47. Wahrhaftig AL (1959) Ion dissociations in the mass spectrometer. In: Waldron JD (ed) Advances in Mass Spectrometry. Pergamon Press, Oxford
48. Wahrhaftig AL (1986) Unimolecular dissociations of gaseous ions. In: Futrell JH (ed) Gaseous Ion Chemistry and Mass Spectrometry. Wiley, New York
49. Rosenstock HM, Krauss M (1963) Quasi-equilibrium theory of mass spectra. In: McLafferty FW (ed) Mass Spectrometry of Organic Ions. Academic Press, London
50. Bohme DK, Mackay GI (1981) Bridging the Gap Between the Gas Phase and Solution: Transition in the Kinetics of Nucleophilic Displacement Reactions. J Am Chem Soc 103:978–979. doi:10.1021/ja00394a062
51. Speranza M (1992) Gas Phase Ion Chemistry Versus Solution Chemistry. Int J Mass Spectrom Ion Proc 118(119):395–447. doi:10.1016/0168-1176(92)85071-7
52. Rosenstock HM, Wallenstein MB, Wahrhaftig AL, Eyring H (1952) Absolute Rate Theory for Isolated Systems and the Mass Spectra of Polyatomic Molecules. Proc Natl Acad Sci USA 38:667–678. doi:10.1073/pnas.38.8.667
53. McAdoo DJ, Bente PFI, Gross ML, McLafferty FW (1974) Metastable Ion Characteristics. XXIII. Internal Energy of Product Ions Formed in Mass Spectral Reactions. Org Mass Spectrom 9:525–535. doi:10.1002/oms.1210090510
54. Meier K, Seibl J (1974) Measurement of Ion Residence Times in a Commercial Electron Impact Ion Source. Int J Mass Spectrom Ion Phys 14:99–106. doi:10.1016/0020-7381(74)80065-3
55. Chupka WA (1959) Effect of Unimolecular Decay Kinetics on the Interpretation of Appearance Potentials. J Chem Phys 30:191–211. doi:10.1063/1.1729875
56. Holmes JL, Terlouw JK (1980) The Scope of Metastable Peak Shape Observations. Org Mass Spectrom 15:383–396. doi:10.1002/oms.1210150802
57. Williams DH (1977) A Transition State Probe. Acc Chem Res 10:280–286. doi:10.1021/ar50116a002
58. Williams DH, Hvistendahl G (1974) Kinetic Energy Release in Relation to Symmetry-Forbidden Reactions. J Am Chem Soc 96:6753–6755. doi:10.1021/ja00828a034
59. Williams DH, Hvistendahl G (1974) Kinetic Energy Release as a Mechanistic Probe. The Role of Orbital Symmetry. J Am Chem Soc 96:6755–6757. doi:10.1021/ja00828a035
60. Hvistendahl G, Williams DH (1975) Partitioning of Reverse Activation Energy Between Kinetic and Internal Energy in Reactions of Simple Organic Ions. J Chem Soc Perkin Trans 2:881–885. doi:10.1039/P29750000881
61. Hvistendahl G, Uggerud E (1985) Secondary Isotope Effect on Kinetic Energy Release and Reaction Symmetry. Org Mass Spectrom 20:541–542. doi:10.1002/oms.1210200902
62. Kim KC, Beynon JH, Cooks RG (1974) Energy Partitioning by Mass Spectrometry. Chloroalkanes and Chloroalkenes. J Chem Phys 61:1305–1314. doi:10.1063/1.1682054
63. Haney MA, Franklin JL (1968) Correlation of Excess Energies of Electron Impact Dissociations with the Translational Energies of the Products. J Chem Phys 48:4093–4097. doi:10.1063/1.1669743
64. Cooks RG, Williams DH (1968) The Relative Rates of Fragmentation of Benzoyl Ions Generated upon Electron Impact From Different Precursors. Chem Commun:627–629. doi:10.1039/C19680000627
65. Lin YN, Rabinovitch BS (1970) Degrees of Freedom Effect and Internal Energy Partitioning Upon Ion Decomposition. J Phys Chem 74:1769–1775. doi:10.1021/j100703a019

66. Bente PF III, McLafferty FW, McAdoo DJ, Lifshitz C (1975) Internal Energy of Product Ions Formed in Mass Spectral Reactions. The Degrees of Freedom Effect. J Phys Chem 79:713–721. doi:10.1021/j100574a011
67. Todd JFJ (1995) Recommendations for Nomenclature and Symbolism for Mass Spectroscopy Including an Appendix of Terms Used in Vacuum Technology. Int J Mass Spectrom Ion Proc 142:211–240. doi:10.1016/0168-1176(95)93811-F
68. Robinson PJ, Holbrook KA (1972) Unimolecular Reactions. In: Unimolecular Reactions. Wiley, London
69. Ingemann S, Hammerum S, Derrick PJ, Fokkens RH, Nibbering NMM (1989) Energy-Dependent Reversal of Secondary Isotope Effects on Simple Cleavage Reactions: Tertiary Amine Radical Cations with Deuterium at Remote Positions. Org Mass Spectrom 24:885–889. doi:10.1002/oms.1210241006
70. Lowry TH, Schueller-Richardson K (1976) Isotope Effects. In: Mechanism and Theory in Organic Chemistry. Harper and Row, New York
71. Stringer MB, Underwood DJ, Bowie JH, Allison CE, Donchi KF, Derrick PJ (1992) Is the McLafferty Rearrangement of Ketones Concerted or Stepwise? The Application of Kinetic Isotope Effects. Org Mass Spectrom 27:270–276. doi:10.1002/oms.1210270319
72. Derrick PJ (1983) Isotope Effects in Fragmentation. Mass Spectrom Rev 2:285–298. doi:10.1002/mas.1280020204
73. Hvistendahl G, Uggerud E (1986) Deuterium Isotope Effects and Mechanism of the Gas-Phase Reaction $[C_3H_7]^+$ -> $[C_3H_5]^+ + H_2$. Org Mass Spectrom 21:347–350. doi:10.1002/oms.1210210609
74. Howe I, McLafferty FW (1971) Unimolecular Decomposition of Toluene and Cycloheptatriene Molecular Ions. Variation of the Degree of Scrambling and Isotope Effect with Internal Energy. J Am Chem Soc 93:99–105. doi:10.1021/ja00730a019
75. Bertrand M, Beynon JH, Cooks RG (1973) Isotope Effects Upon Hydrogen Atom Loss from Molecular Ions. Org Mass Spectrom 7:193–201. doi:10.1002/oms.1210070209
76. Lau AYK, Solka BH, Harrison AG (1974) Isotope Effects and H/D Scrambling in the Fragmentation of Labeled Propenes. Org Mass Spectrom 9:555–557. doi:10.1002/oms.1210090602
77. Benoit FM, Harrison AG (1976) Hydrogen Migrations in Mass Spectrometry. I. The Loss of Olefin From Phenyl-*n*-Propyl Ether Following Electron Impact Ionization and Chemical Ionization. Org Mass Spectrom 11:599–608. doi:10.1002/oms.1210110606
78. Veith HJ, Gross JH (1991) Alkene Loss From Metastable Methyleneimmonium Ions: Unusual Inverse Secondary Isotope Effect in Ion-Neutral Complex Intermediate Fragmentations. Org Mass Spectrom 26:1097–1105. doi:10.1002/oms.1210261214
79. Ingemann S, Kluft E, Nibbering NMM, Allison CE, Derrick PJ, Hammerum S (1991) Time-Dependence of the Isotope Effects in the Unimolecular Dissociation of Tertiary Amine Molecular Ions. Org Mass Spectrom 26:875–881. doi:10.1002/oms.1210261013
80. Nacson S, Harrison AG (1985) Dependence of Secondary Hydrogen/Deuterium Isotope Effects on Internal Energy. Org Mass Spectrom 20:429–430
81. Ingemann S, Hammerum S, Derrick PJ (1988) Secondary Hydrogen Isotope Effects on Simple Cleavage Reactions in the Gas Phase: The α-Cleavage of Tertiary Amine Cation Radicals. J Am Chem Soc 110:3869–3873. doi:10.1021/ja00220a024
82. Rosenstock HM (1976) The Measurement of Ionization and Appearance Potentials. Int J Mass Spectrom Ion Phys 20:139–190. doi:10.1016/0020-7381(76)80149-0
83. Urban B, Bondybey VE (2001) Multiphoton Photoelectron Spectroscopy: Watching Molecules Dissociate. Phys Chem Chem Phys 3:1942–1944. doi:10.1039/b102772g
84. Barfield AF, Wahrhaftig AL (1964) Determination of Appearance Potentials by the Critical Slope Method. J Chem Phys 41:2947–2948. doi:10.1063/1.1726381
85. Nicholson AJC (1958) Measurement of Ionization Potentials by Electron Impact. J Chem Phys 29:1312–1318. doi:10.1063/1.1744714

86. Levin RD, Lias SG (1982) Ionization Potential and Appearance Potential Measurements, 1971–1981. National Standard Reference Data Series 71:634 pp
87. Harris FM, Beynon JH (1985) Photodissociation in beams: organic ions. In: Bowers MT (ed) Gas Phase Ion Chemistry – Ions and Light. Academic Press, New York
88. Dunbar RC (1979) Ion photodissociation. In: Bowers MT (ed) Gas Phase Ion Chemistry. Academic Press, New York
89. Maeda K, Semeluk GP, Lossing FP (1968) A Two-Stage Double-Hemispherical Electron Energy Selector. Int J Mass Spectrom Ion Phys 1:395–407. doi:10.1016/0020-7381(68)85015-6
90. Traeger JC, McLoughlin RG (1978) A Photoionization Study of the Energetics of the $C_7H_7^+$ Ion Formed from C_7H_8 Precursors. Int J Mass Spectrom Ion Phys 27:319–333. doi:10.1016/0020-7381(78)80040-0
91. Boesl U (2000) Laser Mass Spectrometry for Environmental and Industrial Chemical Trace Analysis. J Mass Spectrom 35:289–304. doi:10.1002/(SICI)1096-9888(200003)35:3<289::AID-JMS960>3.0.CO;2-Y
92. Wendt KDA (2002) The New Generation of Resonant Laser Ionization Mass Spectrometers: Becoming Competitive for Selective Atomic Ultra-Trace Determination? Eur J Mass Spectrom 8:273–285. doi:10.1255/ejms.501
93. Matsumoto J, Misawa K, Ishiuchi SI, Suzuki T, Hayashi SI, Fujii M (2007) On-Site and Real-Time Mass Spectrometer Utilizing the Resonance-Enhanced Multiphoton Ionization Technique. Shinku 50:241–245. doi:10.3131/jvsj.50.241
94. Thanner R, Oser H, Grotheer HH (1998) Time-Resolved Monitoring of Aromatic Compounds in an Experimental Incinerator Using an Improved Jet-Resonance-Enhanced Multi-Photon Ionization System Jet-REMPI. Eur Mass Spectrom 4:215–222. doi:10.1255/ejms.213
95. Zenobi R, Zhan Q, Voumard P (1996) Multiphoton Ionization Spectroscopy in Surface Analysis and Laser Desorption Mass Spectrometry. Mikrochim Acta 124:273–281. doi:10.1007/BF01242825
96. Weickhardt C, Grun C, Grotemeyer J (1998) Fundamentals and Features of Analytical Laser Mass Spectrometry with Ultrashort Laser Pulses. Eur Mass Spectrom 4:239–244. doi:10.1255/ejms.216
97. Turner DW, Al Jobory MI (1962) Determination of Ionization Potentials by Photoelectron Energy Measurement. J Chem Phys 37:3007–3008. doi:10.1063/1.1733134
98. Müller-Dethlefs K, Sander M, Schlag EW (1984) Two-Color Photoionization Resonance Spectroscopy of Nitric Oxide: Complete Separation of Rotational Levels of Nitrosyl Ion at the Ionization Threshold. Chem Phys Lett 112:291–294. doi:10.1016/0009-2614(84)85743-7
99. Müller-Dethlefs K, Sander M, Schlag EW (1984) A Novel Method Capable of Resolving Rotational Ionic States by the Detection of Threshold Photoelectrons with a Resolution of 1.2 cm^{-1}. Z Naturforsch A 39:1089–1091. doi:10.1515/zna-1984-1112
100. Schlag EW (1998) ZEKE Spectroscopy. Cambridge University Press, Cambridge
101. Edqvist O, Lindholm E, Selin LE, Åsbrink L (1970) Photoelectron Spectrum of Molecular Oxygen. Phys Scr 1:25–30. doi:10.1088/0031-8949/1/1/004
102. Zhu L, Johnson P (1991) Mass Analyzed Threshold Ionization Spectroscopy. J Chem Phys 94:5769–5771. doi:10.1063/1.460460
103. Weickhardt C, Moritz F, Grotemeyer J (1997) Time-of-Flight Mass Spectrometry: State-of-the-Art in Chemical Analysis and Molecular Science. Mass Spectrom Rev 15:139–162. doi:10.1002/(SICI)1098-2787(1996)15:3<139::AID-MAS1>3.0.CO;2-J
104. Gunzer F, Grotemeyer J (2002) New Features in the Mass Analyzed Threshold Ionization (MATI) Spectra of Alkyl Benzenes. Phys Chem Chem Phys 4:5966–5972. doi:10.1039/B208283G
105. Peng X, Kong W (2002) Zero Energy Kinetic Electron and Mass-Analyzed Threshold Ionization Spectroscopy of $Na\times(NH_3)_n$ (n = 1, 2, and 4) Complexes. J Chem Phys 117:9306–9315. doi:10.1063/1.1516796

106. Haines SR, Dessent CEH, Müller-Dethlefs K (1999) Mass Analyzed Threshold Ionization of Phenol×CO: Intermolecular Binding Energies of a Hydrogen-Bonded Complex. J Chem Phys 111:1947–1954. doi:10.1063/1.479463
107. Gleiter R, Heilbronner E, Hornung V (1972) Applications of Photoelectron Spectroscopy. 28. Photoelectron Spectra of Azabenzenes and Azanaphthalenes. I. Pyridine, Diazines, *S*-Triazine, and *S*-Tetrazine. Helv Chim Acta 55:255–274. doi:10.1002/hlca.19720550130
108. Lavanchy A, Houriet R, Gäumann T (1978) The Mass Spectrometric Fragmentation of *N*-Heptane. Org Mass Spectrom 13:410–416. doi:10.1002/oms.1210130709
109. Meisels GG, Chen CT, Giessner BG, Emmel RH (1972) Energy-Deposition Functions in Mass Spectrometry. J Chem Phys 56:793–800. doi:10.1063/1.1677233
110. Herman JA, Li YH, Harrison AG (1982) Energy Dependence of the Fragmentation of Some Isomeric $C_6H_{12}^{+\cdot}$ Ions. Org Mass Spectrom 17:143–150. doi:10.1002/oms.1210170309
111. Lindinger W, Jordan A (1998) Proton-Transfer-Reaction Mass Spectrometry (PTR-MS): On-line Monitoring of Volatile Organic Compounds at pptv Levels. Chem Soc Rev 27:347–354. doi:10.1039/a827347z
112. Blake RS, Monks PS, Ellis AM (2009) Proton-Transfer Reaction Mass Spectrometry. Chem Rev 109:861–896. doi:10.1021/cr800364q
113. Lias SG, Liebman JF, Levin RD (1984) Evaluated Gas Phase Basicities and Proton Affinities of Molecules; Heats of Formation of Protonated Molecules. J Phys Chem Ref Data 13:695–808. doi:10.1063/1.555719
114. Harrison AG (1997) The Gas-Phase Basicities and Proton Affinities of Amino Acids and Peptides. Mass Spectrom Rev 16:201–217. doi:10.1002/(SICI)1098-2787(1997)16:4<201::AID-MAS3>3.0.CO;2-L
115. Kukol A, Strehle F, Thielking G, Grützmacher HF (1993) Methyl Group Effect on the Proton Affinity of Methylated Acetophenones Studied by Two Mass Spectrometric Techniques. Org Mass Spectrom 28:1107–1110. doi:10.1002/oms.1210281021
116. McMahon TB (2000) Thermochemical Ladders: Scaling the Ramparts of Gaseous Ion Energetics. Int J Mass Spectrom 200:187–199. doi:10.1016/S1387-3806(00)00308-0
117. Lias SG, Bartmess JE, Liebman JF, Holmes JL, Levin RD, Mallard WG (1988) Gas-Phase Ion and Neutral Thermochemistry. J Phys Chem Ref Data 17(Suppl 1):861pp
118. Talrose VL, Ljubimova AK (1998) Secondary Processes in the Ion Source of a Mass Spectrometer (Presented by Academician NN Semenov 27 VIII 1952) – Reprinted from Report of the Soviet Academy of Sciences, Vol LXXXVI, -N5 (1952). J Mass Spectrom 33:502–504
119. Munson MSB (2000) Development of Chemical Ionization Mass Spectrometry. Int J Mass Spectrom 200:243–251. doi:10.1016/S1387-3806(00)00301-8
120. Schalley CA, Springer A (2009) Mass Spectrometry and Gas-Phase Chemistry of Non-Covalent Complexes. Wiley, Hoboken

3 Isotopic Composition and Accurate Mass

Learning Objectives

- Isotopic composition of elements and their effect on mass spectra
- Translation of isotopic abundances into mass spectral patterns
- Analytical information from isotopic patterns
- Nominal and accurate mass of molecules and ions
- Mass resolution and its effects on isotopic patterns and mass accuracy
- Accurate mass as a tool for determining molecular formulas
- Ultrahigh resolution – aspects and applications
- Relevance of these topics for all types of mass spectral analyses

In the context of general chemistry we rarely pay attention to the different isotopes of the individual elements involved in a reaction. For instance, the molecular mass of tribromomethane, $CHBr_3$, is usually calculated as 252.73 g mol^{-1} on the basis of relative atomic mass from the Periodic Table. In mass spectrometry, however, we need to more accurately consider individual isotopes, because mass spectrometry is based upon the separation of ions by mass-to-charge ratio, *m/z* [1–3]. Thus, there actually is no molecular ion peak at *m/z* 252.73 in the mass spectrum of tribromomethane. Instead, major peaks occur at *m/z* 250, 252, 254, and 256 accompanied by some minor other ones.

In order to successfully interpret a mass spectrum, one needs to understand isotopic masses and their relation to the atomic weights, isotopic abundances, and the resulting isotopic patterns, and finally, high-resolution and accurate mass measurements. These issues are closely related to each other, offer a wealth of analytical information, and are valid for any type of mass spectrometer and any ionization method employed. Therefore, the content of this chapter is of highest relevance for the interpretation of any kind of mass spectral data.

J.H. Gross, *Mass Spectrometry*, DOI 10.1007/978-3-319-54398-7_3

3.1 Isotopic Classification of the Elements

An element is specified by the number of protons in its nucleus. This equals the *atomic number* Z of the respective element and determines its place within the periodic table of the elements. The atomic number is given as a subscript preceding the elemental symbol, e.g., $_6$C in case of carbon. Atoms with nuclei of the same atomic number differing in the number of neutrons are termed *isotopes*. One isotope differs from another isotope of the same element in that it possesses a different *number of neutrons* N, i.e., by the *mass number* A or *nucleon number*. The mass number of an isotope is given as a superscript preceding the elemental symbol, e.g., ^{12}C. The mass number A is the sum of the total number of protons and neutrons in an atom, molecule, or ion [4].

$$A = Z + N \tag{3.1}$$

Mass and order

The *mass number* must not be confused with the *atomic number* of an element. For the heavier atoms there can be isotopes of the same mass number belonging to different elements, e.g., the most abundant isotopes of both $_{18}$Ar and $_{20}$Ca have mass number 40.

3.1.1 Monoisotopic Elements

Among 83 naturally occurring stable elements, 20 elements do exist in the form of only one single naturally occurring stable isotope. Therefore, they are termed *monoisotopic elements*, i.e., all of their atoms have equal A. Among the monoisotopic elements, fluorine (^{19}F), sodium (^{23}Na), phosphorus (^{31}P), and iodine (^{127}I) belong to the more prominent examples in organic mass spectrometry. Nonetheless, there are many more such as beryllium (^{9}Be), aluminum (^{27}Al), manganese (^{55}Mn), cobalt (^{59}Co), arsenic (^{75}As), niobium (^{93}Nb), rhodium (^{103}Rh), cesium (^{133}Cs), and gold (^{197}Au). The monoisotopic elements are also referred to as A or X elements [5, 6]. If radioactive isotopes were also taken into account, not a single monoisotopic element would remain.

3.1.2 Di-isotopic Elements

Several elements exist naturally in two isotopes and within the context of mass spectrometry it is useful to deal with them as a class of their own. Nevertheless, the term *di-isotopic element* is not an official one, i.e., not part of IUPAC nomenclature. These elements can even be sub-classified into those having one isotope that is 1 u heavier than the most abundant isotope and those having one isotope that is 2 u heavier than the most abundant isotope. The first group has been termed A + 1 or

X + 1 elements, the latter ones have been termed A + 2 or X + 2 elements, respectively [5, 6]. If we do not restrict our view to the elements typically encountered in organic mass spectrometry, one should add the class of X–1 elements with one minor isotope of 1 u lower mass than the most abundant one.

Prominent examples of X + 1 elements are hydrogen (^{1}H, $^{2}H \equiv D$), carbon (^{12}C, ^{13}C), and nitrogen (^{14}N, ^{15}N). Deuterium (D) is of low abundance (0.0115%) and therefore, hydrogen is usually treated as a monoisotopic or as an X element, which is a valid approximation, even if a hundred hydrogens are contained in a molecule.

Among the X + 2 elements, chlorine (^{35}Cl, ^{37}Cl) and bromine (^{79}Br, ^{81}Br) are relatively common, but copper (^{63}Cu, ^{65}Cu), gallium (^{69}Ga, ^{71}Ga), silver (^{107}Ag, ^{109}Ag), indium (^{113}In, ^{115}In), and antimony (^{121}Sb, ^{123}Sb) also belong to this group. Even though occurring in more than two isotopes, some other elements such as oxygen, sulfur, and silicon, can be dealt with as X + 2 elements for practical reasons. As long as only a few oxygens are part of a formula, oxygen might even be treated as an X element because of the low abundances of ^{17}O and ^{18}O.

Finally, the elements lithium (^{6}Li, ^{7}Li), boron (^{10}B, ^{11}B), and vanadium (^{50}V, ^{51}V) come along with a lighter isotope of lower abundance than the heavier one and thus, they can be grouped together as X–1 elements.

Atomic numbers, mass numbers, and isotopes Let us apply the notation of Eq. (3.1) to the elements contributing to a molecule of tribromomethane that has already been mentioned in the introductory paragraph of this chapter. The molecule is composed of carbon, hydrogen, and bromine, the latter occurs naturally as two isotopes of almost equal abundance. Thus, these four species are most relevant for the $CHBr_3$ molecule (Fig. 3.1). Now we get an idea of why tribromomethane molecular ions appear split into several peaks in a mass spectrum. We will return to this topic shortly.

3.1.3 Polyisotopic Elements

The majority of elements are grouped as *polyisotopic elements* because they consist of three or more isotopes showing a wide variety of isotopic distributions.

3.1.4 Representation of Isotopic Abundances

Isotopic abundances are listed either as their sum being 100% or with the abundance of the most abundant isotope normalized to 100%. The first normalization is

$$^{A}_{Z} \quad ^{1}_{1}\mathrm{H} \quad ^{12}_{6}\mathrm{C} \quad ^{79}_{35}\mathrm{Br} \quad ^{81}_{35}\mathrm{Br}$$

Fig. 3.1 Atomic numbers and mass numbers relevant for the elements contributing to tribromomethane, $CHBr_3$

obvious as it reflects all isotopes as contributing to 100% of an element. The second normalization (also used throughout this book) is commonly applied in mass spectrometry: mass spectra are customarily reported as normalized to the base peak or at least to the most intensive peak within the *m/z* range of interest (Chap. 1). The isotopic classifications and *isotopic compositions* of some common elements are listed below (Table 3.1).

Check mode of normalization
Care has to be taken when comparing isotopic abundances from different sources as they might be compiled using one *or* the other procedure of normalization. Never mix normalization modes in your calculations!

Bar graph representations are much better suited for visualization of isotopic compositions than tables, and in fact they exactly show how such a distribution would appear in a mass spectrum (Fig. 3.2). This appearance coined the term *isotopic pattern* or *isotope pattern*.

Note
Some authors use the term *isotopic cluster*, which is incorrect, as *cluster* refers to an associate of more atoms, molecules, or ions of the same species, sometimes associated with one other species, e.g., $[Ar_n]^{+\bullet}$, $[(H_2O)_nH]^+$, and $[I(CsI)_n]^-$ are cluster ions.

3.1.5 Calculation of Atomic, Molecular, and Ionic Mass

3.1.5.1 Nominal Mass

In order to calculate the approximate mass of a molecule we usually sum up integer masses of the elements encountered, e.g., for CO_2 we calculate the mass as $12\ u + 2 \times 16\ u = 44\ u$. The result of this simple procedure is not particularly precise but provides acceptable values for simple molecules. This is called *nominal mass* [6].

More precisely, the nominal mass of an element is defined as the *integer mass* of its most abundant naturally occurring stable isotope [6]. The nominal mass of an element is often equal to the integer mass of the lowest mass isotope of that element, e.g., for H, C, N, O, S, Si, P, F, Cl, Br, I (Table 3.1). The nominal mass of an ion is the sum of the nominal masses of its constituent elements.

Nominal mass of trifluoroacetic acid The nominal mass of trifluoroacetic acid, CF_3COOH, is calculated based on the mass number of the most abundant isotopes of the contributing elements. Using ^1H, ^{12}C, ^{16}O, and ^{19}F we obtain $1\ u + 2 \times 12\ u + 2 \times 16\ u + 3 \times 19\ u = 114\ u$.

Table 3.1 Isotopic classifications and isotopic compositions of some common elements

Classification	Atomic symbol	Atomic number Z	Mass number A	Isotopic composition	Isotopic mass [u]	Relative atomic mass [u]
(X)[a]	H	1	1	100	1.007825	1.00795
			2	0.0115	2.014101	
X	F	9	19	100	18.998403	18.998403
X	Na	11	23	100	22.989769	22.989769
X	P	15	31	100	30.973762	30.973762
X	I	53	127	100	126.904468	126.904468
X + 1	C	6	12	100	12.000000[b]	12.0108
			13	1.08	13.003355	
X + 1	N	7	14	100	14.003074	14.00675
			15	0.369	15.000109	
(X + 2)[a]	O	8	16	100	15.994915	15.9994
			17	0.038	16.999132	
			18	0.205	17.999161	
(X + 2)[a]	Si	14	28	100	27.976927	28.0855
			29	5.0778	28.976495	
			30	3.3473	29.973770	
(X + 2)[a]	S	16	32	100	31.972071	32.067
			33	0.80	32.971459	
			34	4.52	33.967867	
			36	0.02	35.967081	
X + 2	Cl	17	35	100	34.968853	35.4528
			37	31.96	36.965903	
X + 2	Br	35	79	100	78.918338	79.904
			81	97.28	80.916291	
X–1	Li	3	6	8.21	6.015122	6.941
			7	100	7.016004	
X–1	B	5	10	24.8	10.012937	10.812
			11	100	11.009306	
poly	Xe	54	124	0.33	123.905896	131.29
			126	0.33	125.904270	
			128	7.14	127.903530	
			129	98.33	128.904779	
			130	15.17	129.903508	
			131	78.77	130.905082	
			132	100	131.904154	
			134	38.82	133.905395	
			136	32.99	135.907221	

A complete table is provided in the Appendix. © IUPAC 2001 [7, 8]
[a]Classification in parentheses means "not in the strict sense"
[b]Standard of atomic mass scale

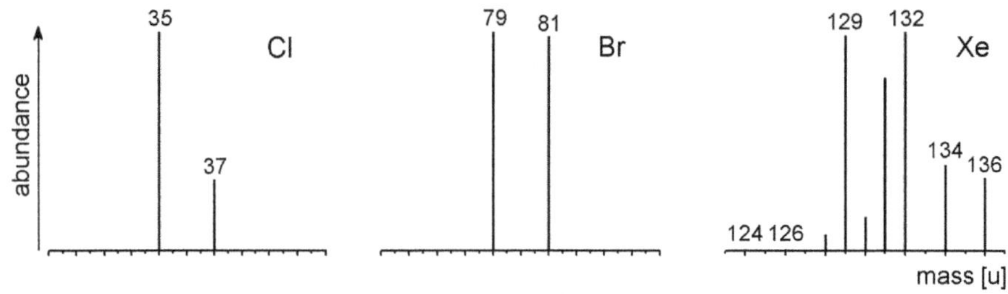

Fig. 3.2 Isotopic patterns of chlorine, bromine, and xenon. The bar graph representations of the isotopic distributions have the same optical appearance as mass spectra. You should compare these graphical representations to the compositions listed in Table 3.1. Afterwards, you may decide for yourself which type you would consider to be easier to perceive and to compare

Nominal mass of $SnCl_2$ To calculate the nominal mass of $SnCl_2$, the masses of ^{120}Sn and ^{35}Cl have to be used, i.e., 120 u + 2 × 35 u = 190 u. While the ^{35}Cl isotope represents the most abundant as well as the lowest mass isotope of chlorine, ^{120}Sn is the most abundant but not the lowest mass isotope of tin which is ^{112}Sn.

Mass versus mass number

When dealing with nominal mass, mass number and nominal mass both have the same numerical value. However, the *mass number* is dimensionless and must not be confused with *nominal mass* in units of u.

3.1.5.2 Isotopic Mass

The *isotopic mass* is the exact mass of an isotope. It is very close to but not equal to the nominal mass of the isotope (Table 3.1). The only exception is the carbon isotope ^{12}C which has an isotopic mass of 12.000000 u.

The *unified atomic mass* [u] is defined as $^{1}/_{12}$ of the mass of one atom of nuclide ^{12}C which has been assigned precisely 12 u, where 1 u = 1.660538 × 10^{-27} kg [4, 6, 9, 10]. This convention dates back to 1961 [2].

Avoid using outdated masses

The *unified atomic mass* [u], defined as $^{1}/_{12}$ of the mass of one atom of nuclide ^{12}C is the only valid unit for atomic mass. Mass values from dated literature can be ambiguous. Prior to 1961, physicists defined the *atomic mass unit* [amu] based on $^{1}/_{16}$ of the mass of one atom of nuclide ^{16}O. The definition of chemists was based on the relative atomic mass of oxygen which is somewhat higher due to the nuclides ^{17}O and ^{18}O that also occur in natural oxygen [2]. Thus, the oxygen-based mass scales are neither compatible among each other nor are the mass values equal to the actual ^{12}C–based scale. You *always* should be using u and *never* amu.

3.1.5.3 Relative Atomic Mass

The *relative atomic mass* or the *atomic weight* as it is also often imprecisely termed is calculated as the weighted average of the naturally occurring isotopes of an element [6]. The weighted average $M_{r.}$ is calculated from

$$M_r = \frac{\sum_{i=1}^{i} A_i \times m_i}{\sum_{i=1}^{i} A_i} \tag{3.2}$$

with A_i being the abundances of the isotopes and m_i their respective isotopic masses [11]. For this purpose, the abundances can be used in any numerical form or normalization as long as they are used consistently.

Atomic mass of chlorine The relative atomic mass of chlorine is 35.4528 u. However, there is such atom. Instead, chlorine is composed of ^{35}Cl (34.968853 u) and ^{37}Cl (36.965903 u), the former making up 75.78% and the latter 24.22% – or having relative abundances of 100% and 31.96%, respectively (Table 3.1 and Fig. 3.2). According to Eq. (3.2), we would calculate the relative atomic mass of chlorine as $M_{r.}$ = (100 × 34.968853 u + 31.96 × 36.965903 u)/(100 + 31.96) = 35.4528 u.

3.1.5.4 Monoisotopic Mass

The exact mass of the most abundant isotope of an element is termed *monoisotopic mass* [6]. The monoisotopic mass of a molecule is the sum of the monoisotopic masses of the elements in its empirical formula. As mentioned before, the monoisotopic mass is not necessarily the naturally occurring isotope of lowest mass. However, for the common elements in organic mass spectrometry the monoisotopic mass is obtained using the mass of the lowest mass isotope of that element, because this is also the most abundant isotope of the respective element (Sect. 3.1.5.1).

Monoisotopic mass of trifluoroacetic acid The monoisotopic mass of trifluoroacetic acid, CF_3COOH, is calculated based on the isotopic masses of the most abundant isotopes of the contributing elements. Using ^{1}H, ^{12}C, ^{16}O, and ^{19}F we obtain 1.007825 u + 2 × 12.000000 u + 2 × 15.994915 u + 3 × 18.998403 u = 113.992864 u. While the result is very close to the nominal mass 114 u, it still differs by 0.007136 u from that value.

3.1.5.5 Relative Molecular Mass

The *relative molecular mass*, M_r, or *molecular weight* is calculated from the relative atomic masses of the elements contributing to the empirical formula [6]. With the exception of very large molecules of say $>10^3$ u the relative molecular mass is rarely useful in mass spectrometry.

Molecular weight of tribromomethane Let's once more revisit tribromomethane. Using the relative atomic mass of H, C, and Br from Table 3.1 the molecular mass of $CHBr_3$ is calculated as 1.0079 u + 12.0108 u + 3 × 79.9040 u = 252.7307 u.

3.1.5.6 Exact Ionic Mass

The *exact mass of a positive ion* formed by the removal of one or more electrons from a molecule is equal to its monoisotopic mass minus the mass of the electron(s), m_e [4]. For negative ions, the electron mass (0.000548 u) has to be added accordingly.

Exact mass of a $CO_2^{+\bullet}$ ion The exact mass of the carbon dioxide molecular ion, $CO_2^{+\bullet}$, is calculated as 12.000000 u + 2 × 15.994915 u − 0.000548 u = 43.989282 u.

3.1.5.7 Role of the Electron Mass When Calculating Exact Mass

The question remains whether the mass of the electron m_e (5.48×10^{-4} u) has really to be taken into account. This issue was of almost pure academic interest as long as mass spectrometry was limited to mass accuracies of several 10^{-3} u. As FT-ICR, Orbitrap, and even recent oaTOF instruments deliver mass accuracies in the order of $<10^{-3}$ u, one should routinely include the electron mass in calculations [12, 13]. Here, neglecting the electron mass would cause a systematic error of the size of m_e, which is unacceptable when mass measurement accuracies in the order of $<10^{-3}$ u are to be achieved.

3.1.5.8 Number of Decimals When Calculating Exact Mass

The isotopic masses provided in this book are listed with six decimal places corresponding to an accuracy of 10^{-6} u (Table 3.1 and Appendix A.2), which is about three orders of magnitude below typical mass errors in mass spectrometry (± 0.001 u).

The number of decimal places one should employ in mass calculations depends on the purpose they are used for. In the *m*/*z* range of up to about 500 u, the use of isotopic mass with four decimal places may provide sufficient accuracy. Above that, at least five decimal places are required, because the increasing number of atoms results in an unacceptable multiplication of many small mass errors. The results of those calculations may again be reported with only four decimal places (± 0.0001 u), because this is sufficient for most applications.

Exact mass of mellitin $[M + H]^+$ ions Mellitin is the major active component of the honey bee venom. Mellitin is a peptide consisting of 26 amino acids with a molecular formula of $C_{131}H_{229}N_{39}O_{31}$. Let us calculate the exact mass of the protonated molecule, $[M + H]^+$, based on isotopic masses rounded to three and four decimals, respectively, and finally, based on full six decimals (Table 3.2). The resulting mass based on four decimals already deviates from the accurate result by 0.0051 u, the mass based on only three decimals is off by unacceptable 0.0405 u.

Table 3.2 Calculation of the exact mass of $[M + H]^+$ ions of the peptide mellitin based on different levels of accuracy

Element	Mass, three decimals [u]	Mass, four decimals [u]	Mass exact [u]	Number of atoms
C	12.000	12.0000	12.000000	131
H	1.008	1.0078	1.007825	230
N	14.003	14.0031	14.003074	39
O	15.995	15.9949	15.994915	31
Summed mass minus m_e	2845.802	2845.7563	2845.761453	

3.1.6 Natural Variations in Relative Atomic Mass

The masses of isotopes can be measured with accuracies better than *parts per billion* (ppb), e.g., $m_{40\mathrm{Ar}} = 39.9623831235 \pm 0.000000005$ u. Unfortunately, determinations of abundance ratios are less accurate, causing errors of several *parts per million* (ppm) in relative atomic mass. The real limiting factor, however, comes from the variation of isotopic abundances from natural samples, e.g., in case of lead (Pb) which is the final product of radioactive decay of uranium, the atomic weight varies by 500 ppm depending on the Pb/U ratios in the lead ore [11]. Variations in natural isotopic distributions are also responsible for the varying number of decimal places stated with the relative atomic masses in Table 3.1.

For organic mass spectrometry the case of carbon is of highest relevance. Carbon is ubiquitous in metabolic processes and the most prominent example of variations in the $^{13}C/^{12}C$ isotopic ratio is presented by the different pathways of CO_2 fixation during photosynthesis, causing $^{13}C/^{12}C$ ratios of 0.01085–0.01115. Petroleum, coal, and natural gas yield very low $^{13}C/^{12}C$ ratios of 0.01068–0.01099 and carbonate minerals, on the other side, set the upper limit at about 0.01125 [11]. Even proteins of different origin (plants, fish, mammals) can be distinguished by their $^{13}C/^{12}C$ ratios [14, 15].

Isotope ratio mass spectrometry (IR-MS) makes use of these facts to determine the origin or the age of a sample (Chap. 15). For convenience, the minor changes in isotopic ratios are expressed using the *delta notation* stating the deviation of the isotopic ratio from a defined standard in parts per thousand (‰) [11, 16]. The delta value of carbon, $\delta^{13}C$, for example, is calculated from:

$$\delta^{13}\mathrm{C}(‰) = \left[\left({}^{13}\mathrm{C}/{}^{12}\mathrm{C}_{\mathrm{sample}}\right)/\left({}^{13}\mathrm{C}/{}^{12}\mathrm{C}_{\mathrm{standard}}\right) - 1\right] \times 1000 \qquad (3.3)$$

The internationally accepted standard value for $^{13}C/^{12}C_{standard}$ is 0.0112372 as represented by belemnite from the Pee Dee formation, i.e., for PDP $\delta^{13}C = 0‰$ (PDB standard). PDB is a well-defined belemnite fossil from the Pee Dee formation of South Carolina, USA. For example, to calculate $\delta^{13}C$ by use of Eq. (3.3) for a compound having $^{13}C/^{12}C_{sample} = 0.0109800$ we obtain $\delta^{13}C = [(0.0109800/0.0112372) - 1] \times 1000 = -22.88‰$.

Stable carbon isotope ratios of most natural materials of biological interest range from $\delta^{13}C = -100‰$ to about $\delta^{13}C = 0‰$ versus PDB (Fig. 3.3). These natural variations result from isotopic fractionation during physical, chemical, and biological processes. Inorganic carbon in seawater, freshwater, and carbonates has a rather high proportion of ^{13}C. Organic carbon, on the other side, is generally depleted of ^{13}C as a result of biological isotope fractionation, mostly due to kinetic isotope effects during photosynthesis [17]. Thus, the origin of food can be determined by employing $\delta^{13}C$ measurements, e.g., fruit/vegetables by country or whether the source of ethanol in alcoholic beverages is sugar cane, sugar beet, cereal starch, or obtained by synthetic processes [14, 16, 18].

Wool from western or eastern Ireland? Among numerous other applications, the $^{34}S/^{32}S$ isotope ratio has been exploited to determine whether wool originated from sheep living at or close to the west or east coast of Ireland [19]. The distance from the west coast at which Irish farm sheep were kept was found to be negatively correlated to the $\delta^{34}S$ values. The values changed from +15.8‰ for west coast wool to as low as +5.3‰ for east coast wool. In IR-MS, differences of >10‰ $\delta^{34}S$ are considered highly significant.

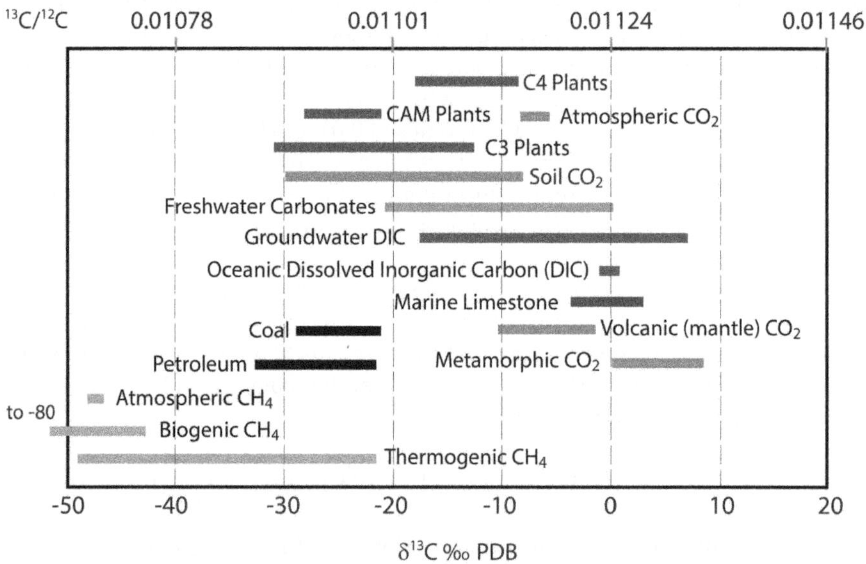

Fig. 3.3 Compilation of $\delta^{13}C$ values of different sources of carbon relative to PDB. The ratios of $^{13}C/^{12}C$ (rounded to five decimals) at $\delta^{13}C = -40‰, -20‰, 0‰, 20‰$ are shown for comparison to a more common scale (Adapted with kind permission from a figure by James Wittke, Northern Arizona University)

Common practice
Assuming an average ^{13}C content of 1.1%, equaling a $^{13}C/^{12}C$ ratio of 0.0111 has proven to be most useful in the majority of mass spectrometric applications.

3.2 Calculation of Isotopic Distributions

As long as we are dealing with molecular masses in a range of up to some 10^3 u, it is possible to separate ions which differ by 1 u in mass. The upper mass limit for their separation depends on the resolution of the instrument employed. Consequently, the isotopic composition of the analyte is directly reflected in the mass spectrum – it can be regarded as an elemental fingerprint.

Even if the analyte is chemically perfectly pure it represents a mixture of different isotopic compositions, provided it is not solely composed of monoisotopic elements. Therefore, a mass spectrum normally superimposes the mass spectra of all isotopic species involved [20]. The *isotopic distribution* or *isotopic pattern* of molecules containing one chlorine or bromine atom is listed in Table 3.1. But what about molecules containing two or more di-isotopic or even polyisotopic elements? While it may seem, at the first glance, to complicate the interpretation of mass spectra, isotopic patterns are in fact an ideal source of analytical information.

3.2.1 Carbon: An X + 1 Element

In the mass spectrum of methane (Fig. 1.6), there is a tiny peak at m/z 17 that has not been mentioned in the introduction. As one can infer from Table 3.1 this should result from the ^{13}C content of natural carbon which is an X + 1 element according to our classification.

How isotope patterns come about Imagine a total of 1000 methane molecules, CH_4. Due to a content of 1.1% ^{13}C, there will be 11 molecules containing ^{13}C instead of ^{12}C; the remaining 989 molecules are $^{12}CH_4$. Therefore, the ratio of relative intensities of the peaks at m/z 16 and m/z 17 is defined by the ratio 989/11 or by usual normalization 100/1.1.

In a more general way, carbon consists of ^{13}C and ^{12}C in a ratio r that can be written as $r = c/(100 - c)$ where c is the abundance of ^{13}C. Then, the probability to have only ^{12}C in a molecular ion M consisting of w carbons, i.e., the probability of monoisotopic ions P_M is given by [21]:

$$P_M = \left(\frac{100-c}{100}\right)^w \tag{3.4}$$

The probability of having exactly one ^{13}C atom in an ion with w carbon atoms is therefore

$$P_{M+1} = w\left(\frac{c}{100-c}\right)\left(\frac{100-c}{100}\right)^w \tag{3.5}$$

and the ratio P_{M+1}/P_M is given as

$$\frac{P_{M+1}}{P_M} = w\left(\frac{c}{100-c}\right) \tag{3.6}$$

In case of a carbon-only molecule such as the buckminster fullerene C_{60}, the ratio P_{M+1}/P_M becomes $60 \times 1.1/98.9 = 0.667$. If the monoisotopic peak at *m/z* 720 due to $^{12}C_{60}$ is regarded as 100%, the M + 1 peak due to $^{12}C_{59}{}^{13}C$ will have 66.7% relative intensity.

Estimate the intensity of the ^{13}C peak

For the $^{13}C/^{12}C$ ratio, the M + 1 peak intensity can be easily estimated in percent in a simplified manner, and with an insignificant error, by multiplying the number of carbon atoms by 1.1%, e.g., 60 × 1.1% = 66%.

There is again a certain probability for one of the remaining 59 carbon atoms to be ^{13}C rather than ^{12}C. After simplification of Beynon's approach [21] to be used for one atomic species only, the probability that there will be an ion containing two ^{13}C atoms is expressed by:

$$\frac{P_{M+2}}{P_M} = \frac{w}{2}\left(\frac{c}{100-c}\right)(w-1)\left(\frac{c}{100-c}\right) = \frac{w(w-1)c^2}{2(100-c)^2} \tag{3.7}$$

For C_{60} the ratio P_{M+2}/P_M now becomes $(60 \times 59 \times 1.1^2)/(2 \times 98.9^2) = 0.219$, i.e., the M + 2 peak at *m/z* 722 due to $^{12}C_{58}{}^{13}C_2$ ions will show as 21.9% relative to the M peak, which definitely cannot be neglected. By extension of this principle, equations for the P_{M+3}/P_M ratio representing the third isotopic peak can be derived and so forth.

The calculation of isotopic patterns as just shown for the carbon-only molecule C_{60} can be done analogously for any X + 1 element. Furthermore, the application of this scheme is not restricted to molecular ions, but can also be used for fragment ions (Fig. 3.4). Nevertheless, care should be taken to assure that the presumed isotopic peak is not partially or even completely due to a different fragment ion, e.g., an ion containing one hydrogen more than the presumed X + 1 composition.

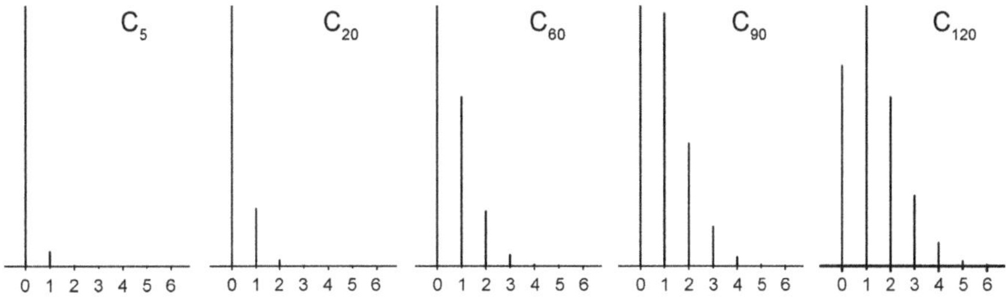

Fig. 3.4 Calculated isotopic patterns for carbon. Note the steadily expanding width of the pattern as X + 2, X + 3, X + 4,... become visible. At about C_{90} the X + 1 peak reaches the same intensity as the X peak. At higher carbon numbers it becomes the base peak of the pattern

Estimate the number of carbon atoms

It is very helpful to read out the P_{M+1}/P_M ratio from a mass spectrum to calculate the approximate number of carbon atoms. Provided no other element contributing to M + 1 is present, an M + 1 intensity of 15%, for example, indicates the presence of 14 carbons. (For possible overestimation due to autoprotonation cf. Sect. 7.2).

It is interesting how the width of the isotopic pattern increases as X + 2, X + 3, X + 4, ... become detectable. In principle, the isotopic pattern of C_w expands up to X + *w*, because even the composition $^{13}C_w$ is possible. As a result, the isotopic pattern of *w* atoms of a di-isotopic element consists at least theoretically of *w* + 1 peaks. However, the probability of extreme combinations is negligible and even somewhat more probable combinations are of no importance as long they are below about 0.1%. In practice, the interpretation of the carbon isotopic pattern is limited by experimental errors in relative intensities rather than by detection limits for peaks of low intensity. Such experimental errors can be due to poor signal-to-noise ratios (Sect. 1.6.3), autoprotonation (Sect. 7.2), or interference with other peaks.

At about C_{90} the X + 1 peak reaches the same intensity as the X peak, and at higher carbon number *w*, it becomes the base peak of the pattern, because the probability that an ion contains at least one ^{13}C becomes larger than that for the monoisotopic ion. A further increase in *w* makes the X + 2 signal stronger than the X and X + 1 peak and so on. A table with representative carbon isotopic abundances is provided in the Appendix.

3.2.2 Terms Related to Isotopic Composition

Molecules and ions of identical elemental composition but differing in isotopic composition are termed *isotopic homologs* or simply *isotopologs*. For example, $H_3C\text{-}CH_3$ and $H_3C\text{-}^{13}CH_3$ are isotopologs. Molecules and ions of identical isotopic composition but differing in position of the isotopes are termed *isotopomers*. For example, $H_2C = CD_2$ and HDC = CHD are isotopomers.

The *isotopic molecular ion* (M + 1, M + 2, ...) is a molecular ion containing one or more of the less abundant naturally occurring isotopes of the atoms that make up the molecular structure [4]. This term can be generalized for any non-monoisotopic ion. Thus, *isotopic ions* are those ions containing one or more of the less abundant naturally occurring isotopes of the atoms that make up the ion.

The position of the most intensive peak of an isotopic pattern is termed *most abundant mass* [6], and the corresponding ion should be named *most abundant isotopolog (ion)*. For example, the most abundant mass in case of C_{120} is 1441 u corresponding to M + 1 (Fig. 3.4). The most abundant mass is relevant in the case of large ions (Sect. 3.4.3).

3.2.3 Binomial Approach

The above stepwise treatment of X + 1, X + 2, and X + 3 peaks has the advantage that it can be followed easier, but it bears the disadvantage that an equation needs to be solved for each individual peak. Alternatively, one can calculate the relative abundances of the isotopic species for a di-isotopic element from a binomial expression [5, 22, 23]. In the term $(a + b)^n$ the isotopic abundances of both isotopes are given as a and b, respectively, and n is the number of this species in the molecule.

$$\begin{aligned}(a+b)^n &= a^n + na^{n-1}b + n\,(n-1)\,a^{n-2}b^2/(2!)\\ &\quad + n\,(n-1)\,(n-2)\,a^{n-3}b^3/(3!) + \ldots\end{aligned} \tag{3.8}$$

For $n = 1$ the isotopic distribution can of course be directly obtained from the isotopic abundance table (Table 3.1 and Fig. 3.2) and in case of $n = 2$, 3, or 4 the expression can easily be solved by simple multiplication, e.g.,

$$\begin{aligned}(a+b)^2 &= a^2 + 2ab + b^2\\ (a+b)^3 &= a^3 + 3a^2b + 3ab^2 + b^3\\ (a+b)^4 &= a^4 + 4a^3b + 6a^2b^2 + 4ab^3 + b^4\end{aligned} \tag{3.9}$$

Again, we obtain $w + 1$ terms for the isotopic pattern of w atoms. The binomial approach works for any di-isotopic element, regardless of whether it is of X + 1, X + 2, or X–1 type. However, as the number of atoms increases, any manual calculation will grow more tedious and become more prone to error.

3.2.4 Halogens

The halogens Cl and Br occur in two isotopic forms, each of them being of significant abundance, whereas F and I are monoisotopic (Table 3.1). In most cases there are only a few Cl and/or Br atoms in a molecule and this predestinates the binomial approach for this purpose.

Isotopic pattern by two chlorines The isotopic pattern of Cl_2 is calculated from Eq. (3.9) with the abundances $a = 100$ and $b = 31.96$ as $(100 + 31.96)^2 = 10{,}000 + 6392 + 1019$. After normalization we obtain 100 : 63.9 : 10.2 as the relative intensities of the three peaks. Any other normalization for the isotopic abundances would give the same result, e.g., $a = 0.7578$, $b = 0.2422$. The calculated isotopic pattern of Cl_2 can be understood from the following practical consideration: The two isotopes ^{35}Cl and ^{37}Cl can be combined in three different ways: (*i*) $^{35}Cl_2$ giving rise to the monoisotopic composition, (*ii*) $^{35}Cl^{37}Cl$ yielding the first isotopic peak which is here X + 2, and finally (*iii*) $^{37}Cl_2$ giving the second isotopic peak X + 4. Thus, two chlorines cause three peaks in total. The combinations with a higher number of chlorine atoms can be explained accordingly.

Expect *w* + 1 peaks

As already mentioned, the isotopic pattern of C_w expands up to X + *w*, because in theory even the composition $^{13}C_w$ is possible. In fact, for any di-isotopic element, the isotopic pattern of *w* atoms comprises *w* + 1 peaks, e.g., C_{10} yields 11 peaks, Cl_2 yields 3 peaks, and Br_4 yields 5 peaks (check by yourself in Figs. 3.4 and 3.5). Not all peaks may be clearly visible in the spectrum because the probability of some isotopic combinations can be negligible.

It is helpful to have frequent isotopic distributions at hand. For some Cl_x, Br_y, and Cl_xBr_y combinations these are tabulated in the Appendix. Tables are useful for the construction of isotopic patterns from "building blocks". Nevertheless, as visual information is easier to compare with a plotted spectrum, these patterns are also shown below (Fig. 3.5). In case of Cl and Br the peaks are always separated from each other by 2 u, i.e., the isotopic peaks are located at X + 2, 4, 6 and so on.

If there are two bromine or four chlorine atoms contained in the formula, the isotopic peaks become stronger than the monoisotopic peak, because the second isotope is of much higher abundance than in case of the ^{13}C isotope.

Quick estimate of Cl and Br patterns

Rapid estimation of the isotopic patterns of chlorine and bromine can be achieved with good results by using the approximate isotope ratios $^{35}Cl/^{37}Cl = 3:1$ and $^{79}Br/^{81}Br = 1:1$. Visual comparison with calculated patterns is also suitable (Fig. 3.5).

Decision-making help One may want to seek advice on how to distinguish between those patterns. For example, the patterns of Cl_2Br and Cl_3Br or of

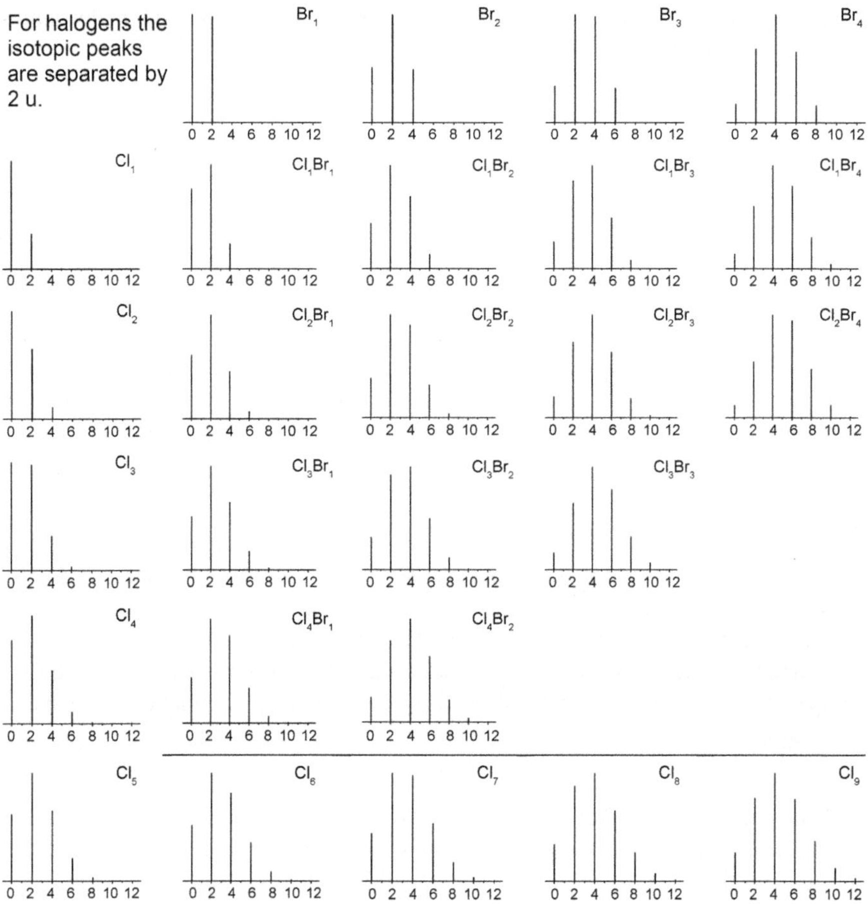

Fig. 3.5 Calculated isotopic patterns for combinations of bromine and chlorine. The peak shown at zero position corresponds to the monoisotopic ion at *m/z* X. The isotopic peaks are then located at *m/z* = X + 2, 4, 6, ... The numerical value of X is given by the mass number of the monoisotopic combination, e.g., 70 u for Cl_2

Cl_2Br_3 and Cl_3Br_3 closely resemble each other. To distinguish such pairs it is helpful to construct orientation lines between signal peak tips of comparable intensity. Generally these will decline with one pattern but can be positively inclined or even close to horizontal in others (Fig. 3.6).

Six bromine patterns united The EI mass spectrum of hexabromobenzene, C_6Br_6, is particularly illustrative in that it provides the complete series of isotope patterns from Br_1 to Br_6 in a row (Fig. 3.7). The series starts with the molecular ion, $[C_6Br_6]^{+\bullet}$, and proceeds via $[M–Br]^+$ and $[M–Br_2]^{+\bullet}$ down to the signals for $[C_6Br]^+$. This also shows that such patterns are not rare exceptions but have to be expected in real-world samples. For practicing purposes, you might want to compare the patterns in

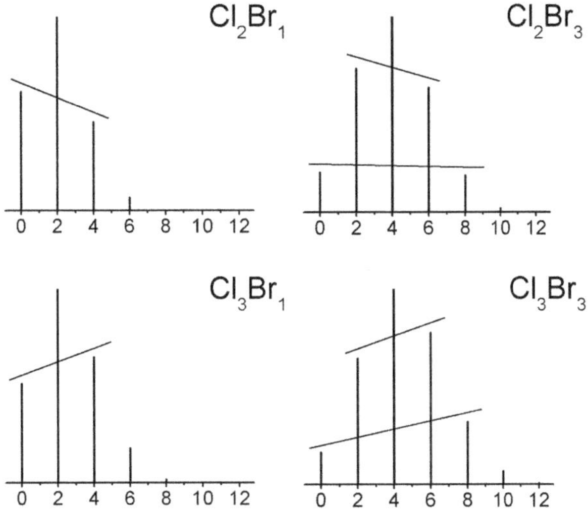

Fig. 3.6 Aid in distinguishing isotopic patterns by using orientation lines. *Left side:* patterns with four peaks each; *right side*: patterns with six peaks

the spectrum to those in Fig. 3.5. (For explanations on how these numerous ions come about refer to Chap. 6.)

3.2.5 Combinations of Carbon and Halogens

So far we have treated the X + 1 and the X + 2 elements separately, admittedly a rather artificial approach. The combination of C, H, N, and O with the halogens F, Cl, Br, and I covers a large fraction of the molecules one usually has to deal with. When regarding H, O, and N as X elements, which is a valid approximation for not too large molecules, the construction of isotopic patterns can be conveniently accomplished. By use of the isotopic abundance tables of the elements or of tables of frequent combinations of these as provided in this chapter or in the Appendix, the building blocks can be combined to obtain more complex isotopic patterns.

Construction of an isotopic pattern Let us construct the isotopic pattern of $C_9N_3Cl_3$ restricting ourselves to the isotopic contributions of C and Cl, i.e., with N as an X element. Here, the isotopic pattern of chlorine can be expected to be dominant over that of carbon. First, from the cubic form of Eq. (3.9) the Cl_3 pattern is calculated as follows: $(0.7578 + 0.2422)^3 = 0.435 + 0.417 + 0.133 + 0.014$ and after normalization this becomes 100 : 95.9 : 30.7 : 3.3. Of course, using the tabulated abundances of the Cl_3 distribution (Appendix) would be faster. The result is then plotted with 2 u distance, beginning at the nominal mass of the monoisotopic ion, i.e., 9×12 u + 3×14 u + 3×35 u = 255 u. The contribution of C_9 to the pattern is mainly at X + 1 where we have $9 \times 1.1\% = 9.9\%$, whereas its contribution to X + 2 (0.4%, Appendix) is negligible in this simple estimation. Finally, the

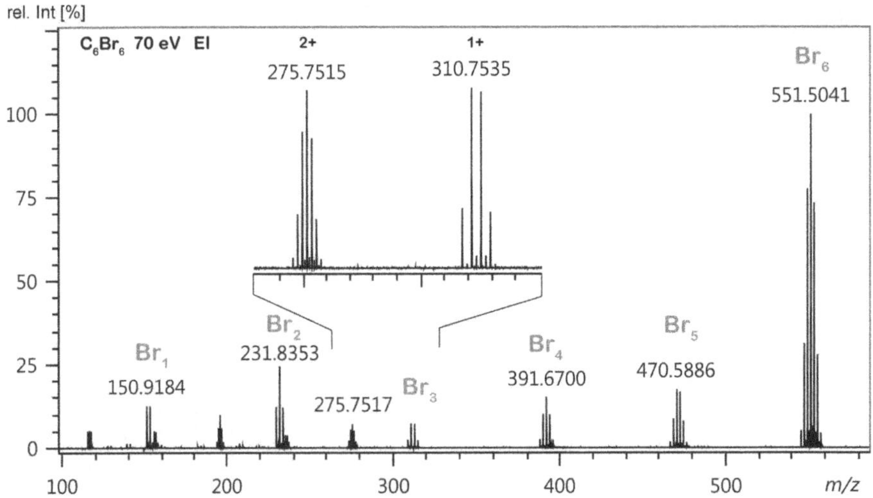

Fig. 3.7 70-eV EI mass spectrum of hexabromobenzene in the range *m/z* 100–580. The lower *m/z* range is omitted to allow for a clearer presentation of the bromine patterns. The number of bromines is annotated for convenience. The *m/z* labels provide accurate mass (Sect. 3.5) and refer to the most abundant signal of the respective isotope pattern. Watch how and where the pattern of the doubly charged molecular ion, M^{2+}, is displayed on the *m/z* scale next to the singly charged ion with a Br_3 pattern (*inset*)

X + 1 contribution of C_9 is placed into the gaps of the Cl_3 pattern each with 9.9% relative to the preceding peak of the chlorine isotopic distribution (Fig. 3.8).

3.2.6 Polynomial Approach

The polynomial approach is the logical expansion of the binomial approach. It is useful for the calculation of isotopic distributions of polyisotopic elements or for formulas composed of several non-monoisotopic elements [22, 23]. In general, the isotopic distribution of a molecule can be described by a product of polynominals

$$(a_1 + a_2 + a_3 + \ldots)^m \ (b_1 + b_2 + b_3 + \ldots)^n \, (c_1 + c_2 + c_3 + \ldots)^o + \ldots \qquad (3.10)$$

where a_1, a_2, a_3 etc. represent the individual isotopes of one element, b_1, b_2, b_3 etc. represent those of another and so on until all elements are included. The exponents m, n, o etc. give the number of atoms of these elements as contained in the empirical formula.

Calculating a complete pattern The complete isotopic distribution of stearic acid trichloromethylester, $C_{19}H_{35}O_2Cl_3$ is obtained according to Eq. (3.10) from polynomial expression

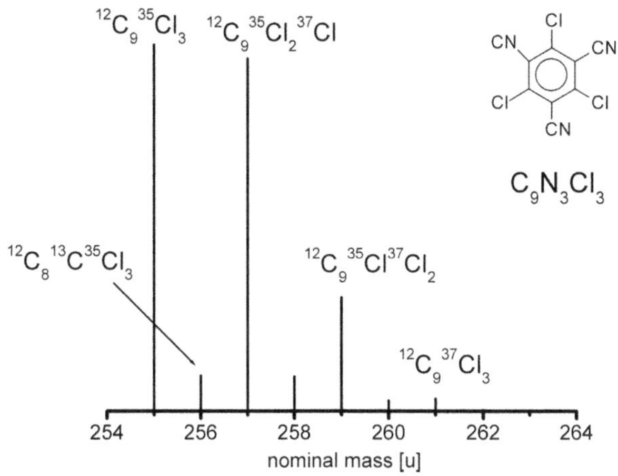

Fig. 3.8 The isotopic pattern of $C_9N_3Cl_3$ as constructed in the example above. The first ^{13}C isotopic peaks are located between the X + 2, 4, and 6 peaks of the dominant Cl_3 pattern. Nitrogen is treated as an X element and has been omitted from the peak labels for clarity

$$(A_{12C} + A_{13C})^{19} (A_{1H} + A_{2H})^{35} (A_{16O} + A_{17O} + A_{18O})^2 (A_{35Cl} + A_{37Cl})^3$$

with A_x representing the relative abundances of the isotopes involved for each element. The problem with the calculation of isotopic patterns resides in the enormous number of terms obtained for larger molecules. Even for this simple example, the number of terms would be $(2)^{19} \times (2)^{35} \times (3)^2 \times (2)^3 = 1.297 \times 10^{18}$. The number is dramatically reduced if like terms are combined which describe the same isotopic composition regardless where the isotopes are located in the molecule. However, manual calculations are prone to become tedious if not impractical; computer programs now simplify the process [24, 25].

Software-based calculation of $C_{19}H_{35}O_2Cl_3$ isotope pattern Let us apply IsoPro 3.1, a freely available software program, to calculate the isotopic pattern of stearic acid trichloromethylester, $C_{19}H_{35}O_2Cl_3$. After entering the composition, it is just a matter of a mouse click to get the pattern either as a graphical display or as a mass list (Fig. 3.9). Obviously, the three chlorine atoms are dominating the appearance of the pattern and it is thus not surprising that the relative intensities are very similar to what we had in the case of $C_9N_3Cl_3$ (Fig. 3.8).

Knowing your software

Mass spectrometers usually are delivered with the software for calculating isotopic distributions. Similar programs are also offered as internet-based or shareware solutions [26, 27]. While such software is readily accessible, it is still necessary to obtain a thorough understanding of isotopic patterns as a prerequisite for adequately interpreting mass spectra.

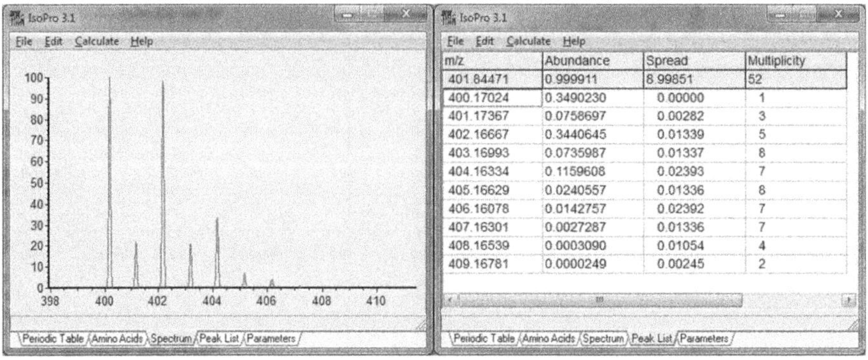

Fig. 3.9 Results from entering the formula $C_{19}H_{35}O_2Cl_3$ into IsoPro 3.1 isotopic distribution calculator [26]. The program provides either a customizable plot *(left)* or a peak list (*right*). Note that the list is normalized to 100% as equal to all species and that the *m*/*z* values provide accurate mass (Sect. 3.5)

3.2.7 Oxygen, Silicon, and Sulfur

Oxygen, silicon, and sulfur are polyisotopic elements in the strict sense – oxygen as ^{16}O, ^{17}O, and ^{18}O, sulfur as ^{32}S, ^{33}S, ^{34}S, and ^{36}S, and silicon as ^{28}Si, ^{29}Si, and ^{30}Si. The isotopic patterns of sulfur and silicon are by far not as prominent as those of chlorine and bromine, but still important.

^{17}O (0.038%) and ^{18}O (0.205%) are so rare that the occurrence of oxygen usually cannot be detected from the isotopic pattern in routine spectra because the experimental error in relative intensities tends to be larger than the contribution of ^{18}O. Therefore, oxygen is frequently treated as an X type element although X + 2 would be a more appropriate but practically rather useless classification. In oligosaccharides, for instance, a substantial number of oxygen atoms contribute to the X + 2 signal.

Sulfur can be classified as an X + 2 element as long as only a few sulfur atoms are present in a molecule. However, the 0.8% contributed by ^{33}S to the X + 1 is almost comparable to the situation with ^{13}C (1.1% per atom). If the X + 1 peak is used for estimating the number of carbons present, then for ^{33}S this would cause an overestimation of the number of carbon atoms by roughly one carbon per sulfur (Fig. 3.10).

In the case of silicon the ^{30}Si isotope contributes a "mere" 3.4% to the X + 2 signal, and ^{29}Si even 5.1% to X + 1. So, neglecting ^{29}Si would cause an overestimation of the carbon number by 5 per Si present, which is unacceptable (Fig. 3.11).

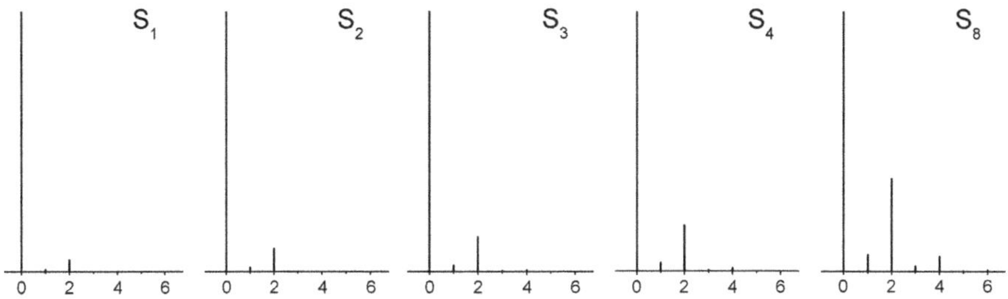

Fig. 3.10 Calculated isotopic patterns for combinations of elemental sulfur. The peak shown at zero position corresponds to the monoisotopic ion at *m/z* X. The isotopic peaks are then located at *m/z* = X + 1, 2, 3, ...

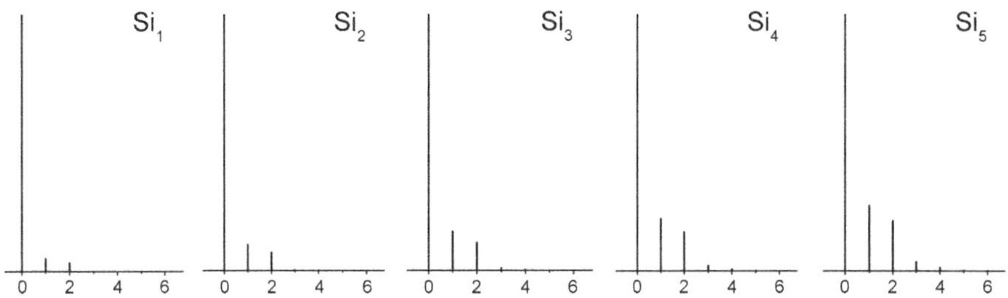

Fig. 3.11 Calculated isotopic patterns for combinations of elemental silicon. The peak shown at zero position corresponds to the monoisotopic ion at *m/z* X. The isotopic peaks are then located at *m/z* = X + 1, 2, 3, ...

Identifying S and Si

The presence of S and Si in a mass spectrum is best revealed by carefully examining the X + 2 intensity: this signal's intensity will be too high to be caused by the contribution of $^{13}C_2$ alone, even if the number of carbons has been obtained from X + 1 without prior subtraction of the S or Si contribution.

Isotopic pattern of a thioether The isotopic pattern calculated for ethyl propyl thioether, $C_5H_{12}S$, with the relative contributions of ^{33}S and ^{13}C to the M + 1 and of ^{34}S and $^{13}C_2$ to the M + 2 signal are shown below (Fig. 3.12 and Sect. 6.13). If the M + 1 peak resulted from ^{13}C alone, this would rather indicate the presence of 6 carbon atoms, which in turn would imply an M + 2 intensity of only 0.1% instead of the actually observed 4.6%. Consideration of Si for explaining the isotopic pattern would still fit the M + 2 intensity, however with relatively low accuracy, while for M + 1 the situation would be quite different. As ^{29}Si itself demands 5.1% at M + 1, there would be no or one carbon maximum allowed to explain the observed M + 1 intensity.

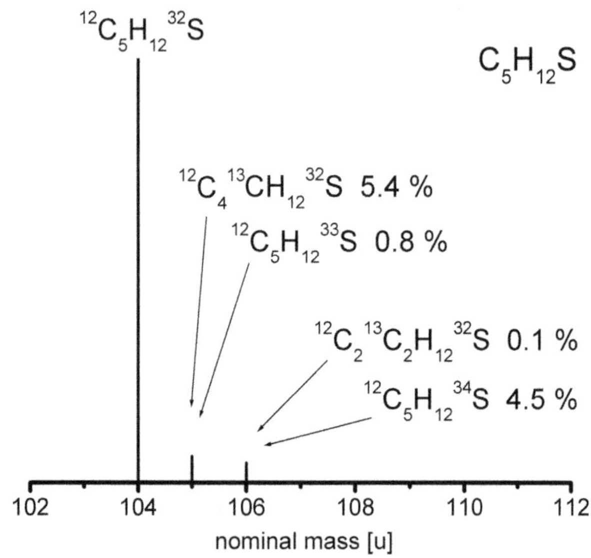

Fig. 3.12 Ethyl propyl thioether, $C_5H_{12}S$ – calculated isotopic pattern of the molecular ion indicating the respective contributions of ^{33}S and ^{13}C to the M + 1 and of ^{34}S and $^{13}C_2$ to the M + 2 signal

3.2.8 Polyisotopic Elements

The treatment of polyisotopic elements does not require other techniques as far as calculation or construction of isotopic patterns are concerned. However, isotopic patterns can differ largely from what has been considered so far and it is worth mentioning their peculiarities.

The polyisotopic element tin The presence or absence of tin, a polyisotopic element, can readily be detected from its characteristic isotopic pattern. For tetrabutyltin, $C_{16}H_{36}Sn$, the lowest mass isotopic composition is $^{12}C_{16}H_{36}{}^{112}Sn$, 340 u. Regarding the 16 carbon atoms, the ^{13}C isotopic abundance is about 17.5%. This is superimposed on the isotopic pattern of elemental Sn, which becomes especially obvious at 345 and 347 u (Fig. 3.13). The bars labeled with a tin isotope alone are almost solely due to $^{x}Sn^{12}C$ species. Tin neither has an isotope ^{121}Sn nor ^{123}Sn, and therefore the contributions at 349 and 351 u must be due to $^{120}Sn^{13}C$ and $^{122}Sn^{13}C$, respectively.

3.2.9 Practical Aspects of Isotopic Patterns

The recognition of isotopic patterns bears some potential pitfalls. Particularly, if signals from compounds differing by two or four hydrogens are superimposed or if such a superimposition can not a priori be excluded, the observed pattern has to be stepwise carefully checked to avoid misinterpretation of mass spectral data. When isotopically labeled compounds are involved similar care also becomes necessary.

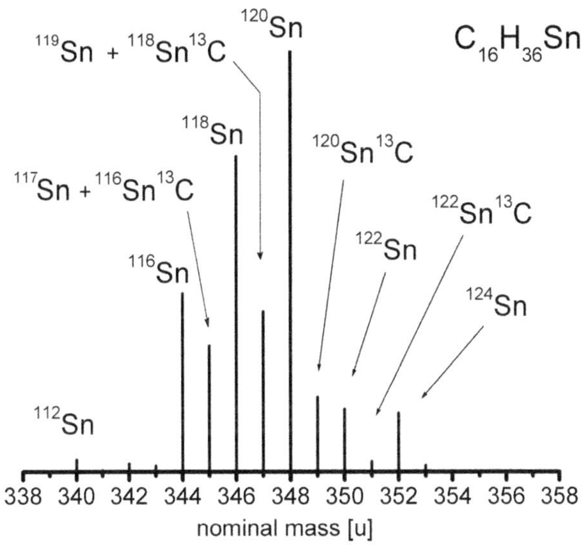

Fig. 3.13 Tetrabutyltin, $C_{16}H_{36}Sn$. Calculated isotopic pattern and isotopic compositions of the major contributions to the peaks

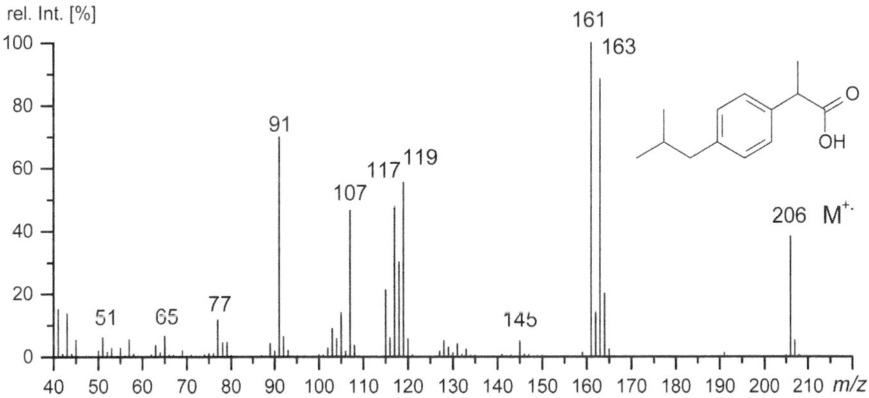

Fig. 3.14 EI mass spectrum of ibuprofen showing some signals that can be misinterpreted as a bromine isotopic pattern (Adapted with permission. © NIST, 2011)

A clear-cut bromine pattern! Or maybe not? The EI spectrum of ibuprofen shows some "fake" isotopic patterns. Supposing it to be an unknown, the peak pairs at *m/z* 161, 163 and also at *m/z* 117, 119 could easily be misinterpreted as isotopic patterns due to bromine, more exactly Br_1 (Fig. 3.14). However, a closer examination reveals that both pairs do not have the required intensity ratio of about 100 : 98. Instead, the peak at *m/z* 163 is merely at a relative intensity of 89% of *m/z* 161. In case of the *m/z* 117, 119 pair the intensity ratio is even reversed. Also, a look at the molecular ion peak at *m/z* 206 reveals that there is no bromine isotopic pattern at all.

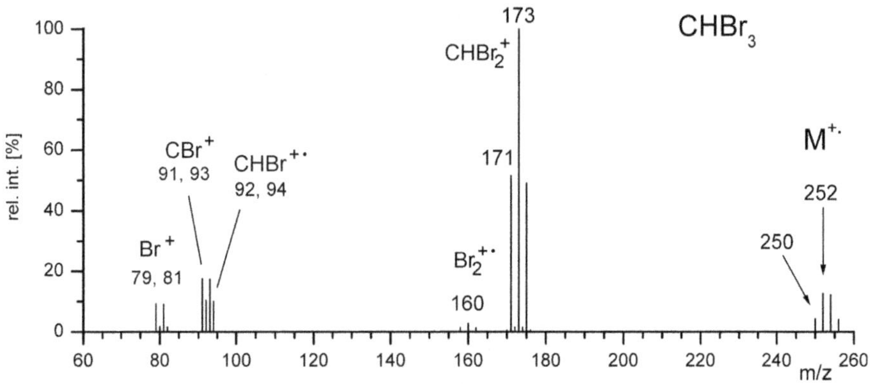

Fig. 3.15 Tribromomethane EI mass spectrum (Adapted with permission. © NIST, 2011)

If bromine was present, it necessarily had to cause the isotopic pattern for the $M^{+\bullet}$ ion, too. The true reason for ions of *m/z* 163 is loss of $C_3H_7^{\bullet}$, 43 u, from $M^{+\bullet}$ ions whereas ions at *m/z* 161 are due to a loss of $COOH^{\bullet}$, 45 u. Furthermore, there should be some peaks by Br^+ at *m/z* 79, 81 and by $HBr^{+\bullet}$, *m/z* 80, 82, which are absent, however. This case shows us that many patterns that superficially appear to be clear-cut and straight forward at first sight may require reinterpretation. Relative intensities need to be compared with tabulated data and all information of a spectrum needs to be considered.

3.2.10 Bookkeeping with Isotopic Patterns in Mass Spectra

Proving the identity of isotopic patterns requires careful comparison with calculated patterns. The mass differences must be consistent with the mass of the presumed neutral losses. In order to hold true, a pattern can only be assigned to signals at or above the mass given by the sum of all contributing atoms.

In calculating the mass differences between peaks from different isotopic patterns it is strongly recommended to proceed from the monoisotopic peak of one group to the monoisotopic peak of the next. Accordingly, the mass difference obtained also owes to the loss of a monoisotopic fragment. Otherwise, one bears the risk of erroneously omitting or adding hydrogens in a formula.

Tricky tribromomethane The EI mass spectrum of tribromomethane is dominated by the bromine isotopic distribution (Fig. 3.15). At first, there is no need to wonder *why* tribromomethane fragments like it does upon EI (Sect. 6.1). Let us simply accept this fragmentation and focus on the isotopic patterns. By referring to Fig. 3.5 one can identify the patterns of Br_3, Br_2, and Br. As a matter of fact, the molecular ion must contain the full number of bromine atoms (*m/z* 250, 252, 254, 256).

The primary fragment ion due to $Br^{\bullet}$ loss will then show a Br_2 pattern (*m/z* 171, 173, 175). A mass difference of 79 u is calculated between *m/z* 250 and *m/z*

171, owing to ^{79}Br, and thus identifying the process as a loss of $Br^{\bullet}$. Starting from the $CH^{79}Br_2{}^{81}Br$ isotopic ion at *m/z* 252 would yield the same information if ^{81}Br was used for the calculation. Here, ^{79}Br would wrongly indicate loss of H_2Br.

Subsequent elimination of HBr leads to CBr^+ at *m/z* 91, 93. Alternatively, the molecular ion can eliminate Br_2 to form $CHBr^{+\bullet}$, *m/z* 92, 94, overlapping with the *m/z* 91, 93 doublet, or it may lose CHBr to yield $Br_2{}^{+\bullet}$, causing the peaks at *m/z* 158, 160, 162. The peaks at *m/z* 79, 81 are due to Br^+ and those at *m/z* 80, 82 result from $HBr^{+\bullet}$ formed by CBr_2 loss from the molecular ion.

3.2.11 Information from Complex Isotopic Patterns

If the isotopic distribution is very broad and/or there are elements encountered that have a lowest mass isotope of very low abundance, recognition of the monoisotopic peak would become rather uncertain. However, there are ways to cope with that situation.

Find a checkpoint The ^{112}Sn isotopic peak of tin compounds can easily be overlooked or simply could be superimposed by background signals (Fig. 3.13). Here, one should identify the ^{120}Sn peak from its unique position within the characteristic pattern before screening the spectrum for Sn patterns from peak to peak. For all other elements contained in the respective ions still the lowest mass isotope would be used in calculations.

Assign a marker isotope Ruthenium exhibits a wide isotopic distribution of which the ^{102}Ru isotope can be used as a marker during assignment of mass differences. Moreover, the strong isotopic fingerprint of Ru makes it easily detectable from mass spectra and even compensates for a lack of information resulting from moderate mass accuracy (Fig. 3.16).

> **Refer to an abundant isotope**
> If the isotopic distribution is broad and/or there are elements encountered that have a lowest mass isotope of very low abundance, it is recommended to base calculations on the most abundant isotope of the respective element.

3.2.12 Systematic Approach to Reading Isotopic Patterns

Most mass spectra exhibit some sort of isotopic pattern. Especially those of organic molecules never come without at least a contribution from ^{13}C. It is thus good practice to carefully examine mass spectra for isotopic patterns, some of which may be obvious like those of Br and Cl, while others can be less apparent like those from Si, S, or Li, for example. When starting to interpret a mass spectrum, you are well

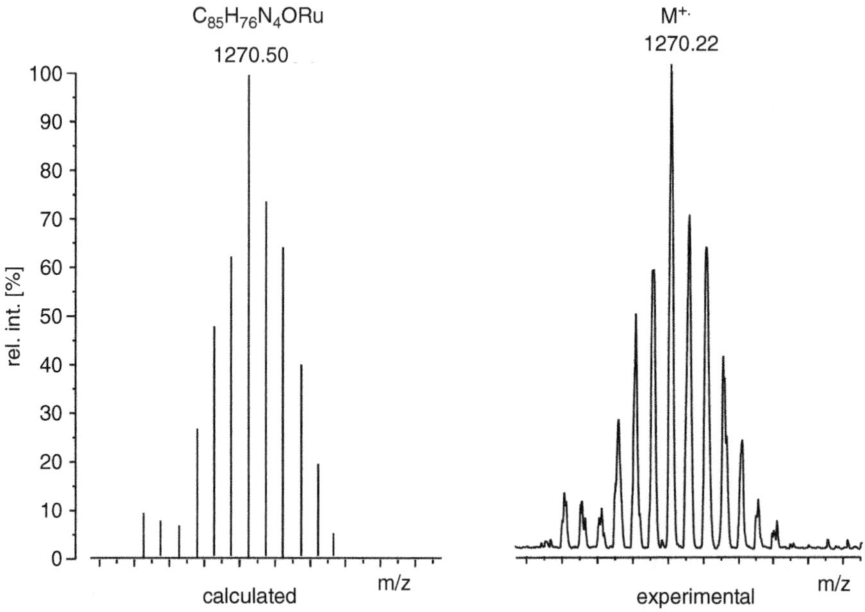

Fig. 3.16 Ruthenium carbonyl porphyrin complex – calculated and experimental isotopic pattern (FD-MS, cf. Sect. 8.6). The isotopic pattern supports the presumed molecular composition. The labeled peak corresponds to the ^{102}Ru-containing ion (Adapted from Ref. [28] with permission. © IM Publications, 1997)

advised to begin by carefully looking for isotopic patterns. A guideline is provided below (Fig. 3.17).

3.3 Isotopic Enrichment and Isotopic Labeling

3.3.1 Isotopic Enrichment

If the abundance of a particular nuclide is higher than the natural level in an ion, the term *isotopically enriched ion* is used to describe any ion enriched in the isotope [4]. The degree of *isotopic enrichment* is best determined by mass spectrometry.

Fullerenes enriched in ^{13}C Isotopic enrichment is a standard means to enhance the response of an analyte in nuclear magnetic resonance (NMR). Such measures gain importance if extremely low solubility is combined with a large number of carbons, as is often the case with [60]fullerene compounds [29]. The molecular ion signals, $M^{+\bullet}$, of C_{60} with natural isotopic abundance and of ^{13}C–enriched C_{60} are shown below (Fig. 3.18); for EI-MS of [60]fullerenes cf. Refs. [30–32]). From these mass spectra, the ^{13}C enrichment can be determined by use of Eq. (3.2). For C_{60} of natural isotopic abundance we obtain $M_{rC60} = 60 \times 12.0108\ \text{u} = 720.65\ \text{u}$. Applying

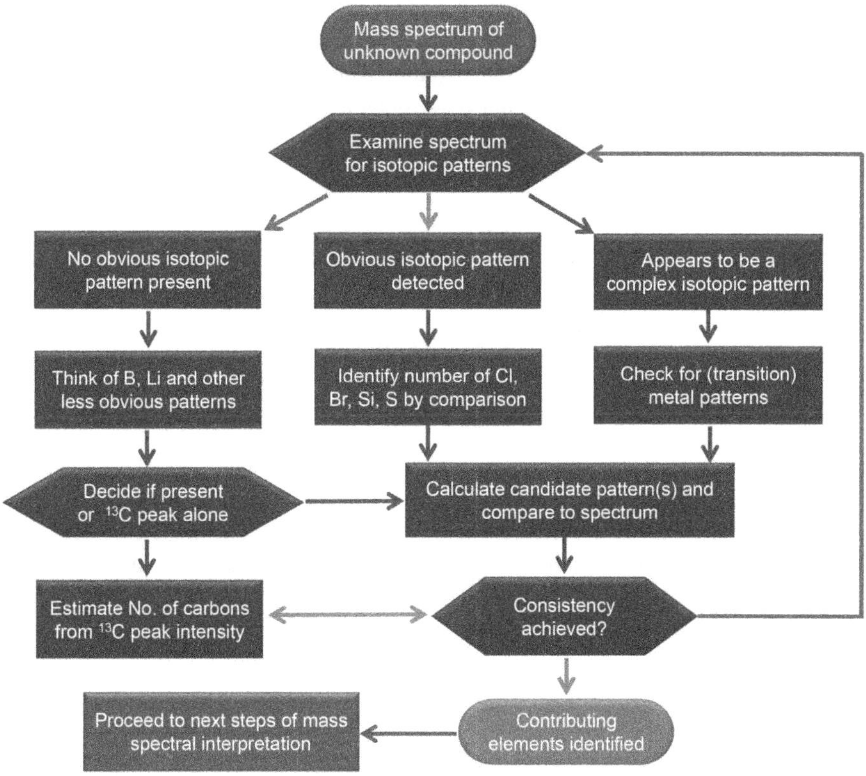

Fig. 3.17 Guideline for the identification of contributing elements based on isotopic pattern analysis

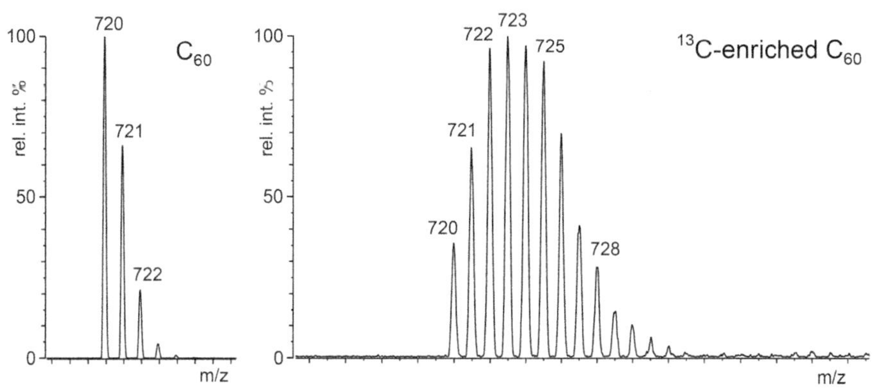

Fig. 3.18 [60]Fullerene – comparison of the molecular ion signals, $M^{+\bullet}$, with natural isotopic abundance and of ^{13}C–enriched C_{60} (By courtesy of W. Krätschmer, Max Planck Institute for Nuclear Physics, Heidelberg)

Eq. (3.2) to the isotopically enriched compound yields $M_{r13C\text{-}C60}$ = (35 × 720 + 65 × 721 + 98 × 722 + 100 × 723 + 99 × 724 + 93 × 725 + ...) u/(35 + 65 + 98 + 100 + 99 + 93 + ...) = 724.10 u. (Integer mass and intensity values are used here for clarity.) This result is equivalent to an average content of 4.1 ^{13}C atoms per [60]fullerene molecule which on the average means 3.45 ^{13}C atoms more than the natural content of 0.65 ^{13}C atoms per molecule.

3.3.2 Isotopic Labeling

If the abundance of a particular nuclide is higher than the natural level at one or more (specific) positions within an ion, the term *isotopically labeled ion* is used to describe such an ion. Among other applications, *isotopic labeling* is used in order to track metabolic pathways, to serve as internal standard for quantitative analysis, or to elucidate fragmentation mechanisms of ions in the gas phase. In mass spectrometry, the nonradiating isotopes ^{2}H (deuterium, D), ^{13}C, and ^{18}O are preferably employed and thus, a rich methodology to incorporate isotopic labels has been developed [33]. Isotopic labeling is rather a mass spectrometric research tool [34] than mass spectrometry being a tool to control the quality of isotopic labeling. As a result, isotopic labeling is used in many applications; examples are given throughout the book.

3.4 Resolution and Resolving Power

3.4.1 Definitions

So far, we have taken for granted that mass spectra separate isotopic patterns; now we want to quantify this degree of separation. The separation observed in a mass spectrum is termed *mass resolution, R*, or simply *resolution* [35]. Mass resolution is given as the smallest difference in m/z , i.e., $\Delta(m/z)$ that can be separated for a given signal, i.e., at a given m/z value:

$$R = \frac{m}{\Delta m} = \frac{m/z}{\Delta(m/z)} \tag{3.11}$$

Accordingly resolution is dimensionless. The ability of an instrument to resolve neighboring peaks is called its *mass resolving power* or simply *resolving power*. It is obtained from the peak width at a specific percentage of the peak height expressed as a function of mass [4, 35].

Two neighboring peaks are assumed to be sufficiently separated when the valley separating their maxima has decreased to 10% of their intensity. Hence, this is known as *10% valley definition of resolution*, $R_{10\%}$. The 10% valley conditions are fulfilled if the peak width at 5% relative height equals the mass difference of the corresponding ions, because then the 5% contribution of each peak to the same point of the m/z axis adds up to 10% (Fig. 3.19).

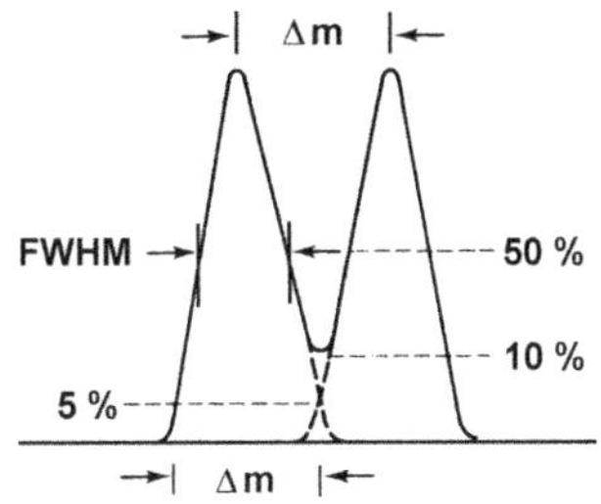

Fig. 3.19 The 10% valley and full width at half maximum (FWHM) definitions of resolution. Peak heights are not to scale

With the advent of linear quadrupole analyzers the *full width at half maximum (FWHM) definition* of resolution became widespread especially among instruments manufacturers. It is also commonly used for time-of-flight and quadrupole ion trap mass analyzers. With Gaussian peak shapes, the ratio of R_{FWHM} to $R_{10\%}$ is 1.8. The resolution for a pair of peaks at different *m/z* and its practical implications are illustrated below (Fig. 3.20).

Resolution affects spectrum of residual air The changes in the electron ionization spectra of residual air nicely show the effect of higher resolution (Fig. 3.21). Setting $R = 1000$ yields a peak width of 0.028 u for the signal at *m/z* 28. An increase to $R = 7000$ perfectly separates the minor contribution of CO^+, *m/z* 27.995, from the predominating $N_2^{+\bullet}$ at *m/z* 28.006 (The CO^+ ion rather results from fragmenting $CO_2^{+\bullet}$ ions than from carbon monoxide in laboratory air.)

LR and HR
The attributive *low resolution* (LR) is generally used to describe spectra obtained at $R < 3000$. *High resolution* (HR) is appropriate for $R > 5000$. However, there is no exact definition of these terms.

3.4.2 Resolution and Its Experimental Determination

In principle, resolution is always determined from the peak width of some signal at a certain relative height and therefore, any peak can serve this purpose. As the exact determination of a peak width is not always easy to perform, certain doublets of known Δm are being used.

The minimum resolution to separate CO^+ from $N_2^{+\bullet}$ is $28/0.011 \approx 2500$. The doublet from the pyridine molecular ion, $C_5H_5N^{+\bullet}$, *m/z* 79.0422, and from the first isotopic peak of the benzene molecular ion, $^{13}CC_5H_6^{+\bullet}$, *m/z* 79.0503, necessitates $R = 9750$ to be separated. Finally, the doublet composed of the first isotopic ion of $[M–CH_3]^{+\bullet}$ from xylene, $^{13}CC_6H_7^{+}$, *m/z* 92.0581, and toluene molecular ion, $C_7H_8^{+\bullet}$, *m/z* 92.0626, requires $R = 20{,}600$ for separation (Fig. 3.22).

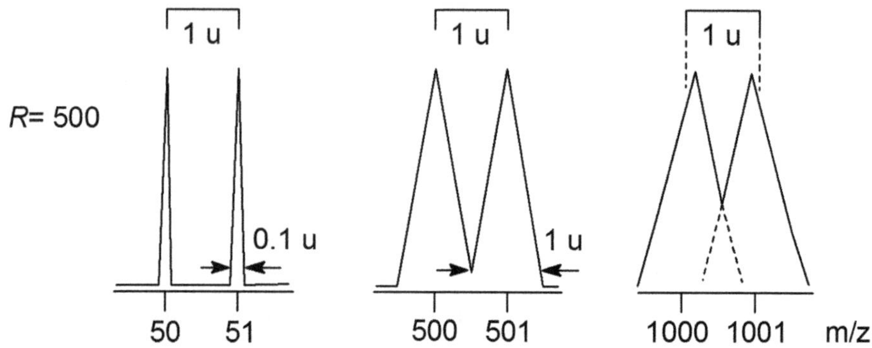

Fig. 3.20 Simulated signals of simplified triangular shape at *m/z* 50, 500, and 1000 as obtained at $R = 500$. At *m/z* 1000 the peak maxima shift towards each other due to superimposing peaks; this also approximates the result of $R_{FWHM} = 900$

Report resolution rounded
There is no need to use a more accurate value of *m/z* than nominal and likewise, there is no use of reporting $R = 2522.52$ exactly as obtained for the $CO^+/N_2^{+\bullet}$ pair. It is fully sufficient to know that setting $R = 3000$ is sufficient for one specific task or that $R = 10{,}000$ is suitable for another.

With magnetic sector instruments a resolving power of up to $R = 10{,}000$ can routinely be employed, even $R = 15{,}000$. In practice, those instruments are rarely adjusted to resolve beyond $R = 10{,}000$, e.g., only when interferences of ions of the same nominal *m/z* need to be excluded. With an instrument in perfect condition, it is possible to achieve higher resolving power; typically they are specified to deliver about $R \approx 60{,}000$ (on intensive peaks).

3.4.3 Resolving Power and Its Effect on Relative Peak Intensity

Increasing resolution does not affect the relative intensities of the peaks, i.e., the intensity ratios for *m/z* 28 : 32 : 40 : 44 in the spectrum of air generally remain constant (Fig. 3.22). However, increased settings of resolving power are often obtained at the cost of transmission of the mass analyzer, thereby reducing the absolute signal intensity. Accordingly, isotopic patterns are not affected by increasing resolution up to $R \approx 10{,}000$; beyond, there can be changes in isotopic patterns due to the separation of different isotopic species of the same nominal mass (Sect. 3.7).

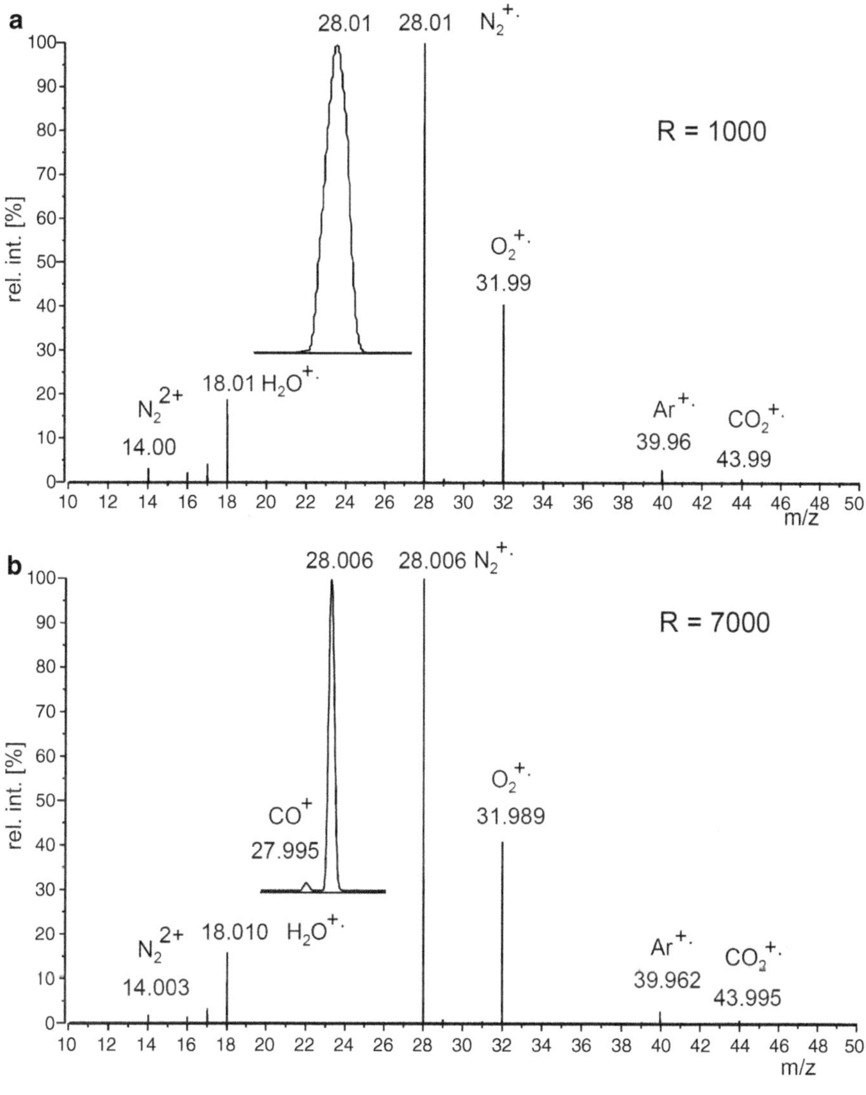

Fig. 3.21 EI mass spectra of residual air (**a**) at $R = 1000$ and (**b**) at $R = 7000$. The relative intensities are not affected by different resolution. The decimal digits of the mass labels indicate achievable mass accuracies under the respective conditions

3.5 Accurate Mass

The section on high resolution (HR) already anticipated *accurate mass* to a certain extent. In fact, HR and accurate mass measurements are closely related and depend on each other, because mass accuracy tends to improve as peak resolution is

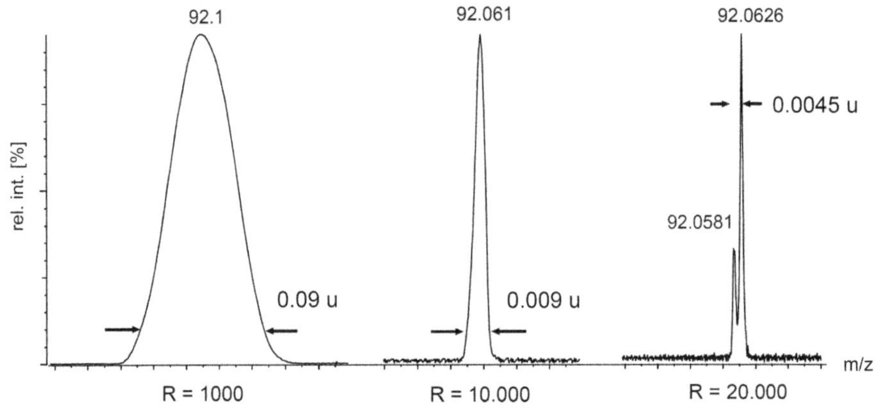

Fig. 3.22 The *m/z* 92 peak from a mixture of xylene and toluene at different resolving power. At $R = 10{,}000$ some separation of the lower mass ion can already be presumed from a slight asymmetry of the peak. $R = 20{,}600$ is needed to fully separate $^{13}CC_6H_7^+$, *m/z* 92.0581, from $C_7H_8^{+\bullet}$, *m/z* 92.0626. The *m/z* scale is the same for all of the signals

improved. Nevertheless, they should not be confused, as performing a measurement at *high resolution* alone does not equally imply measuring the *accurate mass*. High resolution separates adjacent signals, accurate mass can deliver molecular formulas [36–38].

Until the early 1980s, accurate mass measurements were nearly restricted to electron ionization, and for a while, the technique even seemed to become abandoned. New options available through FT-ICR instrumentation then revived the value of accurate mass measurements. The newly developed Orbitrap and a new generation of oaTOF analyzers contributed to an increased demand for accurate mass data. Nowadays, formula elucidation can be performed using any ionization method [39], their widespread application thus demanding a thorough understanding of their potential and limitations [37].

3.5.1 Exact Mass and Molecular Formulas

Let us briefly summarize some important definitions and terms related to ionic mass:

- The *isotopic mass* is the *exact mass* of an isotope.
- The isotopic mass is very close but not equal to the *nominal mass* of that isotope.
- The calculated exact mass of a molecule or of a monoisotopic ion equals its monoisotopic mass.
- The definition of our mass scale will imply that the isotope ^{12}C represents the only exception from non-integer isotopic mass.

As a consequence of these individual non-integer isotopic masses, no combination of elements in a molecular or ionic formula has the same *calculated exact mass*, or simply *exact mass* as it is often referred to, as any other one [40]. In other words, any elemental composition has its unique exact mass. Infinite accuracy provided, any formula can be identified by the accurate mass of the ions.

Isobaric ions of *m*/*z* 28 The molecular ions of nitrogen, $N_2^{+\bullet}$, carbon monoxide, $CO^{+\bullet}$, and ethene, $C_2H_4^{+\bullet}$, have the same nominal mass of 28 u, i.e., they are so-called *isobaric ions*. The isotopic masses of the most abundant isotopes of hydrogen, carbon, nitrogen, and oxygen are 1.007825 u, 12.000000 u, 14.003074 u, and 15.994915 u, respectively. Thus, the calculated ionic masses are 28.00559 u for $N_2^{+\bullet}$, 27.99437 u for $CO^{+\bullet}$, and 28.03075 u for $C_2H_4^{+\bullet}$. This means they differ by several 10^{-3} u, and none of these isobaric ions has precisely 28.00000 u (Sects. 3.1.5 and 6.10.6).

The "mmu"
Historically, 10^{-3} u was referred to as 1 *millimass unit* (mmu). There is still some use of mmu in the MS community because of its convenience in dealing with small differences in mass. However, using the SI prefix m for milli, the correct way of writing 10^{-3} u would be as 1 mu or 1 mDa (non IUPAC).

3.5.2 Relativistic Mass Defect

Mass–energy equivalence is a key postulate of Einstein's theory of relativity as expressed by his famous eq. $E = mc^2$. It describes the conversion of mass into energy during nucleation. The binding energy per nucleon steeply increases along the mass numbers from ^2H to its maximum around ^{56}Fe and then decreases again somewhat up to ^{238}U (Fig. 3.23). Translation into isotopic mass reveals that mass is by some 10^{-3} u above the nominal value for light elements (^1H, ^4He, ^7Li, ^{11}B, ^{14}N), while being some 10^{-3} u (^{19}F) to almost 10^{-1} u (^{127}I) below that for heavier elements [38]. This also complies with the fact that the radioactive isotopes of thorium and uranium have isotopic masses above the nominal value, thus reflecting their comparatively unstable nuclei (Appendix).

3.5.3 Role of Mass Defect in Mass Spectrometry

The term *mass defect*, m_{defect}, is defined as the difference between integer mass, $m_{nominal}$, and exact mass, m_{exact}, and is used to describe this deviation [6].

$$m_{defect} = m_{nominal} - m_{exact} \tag{3.12}$$

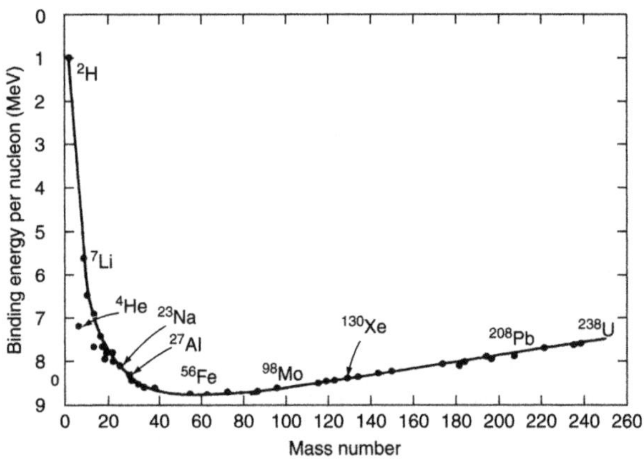

Fig. 3.23 Plot of binding energy per nucleon vs. mass number (Reproduced from Ref. [1] by permission. © John Wiley & Sons, 1992)

Application of this concept leads to *positive* and *negative mass* defects. The hydrogen atom, for example, has a negative mass defect, $m_{\text{defectH}} = -7.825 \times 10^{-3}$ u. In addition, the assumption that things appearing to be "defective" are associated with certain isotopic masses can be misleading. The mass defect was unveiled by Aston [2, 3] who already had discovered 212 of the total 287 stable isotopes. Obviously, the deviation of exact mass from nominal mass can be either to the higher or lower side, depending on the isotopes encountered. While the issue itself is easy to understand, the current terminology here can be somewhat deceptive.

The term *mass deficiency* better describes the fact that the exact mass of an isotope or a complete molecule is lower than the corresponding nominal mass. In case of ^{16}O, for example, the isotopic mass is 15.994915 u, being 5.085×10^{-3} u deficient as compared to the nominal value ($m_{\text{defectO}} = 5.085 \times 10^{-3}$ u). Most isotopes are more or less mass deficient with a tendency towards larger mass defect for the heavier isotopes, e.g., $M_{35\text{Cl}} = 34.96885$ u (-3.115×10^{-2} u) and $M_{127\text{I}} = 129.90447$ u (-9.553×10^{-2} u).

Among the elements frequently encountered in mass spectrometry, only H, He, Li, Be, B, and N exhibit isotopic masses larger than their nominal value. Among the isotopes with negative mass defect, ^{1}H is the most important one, because each hydrogen adds 7.825×10^{-3} u. Thereby, it significantly contributes to the mass of larger hydrocarbon molecules [41]. In general, the ubiquitous occurrence of hydrogen in organic molecules causes most of them to exhibit considerable negative mass defects, which again decreases with the number of mass-deficient isotopes, e.g., from halogens, oxygen, or metals.

Mass deficiency as first indication Plotting the deviations from nominal mass of different oligomers as a function of nominal mass, one finds only pure carbon molecules (such as fullerenes) to be located on the *x*-axis. Hydrocarbons, due to their large number of hydrogens, receive roughly 1 u from negative mass defect per 1000 u in molecular mass. Halogenated oligomers, on the other hand, are more or

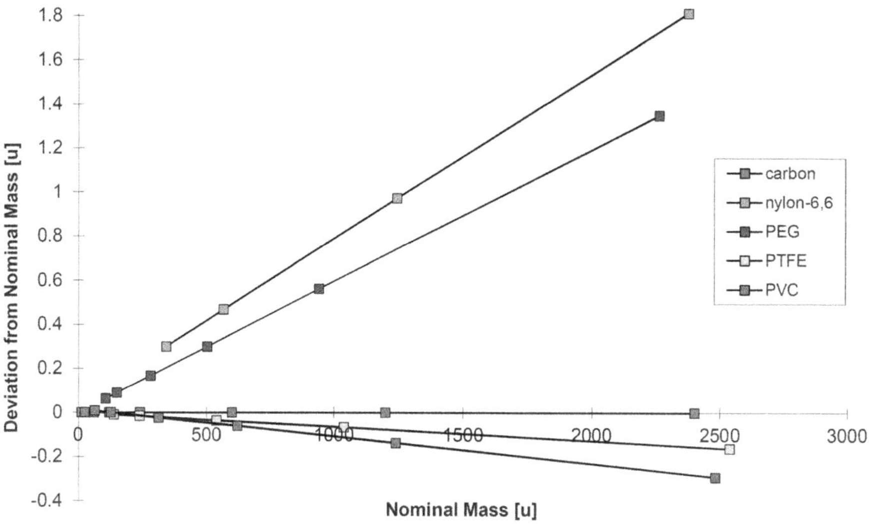

Fig. 3.24 Deviation from nominal mass for some oligomers as a function of nominal mass. *PE* polyethylene, *PEG* polyethyleneglycol, *PTFE* polytetrafluoroethylene, *PVC* polyvinylchloride

less mass deficient and those oligomers containing some oxygen are located in between (Fig. 3.24).

Limits of nominal mass

The use of nominal mass is limited to the low mass range. Above about 400–500 u the first decimal of isotopic mass can be larger than 0.5 causing it to be rounded up, e.g., to 501 u instead of the expected value of 500 u. This, in turn, will lead to severe misinterpretation of a mass spectrum (Chap. 6). One should write *m*/*z* values above *m*/*z* 400 with at least one decimal, e.g., as *m*/*z* 474.5 for $[C_{34}H_{66}]^{+\bullet}$.

3.5.4 Mass Accuracy

The *absolute mass accuracy*, Δ(*m*/*z*), is defined as the difference between *measured accurate mass* and *calculated exact mass*:

$$\Delta(m/z) = m/z_{\text{experimental}} - m/z_{\text{calculated}} \tag{3.13}$$

Instead of stating the absolute mass accuracy in units of u, it can also be given as *relative mass accuracy*, δ*m*/*m*, i.e., absolute mass accuracy divided by the mass it is determined for:

$$\delta m/m = \Delta(m/z)/(m/z) \tag{3.14}$$

The *relative mass accuracy*, δ*m*/*m*, is normally given in *parts per million* (ppm). As mass spectrometers tend to have similar absolute mass accuracies over a comparatively wide range, absolute mass accuracy represents a more meaningful way of stating mass accuracies than the use of ppm.

Use of ppm and ppb
Part per million (1 ppm = 10^{-6}) is simply a relative measure as are percent (%) or permill (parts per thousand, ‰). In addition, *parts per billion* (1 ppb = 10^{-9}), and *parts per trillion* (1 ppt = 10^{-12}) are in use.

Accuracy or just the impression thereof A magnetic sector mass spectrometer allows for an absolute mass accuracy of Δ(*m*/*z*) = 0.002–0.005 u in scanning mode over a range of about *m*/*z* 50–1500. At *m*/*z* 1200 an error of Δ(*m*/*z*) = 0.003 u corresponds to inconspicuous δ*m*/*m* = 2.5 ppm, whereas the same error yields 60 ppm at *m*/*z* 50, which appears to be unacceptably high.

3.5.5 Accuracy and Precision

The concepts of *accuracy* and *precision* can best be illustrated using the analogy to a target where the center represents the true value of some physical quantity [42]. Accuracy describes the deviation of the experimental value from the true value, which normally is rather an accepted reference value than a "true" one in the strict sense. Accuracy is high (A+ in Fig. 3.25) if the values from several measurements are close to the reference value. Accuracy depends on systematic errors of an experiment. Precision describes the deviation within a group of determinations and it is high (P+ in Fig. 3.25) if the values from several measurements are in close proximity to but not necessarily identical with the reference value. Precision is an expression of random error, e.g., as introduced by noise, variation in injection volumes or times. *Repeatability* and *reproducibility* are two aspects of precision. Repeatability is connected to the repetition of the same measurement on the same setup within a short time frame while reproducibility is related to long term stability of a setup and inter-platform or inter-operator effects. Suitable statistical evaluation of a widespread dataset can result in an accurate determination of a quantity at the cost of lower precision (P– A?), e.g., root-mean-square deviation (Sect. 3.6.4) [43, 44].

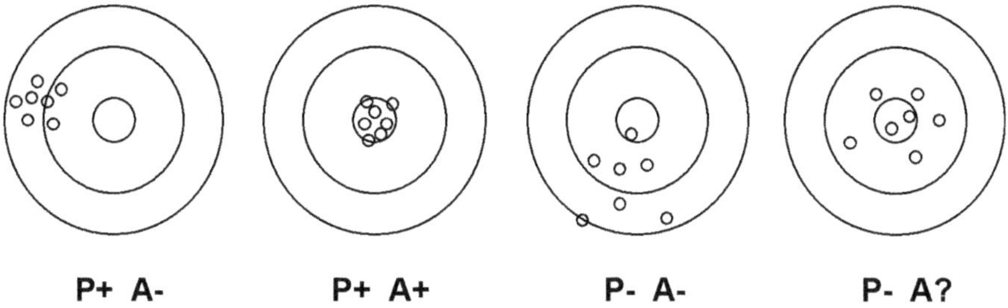

Fig. 3.25 Precision (*P*) and accuracy (*A*), along with seven hits on a target

3.5.6 Mass Accuracy and the Determination of Molecular Formulas

Assuming infinite mass accuracy, we should be able to identify the molecular formula of any ion merely on the basis of its exact mass – the emphasis is on *infinite* mass accuracy (Sect. 3.5.1). In reality we are dealing with errors in the order of one to several ppm depending on the type of instrument and the mode of its operation.

Number of formulas to be considered The number of possible even-electron ionic formulas based on an unrestricted selection among the elements C, H, N, and O as a function of relative mass error strongly depends on the *m*/*z* value of the ion. Here, the formulas proposed for the measured signals from $[(\text{arginine})_{1-5} + \text{H}]^+$ cluster ions, *m*/*z* 175.1189, 349.2309, 523.3427, 697.4548, and 871.5666 were counted for different relative mass error. While the lowest-mass ion is undoubtedly identified up to 5 ppm, the second ion is only unambiguously identified up to 2 ppm (Fig. 3.26). Allowing sulfur (S_{0-2}) in addition would already result in 18 rather than the 7 hits shown for the $[(\text{arginine})_3 + \text{H}]^+$ ion, *m*/*z* 523.3427, at 2 ppm error. Taking also odd-electron ions into account would contribute another 15 compositions to this selection. In case of the $[(\text{arginine})_5 + \text{H}]^+$ ion, *m*/*z* 871.5666, the number of C, H, N, O hits reaches 26 at 1 ppm error and even 232 at 10 ppm.

Unequivocal formula assignment by accurate mass alone only works in a range up to about *m*/*z* 500 depending on the particular restrictions [45]. Obviously, for ions of larger *m*/*z* the number of hits rapidly increases beyond a reasonable limit. Even at a high mass accuracy of 1 ppm and with the particular case of peptides the elemental composition can only be unambiguously identified up to about 800 u [46–48]. Determining the formula of a peptide among all natural peptide compositions possible at *m*/*z* 1005.4433 requires $\delta m/m = 0.1$ ppm [49].

The situation becomes more complicated as more elements and fewer limitations of their number must be taken into account. In practice, one must try to restrict oneself to certain elements and a maximum and/or minimum number of certain isotopes to assure a high degree of confidence in the assignment of formulas. Isotopic patterns provide a prime source of such additional information. Combining the information from accurate mass data and experimental peak intensities with

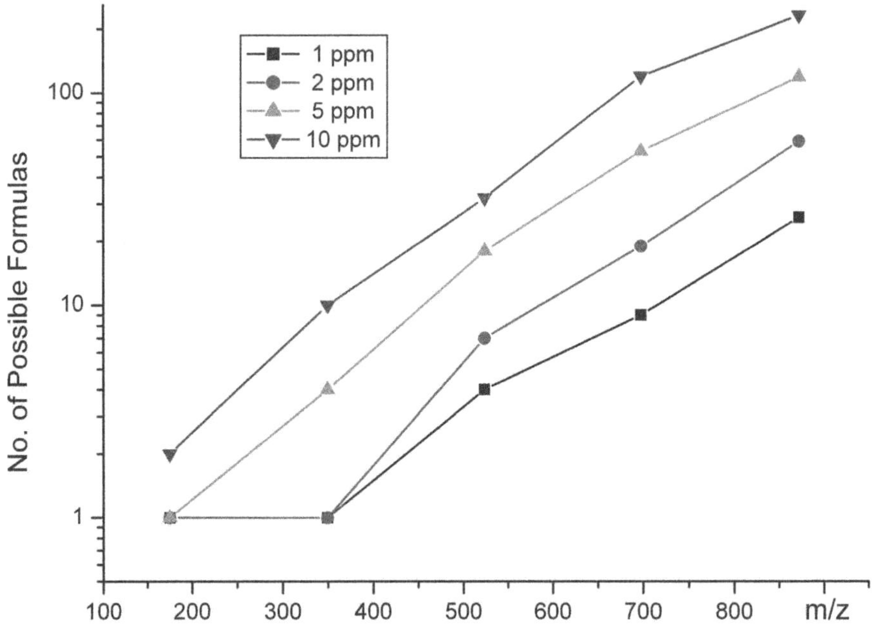

Fig. 3.26 Number of possible even-electron ionic formulas based on a free selection among the elements C, H, N, O as a function of relative mass error vs. *m/z*. The data points correspond to $[(\text{arginine})_{1\text{–}5} + \text{H}]^+$ cluster ions, *m/z* 175.1189, 349.2309, 523.3427, 697.4548, and 871.5666. The lines are meant as visual guides

calculated isotopic patterns allows to significantly reduce the number of potential elemental compositions of a particular ion [50, 51].

3.5.7 Extreme Mass Accuracy: Special Considerations

Even when we have determined a molecular formula, it does not tell us much about the structure of the molecule. According to the mass–energy equivalence (1 u = 931.5 MeV), a mass accuracy of 1 ppm ($\delta m/m = 10^{-6}$) roughly corresponds to an energy of 100 keV if an ion of *m/z* 100 is considered. A mass accuracy of 1 ppb ($\delta m/m = 10^{-9}$) still corresponds to an energy of 100 eV, and thus, 1 ppt ($\delta m/m = 10^{-12}$) would be required to approach energy differences of 0.1 eV, i.e., between isomers. Obviously, isomers are (almost) perfect isobars [52]. Nonetheless, it is worth noting that physicist are approaching 10 ppt, at least in the case of single atomic species (Fig. 3.27).

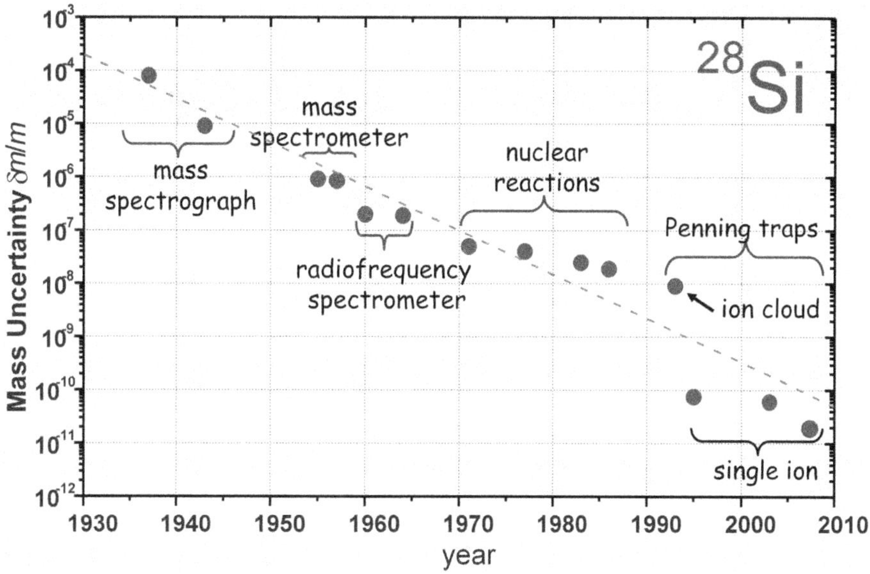

Fig. 3.27 Relative mass uncertainty $\delta m/m$ for ^{28}Si as a function of time. The most accurate mass of ^{28}Si so far is $m_{(28\text{Si})} = 27.876926534\ 96(62)$ u corresponding to an uncertainty of 0.2 ppt. The *dashed line* serves as a visual orientation and reveals an improvement in accuracy by about one order of magnitude per decade (By courtesy of H.-J. Kluge, GSI Helmholtz Centre for Heavy Ion Research GmbH, Darmstadt, Germany)

3.6 Applied High-Resolution Mass Spectrometry

Generally, *high-resolution mass spectrometry* (HR-MS) aims to achieve both high mass resolution and high mass accuracy. These quantities have been introduced without considering the means by which they can be measured. The key to this problem is *mass calibration*. Resolution alone can separate ions with *m/z* in close proximity, but it does not automatically reveal where on the *m/z* axis the respective signals are located. This section deals with the techniques for establishing accurate mass data and their analytical evaluation [36, 37].

3.6.1 Mass Calibration

All mass spectrometers require *mass calibration* before they are put to use. However, proper procedures and the number of required calibration points may largely differ between different types of mass analyzers. Typically, a robust mass calibration necessitates several peaks of well-known *m/z* values evenly distributed over the mass range of interest. These are supplied from a well-known *mass calibration compound* or *mass reference compound*.

3.6.1.1 Compiling Mass Reference Lists

A mass reference list can be compiled once the mass spectrum of a calibration standard is known and the elemental composition of the ions that are to be included in the mass reference list are established by an independent measurement. For this purpose, the listed reference masses should be calculated down to six decimals. Otherwise, one runs a chance of obtaining erroneous reference values, especially when masses of ion series are calculated by multiplication of a subunit. This can easily be done using conventional spreadsheet applications.

Cluster ions as mass reference Cluster ions are frequently employed for mass calibration as they provide series of ions that are equidistant on the *m/z* axis [53–58]. For example, CsI and CsI_3, respectively, can be used for mass calibration in fast atom bombardment (FAB, Chap. 10) and matrix-assisted laser desorption/ionization (MALDI, Chap. 11) mass spectrometry because they yield cluster ions of the general formula $[Cs(CsI)_n]^+$ in positive-ion and $[I(CsI)_n]^-$ in negative-ion mode.

3.6.2 Performing an External Mass Calibration

Mass calibration is performed by recording a mass spectrum of the *calibration compound* and subsequent correlation of experimental *m/z* values to the *mass reference list* [37, 59, 60]. Usually, this conversion of the mass reference list to a calibration is accomplished by the mass spectrometer's software. Thus, the mass spectrum is recalibrated by interpolation of the *m/z* scale between the assigned calibration peaks to obtain the best match. The mass calibration obtained may then be stored in a *calibration file* and used for future measurements without the presence of a calibration compound. This procedure is termed *external mass calibration.*

The numerous ionization methods and mass analyzers in use have created a demand for a large number of calibration compounds to suit their specific needs. Therefore, mass calibration will variously be addressed at the end of the chapters on ionization methods.

Classical standard PFK *Perfluorokerosene* (PFK) is a well-established mass calibration standard in electron ionization. It provides evenly spaced $C_xF_y^+$ fragment ions over a wide mass range (Figs. 3.28 and 3.29). The major ions are all mass deficient, with CHF_2^+, *m/z* 51.0046, being the only exception. PFK mixtures are available from low-boiling to high-boiling grades which may be used up to *m/z* 700–1100. Apart from the highest boiling grades, PFK is suitable to be introduced by the reference inlet (Sect. 5.2.1), a property making it very attractive for internal calibration as well.

Calibration with perfluorotributylamine Perfluorotributylamine (PFTBA, also termed FC-43), is another frequently used calibrant in EI-MS. This single

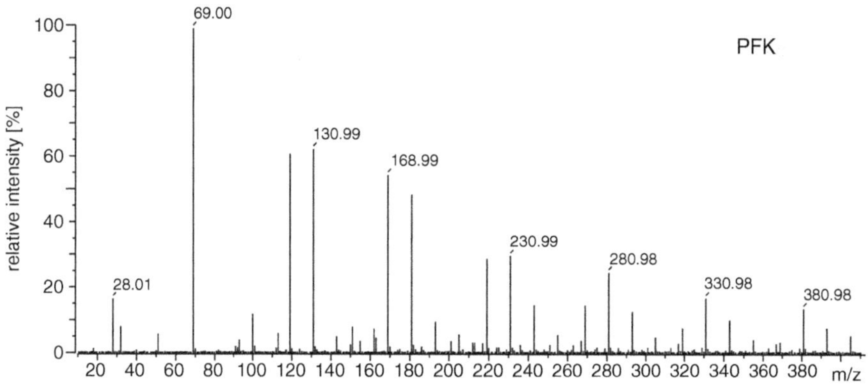

Fig. 3.28 Perfluorokerosene, PFK: partial 70-eV EI mass spectrum. The peaks are evenly distributed over a wide *m/z* range. Also, peaks from residual air occur in the low *m/z* range

No.	STD–m/z	Int .	Pos.
1	1 . 0078	0 . 0	0
2	4 . 0026	0 . 0	0
3	18 . 0106	1 . 1	155289
4	28 . 0061	12 . 4	307693
5	31 . 9898	6 . 1	360716
6	39 . 9624	0 . 8	457947
7	43 . 9898	0 . 0	0
8	51 . 0046	4 . 4	578153
9	68 . 9952	100 . 0	749596
10	92 . 9952	3 . 1	947601
11	99 . 9936	8 . 9	1000568
12	118 . 9920	45 . 4	1136056
13	130 . 9920	46 . 5	1216350
14	142 . 9920	3 . 8	1293209
15	154 . 9920	2 . 8	1367064
16	168 . 9888	40 . 6	1449851
17	180 . 9888	36 . 1	1518276
18	192 . 9888	7 . 2	1584564
19	204 . 9888	4 . 3	1648914
20	218 . 9888	21 . 5	1721755
21	230 . 9856	22 . 2	1782476
22	242 . 9856	11 . 0	1841691
23	254 . 9856	4 . 2	1899529
24	268 . 9824	10 . 9	1965392
25	280 . 9824	18 . 4	2020563
26	292 . 9824	9 . 5	2074630
27	304 . 9824	3 . 7	2127653
28	318 . 9792	5 . 8	2188219
29	330 . 9792	12 . 6	2239166
30	342 . 9792	7 . 5	2289210
31	354 . 9792	3 . 1	2338447
32	366 . 9792	2 . 2	2386888
33	380 . 9760	10 . 1	2442422
34	392 . 9760	5 . 8	2489260
35	404 . 9760	4 . 0	2535438

calculated m/z of mass reference

relative intensity of peaks

not assignes as reference masses

assigned value of magnet current in arbitrary units

Fig. 3.29 Reproduction of a partial PFK calibration table (*m/z* 1–305 range) of a magnetic sector instrument. In order to expand the PFK reference peak list to the low *m/z* range, ^{1}H, ^{4}He, and peaks from residual air are included, but for intensity reasons ^{1}H, ^{4}He, and CO_2 have not been assigned in this particular case

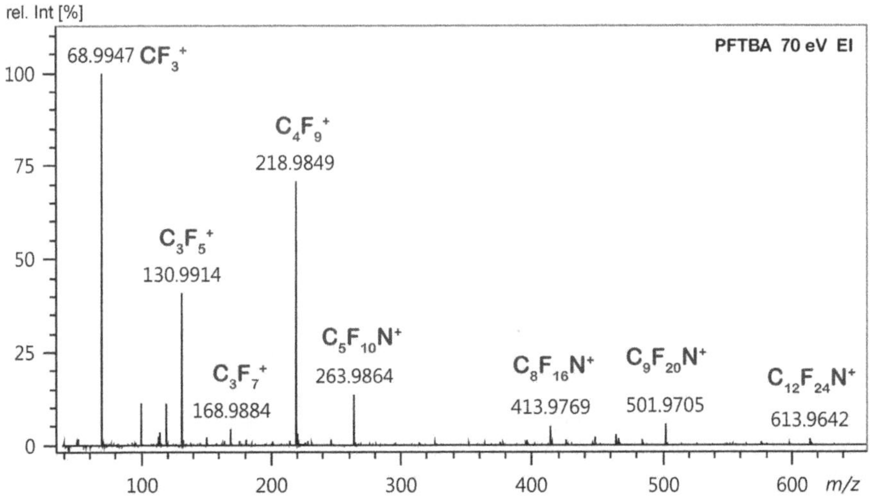

Fig. 3.30 EI mass spectrum of PFTBA with the composition of the most significant reference ions assigned. The calibration has already been performed, and thus, the *m/z* values are accurate

compound yields peaks up to *m/z* 614 [44, 60]. Like PFK, PFTBA is admitted via the reference inlet. The spectrum of PFTBA shows a reasonable number of peaks to be used for mass calibration (Fig. 3.30). How many of them are actually being used depends on the mass reference list. Also, the operator will normally check the automated assignment of reference peaks and may remove outliers. Such outliers are often due to overlap with background or sample peaks, e.g., in case of internal calibration (next paragraph). Their deletion can substantially improve the final calibration curve in that it reduces the average mass error of the calibration points, i.e., this measure reduces the standard deviation of the curve. While calibration curves can in principle be straight lines, actual instrument characteristics are often better approximated by using higher-order polynomials to fit the data. For example, based on the same spectrum of PFTBA a 3rd-order polynomial calibration yielded a gently bent curve (Fig. 3.31a). Among 19 assigned peaks, three outliers were identified and deleted. Repetition of the calibration using the corrected set of 16 peaks and a 4th-order polynomial (Fig. 3.31b) resulted in a notable reduction of average error.

3.6.2.1 Mass Accuracy Depends on Many Variables

Mass accuracy strongly depends on various parameters such as resolving power, scan rate, scanning method, signal-to-noise ratio of the peaks, peak shapes, overlap of isotopic peaks at same nominal mass, mass difference between adjacent reference peaks, calibration method etc. For instance, there is a marked effect of ion statistics on mass accuracy (Fig. 3.32). While peaks based on 10^3 to 10^5 ions yield results in a 1–5 ppm window, losses in accuracy occur due to Coulombic repulsion above 10^5 ions and due to poor ion statistics below 10^3 ions. Even though

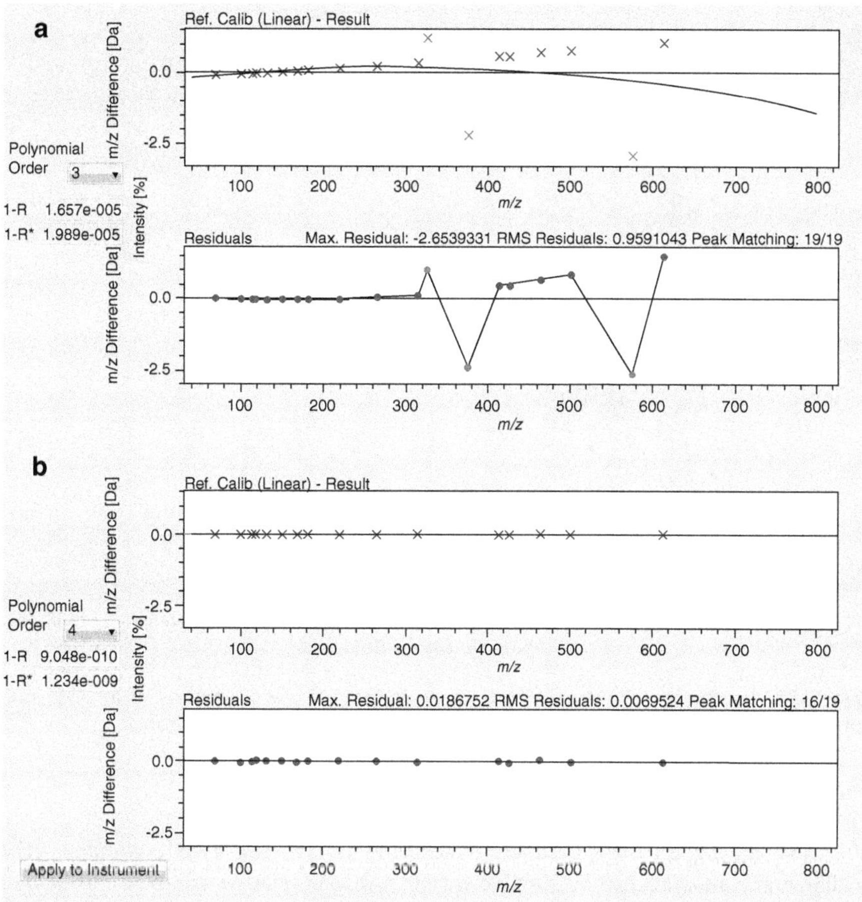

Fig. 3.31 Calibrations based on PFTBA. (**a**) 3rd-order polynomial calibration yields a gently bent curve. Three outliers (*red*) were identified and deleted. (**b**) Repetition of calibration using the corrected set of peaks and a 4th-order polynomial. Upon these measures, the correlation coefficients improve from the order of 10^{-5} to 10^{-9}. Figure composed of screenshots of JEOL AccuTOF GCx calibration software

determined for a specific Agilent GC-Q-TOF mass spectrometer, the basic characteristics of this graph can be assumed to be representative for most instruments.

It is also not possible to specify a general level of mass accuracy with external calibration. Depending on the type of mass analyzer and on the frequency of recalibration (monthly, weekly, daily, per sample), mass accuracy can vary from mediocre 0.5 u to perfect 10^{-3} u.

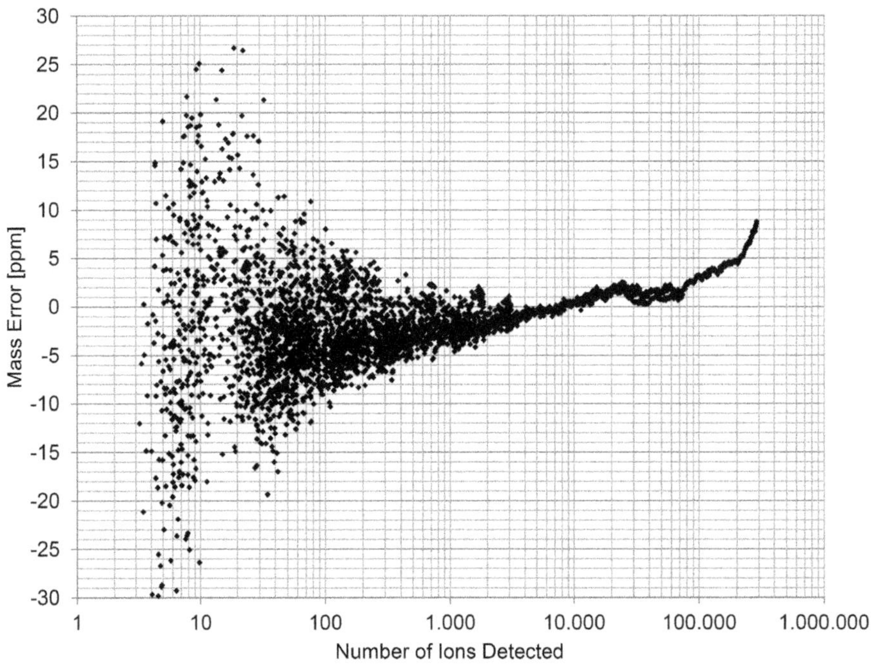

Fig. 3.32 Dependence of mass accuracy versus ion statistics as determined of a GC-Q-TOF instrument (Reproduced with kind permission of Bill Russ, Agilent Technologies)

3.6.3 Internal Mass Calibration

In principle, highest mass accuracy is achieved via *internal mass calibration.* The calibration compound can be introduced from a second inlet system or be mixed with the analyte prior to analysis. Mixing calibration compounds with the analyte requires some operational skills in order for it not to modify the analyte or to be modified itself. Therefore, a separate inlet for introducing the calibration compound is preferred. This can be done by introducing volatile standards such as PFK from a reference inlet system in electron ionization, by use of a dual-target probe in fast atom bombardment, or by use of a second sprayer in electrospray ionization. Internal mass calibration typically affords mass accuracies in the order of 0.1–0.5 ppm with FT-ICR, 0.5–1 ppm with Orbitrap, 0.5–5 ppm with magnetic sector, and 1–10 ppm with time-of-flight analyzers.

Overlap of PFK and sample For zirconium complexes the molecular ion range of an HR-EI spectrum is typified by the isotopic pattern of zirconium and chlorine (Fig. 3.33). ^{90}Zr represents the most abundant zirconium isotope which is accompanied by ^{91}Zr, ^{92}Zr, ^{94}Zr, and ^{96}Zr, all of them having considerable abundances. If the peak at *m/z* 414.9223 represents the monoisotopic ion, then the elemental composition containing ^{90}Zr and ^{35}Cl is the only correct interpretation. Thus, the formula $C_{16}H_{14}NCl_3Zr$ can be identified from the composition list (Fig. 3.34). Next, the X + 2 and X + 4 compositions should mainly be due to $^{35}Cl_2$

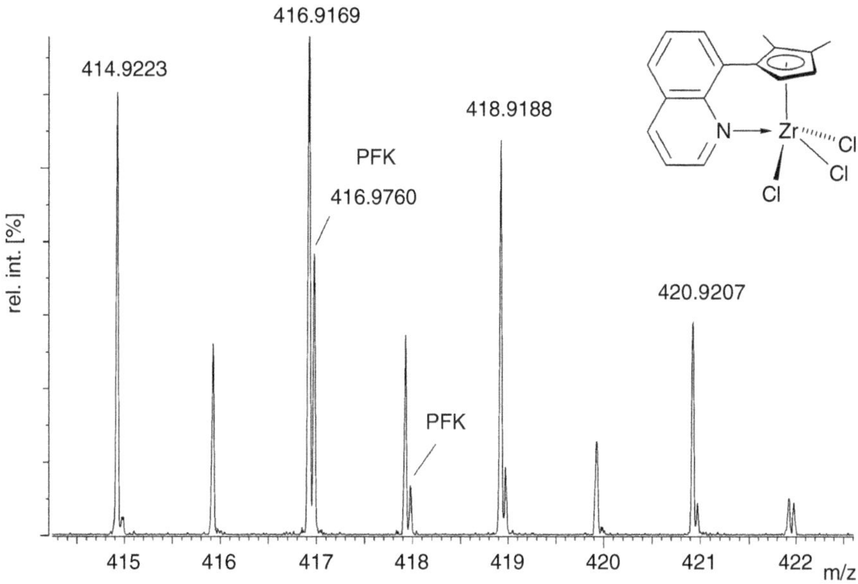

Fig. 3.33 Partial high-resolution EI mass spectrum in the molecular ion region of a zirconium complex. At $R = 8000$ the PFK ion can barely be separated from the slightly more mass-deficient analyte ion (By courtesy of M. Enders, Heidelberg University)

^{37}Cl and $^{35}Cl_{37}Cl_2$, respectively, leading to their identification. All formulas must have a remainder of $C_{16}H_{14}N$ in common. In this example, $R = 8000$ is the minimum to separate the PFK reference peak at *m/z* 417 from that of the analyte. Otherwise, the mass assignment would have been wrong because the peak at *m/z* 417 would then be centered at a weighted mass average of its two contributors. Alternatively, such a peak may be omitted from both reference list and composition list.

3.6.4 Specification of Mass Accuracy

Measured accurate masses, when used to assign molecular formulas, should always be accompanied by their mass accuracies [61]. Ideally, this can be done by giving the mean mass value and the corresponding error in terms of standard deviation through several repeated measurements of the same ion [44]. This is definitely not identical to the error usually provided with a mass spectrometer's software, where the error is based on the difference of a single pair of calculated and measured values. The reduction of the average mass error goes with the square root of the number of determinations (Sect. 3.5.4) [43].

Identifying the [M-Cl]$^+$ ion of chloroform The [M-Cl]$^+$ ion, $[CHCl_2]^+$, represents the base peak in the EI spectrum of chloroform. The results of three

```
Inlet : Direct                               Ion Mode : EI+
RT : 1.94 min                                Scan#: 5
Elements : C 40/0, H 40/0, N 2/0, Cl 3/0(35Cl 3/0, 37Cl 3/0), Zr 1/0
Mass Tolerance        : 5mmu
Unsaturation (U.S.) : 0.0 - 100.0

Observed m/z Int%    Err[ppm / mmu]    U.S.   Composition
  414.9223     7.5       -0.4 /  -0.2    22.5   C 23 H 2 N 2 35Cl 37Cl 2
               ----->    -3.9 /  -1.6    10.0   C 16 H 14 N 35Cl 3 Zr
                        -15.3 /  -6.3    15.0   C 19 H 11 N 35Cl 37Cl Zr
                         -0.8 /  -0.3    15.5   C 20 H 11 37Cl 2 Zr

  416.9169     8.9       -6.2 /  -2.6    22.5   C 23 H 2 N 2 37Cl 3
                         +3.1 /  +1.3    28.0   C 26 H N Zr
               ----->    -9.7 /  -4.0    10.0   C 16 H 14 N 35Cl 2 37Cl Zr
                         +9.1 /  +3.8    15.5   C 18 H 9 N 2 37Cl 2 Zr
                         +4.8 /  +2.0    10.5   C 17 H 14 35Cl 37Cl 2 Zr

  418.9188     7.5       -8.2 /  -3.4    24.5   C 26 H 2 35Cl 3
                         +0.2 /  +0.1    27.5   C 25 H N 2 Zr
                         -4.2 /  -1.7    22.5   C 24 H 6 35Cl Zr
               ----->    +1.8 /  +0.8    10.0   C 16 H 14 N 35Cl 37Cl 2 Zr
```

Fig. 3.34 Possible elemental compositions of the zirconium complex shown in the preceding figure. The error for each proposal is listed in units of ppm and "mmu" (0.001 u). U.S. = "unsaturation", i.e., the number of rings and/or double bonds (Sect. 6.4.4). For simplicity, here the correct assignments are highlighted with an *arrow* (By courtesy of M. Enders, Heidelberg University)

subsequent determinations for the major peaks of the isotopic pattern are listed below (Fig. 3.35). The typical printout of a mass spectrometer's data system provides experimental accurate mass and relative intensity of the signal along with absolute and relative mass error as calculated for a set of suggested formulas. Here, the experimentally accurate mass values yield a root-mean-square of 82.9442 ± 0.0006 u for the $[^{12}CH^{35}Cl_2]^+$ ion. The comparatively small standard deviation of 0.0006 u corresponds to a relative error of 7.5 ppm.

Balanced settings for best results

There is always a trade-off between resolving power, signal intensity, and mass accuracy. Mass accuracy may even suffer from overly ambitious settings of resolving power if this ends up in causing noisy peaks. Often, centroids are determined more accurately from smooth and symmetrically shaped peaks at somewhat lower resolving power. One should be aware of the fact that the position of a peak of 0.1 u width, for example, has to be determined to $^1/_{50}$ of its width to obtain 0.002 u accuracy [36].

```
[ Elemental Composition ]
Data   : JMS18120_009                     Date : 14-May-2002 08:20
Sample: CHCl3
Elements : C 10/1(12C 10/0, 13C 1/0), H 10/0, Cl 4/0(35Cl 4/0, 37Cl 4/0)
Mass Tolerance         : 10mmu
Unsaturation (U.S.) : -200.0 - 200.0

Observed m/z Int%    Err[ppm / mmu]    U.S.  Composition
   82.9433   100.0     +27.5 /  +2.3    1.0  13C 35Cl 2
                       -26.4 /  -2.2    0.5  12C H 35Cl 2

   84.9406    62.5     +29.5 /  +2.5    1.0  13C 35Cl 37Cl
                       -23.2 /  -2.0    0.5  12C H 35Cl 37Cl

   86.9379    10.1     +31.6 /  +2.7    1.0  13C 37Cl 2
                       -19.9 /  -1.7    0.5  12C H 37Cl 2
Observed m/z Int%    Err[ppm / mmu]    U.S.  Composition
   82.9449   100.0     +45.8 /  +3.8    1.0  13C 35Cl 2
                        -8.1 /  -0.7    0.5  12C H 35Cl 2

   84.9422    66.0     +48.0 /  +4.1    1.0  13C 35Cl 37Cl
                        -4.7 /  -0.4    0.5  12C H 35Cl 37Cl

   86.9404    11.2     +60.3 /  +5.2    1.0  13C 37Cl 2
                        +8.9 /  +0.8    0.5  12C H 37Cl 2
Observed m/z Int%    Err[ppm / mmu]    U.S.  Composition
   82.9447   100.0     +43.7 /  +3.6    1.0  13C 35Cl 2
                       -10.2 /  -0.8    0.5  12C H 35Cl 2

   84.9419    65.1     +44.6 /  +3.8    1.0  13C 35Cl 37Cl
                        -8.1 /  -0.7    0.5  12C H 35Cl 37Cl

   86.9391    10.8     +45.1 /  +3.9    1.0  13C 37Cl 2
                        -6.3 /  -0.6    0.5  12C H 37Cl 2
```

Fig. 3.35 Printout of elemental compositions of the $[M–Cl]^+$ ion of chloroform as obtained from three subsequent measurements (70 eV EI, $R = 8000$). The error for each proposal is listed in units of ppm and "mmu" (outdated for mu). U.S. ("unsaturation") is the number of rings and/or double bonds (Sect. 6.4.4)

3.6.5 Identification of Formulas from HR-MS Data

The experimentally determined accurate mass of an ion should lie within a reasonable error range independent of the ionization method and the instrument used [62]. The correct (expected) composition is not necessarily the one with the least error but just one within the experimental error interval. You should examine the examples in Figs. 3.34 and 3.35 to verify that the correct formulas can have a larger mass error than illogical ones.

Often, computer-generated formula lists contain suggested formulas that are not reasonable from a chemical point of view or are in contradiction to mass spectrometric rules. When searching for the correct formula of an ion you need to consider some basic rules:

- All elements that have to be taken into account have to be admitted in suitable numbers when the list is being created.
- Depending on the ionization method, even-electron or odd-electron ions may be formed. This criterion can rule out some compositions.
- Also, dependent on the ionization method, molecules may form $M^{+\bullet}$, $[M + H]^+$, $[M + NH_4]^+$, $[M + alkali]^+$ ions and others. Therefore, reasonable adducts have to be taken into account.
- The assigned formula must be in accordance with the experimentally observed and the calculated isotopic pattern for the assumed composition.
- The formula has to obey the nitrogen rule (Sect. 6.2.7)
- Formulas in contradiction to one of these points are erroneous.

The latest software packages for formula generation from accurate mass tend to imply such rules by offering selections not only on error interval, elements, and number thereof to be taken into account but also of odd-electron and/or even-electron species, ranges of H/C ratio, ranking by correlation to calculated isotopic pattern etc. [63]. Additionally, $\Delta(m/z)$ between isotopic peaks of the same element should be used as a source of information [64] (Sect. 3.7.2.1). Whatever the level of sophistication of such software tools, obtaining correct results still requires knowledgeable operator input and eventually refinement after communicating with the person who provided the sample.

Formula calculation for a silicone Silicone oligomers as present in silicone oil and rubber can readily be analyzed using direct analysis in real time (DART) mass spectrometry in positive-ion mode on a Fourier transform-ion cyclotron resonance (FT-ICR) instrument [65, 66]. Under these conditions, the silicone oligomers form ammonium adduct ions where the number of O atoms equals that of Si atoms. The signals also exhibit marked Si isotope patterns (Fig. 3.11). The example shows a screenshot of a formula calculation for a 13mer silicone ion with the monoisotopic ion at *m/z* 980.27736 (Fig. 3.36). The formula list is calculated within restrictive limits for elemental composition $C_{20–30}H_{60–90}O_{10–14}Si_{10–14}$, mass error of 5 ppm, and for even-electron ions only. Nonetheless, there is still a selection among ten candidates; a tighter error interval would have further reduced the number (Sect. 3.5.6). In this case, the assignment was assisted by the fact that the ion belongs to a homologous series. The correct composition, $[C_{26}H_{82}O_{13}Si_{13}]^+$, is highlighted by a blue bar [66].

3.7 Resolution Interacting with Isotopic Patterns

3.7.1 Multiple Isotopic Compositions at Very High Resolution

We started our lesson on isotopic patterns with the unspoken assumption of nominal mass resolution, which makes it much easier to understand how isotopic patterns are formed. The procedure of summing up all isotopic abundances contributing to

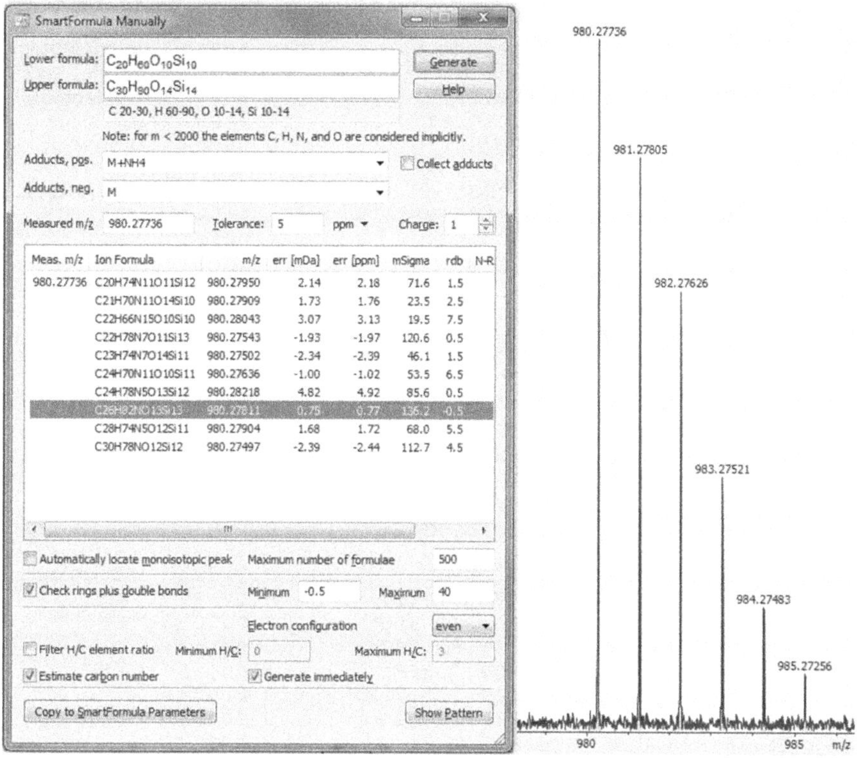

Fig. 3.36 Screenshot of formula calculation for a silicone ion using Bruker SmartFormula software (*left*) and the corresponding signal (*right*) as obtained by DART-FT-ICR-MS. The formula list is calculated within restrictive limits for elemental composition $C_{20-30}H_{60-90}O_{10-14}Si_{10-14}$, mass error of 5 ppm, and even-electron ions only. The correct composition of the NH_4^+ adduct ion, *m/z* 980.27736, is highlighted by a blue bar

the same nominal mass is correct as long as very high resolution is not employed. In that case, following such a simplified protocol is acceptable, because generally isobaric isotopolog ions are very similar in mass [25].

In the earlier introduction of resolution it should have become clear that very high resolution is capable of separating different isotopic compositions of the same nominal mass, thereby giving rise to multiple peaks on the same nominal *m/z* (Figs. 3.21, 3.22, and 3.32). In molecules with masses of around 10,000 u, a single unresolved isotopic peak may consist of as many as 20 different isotopic compositions (also cf. Fig. 3.39) [67, 68].

Imagine infinite resolution Numerous isotopologs contribute to the isotopic pattern of $C_{16}H_{20}OSi$. Among them the monoisotopic ion at *m/z* 256.1283 is the most abundant (Fig. 3.37). For the first isotopic peak at *m/z* 257 the major contribution derives from ^{13}C, but ^{29}Si and ^{17}O also play a role. Actually, ^{2}H should also be

m/z	composition	rel. int. [%]	
256.12836	C16.H20.O.Si	100.00000	monoisotopic
257.12790	C16.H20.O.29Si	5.10957	1st isotopic
257.13171	C15.13C.H20.O.Si	17.92663	
257.13257	C16.H20.17O.Si	0.03709	
258.12518	C16.H20.O.30Si	3.38468	2nd isotopic
258.13126	C15.13C.H20.O.29Si	0.91597	
258.13214	C16.H20.17O.29Si	0.00190	
258.13260	C16.H20.18O.Si	0.20449	
258.13507	C14.13C2.H20.O.Si	1.50639	
258.13593	C15.13C.H20.17O.Si	0.00665	
259.12854	C15.13C.H20.O.30Si	0.60676	3rd isotopic
259.12939	C16.H20.17O.30Si	0.00126	
259.13214	C16.H20.18O.29Si	0.01045	
259.13461	C14.13C2.H20.O.29Si	0.07697	
259.13550	C15.13C.H20.17O.29Si	0.00034	
259.13596	C15.13C.H20.18O.Si	0.03666	
259.13843	C13.13C3.H20.O.Si	0.07876	
259.13928	C14.13C2.H20.17O.Si	0.00056	
260.12943	C16.H20.18O.30Si	0.00692	4th isotopic
260.13190	C14.13C2.H20.O.30Si	0.05099	
260.13275	C15.13C.H20.17O.30Si	0.00023	
260.13550	C15.13C.H20.18O.29Si	0.00187	
260.13797	C13.13C3.H20.O.29Si	0.00402	
260.13885	C14.13C2.H20.17O.29Si	0.00003	
260.13931	C14.13C2.H20.18O.Si	0.00308	
260.14175	C12.13C4.H20.O.Si	0.00287	
260.14264	C13.13C3.H20.17O.Si	0.00003	

Fig. 3.37 Tabular representation of the theoretical isotopic distribution of $C_{16}H_{20}OSi$ at infinite resolution. The contribution of ^{2}H is not considered, and isotopic peaks above *m/z* 260 are omitted due to their minor intensities

considered, but has been omitted due to its extremely low isotopic abundance. As the isotopologs of the same nominal *m/z* are not true isobars, their intensities will not sum up in one common peak. Instead, they are detected side by side provided sufficient resolving power is available. The pair $^{13}C^{12}C_{15}H_{20}{}^{16}OSi$, *m/z* 257.13171, and $^{12}C_{16}H_{20}{}^{17}OSi$, *m/z* 257.13257, roughly necessitates 3×10^5 resolution ($R = 257/0.00086 = 299{,}000$). There are six different compositions contributing to the second isotopic peak at *m/z* 258 and even eight for the third isotopic peak at *m/z* 259. Again, it is the merit of FT-ICR-MS that resolutions in the order of several 10^5 are now available although *ultrahigh resolution*, as this is termed, is still not fully routine on those instruments (Sect. 4.7).

Telling $^{13}C_2$ and ^{34}S peaks apart Peptides often contain sulfur from cysteine. Provided there are at least two cysteines in the peptide molecule, sulfur can be in the form of thiol group (SH, reduced) or sulfur bridges (S–S, oxidized). Often, both forms are contained in the same sample. At ultrahigh resolution, the contributions

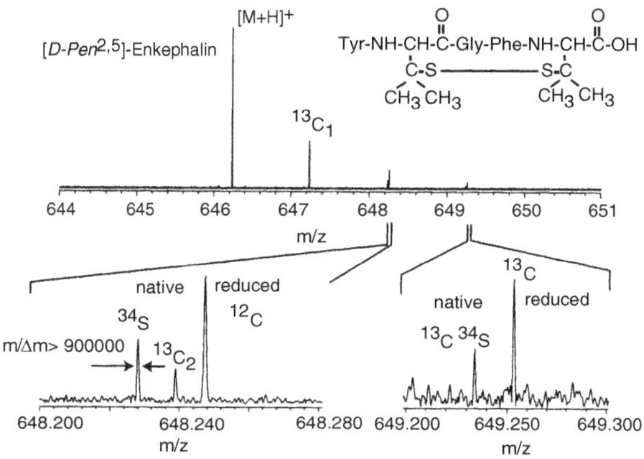

Fig. 3.38 [D-Pen^{2,5}] Enkephalin – Ultrahigh-resolution MALDI-FT-ICR mass spectrum of native (S–S) and reduced (2 × SH) forms. The expanded *m/z* views of the second and third isotopic peak show fully mass-resolved signals (Reproduced from Ref. [69] with permission. © American Chemical Society, 1997)

of these compositions to the same nominal *m/z* can be distinguished. The ultrahigh-resolution matrix-assisted laser desorption/ionization (MALDI) FT-ICR mass spectrum of native and reduced [D-Pen^{2,5}]enkephalin is an example of such a separation (Fig. 3.38) [69]. The left expanded view shows fully resolved peaks due to ^{34}S and $^{13}C_2$ isotopologs of the native and the all-^{12}C peak of the reduced compound at *m/z* 648. The right expansion reveals the $^{13}C_1{}^{34}S$ peak of the native plus the $^{13}C_1$ signal of the reduced form at *m/z* 649. Here, R_{FWHM} is more than 9×10^5.

3.7.2 Isotopologs and Accurate Mass

It has been pointed out that routine accurate mass measurements are conducted at resolutions which are normally too low to separate isobaric isotopologs. Unfortunately, multiple isotopic compositions under the same signal tend to distort the peak shape (Fig. 3.39) [68]. This effect causes problems when elemental compositions have to be determined from such multi-isotopolog peaks, e.g., if the mono- isotopic peak is too weak as in case of many transition metals. Generally, the observed decrease in mass accuracy is not dramatic and is somewhat counterbalanced by the information derived from the isotopic pattern. However, it can be observed that mass accuracy decreases by about 50% on such unresolved signals.

3.7.2.1 Information from Accurate Mass Differences Between Isotopes

If isotopolog ions are resolved or if certain isotopologs are free from interference, and provided sufficient mass accuracy is available, Δ(*m/z*) between isotopic peaks can yield adequate analytical information [64]. As are the isotopic masses themselves, the differences between isotopic masses are characteristic for certain elements. Boron for example, has a small mass difference of just 0.9964 u between ^{10}B and ^{11}B, whereas the pair of ^{191}Ir and ^{193}Ir presents a rare example of a difference clearly above 2 u, which is still distinguishable from hydrogenation. Determination of Δ(*m/z*) values can thus help to distinguish between hydrogenation

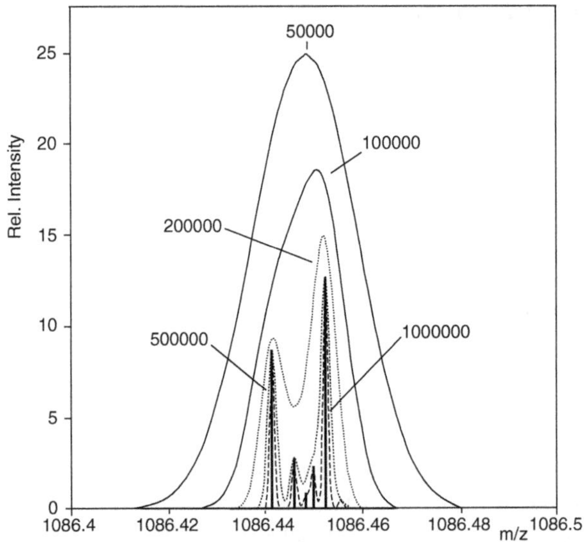

Fig. 3.39 Arg^8 vasopressin – Theoretical effect of resolution on the shape of the M + 2 peak at *m/z* 1086.4. Theoretical mass spectra of the [vasopressin + H]$^+$ ion and the five indicated resolution values (FWHM) have been superimposed and the bar spectrum corresponds to infinite resolution (Adapted from Ref. [68] with permission. © John Wiley and Sons Ltd., 1994)

and X + 2 element isotopic peaks can ascertain the presence of boron vs. loss of a hydrogen radical etc. Some helpful values are compiled in Table 3.3. Obviously, there are also limits to this approach, for example, when a decision between M + 2 due to ^{37}Cl or ^{65}Cu is called for, in particular, as their isotopic abundances are also similar.

Isotopic pattern of substance P at R = 4 million Werlen (Fig. 3.39) [68] had anticipated that ultrahigh resolution would reveal multiple peaks. Modern FT-ICR instruments are, in fact, able to resolve these peaks [70, 71]. The peaks contributing to the isotopic pattern of doubly protonated substance P, a peptide ion of the composition $[C_{63}H_{100}O_{13}N_{18}S]^{2+}$, have been measured one by one at $R = 4{,}000{,}000$. (To avoid space charge effects and to operate at optimum ion population – a limitation inherent to FT-ICR-MS – the ultimate resolving power was achieved via the measurement of isolated isotopologs.)

The set of four partial spectra in Fig. 3.40 reflects the increasing complexity of the isotopic composition as one moves from [M + 1] (Fig. 3.40a) to [M + 4] (Fig. 3.40d). The most relevant contributions to the [M + 4] ion in order of rising mass are formed by combinations of $^{13}C^{15}N^{34}S$, $^{34}S^{18}O$, $^{13}C_2{}^{34}S$, $^{13}C^{15}N^{18}O$, $^{13}C_3{}^{15}N$, $^{13}C_3{}^{33}S$, $^{13}C_2{}^{18}O$, and finally $^{13}C_4$. The masses of these ions spread across just 8.63 mu between the lightest and the heaviest of the group. Note that the pure $^{13}C_X$ isotopic ion is always that of highest *m/z* within the respective [M + X] ion provided that only C, H, N, O, and S are involved (some peaks of very low intensity may occur above).

Ultrahigh resolving power alone is merely able to separate the various isotopic contributions belonging to [M + 1] to [M + 4] ions. Key to the assignment of these compositions is the knowledge of the accurate mass differences between certain

Table 3.3 Characteristic mass differences to identify the presence of elements

Pair of isotopes or modification	Δm [u]
^{6}Li vs. ^{7}Li	1.0009
^{10}B vs. ^{11}B	0.9964
^{12}C vs. ^{13}C	1.0033
^{32}S vs. ^{34}S	1.9958
^{35}Cl vs. ^{37}Cl	1.9970
^{58}Ni vs. ^{60}Ni	1.9955
^{63}Cu vs. ^{65}Cu	1.9982
^{79}Br vs. ^{81}Br	1.9980
^{191}Ir vs. ^{193}Ir	2.0023
gain or loss of H	1.0078
gain or loss of H_2	2.0156

pairs of isotopologs (Table 3.3). The $^{13}C_X$ peak, for example, will be located at $m/z_{monoisotopic} + 1.0033 \times X$ (note that $\Delta m/z$ is half of the mass difference in case of a doubly charged ion as $z = 2$, Sect. 3.8). Thus, assignment of isotopic peaks is achieved by their accurate mass differences. Vice versa, the reliability of the assignment of elemental compositions increases the better the suggested formula complies with the measured isotopic fine structure; modern data analysis software packages exploit this to their advantage.

3.7.3 Large Molecules – Isotopic Patterns at Sufficient Resolution

Terms such as *large molecules* or *high mass* are subject to steady change in mass spectrometry as new techniques for analyzing high-mass ions are being developed or improved [72]. Here, the focus is on masses in the range of 10^3–10^4 u.

With increasing *m*/*z* the center of the isotopic pattern, i.e., the *average molecular mass*, is shifted to values higher than the *monoisotopic mass*. The center, i.e., the average mass, may not be represented by a real peak, but it tends to be close to the peak of *most abundant* mass (Fig. 3.41). The monoisotopic mass is of course still related to a real signal, but it may be of such a low intensity that it is difficult to recognize. Finally, the *nominal mass* becomes a mere number which is no longer useful to describe the molecular weight [41, 67].

The calculation of isotopic patterns of molecules of several 10^3 u is not a trivial task, because slight variations in the relative abundances of the isotopes encountered gain relevance and may shift the most abundant mass and the average mass up or down by 1 u. In a similar fashion the algorithm and the number of iterations employed to perform the actual calculation affect the final result [25].

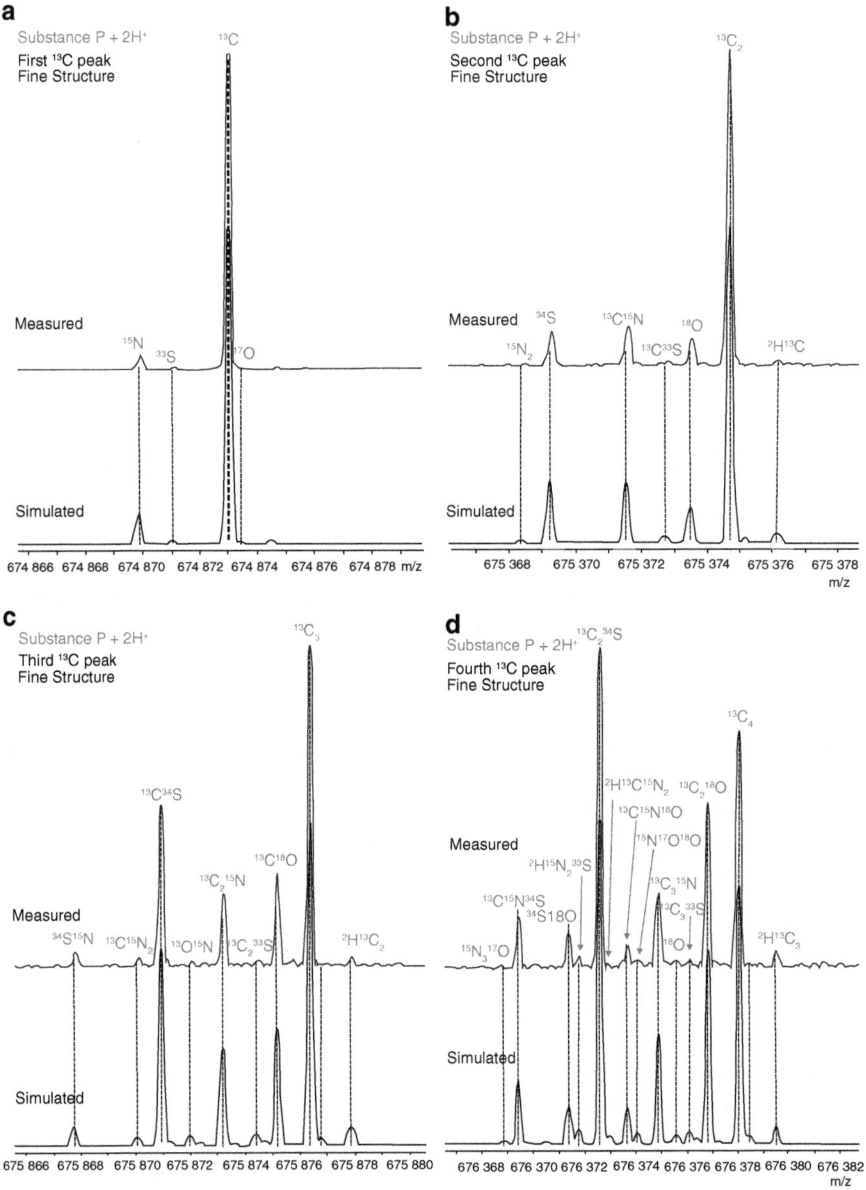

Fig. 3.40 Isotope peaks of doubly protonated substance P, $[C_{63}H_{100}O_{13}N_{18}S]^{2+}$, as measured individually by FT-ICR-MS at R = 4,000,000. (**a**) First isotopic peak, [M + 1], (**b**) [M + 2], (**c**) [M + 3], and (**d**) [M + 4]. The most relevant contributions are due to ^{13}C, ^{34}S, and ^{18}O. The [M + 4] signal splits into eight major and several very minor peaks (Reproduced from Ref. [70] by permission. © American Chemical Society, 2012)

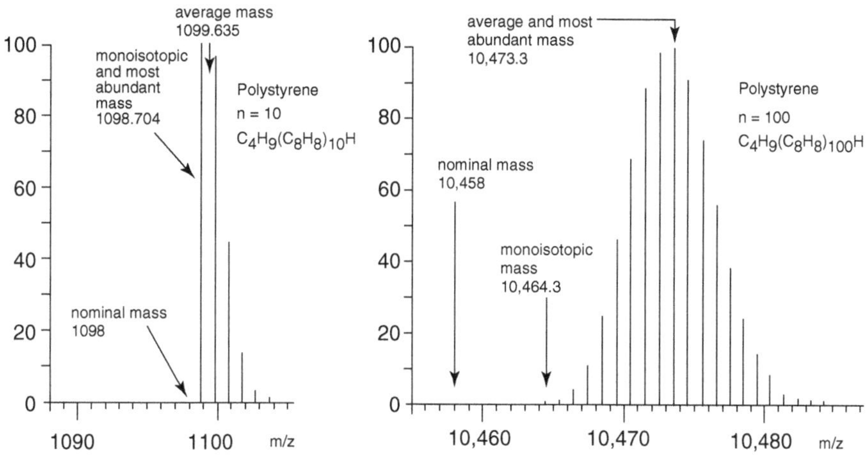

Fig. 3.41 Polystyrene. Calculated isotopic patterns of large ions (Adapted from Ref. [67] with permission. © American Chemical Society, 1983)

Mass of large molecules

The calculation of relative molecular mass, M_r, of organic molecules exceeding 2000 u is significantly influenced by the basis it is performed on. Both the atomic weights of the constituent elements and the natural variations in isotopic abundance contribute to the differences between *monoisotopic*- and *relative atomic mass-based* M_r values. In addition, they tend to characteristically differ between major classes of biomolecules. This is primarily because of molar carbon content, e.g., the difference between polypeptides and nucleic acids is about 4 u at $M_r = 25{,}000$ u. Considering terrestrial sources alone, variations in the isotopic abundance of carbon lead to differences of about 10–25 ppm in M_r which is significant with respect to mass measurement accuracy in the region up to several 10^3 u [41].

3.7.4 Isotopic Patterns of Macromolecules Versus Resolution

It is certainly desirable to have at least sufficient resolution to resolve isotopic patterns to their nominal mass contributions. However, not every mass analyzer is capable of doing so with any ion it can pass through. Such conditions often occur when ions of several thousand u are being analyzed by quadrupole, time-of-flight or quadrupole ion trap analyzers, and hence it is useful to know about the changes in spectral appearance and their effect on peak width and detected mass [68].

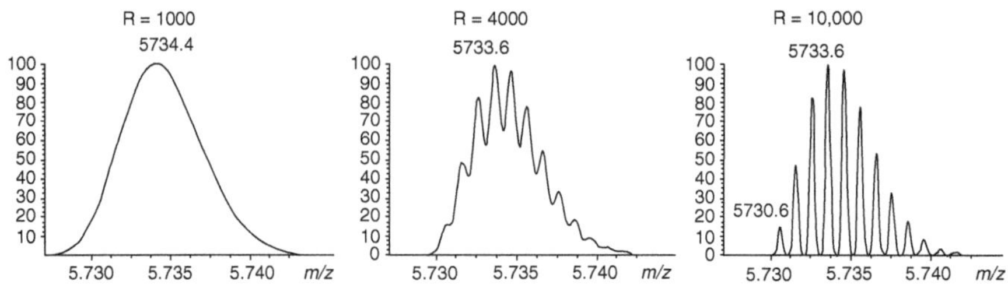

Fig. 3.42 Bovine insulin – the isotopic pattern calculated for $[M + H]^+$ at different resolutions ($R_{10\%}$). Note that the envelope at $R = 1000$ is wider than the real isotopic pattern

Isotopic pattern of bovine insulin The isotopic pattern of the $[M + H]^+$ ion of bovine insulin, $[C_{254}H_{378}N_{65}O_{75}S_6]^+$, has been calculated for $R_{10\%} = 1000$, 4000, and 10,000. At $R = 1000$ the isotopic peaks are not resolved (Fig. 3.42) and an envelope smoothly covering the isotopic peaks is observed instead; it is even slightly wider than the real isotopic pattern. The maximum of this envelope is in good agreement with the calculated average mass, i.e., the molecular weight (Eq. 3.2). At $R = 4000$ the isotopic peaks become sufficiently resolved to be recognized as such. The *m/z* values are very close to the corresponding isotopic masses; however, there can be some minor shifts due to their still significant overlap. Finally, at $R = 10{,}000$ the isotopic pattern is well resolved and interferences between isotopic peaks are avoided. The next step, i.e., to resolve the multiple isotopic contributions to each of the peaks would require $R > 10^6$.

Fading separation at high *m/z* Dendrimers are a class of synthetic macromolecules that can be synthesized at various sizes. A special set of monodisperse dendrimers has thus been developed for mass calibration in MALDI-MS, in particular with time-of-flight (TOF) analyzers in mind [73]. Depending on the actual MALDI-TOF instrument some of the higher *m/z* dendrimers are at or just beyond the limits of resolving power, i.e., the isotopic separation is fading away as one moves along the series of peaks. The positive-ion MALDI-TOF spectrum of such a SpheriCal mixture ($C_{398}H_{468}O_{138}$, $C_{529}H_{620}O_{184}$, $C_{660}H_{772}O_{230}$, $C_{796}H_{934}O_{277}$) exemplifies this behavior upon transition from about *m/z* 7600 to 15,000 (Fig. 3.43) [74].

3.8 Charge State and Interaction with Isotopic Patterns

Even though singly charged ions seem to be the dominant species in mass spectrometry at first sight, there are many applications where doubly and multiply charged ions are of utmost importance. In electrospray ionization (Chap. 12) even extremely high *charge states* can be observed, e.g., up to 60-fold in case of proteins of about 60,000 u molecular weight. Doubly and triply charged ions are also common in electron ionization (Chaps. 5 and 6) and field desorption (Chap. 8).

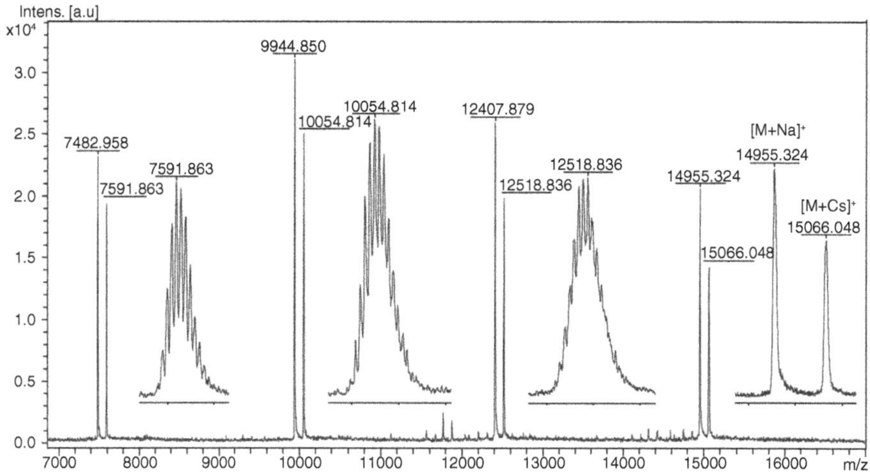

Fig. 3.43 Positive-ion MALDI-TOF spectrum of a SpheriCal kit (PFS-14) as obtained in the presence of Na^+ and Cs^+ ions where each of the four dendrimers forms $[M + Na]^+$ and $[M + Cs]^+$ ions leading to eight reference peaks in total. The insets show expanded views of the isotopic patterns of the respective $[M + Cs]^+$ ion signals. As *m*/*z* increases, resolution of isotopic peaks can no longer be achieved (Adapted from Ref. [74] with permission. © Springer-Verlag, Heidelberg, 2016)

The effect of higher charge states are worth considering. As z increases from 1 to 2, 3 etc., the numerical value of m/z is reduced by a factor of 2, 3 etc., i.e., the ion will be detected at lower m/z than the corresponding singly charged ion of the same mass. In general, the entire m/z scale is compressed by a factor of z if $z > 1$.

Consequently, the isotopic peaks are then located at $\Delta(m/z) = {}^1/_z$. Vice versa, the charge state is obtained from the reciprocal value of the distance between adjacent peaks, e.g., peaks at $\Delta m/z = {}^1/_3$ correspond to $z = 3$, i.e., triply charged ions. The reasons for the compression of the m/z scale are discussed later (Sect. 4.2).

Isotopic patterns of $M^{+\bullet}$, M^{2+}, and $M^{3+\bullet}$ The EI mass spectrum of C_{60} also shows an abundant doubly charged molecular ion, $C_{60}{}^{2+}$, at m/z 360 with its isotopic peaks located at $\Delta(m/z) = 0.5$ and a $C_{60}{}^{3+\bullet}$ signal at m/z 240 of very low intensity (Fig. 3.44) [32]. The isotopic pattern remains unaffected by the charge state. As a consequence of the compressed m/z scale, the doubly charged $C_{58}{}^{2+}$ fragment ion is detected at m/z 348.

Isotopic distribution and charge state

Isotopic distributions are of course not affected by the charge state of an ion. Therefore, the relative intensities of the isotopic peaks are independent of the charge state. However, $\Delta m/z$ between the isotopic peaks is reduced by ${}^1/_z$,

(continued)

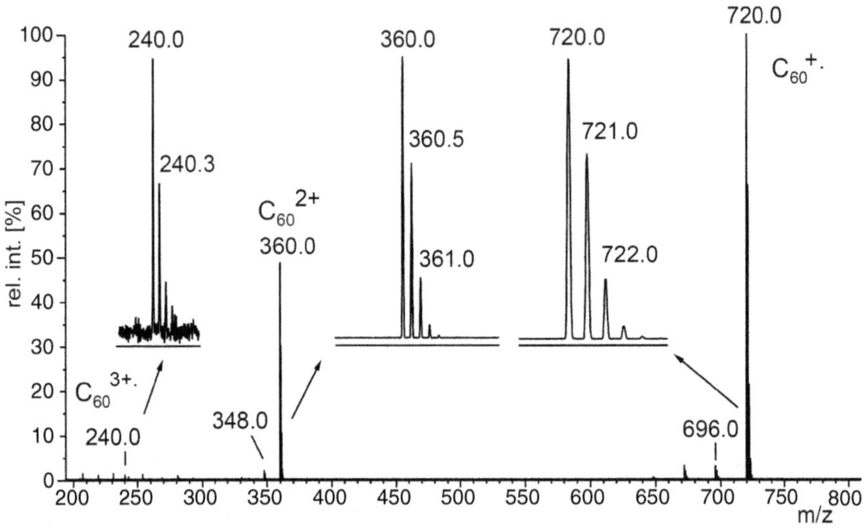

Fig. 3.44 EI mass spectrum of [60]Fullerene. The insets show the expanded signals of $M^{+\bullet}$, M^{2+}, and $M^{3+\bullet}$ ions. The signals of the patterns are at $\Delta m/z = 1, 0.5$, and 0.33, respectively. The intensity scale has been normalized in the insets to allow for easier comparison of the isotopic patterns (By courtesy of W. Krätschmer, Max Planck Institute for Nuclear Physics, Heidelberg)

thus allowing multiply charged ions to be easily distinguished from singly charged ions. Furthermore, the charge state can be directly determined from the reciprocal value of $^{1}/_{z}$.

3.9 Approaches to Visualize Complex HR-MS Data Sets

3.9.1 Deltamass

The term *deltamass* has been coined to define the mass value following the decimal point [75] thereby elegantly circumventing the somewhat unfortunate terminology related to the mass defect. The deltamass concept is only valid in the context for which it has been developed, i.e., to describe mass deviations of peptides from average values. Beyond this context, ambiguities arise from its rigorous application because *i*) a mass defect would then be expressed the same way as larger values of negative mass defect, e.g., in case of $^{127}I^+$ as 0.9045 u and in case of $C_{54}H_{110}^{+\bullet}$ as 0.8608 u, respectively, and *ii*) deviations of more than 1 u would be expressed by the same numerical value as those of less than 1 u.

Peptide modifications by deltamass The magnitude of mass defect can provide an idea of what compound class is being analyzed (Sect. 3.5.2). At a sufficient level of sophistication, mass defect can even reveal more detail [47]. Peptides consist of amino acids and therefore, their elemental compositions are rather similar independent of their size or sequence. This results in a characteristic relationship of formulas and deltamass values. Phosphorylation and more pronounced glycosylation cause lower deltamass, because they introduce mass-deficient atoms (P, O) into the molecule. The large number of hydrogens associated with lipidation, on the other side, contributes to a deltamass above normal level. On the average, an unmodified peptide of 1968 u, for example, shows a deltamass of 0.99 u, whereas a glycosylated peptide of the same nominal mass will have a value of 0.76 u. Therefore, the deltamass can be employed to obtain information on the type of covalent protein modification [75].

3.9.2 Kendrick Mass Scale

The intention of the *Kendrick mass scale* is to provide data reduction in a way that homologs can be recognized by their identical *Kendrick mass defect* (KMD). Due to the steadily increasing resolution and mass accuracy of modern instrumentation this issue is again gaining importance for complex mixture analysis by MS. The Kendrick mass scale is based on the definition $M_{(CH2)} = 14.0000$ u [76]. The conversion factor from the IUPAC mass scale, m_{IUPAC}, to the Kendrick mass scale, $m_{Kendrick}$, is therefore 14.000000/14.015650 = 0.9988834:

$$m_{Kendrick} = 0.9988834\, m_{IUPAC} \tag{3.15}$$

Next, we define the *Kendrick mass defect*, $m_{defectKendrick}$, as

$$m_{defectKendrick} = m_{nomKendrick} - m_{Kendrick} = \text{KMD} \tag{3.16}$$

where $m_{nomKendrick}$ is the *nominal Kendrick mass*, the closest integer to Kendrick mass.

Kendrick mass of $[C_{30}H_{49}O_3]^-$ The IUPAC mass of $[C_{30}H_{49}O_3]^-$ is 457.3687 u. The Kendrick mass of this ion is calculated as 457.3687 u × 0.9988834 = 456.8580 u. From this it follows that $m_{nomKendrick} = 457$ u. The Kendrick mass defect of this ion is thus obtained as $m_{defectKendrick} = 457$ u − 456.8580 u = 0.1419 u.

To translate spectral data into a useful *Kendrick mass plot*, a high-resolution mass spectrum is broken into segments of 1 u, which are aligned on the abscissa. Then, the Kendrick mass defect of the isobaric ions contained in the respective segment is plotted onto the ordinate. The resulting graph preserves not only the "coarse" spacing, e.g., about 1 u between odd and even mass values, but also the "fine structure", i.e., different Kendrick mass defects (KMDs) for different

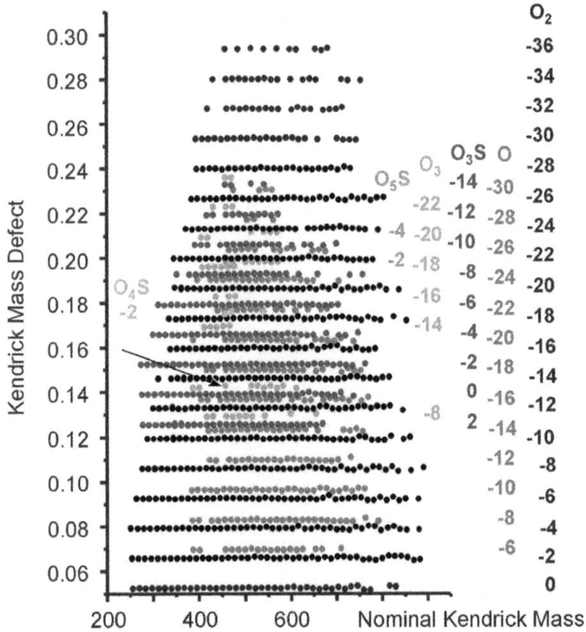

Fig. 3.45 Kendrick mass defect vs. nominal Kendrick mass for odd-mass $^{12}C_x$ ions ($[M-H]^-$ ions). The compound classes (O, O_2, O_3S, and O_4S) and the different numbers of rings plus double bonds (Sect. 6.4.4) are separated vertically. Horizontally, the points are spaced by CH_2 groups along a homologous series [77] (By courtesy of A.G. Marshall, NHFL, Tallahassee)

elemental compositions across each segment. Homologs are now easily recognized as horizontal rows in the plot [77].

Kendrick plots are becoming increasingly important as more instruments are able to provide ultrahigh resolution spectra of complex mixtures, and thus, create a demand for tools to retrieve analytically useful information from such large data sets [78–80]. Recently, Kendrick plots have been introduced as a tool for the convenient visualization of tandem mass spectral data of synthetic polymers, e.g., by referring to the monomeric building block as the base unit upon which the Kendrick mass defect is calculated [81].

Crude oil and diesel fuel In a Kendrick plot the composition of complex systems can be conveniently displayed. Several thousand elemental compositions in the ultrahigh resolution spectrum of petroleum crude oil [77] or diesel fuel [82] may be resolved. Such samples consist of numerous compound classes and/or alkylation series with some 30 homologs each that can be visually identified (Fig. 3.45). The formula employed for the preceding example is marked in the plot by an arrow.

3.9.3 Van Krevelen Diagrams

There is yet another tool for the display of composition characteristics of complex mixtures, the *van Krevelen diagram* [83]. The van Krevelen diagram is a plot of the atomic H/C ratio against the atomic O/C ratio. This plot causes the products related

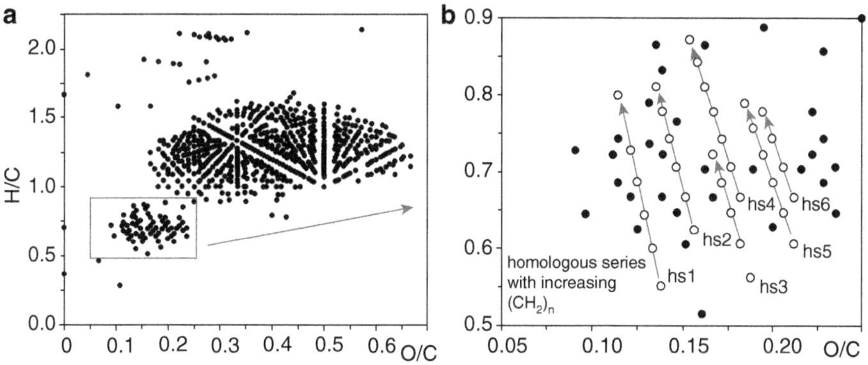

Fig. 3.46 Van Krevelen diagrams of deep-sea DOM. (**a**) Presentation of all molecules in 3500 m and 4600 m water depth. (**b**) Enlarged region of condensed polyaromatics where the members of the homologous series $(CH_2)_n$ with $n \geq 4$ are shown as *white circles* and connected along a *gray line* (Reproduced from Ref. [87] with permission. © Elsevier Science Publishers, 2006)

by reactions such as decarboxylation, dehydration, dehydrogenation, or oxidation to be displayed along straight lines. Along with KMD plots, the van Krevelen plot is therefore a major tool for the assessment of complex organic mixtures such as crude oil and its refinery products or the wide field of *natural organic matter* (NOM) that represents the largest share of biomass on earth [84–88].

Dissolved organic matter (DOM) The van Krevelen diagrams of HR-MS data obtained of deep-sea *dissolved organic matter* (DOM) show a group of molecules having low H/C (<0.9) and low O/C (<0.25) ratios clearly separated from each other (Fig. 3.46) [87]. An enlarged view of this group shows that it comprises 224 different molecular formulas corresponding to molecules that contain up to 35 rings and/or double bonds (r + d, Sect. 6.4.4). Homologous series can be identified along straight lines. Still this does not tell the complete structure of those molecules, but it delivers much more insight into the composition of DOM than pure accurate mass data alone.

3.10 Vantage Point on the World of Isotopes and Masses

Isotopes

Atoms belonging to the same element but different in mass due to a different number of neutrons in their nuclei are termed isotopes. Most elements occur naturally in two or three isotopes, others are monoisotopic and many are polyisotopic.

Isotopic Patterns

Mass spectrometry resolves matter by mass, and thus, separates atoms and molecules of different isotopic composition due to their difference in mass.

Consequently, the isotopic distribution is reflected by a mass spectrum as a set of peaks at neighboring *m/z* values.

Resolution
Separation of peaks relies on the ability of a mass spectrometer to resolve the signals corresponding to individual masses by virtue of its resolving power. Higher resolution provides additional information as species close in *m/z* can be separated in the spectrum. High resolution also results in more narrow peaks that can potentially be located more accurately on the *m/z* scale.

Accurate Mass
Accurate mass enables the assignment of molecular formulas due to the individual exact isotopic masses and the resulting distinguished masses of ions of given elemental composition. Besides sufficient resolving power to deliver sharp peaks, accurate mass measurements require careful mass calibration. Mass calibration can either be performed externally, i.e., prior to the analytical measurement, or internally by simultaneous admission of analyte and reference.

Ultrahigh Resolving Power
At ultrahigh resolving power, isotopic fine structure is resolved and different isotopic compositions of equal nominal mass, i.e., isotopolog ions, become separated. In addition, isobaric ions of different molecular formulas as present in complex mixtures become separated. Ultrahigh resolving power is therefore useful, or even a prerequisite, to analyze complex mixtures by MS.

Global Relevance of Mass Spectrometry
Understanding isotopic compositions of the elements, the way they are causing isotopic distributions and how they become expressed as isotopic patterns in mass spectra is absolutely essential for any use of mass spectral data. This also applies to accurate masses and the process of their translation into molecular formulas.

References

1. de Laeter JR, De Bièvre P, Peiser HS (1992) Isotope Mass Spectrometry in Metrology. Mass Spectrom Rev 11:193–245. doi:10.1002/mas.1280110303
2. Audi G (2006) The History of Nuclidic Masses and of Their Evaluation. Int J Mass Spectrom 251:85–94. doi:10.1016/j.ijms.2006.01.048
3. Budzikiewicz H, Grigsby RD (2006) Mass Spectrometry and Isotopes: A Century of Research and Discussion. Mass Spectrom Rev 25:146–157. doi:10.1002/mas.20061
4. Todd JFJ (1995) Recommendations for Nomenclature and Symbolism for Mass Spectroscopy Including an Appendix of Terms Used in Vacuum Technology. Int J Mass Spectrom Ion Proc 142:211–240. doi:10.1016/0168-1176(95)93811-F
5. McLafferty FW, Turecek F (1993) Interpretation of Mass Spectra. University Science Books, Mill Valley
6. Sparkman OD (2006) Mass Spectrometry Desk Reference. Global View Publishing, Pittsburgh
7. IUPAC (1998) Isotopic Composition of the Elements 1997. Pure Appl Chem 70:217–235

8. IUPAC, Coplen TP (2001) Atomic Weights of the Elements 1999. Pure Appl Chem 73:667–683
9. Price P (1991) Standard Definitions of Terms Relating to Mass Spectrometry. A Report From the Committee on Measurements and Standards of the Amercian Society for Mass Spectrometry. J Am Soc Mass Spectrom 2:336–348. doi:10.1016/1044-0305(91)80025-3
10. Busch KL (2001) Units in Mass Spectrometry. Spectroscopy 16:28–31
11. Platzner IT (1997) Applications of isotope ratio mass spectrometry. In: Modern Isotope Ratio Mass Spectrometry. Wiley, Chichester
12. Ferrer I, Thurman EM (2005) Measuring the Mass of an Electron by LC/TOF-MS: A Study of "Twin Ions". Anal Chem 77:3394–3400. doi:10.1021/ac0485942
13. Ferrer I, Thurman EM (2007) Importance of the Electron Mass in the Calculations of Exact Mass by Time-of-Flight Mass Spectrometry. Rapid Commun Mass Spectrom 21:2538–2539. doi:10.1002/rcm.3102
14. Schmidt HL (1986) Food Quality Control and Studies on Human Nutrition by Mass Spectrometric and Nuclear Magnetic Resonance Isotope Ratio Determination. Fresenius Z Anal Chem 324:760–766. doi:10.1007/BF00468387
15. Beavis RC (1993) Chemical Mass of Carbon in Proteins. Anal Chem 65:496–497. doi:10.1021/ac00052a030
16. Carle R (1991) Isotopen-Massenspektrometrie: Grundlagen und Anwendungsmöglichkeiten. Pharm Unserer Zeit 20:75–82. doi:10.1002/pauz.19910200208
17. Ghosh P, Brand WA (2003) Stable Isotope Ratio Mass Spectrometry in Global Climate Change Research. Int J Mass Spectrom 228:1–33. doi:10.1016/S1387-3806(03)00289-6
18. Förstel H (2007) The Natural Fingerprint of Stable Isotopes-Use of IRMS to Test Food Authenticity. Anal Bioanal Chem 388:541–544. doi:10.1007/s00216-007-1241-z
19. Zazzo A, Monahan FJ, Moloney AP, Green S, Schmidt O (2011) Sulphur Isotopes in Animal Hair Track Distance to Sea. Rapid Commun Mass Spectrom 25:2371–2378. doi:10.1002/rcm.5131
20. Busch KL (1997) Isotopes and Mass Spectrometry. Spectroscopy 12:22–26
21. Beynon JH (1960) The compilation of a table of mass and abundance values. In: Mass Spectrometry and Its Applications to Organic Chemistry. Elsevier, Amsterdam
22. Margrave JL, Polansky RB (1962) Relative Abundance Calculations for Isotopic Molecular Species. J Chem Educ 39:335–337. doi:10.1021/ed039p335
23. Yergey JA (1983) A General Approach to Calculating Isotopic Distributions for Mass Spectrometry. Int J Mass Spectrom Ion Phys 52:337–349. doi:10.1016/0020-7381(83)85053-0
24. Hsu CS (1984) Diophantine Approach to Isotopic Abundance Calculations. Anal Chem 56:1356–1361. doi:10.1021/ac00272a035
25. Kubinyi H (1991) Calculation of Isotope Distributions in Mass Spectrometry. A Trivial Solution for a Non-Trivial Problem. Anal Chim Acta 247:107–119. doi:10.1016/S0003-2670(00)83059-7
26. https://sites.google.com/site/isoproms/home
27. http://www.sisweb.com/mstools/isotope.htm
28. Frauenkron M, Berkessel A, Gross JH (1997) Analysis of Ruthenium Carbonyl-Porphyrin Complexes: a Comparison of Matrix-Assisted Laser Desorption/Ionization Time-of-Flight, Fast-Atom Bombardment and Field Desorption Mass Spectrometry. Eur Mass Spectrom 3:427–438. doi:10.1255/ejms.177
29. Giesa S, Gross JH, Hull WE, Lebedkin S, Gromov A, Krätschmer W, Gleiter R (1999) $C_{120}OS$: the First Sulfur-Containing Dimeric [60]Fullerene Derivative. Chem Commun:465–466. doi:10.1039/a809831j
30. Luffer DR, Schram KH (1990) Electron Ionization Mass Spectrometry of Synthetic C_{60}. Rapid Commun Mass Spectrom 4:552–556. doi:10.1002/rcm.1290041218
31. Srivastava SK, Saunders W (1993) Ionization of C_{60} (Buckminsterfullerene) by Electron Impact. Rapid Commun Mass Spectrom 7:610–613. doi:10.1002/rcm.1290070711
32. Scheier P, Dünser B, Märk TD (1995) Production and Stability of Multiply-Charged C_{60}. Electrochem Soc Proc 95:1378–1394

33. Thomas AF (1971) Deuterium Labeling in Organic Chemistry. Appleton-Century-Crofts, New York
34. Kaltashov IA, Eyles SJ (2005) Mass Spectrometry in Biophysics: Conformation and Dynamics of Biomolecules. Wiley, Hoboken
35. Murray KK, Boyd RK, Eberlin MN, Langley GJ, Li L, Naito Y (2013) Definitions of Terms Relating to Mass Spectrometry (IUPAC Recommendations 2013). Pure Appl Chem 85:1515–1609. doi:10.1351/PAC-REC-06-04-06
36. Balogh MP (2004) Debating Resolution and Mass Accuracy in Mass Spectrometry. Spectroscopy 19:34–38,40
37. Bristow AWT (2006) Accurate Mass Measurement for the Determination of Elemental Formula – A Tutorial. Mass Spectrom Rev 25:99–111. doi:10.1002/mas.20058
38. Leslie AD, Volmer DA (2007) Dealing With the Masses: A Tutorial on Accurate Masses, Mass Uncertainties, and Mass Defects. Spectroscopy 22:32,34–32,39
39. Busch KL (2000) The Resurgence of Exact Mass Measurement With FTMS. Spectroscopy 15:22–27
40. Beynon JH (1954) Qualitative Analysis of Organic Compounds by Mass Spectrometry. Nature 174:735–737. doi:10.1038/174735a0
41. Pomerantz SC, McCloskey JA (1987) Fractional Mass Values of Large Molecules. Org Mass Spectrom 22:251–253. doi:10.1002/oms.1210220505
42. Boyd RK, Basic C, Bethem RA (2008) Trace Quantitative Analysis by Mass Spectrometry. Wiley, Chichester
43. Kilburn KD, Lewis PH, Underwood JG, Evans S, Holmes J, Dean M (1979) Quality of Mass and Intensity Measurements from a High Performance Mass Spectrometer. Anal Chem 51:1420–1425. doi:10.1021/ac50045a017
44. Sack TM, Lapp RL, Gross ML, Kimble BJ (1984) A Method for the Statistical Evaluation of Accurate Mass Measurement Quality. Int J Mass Spectrom Ion Proc 61:191–213. doi:10.1016/0168-1176(84)85129-0
45. Kim S, Rodgers RP, Marshall AG (2006) Truly "Exact" Mass: Elemental Composition Can Be Determined Uniquely from Molecular Mass Measurement at Approximately 0.1 MDa Accuracy for Molecules Up to Approximately 500 Da. Int J Mass Spectrom 251:260–265. doi:10.1016/j.ijms.2006.02.001
46. Zubarev RA, Demirev PA, Håkansson P, Sundqvist BUR (1995) Approaches and Limits for Accurate Mass Characterization of Large Biomolecules. Anal Chem 67:3793–3798. doi:10.1021/ac00116a028
47. Zubarev RA, Håkansson P, Sundqvist B (1996) Accuracy Requirements for Peptide Characterization by Monoisotopic Molecular Mass Measurements. Anal Chem 68:4060–4063. doi:10.1021/ac9604651
48. Clauser KR, Baker P, Burlingame A (1999) Role of Accurate Mass Measurement ($\pm$10 ppm) in Protein Identification Strategies Employing MS or MS/MS and Database Searching. Anal Chem 71:2871–2882. doi:10.1021/ac9810516
49. Spengler B (2004) De Novo Sequencing, Peptide Composition Analysis, and Composition-Based Sequencing: A New Strategy Employing Accurate Mass Determination by Fourier Transform Ion Cyclotron Resonance Mass Spectrometry. J Am Soc Mass Spectrom 15:703–714. doi:10.1016/j.jasms.2004.01.007
50. Roussis SG, Proulx R (2003) Reduction of Chemical Formulas from the Isotopic Peak Distributions of High-Resolution Mass Spectra. Anal Chem 75:1470–1482. doi:10.1021/ac020516w
51. Stoll N, Schmidt E, Thurow K (2006) Isotope Pattern Evaluation for the Reduction of Elemental Compositions Assigned to High-Resolution Mass Spectral Data from Electrospray Ionization Fourier Transform Ion Cyclotron Resonance Mass Spectrometry. J Am Soc Mass Spectrom 17:1692–1699. doi:10.1016/j.jasms.2006.07.022
52. Marshall AG, Hendrickson CL, Shi SDH (2002) Scaling MS Plateaus with High-Resolution FT-ICR-MS. Anal Chem 74:252A–259A. doi:10.1021/ac022010j

53. Sim PG, Boyd RK (1991) Calibration and Mass Measurement in Negative-Ion Fast-Atom Bombardment Mass Spectrometry. Rapid Commun Mass Spectrom 5:538–542. doi:10.1002/rcm.1290051111
54. Anacleto JF, Pleasance S, Boyd RK (1992) Calibration of Ion Spray Mass Spectra Using Cluster Ions. Org Mass Spectrom 27:660–666. doi:10.1002/oms.1210270603
55. Hop CECA (1996) Generation of High Molecular Weight Cluster Ions by Electrospray Ionization; Implications for Mass Calibration. J Mass Spectrom 31:1314–1316. doi:10.1002/(SICI)1096-9888(199611)31:11<1314::AID-JMS429>3.0.CO;2-N
56. Moini M, Jones BL, Rogers RM, Jiang L (1998) Sodium Trifluoroacetate as a Tune/Calibration Compound for Positive- and Negative-Ion Electrospray Ionization Mass Spectrometry in the Mass Range of 100–4000 Da. J Am Soc Mass Spectrom 9:977–980. doi:10.1016/S1044-0305(98)00079-8
57. Lou X, van Dongen JLJ, Meijer EW (2010) Generation of CsI Cluster Ions for Mass Calibration in Matrix-Assisted Laser Desorption/Ionization Mass Spectrometry. J Am Soc Mass Spectrom 21:1223–1226. doi:10.1016/j.jasms.2010.02.029
58. Gross JH (2014) High-Mass Cluster Ions of Ionic Liquids in Positive-Ion and Negative-Ion DART-MS and Their Application for Wide Range Mass Calibrations. Anal Bioanal Chem 406:2853–2862. doi:10.1007/s00216-014-7720-0
59. Busch KL (2004) Masses in Mass Spectrometry: Balancing the Analytical Scales. Spectroscopy 19:32–34
60. Busch KL (2005) Masses in Mass Spectrometry: Perfluors and More. Part II. Spectroscopy 20:76–81
61. Gross ML (1994) Accurate Masses for Structure Confirmation. J Am Soc Mass Spectrom 5:57. doi:10.1016/1044-0305(94)85036-4
62. Bristow AWT, Webb KS (2003) Intercomparison Study on Accurate Mass Measurement of Small Molecules in Mass Spectrometry. J Am Soc Mass Spectrom 14:1086–1098. doi:10.1016/S1044-0305(03)00403-3
63. Pluskal T, Uehara T, Yanagida M (2012) Highly Accurate Chemical Formula Prediction Tool Utilizing High-Resolution Mass Spectra, MS/MS Fragmentation, Heuristic Rules, and Isotope Pattern Matching. Anal Chem 84:4396–4403. doi:10.1021/ac3000418
64. Thurman EM, Ferrer I (2010) The Isotopic Mass Defect: a Tool for Limiting Molecular Formulas by Accurate Mass. Anal Bioanal Chem 397:2807–2816. doi:10.1007/s00216-010-3562-6
65. Gross JH (2013) Polydimethylsiloxane-Based Wide Range Mass Calibration for Direct Analysis in Real Time Mass Spectrometry. Anal Bioanal Chem 405:8663–8668. doi:10.1007/s00216-013-7287-1
66. Gross JH (2015) Polydimethylsiloxane Extraction from Silicone Rubber into Baked Goods Detected by Direct Analysis in Real Time Mass Spectrometry. Eur J Mass Spectrom 21:313–319. doi:10.1255/ejms.1333
67. Yergey J, Heller D, Hansen G, Cotter RJ, Fenselau C (1983) Isotopic Distributions in Mass Spectra of Large Molecules. Anal Chem 55:353–356. doi:10.1021/ac00253a037
68. Werlen RC (1994) Effect of Resolution on the Shape of Mass Spectra of Proteins: Some Theoretical Considerations. Rapid Commun Mass Spectrom 8:976–980. doi:10.1002/rcm.1290081214
69. Solouki T, Emmet MR, Guan S, Marshall AG (1997) Detection, Number, and Sequence Location of Sulfur-Containing Amino Acids and Disulfide Bridges in Peptides by Ultrahigh-Resolution MALDI-FTICR Mass Spectrometry. Anal Chem 69:1163–1168. doi:10.1021/ac960885q
70. Nikolaev EN, Jertz R, Grigoryev A, Baykut G (2012) Fine Structure in Isotopic Peak Distributions Measured Using a Dynamically Harmonized Fourier Transform Ion Cyclotron Resonance Cell at 7 T. Anal Chem 84:2275–2283. doi:10.1021/ac202804f
71. Popov IA, Nagornov K, Vladimirov GN, Kostyukevich YI, Nikolaev EN (2014) Twelve Million Resolving Power on 4.7 T Fourier Transform Ion Cyclotron Resonance Instrument

With Dynamically Harmonized Cell-Observation of Fine Structure in Peptide Mass Spectra. J Am Soc Mass Spectrom 25:790–799. doi:10.1007/s13361-014-0846-7

72. Matsuo T, Sakurai T, Ito H, Wada Y (1991) High Masses. Int J Mass Spectrom Ion Proc 118 (119):635–659. doi:10.1016/0168-1176(92)85079-F
73. Grayson SM, Myers BK, Bengtsson J, Malkoch M (2014) Advantages of Monodisperse and Chemically Robust "SpheriCal" Polyester Dendrimers as a "Universal" MS Calibrant. J Am Soc Mass Spectrom 25:303–309. doi:10.1007/s13361-013-0777-8
74. Gross JH (2016) Improved Procedure for Dendrimer-Based Mass Calibration in Matrix-Assisted Laser Desorption/Ionization-Time-of-Flight–Mass Spectrometry. Anal Bioanal Chem 408:5945–5951. doi:10.1007/s00216-016-9714-6
75. Lehmann WD, Bohne A, von der Lieth CW (2000) The Information Encrypted in Accurate Peptide Masses – Improved Protein Identification and Assistance in Glycopeptide Identification and Characterization. J Mass Spectrom 35:1335–1341. doi:10.1002/1096-9888(200011)35:11<1335::AID-JMS70>3.0.CO;2-0
76. Kendrick E (1963) Mass Scale Based on $CH_2 = 14.0000$ for High-Resolution Mass Spectrometry of Organic Compounds. Anal Chem 35:2146–2154. doi:10.1021/ac60206a048
77. Hughey CA, Hendrickson CL, Rodgers RP, Marshall AG, Qian K (2001) Kendrick Mass Defect Spectrum: A Compact Visual Analysis for Ultrahigh-Resolution Broadband Mass Spectra. Anal Chem 73:4676–4681. doi:10.1021/ac010560w
78. Jobst KJ, Shen L, Reiner EJ, Taguchi VY, Helm PA, McCrindle R, Backus S (2013) The Use of Mass Defect Plots for the Identification of (Novel) Halogenated Contaminants in the Environment. Anal Bioanal Chem 405:3289–3297. doi:10.1007/s00216-013-6735-2
79. Myers AL, Jobst KJ, Mabury SA, Reiner EJ (2014) Using Mass Defect Plots As a Discovery Tool to Identify Novel Fluoropolymer Thermal Decomposition Products. J Mass Spectrom 49:291–296. doi:10.1002/jms.3340
80. Ibanez C, Simo C, Garcia-Canas V, Acunha T, Cifuentes A (2015) The Role of Direct High-Resolution Mass Spectrometry in Foodomics. Anal Bioanal Chem 407:6275–6287. doi:10.1007/s00216-015-8812-1
81. Fouquet T, Sato H (2016) Convenient Visualization of High-Resolution Tandem Mass Spectra of Synthetic Polymer Ions Using Kendrick Mass Defect Analysis – The Case of Polysiloxanes. Rapid Commun Mass Spectrom 30:1361–1364. doi:10.1002/rcm.7560
82. Hughey CA, Hendrickson CL, Rodgers RP, Marshall AG (2001) Elemental Composition Analysis of Processed and Unprocessed Diesel Fuel by Electrospray Ionization Fourier Transform Ion Cyclotron Resonance Mass Spectrometry. Energy & Fuels 15:1186–1193. doi:10.1021/ef010028b
83. van Krevelen DW (1950) Graphical-Statistical Method for the Study of Structure and Reaction Processes of Coal. Fuel 29:269–284
84. Wu Z, Rodgers RP, Marshall AG (2004) Two- and Three-Dimensional Van Krevelen Diagrams: A Graphical Analysis Complementary to the Kendrick Mass Plot for Sorting Elemental Compositions of Complex Organic Mixtures Based on Ultrahigh-Resolution Broadband Fourier Transform Ion Cyclotron Resonance Mass Measurements. Anal Chem 76:2511–2516. doi:10.1021/ac0355449
85. Kim S, Kramer RW, Hatcher PG (2003) Graphical Method for Analysis of Ultrahigh-Resolution Broadband Mass Spectra of Natural Organic Matter, the Van Krevelen Diagram. Anal Chem 75:5336–5344. doi:10.1021/ac034415p
86. Hertkorn N, Benner R, Frommberger M, Schmitt-Kopplin P, Witt M, Kaiser K, Kettrup A, Hedges JI (2006) Characterization of a Major Refractory Component of Marine Dissolved Organic Matter. Geochim Cosmochim Acta 70:2990–3010. doi:10.1016/j.gca.2006.03.021
87. Dittmar T, Koch BP (2006) Thermogenic Organic Matter Dissolved in the Abyssal Ocean. Marine Chem 102:208–217. doi:10.1016/j.marchem.2006.04.003
88. Koch BP, Dittmar T (2005) From Mass to Structure: an Aromaticity Index for High-Resolution Mass Data of Natural Organic Matter. Rapid Commun Mass Spectrom 20:926–932. doi:10.1002/rcm.2386

Instrumentation

4

Learning Objectives

- Separating ions by *m*/*z* – basic principles
- Mass analyzers as designed from basic principles
- Types of mass analyzers and their modes of operation
- Guiding, collimating, and focusing ions along a path
- Hybrid instruments including ion mobility-mass spectrometry
- Detectors for mass-analyzed ions
- Vacuum generation for mass spectrometry
- Ability to judge fitness for purpose of commercial instruments

"A modern mass spectrometer is constructed from elements which approach the state-of-the-art in solid-state electronics, vacuum systems, magnet design, precision machining, and computerized data acquisition and processing" [1]. This statement published in 1979 has always been and still is absolutely true in the context of mass spectrometers.

Under the headline of instrumentation we shall mainly discuss the different types of mass analyzers in order to understand their basic principles of operation, their specific properties, and their performance characteristics. The order of treatment in this chapter neither reflects their ever-changing individual predominance in mass spectrometry nor does it follow a strictly historic time line. Rather, an attempt is made to follow a trail of easiest understanding. Of course, this is only one aspect of instrumentation; hence topics such as ion detection and vacuum generation will also be addressed in brief. As a matter of fact, sample introduction is more closely related to particular ionization methods than to the type of mass analyzer employed, and therefore, this issue is treated in the corresponding chapters on ionization methods.

J.H. Gross, *Mass Spectrometry*, DOI 10.1007/978-3-319-54398-7_4

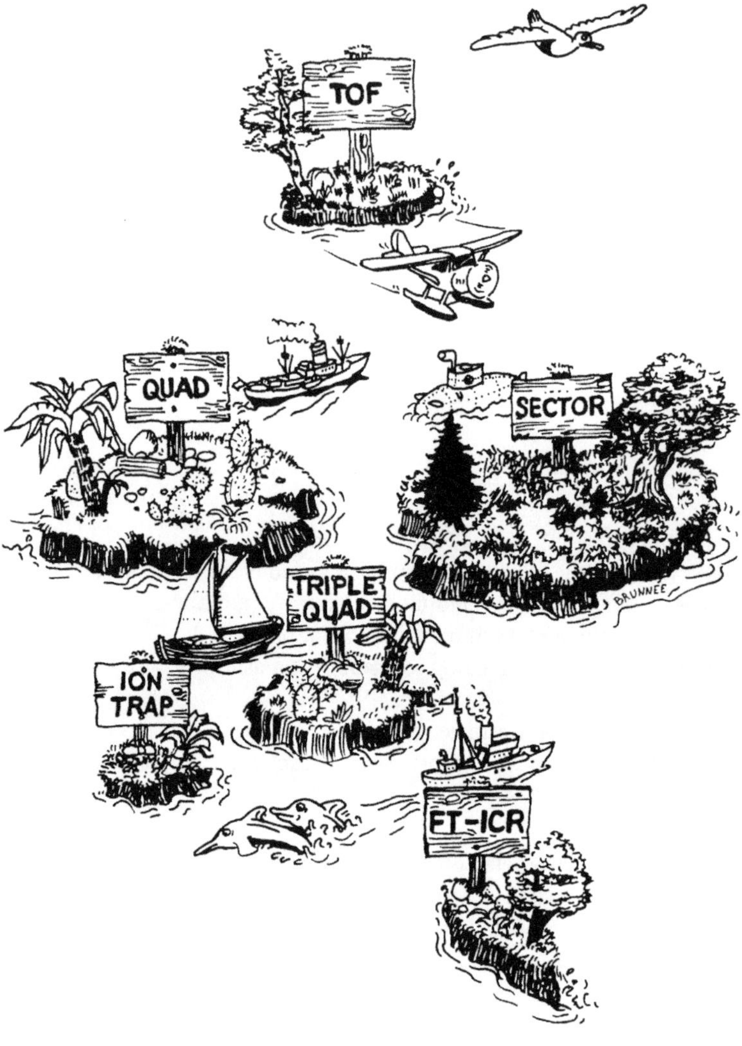

Fig. 4.1 Mass spectrometer islands as presented in a cartoon by C. Brunnée in 1987. The actual situation is quite different, however: much of the cliffs of the sector and quad islands have vanished in the sea while all others have gained new land, and moreover, the Orbitrap island has been given birth in the south east (Reproduced from Ref. [2] with permission. © Elsevier Science, 1987)

From the very beginning to the present almost any physical principle ranging from time-of-flight to cyclotron motion has been employed to construct mass-analyzing devices (Fig. 4.1). Some were extremely successful at the time of their

Table 4.1 Common mass analyzers

Type	Acronym	Principle
Time-of-flight	TOF	Time dispersion of a pulsed ion beam; separation by time-of-flight
Magnetic sector	B	Deflection of a continuous ion beam; separation by momentum in magnetic field due to Lorentz force
Linear quadrupole	Q	Continuous ion beam in linear radio frequency quadrupole field; s due to instability of ion trajectories
Linear quadrupole ion trap	LIT	Continuous ion beam delivers ions for trapping; storage, and eventually separation in linear radio frequency quadrupole field by resonant excitation
Quadrupole ion trap	QIT	Trapped ions; separation in three-dimensional radio frequency quadrupole field by resonant excitation
Fourier transform-ion cyclotron resonance	FT-ICR	Trapped ions in magnetic field (Lorentz force); separation by cyclotron frequency, image current detection and Fourier transformation of a transient signal
Orbitrap	Orbitrap	Axial oscillation in inhomogeneous electric field; detection of frequency after Fourier transformation of a transient signal

invention, for others it took decades until their potential had fully been recognized. The basic types of mass analyzers employed for analytical mass spectrometry are summarized in Table 4.1.

A comparison of Brunnée's cartoon with Table 4.1 reveals that linear ion traps and Orbitraps had not yet been invented at the time of his writing said review. An "updated version" of Brunnée's map was presented 2014 in Geneva at the International Mass Spectrometry Conference (IMSC) during the Brunnée Award lecture by Dimitris Papanastasiou (Fig. 4.2).

The properties of an ideal mass analyzer are well described [2], but despite the tremendous improvements made, still no mass analyzer is perfect. There is a wealth of articles and books that are highly recommended for those seeking a deeper look at the evolution of mass spectrometers [3–13]. In recent years, there has been a growing interest in employing miniature mass analyzers for *in situ* analysis [14, 15], for instance in environmental [16] and biochemical applications [17], for process monitoring, for detection of chemical warfare agents, and for space missions [18, 19]. The most recent completely new type of mass analyzer, the Orbitrap, was introduced in 2005 by Makarov [20].

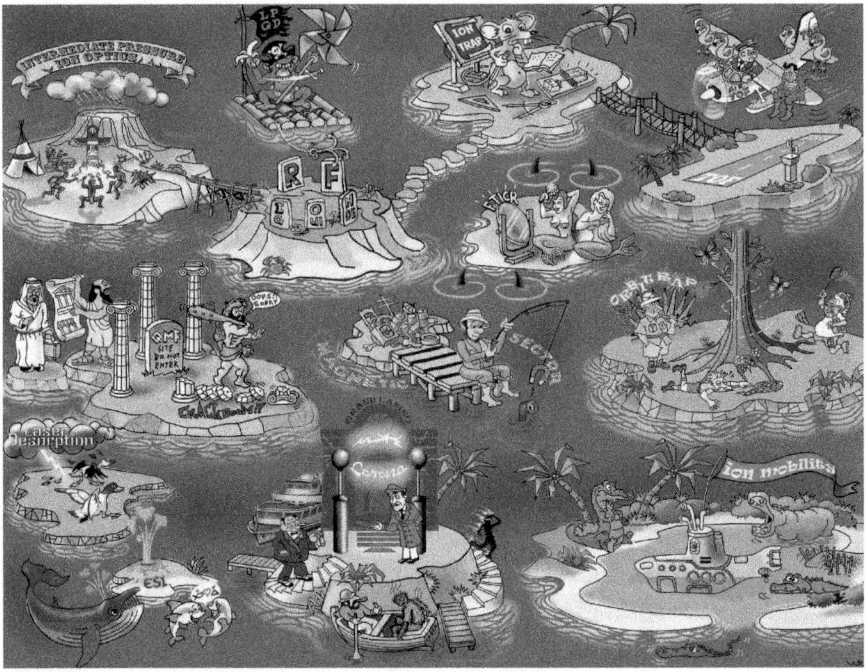

Fig. 4.2 The treasure islands of MS: The Brunnée map expanded to reflect latest advancements in mass analyzers like Orbitrap, ionization methods such as ESI, MALDI and discharge-based techniques, ion mobility spectrometry instrumentation, and the emerging role of intermediate pressure RF ion optics. Low-pressure gas dynamics (LPGD) provides a new tool for atmospheric pressure interface design. The expanded Brunnée map was presented at the IMSC 2014 Brunnée Award lecture by Dimitris Papanastasiou

4.1 How to Create a Beam of Ions

Consider an ion that is brought into or generated within an electric field between two oppositely charged plates of a capacitor. Such an ion will be accelerated towards the plate of opposite charge. If the attracting plate has a (round) orifice or a slit, an ion beam is produced by this simple ion source. Assuming the spread in ion kinetic energy to be small as compared to the total ion kinetic energy, i.e., $\Delta E_{kin} << E_{kin}$, the beam can be considered to be monoenergetic. The actual charge of an ion may be either positive or negative depending on the ionization method employed. Changing the polarity of the plates causes a switch from the extraction of positive ions to negative ions or vice versa. For practical reasons, the attracting electrode is usually grounded and the pushing plate is set to high voltage. Doing so allows to keep the entire mass analyzer grounded, thereby contributing substantially to safety of operation (Fig. 4.3). The extraction of ions and the shape of the ion beam can largely be improved if the acceleration voltage is applied in two [21] or

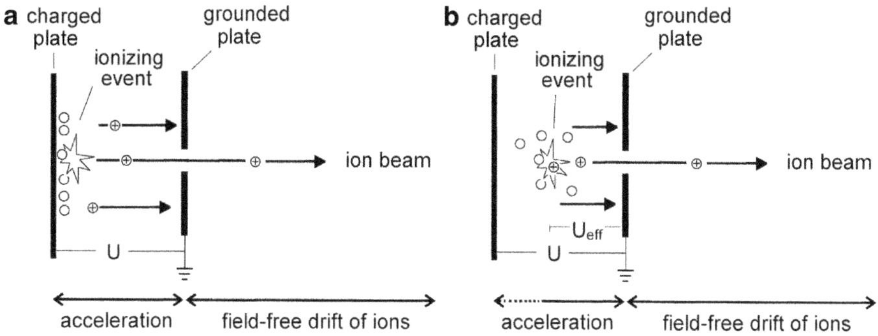

Fig. 4.3 Simple single-stage ion sources. (**a**) Ionization from a surface or probe where the ionizing event is located on the charged plate; in reality ionizing events in a spatially confined volume above the surface have to be taken into account. (**b**) Gas phase ionization, where the effective accelerating voltage U_{eff} depends on the actual position of the ion between the plates. After a neutral has been ionized (positive in this illustration), it is attracted by the opposite grounded plate. Those ions passing through a hole of the grounded electrode create an ion beam emerging into the field-free region behind. The ion beam produced by such a primitive ion source is not parallel, but has some angular spread

more successive stages instead of a single one and if ion optical lenses are part of the ion acceleration assembly.

Keep it grounded
Apart from a few exotic exceptions, all mass spectrometers are – and always have been – constructed in a way to ensure that most parts are electrically grounded. Voltage, especially because this often means high voltage, is only applied to comparatively small parts inside. This ensures safety of operation, and in addition, low capacitive load simplifies rapid DC voltage changes, enables high RF frequencies, and allows for quick polarity switching.

4.2 Time-of-Flight Instruments

4.2.1 Time-of-Flight: Basic Principles

The first *time-of-flight* (TOF) analyzer was constructed and published in 1946 by W. E. Stephens [22]. The principle of TOF is quite simple: ions of different *m*/*z* are dispersed in time during their flight along a field-free drift path of known length. Provided all the ions start their journey at the same time or at least within a sufficiently short time interval, the lighter ones will arrive earlier at the detector than the heavier ones. This demands that they emerge from a pulsed ion source

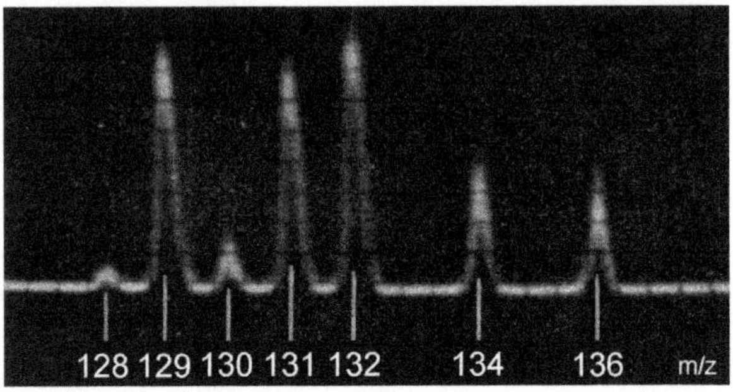

Fig. 4.4 Oscilloscope output of the electron ionization TOF spectrum of xenon on a Bendix TOF-MS. The *dark horizontal lines* are a grid on the oscilloscopic screen. (For the isotopic pattern of Xe cf. Fig. 3.2.) (Adapted from Ref. [26] with permission. © Pergamon Press, 1959)

which can be realized either by pulsing ion packages out of a continuous beam or more conveniently by employing a true pulsed ionization method.

Soon, other groups embarked on Stephens' concept [23] and increasingly useful TOF instruments were designed and constructed [21, 24, 25] leading to their first commercialization by Bendix in the mid-1950s. These first-generation TOF instruments were designed for gas chromatography-mass spectrometry (GC-MS) coupling [26, 27]. Resolution-wise, their performance was poor as compared to modern TOF analyzers, but the specific advantage of TOFs over magnetic sector instruments was the rate of spectral acquisition, i.e., the number of spectra per second they provided (Fig. 4.4). In GC-MS the TOF analyzer soon became superseded by linear quadrupole analyzers and it was not until the late 1980s that development of TOF analyzers encountered a revival [28, 29] – the success of pulsed ionization methods, especially of matrix-assisted laser desorption/ionization (MALDI), made this possible (Chap. 11). Therefore, we will repeatedly refer to MALDI in our discussion of TOF analyzers.

MALDI generated a great demand for mass analyzers which are suitable to be used in conjunction with a naturally pulsed ion source and capable of transmitting ions of extremely high mass up to several 10^5 u [30]. Since then, the performance of TOF instruments has tremendously increased [31, 32]. TOF analyzers have been adapted for use with other ionization methods and – together with Orbitraps and FT-ICR instruments – have superseded the established magnetic sector instruments in most applications [31, 33].

The main advantages of TOF instruments are:

- In principle, the *m*/*z* range of a TOF analyzer is unlimited [34, 35].
- Complete mass spectra are obtained of ions created during a short (nanoseconds) ionizing event, e.g., from a laser shot in LDI or MALDI.
- TOF analyzers offer high ion transmission and thus contribute to high sensitivity.
- The mass spectral acquisition rate of TOFs is very high, essentially $>10^3$ Hz.
- TOF instrument design and construction is comparatively straightforward.
- Modern TOF instruments allow for accurate mass measurements and tandem MS experiments [36].

4.2.2 TOF Instruments: Velocity of Ions and Time-of-Flight

Independent of the ionization method, the electric charge q of an ion of mass m_i is equal to an integer number z of electron charges e, and thus $q = ez$. The energy uptake E_{el} by moving through a voltage U is given by

$$E_{el} = qU = ezU \tag{4.1}$$

Thereby, the former potential energy of a charged particle in an electric field is converted into kinetic energy E_{kin}, i.e., into translational motion

$$E_{el} = ezU = \frac{1}{2} m_i v^2 = E_{kin} \tag{4.2}$$

Assuming that the ion was initially at rest, which holds by first approximation, the velocity attained is calculated by rearranging Eq. (4.2) into

$$v = \sqrt{\frac{2ezU}{m_i}} \tag{4.3}$$

i.e., v is inversely proportional to the square root of mass.

A racing soccer ball The velocity of the [60]fullerene molecular ion, $C_{60}^{+\bullet}$, after acceleration by 19.5 kV is obtained from Eq. (4.3) as

$$v = \sqrt{\frac{2 \cdot 1.6022 \times 10^{-19}\mathrm{C} \times 19{,}500\mathrm{V}}{1.1956 \times 10^{-24}\mathrm{kg}}} = 72{,}294\,\mathrm{m\ s^{-1}}$$

An ion velocity of 72,294 m s^{-1} appears rather high, but merely is 0.0024% of the speed of light. The acceleration voltages and thus, the ion velocities are the highest in TOF-MS, although magnetic sector instruments are operated with kilo-electron-volt ion beams, too (Sect. 4.3). The other types of mass analyzers require ions to enter at much lower kinetic energies.

Valid for any mass analyzer
Equation (4.3) describes the velocity of any ion after acceleration in an electric field, and therefore it is valid not only for TOF-MS, but for any part of a mass spectrometer handling beams of ions.

One now can quite easily imagine measuring the time for an ion of unknown m/z in traveling a distance s after being accelerated by a voltage U. The relationship between velocity and time t needed for traveling the distance s is

$$t = \frac{s}{v} \tag{4.4}$$

which upon substitution of v by Eq. (4.3) becomes

$$t = \frac{s}{\sqrt{\frac{2ezU}{m_i}}} \tag{4.5}$$

Equation (4.5) yields the time needed for the ion to travel the distance s at constant velocity, i.e., in a *field-free* environment after the process of acceleration has been completed. Rearrangement of Eq. (4.5) reveals the relationship between the instrumental parameters s and U, the experimental value of t and the ratio m_i/z

$$\frac{m_i}{z} = \frac{2\,e\,U t^2}{s^2} \tag{4.6}$$

It is also obvious from Eq. (4.5) that the time to drift through a fixed length of field-free space is proportional to the square root of m_i/z

$$t = \frac{s}{\sqrt{2eU}} \sqrt{\frac{m_i}{z}} \tag{4.7}$$

and thus, the time interval Δt between the arrival times of ions of different m/z is proportional to $s \times ((m_i/z_1)^{½} - (m_i/z_2)^{½})$.

Mass, not *m/z*
Here, the ratio m_i/z denotes ion mass [kg] per number of electron charges. The index i at the mass symbol is used to avoid confusion with the *mass-to-charge ratio*, *m/z*, as used to specify the position of a peak on the abscissa of a mass spectrum (Sect. 1.4.3).

Small differences in time-of-flight According to Eq. (4.7) the $C_{60}^{+\bullet}$ ion, *m/z* 720, dealt with in the preceding example will travel through a field-free flight path of 2.0 m in 27.665 µs, while it takes slightly longer for its isotopolog $^{13}C^{12}C_{59}^{+\bullet}$, *m/z* 721. The proportionality to the square root of *m/z* gives (use of m_i/z values yields identical results as the dimension is cancelled):

$$\frac{t_{721}}{t_{720}} = \frac{\sqrt{721}}{\sqrt{720}} = 1.000694$$

Thus, $t_{721} = 27.684$ µs. This corresponds to a difference in time-of-flight of 19 ns under these conditions (cf. Fig. 4.9).

The proportionality of time-of-flight to the square root of m/z causes Δt for a given $\Delta(m/z)$ to decrease with increasing m/z: under otherwise the same conditions Δt per 1 u is calculated as 114 ns at m/z 20, 36 ns at m/z 200, and just 11 ns at m/z 2000. Therefore, the realization of a time-of-flight mass analyzer depends on the ability to measure short time intervals with sufficient accuracy [37–39]. At this point it becomes clear that the performance of the early TOF analyzers – among other reasons – suffered from the low-efficiency electronics of their time. It took until the mid-1990s to overcome this barrier [32].

"Compressed" isotopic patterns of multiply charged ions The time-of-flight of multiply charged ions ($z > 1$) explains the position and appearance of signals caused by ions of higher charge states (Sect. 3.8). As z increases to 2, 3 etc., the numerical value of m/z is reduced by a factor of 2, 3 etc., i.e., the ion will be detected at lower m/z than the corresponding singly charged ion of the same mass. According to Eq. (4.7), the time-of-flight is reduced by a factor of 1.414 (the square root of 2) for doubly charged ions which is the same time-of-flight as for a singly-charged ion of half of its mass. Accordingly, the time-of-flight is reduced by a factor of 1.732 (the square root of 3), for triply charged ions corresponding to a single-charged ion of one third of its mass, and so on for higher charge states.

Inferring the charge state
For multiply charged ions, the m/z scale is compressed by a factor of z equal to the charge state of the ion. Isotopic patterns remain unaffected as far as the relative intensities are concerned. As $\Delta(m/z)$ between isotopic peaks is reduced inversely proportional to z, the charge state can readily be assigned, e.g., doubly charged ions cause isotopic peaks at $\Delta(m/z) = 0.5$, triply charged ions cause them at $\Delta(m/z) = 0.333$, and so on.

4.2.3 Linear Time-of-Flight Analyzer

Restricting its use to laser desorption/ionization (LDI) and matrix-assisted laser desorption/ionization (MALDI, Chap. 11), a simple TOF instrument can be set up as follows (Fig. 4.5): The analyte is supplied as a thin layer on a *sample holder* or *target* upon which a pulsed laser is focused. The acceleration voltage U is applied between this target and a grounded counter electrode. Ions formed and desorbed during the laser pulse are continuously extracted and accelerated as they emerge from the target into the gas phase. When leaving the acceleration region s_0 the ions should possess equal kinetic energies. They drift down a field-free flight path s in the order of 1–2 m and finally hit the detector. Typically, *microchannel plate* (MCP) detectors are employed to compensate for the angular spread of the ion beam (Sect. 4.12). A fast *analog-to-digital converter* (8 bit or 10 bit ADC)

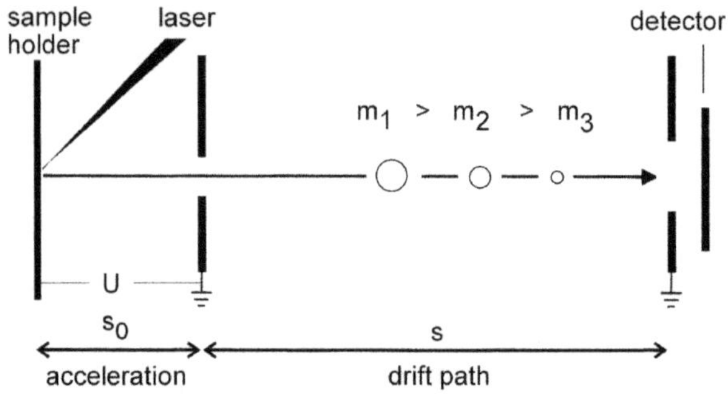

Fig. 4.5 Scheme of a linear TOF instrument designed for use in combination with a laser desorption ion source. Once created during a laser pulse onto the sample layer, ions are continuously accelerated by a voltage U. While drifting along the field-free drift path s, they are dispersed in time. Lighter ions reach the detector first

transforms the analog output of the detector for computer-based data storage and data processing. Such an instrumental setup where the ions are traveling on a straight line from the point of their creation to the detector is called *linear TOF*.

In principle, any other ionization method can be combined with a TOF analyzer even if it is not an intrinsically pulsed technique, provided there are means to extract ions in a pulsed manner from such an ion source (Sect. 4.2.6).

The drift time t_d as calculated by means of Eq. (4.7) is not fully identical to the total time-of-flight. Obviously, the time needed for acceleration of the ions t_a has to be added. Furthermore, a short period of time t_0 may be attributed to the laser pulse width and the process of desorption/ionization, which is typically in the order of a few nanoseconds. Thus, the total time-of-flight t_{total} is given by

$$t_{total} = t_0 + t_a + t_d \tag{4.8}$$

A rigorous mathematical treatment of the TOF analyzers as needed for the construction of such instruments of course has to include all contributions to the total time-of-flight [32, 36–38, 40–42].

The transmittance of a linear TOF analyzer approaches 90% because ion losses are solely caused by collisional scattering due to residual gas or by poor spatial focusing of the ion source. With a sufficiently large detector surface located at a short distance from the ion source exit, a very high fraction of the ions will be collected by the detector.

Even metastable decompositions during the flight do not reduce the intensity of a molecular ion signal, because the fragments formed conserve the velocity of the fragmenting ion and are therefore detected simultaneously with their intact precursors. In such a case, the ionic *and* the neutral fragment cause a response at the detector. These properties make the linear TOF analyzer the ideal device for analyzing easily fragmenting and/or high-mass analytes [43].

Detection of neutrals
In linear TOF analyzers, neutrals formed by metastable fragmentation also give rise to a signal. This is because they impinge on the detector after having travelled down the flight tube side-by-side with the ionic product of ion dissociation. As a result, nonfragmenting intact precursor ions plus both ionic and neutral products of the metastable dissociation of precursor ions will hit the detector simultaneously. Therefore, linear TOF analyzers are best suited for the analysis of large and labile molecules, e.g., oligonucleotides (Sect. 11.5). This presents a rare case where neutrals contribute to a useful signal in mass spectrometry.

The example in Sect. 4.2.2 demonstrates that the differences in time-of-flight of ions differing by 1 u in mass are in the order of about 10 ns at about *m/z* 1000. The time elapsing during desorption/ionization is roughly 10–50 ns in case of standard UV lasers, but can be longer with IR lasers. Consequently, the variation in starting times for ions of the same *m/z* value is often larger than the difference in time-of-flight of neighboring *m/z* values, thereby limiting the resolution.

4.2.4 Better Vacuum Improves Resolving Power

The mass resolution of a TOF analyzer is directly proportional to its total flight path length [44]. Improved vacuum conditions result in an elongated mean free path for the ions and thus reduce the risk of collisions in transit through the analyzer. The resolving power of a TOF analyzer clearly depends on the background pressure [45]. Despite improvements of resolving power in the order of a factor of two can be realized (Fig. 4.6), enhanced pumping systems alone are not able to effect a breakthrough in resolving power.

Only QITs use buffer gas
The quadrupole ion trap (Sect. 4.5) is the only type of mass analyzer that uses buffer gas to damp ion trajectories. All other mass analyzers require the highest possible vacuum for optimum performance.

4.2.5 Energy Spread of Laser-Desorbed Ions

Laser-desorbed ions possess comparatively large initial kinetic energies of some 10 eV that are superimposed on the kinetic energy provided by the acceleration voltage, which is typically in the order of 10–30 kV. Obviously, higher acceleration

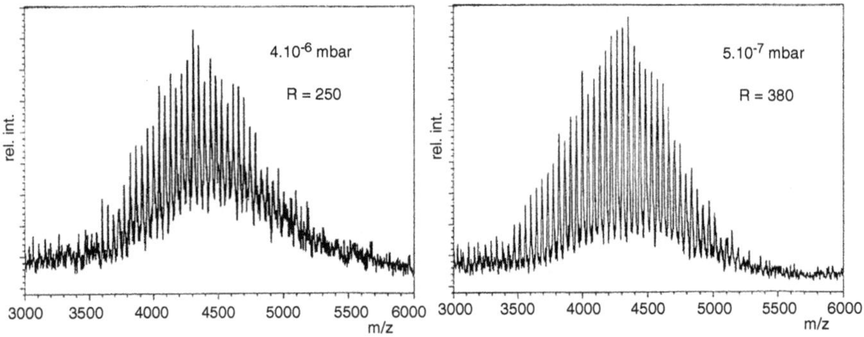

Fig. 4.6 Dependence of resolution on analyzer pressure: linear MALDI-TOF spectra of polyethylene glycol 4000 recorded at a pressure of 4×10^{-4} Pa (*left*) and 5×10^{-5} Pa (*right*) (Adapted from Ref. [45] with permission. © John Wiley & Sons, 1994)

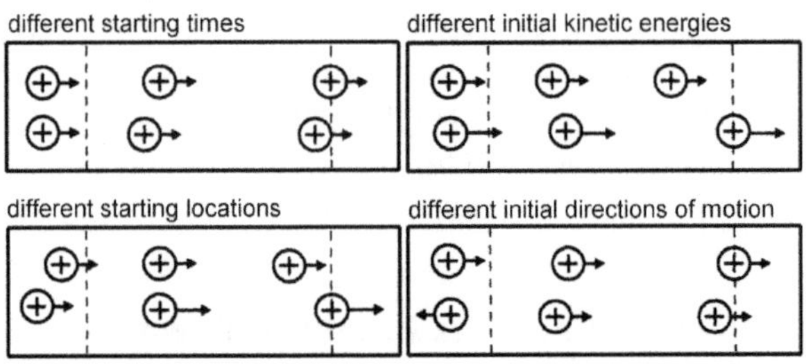

Fig. 4.7 Effects of initial time, space, and kinetic energy distributions on mass resolution in TOF-MS (Adapted from Ref. [39] with permission. © American Chemical Society, 1992)

voltages are advantageous in that they diminish the relative contribution of the energy distribution caused by the ionization process. Figure 4.7 illustrates the possible effects of deviations from the assumption that ions initially are at rest on an equipotential surface [39]. All these effects together limit resolution to $R \approx 500$ for continuous extraction linear TOF analyzers.

Bothersome energy spread

The spread in ion kinetic energies from thermal energy as well as from inhomogeneous acceleration presents a general problem in the construction of mass analyzers. Accordingly, there are numerous approaches to narrow down the kinetic energy distributions of ions or to compensate for their effects.

4.2.6 Reflector Time-of-Flight Analyzer

The *reflector* or *reflectron* was devised by Mamyrin in 1994 [46]. In the reflector TOF analyzer – often abbreviated *ReTOF* – the reflector acts as an ion mirror that focuses ions of different kinetic energies in time. Its performance is improved by using two-stage or even multistage reflector designs.

Commonly, reflector instruments are also equipped with a detector behind the reflector allowing linear mode operation simply by switching off the reflector voltage. A complete mathematical treatment of single-stage and two-stage reflectors is found in the literature [36–38, 42]. Here, we will restrict ourselves to a qualitative explanation of the reflector.

A simple reflector consist of a retarding electric field located behind the field-free drift region opposed to the ion source. In practice, a reflector is comprised of a series of ring-shaped electrodes at increasing potential. The reflection voltage U_r is set to about 1.05–1.10 times the acceleration voltage U in order to ensure that all ions are reflected within the homogeneous portion of the electric field of the device

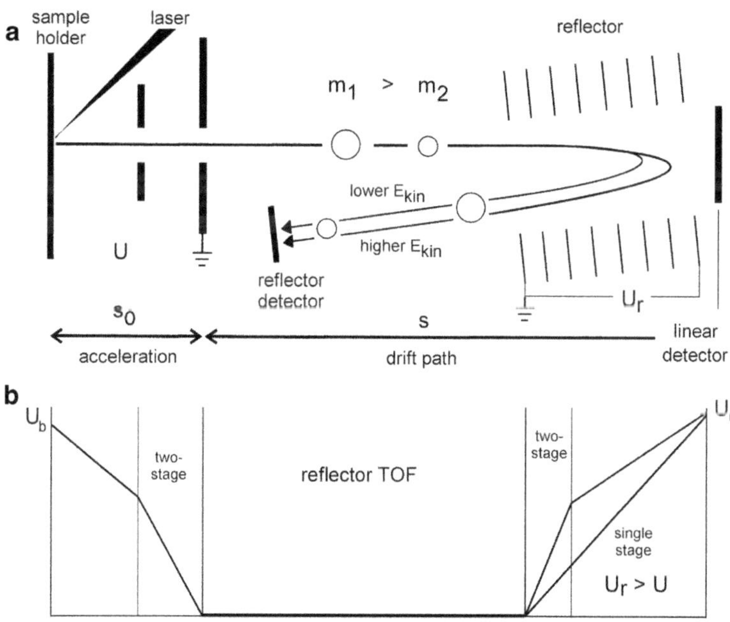

Fig. 4.8 ReTOF analyzer. (**a**) Principle of operation, (**b**) potentials along the instrument. Ions of different kinetic energy penetrate the reflector to different depths before they come to a halt and get ejected into the opposite direction. Faster ions have to travel a longer path than slower ones, and thus, time focus is achieved at some point on the return path. There, the detector receives ions of the same mass at (about) the same time. A small angle between the axis of the flight path and the reflector allows the detector to be placed beside the ion source

(Fig. 4.8). The ions penetrate the reflectron until they reach zero kinetic energy and are then expelled from the reflector in opposite direction. The kinetic energy of the leaving ions remains unaffected, however their flight paths vary according to their differences in kinetic energy. Ions carrying more kinetic energy will fly deeper into the decelerating field, and thus spend more time within the reflector than less energetic ions. Thereby, the reflector achieves a correction in time-of-flight that substantially improves the resolving power of the TOF analyzer [32, 37–39]. In addition, the reflector provides (imperfect) focusing with respect to angular spread of the ions leaving the source and it corrects for their spatial distribution [37, 46]. Adjusting the reflector at a small angle with respect to the ions exiting from the source allows the reflector–detector to be placed adjacent to the ion source (Mamyrin design). Alternatively, a detector with a central hole to transmit the ions leaving the ion source has to be used in *coaxial reflectrons* (cf. Sect. 9.5).

Although the reflector elongates the flight path and hence the dispersion in time-of-flight, this effect is of lower importance than its capability to compensate for initial energy spread. Simple elongation of the flight path can also be achieved with longer flight tubes in linear instruments. However, too long flight paths may even decrease the overall performance of TOF analyzers due to loss of ions by angular spread of the ion beam and scattering of ions after collisions with residual gas.

Nonetheless, the remarkable improvements of resolving power delivered by TOF analyzers with their very long flight paths have more recently led to the development of TOF analyzers with folded ion paths and sophisticated ion optics (Sect. 4.2.11).

The ability of the ReTOF to compensate for the initial energy spread of ions largely increases the resolving power of TOF instruments. While a typical continuous extraction TOF instrument in linear mode cannot resolve isotopic patterns of analytes above about *m*/*z* 500, it will do when operated in reflector mode (Fig. 4.9). At substantially higher *m*/*z*, the ReTOF still fails to resolve isotopic patterns, even though its resolution is still better than that of a linear TOF analyzer.

Metastable ions in a ReTOF

In case of metastable fragmentations, ReTOF analyzers behave differently from linear TOF analyzers. If fragmentation occurs between ion source and reflector, the ions will be lost by the reflector due to their change in kinetic energy. Transmission occurs only for fragments still having kinetic energies close to that of the precursor due to the energy tolerance of the reflector, as, for instance, $[M + H–NH_3]^+$ in case of a peptide of about *m*/*z* 2000. However, such ions are not detected at correct *m*/*z*, thereby giving rise to a "tailing" of the signal. Ions fragmenting in transit from reflector to detector are treated the same way as ions in the linear TOF. Thus, the elongated flight path of the ReTOF analyzer also allows more time for fragmentation. This can complicate the detection of very labile analytes in reflector mode.

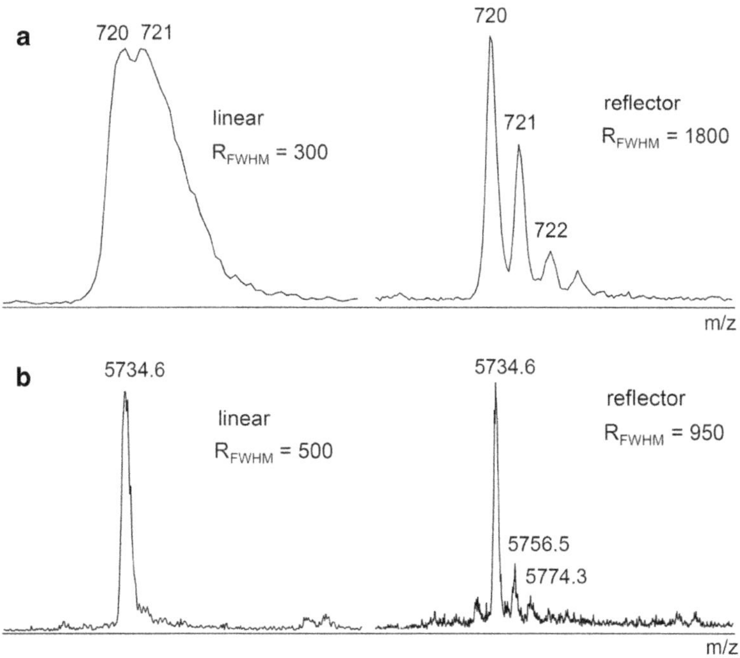

Fig. 4.9 C_{60} molecular ion signal of at *m/z* 720 (**a**) and the $[M + H]^+$ ion signal of bovine insulin, *m/z* 5734.6 (**b**), as obtained on a TOF instrument in linear mode (*left*) and reflector mode (*right*). All other experimental parameters remained unchanged

4.2.7 Delay Before Extraction to Improve Resolving Power

In MALDI-TOF-MS, the energy spread of the emerging ions is of significant magnitude as a result of the MALDI process, which in addition, creates a temporal distribution of ion formation. The most successful approach of handling such conditions is presented by ion sources allowing a delay between generation and extraction/acceleration of the ions. *Time-lag focusing* dates back to 1955 [21] and since then has been adapted to the needs of MALDI-TOF-MS by several groups [47–50].

The advantage of pulsed acceleration is its capability to focus the ions in time thereby reducing the effect of initial position and initial velocity on resolution. In addition, the delay permits the plume generated upon laser irradiation to disperse while still in a field-free region prior to acceleration. This avoids collisions of energetic ions with neutrals in the initially dense plume that could broaden the translational energy distribution and cause fragmentation due to CID (Sect. 9.3). Continuous extraction MALDI ion sources had to be operated with laser fluences close to the threshold for ion formation in order not to sacrifice the limited resolution any further. With pulsed acceleration, this effect is greatly reduced.

After allowing the ions to separate in space according to their different initial velocities during a delay of some hundreds of nanoseconds the acceleration voltage is switched on with a fast pulse. This procedure also ensures that laser-induced reactions have terminated before ion acceleration begins. A delay of about 200 ns was empirically found to be required to realize the desired effect [36, 42].

Longer delays allow to achieve very high resolving power at the focused mass, but outside the optimized m/z range resolution remains limited. More recently, the so-called *panoramic pulsed ion extraction* (PAN) was introduced (Bruker Daltonik) that makes use of a time-modulated extraction pulse to stretch the optimum resolution over a wide m/z range.

Many names

Unfortunately, establishing patents and trademarks has caused redundant names for almost the same thing: *time lag focusing* (TLF, Micromass); *delayed extraction* (DE, Applied Biosystems); *pulsed ion extraction* (PIE), and more recently *panoramic pulsed ion extraction* (PAN, Bruker Daltonik).

Using a two-stage acceleration ion source allows the electric field between target (repeller) and extraction plate P_1 to be varied. The remaining fraction of the acceleration voltage is applied in the second stage. At the onset of extraction, ions with high initial velocities have traveled farther than slower ones, and therefore experience only a fraction of the extraction voltage dV between target and extraction plate P_1. The voltage of the second stage is the same for all ions. As a result, the fastest ions receive less energy from the accelerating field than the slowest. Thereby, such ion sources compensate for the initial energy distribution [50].

The optimum settings of the delay time and of the ratio of pulsed to fixed voltage (V_1/V_2) depend on m/z with a tendency towards longer delays and/or a larger V_1/V_2 ratio for heavier ions. In practice, the variation of potentials in pulsed ion extraction with time can be handled as follows (Fig. 4.10): target and extraction plate P_1 are maintained at the same potential during the delay time, thereby creating a field-free region d_1. After the delay has passed, P_1 switches from V_1 by a variable value dV to V_2 causing extraction of the ions.

Impressive gain in resolving power Regardless of the manufacturer of the hardware, the effect of a time lag on resolution is quite dramatic. The resolving power of linear instruments is improved by a factor of 3–4 and reflector instruments become better by a factor of about 2–3 [50]. The advantages are obvious by comparison of MALDI-TOF spectra of substance P, a low mass peptide, as obtained in continuous extraction mode and after PIE upgrade of the same instrument (Fig. 4.11). Modern mid-class MALDI-TOF instruments easily deliver twice that resolution.

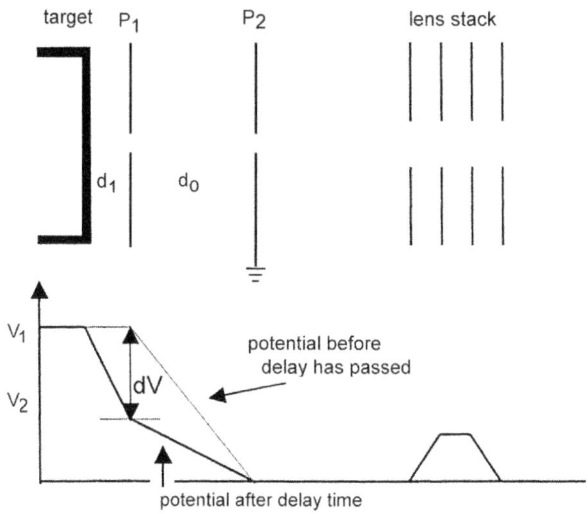

Fig. 4.10 Variation of potentials in pulsed ion extraction with time. The lens stack acts as angular focusing device for the ion beam (By courtesy of Bruker Daltonik, Bremen)

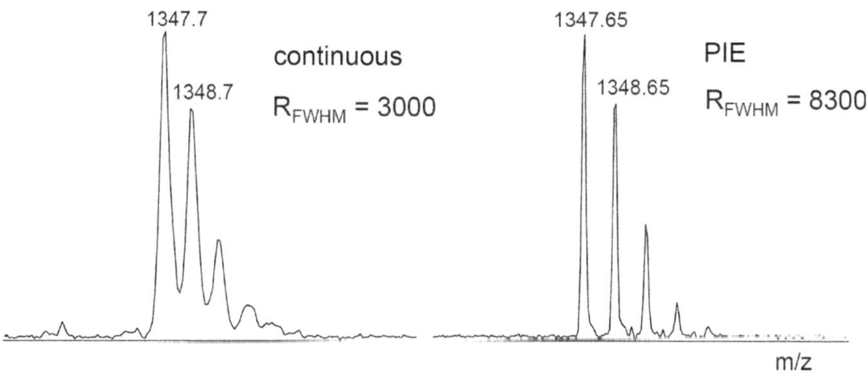

Fig. 4.11 MALDI-TOF spectra of substance P, a low-mass peptide, as obtained from a Bruker Biflex ReTOF in continuous extraction reflector mode (in 1995, *left*) and after PIE upgrade of this instrument (in 2001, *right*)

4.2.8 Orthogonal Acceleration TOF Analyzers

Up to here, the TOF analyzer has been under consideration bearing MALDI-TOF equipment in mind, just because MALDI as a pulsed ionization method delivers ions to a TOF analyzer in an ideal manner. In fact, MALDI initiated such tremendous improvements of TOF analyzers that it became attractive to combine these compact but powerful analyzers with other, inherently nonpulsed, ionization methods. The major breakthrough for generalized use of TOF analyzers arose from the design of the *orthogonal acceleration* TOF analyzer (oaTOF). In an

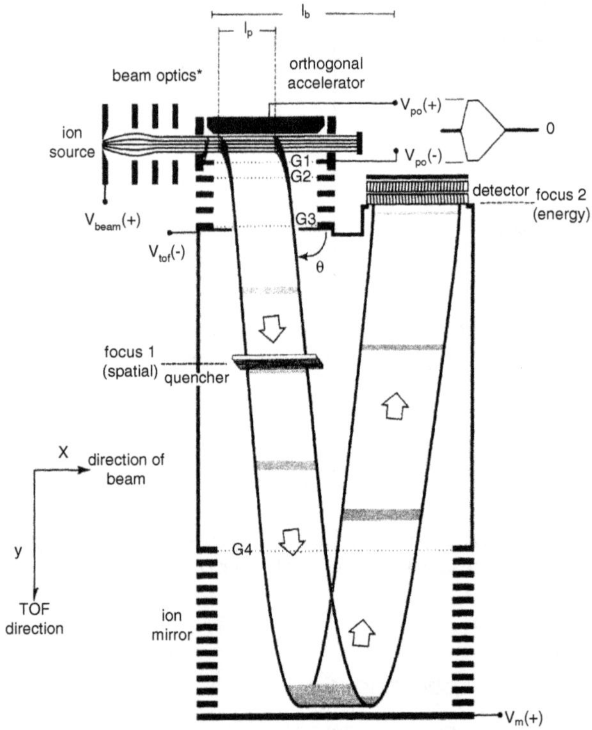

Fig. 4.12 An orthogonal acceleration reflector TOF instrument. See text for discussion (Reproduced from Ref. [55] by permission. © John Wiley & Sons, 2000)

oaTOF analyzer, pulses of ions are extracted orthogonally from a continuous ion beam (Fig. 4.12) [51, 52]. The oaTOF analyzer can be of linear or ReTOF type. Although different problems have to be overcome for each ionization method, the oaTOF analyzer is in principle suited for any of them [29, 53–55].

The main advantages of oaTOF analyzers are:

- High sensitivity due to good duty cycle and high transmission of TOF analyzers.
- High spectral acquisition rate (spectra per second) even after pre-averaging.
- High mass-resolving power.
- Mass accuracies as good as 1 ppm for formula determination.
- Compact design and small footprint.

Therefore, it is not astonishing that oaTOF instruments are currently widespread in use for numerous kinds of applications. Electrospray ionization (ESI) oaTOF instruments with accurate mass capabilities represent the majority of these systems [56–58], but gas chromatography–mass spectrometry (GC-MS) instruments are also available. In particular for *fast GC* applications [59, 60] and for HR-GC-MS [61] oaTOF systems are advantageous. Today, a large portion of the instruments incorporating oaTOF analyzers are hybrids mostly of the quadrupole-oaTOF type. We will therefore deal with them in the section on hybrid instruments.

4.2.9 Operation of the oaTOF Analyzer

Ions leaving the ion source are focused to form an almost parallel ion beam, i.e., to minimize ion motion orthogonal to the ion beam axis. Then, the ion beam enters the orthogonal accelerator (x-axis) [29, 53, 55]. The ion kinetic energy in this beam is only in the range of 10–20 eV. A package of ions of length l_p is pushed out orthogonally from its initial direction by a sharp pulse, and is thus accelerated into the TOF analyzer (y-axis) by a voltage of 5–10 kV. From the TOF analyzer's point of view the orthogonal acceleration unit can be regarded as the ion source. Usually, ions are accelerated through a two-stage setup analogous to the Wiley-McLaren ion source [21].

The design of the TOF analyzer itself is similar to those discussed before, but its diameter is much wider because the velocity of the ions in x-direction, v_{beam}, is not affected by the orthogonal push-out process. Therefore, the detector needs to be comparatively wide in x-direction to enable ions extracted anywhere from the whole path l_p to hit its surface. In practice, the detector needs to be several centimeters in length. The angle θ between the x-direction and the flight axis into the TOF analyzer is given by

$$\theta = \tan^{-1}\sqrt{\frac{-V_{tof}}{V_{beam}}} = \tan^{-1}\left(\frac{v_{tof}}{v_{beam}}\right) \tag{4.9}$$

where V_{tof} and V_{beam} are the acceleration voltages for ion beam and orthogonal accelerator, respectively, and v_{tof} and v_{beam} are the corresponding ion velocities.

While one ion package travels through the TOF analyzer and is being dispersed in time, the accelerator is refilled with new ions from the ion source (the time-of-flight to cover an m/z range up to about 5000 by the oaTOF is about 100 μs). During the drift time of an ion through the oaTOF, it travels a distance l_b. The ratio of the length of the orthogonal accelerator l_p to l_b determines the efficiency of the mass analyzer in terms of the ratio of ions used to ions created. This efficiency is known as the *duty cycle* of an instrument (next paragraph). The duty cycle of an oaTOF instrument is at an optimum if the time-of-flight to pass the TOF analyzer is slightly longer than the time needed for the continuous ion beam to refill the orthogonal accelerator. As soon as the heaviest ions have reached the detector, the next package is pulsed into the analyzer, giving rise to 10,000 complete mass spectra per second. In order to reduce the amount of data and to improve the signal-to-noise ratio, summation of several single spectra is done by an acquisition processing unit before the spectra are passed to a computer for data storage and post-processing.

4.2.10 Duty Cycle

In mass spectrometry the term *duty cycle* is used to specify the fraction of time of an ion current as continuously delivered from an ion source that is finally used for mass analysis. The duty cycle of scanning instruments is intrinsically low as only ions of one *m/z* value hit the detector at a time while all others are discarded by the analyzer, e.g., at $R = 1000$ only a fraction of 10^{-3} of the *m/z* range reaches the detector corresponding to a duty cycle of just 10^{-3}. Linear and ReTOF analyzers, on the other side, are capable of using almost all ions that are created from a pulsed ionizing event, and thus, these allow duty cycles in the order of 0.9. Although the oaTOF analyzer is by far better than scanning devices, it has to deal with a batch operation of the ion pulser. Fast (low-mass) ions traverse the orthogonal accelerator in a shorter time span than slow (high-mass) ions, thereby causing discrimination of low-mass ions. This behavior poses limitations on the mass range that can be simultaneously pulsed into the TOF analyzer. Depending on the axial velocity distribution of the ions and on the *m/z* range to be analyzed, the duty cycle of oaTOF analyzers is in the 3–30% range.

Determination of the duty cycle In oaTOF operation, the frequency between acceleration pulses is selected as to avoid spectral overlap due to mixing of subsequent ion packages traveling along the TOF analyzer. The slowest ions arrive at the detector at a time that is determined by the ratio of the length of the ion entrance window, l_p, to the distance between the midpoints of this window and the detector, l_b. The duty cycle (*Du*) for the heaviest ion at m/z_{max} is therefore given by $Du = l_p / l_b$. (Fig. 4.12) [62]. Furthermore, as the velocity of ions is proportional $(m/z)^{-2}$ (Eq. 4.3) the duty cycle for low-mass ions at m/z_{low} is given by

$$Du = \frac{l_p}{l_b}\sqrt{\frac{m/z_{low}}{m/z_{max}}} \qquad (4.10)$$

In practice, the ratio l_p / l_b. is about 0.25, and thus, for $m/z_{low} = 100$ and $m/z_{max} = 2000$ we obtain $Du = 0.056$ for the low-mass ion.

Nonetheless, it is not the duty cycle alone that defines the transmission of oaTOF analyzers. Actually, the overall sensitivity of instruments is also influenced by ion losses during entrance into the orthogonal accelerator, divergence of ions prior to pulsing, eventual grids in the flight path, etc.

4.2.11 TOF Analyzers with a Folded Eight-Shaped Flight Path

It should have become clear that elongated flight paths could provide an effective means of increasing the resolving power of a TOF analyzer if it were not for the ion losses due to spreading of the beam by Coulombic repulsion and by scattering of ions upon collision with residual gas. Apart from these considerations, a flight tube of say 10 m in length would be impracticable for any commercial instrument. On the next few pages we will therefore take a – hopefully instructive – view of some extraordinary TOF analyzer designs to get a perspective on what can be done.

Folding the flight path into compact dimensions presents an elegant concept to build a TOF analyzer featuring a very long flight path. An approach by M. Toyoda makes use of four electrostatic sectors that enable eight-shaped ion optical geometries for multi-turn and multi-passage ion paths [44]. While electrostatic sectors enable curved ion paths, they still cannot provide angular focusing of the ion beam to a level required for multiple passages through the analyzer. Therefore, additional ion optical elements such as electrostatic lenses and/or DC quadrupoles are incorporated, leading to a rather complex ion optical system. Additionally, ion injection from an external ion source into this "race track" has to be incorporated into the design if the final instrument is intended to be of practical use.

One representative of this TOF geometry is the MULTUM Linear plus instrument [44, 63], which consists of four cylindrical electrostatic sectors and 28 DC quadrupole lenses. The setup of this TOF analyzer is shown in Fig. 4.13 and the corresponding ion trajectories as visualized by a computer simulation are depicted in Fig. 4.14. The ions are injected at moderate kinetic energy of 1.5 keV and one cycle, a "full eight", corresponds to 1.284 m. Thus, the analyzer fits into a suitcase-sized housing (60 × 70 × 20 cm).

Outstanding resolving power The mass resolving power of the MULTUM Linear plus instrument increases as more repetitive cycles are employed. This has been demonstrated for the doublet of $CO^{+\bullet}$ and $N_2^{+\bullet}$ ions at *m/z* 28 (Fig. 4.15). It is remarkable that the time interval to the neighboring peak increases while the peak width in the spectra corresponding to 25.5, 101.5, 301.5, and 501.5 cycles or about 33, 130, 387, and 644 m path length, respectively, remains almost constant at 8 ± 1 ns. Finally, a mass resolution of $R_{FWHM} = 350{,}000$ is achieved after 501.5 cycles equaling a flight path of 644 m and a flight time of 6.3 ms.

It is an inherent weakness of this design that the next injection of ions has to wait until the preceding ion package has completed its journey through the TOF analyzer. Otherwise, fast ions of the following ion injection could overtake the slower ones of the previous one. The design does, however, not permit to distinguish this sort of interference, and thus, suffers from very low duty cycle as it takes several milliseconds to complete a single run. The *m/z* range per analysis is also limited due

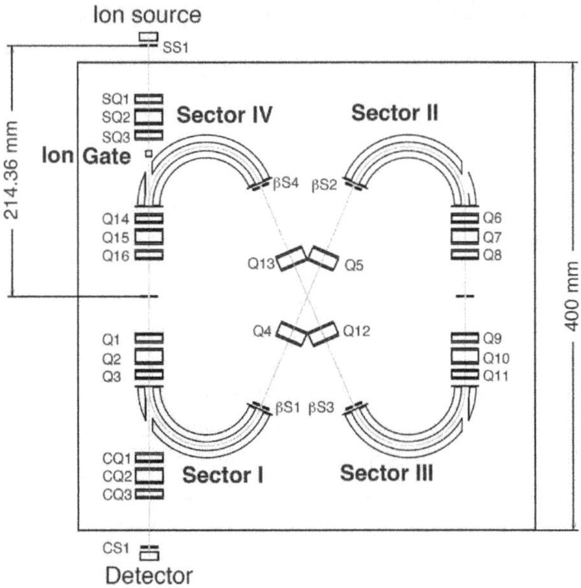

Fig. 4.13 Complex but compact ion optical design of the MULTUM Linear plus TOF analyzer. The eight-shaped path is realized by electrostatic sectors and numerous DC quadrupole lenses (*SQ*, *Q*, and *CQ*) (Reproduced from Ref. [63] by permission. © IM Publications, 2010)

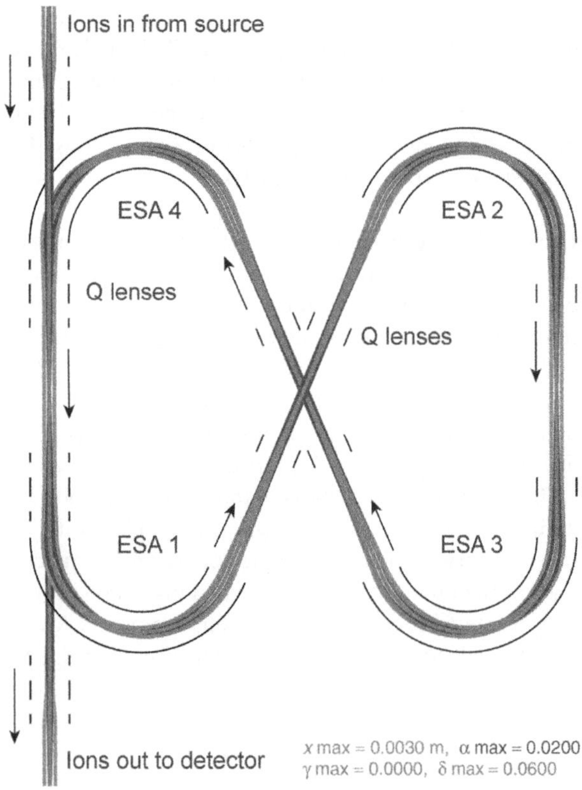

Fig. 4.14 Simulated ion trajectories in the MULTUM Linear plus (cf. Fig. 4.13). The *arrows* indicate the direction of ion motion (Adapted from Ref. [44] by permission. © John Wiley & Sons, 2003)

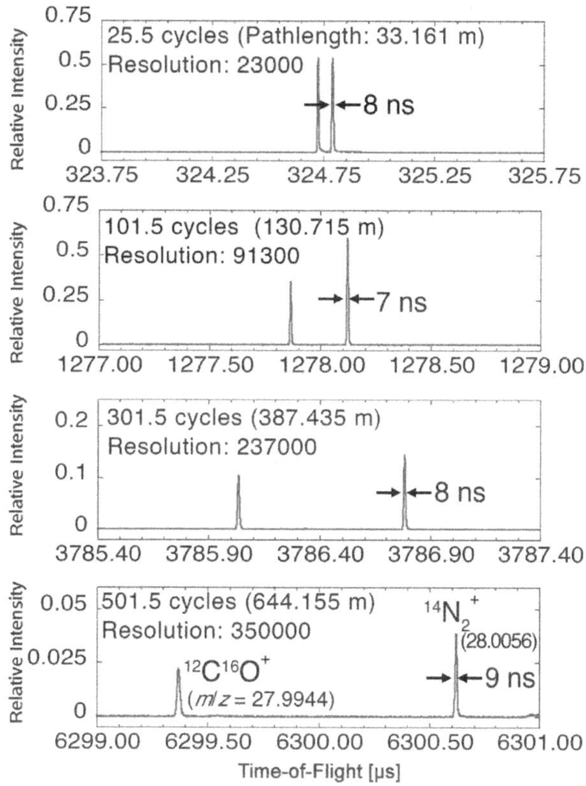

Fig. 4.15 Gain of resolution upon increasing ion flight path through the MULTUM Linear plus as demonstrated for the doublet of $CO^{+\bullet}$ and $N_2^{+\bullet}$ at *m*/*z* 28. From *top* to *bottom* the spectra correspond to 25.5, 101.5, 301.5, and 501.5 cycles or about 33, 130, 387, and 644 m path length, respectively (Reproduced from Ref. [63] by permission.)

to this phenomenon: lighter ions would overtake the heavier ones after some cycles. In other words, only ions traveling the same number of cycles can be reliably analyzed.

Space mission From the commercial point of view, this unconventional yet impressive design still possesses some prototype character. Nonetheless, it has seen an application on the ROSETTA space mission. In fact, the lander Philae carried a miniature instrument of this design for the COSAC project [64, 65]. The lander was dropped on the surface of the comet 67P/Churyumov-Gerasimenko on November 12, 2014 after a 10-year journey of some seven billion kilometers. After some difficulties due to an unlucky touch down, it finally managed to acquire a mass spectrum on the comet's surface [66].

The problems of indistinguishable ion packages and of overtaking lighter ions can be resolved by tilting the axis of ion injection out of the x,y plane to introduce a translational motion in z direction. This way, ions are moving through a stack of eight-shaped paths. While the number of cycles is then defined by the analyzer hardware, the design allows to cover a large *m*/*z* range as required in analytical mass spectrometry [67–69].

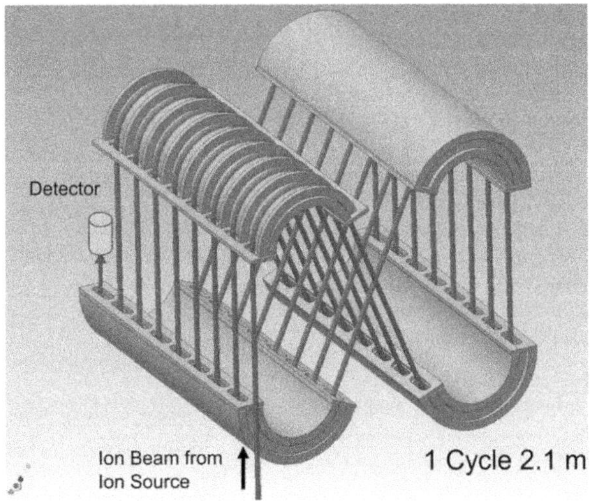

Fig. 4.16 SpiralTOF analyzer using four arrays of electrostatic analyzers (*gray*). The outer electrode of the top left ESA has been omitted. The ion flight path is visualized as a *red line* (Reproduced with permission from Ref. [71] © Mass Spectrometry Society of Japan, 2014)

JEOL has developed a MALDI-TOF instrument incorporating the so-called "SpiralTOF" analyzer. The geometry comprises eight loops of 2.1 m each resulting in a total flight path of about 17 m (Fig. 4.16). While not actually flat, the entire analyzer fits into a compact almost cubic housing. As the ion source uses delayed extraction (Sect. 4.2.7) to minimize the translational energy spread of the ions prior to entering the SpiralTOF assembly, this instrument can deliver 80,000 resolving power [70–72]. An application of this instrument to MALDI analysis of a synthetic polymer is shown in Sect. 11.5.

4.2.12 Multi-reflecting TOFs

Alternatively, TOF analyzers can be compacted by folding the flight path via multiple reflection of the ions. The concept of multi-pass and multi-reflecting TOF analyzers has been explored by H. Wollnik [73, 74]. Following the line of thought that leads from the MULTUM design to the SpiralTOF, it appears logical to employ an array of reflectors and some tilt of the direction of motion to avoid overtaking of lighter ions. Rather than using the same pair of reflectors to oscillate ion packages back and forth as many times as possible, such a multi-reflector design with a defined number of cycles offers free selection of the m/z range to be covered. The setup that has finally been commercialized employs an array of multi-stage reflectors that are aligned in a way as to effect a "zig-zag" or "jig-saw" ion path [75]. To avoid ion loss by scattering, a set of electrostatic lenses is positioned halfway between the opposed reflectors. It requires carefully tuned spatial focusing of both reflector stages and lenses to keep ions on track along such a flight path.

Ions leaving the source are injected into the first reflector at an angle and then pass a switchable deflector electrode. With the deflector electrode switched on, ions are sent into the second reflector stage and leave from there to hit the detector after

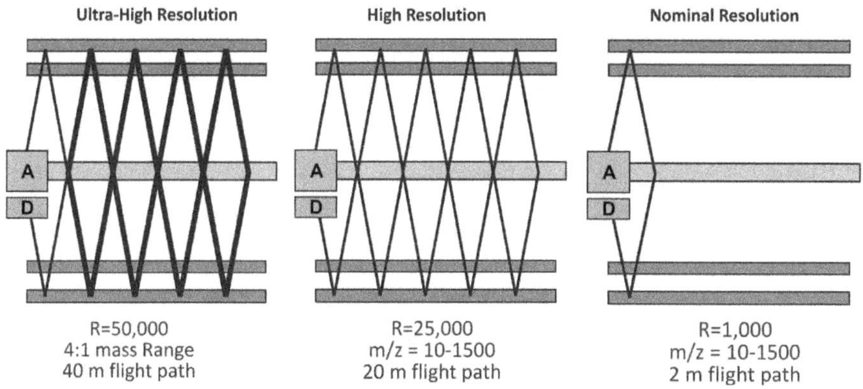

Fig. 4.17 Scheme of multi-reflecting TOF operational modes (*A* ion source, *D* detector). By using a switchable deflector ions can either be passed through one double reflection to deliver $R = 1000$, to five double reflection to achieve $R = 25{,}000$, or even to have a second full passage enabling $R = 50{,}000$ (Courtesy of LECO, Germany)

having gone through a rhombic flight path of just 2 m (Fig. 4.17). In this mode, the instrument can deliver $R = 1000$. When no potential is applied to the deflector, ions move on to start their zig-zag journey until they are reflected at the end of the array to send them back on a path leading to the detector. Providing a flight path of 20 m, this mode delivers $R = 25{,}000$. By using the deflector to send ions back, the ions are going for second passage through the mass analyzer to enable $R = 50{,}000$ after 40 m of flight. The latter mode limits the m/z range to a ratio of 1:4, e.g., m/z 200–800, because ions of the first and second passage are simultaneously traveling on the track.

A better idea of the dimensions of this compact analyzer and of the penetration depth of the multi-stage reflectors is conveyed by Fig. 4.18. This multi-reflecting TOF analyzer is commercialized by LECO as Pegasus HRT series of instruments [76, 77].

Multi-reflecting TOF at CERN At CERN, the online precision mass spectrometer ISOLTRAP uses a dedicated multi-reflecting TOF analyzer between the linear RF ion trap and two Penning traps for precision mass measurement of exotic nuclei [78]. The MR-TOF analyzer comprises two ion-optical mirrors between which oscillating ions are separated according to their different mass-to-charge ratios. By the multiple reflections, the analyzer of less than 1 m in length allows for total ion flight paths of several hundreds of meters. Tests of an offline version of this device delivered a resolving power of up to $R = 80{,}000$ [79]. As part of the highly specialized setup of ISOLTRAP at CERN, the MR-TOF serves for purification of contaminated ion beams. Furthermore, the MR-TOF can be operated as a mass spectrometer on its own, in particular for precision mass measurements of nuclides that are shorter-lived or that have lower yields than those accessible for Penning trap mass spectrometry [78–80].

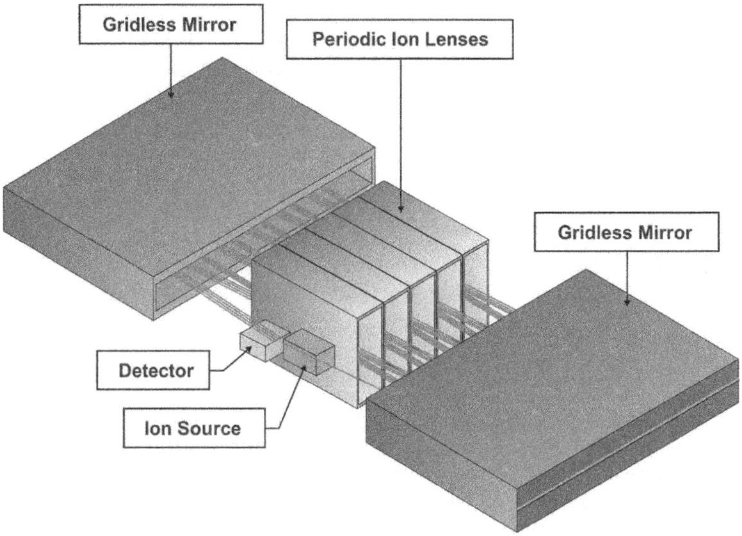

Fig. 4.18 Schematic of the multi-reflecting TOF analyzer. During the most part of their journey, ions are traveling either within reflectors or are passing electrostatic lenses (Courtesy of LECO, Germany)

4.2.13 Essence of TOF Instruments

Principle of Operation

Ions of equal kinetic energy but different in mass are moving at different velocities. When such ions are traveling down a field-free drift path of given length, their flight times depend on mass, more precisely on the square root of m/z. Measuring the time-of-flight (TOF) allows to calculate the ionic mass. The mass resolving power of a TOF analyzer is proportional to its length.

TOF Configurations

The simplest form of a TOF analyzer is presented by the linear TOF with continuous ion extraction from the source. The reflector TOF (ReTOF) design offers 2–4-fold improved resolving power that can be further boosted by implementation of a delay between ion creation and onset of ion acceleration. Typically, such TOF analyzers, generally of reflector design, are attached on-axis to MALDI sources featuring some sort of pulsed ion extraction.

Continuous ion sources can be used in combination with orthogonal-acceleration (oaTOF) analyzers. For m/z analysis in oaTOFs, ions are deflected from an ion beam orthogonal to its direction. Commonly, the TOF analyzer of these instruments is also of reflector design. Furthermore, oaTOFs are well-suited for combination with other mass-analyzing devices.

Performance Characteristics

The performance of TOF analyzers in terms of mass range, resolving power, and mass accuracy varies widely in accordance with their design (on-axis TOF versus oaTOF), mode of operation (linear or reflector mode), and intended use (MALDI versus ESI, APCI versus EI, CI) of the instrument. Thus, TOFs may cover ranges of up to *m/z* 1000 (GC-MS), to *m/z* 5000 (ESI, APCI sources), and even to far beyond *m/z* 100,000 (MALDI). TOFs can deliver resolving power of $R = 1000$ (GC-MS, GC × GC-MS) to R > 30,000. Accordingly, mass accuracies range from just 0.2 u to 0.001 u.

TOF Analyzers in the Laboratory

TOF analyzers are widely used in modern instrumentation. Their success is based on a balance between performance in terms of resolving power, mass accuracy, mass range, speed, and sensitivity on the one side and of reasonable investment on the other. Their compact footprint in the laboratory and moderate power consumption also contribute to their success. On-axis TOF and oaTOF analyzers make up the majority of today's TOF instrumentation, while the more complex folded ion path layouts are less common.

4.3 Magnetic Sector Instruments

4.3.1 Evolution of Magnetic Sector Instruments

Magnetic sector instruments paved the road to organic mass spectrometry. "Whereas mass spectrometry was still very an art rather than a science in 1940, the picture changed drastically during the war years. Vacuum and electronic techniques had matured" [81]. It took until the 1950s for magnetic sector instruments to become commercially available [7, 8]. These pioneering instruments were fairly bulky and not very easy to use [81 83]. Nevertheless, they provided analytical information of a kind that chemists had long been seeking for. They continuously became faster, more accurate, with higher resolving power [3, 5, 9, 84]. The first instruments used a single magnetic sector (symbol B) to effect separation of the ions. Later, the introduction of *double-focusing instruments* which in addition were equipped with an *electrostatic sector* or *electrostatic analyzer* (ESA, symbol E) in addition defined a standard which is still valid. With few exceptions, magnetic sector instruments are comparatively large devices capable of high resolution and accurate mass determination, and suited for a wide variety of ionization methods.

Trends in instrumentation

Two decades ago, double-focusing sector instruments were commonly used with a large chemical diversity of samples. Within the last decade, however, there has been a strong tendency to replace sector instruments with TOF, Orbitrap, or FT-ICR instruments, and moreover, to even substitute classical ionization methods such as EI, CI, or FAB with APCI or ESI just to redirect the stream of samples to those preferable modern mass analyzers. Recently, manufacturers have "rediscovered" the utility of EI and CI and started to offer TOF and Orbitrap analyzers adapted to these ionization methods. These instruments often are dedicated to gas chromatography-mass spectrometry (GC-MS), but direct insertion probes are also having a renaissance (Sect. 5.2).

4.3.2 Principle of the Magnetic Sector

The *Lorentz Force Law* can be used to describe the effects exerted onto a charged particle entering a constant magnetic field. The Lorentz force F_L depends on the velocity v, the magnetic field B, and the charge q of an ion. In the simplest form the force is given by the scalar equation [3, 4, 85, 86]

$$F_L = qvB \tag{4.11}$$

which is valid if v and B (both are vectors) are perpendicular to each other. Otherwise, the relationship becomes

$$F_L = qvB(\sin\alpha) \tag{4.11a}$$

where α is the angle between v and B. Figure 4.19 demonstrates the relationship between the direction of the magnetic field, the direction of the ionic motion, and the direction of the resulting Lorentz force. Each of them is at right angles to the others. An ion of mass m and charge q traveling at a velocity v in a direction perpendicular to an homogeneous magnetic field will follow a circular path of radius r_m that fulfills the condition of equilibrium of F_L and centripetal force F_c

$$F_L = qvB = \frac{m_i v^2}{r_m} = F_c \tag{4.12}$$

Upon rearrangement we obtain the radius r_m of this circular motion

$$r_m = \frac{m_i v}{qB} \tag{4.13}$$

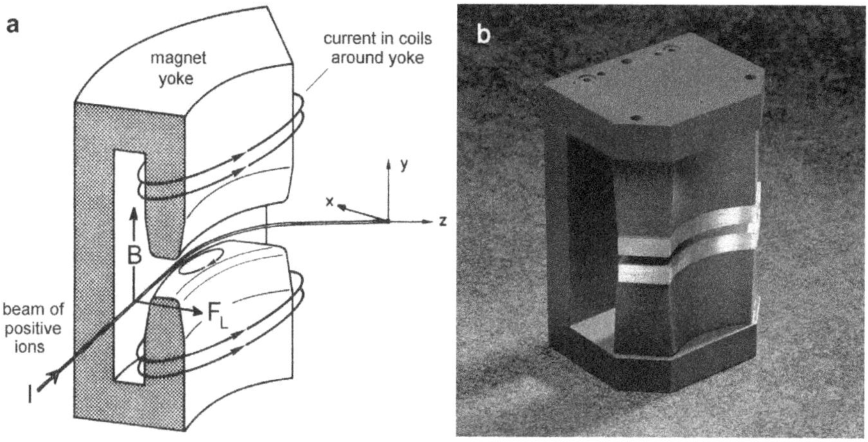

Fig. 4.19 The Right Hand Rule (*I* thumb, *B* index finger, F_L middle finger) to determine the direction of the Lorentz force (**a**), where the current corresponds to the direction where positive charges move, i.e., the figure directly applies for positive ions. (**b**) A real magnet yoke without coils and flight tube. With kind permission of Thermo Electron (Bremen) GmbH, (*left*) and Waters Corporation, MS Technologies, Manchester, UK (*right*)

This shows the working principle of a magnetic sector where the radius r_m depends on the momentum mv of an ion, which itself depends on m/z.

Momentum analyzer
The magnetic sector does not directly separate ions by mass. Rather it effects ion separation by their momentum and this feature can be used as a measure of mass provided all ions possess equal kinetic energy.

Finally, dispersion in momentum causes a dependence of r_m on the square root of mass becoming obvious by substitution of v from Eq. (4.3) and $q = ez$

$$r_m = \frac{m_i}{ezB}\sqrt{\frac{2ezU}{m_i}} = \frac{1}{B}\sqrt{\frac{2m_iU}{ez}} \tag{4.13a}$$

Alternatively, the ratio m_i/q can be expressed by rearranging Eq. (4.13)

$$\frac{m_i}{q} = \frac{r_m B}{v} \tag{4.14}$$

which upon substitution of v as performed above becomes

$$\frac{m_i}{q} = \frac{r_m B}{\sqrt{\frac{2qU}{m_i}}} \quad \Rightarrow \quad \frac{m_i}{q} = \frac{{r_m}^2 B^2}{2U} \tag{4.14a}$$

For singly charged ions ($z = 1$, $q = e$) we obtain the more widespread form

$$\frac{m_i}{e} = \frac{{r_m}^2 B^2}{2U} \tag{4.14b}$$

Basic equation of MS
Equation (4.14b) has become known as the *basic equation of mass spectrometry*. Nowadays, there is no more justification for a single basic equation of mass spectrometry because of the large variety of mass analyzers employed.

4.3.3 Focusing Action of the Magnetic Field

The focusing action of an homogeneous magnetic field on a beam of ions having the same m/z and the same kinetic energy can best be illustrated by a 180° sector (Fig. 4.20). If the beam is divergent by a half-angle α, the collector slit must be $\alpha^2 r_m$ wide to pass all ions after suffering 180° deflection. This is because the ions come to a first order, i.e., imperfect, focus as they all traverse the magnetic field at the same radius but not all of them entered the field at right angles. Ions of different m/z fly at a different radius, e.g., the lighter ions of m/z_1 hit the wall while ions of m/z_2 reach the collector slit. To allow for detection of various masses, such an analyzer could either be equipped with a photographic plate in the focal plane to become a so-called *mass spectrograph*, or it could be designed with variable magnetic field to detect different masses at the same point by bringing them subsequently to the collector slit. Indeed, such a 180° geometry with *scanning* magnetic field has been used by Dempster [87]. Later, the term *mass spectrometer* was coined for this type of instruments [83].

Among other complications, the 180° design requires large and heavy magnetic sectors. It is by far more elegant to employ magnetic sectors of smaller angles (Fig. 4.21). An optimized magnetic sector alone can provide a resolving power of $R = 2000–5000$ depending on its radius. The limitation arises from the fact that ions emerging from the ion source are not really monoenergetic. This way, ions of different m/z can have equal momentum and thus cause overlap of adjacent ion beams at the detector.

Energy spread limits resolving power Equation (4.13a) describes the radius r_m in the magnetic field. Obviously, the value r_m remains constant as long as $m_i U = const.$ If the instrument is set to pass an ion of say m/z 500 and 3000 eV kinetic energy, it

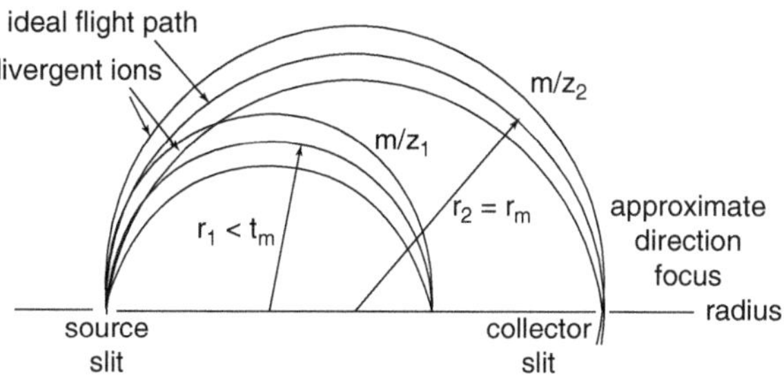

Fig. 4.20 Direction focusing properties of a 180° magnetic sector on a diverging beam of ions of the same *m*/*z* and the same kinetic energy and effect on ions of different *m*/*z*. In this illustration, *B* has to come out of the plane towards the reader for positive ions

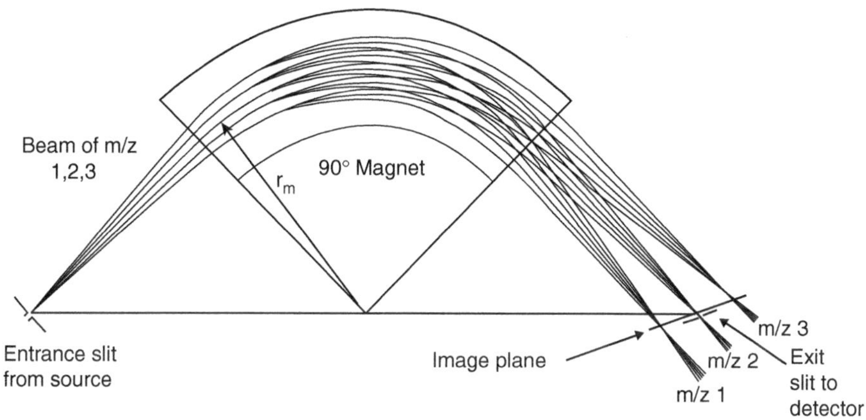

Fig. 4.21 Ion separation and direction focusing in a plane by a 90° magnetic sector. A divergent beam of ions of *m*/*z* 1, 2, 3 is separated into three beams and focused to a point on the image plane (divergence shown exaggerated). Only ions of *m*/*z* 2 are passing the exit slit and eventually hit the detector (Adapted from Ref. [88] with permission. © Wiley-VCH, 1999–2014)

will simultaneously allow the passage for ions of *m*/*z* 501 having 2994 eV or of *m*/*z* 499 having 3006 eV of kinetic energy. This is why high resolving power demands narrow kinetic energy distributions.

4.3.4 Double-Focusing Sector Instruments

The *electrostatic sector* or *electrostatic analyzer* (ESA) produces a radial electric field between two oppositely charged plates extending over the ESA angle ϕ (Fig. 4.23). An ion passes the ESA midway on a circular path if

$$F_e = qE = \frac{m_i v^2}{r_e} = F_c \tag{4.15}$$

where F_e represents the electric force, E the electric field strength, and r_e the radius of the ESA. Rearrangement of Eq. (4.15) demonstrates that the ESA acts as an energy dispersive device

$$r_e = \frac{m_i v^2}{qE} = \frac{m_i v^2}{ezE} \tag{4.16}$$

Energy filter

The ESA effects energy dispersion. Thus, the kinetic energy distribution of an ion beam can be reduced. The ESA does not allow for mass separation among monoenergetic ions.

Upon substitution of Eq. (4.3) for v one obtains the simple relationship

$$r_e = \frac{2U}{E} \tag{4.17}$$

to describe the radius of the ESA. As with the magnetic sector before, the ESA has direction-focusing properties in one plane (Fig. 4.22). Ions entering the ESA in the middle and at right angles to the field boundaries pass through on a path of equipotential, whereas ions with a velocity component towards one of the capacitor

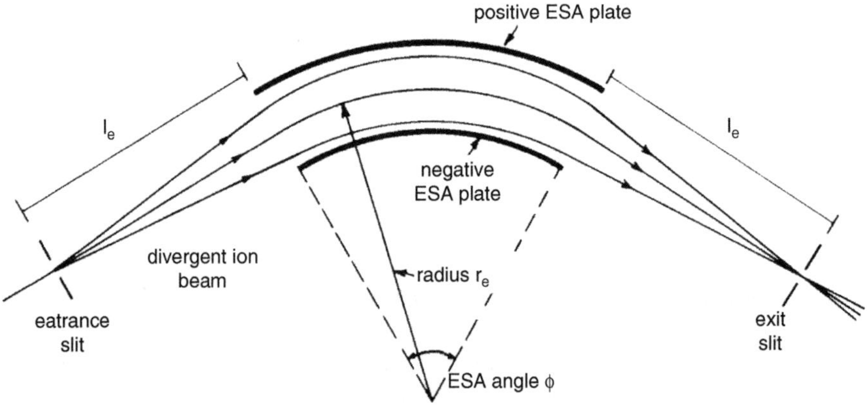

Fig. 4.22 Direction focusing of a radial electric field. Ions of appropriate kinetic energy are focused at the exit slit. Divergent ions pass the ESA close to either plate. Here, the electric potentials are set to transmit positive ions. The image distance l_e depends on the ESA angle

plates are brought into focus at the focal length l_e. To understand this, imagine an ion drifting towards the outer plate having the same charge sign as the ion. As it approaches the plate it is decelerated by the opposed electric field and finally reflected towards the center of the beam. With its radial component of v inverted it crosses the ideal path at l_e. In an analogous fashion an ion approaching the inner plate becomes accelerated by the attractive force. The resulting higher velocity causes an increase in centripetal force, and thereby effects a correction of the flight path in the appropriate sense.

Energy focusing is achieved by combining a magnetic sector and an electric sector in a way that the energy dispersion of the magnetic field is just compensated by the energy dispersion of the electric field. Additional direction focusing is obtained if the radii and angles of these fields and their mutual alignment does not diminish the focusing properties of each of them. Then, an ion optical system is obtained that is able to focus ions onto a single image point, although these were emerging from the ion source in (slightly) different directions and with (slightly) different kinetic energies. This is called *double focusing*. Double focusing can improve the resolving power of a magnetic sector instrument more than ten times.

4.3.5 Geometries of Double-Focusing Sector Instruments

The following passages present examples of particular double-focusing geometries that either have been milestones in instrument design [3, 5] or still are incorporated in modern mass spectrometers.

The EB design by Mattauch and Herzog combines a 31° 50′ ESA with a 90° magnetic sector producing an image plane that allows for simultaneous photographic detection of a comparatively large *m*/*z* range [89]. This mass spectrograph attains double-focusing over the total image plane resulting in resolving powers of $R > 10{,}000$. Thus, it became the basis for numerous commercial instruments (Fig. 4.23). The *Mattauch-Herzog geometry* has survived until today in dedicated instruments for spark source (SS)-MS and isotope ration (IR)-MS (Sect. 15.2) [90].

An EB design effecting an image plane of 140 mm in length with a linear mass scale for detection on a photographic plate has been published by Bainbridge and Jordan (*Bainbridge-Jordan geometry*) [92]. Their paper is especially recommended as it also nicely illustrates the use of photographic plates in those days.

The third famous type of EB arrangement has become known as *Nier-Johnson geometry* (Fig. 4.24) [93]. Here, the ion beam first passes through the electrostatic analyzer producing energy-resolved beams without mass dispersion in the plane of an intermediate slit located at the focal point of the ESA. It then passes through a magnetic analyzer to achieve mass dispersion of the ions. Different from the Mattauch-Herzog *mass spectrograph*, the Nier-Johnson *mass spectrometer* was constructed to be used in conjunction with a *scanning magnet* to focus one specific *m*/*z* after the other onto a point detector. This presented a major advantage for the use of UV recorders or electronic data acquisition as well as for the achievement of better ion optics.

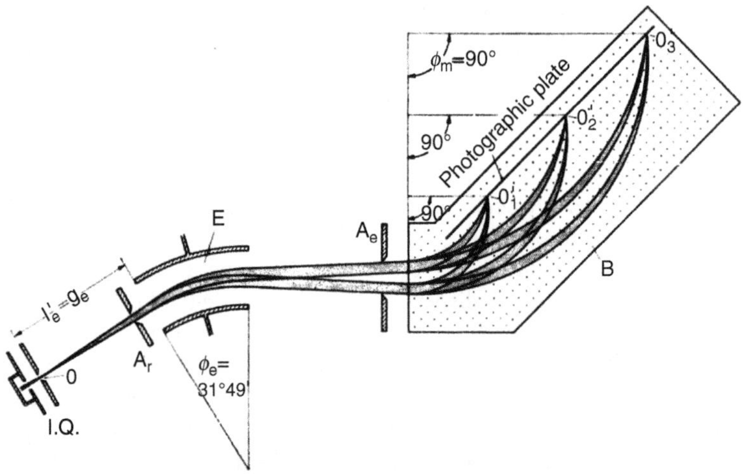

Fig. 4.23 Mattauch-Herzog double-focusing mass spectrograph providing direction and momentum focusing of ions on a plane [89]. The ESA precedes the magnet. Placing a photographic plate in the image plane allows simultaneous recording of a *m/z* range (Reproduced from Ref. [91] with kind permission of Curt Brunnée)

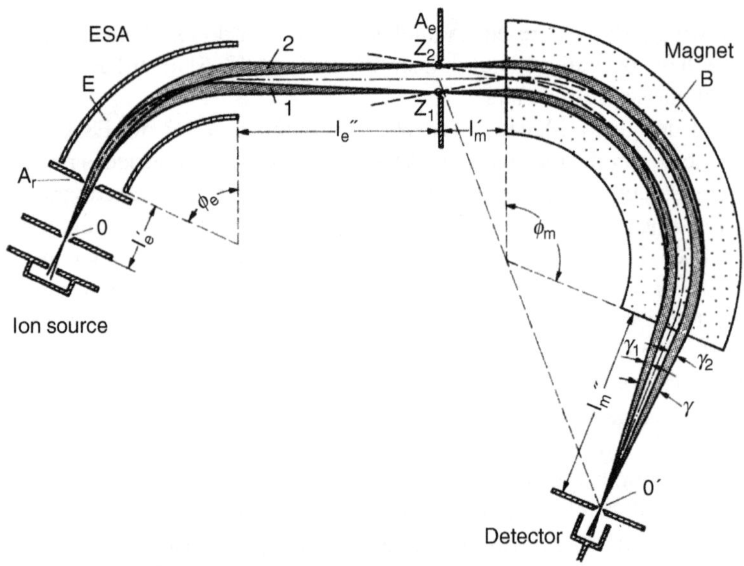

Fig. 4.24 Double-focusing mass spectrometer of EB geometry, basically a Nier–Johnson type instrument. Direction and velocity focusing are shown exaggerated. After exiting the ESA, the energy-resolved beam passes through a wide intermediate slit into the magnetic sector. The large aperture ensures good overall transmission (Reproduced from Ref. [91] with kind permission of Curt Brunnée)

Scan

Typically, on magnetic sector mass spectrometers a spectrum is produced by varying the strength of the magnetic field to successively pass through ions of different *m/z*. This is termed *magnetic field scan* [94]. For scans *linear in time*, the *scan rate* is given in units of *m/z* s^{-1}, e.g., 500 *m/z* s^{-1}. For scans *exponential in time*, the *scan rate* is reported in units of s per decade, e.g., 10 s/decade means 10 s from *m/z* 30 to 300 or from *m/z* 100 to 1000.

Some later EB instrument models were constructed to be used in combination with an (optional) array detector, e.g., the JEOL HX-110 (EB), the Thermo Finnigan MAT 900 (EB), and the Micromass Autospec (EBE) instruments could be equipped in that way. The array detector was located at the focus plane of the magnet.

Successful constructions of *reversed geometry*, i.e., BE instead of *forward* EB design, have been presented in the form of the MAT 311 in the mid-1970s and shortly after by the VG Analytical ZAB-2F instrument [95] based on a proposal by Hintenberger and König [96].

More recent BE geometry instruments are presented by the Thermo Finnigan MAT 90 and 95 series (Fig. 4.25), the JEOL JMS-700, and although not strictly due to its EBE geometry [97], the Micromass Autospec. However, the only instrument of this millennium incorporating a redesigned BE geometry has been the Thermo Scientific DSF introduced in 2005. In contrast to organic and biomedical MS, double-focusing designs are still highly relevant in inorganic MS (Chap. 15) [90].

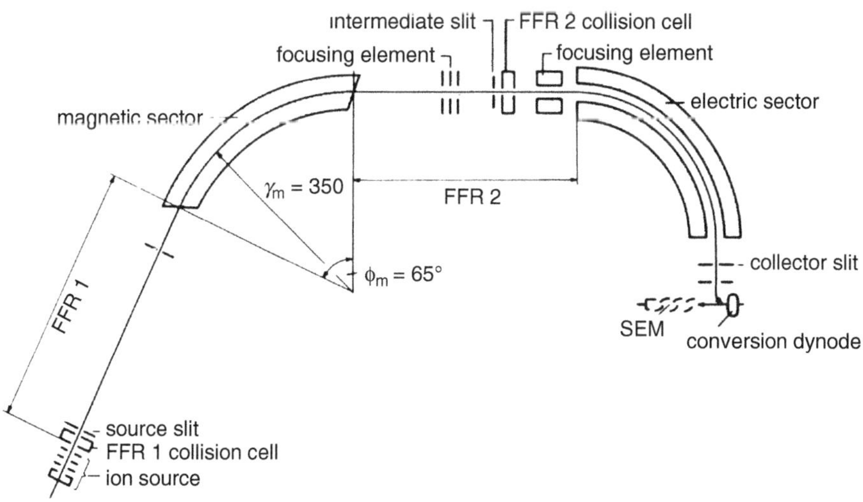

Fig. 4.25 The Finnigan MAT 90 double-focusing mass spectrometer with rotated pole faces of the magnetic sector (Reproduced from Ref. [2] with permission. © Elsevier Science, 1987)

4.3.6 Adjusting the Resolving Power of a Sector Instrument

The ion optics of a sector instrument are the analog to a cylindrical lens in light optics. Accordingly, the reduction of an aperture can be used to obtain a sharper image, i.e., to increase resolving power (Sect. 3.4). Slits are used instead of circular apertures to comply with the cylindrical properties of the ion optical system. Most important are the settings of the *object slit* (*source slit*, *entrance slit*) and the *image slit* (*collector slit*, *exit slit*, *detector slit*). Intermediate slits may be used in addition. Unfortunately, closing slits also means cutting off ions from the beam, and thus reduction of the transmission of the mass analyzer. In the ideal case, the improvement of resolution by a factor of 10 goes along with a reduction in transmission to 10%, in reality the effect is often worse.

Setting the slits The influence of relative slit width on peak shape and resolution is demonstrated on the second isotopic peak of toluene molecular ion, $^{13}C_2{}^{12}C_5H_8{}^{+\bullet}$, *m/z* 94 (Fig. 4.26). With the entrance slit at 50 μm and the exit slit at 500 μm the peak is flat-topped (*left*), because a narrow beam from the entrance sweeps over the wide open detector slit keeping the intensity constant as the scan proceeds until the beam passes over the other edge of the slit. Closing the exit slit to 100 μm increases resolution to 2000 without affecting the peak height (*center*), but reduces the peak area by a factor of 4 in accordance with an increase in resolution by the same factor. Further reduction of the exit slit width to 30 μm improves resolution at the cost of peak height (*right*). (Any sector instrument must behave alike, otherwise, cleaning or other maintenance are required.)

Operate to fit your needs
The ultimate resolution of a magnetic sector mass spectrometer is reached when the slits are closed to a width of a few micrometers. Often, the slit height is also reduced, e.g., from 5 to 1 mm. In daily work, the resolution will be set to fit the actual task, e.g., $R = 1000–2000$ for low-resolution work, $R = 3000–5000$ if accurate mass determination at high scan rates is needed (GC-MS, Chap. 14) or isotopic patterns of high mass analytes have to be resolved, or $R = 7000–15{,}000$ in slow-scanning accurate mass measurements.

4.3.7 Optimization of Sector Instruments

To improve the performance of sector instruments in terms of scan speed, resolving power, transmission, and mass range, the construction, in particular that of the magnet, needs some additional refining.

The rapid change of a magnetic field suffers from hysteresis, i.e., the magnetic flux does not exactly follow the change of the electric current through the coils in

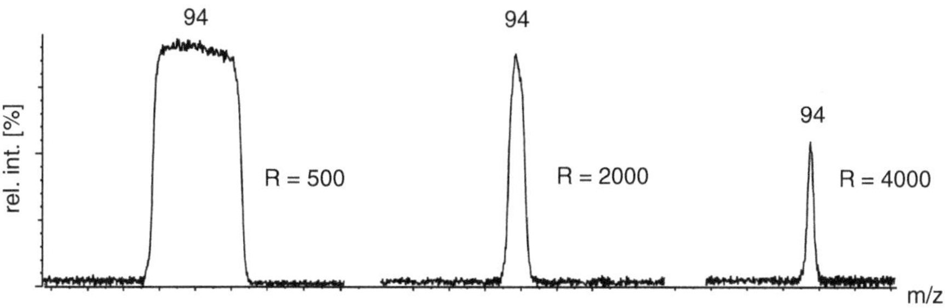

Fig. 4.26 The influence of relative slit width settings on peak shape and resolution on a magnetic sector instrument. The peak shape first changes from flat-topped (*left*) to Gaussian (*center*) and finally resolution improves at cost of peak height (*right*)

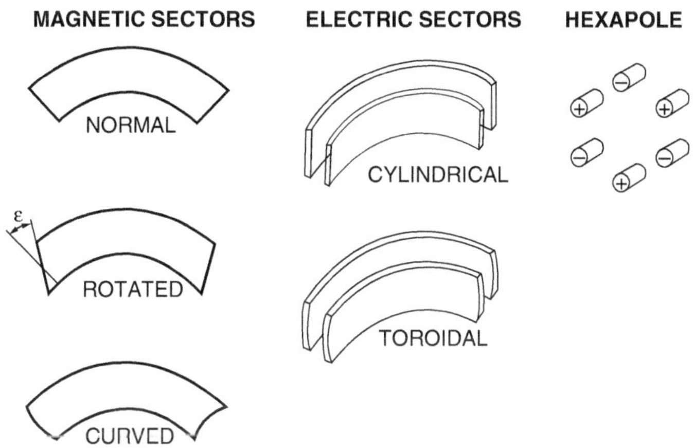

Fig. 4.27 Types and shapes of ion optical elements used in magnetic sector instrument design (By courtesy of Thermo Fisher Scientific, Bremen)

time, but lags behind due to the induction of eddy currents. On one side, this causes problems in creating a scan perfectly linear in time, on the other this prevents high scan rates as required for GC-MS. Lamination of the yoke substantially reduces these problems [98] and is employed in all modern sector instruments.

In order to extend the mass range one either has to increase the field strength or the radius of the magnet. However, there are limitations of the field strength with non-superconducting magnets at about 2.4 T. Instead of simply enlarging the radius, the pole faces of the magnet can be rotated to preserve a compact design by reduction of its focal length (Figs. 4.27, 4.28, and 4.29) [2].

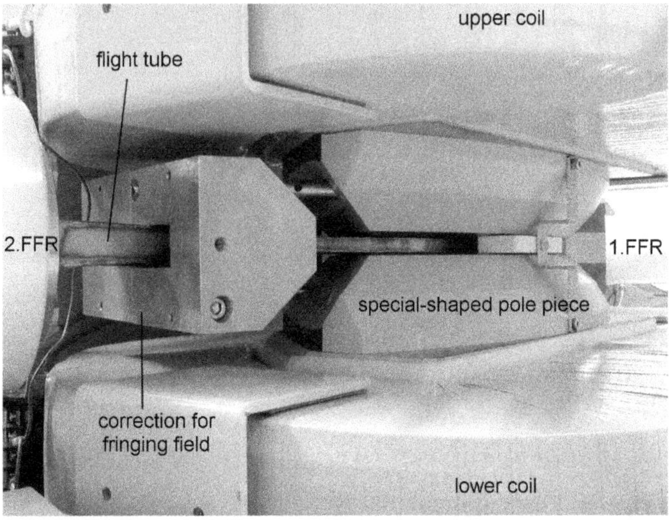

Fig. 4.28 Flight tube passing through the gap of the magnetic sector of a JEOL JMS-700 instrument seen from the ESA side. The shapes of the pole pieces of the yoke and the additional blocks around the tube are designed to minimize fringing fields. In addition the pole faces are rotated to increase the mass range

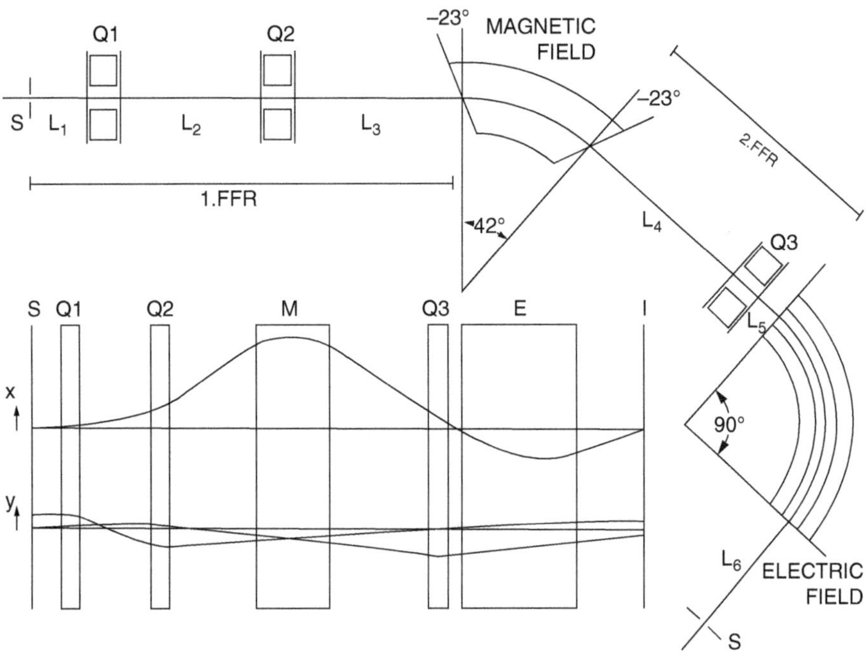

Fig. 4.29 Layout of the JEOL JMS-700. Three DC quadrupole lenses are used to improve the transmission of the magnetic sector. The inset shows horizontal (x) and vertical (y) trajectories where the height of the beam (y) is clearly reduced to pass through a narrow gap between the pole shoes of the magnet (Adapted from Ref. [99] with permission. © Elsevier Science, 1985)

Another problem is due to fringing fields. To reduce these defocusing effects at the entrance and exit of the field, the pole pieces of the yoke of the electromagnet generally have specially shaped edges.

Furthermore, pure EB and BE designs are somewhat limited concerning the transmittance through a narrow magnet gap as compared to instrument designs using some DC quadrupole (q) or DC hexapole (h) lenses to form the ion beam (Fig. 4.29) [99, 100]. However, quadrupole and hexapole lenses do not alter the effective instrument geometry, i.e., such an analyzer behaves like a pure BE analyzer in any mode of operation.

4.3.8 Summary of Magnetic Sector Instruments

Ion Separation

Ions moving perpendicular to a magnetic field are forced on a circular path by action of the Lorentz force. The radius of that motion is determined by a counter-balance of Lorentz force and centripetal force. Ions of equal kinetic energy but different in mass therefore travel on individual radii, and thus, a separation by momentum is effected. The radius of ion motion or the magnetic field strength to achieve a defined radius to hit the detector is then used to derive *m*/*z* values of the ions.

Configurations

Magnetic sector instruments can be built relying on magnetic (B) separation alone. Such single-focusing instruments are limited in resolving power. At least one order of magnitude higher resolving power is achieved when the kinetic energy spread of ions is compensated or filtered by means of an electrostatic sector (E). Designs employing B and E are termed double-focusing. E and B can be combined in numerous ways thereby giving rise to EB, BE, EBE, BEBE, and other designs.

Performance Characteristics

Double-focusing magnetic sector instruments, either in BE or EB configuration, typically can achieve resolving powers in excess of $R = 60{,}000$. However, this requires extremely slow scanning and comes at the expense of very low transmission, as the slits need to be closed down. High transmission at wide-open slits results in $R = 1000$–2000 and allows faster scanning. Accurate mass measurements are typically performed at moderate scan rates and $R = 5000$–$10{,}000$ and require internal mass calibration.

Magnetic Sector Instruments in the Laboratory

In organic and biomedical MS, magnetic sector instruments were most popular in the 1960s to early 2000s. More recently, most have been replaced by TOF, FT-ICR, or Orbitrap mass analyzers. In inorganic MS, in particular for isotope ratio determinations and spark-source MS, magnetic sector instruments are still of high relevance as they can deal with large energy dispersion and allow for multi-collector setups in the image plane of the magnet.

4.4 Linear Quadrupole Instruments

4.4.1 Introduction

Since the Nobel Prize-awarded discovery of the mass-analyzing and ion-trapping properties of two- and three-dimensional electric quadrupole fields [101, 102] and the concomitant construction of a *quadrupole* (Q) *mass spectrometer* [103, 104], this type of instrument has steadily gained importance. Chiefly starting from GC-MS that demanded for rapid scanning analyzers, quadrupole instruments made their way into the MS laboratories [105–108], although those early systems offered poor resolving power and low mass range, e.g., *m*/*z* 1–200. Modern quadrupole instruments cover up to *m*/*z* 2000 or even higher with good resolving power and represent some kind of routine device in LC-MS. The advantages of linear quadrupoles are:

- Linear quadrupoles offer high transmission.
- Quadrupoles are light-weight, very compact, and comparatively low-priced.
- Quadrupoles require low ion acceleration voltages.
- Quadrupoles allow high scan speeds since scanning is realized by solely sweeping electric potentials.

Terminology
Linear quadrupoles were the first to be incorporated in commercial instruments. Thus, these instruments are simply referred to as quadrupole mass spectrometers and the attribute "linear" is often omitted. As we will see later (Sects. 4.5 and 4.6) other electrode shapes are also possible but are forming electric RF quadrupole fields of other geometries. These designs are also available in commercial mass spectrometers.

4.4.2 The Linear Quadrupole

A linear quadrupole mass analyzer consists of four hyperbolically or cylindrically shaped rod electrodes extending in the *z*-direction and mounted in a square configuration (*xy*-plane, Figs. 4.30 and 4.31). The pairs of opposite rods are each held at the same potential which is composed of a DC and an AC component.

As an ion enters the quadrupole assembly in the *z*-direction, an attractive force is exerted on it by one of the rods with its charge actually opposite to the ionic charge. If the voltage applied to the rods is periodic, attraction and repulsion in both the *x*-

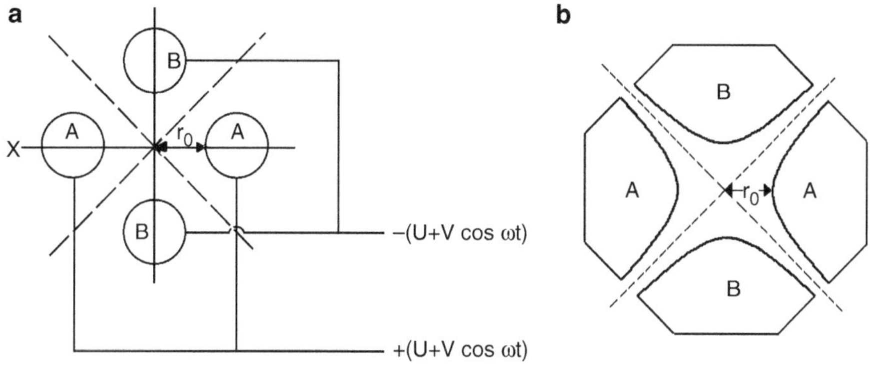

Fig. 4.30 Cross section of a quadrupole (**a**) for the cylindrical approximation and (**b**) for the hyperbolic profile of the rods. The electric field is zero along the *dotted lines*, i.e., along the asymptotes in (**b**) ((**a**) Courtesy of Waters Corp., MS Technologies, Manchester, UK)

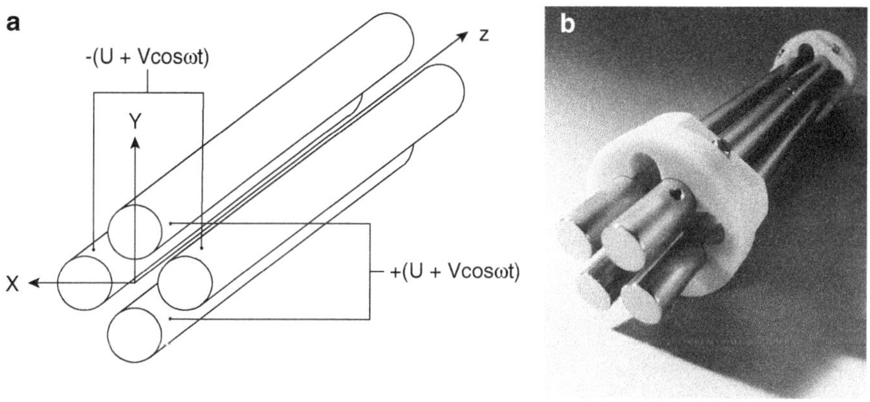

Fig. 4.31 Linear quadrupole mass analyzer: schematic (**a**) and photograph (**b**) (By courtesy of (**a**) JEOL, Tokyo and (**b**) Waters Corp., MS Technologies, Manchester, UK)

and *y*-directions will alternate in time, because the sign of the electric force also changes periodically in time. If the applied voltage is composed of a DC voltage U and a radiofrequency (RF) voltage V with the frequency ω the total potential Φ_0 is given by

$$\Phi_0 = U + V \cos \omega t \tag{4.18}$$

Thus, the equations of motion are

$$
\begin{aligned}
\frac{d^2x}{dt^2} + \frac{ez}{m_i r_0^2}(U + V\cos\omega t)x = 0 \\
\frac{d^2y}{dt^2} - \frac{ez}{m_i r_0^2}(U + V\cos\omega t)y = 0
\end{aligned}
\tag{4.19}
$$

Remember that m_i denotes ion mass [kg] and charge is $q = ez$, where e is the electron charge [C] and z the charge number. In case of an inhomogeneous periodic field such as the above quadrupole field, there is a small average force which is always in the direction of the lower field. The electric field is zero along the dotted lines in Fig. 4.30, i.e., along the asymptotes in case of the hyperbolic electrodes. It is therefore possible that an ion may traverse the quadrupole without hitting the rods, provided its motion around the z-axis is stable with limited amplitudes in the xy-plane. Such conditions can be derived from the theory of the *Mathieu equations.*

Mathieu equations
The Mathieu functions were originally derived in 1868 by Émile Léonard Mathieu, a French mathematician, to describe the vibrations of elliptical drumheads. It turned out that they are also useful to treat quadrupole mass filters and several other physical phenomena.

Now, writing Eq. (4.19) in dimensionless form yields

$$
\begin{aligned}
\frac{d^2x}{d\tau^2} + (a_x + 2q_x\cos 2\tau)x = 0 \\
\frac{d^2y}{d\tau^2} + (a_y + 2q_y\cos 2\tau)y = 0
\end{aligned}
\tag{4.20}
$$

The parameters a and q can now be obtained by comparing with Eq. (4.19)

$$
a_x = -a_y = \frac{4qU}{m_i r_0^2 \omega^2}, \quad q_x = -q_y = \frac{2qV}{m_i r_0^2 \omega^2}, \quad \tau = \frac{\omega t}{2}
\tag{4.21}
$$

For a given set of U, V, and ω the overall ion motion can result in a stable trajectory causing ions of a certain m/z value or m/z range to pass the quadrupole. Ions oscillating within the distance $2r_0$ between the electrodes will have stable trajectories. These are transmitted through the quadrupole and detected thereafter. The path stability of a particular ion is defined by the magnitude of the RF voltage V and by the ratio U/V.

By plotting the parameter a (ordinate, time invariant field) vs. q (abscissa, time variant field) we obtain the stability diagram of the two-dimensional quadrupole field. This reveals the existence of regions where (*i*) both x- and y-trajectories are stable, (*ii*) either x- or y-trajectories are stable, and (*iii*) no stable ion motion occurs

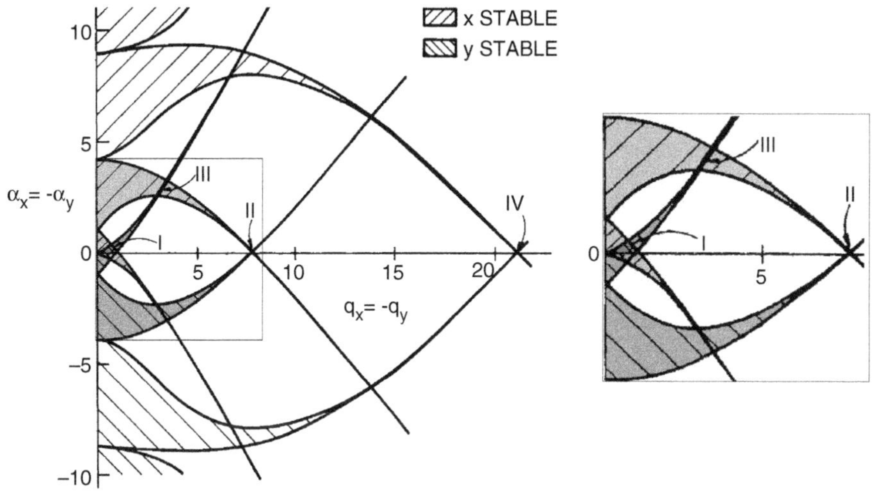

Fig. 4.32 Stability diagram for a linear quadrupole analyzer showing four stability regions (I–IV) for *x*- and *y*-motion. The portion within the *square frame* is zoomed to double size on the *right*. Stability region I only covers the small *red region* in the center (Adapted from Ref. [107] with permission.

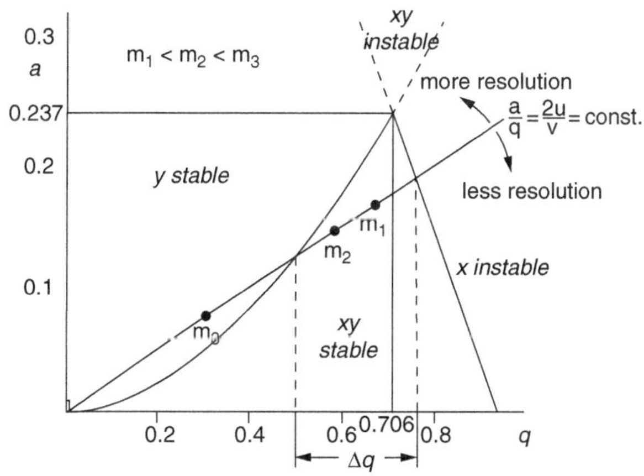

Fig. 4.33 Detail of the upper half of region I of the stability diagram for a linear quadrupole analyzer (Reproduced from Ref. [102] with permission.

(Fig. 4.32) [107]. Among the four stability regions of the first category, the tiny central region I is of special interest for the normal mass-separating operation of the linear quadrupole. Zooming in to region I (*x*- and *y*-trajectories stable) yields what is commonly referred to as the *stability diagram of the linear quadrupole* (Fig. 4.33) [101, 102].

If the ratio a/q is chosen so that $2\ U/V = 0.237/0.706 = 0.336$, the *xy*-stability region shrinks to one point, the apex, of the diagram (cf. Eq. 4.21, Fig. 4.33).

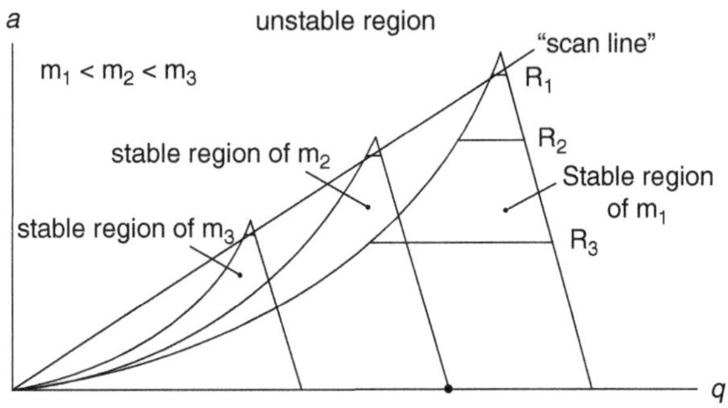

Fig. 4.34 Scanning of linear quadrupoles means performing a $U/V = constant$ linked scan. Resolution is adjusted by variation of the a/q ratio: higher a/q ratio means higher resolving power and is represented by a steeper "scan line"; $R_1 > R_2 > R_3$

By reducing a at constant q, i.e., reducing U relative to V, an increasingly wider m/z range can be transmitted simultaneously. Sufficient resolving power is achieved as long as only a small m/z range remains stable, e.g., one specific $m/z \pm 0.5$ for *unit resolution* (Sect. 4.4.3). Thus, the width (Δq) of the stable region determines the resolving power (Fig. 4.34). By varying the magnitude of U and V at constant U/V ratio an $U/V = constant$ linked scan is obtained allowing ions of increasingly higher m/z to pass the quadrupole.

Overall, the quadrupole analyzer rather acts as a mass filter than as a momentum (B sector) or energy (ESA) spectrometer; hence the widespread use of the term *quadrupole mass filter*.

Scanning a quadrupole
Scanning of any linear quadrupole means shifting the whole stability diagram along a "scan line", because each m/z value has a stability diagram of its own (Figs. 4.33 and 4.34). The representation of a scan by a "scan line" would only be correct in case of infinite resolving power, i.e., if the apices were connected. Any real resolving power is represented by a horizontal line across the stability region, where only ions falling in the region above that line are transmitted.

Ion trajectory simulations allow for the visualization of the ion motions while traveling through a quadrupole mass analyzer (Fig. 4.35). Furthermore, the optimum number of oscillations to achieve a certain level of performance can be determined. It turns out that best performance is obtained when ions of about 10 eV kinetic energy undergo approximately a hundred oscillations (Fig. 4.36) [109].

Typical quadrupoles
Standard quadrupole analyzers have rods of 10–20 mm in diameter and 15–25 cm in length. The radiofrequency is in the order of 1–4 MHz, and the DC and RF voltages are in the range of some 10^2–10^3 V. Thus, ions of about 10 eV kinetic energy undergo about 100 oscillations during their passage.

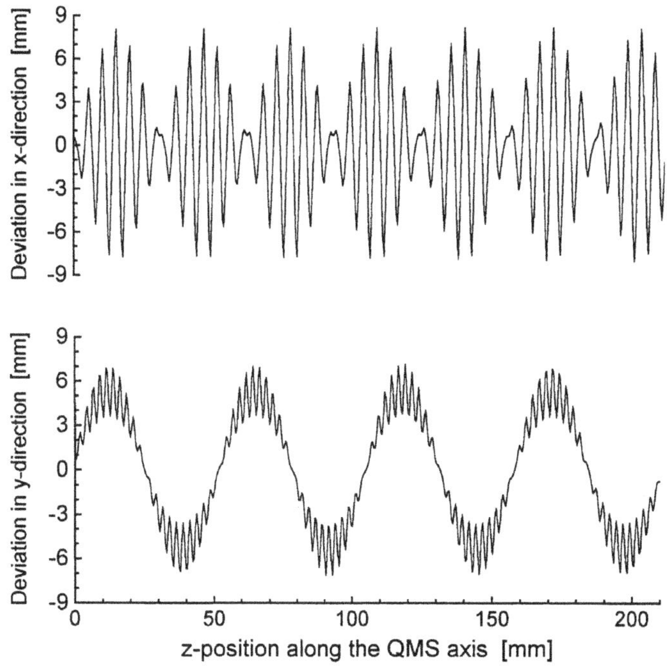

Fig. 4.35 Projection of a 3D trajectory simulation of a stable ion onto the *x*- and *y*-coordinates (Reproduced from Ref. [109] with permission. © Elsevier Science, 1998)

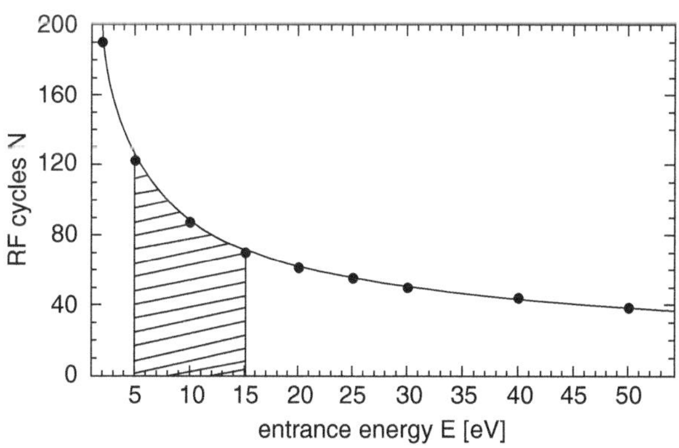

Fig. 4.36 Relation of RF cycles experienced by the ions as a function of entrance energy. The *shaded area* marks the region of optimized performance (Reproduced from Ref. [109] with permission. © Elsevier Science, 1998)

4.4.3 Resolving Power of Linear Quadrupoles

Quadrupole analyzers generally are operated at so-called *unit resolution*, normally restricting their use to typical low resolution (LR) applications [110, 111]. At unit resolution adjacent peaks are just separated from each other over the entire *m*/*z* range, i.e., $R = 20$ at *m*/*z* 20, $R = 200$ at *m*/*z* 200, and $R = 2000$ at *m*/*z* 2000. An example of unit resolution is presented in Sect. 4.5.3.

The resolution as adjusted by the *U*/*V* ratio cannot arbitrarily be increased, but is ultimately limited by the mechanical accuracy with which the rods are constructed and supported (±10 μm) [110]. Above an *m*/*z* value characteristic of each quadrupole assembly, any further improvement of resolution can only be achieved at the cost of significantly reduced transmission. Nonetheless, high-performance quadrupoles allowing for about tenfold unit resolution can be built [111].

Theoretically, the electrodes of a quadrupole mass filter should have a hyperbolic cross section for optimized geometry of the resulting quadrupole field, and thus for optimized performance (Fig. 4.37) [101, 102]. However, for ease of manufacture, cylindrical rods are often employed instead. By adjusting the radius of the rods carefully ($r = 1.1468 \times r_0$), a hyperbolic field may be approximated [112]. However, even slight distortions of the ideal quadrupole field either from interference with external fields or due to low mechanical precision or inadequate shape of the device cause severe losses of transmission and resolution [113]. The expected advantages of hyperbolic rods [114] have been demonstrated by ion trajectory calculations [109, 115]: circular rods cause a reduction in macromotion frequency because of an increased residence time of the ions in close vicinity to the rods (Fig. 4.38); this in turn means reduced resolution.

Besides optimization of mechanical accuracy, the resolving power of quadrupoles can be improved by innovative modes of operation. The operation as a multiple pass system with ion reflection at either end extends the flight path and

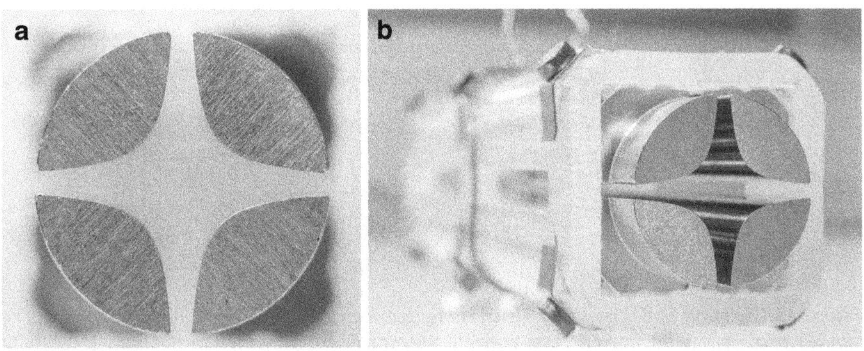

Fig. 4.37 Linear quadrupole with hyperbolic rods. (**a**) Head on view showing the cross section of the rods and (**b**) whole device partially revealing the polished inner surfaces. The rods are mounted in a precision-machined quartz frame. This particular quadrupole once belonged to a Finnigan TSQ 700 instrument

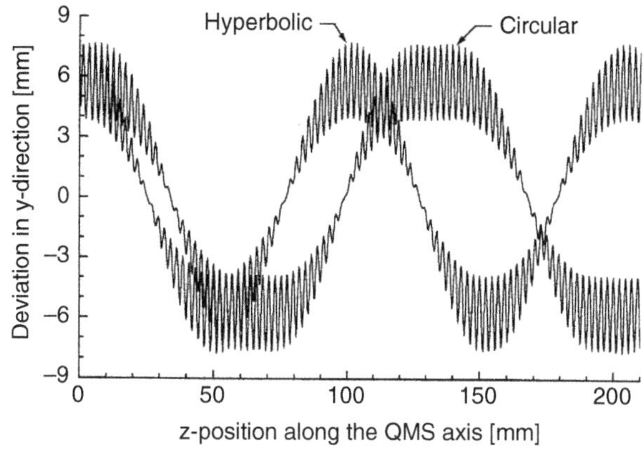

Fig. 4.38 Motion in the y-coordinate of ions traveling along a quadrupole with circular rods compared to ions in a quadrupole with ideal hyperbolic field. Circular rods cause a reduced macromotional frequency and longer residence time in the close vicinity to the (non-ideal) rod surfaces (Reproduced from Ref. [109] with permission. © Elsevier Science, 1998)

thus the number of RF cycles. The same effect can be obtained from increased radiofrequency and for ions traveling slower through the device [110]. Alternatively, the quadrupole may be operated in stability regions other than the first, e.g., in the second or fourth [110, 116]; doing so requires higher ion kinetic energies of about 750 eV.

4.4.4 RF-Only Quadrupoles, Hexapoles, and Octopoles

Setting the DC voltage U to zero transforms the quadrupole into a wide band pass for ions. In the stability diagram this mode of operation is represented by an operation line equivalent to the q-axis (Figs. 4.33 and 4.34). Such devices are commonly known as *RF-only quadrupoles* (q). *RF-only hexapoles* (h) and *RF-only octopoles* (o) are used analogously. Generally, higher-order RF 2 N–multipoles differ from quadrupoles in that they do not exhibit a sharp m/z cutoff in transmission, because x and y motions are strongly coupled, which causes the boundaries of ion stability to become rather diffuse. For low trapping voltages, the ion trajectories in an RF 2 N–multipole are approximated by an effective mechanical potential, $U_{\mathrm{eff(r)}}$, given by [108, 117]:

$$U_{\mathrm{eff(r)}} = \frac{N^2}{4}\,\frac{(ze)^2}{m_i\Omega^2}\,\frac{V^2}{r_0^2}\left(\frac{r}{r_0}\right)^{2N-2} \tag{4.22}$$

where N is the order of the multipole, e.g., $N = 3$ for a hexapole. According to Eq. (4.22), higher-order multipoles exhibit increasingly steeper potential wells, offer better ion-guiding capabilities and better wide-band pass characteristics, i.e., wider m/z range acceptance (Fig. 4.39). This property led to the widespread application of RF quadrupoles, RF hexapoles, and RF octopoles as *ion guides* and *collision cells* [118].

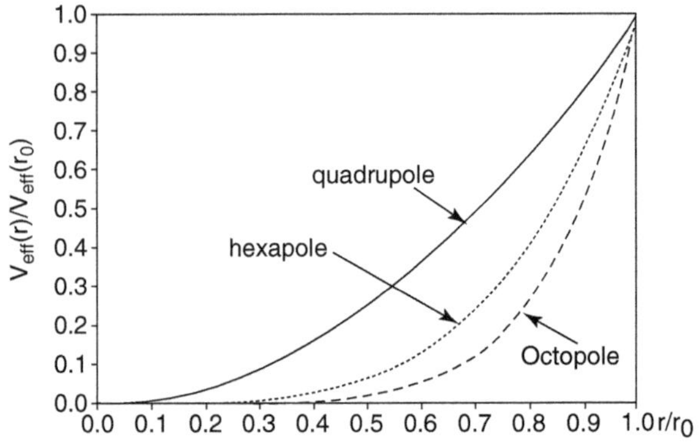

Fig. 4.39 Comparison of effective potentials for quadrupole (r^2), hexapole (r^4) and octopole fields (r^6) (Reproduced from Ref. [117] with permission. © Wiley Periodicals, Inc., 2005)

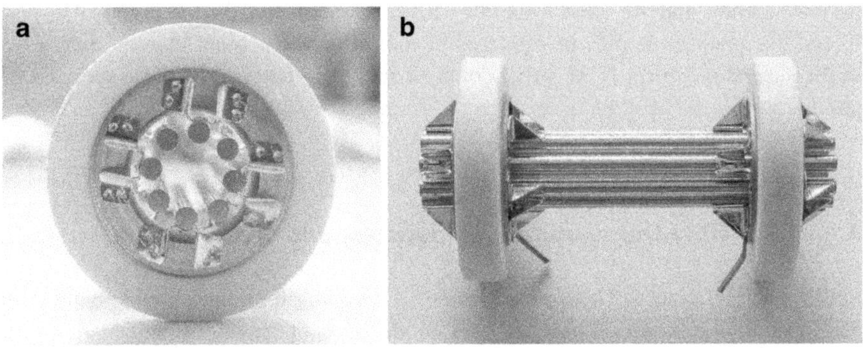

Fig. 4.40 RF octopole ion guide used to bridge a differential pumping stage of an ESI interface in a Finnigan LCQ instrument. (**a**) Head-on view to show the octopole alignment and (**b**) side view. Each of the two pins pointing down is connected to supply the RF voltage to four of the rods in alternation. The round rods are ca. 3 mm in diameter and the length of this device is about 7 cm

RF ion guides are employed in many ways to transfer ions of low kinetic energy, typically of 1–50 eV, from one functional unit to another without substantial losses [117, 119]. Ion guides are used to adapt atmospheric pressure ion sources to mass analyzers, e.g., for APCI, ESI, and ambient MS (Fig. 4.40; Chaps. 7, 8, 12, and 13). From the viewpoint of the ions, they act like a hose or pipe while being fully permeable for neutrals. Thus, the RF ion guide allows residual gas to effuse through the gaps between the rods into the vacuum pumps, whereas ions are escorted into the mass analyzer. Examples for RF ion guide usage will be given in the instrument schemes to follow later in this chapter.

In contrast to expectations based on scattering by collisions with residual gas, RF-only multipoles deliver even improved transmission at moderate vacuum conditions in the range of 10^{-3}–10^{-2} mbar. This is due to a reduction in ion kinetic energy and concomitant collisional damping of ion motion toward the central axis of the device, so-called *collisional cooling* [108, 120–122]. It has been shown that

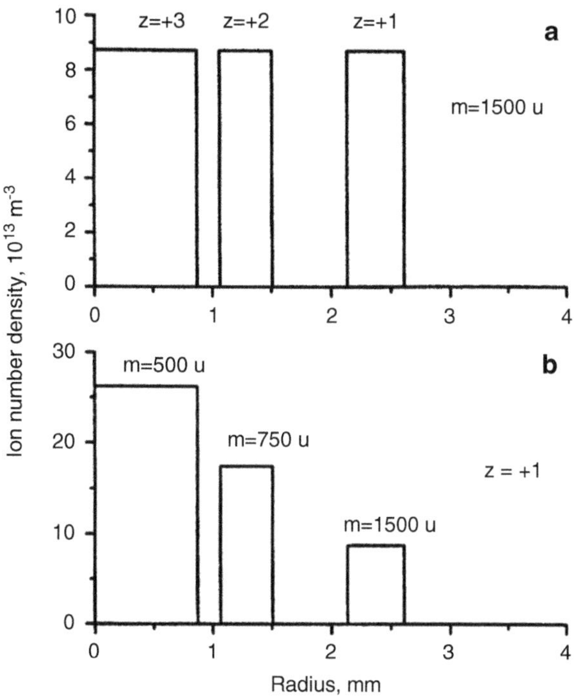

Fig. 4.41 Calculated number density distributions of ions stored in a collisional cooling RF-only quadrupole ion guide having an inner radius of 4 mm and being operated at 1 MHz. (**a**) Radial positions of ions of 1500 u bearing 1, 2, and 3 positive charges. (**b**) Radial position of ion clouds of singly charged ions of *m*/*z* 500, 1000, and 1500 (Reproduced from Ref. [121] with permission. © John Wiley & Sons, Ltd., 2000)

ions of 25 eV kinetic energy are slowed down to 0–2 eV upon passing through a 15-cm-long RF-only quadrupole ion guide at 8×10^{-3} mbar [120, 123]. Ions of higher mass (not higher *m*/*z*) are more prone to this effect, e.g., a sevenfold increase was found for ions of about 200 u, whereas ions of about 17,000 u showed 80-fold improvement in transmission [120]. Here, collisional cooling causes a confinement of the ion beam towards the central axis of the quadrupole which in turn increases the transmission efficiency through an exit aperture. This phenomenon is known as *collisional focusing* (cf. Fig. 4.43 in Sect. 4.5.1) [108, 122, 124].

It is even more interesting that the cooled ion cloud forms concentric cylindrical layers inside the RF-only multipole, each of those layers being composed of ions of the same *m*/*z* value with higher *m*/*z* ions gathering in more outward radial layers. This behavior is due to more effective RF focusing for ions of lower *m*/*z* that pushes these ions closer towards the center. Multiply charged ions form more distinct radial boundaries of the layers as compared to singly charged ion clouds of the same *m*/*z* and charge density (Fig. 4.41). The gaps of low ion population between the layers result from space charge repulsion [121]. Formation of such *m*/*z*-stratified structures requires sufficiently high charge density and effective collisional damping. Both RF-only collision multipoles and linear quadrupole ion traps as employed for external ion accumulation fulfill those criteria. When the linear ion density increases, the maximum ion cloud radius also increases. Overfilling of the multipole capacity results in a strong discrimination against high *m*/*z* ions, because the ion clouds expand to larger radii causing outer layers (high-*m*/*z* ions) to hit the multipole rods [121].

Conditions for thermalization

From the work by Douglas [120] a rule of thumb can be derived to judge whether thermalization occurs. This $p \times d$ *rule* demands the product of pressure (p in Torr) times path length (l in mm) to be larger than 0.2 mTorr. For example, at 2×10^{-3} Torr a RF-only device of 100 mm length is just sufficient for effective ion cooling as we have 2×10^{-3} Torr × 100 mm = 0.2 mTorr.

RF-only *quadrupole, hexapole*, or *octopole collision cells* [117, 125, 126] are part of so-called *triple quadrupole mass spectrometers*, which essentially represent QqQ, QhQ, or QoQ instruments, respectively, depending on the type of RF-only collision cell actually in place. They are efficient tools for tandem mass spectrometry (Chap. 9).

Different from magnetic sector or TOF instruments having collimated beams of energetic ions, the ions are exiting from quadrupoles in almost any direction on the *xy*-plane. Thus, real field-free regions as employed in sector or TOF instruments have to be replaced by ion-guiding collision cells to allow CID of ions of 5–100 eV kinetic energy. RF-only collision cells need not to be straight: starting from the Finnigan TSQ700 bent geometries were introduced, and 90° cells or 180° cells are nowadays common. Besides a reduced footprint of the instrument, the bent geometries have other beneficial effects such as the elongation of the flight path through the collision region for improved fragmentation efficiency and the exclusion of neutrals or photons from hitting the detector, and thus, reduced noise levels.

Ions can even stop

The initial kinetic energy of slow ions can be lost upon several collisions. At 5×10^{-3} mbar (0.5 Pa) fragment ion kinetic energies are reduced to about 1 eV [123]. The ions may even stop their motion along the cell [121, 124]. Under such conditions, the continuous ion current into the cell is the only impetus to push the ions through as a result of space-charge effects. The resulting dwell time of about 10 ms allows up to about 5000 (reactive) collisions to take place at about 5×10^{-2} mbar (5 Pa) collision gas (or reagent gas) pressure in an octopole collision cell [127].

Within the last decade, RF quadrupole ion guides with square or at least rectangular rod cross sections have also been used. Most of this development has been done by instrument manufacturers and few has been published on this topic. However, it appears that these square-rod quadrupoles offer the same level of performance as round-rod higher-order RF ion guides at reduced cost of manufacture. We will get back to square rods in the context of linear quadrupole ion traps in the next section.

Postponed summary A summary of RF quadrupole devices will be given in Sect. 4.6.12. As we will see during the next two sections dealing with linear quadrupole ions traps and ion traps with three-dimensional quadrupole fields these devices have much in common, suggesting to summarize and compare them together later.

4.5 Linear Quadrupole Ion Traps

4.5.1 Linear RF-Only Multipole Ion Traps

As we have just learned, collisional cooling may bring translational ion motion along the axis of an RF-only multipole almost to a halt, thereby transforming such an RF-only multipole ion guide into an ion storage device [121]. To prevent ions inside the multipole from escaping via either open end, one creates a trapping potential well by placing electrodes of slightly higher potential adjacent to the front and rear ends of the multipole [128]. Such devices are known as *linear (quadrupole) ion traps* (LIT).

Only quadrupoles are mass-selective
Quadrupoles are the only devices capable of mass-selective operation, whereas higher-order RF ion guides or higher-order LITs can only guide, accumulate, store, and finally release ions for subsequent *m/z* analysis.

While the entrance plate of the LIT is held at low potential, ions may enter the radially ion-confining RF field. The time span for ion accumulation is limited by

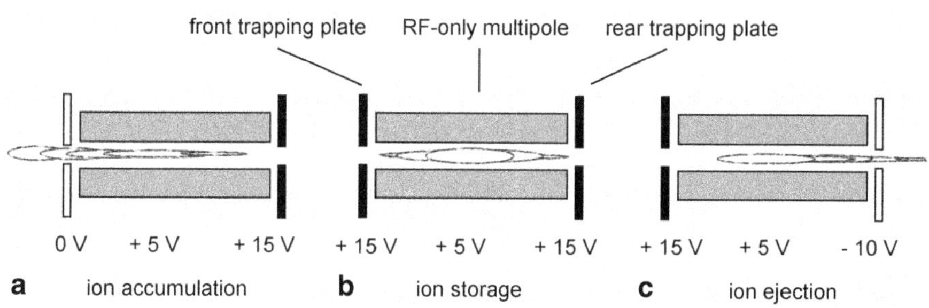

Fig. 4.42 Operation of a linear RF multipole ion trap illustrated using typical DC voltage offsets for positive ions. (**a**) Ion accumulation with backside potential wall up, (**b**) storage of ions with both trapping potentials up, and (**c**) axial ejection of ions from trap using an attractive exit plate potential. The trapping RF multipole section is held at constant DC offset of +5 V in this example

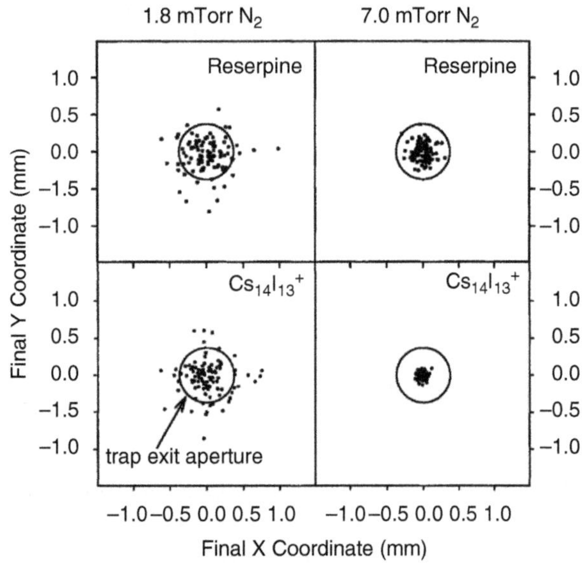

Fig. 4.43 Radial distribution of 100 ion trajectories at the LIT exit aperture (*circle* indicates 0.7 mm aperture hole) for ions of reserpine and $Cs_{14}I_{13}^+$ cluster ions. Collisional focusing is well improved when raising the LIT pressure from 1.8 mTorr (2.4×10^{-3} mbar) to 7.0 mTorr (9.3×10^{-3} mbar) (Adapted from Ref. [122] with permission. © John Wiley & Sons, Ltd., 2001)

reflection of the fast ions at the backside potential wall affording that the entrance gate has to be closed before the lightest ions to be stored can exit the trap via the entrance (Fig. 4.42). Storage of ions in the presence of some buffer gas, e.g., argon or nitrogen at 10^{-3}–10^{-2} mbar, then allows for their thermalization and collisional focusing towards the LIT axis (Fig. 4.43). Both actual ion kinetic energy of the entering ion beam and the degree of thermalization directly influence the potential required to stop axial ion motion [122]. Vice versa, the trapping efficiency of an LIT for faster ions improves with rising pressure (Fig. 4.44) [129]. Finally, the ions can be axially ejected at any convenient point in time. Alternatively, the RF multipole may be segmented, typically into a longer middle and two shorter ends, which are operated at the same RF drive frequency and amplitude but at a DC offset voltage to create the switchable trapping potential well analogous to the trapping plates [130].

LITs present a rapidly expanding field of instrumentation; they have been established to collect ions externally before injecting them in bunches into an FT-ICR [131] or oaTOF analyzer [122, 128]. LITs capable of scanning by either axial or radial excitation of the ions and even capable of precursor ion selection for MS/MS experiments [129, 130, 132] and have been incorporated in commercial mass spectrometers [117, 133–135]. LITs can be built to store ions of very high *m/z*, e.g., singly charged ions of bovine serum albumine, *m/z* 66.000, or even charged particulate matter [136].

This tells us that LITs are highly versatile devices:

- LITs may thermalize ions during their passage to provide narrow kinetic energy distributions before the next step of ion manipulation.

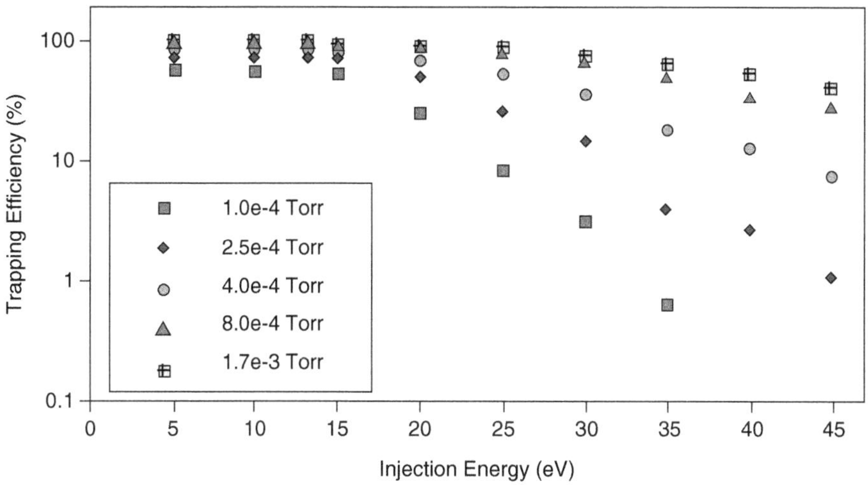

Fig. 4.44 Dependence of the trapping efficiency of an LIT on ion injection energy (reserpine $[M + H]^+$ ions, *m/z* 609) for varying LIT pressures (from the top 1.3×10^{-4} mbar, 3.3×10^{-4} mbar, 5.3×10^{-4} mbar, 1.1×10^{-3} mbar, 2.3×10^{-3} mbar) (Adapted from Ref. [129] with permission. © John Wiley & Sons, Ltd., 2002)

- LITs can accumulate ions until a population suitable for the respective next step of mass analysis is reached.
- LITs can deliver packages of ions for a mass analyzer operating in batch mode.
- LITs themselves are capable of mass-selective operation and scanning to serve as mass analyzers on their own (Sect. 4.5.2).
- LITs are even capable of precursor ion selection and subsequent ion fragmentation by collisions with buffer gas for MS/MS experiments.

A new time scale
With RF multipoles and even more so with LITs, we have definitely gone beyond the domain of the classical mass spectrometric time scale (Sect. 2.6.2). In ion trapping devices, ions are stored for milliseconds to seconds, i.e., 10^3–10^6 times longer than their lifetimes in beam instruments.

4.5.2 Mass-Analyzing Linear Quadrupole Ion Trap with Axial Ejection

Linear ion traps provide high capacities as far as the number of trapped ions is concerned, because the ion cloud can expand along the entire device. It is thus desirable to operate such an LIT not only for ion thermalization and ion accumulation but also as a mass analyzer. In principle, there are two modes possible: one employs excitation of the ions to achieve mass-selective ejection in radial direction

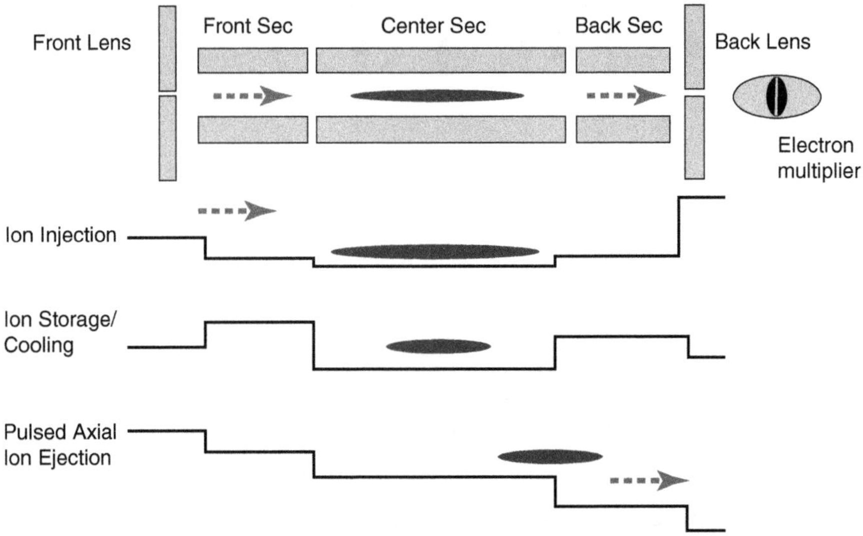

Fig. 4.45 Sequence of DC voltages applied of the lenses and sections of a segmented linear ion trap to achieve mass-selective isolation and axial pulse-out of trapped ions from the mass analyzer. The reasons for segmenting of the LIT are explained in Sect. 4.5.3 and Fig. 4.49 (Reproduced from Ref. [140] with permission. © American Chemical Society, 2004)

[137], the other uses mass-selective axial ejection by application of an auxiliary AC field to the rods of the LIT [129]. The latter mode makes use of the fact that near the exit of the LIT radial ion motion (RF-controlled) and axial ion motion (trapping potential-controlled) are coupled via the fringing fields. When the ion radial secular frequency (governed by the stability parameters and the drive RF) matches that of the auxiliary AC field, ion excitation is effected in a way that also enhances its axial kinetic energy, and thus, leads to ejection from the LIT (Fig. 4.45) [138] and Chap. 5 in [139]).

An instrument incorporating a LIT with mass-selective axial ejection has been developed by Hager by replacing either the RF-only collision quadrupole or the second mass-analyzing quadrupole of a QqQ instrument with a LIT. The attained configurations are Q-LIT-Q (Fig. 4.46) and QqLIT, respectively [129, 134, 135]. The QqLIT offers enhanced sensitivity as compared to its QqQ precursor model and offers new modes of operation [134] and Chap. 3 in [141]). The QqLIT has been commercialized by AB Sciex as their Q-Trap series.

As with the linear quadrupole before, the potential $\Phi_{(x,y,z,t)}$ in the two-dimensional quadrupole field of the LIT is expressed by a DC voltage U and an RF drive voltage V with the frequency Ω [129, 138] and Chap. 5 in [139])

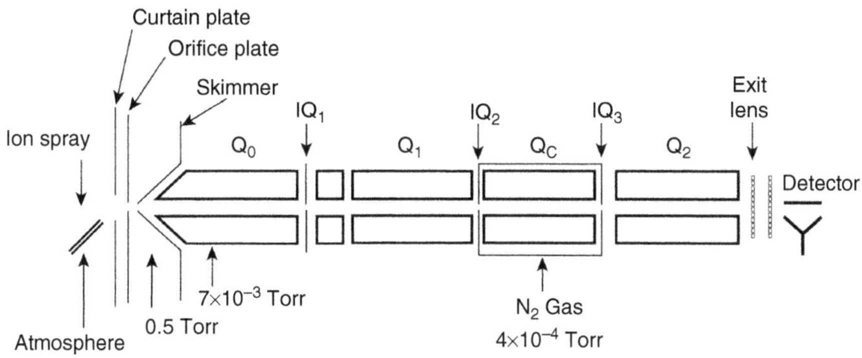

Fig. 4.46 A quadrupole-LIT hybrid instrument. In this scheme, the RF-only collision quadrupole has been replaced by the LIT. The other option, replacement of Q2 by a LIT, is finally in commercial use (Adapted from Ref. [129] with permission. © John Wiley & Sons, Ltd., 2002)

$$\Phi_{(x,y,z,t)} = (U - V\cos\Omega t)\frac{(x^2 - y^2)}{r_0^2} \tag{4.23}$$

from which the equations of motion can be derived. Assuming singly charged ions, i.e., $q = e$, we have

$$\begin{aligned} &\frac{d^2x}{dt^2} + \frac{e}{m_i r_0{}^2}\ (U - V\cos\Omega t)x = 0 \\ &\frac{d^2y}{dt^2} - \frac{e}{m_i r_0{}^2}\ (U - V\cos\Omega t)y = 0 \\ &\frac{d^2z}{dt^2} = 0 \end{aligned} \tag{4.24}$$

where m_i is the mass of the ion, r_o is the distance between the central axis of the LIT and the surface of the rod. At least, these relationships hold valid as long as ions are sufficiently distant to the fringing fields at the end of the rods.

In practice, there is no DC component, and thus, only the Mathieu parameter q is required, which is obtained by solving the above equations

$$q_x = \frac{4eV}{m_i r_0{}^2\Omega^2} \tag{4.25}$$

The voltage V is the zero-to-peak amplitude of the RF drive voltage. For an ion inside the quadrupole field the fundamental resonant frequency ω_n is obtained as

$$\omega_n = (2n + \beta)\left(\frac{\Omega}{2}\right) \tag{4.26}$$

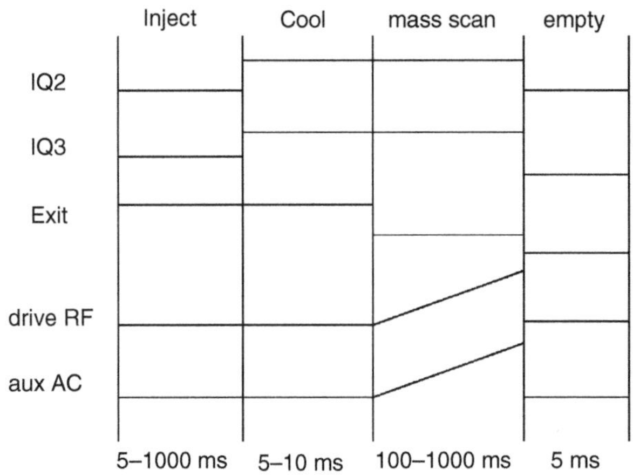

Fig. 4.47 Scan function as used in the QqLIT instrument. IQ2, IQ3, and Exit belong to the trapping plates and the exit lens. Vertical displacements of lines indicate changes of the respective voltages. Note that the time slices are not to scale and that the duration of ion accumulation and mass scan may vary substantially (Adapted from Ref. [129] with permission. © John Wiley & Sons, Ltd., 2002)

For $n = 0$ Eq. (4.26) simplifies to become

$$\omega = \frac{\beta\Omega}{2} \tag{4.26a}$$

which for $q_x < 0.4$ can be approximated by the relationship

$$\omega \approx \frac{q_x}{\sqrt{8}}\Omega \tag{4.27}$$

The stability diagram for the LIT is analogous to that of the linear quadrupole (Figs. 4.32 and 4.33). While a description of the scanning of the LIT to achieve mass-selective axial ejection requires complex mathematics [138] far beyond the scope of this book, the practical application of LIT can easier be understood.

The scan function of such an instrument can be displayed in four time slices comprising:

1. ion injection until enough ions are accumulated,
2. trapping and thermalization,
3. mass scan by linear alteration of RF drive and auxiliary AC voltage,
4. a short blanking pulse to reset the LIT prior to the next scan cycle (Fig. 4.47).

Combination of two analyzer concepts

The QqLIT setup combines into one single instrument different types of mass analyzers, a scanning linear quadrupole, and a scanning linear quadrupole ion trap all connected via an RF-only ion guide. Instruments combining different types of mass analyzers are termed *hybrid instruments*. Most modern mass spectrometers are assembled from different elements to achieve optimum capabilities in the sense of creating instruments uniting the best of two worlds [133]. An overview of hybrids is presented at the end of the analyzer section.

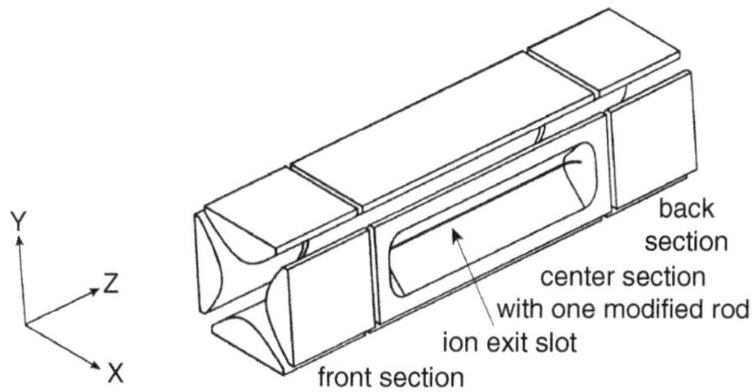

Fig. 4.48 A segmented linear quadrupole ion trap with mass-selective radial ejection capability. Applying higher potential to the front and back sections creates an axial trapping potential for ions in the center section. Radial trapping is again provided by the RF quadrupolar field. Ions are exiting through the slot in one of the four rods. The commercial design offers doubled sensitivity by using two detectors at opposite rods (Adapted from Ref. [130] by permission. © Elsevier Science, 2002)

4.5.3 Mass-Analyzing Linear Ion Trap with Radial Ejection

A scanning LIT [130] can alternatively be realized using a mass-selective radial ejection mode of operation. Such a LIT can either serve as a stand-alone mass analyzer (Thermo Scientific LTQ™ series) or can be combined into a hybrid LIT-FT-ICR instrument (Thermo Scientific LTQ-FT™ series). In the LTQ-FT instruments, the LIT shields the ultrahigh vacuum of the FT-ICR from collision gas and decomposition products in order to operate under optimum conditions. More importantly from the analytical point of view, the LIT can accumulate, mass-select and fragment selected ions prior to the next FT-ICR cycle while the ICR cell is still busy with the previous ion package (FT-ICR cf. Sect. 4.7). By using an Orbitrap analyzer (Sect. 4.8) in place of the FT-ICR cell, the same company offers the Thermo Scientific LTQ-Orbitrap™ series as an economical nonetheless powerful alternative to their LTQ-FT.

The LIT is composed of a quadrupole with hyperbolic rods that is cut into three segments of 12 mm in length for both trapping sections and 37 mm in length for the ion storage compartment (Fig. 4.48) [130]. The segmented design avoids fringing fields from the trapping plates as obvious from the electric field calculations using the SIMION software package (Fig. 4.49) [142, 143]. Although necessary for the axial ejection scan mode discussed in the preceding section, the radial excitation scanning requires the absence of fringing fields in the trapping zone. One pair of opposite storage compartment rods has cut a slit of 0.25 mm width and 30 mm length to allow for radial ejection of ions onto a conversion dynode. The conversion dynode is held at -15 kV (for positive-ion operation), and upon ion impact it delivers secondary electrons to an electron multiplier. In the commercial variant of the instrument, two detectors are in use to double the sensitivity of the device. The field inhomogeneity introduced by cutting slits into the rods is counterbalanced by

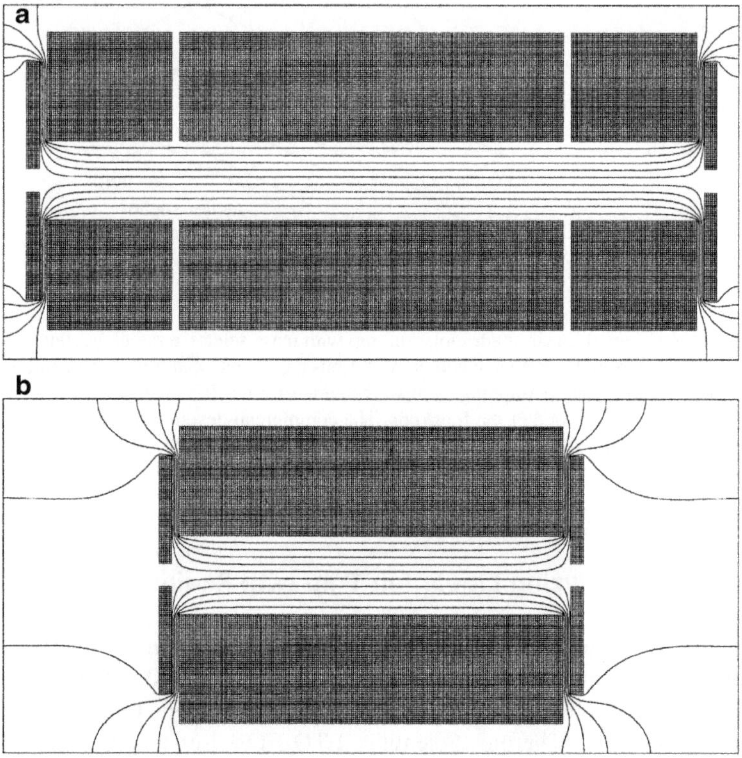

Fig. 4.49 SIMION simulation of the resonance excitation field comparing (**a**) a three-section ion trap and (**b**) a single-section device with end plates for trapping. In (**a**) the field inside the trapping compartment remains unperturbed from fringing fields (Adapted with permission from Ref. [130]. © Elsevier Science Publishers, 2002)

aligning them slightly outward from their theoretical *x*-position [130]. To operate as an *m*/*z* analyzer, the assembly of rods needs (*i*) a DC voltage supply to create the axial trapping field (*z*-coordinate), (*ii*) an RF voltage supply (1 MHz, ± 5 kV rod to ground) to deliver the radial quadrupolar trapping field (*x*,*y*-plane), and (*iii*) two phases of supplemental AC voltage (5–500 kHz, ± 80 V) that is applied across the *x*-rods for ion isolation, activation, and mass-selective ejection.

4.5.4 Constructing an Instrument Around the LIT

It takes more than just a nicely working *m*/*z* analyzer to put together an instrument suitable for real-world use and commercial success. Thus, the elaboration in this short paragraph presents an example of what is relevant for any type of mass spectrometer.

To build a useful mass spectrometer, the above LIT is connected to an electrospray ionization (ESI, Chap. 12) source using RF-only ion guides to bridge the distance from the source orifice to the entrance of the LIT. As the ESI process starts at atmospheric pressure, the incipient ions need to be continuously transferred from outside the mass spectrometer into the high vacuum of the *m*/*z* analyzer. This can be achieved by so-called *differential pumping* (Sect. 4.13). Differential pumping makes use of the fact that macroscopic flow is only sustained as long as the mean free path of a molecule is shorter than the average dimension of the aperture it has to pass or of the vessel where it is contained. In practice, a powerful rotary pump (30 $m^3\ h^{-1}$) maintains a pressure in the order of 1 mbar behind a 0.4–0.5 mm orifice. The next stages of the differentially pumped system are usually pumped by turbomolecular pumps. In modern instruments one split-flow turbomolecular pump often serves for both ports. In case of the LIT instrument the intermediate region is thus evacuated to about 2×10^{-3} mbar and the LIT itself to 2.6×10^{-5} mbar (Fig. 4.50).

The resulting mass spectrometer is able to deliver unit resolution over an *m*/*z* 150–2000 range at about 3 scans per second (Fig. 4.51) and even to provide higher resolution at lower scan rates ([130, 144] and Chap. 5 in [139]).

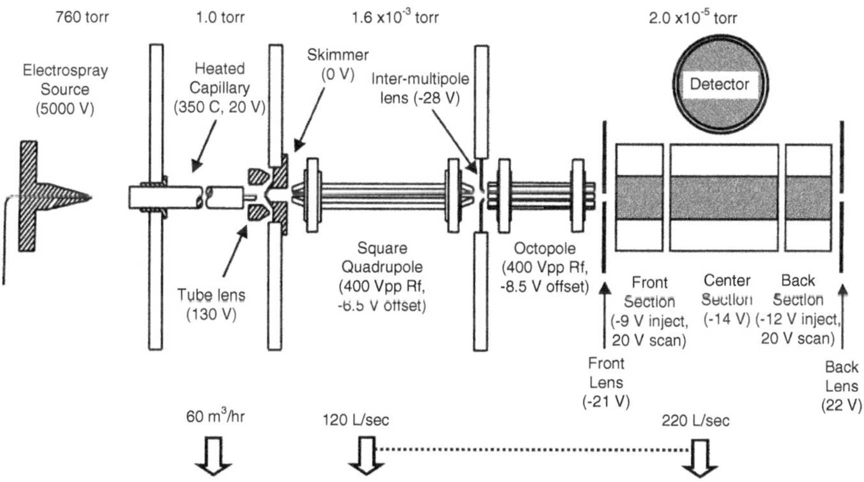

Fig. 4.50 Radial ejection LIT mass spectrometer with ESI source, more precisely the Thermo Fisher LTQ as of 2002. A square RF quadrupole is used to bridge the second pumping stage while an RF octopole like the one shown in Fig. 4.40 is used in the third pumping state. Typical operating voltages and pressures are given (Reprinted with permission from Ref. [130]. © Elsevier Science Publishers, 2002)

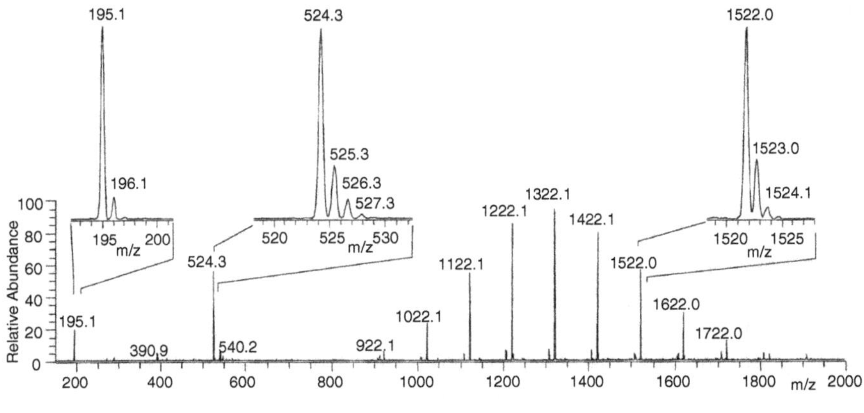

Fig. 4.51 Full scan mass spectrum of a calibration mixture containing caffeine, $[M + H]^+$ at *m/z* 195, the peptide MRFA, $[M + H]^+$ at *m/z* 524, and Ultramark 1621 yielding a series of ions from *m/z* 922 to 1722. The expanded views of selected signals show unit resolution, i.e., uniform resolution over the whole range (Adapted with permission from Ref. [130]. © Elsevier Science Publishers, 2002)

Just a reminder As already pointed out at the end of the linear quadrupole section, a summary of all RF quadrupole devices will be given in Sect. 4.6.12.

4.6 Ion Trap with Three-Dimensional Quadrupole Field

4.6.1 Introduction

In contrast to the linear two-dimensional quadrupole field of the LIT, the *quadrupole ion trap* (QIT) originally developed by Wolfgang Paul creates a three-dimensional RF quadrupole field of rotational symmetry to store ions within defined boundaries. The invention of the QIT goes back to 1953 [101–103]; however, it took until the mid-1980s to access the full analytical potential of quadrupole ion traps [139, 145–149].

Naming

Wolfgang Paul himself preferred to call the device "*Ionenkäfig*" (ion cage) because it does not actively act to catch ions from the outside. The acronym QUISTOR derived from *quadrupole ion store* was also in use for a while. To be precise, we would have to call it *ion trap with three-dimensional quadrupole field*, as used in the title of this section. Rather than insisting on this lengthy term we will be using the commonly accepted term *quadrupole ion trap* (QIT).

The first commercial quadrupole ion traps were incorporated in GC-MS benchtop instruments in the late 1980s (Finnigan MAT ITD and ITMS). Electron ionization was effected inside the trap by admitting the GC effluent and a beam of electrons directly into the storage volume of the trap. Later, external ion sources became available, and soon a large number of ionization methods could be fitted to the QIT analyzer [150–152]. Modern QITs cover ranges up to about *m/z* 3000 with fast scanning at unit resolution, and in addition, offer *"zoom scans"* over smaller *m/z* ranges at higher resolution; instruments delivering resolving power up to 5-fold unit resolution are commercially available. Accurate mass measurements with QITs were expected [148] but not realized so far. The tandem-in-time capabilities of QITs can be employed to conveniently perform MS^n experiments [146, 147], and their compact size is ideal for field applications [16].

Historical versus didactical

Historically, both the linear quadrupole analyzer and the quadrupole ion trap originate from the early 1950s (even from the same inventor), whereas the scanning linear ion trap is a design of the 1990s. A detailed timeline of the development of quadrupole ion traps can be found in the comprehensive monographs by March and Todd [139, 145]. However, from a teaching perspective, it appears advisable to align the explanations in the logical order as presented here. Once the concepts of trapping and mass-selective release from a quadrupole ion trap have been understood, the step from linear to rotational symmetry should be comparatively easy.

4.6.2 Principle of the Quadrupole Ion Trap

The *quadrupole ion trap* (QIT) consists of two hyperbolic electrodes serving as end caps along with a ring electrode that replaces two of the linear quadrupole rods, i.e., it could theoretically be obtained by rotating the axial cross section of a linear quadrupole with hyperbolic rods by 360° around an axis that traverses the apices of two opposed rods (Figs. 4.52 and 4.53). Thus, a section through the *rz*-plane of the QIT closely resembles that of the entrance of a linear quadrupole with hyperbolic rods (cf. Figs. 4.30 and 4.37) [105, 150]. However, the angle between the asymptotes enclosing the ring electrode is 70.5° ($2 \times \arctan(1/\sqrt{2})$) instead of 90°. The end caps are electrically connected and the DC and RF potentials are applied between them and the ring electrode. The working principle of the QIT is based on creating stable trajectories for ions of a certain *m/z* or *m/z* range while removing unwanted ions by letting them collide with the walls or by axial ejection from the trap due to their unstable trajectories [139, 145, 149].

For the QIT, the electric field has to be considered in three dimensions. Let the potential Φ_0 be applied to the ring electrode while the hyperbolic end caps are grounded. The axial coordinate of the trap is designated as the *z*-axis, the value z_0

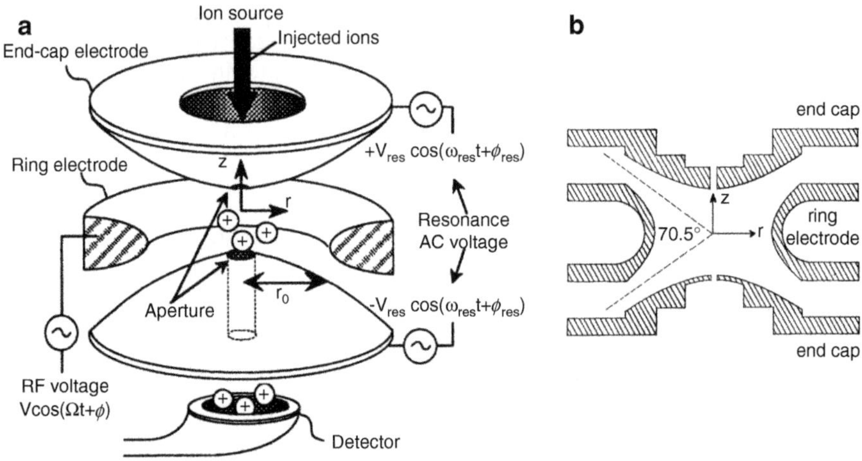

Fig. 4.52 A quadrupole ion trap. (**a**) QIT with external ion source (illustration stretched in z-direction) and (**b**) section in the rz-plane (in scale). (**a**) (Reproduced from Ref. [153] by permission. © John Wiley & Sons, 2000)

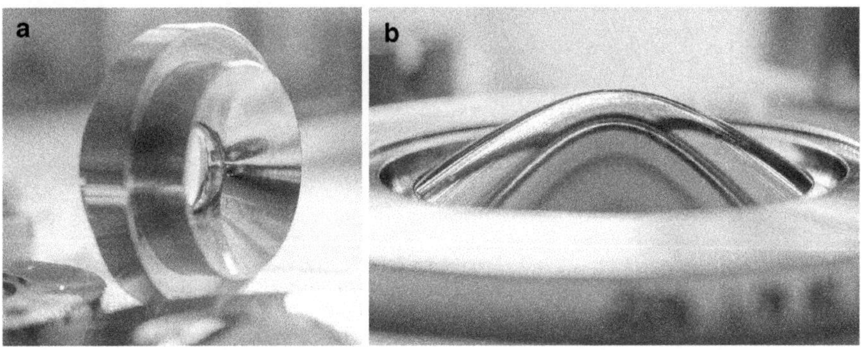

Fig. 4.53 Electrodes of the Finnigan LCQ quadrupole ion trap analyzer. (**a**) Ring electrode with symmetrical hyperbolic cross section of the inner walls of the ring. (**b**) One of the pair of hyperbolic end cap electrodes

defines the physical dimension of the trap (center to cap), and z presents the actual position of an ion with respect to the z-axis. The x,y-plane is resolved into the cell radius r_0 where r analogously defines the actual radial position of an ion. With the pair of end caps grounded the potential inside the trap is given as

$$\Phi_0 = U + V\cos\Omega t \tag{4.28}$$

Then, the field can be described in cylindrical coordinates (using the standard transformations $x = r\cos\theta$, $y = r\sin\theta$, *and* $z = z$) by the expression [145, 150]

$$\Phi_{x,y,z} = \frac{\Phi_0}{{r_0}^2}\left(r^2\cos^2\theta + r^2\sin^2\theta - 2z^2\right) \tag{4.29}$$

Because of $\cos^2 + \sin^2 = 1$ this reduces to

$$\Phi_{r,z} = \frac{\Phi_0}{{r_0}^2}\left(r^2 - 2z^2\right) \tag{4.30}$$

The equations of motion of a singly charged ion of $q = e$ in such a field are

$$\begin{aligned} &\frac{d^2z}{dt^2} - \frac{4e}{m_i\left(r_0^2 + 2z_0^2\right)}\quad (U - V\cos\Omega t)z = 0 \\ &\frac{d^2r}{dt^2} + \frac{2e}{m_i\left(r_0^2 + 2z_0^2\right)}\quad (U - V\cos\Omega t)r = 0 \end{aligned} \tag{4.31}$$

Solving these differential equations which are again of the Mathieu type, finally yields the parameters a_z and q_z

$$\begin{aligned} a_z &= -2a_r = -\frac{16eU}{m_i\left(r_0^2 + 2z_0^2\right)\ \Omega^2} \\ q_z &= -2q_r = \frac{8eV}{m_i\left(r_0^2 + 2z_0^2\right)\ \Omega^2} \end{aligned} \tag{4.32}$$

where $\Omega = 2\pi f$ and f is the fundamental RF frequency of the trap ($\approx$1 MHz). To remain stored in the QIT, an ion has to be simultaneously stable in the r and z directions. The occurrence of stable ion trajectories is determined by the stability parameters β_r and β_z which depend on the parameters a and q. The borders of the first stability region are defined by $0 < \beta_r, \beta_z < 1$ [154].

A stability diagram can be drawn where the stability region closest to its origin is of greatest importance for the operation of the QIT (Fig. 4.54). At a given U/V ratio, ions of different m/z are located along a straight line crossing the stability region; ions of higher m/z are nearer to the origin than lighter ones. The regions of stability as plotted in the a/q plane are represented as envelopes of characteristic shape. Ions with their m/z value inside the boundaries are stored in the QIT. The low-mass limit of the trapped m/z range is strictly defined by $q_z = 0.908$.

Collisional cooling (Sect. 4.4.4) by several tens of soft collisions during the dwell time of the ions inside the QIT significantly enhances its resolving power and sensitivity [155, 156]. The light buffer gas, normally helium at 0.1 Pa, serves to dampen the ion motion towards the center of the trap, and thus, keeps them away from the electrode surfaces and from field inhomogeneities as induced by the entrance and exit holes of the QIT [157].

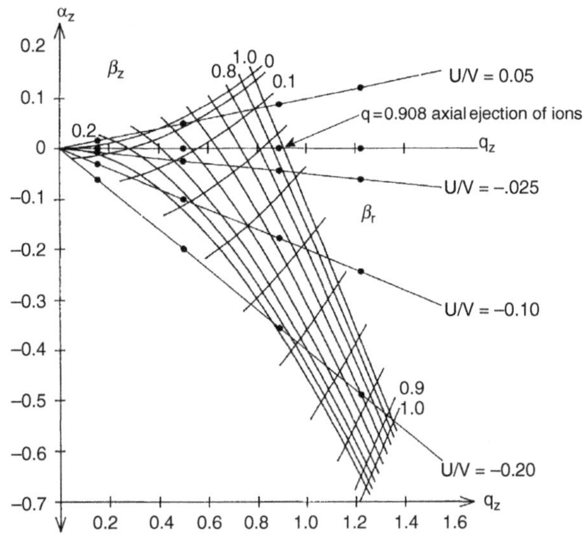

Fig. 4.54 Stability diagram for the quadrupole ion trap. The points collected on a common line mark the *a*/*q* values of a set of ions. Each line results from different settings of the *U*/*V* ratio (Reproduced from Ref. [145] by permission. © John Wiley and Sons, 1989)

4.6.3 Visualization of Ion Motion in the Ion Trap

The way the three-dimensional quadrupole field acts to keep ions within a certain volume, i.e., within a potential well some electron volts in depth, can be illustrated by a mechanical analog: A ball can be prevented from rolling from a saddle by rotating the saddle just right to bring the ball back to the middle before it can leave the surface via one of the steeply falling sides (Fig. 4.55a). Paul demonstrated the dynamic stabilization of up to three steel balls by such a device in his Nobel lecture [101, 102].

The trajectories of low-mass ions in a QIT were shown to be similar to those observed for charged aluminum dust particles [158–161]. Wuerker recorded Lissajous trajectories, superimposed by the RF drive frequency, as a photomicrograph (Fig. 4.55b) [158]. The complex motion of the ions is the result of the two super-imposed secular oscillations in *r* and *z* direction. Calculations of the trajectories yield the same results [162].

4.6.4 Mass-Selective Stability Mode

The whole range of ions is generated within or admitted to the QIT, but solely ions of one particular *m*/*z* are trapped at a time by setting appropriate parameters of the QIT. Then, the stored ions are pulsed out of the storage volume by applying a negative pulse to one of the end caps [163, 164]. Thus, they hit the detector located behind an opening in the center of one of the end caps. A full-scan mass spectrum is obtained by addition of several hundred single steps, one for each nominal *m*/*z* value. This is the so-called *mass-selective stability* mode of the QIT [165, 166]. The mass-selective stability mode is no longer in use, because it is too slow and provides poor sensitivity as most ions are wasted.

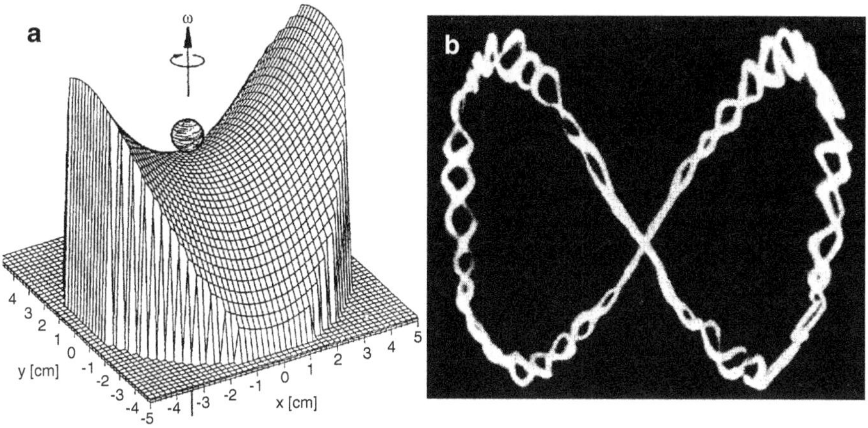

Fig. 4.55 Visualization of ion motion in the ion trap. (**a**) Mechanical analog of the QIT. (**b**) Photograph of ion trajectories of charged aluminum particles in a quadrupole ion trap ((**a**) Reproduced from Ref. [102] with permission. © World Scientific Publishing, 1993. (**b**) Reproduced from Ref. [158] with permission. © American Institute of Physics, 1959)

4.6.5 Mass-Selective Instability Mode

First, the full *m/z* range of interest is trapped within the QIT. The trapped ions may either be created inside the QIT or externally. Then, with the end caps grounded an RF-voltage scan (V) is applied to the ring electrode causing consecutive ejection of ions in the order of their *m/z* values. This is known as *mass-selective instability (ejection)* mode [155, 167]. It can be represented in the stability diagram by a horizontal line from the origin to the point of axial ejection at $q_z = 0.908$. The timing sequence is shown in Fig. 4.56 While easy to understand, this mode is also no longer relevant in QIT operation.

4.6.6 Resonant Ejection

Another technique to operate a QITs employs the effects of *resonant ejection* to remove ions of successively increasing *m/z* value from the storage volume, i.e., to achieve a scan. In an ideal QIT, the motions of the ions in radial and axial directions are mutually independent. Their oscillations can be described by a radial and an axial secular frequency, each of them being a function of the Mathieu trapping parameters a and q. If a supplementary RF voltage which matches the axial secular frequency is applied to the end caps, resonant ejection of ions occurs at $q < 0.908$ (Fig. 4.54) [168]. Excitation occurs when the frequency of a supplementary RF signal matches the secular frequency of a trapped ion in z direction. The secular frequency components in axial direction (ω_z) are given by $\omega_z = (n + \beta_z/2)\Omega$, where Ω represents the angular frequency, n is an integer, and β_z is determined by the working point of an ion within the stability diagram [169]. In the special case when

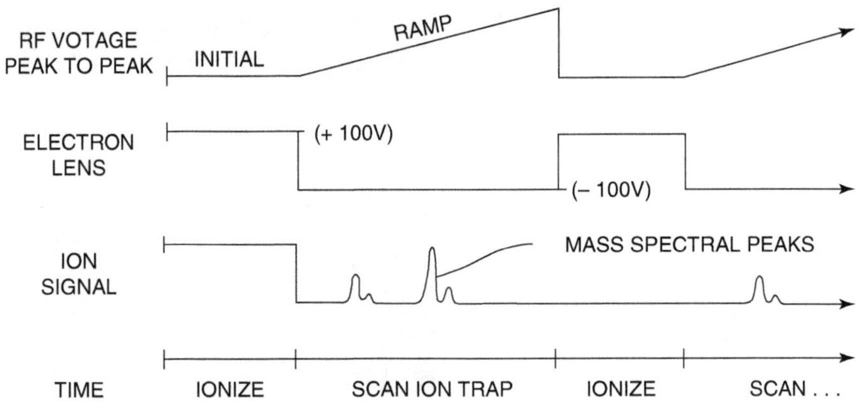

Fig. 4.56 Timing sequence used for mass-selective instability mode (about 1.5 cycles shown). With an external ion source the ionization time is replaced by the ion injection pulse (Reproduced from Ref. [155] by permission. © Elsevier Science, 1984)

$\beta_z = 1$ and $n = 0$, the fundamental secular frequency is exactly half of the RF drive frequency applied between ring electrode and end caps.

Scanning by Resonant Ejection To effect resonant ejection for the set of $\beta_z = 0.5$ and $n = 0$ we have $\omega_z = (0 + 0.5/2) = 0.25\Omega$, i.e., $^1/_4$ of the RF drive frequency has to be applied to eject ions at the $\beta_z = 0.5$ borderline. By scanning the voltage of the RF drive frequency upwards, ions of increasing *m/z* ratio are successively ejected.

Scans based on resonant ejection may either be carried out in a forward, i.e., from low to high mass, or a reverse direction. However, the scan direction has significant influence on the attainable resolving power, the reverse direction being clearly inferior in that respect. [170, 171] The combination of forward and reverse scanning allows for the selective storage of ions of a certain *m/z* value by elimination of ions below and above that *m/z* value from the trap. Thus, it can serve for precursor ion selection in tandem MS experiments [168, 170]. Axial excitation can also be used to cause collision-induced dissociation (CID) of the ions as a result of collisions with the helium buffer gas [155, 168]. A substantial increase of the mass range is realized by reduction of both the RF frequency of the modulation voltage and the physical size of the QIT [166, 172, 173].

4.6.7 Axial Modulation and Control of the Ion Population

Ion trapping devices are sensitive to overload because of the detrimental effects of Coulombic repulsion on the ion trajectories. The maximum number of ions that can be stored in a QIT is about 10^6–10^7, but it reduces to about 10^3–10^4 if unit mass resolution in an RF scan is desired. *Axial modulation*, a subtype of resonant ejection, allows to increase the number of ions stored in the QIT by one order of magnitude while maintaining unit mass resolution [173, 174]. During the RF scan, the modulation voltage with a fixed amplitude and frequency is applied between the end caps. Its frequency is chosen slightly below $^1/_2$ of the fundamental RF frequency, because for $\beta_z \leq 1$, e.g., $\beta_z = 0.98$, we have $\Omega_z = (0 + 0.98/2) \times \Omega = 0.49 \times \Omega$. At the stability boundary, ion motion is in resonance with this modulation voltage, and thus ion ejection is facilitated. Axial modulation basically improves the mass-selective instability mode of operation.

If resolving power is not a major concern, scanning of QITs can be very fast, a property that can be employed to make a *pre-scan*. The actual ion current into the trap is then determined from the pre-scan and the result is used to adjust the number of ions admitted to the QIT by a timed ion gate for the subsequent analytical scan. Thus, the number of ions, and hence, charge density inside the QIT are continuously held close to the optimum. This tool to control the ion population of the QIT has been introduced by Finnigan and referred to as *automatic gain control* (AGC) [146, 175]. AGC gives increased sensitivity at low sample flow and avoids overload of the QIT at high sample flow.

Importance of the ion population in traps
Careful control of the ion population, e.g., as implemented by AGC, is not only relevant for QITs but also for all other types of ion traps. The technique is implemented in LITs that are employed as stand-alone devices and also in LITs serving for ion selection and dosing into FT-ICR or Orbitrap analyzers (Sects. 4.7, 4.8, and 4.9).

Provided sufficiently high scan rates are also available whilst resolution is preserved, the pre-scan can be omitted. Instead, a trend analysis based on a set of two or three preceding analytical scans can be performed. This procedure avoids wasting of ions and results in further optimization of the filling level of the QIT. The exploitation of the phenomenon of nonlinear resonances turned out to be of key importance for the realization of this method.

Tandem MS in a QIT Tandem mass spectrometric experiments in quadrupole ion traps (more in Sect. 9.8) are performed by combining the techniques of resonant ejection, and forward and reverse scanning to achieve an optimum in precursor ion selection, ion activation, and fragment ion scanning (Fig. 4.57) [168].

4.6.8 Nonlinear Resonances

Higher multipole fields, in particular octopole fields, are induced in any real ion trap by deviations from the ideal electrode structure. The trapping potential may then be represented as a sum of an ideal quadrupole field and weak higher order field

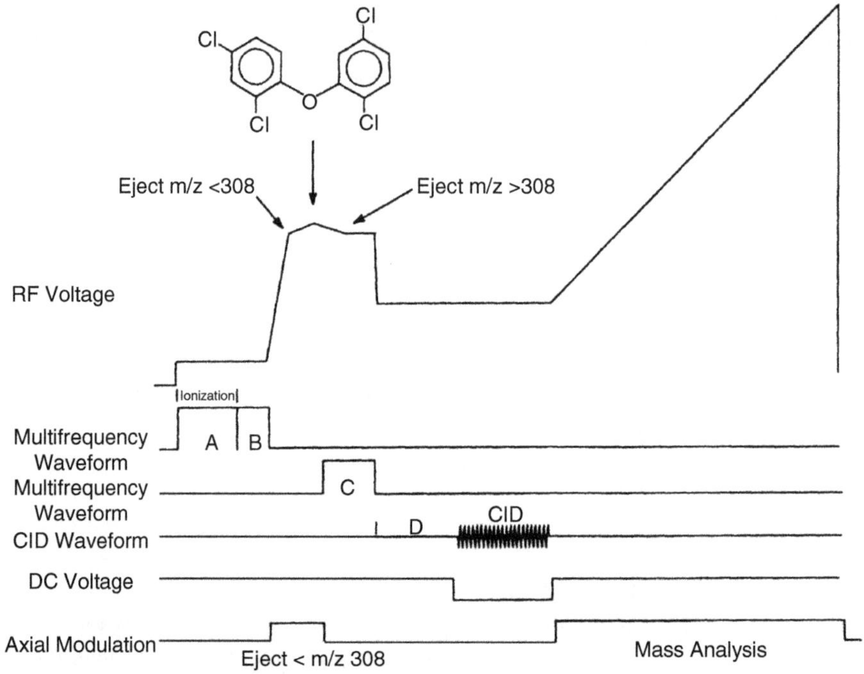

Fig. 4.57 Complex scan function used for a tandem mass spectrometric study of 2,4,3′,6′-tetrachlorodiphenylether (Reproduced from Ref. [168] by permission. © John Wiley and Sons, 1997)

contributions [154, 176, 177]. Application of an excitation voltage across the end caps induces dipole and hexapole fields in addition. Those higher order fields in the QIT may have beneficial effects such as increase in mass resolution in the resonant ejection mode, but may also result in losses of ions due to nonlinear resonances [178]. Nonlinear resonances have been known for long [179, 180], but useful theoretical descriptions were only recently developed [154, 177, 181, 182]. The condition for the appearance of instabilities is related to certain frequencies through the stability parameters β_r and β_z and the integer multiples n_r and n_z. The locations of instability spread like a net over the stability diagram and have been experimentally verified with astonishing accuracy (Fig. 4.58) [154]. Excitation of ions with a suitable frequency can cause their fast ejection from the trap due to the sudden shift to nonlinear stability. Nonlinear resonances can thus be exploited to realize very fast scans of the QIT (26,000 u s^{-1}) while maintaining good resolving power [182], e.g., irradiation of $0.33 \times \Omega$ amplifies hexapole resonances and causes sudden ejection at the $\beta_z = 0.66$ borderline.

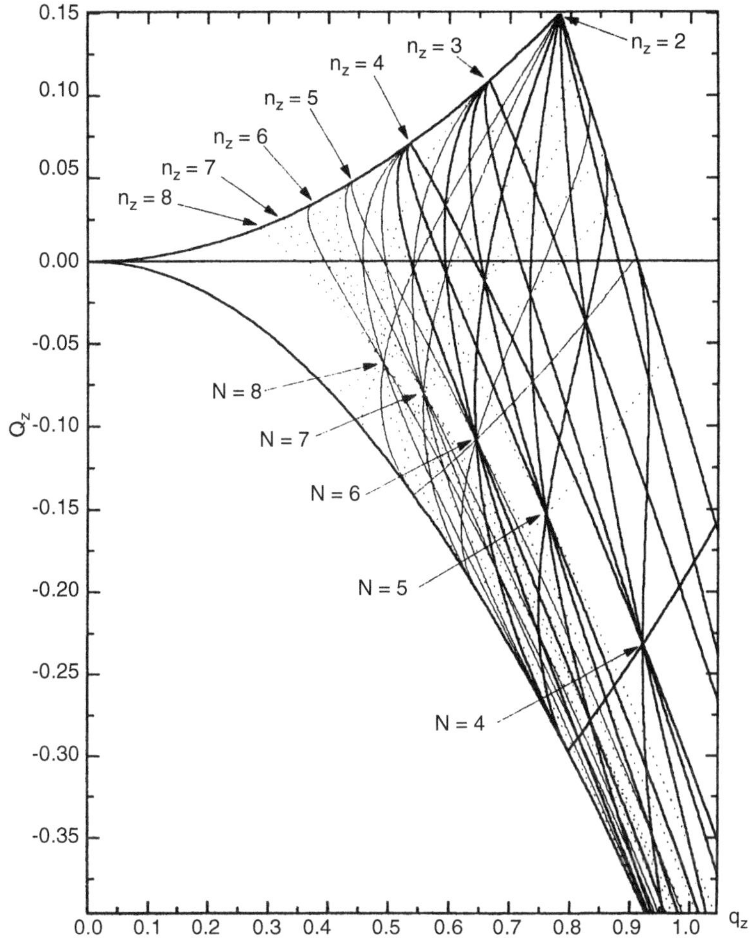

Fig. 4.58 Plot of theoretical lines of instability corresponding to the relation $n_r/2\beta_r + n_z/2\beta_z = 1$ for different orders $N = n_r + n_z$ (strong resonances represented by *solid lines*, weak ones by *dotted lines*) (Reproduced from Ref. [154] by permission. © Elsevier Science, 1996)

4.6.9 Miniaturization and Simplification of Ion Traps

The fabrication of quadrupole mass analyzers of any design necessitates high precision in machining and alignment of the electrodes; the production of hyperbolic electrode surfaces is especially challenging. While quadrupoles are compact, for mobile applications, even smaller and preferably less expensive analyzers are desirable [15, 183, 184]. Additionally, mobile instruments should have reduced vacuum requirements as the generation of high vacuum demands for comparatively heavy and energy-consuming pumps.

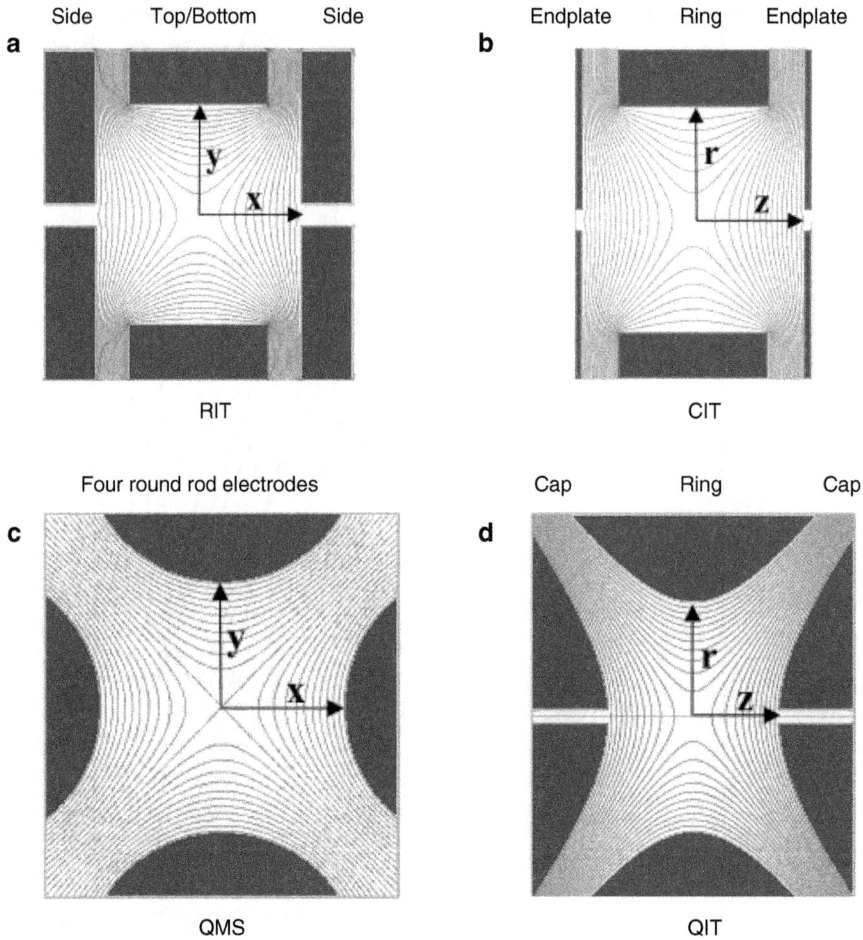

Fig. 4.59 Calculated trapping fields for (**a**) a rectilinear ion trap, (**b**) a cylindrical ion trap with planar endplates, (**c**) a quadrupole mass filter with round rods, and (**d**) a quadrupole ion trap with hyperbolic electrodes (Paul trap). Analyzer views (**a**) and (**c**) are end-on, (**b**) and (**d**) side-on (Adapted from Ref. [185] with permission. © American Chemical Society, 2004)

It turns out that the electrode geometries of LITs and QITs can largely be simplified without sacrificing too much of their performance. Thus, a *rectilinear ion trap* (RIT) can be constructed that has flat rectangular-shaped electrodes, one pair (top and bottom) being smaller than the other (side walls with slits for ion ejection, Fig. 4.59) [185, 186]. Also the geometry of the Paul trap can be transformed into a simple *cylindrical ion trap* (CIT) built of two planar endplates and a cylindrical ring electrode. Such simplified electrode shapes also allow for

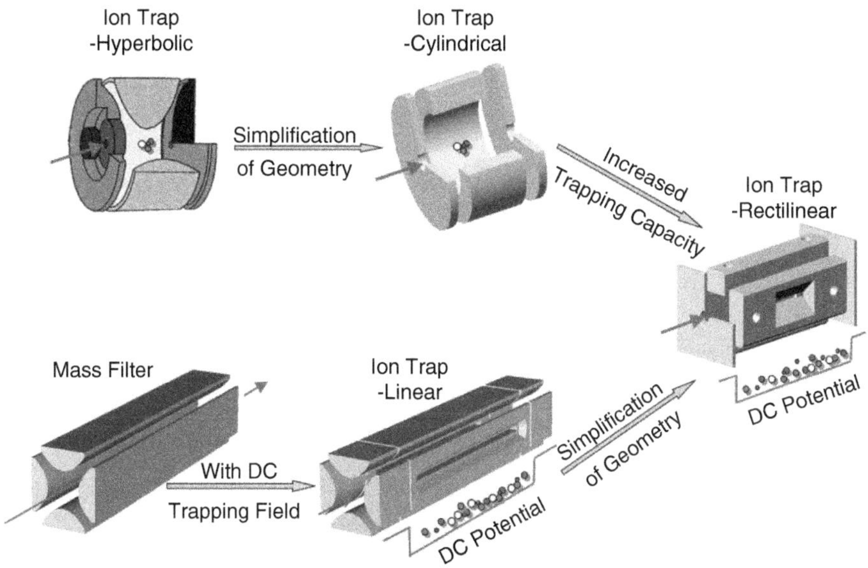

Fig. 4.60 Conceptual evolution of the rectilinear ion trap and interrelationship to other types of ion traps (Reproduced from Ref. [185] with permission. © American Chemical Society, 2004)

more compact traps to be built. The smaller dimensions then result in shorter ion paths, and thus, shorter mean free paths (poorer vacuum) can easily be tolerated. In turn, this allows vacuum generation to be performed by a single stage.

The evolution of ion traps and subsequent combination of characteristics of two "parent lines" that led to the construction of a RIT has instructively been illustrated in a paper by Ouyang et al. (Fig. 4.60) [185].

4.6.10 Digital Waveform Quadrupole Ion Trap

In almost all QITs, the m/z range is extended by lowering the RF drive frequency and/or by resonant ejection at a low q value, e.g., Thermo Fisher Scientific QITs eject the ions at $q = 0.78$–0.80 rather than the classical $q = 0.908$. Alternatively to a scan of the drive voltage at constant RF, a frequency scan at constant voltage can be applied to realize scans over an extended m/z range of up to about m/z 20,000. This demands a waveform generator coupled with a power amplifier, which is associated with excessive power consumption and difficulties in obtaining a high voltage output without waveform distortion [171].

The concept of the *digital ion trap* (DIT) makes use of a digital waveform to trap the ions. In this context, the terms *digital ion trap* and *digital waveform* describe a waveform composed of simple rectangular pulses applied to the ring electrode [171, 187]. In practice, a switching circuit is used to generate a pulsed waveform by rapid alternation between discrete DC high-voltage levels (±250 to ±1000 V).

The digital mode of pulse generation affords precise control of the timing. Furthermore, the AC excitation voltage connected across the end-cap electrodes can be delivered by the same digital circuitry. Interestingly, the ion motion under the influence of a digital waveform may still be expressed in terms of the conventional Mathieu parameters [171, 187, 188].

The development of the DIT has been pursued by Shimadzu and has reached a quite impressive level. Recently, an array of DITs, termed *ion trap array* (ITA), has been developed allowing multiple steps of isolation, activation, or scanning in parallel [189].

4.6.11 External Ion Sources for the Quadrupole Ion Trap

Chemical ionization (CI) mass spectra were first obtained by using the mass-selective instability mode of the QIT [166, 167, 190]. The reagent gas was admitted into the QIT, ionized and then allowed to react with the analyte.

With external ion sources it became feasible to interface any ionization method to the QIT mass analyzer [191]. However, commercial QITs are chiefly offered for two fields of applications: (*i*) GC-MS systems with EI and CI, because they are either inexpensive or capable of MS/MS to improve selectivity of the analysis (Chap. 14); and (*ii*) instruments equipped with atmospheric pressure ionization (API) methods (Chaps. 12 and 13) offering higher mass range, and some fivefold unit resolution to resolve isotopic patterns of multiply charged ions (Fig. 4.61) [161, 175, 192, 193].

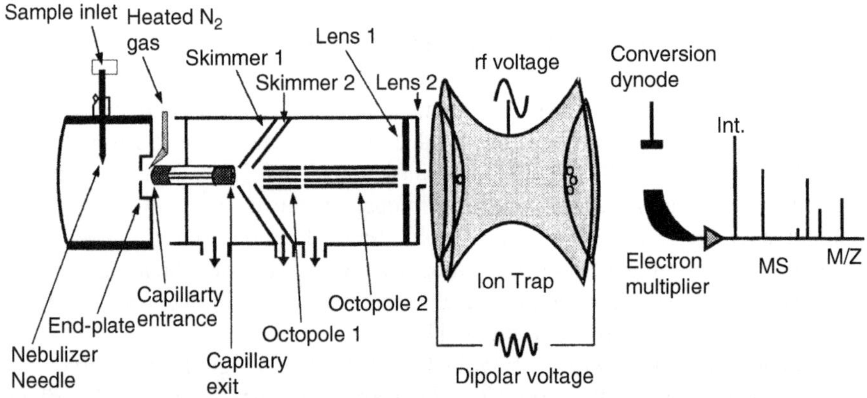

Fig. 4.61 Layout of a quadrupole ion trap instrument equipped with an external ESI ion source. The analogy to the ESI-LIT configuration shown in Fig. 4.50 is striking (Reproduced from Ref. [193] by permission. © John Wiley & Sons, 2000)

4.6.12 Ion Trap Maintenance

The confined volume of quadrupole ion traps and their mode of operation causes a large fraction of the ions to hit the electrodes thereby leading to contamination of their surfaces. Quadrupoles and quadrupole ion traps thus require occasional cleaning, which means that the entire analyzer needs to be disassembled and reassembled afterwards. The photograph in Fig. 4.62a shows the analyzer of a

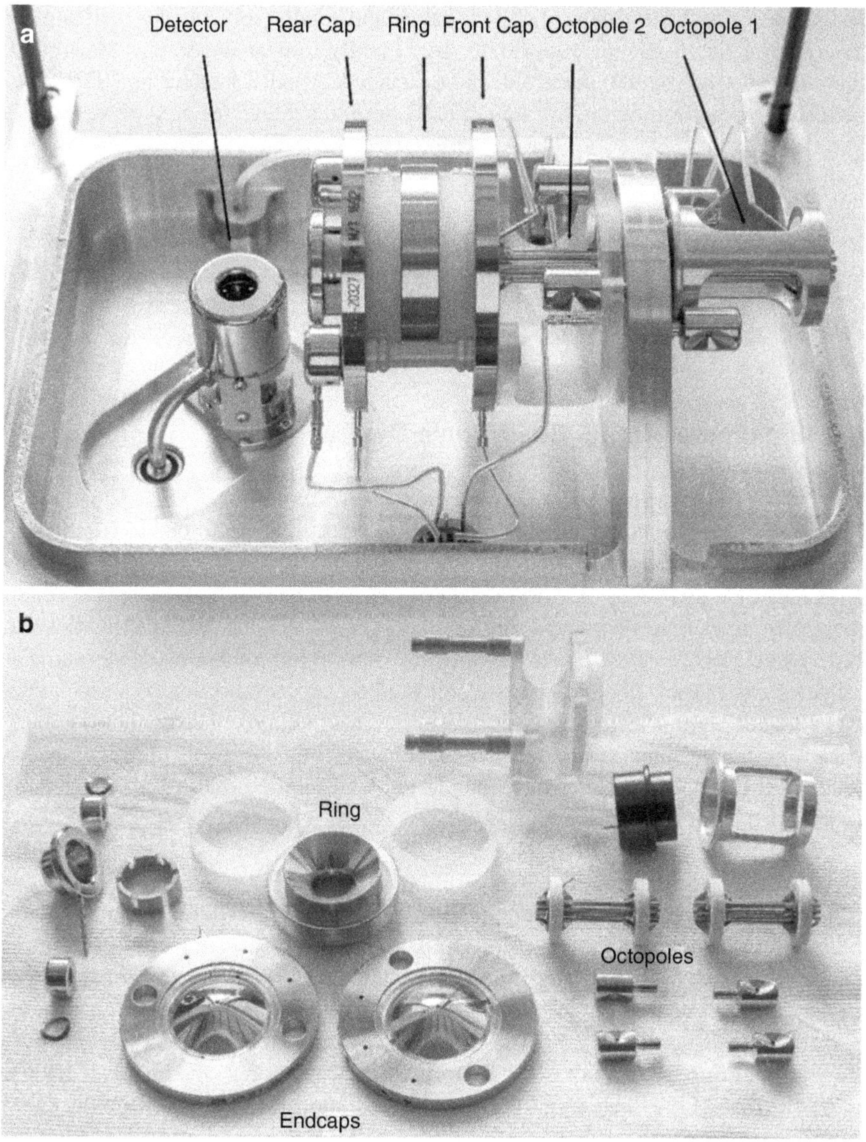

Fig. 4.62 Analyzer maintenance of a QIT; here of the Finnigan LCQ. (**a**) Complete QIT analyzer mounted onto the top cover plate of the vacuum manifold, (**b**) after taking it apart for cleaning

Finnigan LCQ instrument after dismounting the entire unit from the instrument frame. Ions would enter from an ESI source on the right (not shown) and be passed across two stages of differential pumping by means of RF-only octopoles. Here, the second octopole also serves as a linear ion trap to dose ion packages into the QIT under AGC control. The polished electrode on the left below the exit endcap of the QIT is the entrance into the detector.

Figure 4.62b shows the analyzer components spread on a clean sheet of lint-free paper. After gentle cleaning with fine metal polish (only if there are permanent dark spots), water with detergent, distilled water, and finally solvent like methanol or isopropanol the parts are allowed to dry. Finally, the analyzer is reassembled, mounted into the vacuum manifold, and evacuated. About 1 h later, the QIT should be ready for performing the full tuning procedure to achieve restored performance.

Stay grounded
"Ion traps are also the only type of mass spectrometer that most users can disassemble and reassemble without sacrificing instrument performance." [185].

4.6.13 Summary of RF Quadrupole Devices

Principle of Operation
In an electric radiofrequency (RF) quadrupole field, ions are forced to oscillate in the open space between the four electrodes creating this field. Suitable frequency and amplitude provided, this motion can be stable in that the ions never hit one of the electrodes and never escape through the gaps in between. RF quadrupoles can be mass-selective as these conditions are only met for ions of a selected *m/z* value or range of *m/z* values. The *m/z* range is adjusted by superimposition of an RF and a DC voltage. Mass-selective operation also requires that ions to be analyzed experience a sufficient number of oscillations or have sufficient dwell time within this field to eject ions outside the boundaries of stability due to their instable trajectories.

Types of RF Quadrupole Devices
Linear quadrupoles (Q) are operated as mass filters, while linear RF-only multipoles (q, h, o) are used as ion guides and collision cells. In both cases, a beam of ions is passed through the device so that the duration of interaction is determined by the velocity of the ions and the length of the RF device (Q, q, o, h).

Linear quadrupole ion traps (LIT) as well as quadrupole ion traps with three-dimensional quadrupole fields (QIT) are marked by storing ions inside. They are more flexible as they can either serve to accumulate ions to provide ion packages for other analyzer stages or be run to mass analyze a package of ions. During the period of ion storage, ions can also be activated by collisions with residual gas inside the LIT or QIT. Fragment ions arising thereof can be stored and mass-analyzed as well (Chap. 9).

General Characteristics

As Q, LIT, and QIT are purely driven by RF and DC voltages, operational parameters can be changed at very high rates, typically >10,000 u s^{-1}. These analyzers are also very compact (neither requires a long flight tube nor for a heavy magnet), and thus, ideal for use in benchtop instruments. Q, LIT, and QIT are easy to handle and user-friendly. They are typically run at unit resolution but zoom scans to increase the resolving power across a narrow *m/z* window are sometimes enabled. None of these analyzers is adequate for accurate mass measurements.

Use in MS Instrumentation

Most manufacturers offer a variety of Q, LIT, and QIT instruments for use with the different kinds of ionization methods. The majority of stand-alone Q, LIT, and QIT instruments is used in routine gas chromatography (GC)- and liquid chromatography (LC)-mass spectrometry applications. Additionally, Q, LIT, and QIT devices are frequently incorporated into hybrid instruments to serve as the first of the two mass analyzers.

4.7 Fourier Transform Ion Cyclotron Resonance

4.7.1 From Ion Cyclotron Resonance to Mass Spectrometry

The development that led to modern *Fourier transform ion cyclotron resonance* (FT-ICR) mass spectrometers began in 1932 when E. O. Lawrence applied a transverse alternating electric field orthogonally to a magnetic field to build a particle accelerator [194, 195]. It was demonstrated that in *ion cyclotron resonance* (ICR) the angular frequency of the circular motion of ions is independent of the radius they are traveling on.

Later, this principle was applied to construct an ICR mass spectrometer [196, 197]. ICR mass spectrometers measuring the power absorption from the exciting oscillator were commercialized in the mid-1960s by Varian. Starting from their application to gas-phase ion chemistry [198], ICR instruments made their way into analytical mass spectrometry [199]. However, it was the introduction of FT-ICR in 1974 that initiated the major breakthrough [200, 201]. Ever since, the performance of FT-ICR instruments has steadily improved [202, 203] to reach unprecedented levels of resolving power and mass accuracy when superconducting magnets are employed [204–209]. The introduction of a dynamically harmonized ICR cell gave new thrust to the technique [210, 211]. Now, more than 40 years after FT-ICR-MS has been introduced [212], the technique can achieve resolving powers of up to 1.2×10^7 (12 million), and even a 21-Tesla superconducting magnet has been constructed for FT-ICR-MS to obtain ultrahigh resolving power at high spectral acquisition rates and outstanding sensitivity [213].

FT-ICR analyzers are operated in a way that notably differs from what we have dealt with so far. FT-ICR-MS relies on nondestructive ion detection by registering image currents of circulating ions in the time domain. FT is applied to deliver frequency domain data that can then be converted into the intensity versus *m/z* data format. This may appear to be quite complex – and in fact, it is. So let's approach this issue step by step – FT-ICR-MS is well worth the extra effort.

Top-of-the line MS

Todays FT-ICR mass spectrometers offer ultrahigh resolving power ($R = 10^5$ to $>10^6$) [214–217] and highest mass accuracy ($\Delta m = 10^{-4}$–10^{-3} u, cf. Sects. 3.5 and 3.6) [208, 209], attomol detection limits (with nanoESI or MALDI sources), high mass range and MS^n capabilities [218]. Modern FT-ICR instruments actually represent some sort of hybrids with linear quadrupole or LIT front ends.

4.7.2 Ion Cyclotron Motion – Basics

As we know from the discussion of magnetic sectors, an ion of velocity v entering a uniform magnetic field B perpendicular to its direction will, by action of the Lorentz force (Sect. 4.3.2), immediately move on a circular path. Contemplating the path in the direction of the magnetic field reveals that negative ions circulate clockwise while positive ions move counterclockwise (Figs. 4.19 and 4.63).

The radius r_m of the ions' circular motion is determined by Eq. (4.13):

$$r_m = \frac{m_i v}{qB} \tag{4.13}$$

Upon substitution with $v = r_m\omega$ and rearrangement of the resulting term, *the cyclotron angular frequency* ω_c is obtained as:

$$\omega_c = \frac{qB}{m_i} \tag{4.33}$$

and by substituting with the cyclotron frequency ($f_c = \omega_c/2\pi$) Eq. (4.33) becomes

$$f_c = \frac{qB}{2\pi m_i} \tag{4.34}$$

One realizes that the cyclotron frequency is independent of the ions' initial velocity, but proportional to its charge and the magnetic field, and inversely proportional to its mass. Of any physical quantity, frequencies can be measured at

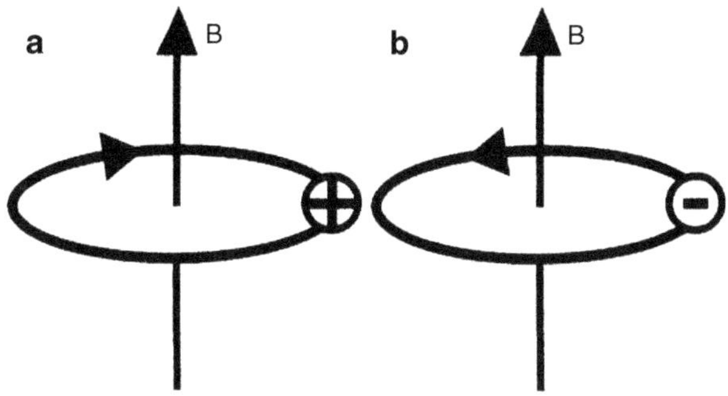

Fig. 4.63 Circular motion of ions in a magnetic field. Viewing along the direction of the magnetic field one observes (**a**) a counterclockwise motion for positive ions and (**b**) a clockwise motion for negative ions (Adapted from Ref. [219] with permission. © Elsevier Science Publishers, 2002)

the highest accuracy, and thus, cyclotron frequency measurements appear as ideal premises for building powerful *m*/*z* analyzers.

4.7.3 Cyclotron Motion: Excitation and Detection

Gaseous ions are not at rest but at least move arbitrarily at their thermal velocities. When such a package of thermal ions is generated within a magnetic field or is injected into it, the resulting small ion cloud contains ions that are all spinning at their respective cyclotron frequencies (circular micromotion) while the cloud as a whole remains stationary provided it has been brought to a halt within the field boundaries. Therefore, the magnetic field not only acts in an *m*/*z*-sensitive way by imposing the cyclotron motion on the ions, but also provides ion trapping in a plane perpendicular to its field lines (*xy*-plane, cf. action of the quadrupolar field in a LIT).

Upon excitation, the circular micromotion is superimposed by the macroscopic cyclotron motion of the whole ion cloud, i.e., the RF excitation field preserves the coherence of ion packages composed of ions of the same *m*/*z* value. As the initial kinetic energy of the ions is small as compared to the energy uptake from the RF field, it is of minor importance for the experiment [220]. Nonetheless, the complexity of the overall motion affects frequency-to-mass calibration if accurate results are required [221].

In practice, mass-selective excitation, so-called *resonant excitation*, is achieved by applying a transverse electric field alternating at the cyclotron frequency f_c ($\omega_c = 2\pi f_c$) to accelerate the ions. Such a field can be applied by a pair of RF electrodes placed on opposite sides of the orbit. As the ions accelerate, the radius of their orbit increases, and the resulting overall motion is a spiral (Fig. 4.64a) [195, 203]. For lighter ions, the spiral reaches the same radius with fewer cycles

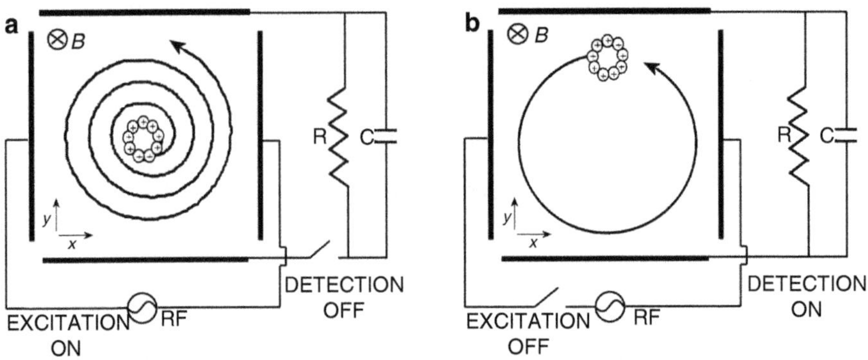

Fig. 4.64 The sequence of (**a**) excitation (**b**) and image current detection in ICR-MS. The ionic micromotion is indicated by the small circle of ions. The cell is shown along the direction of the magnetic field. (**a**) Illustrates the spiral trajectory of the ion cloud as induced by excitation of the ions by an RF electric field oscillating at the cyclotron resonance frequency. Note that the radius is a function of ion velocity, but the frequency f_c of circulation is not and that the radius remains constant during detection

than in case of heavier ones, i.e., the spiral is steeper, because low-mass ions need less energy than high-mass ions to accelerate to a certain velocity.

Ion kinetic energy in ICR Consider a singly charged ion of a mass of 100 u at thermal energy. Assuming a temperature of 300 K, its average velocity (Boltzmann distribution) is about 230 m s^{-1}. In a 3-T magnetic field it will circulate at $r_m \approx 0.08$ mm. To increase the radius to 1 cm, Eq. (4.13) demands the velocity to rise by a factor of 125, i.e., to 28,750 m s^{-1}. Rearranging Eq. (4.3) delivers $eU = v^2 m_i/2$, and thus, we calculate a kinetic energy of about 430 eV. Definitely, the translational energy of ions in an ICR cell is high enough to effect activating collisions (Fig. 4.65 and Chap. 9) [220].

Omegatron The so-called *omegatron* was an early ICR motion-based mass spectrometer. The ions in an omegatron are generated by electron ionization of a gaseous sample inside the cell (Fig. 4.66). The electric RF field causes ions fulfilling the resonance condition, i.e., those of $f_c = f_{RF}$, to accelerate and consequently to increase the radius of their orbit. The m/z value is derived from the number of half cycles (proportional to ion kinetic energy) until the ions strike the electrometer plate at $r = r_{cell}$ [196, 197]. Thus, the omegatron essentially measures ion kinetic energy. To analyze a m/z range either the RF frequency (adaptation of f_{RF} to f_c) or the magnetic field (shifting of f_c to f_{RF}) are varied. Omegatrons were small ($r_{cell} \approx 1$ cm) and mainly used as compact residual gas analyzers.

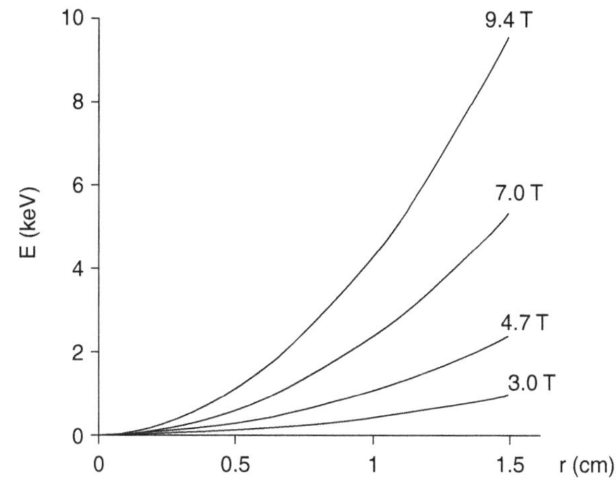

Fig. 4.65 Kinetic energy of *m/z* 100 ions in an ICR cell vs. orbital radius at magnetic field strengths from 3.0 to 9.4 T (Adapted from Ref. [220] with permission. © John Wiley and Sons, Inc., 1998)

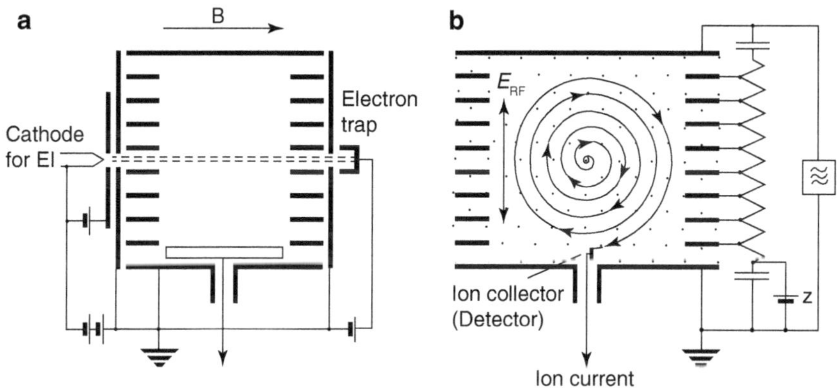

Fig. 4.66 Omegatron. (**a**) View parallel to *B* (*horizontal*) and parallel to the electron beam (*horizontal*) used to generate ions by EI inside the cell. The accelerating electric RF field acts vertical to *B*. (**b**) View on-axis to *B* shows the spiral motion of accelerating ions until the radius of their orbit approaches that of the cell where the ions hit an ion collector for detection (Adapted from Ref. [91] with kind permission of Curt Brunnée)

Mission half-accomplished

The disadvantages of the omegatron for use as a mass analyzer are clear: (*i*) mass accuracy and resolving power are limited to $1/N_c$ (N_c = number of half cycles); (*ii*) the electric signal for ion detection is solely due to neutralization

(continued)

of the ions, and there is no amplification as obtained with multiplier-type detectors used with all other analyzers; and (*iii*) the ions are removed from the cell upon detection precluding the use for MS/MS.

Moving from destructive detection by discharging the ions on the detection plates to nondestructive *image current detection* allows to switch from energy scanning to – indirect – cyclotron frequency measurement (Fig. 4.64b) [222, 223]. Image current detection relies on the fact that an ion cloud repeatedly attracts (positive ions) or repels (negative ions) the electrons of the detection electrodes upon its passage. The resulting minuscule image current can be amplified, transformed into a voltage signal and recorded as long as the ion motion exhibits sufficient coherence. In other words, a transient periodic signal is recorded in the time domain.

Observing swarms in flight
In ICR cells, the ions circulate like separate swarms of birds rather than like matter in the rings of Saturn. If ions of the same *m/z* non-coherently circulated at the same frequency and radius, but occupied the total orbit rather than a small sector of it, there would be no image current induced upon their passage at the detector plates, i.e., coherence of the circulating ion motion is crucial.

4.7.4 Cyclotron Frequency Bandwidth and Energy-Time Uncertainty

The *frequency bandwidth* to be covered by an ICR instrument is governed by the *m/z* range to be analyzed. Assuming a 9.4-T superconducting magnet, which currently represents the "upper-middle class", we may now use Eq. (4.34) to calculate f_c for singly charged ions of *m/z* 50 ($m_i = 8.30 \times 10^{-26}$ kg) as $f_c = (1.66 \times 10^{-19}\ \text{C} \times 9.4\ \text{T})/(2\pi \times 8.30 \times 10^{-26}\ \text{kg}) = 3.00$ MHz. For an ion of *m/z* 500 (8.30×10^{-25} kg) we get a 10 times lower value, $f_c = 300$ kHz, and for an ion of *m/z* 5000 (8.30×10^{-24} kg) we arrive at 30 kHz. To handle ions in the range *m/z* 50–5000, the ICR frequency band has to span from 30 kHz to 3.0 MHz. In other words, an ICR instrument needs to cover a frequency range from several tens of kilohertz to a few megahertz (Fig. 4.67). The tremendous bandwidth has severe implications on both the mode of operation to achieve homogeneous excitation and detection and on the electronics to deliver the required level of performance over the entire range.

Following the above calculation, it takes a frequency resolution of 3 Hz (300 kHz/100,000) to achieve a resolving power of $R = 100{,}000$ at *m/z* 500. The *energy-time uncertainty principle* states that $\Delta E \times \Delta t \approx h$. With $\Delta E = h\Delta \nu$ we

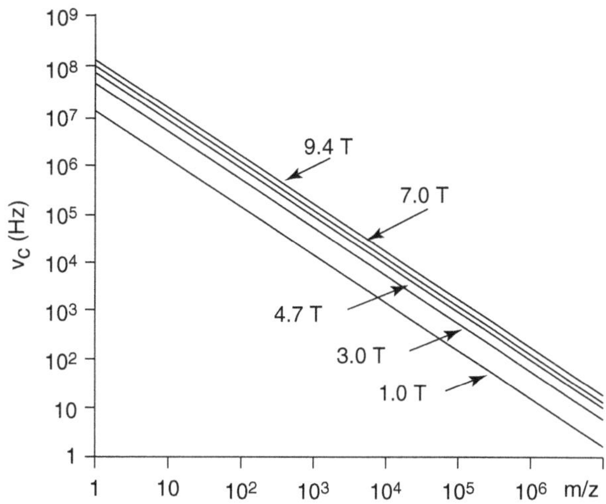

Fig. 4.67 Plot of ICR frequencies vs. *m*/*z* for different magnetic field strengths from 1.0 to 9.4 T (Reproduced from Ref. [220] with permission. © John Wiley and Sons, Inc., 1998)

derive $h\Delta\nu \times \Delta t \approx h$ or $\Delta\nu \times \Delta t \approx 1$. Accordingly, the above frequency resolution of 3 Hz in 0.3 MHz corresponds to a measurement time of 0.33 s per data point of the scan range. Operation of an ICR instrument in *continuous wave mode*, i.e., scanning in the frequency domain, is obviously unrealistic as soon as high resolving power is to be achieved. Therefore, the only practical way to acquire high-resolution ICR spectra would be to realize a broad band detection of all frequencies in parallel.

Although discouraging for ion detection, the energy-time uncertainty principle opens up new perspectives for ion excitation. According to $\Delta\nu \times \Delta t \approx 1$, a rectangular pulse of 1 ms duration covers a frequency bandwidth of 1000 Hz; a pulse of even 1 μs should correspond to a bandwidth (frequency uncertainty) of 1 MHz, i.e., shorter pulses cover increasingly broader ranges. This has been employed in so-called *pulse excitation*.

The "bell model"

To understand pulse excitation, it is helpful to consider a mechanical comparison – a bell, for example, does not require excitation at its resonance frequency. Instead, a short strike with a hammer (pulse excitation) is fully sufficient. The bell takes up the energy with no specified frequency (all potential frequencies are contained) and automatically "finds" its own frequency plus its overtones to resonate and, thus, to sound.

According to the above considerations, the resolving power *R* that can theoretically be achieved depends on the smallest $\Delta\nu$ that can be resolved, and thus, increases the longer Δt used for acquiring the transient, t_{acq}. Further, it depends on *m/z* of the ion and the magnetic field B. A simple numerical-value equation may be used to calculate the theoretical maximum R [220, 224]:

$$R = \frac{\nu}{\Delta \nu} = \frac{m}{\Delta m} = 1.274 \times 10^{7} \frac{zBt_{\mathrm{acq}}}{m} \tag{4.35}$$

For example, for an ion of *m/z* 400, $B = 7$ T, and $t_{\mathrm{acq}} = 1$ s, we obtain $R = 222{,}950 \approx 230{,}000$. A transient of 0.2 s would therefore reduce it to one fifth, $R = 46{,}000$, while recording the transient for 10 s could deliver $R = 2{,}300{,}000$.

Resolving power's interdependence

Obviously, the resolving power of any FT-ICR instrument can only be stated along with *m/z* of the ion of interest, the magnetic field, and the acquisition interval of the transient. A high rate of spectral acquisition sacrifices resolving power, while a long transient can yield ultrahigh resolving power at the expense of speed and duty cycle.

4.7.5 Fourier Transform – Basic Properties

Some knowledge of the basic properties of the *Fourier transform* (FT) will be helpful prior to discussing FT-ICR instrumentation [225]. The Fourier transform is a mathematical operation that transforms one complex-valued function of a real variable into another. The domain of the original function is typically time (as is here) and accordingly is termed the *time domain*. The domain of the function generated upon FT is frequency. The product of FT then is the *frequency domain* representation of the original function. The frequency domain function describes which frequencies are contained in the original function. For example, FT applied to a chord of music comprising several fundamental frequencies (and overtones) as represented by the notes would deliver all contributing frequencies and their amplitudes. The Fourier transform makes the move from a wave and its amplitude to its frequency and its amplitude (Fig. 4.68a, b).

FT of a transient signal, i.e., a signal vanishing to zero amplitude at the end of the observation time span, delivers a Lorentzian curve in the frequency domain (Fig. 4.68c, d). In accordance with the energy-time uncertainty principle, the frequency domain output becomes increasingly sharper the longer the observation time span, because the frequency is more accurately determined the more cycles are recorded in the transient.

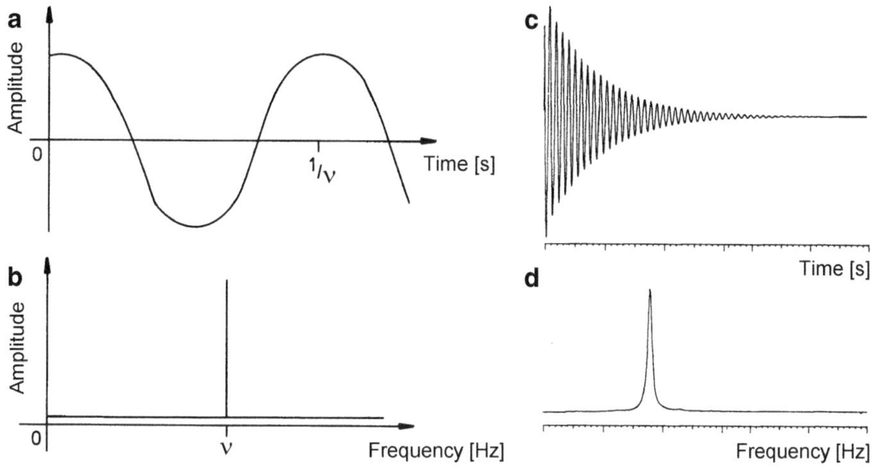

Fig. 4.68 Illustration of the principle of FT. (**a**) A time domain wave, infinite in time, is transformed by FT to (**b**) reveal its frequency. The amplitude is conserved. (**c**) FT of a transient time domain signal into (**d**) a frequency domain signal of Lorentzian shape. FT works equally well if an extremely large number of frequencies and amplitudes is contained in the time domain signal

Jean-Baptiste Joseph Fourier

Fourier was a French mathematician (1768–1830). Besides Fourier transformation, his influential work concerns the mathematical description of the conduction of heat in solids and the development of infinite series (Fourier series). He witnessed the French revolution and accompanied Napoleon on his expedition to Egypt.

In FT-ICR experiments, the observation time span is normally shorter than the time required to damp down the transient to zero. Instead, the detection is abruptly ended when the preset transient length is reached. The duration of the transient is generally determined by the product of the number of data points that is to be recorded and the rate at which those data points are being sampled. The minimum *sampling rate* is in turn determined by the highest cyclotron frequency to be observed. Typical values in FT-ICR-MS are 0.5–2 s transients of 512 k to 2 M (2×10^6) data points at 250 kHz to 1 MHz sampling frequency. Thus, the arbitrary truncation of the transient causes the transient to represent a combination of a step function and a perfectly dampened signal (Fig. 4.69). As FT yields sinc (x) from a step function, the FT output from a truncated signal is a Lorentzian main peak accompanied by side bands, so-called *wiggles*.

To reduce the side band-creating effect of truncation, the transient is normally subjected to *apodization* prior to FT. Apodization means the multiplication of the signal by a mathematical function that causes the values to smooth out to zero.

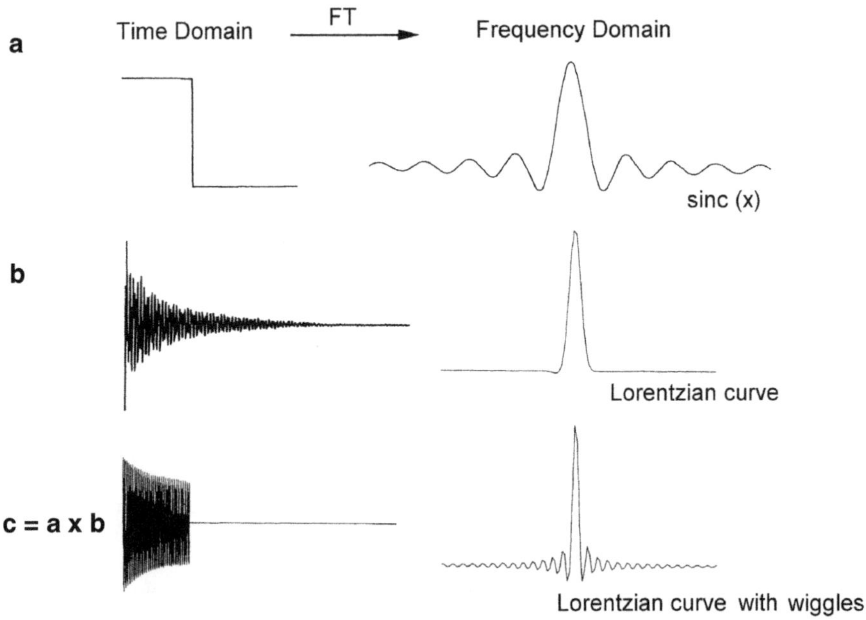

Fig. 4.69 The effects of Fourier transforms on different input signals. (**a**) A step function is converted to sinc (x), (**b**) a fully dampened transient signal containing only one frequency yields a single Lorentzian curve, and (**c**) the truncated transient can be regarded as a combination of (**a**) and (**b**) and yields a Lorentzian curve accompanied by "wiggles"

Some sophisticated apodization methods are in use to deliver the ultimate resolution, nonetheless, simple sin (x) or $\sin^2$ (x) functions work well.

Another feature of FT is to yield better resolved frequency spectra from larger data sets, which not necessarily need to contain real data. Simply adding a row of zeros to the end of the experimental transient is beneficial in that it smoothes the peak shape by increasing the number of data points per m/z interval. This "trick" is known as *zero-filling*. The number of attached zeros normally equals the number of data points, sometimes even twice as many are filled in (*double zero-filling*).

4.7.6 Nyquist Criterion

The actual shape of a peak not only depends on the capabilities of the mass analyzer in use but is also determined by the sampling rate applied to collect the signal (Sects. 4.12 and 11.5). The sampling rate is even more relevant for periodic signals such as from the cyclotron motion in FT-ICR. The minimum sampling rate needed to correctly detect any periodic signal is governed by the *Nyquist criterion*, according to which the sampling rate, ν_{samp}, must have at least twice the frequency of the process, ν_{proc}, that is to be recorded

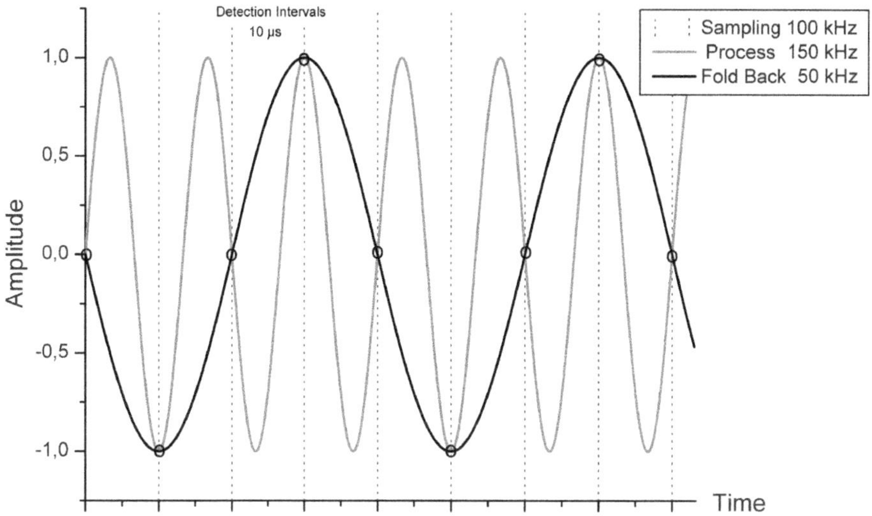

Fig. 4.70 The aliasing phenomenon. Detection points are where the *dotted* verticals cross the *light gray* signal curve (**o**). The process (150 kHz) occurs at $\nu_{proc} = 1.5 \times \nu_{samp}$ (100 kHz or 10 µs per point) instead of $\leq 0.5\ \nu_{samp}$. This causes the output of an aliased signal at $\nu_{fold} = 50$ kHz as determined by Eq. (4.37) (*dark curve*). In this special case setting $n = 1$ just delivers $\nu_{fold} = \nu_{nyq}$

$$\nu_{samp} \geq 2 \times \nu_{proc} \tag{4.36}$$

Vice versa, the Nyquist limit frequency, ν_{nyq}, up to which a process can just be correctly detected is given as

$$\nu_{nyq} = \nu_{samp}/2 \tag{4.37}$$

aliasing (or *folding back*) occurs beyond the Nyquist limit. Then, the detected signal pretends the process to proceed at a foldback frequency, ν_{fold}, described by

$$\nu_{fold} = \left| n \times \nu_{samp} - \nu_{proc} \right| \tag{4.38}$$

where the factor n is an integer selected as to fulfill the condition $0 < \nu_{fold} \leq \nu_{nyq}$ An illustration of the folding back phenomenon is given in Fig. 4.70.

4.7.7 Excitation Modes in FT-ICR-MS

In the ICR cell, there is a stringent correlation of cyclotron frequency f_c and m/z value. For simplicity, the very first FT-ICR experiment was therefore performed with an excitation pulse of a fixed f_c tailored to fit the model analyte, methane molecular ion [200]. However, useful measurements require the simultaneous excitation of all ions in the cell, and this in turn demands for a large RF bandwidth.

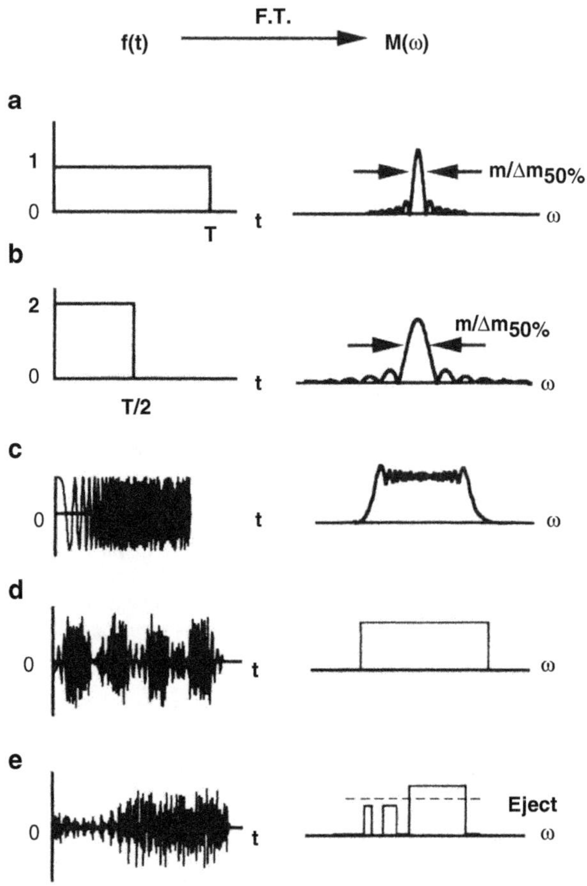

Fig. 4.71 Time-domain (*left*) and frequency-domain (*right*) excitation waveforms: (**a**, **b**) rectangular pulses yield inhomogeneous and rather narrow excitation windows; (**c**) "chirp" excitation; (**d**, **e**) SWIFT excitations, with (**e**) designed to eject a certain mass range from the cell (Reproduced from Ref. [220] by permission. © John Wiley & Sons, 1998)

Several excitation methods have been developed to cope with this technically nontrivial task. The differences between these methods can easily be judged from the shape of the frequency-domain excitation waveforms (Fig. 4.71) [203, 220]. The simplest approach is to irradiate a single frequency (resonant excitation) for some time, i.e., as a *rectangular pulse*, but this selectively excites ions of a single mass [200]. Applying such a narrow band excitation as a short pulse yields some expansion of the range. The effect of a *frequency sweep* or *"chirp" excitation* is much better [201]. Chirp excitation sequentially affects ions across the *m*/*z* range although it never delivers a defined frequency. Instead, the chirp exploits the wide band character of rushing across the frequencies. Chirp excitation is not perfectly homogeneous as it gives some distortions close to the borders of the range, nonetheless is it successfully employed in commercial FT-ICR instruments.

The best results are to be expected from *stored waveform inverse Fourier transform* (SWIFT) excitation [226]. First, the ideal excitation waveform is tailored to the needs of the intended experiment and then produced by an RF generator. SWIFT excitation also allows to remove ions of predefined *m*/*z* ranges from the ICR cell. This results in storage of a small *m*/*z* range, or after repeated SWIFT pulsing of a single nominal mass out of a broad band spectrum. Those ions are then accessible for ultrahigh resolution measurements or as precursors for tandem MS.

4.7.8 Axial Trapping

Our basic considerations of ICR (Sect. 4.7.3 and Fig. 4.64) were so far restricted to the *xy*-plane of a cell. Two of the four side walls (*x*-axis) of the ICR cell are connected to the RF power supply during the period of excitation. Then, the image current induced in the detector plates (*y*-axis) is recorded as transient signal for some period of time (0.5–30 s). The excitation of the ions within the ICR cell has to stop at a level low enough to avoid wall collisions of the lightest ions to be measured [206, 219, 220].

At a first glance, the *z*-dimension of the cell seems to be of no importance for the function of an FT-ICR mass spectrometer. However, the *z*-component of thermal energy and the kinetic energy of ion injection into the ICR cell in case of an external ion source both would lead to rapid loss of the *xy*-trapped ions along that axis, because they would pass through the cell along the *z*-axis on a helical trajectory. It is therefore important to establish a trapping potential in *z*-direction. The simplest way is to place DC trapping electrodes at the open ends [197]. Furthermore, our initial treatment of the ICR cell was also done with the implicit understanding that this would be a cubic cell.

4.7.9 Magnetron Motion and Reduced Cyclotron Frequency

Trapping of ions in a potential well implies reflection of ions between the trapping plates that induces an oscillatory motion along the *z*-axis the frequency ω_z of which is given by

$$\omega_z = \sqrt{\frac{2qV_{\text{trap}}\alpha}{ma^2}} \tag{4.39}$$

where a is the physical *z*-dimension of the trap and α represents a shape parameter that depends on the trap design [220]. The curved electric field close to the borders also produces an outward-bound radial force $F_r = qE_{(r)}$ opposed to the action of the Lorentz force F_L that is given by

$$F_r = qE_{(r)} = \frac{qV_{\text{trap}}\alpha}{a^2} r \tag{4.40}$$

The magnetic field now acts by transforming the radial force component into another circular motion of the trapped ions. The total force on an ion then is

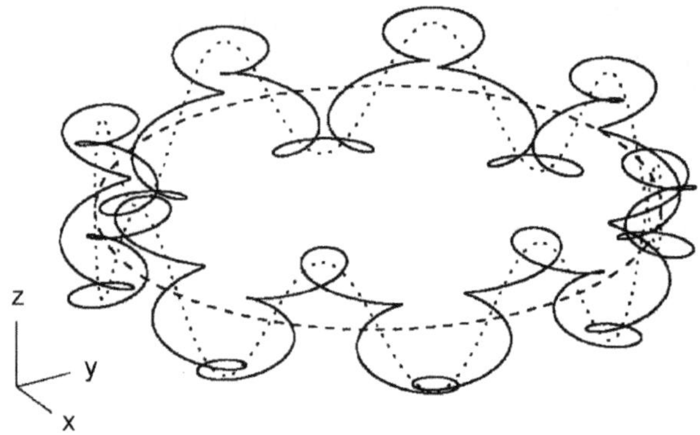

Fig. 4.72 Ion motion for $\omega_+ = 4\omega_z$ and $\omega_z = 8\omega_-$ in an ICR cell. Pure magnetron motion (*dashed*), magnetron plus trapping motion (*dotted*), and the resulting overall motion (*solid*) (Reproduced from Ref. [227] by permission. © Elsevier Science Publishers, 1995)

$$F_{\mathrm{tot}} = F_L - F_r = m_i\omega^2 r = qB\omega r - \frac{qV_{\mathrm{trap}}\alpha}{a^2} r \tag{4.41}$$

which can be rewritten to reveal its character of a quadratic equation in ω

$$\omega^2 - \frac{qB\omega}{m_i} + \frac{qV_{trap}\alpha}{a^2} = 0 \tag{4.42}$$

This quadratic equation has two solutions, the first of them representing the *reduced cyclotron frequency* ω_+

$$\omega_+ = \frac{\omega_c}{2} + \sqrt{\left(\frac{\omega_c}{2}\right)^2 - \frac{\omega_z{}^2}{2}} \tag{4.43}$$

and the second the *magnetron frequency* ω_-

$$\omega_- = \frac{\omega_c}{2} - \sqrt{\left(\frac{\omega_c}{2}\right)^2 - \frac{\omega_z{}^2}{2}} \tag{4.44}$$

where ω_z is obtained from Eq. (4.39) and ω_c from Eq. (4.33). The obvious consequence for the ionic motion in an ICR cell is that the simple description of ω_c by Eq. (4.33) only yields the so-called *unperturbed cyclotron frequency*, whereas the real motion is by far more complex. Figure 4.72 shows the overall motion of ions in an ICR cell taking ω_z, ω_+ and ω_- into account [227]. It should be noted that the radius of the magnetron motion is generally larger than that of the cyclotron motion. In many cases the magnetron motion also causes a small side peak in the vicinity of the main peak.

4.7.10 Detection and Accuracy in FT-ICR-MS

An FT-ICR experiment requires full temporal separation of excitation and subsequent detection of the trapped ions. Detection is based on the measurement

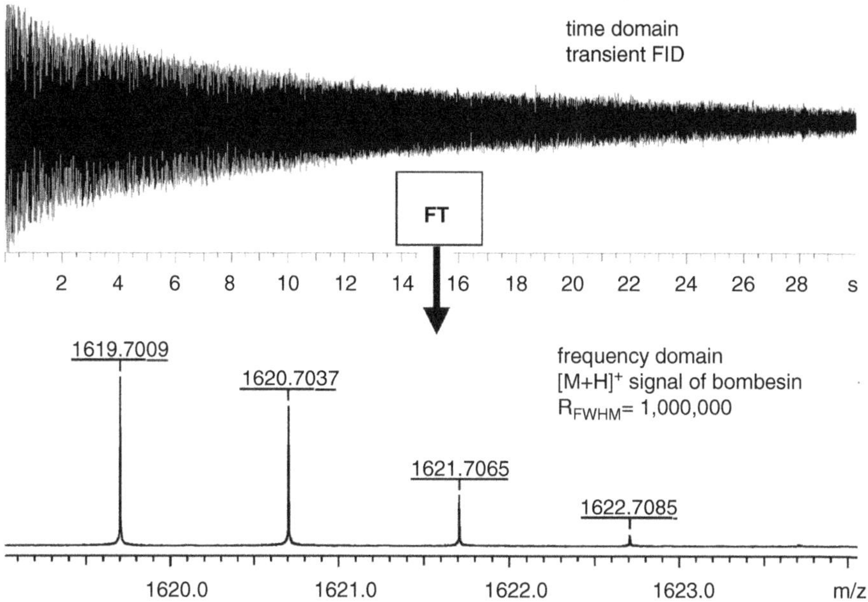

Fig. 4.73 The principle of FT-ICR-MS. In detail, the procedure includes recording the transient, apodization of the transient, zero-filling, FT, and finally the calculation of *m/z* values from the cyclotron frequencies. The longer the detection interval the higher the attainable resolving power. This example shows the $[M + H]^+$ ion of the peptide bombesin, *m/z* 1619.7009, where a 30 s transient resulted in a spectrum at $R = 10^6$ (By courtesy of Bruker Daltonik, Bremen)

of image currents in the detector plates. An image current is induced by each ion package when repeatedly passing the detector plates at its individual cyclotron frequency, i.e., detection in FT-ICR means "listening to the circulating ions". The transient signal or *free induction decay* (FID) is recorded, and afterwards, the FID is converted from the *time domain* to the *frequency domain* by means of Fourier transformation. This means that the complex FID caused by superimposition of many single frequencies is deconvoluted to reveal the single contributing frequencies and their respective amplitudes. Using Eq. (4.34), the frequencies are converted to *m/z* values; their amplitudes now representing the abundances of the corresponding ions (Fig. 4.73) [195, 200, 203, 228, 229].

There is a correlation between the transient signal and the pressure in the ICR cell [220, 228]. In perfect vacuum, the orbiting motion would solely be dampened by induction, whereas in the presence of residual gas collisions will finally slow down the ions to thermal energy. As the resolving power in FT-ICR-MS is also proportional to the acquisition time of the transient signal, ultrahigh vacuum in the range of $\approx 10^{-10}$ mbar is a prerequisite in the ICR cell. Based on a 7-T magnet and Eq. (4.35), the theoretical resolution for the example in Fig. 4.73 is $R \approx 1.6 \times 10^6$, which shows the influence of residual gas and other factors causing loss of coherence on actual resolving power.

Ultrahigh vacuum required
The need for extremely long mean free paths in FT-ICR mass spectrometers arises from the combination of high ion velocities of several 10^3 m s^{-1} and observation intervals in the order of seconds. Coherent swarms of ions thus need to travel hundreds of meters during the detection interval. Collisions would be detrimental for peak shape. The typical ICR cell pressure therefore is 10^{-10} to 10^{-9} mbar.

The detection efficiency is greatly improved for cylindrical cells as compared to cubic cells, because the ions pass the detection electrodes at almost constant distance to their surface. This results in stronger image currents due to on the average closer passages and sharper detection wave forms as their entering and exiting from the detection zone causes more sudden changes.

The ICR voltage signal strength at the detector plates is inversely proportional to ion mass if the monitoring circuit is predominantly resistive, and is independent of ion mass if the circuit is predominantly capacitive [229]. Image current detection at room temperature is typically less sensitive than ion counting techniques in beam instruments. Nonetheless, for modern FT-ICR instruments the detection limit to yield a signal-to-noise ratio of 3:1 corresponds to roughly 200 ions, provided these are excited to travel at half of the maximum cyclotron radius [211, 219].

The advantages of FT-ICR detection over ICR are obvious:

- The $1/N_c$ limit vanishes because every ion undergoes some 10^4–10^8 cycles during the detection interval.
- Sensitivity improves because the ions give rise to a detectable image charge during each passage of a detector plate.
- Ion detection is nondestructive, i.e., ions are not lost upon detection (this enabling MS/MS experiments).
- Elongated recording of the FID provides for extremely precise determination of all cyclotron frequencies, thereby yielding the highest values of resolution and mass accuracy available [214, 215, 230].

External calibration is most effective when the level of excitation and the number of trapped ions of calibrant ions closely approaches that of the analyte ions [219]. The latest FT-ICR instruments can routinely attain mass accuracies of better than 1 ppm. Internal calibration can yield further improvement.

Although resolution and mass accuracy are already high in broadband spectra ($R = 3 \times 10^4$–10^5, $\Delta m < 10^{-3}$ u), the performance of FT-ICR instruments further improves by storing only narrow m/z ranges, because fewer ions in the cell mean less distortion by coulombic interactions.

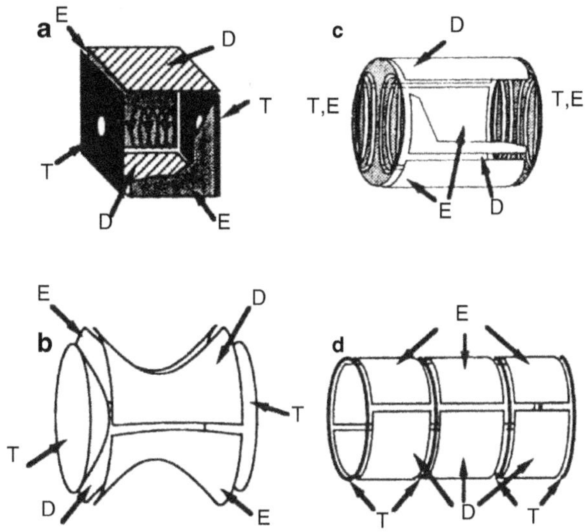

Fig. 4.74 Important ICR cell types; electrodes are labeled with *E* excitation, *D* detection, *T* trapping; (**a**) classic cubic cell, (**b**) Penning cell with hyperbolic electrodes, (**c**) infinity Cell™ with segmented trapping plates, and (**d**) triple cell. The latter two aim at virtually expanding the potentials in the trapping zone along the *z*-axis (Adapted from Ref. [232] with permission. © Elsevier Science Publishers, 1995)

4.7.11 Design of ICR Cells

We have seen that ion motion and detection in FT-ICR are affected by various parameters. Axial trapping oscillation, resulting magnetron motion, and disturbances leading to loss of coherence – or dephasing – strongly depend on the geometry of the ICR cell and on the homogeneity of the magnetic field. The simple cubic cell (the ICR cell of the pioneers) severely suffers from field imperfections. Therefore, numerous other designs have been developed offering remarkable improvements over the cubic cell (Fig. 4.74) [219, 220].

A nearly ideal hyperbolic field is created inside a hyperbolic trap, also known as *Penning trap* or *Penning cell* (Fig. 4.74b). However, this shape requires a small inner volume for the ions to circulate and the performance soon suffers from space charge effects as the number of ions increases. While capable of extremely high performance with 10–1000 ions, Penning cells are not suited for analytical work where a cell has to accommodate large ion populations to offer a high dynamic range and to deal with complex mixtures.

As in the case of segmented LITs with radial ejection (Sect. 4.5.3 and Figs. 4.48 and 4.49), the distortion of the electric field can be avoided when the trapping sections are properly designed and operated; then the ICR cell displays itself to the ions as being of virtually infinite length. Thus, triple-segmented cylindrical cells [231] and many others have been developed [232]. Another approach, the *infinity cell* makes use of segmented end caps on a cylindrical cell (Fig. 4.74c) [233].

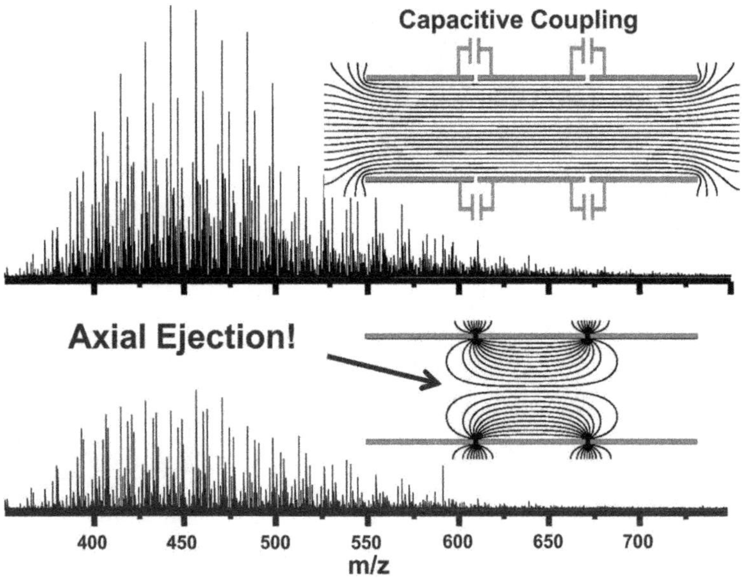

Fig. 4.75 Comparison of a cylindrical cell having both capacitively-coupled (*top*) and noncoupled trapping electrodes (*bottom*) to the resulting spectra of a complex sample. The curvature of the RF excitation isopotentials for the single electrode pair (*bottom*) produces axial RF excitation leading to *m*/*z*-dependent axial ejection. Capacitive coupling of the RF excitation to the end cap electrodes effectively eliminates axial ejection and yields an improved spectrum. (Reproduced with permission from Ref. [212]. © Elsevier Science Publishers, 2015)

The advantageous effect of capacitive coupling of trapping segments in a triple-segmented cylindrical cell are shown in Fig. 4.75. The figure not only depicts the field flattening effect of the capacitive coupling but also shows its correlation to the enhancement of FT-ICR spectra due to this design [212]. ICR cells of this type are used in the Thermo Scientific LTQ-FT Ultra series.

A recently designed cell by E. Nikoleav extends the region of harmonic potential to almost its full volume. This is achieved by subdivision of the walls of a long cylindrical cell (150 × 56 mm) into alternating convexly and concavely shaped segments [210, 224, 234]. The convex segments stay grounded while the trapping potential is applied to the concave parts. The trapping plates are slightly spherical in shape. Overall, this causes ions to experience an on-average harmonic potential per full cycle of cyclotron motion (Fig. 4.76). This fact gives rise to its description as a *dynamically harmonized ICR cell*. For excitation and detection the cylinder is classically divided into four sections of 90° with the dividing cuts slicing every second convex electrode into halves. This design provides a major boost in

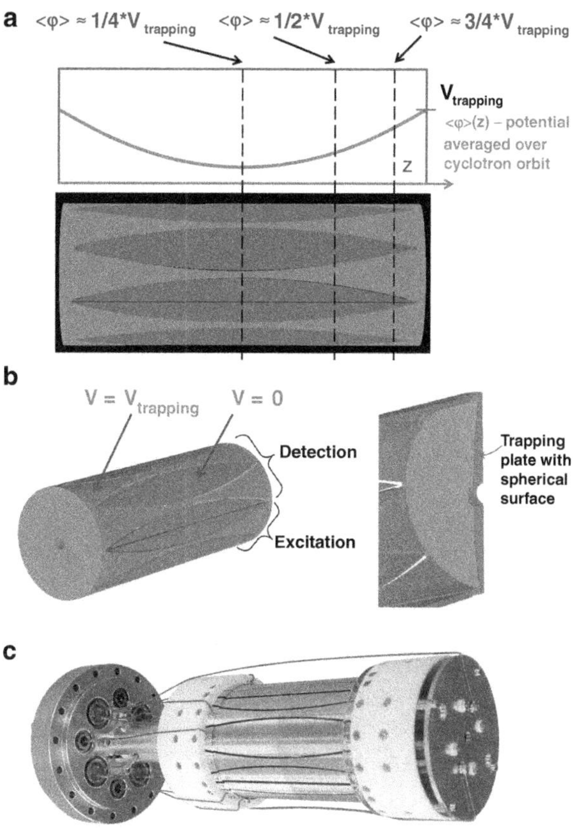

Fig. 4.76 Dynamically harmonized ICR cell. (**a**) Axial cross section showing the segmented cell walls and the hyperbolic trapping potential experienced by ions on average per full cycle. (**b**) Division into four 90° sections to accomplish excitation and detection plus detail of a trapping plate. (**c**) Photograph of the Paracell; gold plating is used to minimize electrode oxidation. (Figure compiled from material by courtesy of Bruker Daltonik, Bremen)

resolving power whilst maintaining high ion capacity and dynamic range [216, 217, 235]. It is commercialized as Paracell by Bruker Daltonik.

4.7.12 FT-ICR Instruments

Ion traps, ICR cells as well as QITs, are best operated with the number of trapped ions close to their respective optimum, because otherwise ion trajectories are distorted by coulombic repulsion. Hence, external ion sources in combination with ion transfer optics capable of controlling the number of injected ions are ideally attached to ion traps. Currently, MALDI [236] and even more so ESI [207, 214, 215, 230, 237] and other atmospheric pressure ionization sources predominate in FT-ICR.

The ion current is not solely regulated by the source but by some device to collect and store the desired amount of ions until the package is ready for injection into the ICR cell. Linear RF-multipole ion traps are normally employed for that purpose (Sect. 4.5.1) [119, 238, 239], but other systems are also in use [218]. RF-only multipoles are commonly used to transfer the ions through the boundaries of the magnetic field into the ICR cell (Sect. 4.4.4) [238]. For their injection, it is important to adjust the conditions so that the ions have low kinetic energy in *z*-direction in order not to overcome the shallow trapping potential. While some buffer gas is beneficial in case of LITs and QITs, ICR cells are operated at the lowest achievable pressure. The typical path from an external ion source into the ICR cell is therefore characterized by multistep differential pumping to achieve some 10^{-8}–10^{-7} Pa inside the ICR cell.

FT-ICR instruments are always equipped with superconducting magnets usually having 7 T and 9.4 T field strength; while 12 T and 15 T is also occasionally available. The advantages of increased field strengths are numerous: resolving power and scan speed, for example, increase linearly with B. Moreover, upper mass limit, ion trapping time, ion energy, and number of trapped ions even increase with B^2.

At the time of writing, FT-ICR instruments as considered here are provided by just two manufacturers: (*i*) the Qh-FT-ICR type as by the Bruker Solarix series (Fig. 4.77) and LIT-FT-ICR hybrid instruments as by the Thermo Scientific LTQ FT Ultra series (Sect. 4.8 and Fig. 4.86).

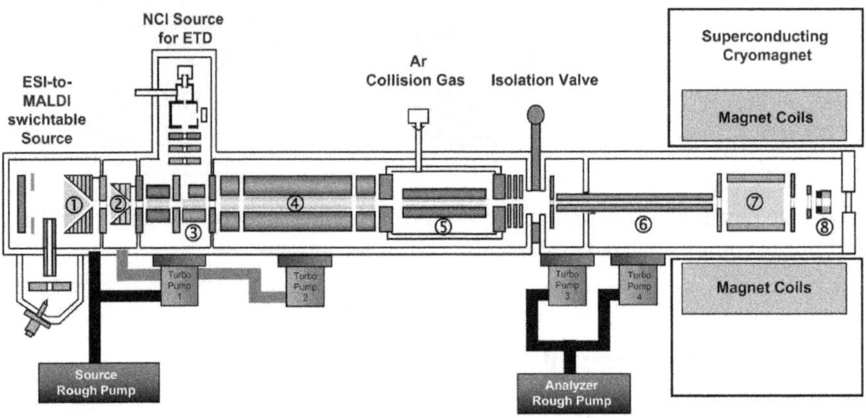

Fig. 4.77 A hQh-ICR hybrid instrument. This instrument is equipped with an ESI-to-MALDI switchable ion source that makes use of a two-stage ion funnel (①, ②) to focus ions into a RF hexapole ion guide (h, ③). The ions then pass a quadrupole (④) that may either be run as band pass (q) or as mass-selective device (Q) and then reach a multifunctional RF hexapole ion trap (h, ⑤) where they can be (*i*) accumulated, (*ii*) collisionally activated, or (*iii*) reacted with radical anions from the NCI source to effect ETD as required. For mass analysis the ions are then guided via an RF-only hexapole (⑥) into the ICR cell (⑦) where a hollow cathode (⑧) is attached for ECD. RF-only hexapole (⑥) and magnet are not to scale but shown relatively much smaller (Schematic of Bruker Solarix instrument series by courtesy of Bruker Daltonik, Bremen)

4.7.13 Summary of FT-ICR Instrumentation

Principle of Operation

Ions moving on a plane orthogonal to the direction of a magnetic field are forced on circular orbits by action of the Lorentz force. The radius of their orbit depends on ion kinetic energy, while the frequency of oscillation – the so-called cyclotron frequency – depends on the mass of the ions. To induce this mass-dependent ion motion, ions that are transferred into a magnetic field need to be excited by an RF electric field of a frequency equaling that of their cyclotron frequency. Once excited, ions of equal *m*/*z* coherently circulate inside the ICR cell. Upon their passage, the ion swarms induce image currents in the detection plates making up about half of the inner wall surface of the ICR cell. The image currents are recorded in the time domain (for 0.2–20 s), transformed into frequency domain by means of Fourier transformation (FT), and finally used to calculate the corresponding *m*/*z* values.

Performance Characteristics

FT-ICR instruments are the best-performing mass spectrometers in terms of resolving power (10^5 to $>10^6$) and mass accuracy (typically 0.1–2 ppm). The level that is achieved depends on the actual instrument, the duration of the transient, and numerous other parameters. Due to the long detection interval and the use of image current detection, FT-ICR-MS offers comparatively low sensitivity. This is counterbalanced by the fact that modern instruments can accommodate different ionization techniques, offer a variety of tandem-MS capabilities, and may even serve for sophisticated experiments in gas-phase ion chemistry. The extraordinary resolving power and mass accuracy enable the analysis of complex mixtures like crude oil or dissolved organic matter. Tandem-MS may serve to solve complex problems in protein analysis.

General Considerations

Mostly due to the prerequisite of using high-field superconducting magnets and the need for ultrahigh vacuum, FT-ICR instruments are large, heavy, and expensive in terms of both investment and cost of operation. While it may be challenging to exploit an instrument's full potential, modern FT-ICR instruments are nonetheless suitable for routine use. In fact, there are problems that can only be solved by FT-ICR-MS.

FT-MS

Occasionally, FT-ICR-MS is referred to as FT-MS or even FTMS. Apparently, FT-MS is most frequently used by mass spectrometrists who have dealt with FT-ICR-MS since the early days of the technique. Of course, ICR-MS without Fourier transformation would never have become as successful, but Fourier transformation alone cannot separate ions according to *m*/*z*. With the advent of the Orbitrap analyzer (Sect. 4.8), there is a second system making use of Fourier transformation of a time domain signal, although the prefix FT finds no mention in that name.

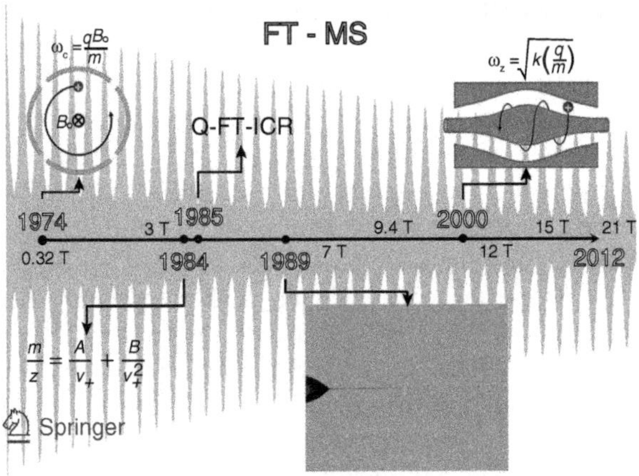

Fig. 4.78 FT-MS timeline as displayed on the journal cover of an issue dedicated to HR-MS. The journey starts with the introduction of FT-ICR and proceeds via *m/z* calibration, introduction of RF quadrupole transfer optics, external ESI source, and the first papers dealing with Orbitrap development. The magnetic fields available for FT-ICR-MS are also included (Adapted from *Analytical and Bioanalytical Chemistry* **403(5)** 2012 with permission. © Springer-Verlag, Heidelberg, 2012)

The acronym FT-MS is hence proposed as a collective term summarizing all FT-based MS techniques, i.e., FT-ICR-MS *and* Orbitrap-MS. Figure 4.78 taken from a journal cover of a special issue dedicated to HR-MS presents a welcome transition from FT-ICR to Orbitraps and also presents a compact timeline of developments.

4.8 Orbitrap Analyzer

The Orbitrap analyzer incorporates a concept of *m/z* analysis of its own [20, 240]. Commercialized by Thermo Fisher Scientific in 2005, the Orbitrap™ delivers high resolving power and accurate mass measurement at a level rivaling FT-ICR to a certain extent [20, 241–245]. It is the special charm of the Orbitrap to operate without a magnetic field, and therefore, to be available at a lower price and having fewer installation room requirements than FT-ICR instruments. Nonetheless, it has one important feature in common with FT-ICR: the Orbitrap also employs image current detection of ion oscillations and Fourier transformation for the conversion of the transient into the frequency domain. As we already have dealt with the very basics of FT in the context of FT-ICR-MS we may now concentrate on design and operation of the Orbitrap analyzer itself.

Orbiting in an electrostatic field

The Orbitrap is also an ion trap, but there is neither a magnet to hold ions inside nor is there any sort of RF excitation to initiate their motion. Instead, moving ions are trapped in a constant radial electrostatic field. The electrostatic attraction towards the central electrode is compensated by a centrifugal force that arises from the initial tangential velocity of ions: very much like a satellite in orbit [241].

4.8.1 Orbitrap – Principle of Operation

In 1923, Kingdon constructed an ion trapping device based on a straight wire along the axis of a surrounding cylindrical electrode having flanges that enclosed the trapping volume. Ions tangentially approaching the wire that is set to attractive electric potential would not hit the wire but become captured in a rotational motion around it. Their trajectory is then defined by an equilibrium of the centrifugal force and the electrostatic force generated by applying a voltage between wire and enclosing cylinder. Axial motion along the wire is confined by the field curvature introduced by the flanges of the cylinder. This became known as the *Kingdon trap* [246]. Later, Knight refined the outer electrode shapes to a design with large radius in the center that continuously decreased toward both ends. The outer electrode was symmetrically split into halves in a fashion similar to the end caps of the QIT. This trap design is often called *ideal Kingdon trap* [247]. Knight's trap could store ions and eject them onto a detector, but did not perform any *m/z* analysis [245]. The first proposal to build a Kingdon trap-based mass analyzer with image current detection addressed the ion rotational frequencies, but it suffered from the poor definition of those frequencies due to the influence of initial ion velocity upon entering the trap [248]. Finally, the concept of Makarov exploited the periodic back and forth motion of ions along the central electrode [240]. This setup requires a precisely defined field composed of a quadrupole field of the ion trap and the logarithmic field of a cylindrical capacitor that is split into two halves. This mass analyzer was termed *Orbitrap* [240] and can be considered as a refined Knight-style Kingdon trap. It has a spindle-like central electrode and a barrel-like outer electrode (Fig. 4.79) [245].

The electric field resulting from the complex shape of the Orbitrap electrodes may be termed quadrologarithmic field and has the potential distribution $U(r,z)$

$$U(r,z) = \frac{k}{2}\left(z^2 - \frac{r^2}{2}\right) + \frac{k}{2}(R_m)^2 \ \ln\left[\frac{r}{R_m}\right] + C \qquad (4.45)$$

where r and z are cylindrical coordinates ($z = 0$ being the plane of symmetry of the field), k is the field curvature, R_m the characteristic radius, and C is a constant [240, 249]. Equation (4.44) determines the electrostatic field experienced by ions inside the Orbitrap that forces them to move in complex spiral patterns. Stable ion trajectories combine rotation around the central axis with axial oscillations, the

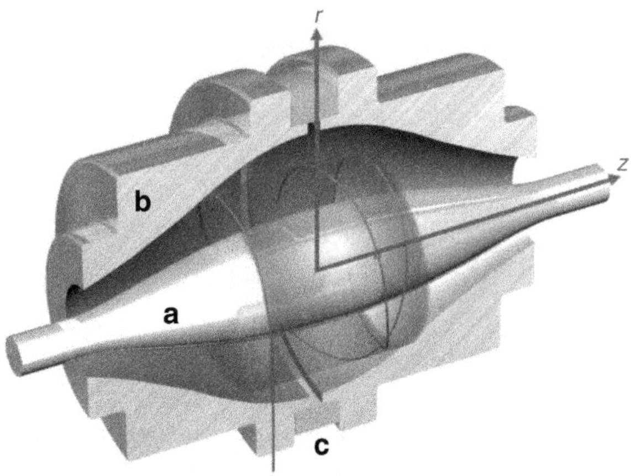

Fig. 4.79 A cut-away view of the Thermo Fisher Orbitrap™ mass analyzer. Ions are moving in spirals around a spindle-like-shaped central electrode (**a**) that creates an axial field gradient. An outer electrode (**b**) is split in half by an insulating ceramic ring (**c**). An image current induced by moving ions is detected via a differential amplifier between the two halves of the outer Orbitrap electrode. The *m/z* of different ions in the Orbitrap can be determined from respective frequencies of oscillation after a Fourier transform (Reproduced from Ref. [241] with permission. © Wiley-VCH, Weinheim, 2006)

frequency ω_z of which solely depends on the ratio of ionic charge q to ionic mass m_i and the field curvature, but is independent of the tangential velocity and spatial spread of the ions [241].

A detailed mathematical treatment of the Orbitrap can be found in Refs. [20, 240]. It delivers this important frequency of axial oscillations ω_z (in rad s^{-1}) as given by

$$\omega_z = \sqrt{k\left(\frac{q}{m_i}\right)} \tag{4.46}$$

The frequency of the harmonic axial oscillation ω_z is inversely proportional to the square root of the mass-to-charge ratio of the ions.

Another two characteristic frequencies can be derived for ions inside the Orbitrap. First the frequency of rotation ω_φ around the central electrode

$$\omega_\phi = \frac{\omega_z}{\sqrt{2}}\sqrt{\left(\frac{R_m}{R}\right)^2 - 1} \tag{4.47}$$

and second, the frequency of radial oscillation ω_r, i.e., the "pumping motion" of the orbit as the ions move along the variable radius of the central electrode:

$$\omega_r = \omega_z \sqrt{\left(\frac{R_m}{R}\right)^2 - 2} \tag{4.48}$$

4.8.2 Ion Detection and Resolving Power of the Orbitrap

The frequency of the harmonic axial oscillation ω_z can be determined by image current detection from a differential amplifier connected to the halves of the outer electrode; for each *m/z* value a sine wave is produced. Analogous to FT-ICR, the image current signal is monitored, stored, and translated into a frequency domain signal by fast Fourier transform resulting in an accurate reading of their *m/z* (Fig. 4.80) [241, 250]. Different from FT-ICR, there is no excitation prior to the detection period. Instead, the electric field gradient induces the axial oscillation when ions are injected tangentially but off-center with respect to plane of symmetry. All ions have exactly the same amplitude whereas the frequency of axial motion is dictated by their *m/z* value. Again, there is an analogy to FT-ICR in that packets of ions of common *m/z* exhibit discrete motions with some interference by interpenetration of ion clouds of different *m/z* that are simultaneously occupying the trapping volume [20].

In an Orbitrap, the mass resolving power *R* is half the frequency resolving power due to the square root in Eq. (4.46) [245, 249]. It can be calculated as

$$R = \frac{m}{\Delta m} = \frac{1}{2\,\Delta\omega_z} \sqrt{\frac{kq}{m}} \tag{4.49}$$

Orbitrap versus FT-ICR While the frequency of the axial oscillation ω_z in an Orbitrap is proportional to $(q/m)^{1/2}$, the cyclotron frequency ω_c in FT-ICR is proportional to *q*/*m*. Accordingly, FT-ICR offers higher resolving power for lower *m/z* ions whereas the Orbitrap may outperform it at high *m/z* values. For example, in case of an FT-ICR instrument with a 7-T magnet, the Orbitrap has an edge over FT-ICR above *m/z* 800 (Fig. 4.81) [241, 245].

4.8.3 Ion Injection into the Orbitrap

The Orbitrap alone does not present a very practical instrument. While it serves as a high performance *m/z* analyzer, its operation demands for proper ion injection and it requires ultra-high vacuum in order to realize sufficiently long transients. Ion injection has to comply with several conditions and restrictions:

- Geometric prerequisites have to be met, such as injection angle, angular spread, and position with respect to the electrodes.

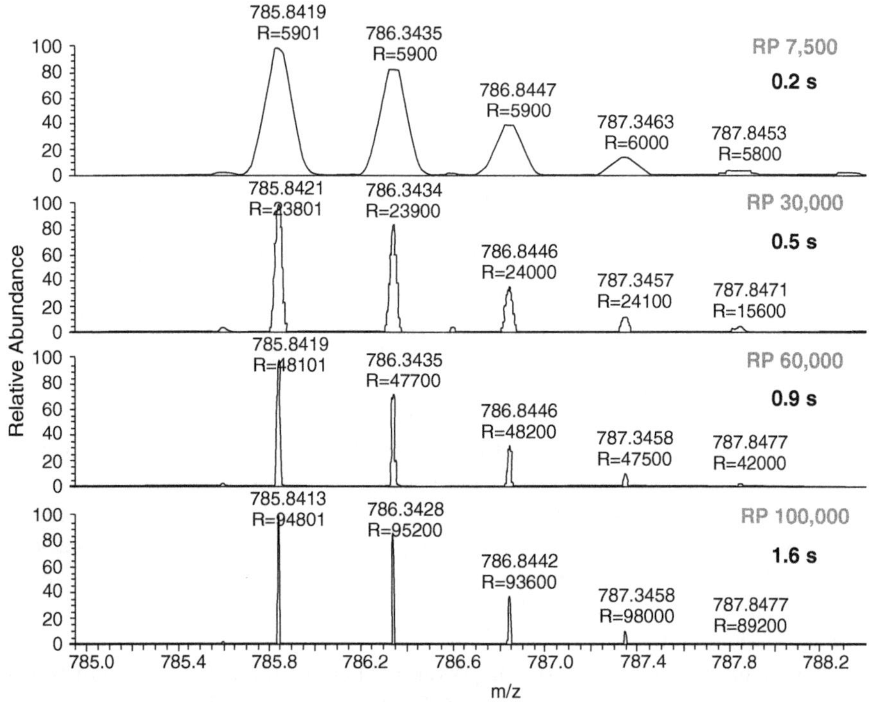

Fig. 4.80 Resolving power of a commercial Orbitrap instrument as achieved for doubly charged peptide ions at detection intervals ranging from 95 to 1267 ms resulting in cycle times from 0.2 to 1.6 s. The cycle times are longer than pure detection intervals due to preparation of ion packets, data processing etc. The values specified are calculated with reference to the manufacturer's standard value of *m/z* 400 (Reproduced from Ref. [241] with permission. © Wiley-VCH, Weinheim, 2006)

- Initial ion velocity and velocity distribution are important.
- Timing of the injection and its duration need to be carefully adjusted.
- Dosage of ions to achieve optimum ion population in the Orbitrap is required.
- Ultrahigh vacuum may not be interrupted to warrant the mean free path for tens to hundreds of thousands of undisturbed revolutions around the central electrode.

Thus, a bent RF-only quadrupole is employed to accumulate, store, and thermalize the ions by a low pressure of nitrogen prior to injection. Derived from the shape of the RF section in the form of the letter "C" this part has been termed the *C-trap*. The C-trap can be filled with about a million elementary charges. Collisional damping is important, because this way the ions are brought to rest in the middle of the C-trap. Nitrogen is used for that purpose as it is already used in the source region of the instrument and it is efficient at capturing and cooling the ions. In other words, the C-trap decouples the Orbitrap from all preceding steps of ion generation, desolvation, and eventually precursor ion selection [250].

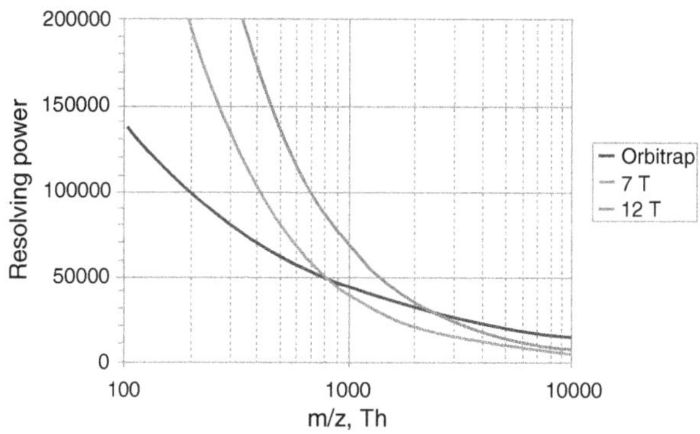

Fig. 4.81 For an Orbitrap analyzer the drop in resolving power with increasing *m/z* is less pronounced than for FT-ICR instruments. While FT-ICR clearly outperforms Orbitraps up to *m/z* 8000 (7 T, *pink line*) or even *m/z* 2500 (12 T, *red line*) the Orbitrap can deliver somewhat better resolving power in the high mass range (*blue line*) (Reproduced from Ref. [241] with permission. © Wiley-VCH, Weinheim, 2006)

High-voltage electric pulses with short rise times in the order of few hundreds of nanoseconds serve to eject the ions from the C-trap through the gap between the inner pair of quadrupole rods along lines converging on the entrance of the Orbitrap. By lowering the electric potential of the central electrode simultaneously with the entry of the ion packets, ions are captured and start circling. Typically, the ions are injected at kinetic energies of about 1.3 keV while the central electrode is set to −3.4 kV (for positive-ion mode) [245]. The initial bunches become reshaped into rings that oscillate axially along the central electrode. The amplitude of these oscillations is determined by the initial offset of ion injection from the Orbitrap center, whereas coherency of axial oscillations, i.e., maintenance of thin rings, is ensured by the short temporal duration of ion packet injection (Fig. 4.82).

One Orbitrap cycle

Ions are collected and thermalized in the C-trap and are injected as a focused beam off-center into the Orbitrap. The electric field of the Orbitrap is increased during the period of injection to compress the ion cloud towards the center. The ions thus are rotating around the central spindle electrode, and in addition, perform radial as well as axial oscillations. After stabilization of the high voltage, the axial oscillation proportional to $(q/m)^{1/2}$ is recorded via image current detection using the pair of outer electrodes.

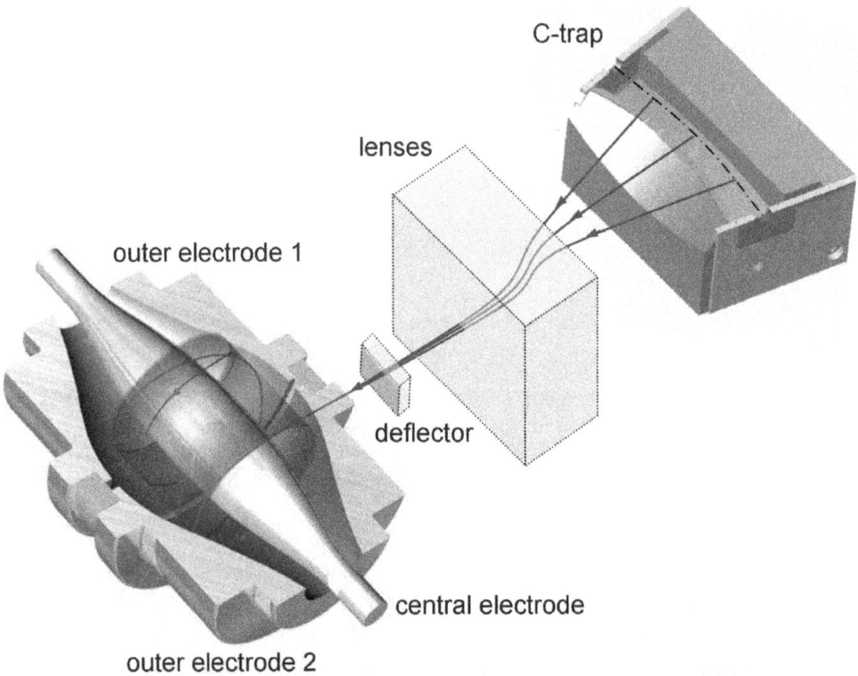

Fig. 4.82 The Orbitrap mass analyzer with ions being injected from the C-trap through lenses and a deflector. During injection, the C-trap acts as a convex lens with the outer rods pushing and the inner short rods pulling the ions by a DC pulse. Trapping voltage is applied to the central electrode (Courtesy of A. Makarov, Thermo Fisher Scientific)

4.8.4 Hybridization with a Linear Quadrupole Ion Trap

To become an analytically useful mass spectrometer, the above combination still needs to be interfaced to an ion source. The prototype implementation of the Orbitrap made use of laser desorption/ionization in the immediate vicinity of the Orbitrap [240], but soon, an external electrospray ion source followed [249]. For highest versatility, the Orbitrap has been attached to the rear of a fully functional Thermo Fisher LTQ instrument (cf. Sect. 4.5.4 and Fig. 4.50). The LIT may either be operated on its own as it still is equipped with SEM detectors or it may be axially emptied into the C-trap via an RF-only transfer octopole. The entire setup, dubbed LTQ-Orbitrap, is shown in Fig. 4.83. This instrument offers both low-resolution MS and MS^n operation in the LTQ section and final high-resolving *m*/*z* analysis at ppm-accuracy of whatever ions decided to be sent into the Orbitrap [241–244, 250]. A differential pumping system reduces the pressure along the instrument to achieve about 2×10^{-10} mbar in the Orbitrap. While Orbitrap technology has strongly advanced, there is still ongoing research for further improvements [251–255].

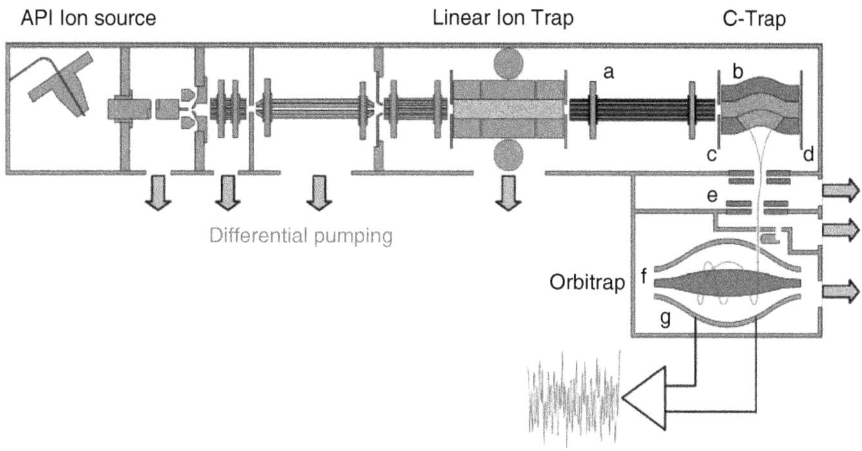

Fig. 4.83 The Thermo Scientific LTQ Orbitrap mass spectrometer. The front end up to the LIT is identical to the LTQ instrument introduced in Sect. 4.5.3 and Fig. 4.41. Ions axially ejected from the LIT are entering (**a**) a transfer octopole to (**b**) a curved RF-only quadrupole known as C-trap, from where they are injected via (**c**) gate electrode, (**d**) trap electrode, and (**e**) ion optics into the Orbitrap comprising (**f**) the inner electrode and (**g**) outer electrodes for detection. Note that there are four ports for differential pumping along the LTQ section and another three sideways to reduce the pressure from the C-trap to the Orbitrap (Adapted from Ref. [243] with permission. © American Chemical Society, 2006)

4.8.5 Orbitrap at a Glance

Mass Analysis in the Orbitrap

In an Orbitrap ions are captured by electrostatic attraction of a spindle-shaped central electrode provided they are entering the trapping field in a tangential direction. Proper ion injection in terms of kinetic energy, spatial focusing, and timing is achieved by radial ejection of ion bunches from a C-shaped quadrupole ion trap. The resulting ionic motion inside the Orbitrap is a superimposition of circulation around the central electrode and oscillation along the axis of the same. The longitudinal oscillation is caused by the electric field gradient along the spindle axis. The oscillation is recorded in the time domain via image current detection by two outer electrodes. The frequency is then obtained by FT of the recorded transient and used to calculate m/z and abundance of the ions in the Orbitrap.

Performance Characteristics

The main features of the Orbitrap are high resolving power and accurate mass. The level of both depends on the actual Orbitrap model and the exact mode of operation. Typically, spectra are acquired at a resolving power of $R = 20{,}000$–$200{,}000$ and mass accuracy is in the order of 0.5–3 ppm.

Growing Orbitrap Family

Since the introduction of the first instrument featuring an Orbitrap mass analyzer, the array of instruments has continuously been growing. In between, the range includes benchtop systems purely offering HR-MS for routine LC-MS and lately also GC-MS plus benchtop systems with tandem MS capabilities due to a Q-Orbitrap design. Instruments of increasing sophistication with LIT and even dual-LIT frontends and other features complement the Orbitrap family of instruments. Some of them will be discussed in the context of tandem MS (Sect. 9.10). The Orbitrap is set apart from all other types of mass analyzers not only by its unique working principle but also by the fact of being exclusively commercialized by a single company, Thermo Fisher.

4.9 Hybrid Instruments

As anticipated in the sections on linear ion traps (Sect. 4.5.4), modern Fourier transform-ion cyclotron resonance (Sect. 4.7.12), and LIT-Orbitrap mass spectrometers (Sect. 4.8.4), instruments can efficiently be designed by combining different types of mass analyzers and ion-guiding devices in a single so-called *hybrid instrument* [256, 257]. By these means one can obtain mass spectrometers that unite the advantageous properties of each mass analyzer they are composed of.

Hybrid mass spectrometers combine the expertise of the various highly developed dedicated devices and mass-analyzing, ion-guiding, ion-accumulating, and ion-focusing elements in a way that ensures the most versatile and yet economic solution. The design of a hybrid instrument may aim at:

- achieving highest resolving power and accuracy,
- boosting speed and sensitivity,
- realizing a compact and versatile yet affordable multi-purpose instrument.

Budgetary aspects are an important issue in favor of hybridization because each stage is selected as to deliver optimum performance at lowest cost. Hybrids are ideally employed for tandem mass spectrometry, for instance. In tandem mass spectrometers the first stage of *m*/*z* analysis (MS1) is used to select ions for further fragmentation and subsequent analysis of the product ions in a second *m*/*z* analyzer (MS2, Chap. 9). It is generally sufficient to combine a low-resolution MS1 unit with a high-resolution MS2.

Table 4.2 Hybrid mass analyzers.

MS1	Properties of MS1	MS2	Properties of MS2
BE or EB	LR and HR	qQ	LR, low energy CID
BE or EB	LR and HR	QIT	LR, low energy CID, MS^n
EB or EBE	LR and HR	oaTOF	LR, low energy CID, high sensitivity
Qq	LR, low-energy CID	oaTOF	high resolution and mass accuracy, high sensitivity
Qq	LR, low-energy CID	LIT	LR, higher sensitivity than QqQ, MS/MS in LIT
Qq	LR, low-energy CID	Orbitrap	High resolution and mass accuracy
QIT	LR, low-energy CID, MS^n	TOF	HR, high sensitivity
LIT	LR, low-energy CID, MS^n	Orbitrap	High to ultrahigh resolution and mass accuracy
Qq	LR, low-energy CID, MS^2	ICR	Ultrahigh resolution and mass accuracy, MS/MS in ICR
LIT	LR, low-energy CID, MS^n	ICR	Ultrahigh resolution and mass accuracy, MS/MS in ICR

4.9.1 Evolution of Hybrid Mass Spectrometers

The development of hybrid instruments started from magnetic sector-quadrupole hybrids, either BqQ [258, 259], EBqQ, [260] or BEqQ [261–263]. Numerous other systems such as magnetic sector-QIT [264], magnetic sector-oaTOF [265, 266], QITTOF [159, 267, 268], QqTOF [55, 269–271], QqLIT [129], LIT-ICR, and QqICR followed. LIT-Orbitraps present the most recent addition [241, 242, 252, 253] (Table 4.2).

The adaptation of conceptually different mass analyzers to each other may demand for sophisticated interfaces, because of the largely differing requirements concerning ion kinetic energies. The magnetic sector-quadrupole or magnetic sector-QIT hybrids, for example, require keV ions exiting the sector to be decelerated to some 10 eV before entering the qQ section, or to be slowed down and pulsed into the QIT, respectively. Due to the bulky and demanding magnetic sector analyzer, hybrids of that type do not anymore play a role.

Geometries composed of an oaTOF as second analyzer bear the advantage that advanced TOFs offer accurate mass measurements equaling the accuracy of magnetic sector instruments. While their linear quadrupole front end serves as MS1 in tandem MS experiments, it is operated in RF-only mode when tandem MS is not intended, because this allows to acquire full-range spectra at high resolution using the TOF analyzer (MS2, Fig. 4.84). It should be noted that the first quadrupole of hybrids with Qq as MS1, i.e., Qq-TOF hybrids, typically offers mass-selective operation covering an m/z range different from the range in RF-only operation, e.g., m/z 50–4000 in mass-selective and m/z 50–10,000 in RF-only transmission mode.

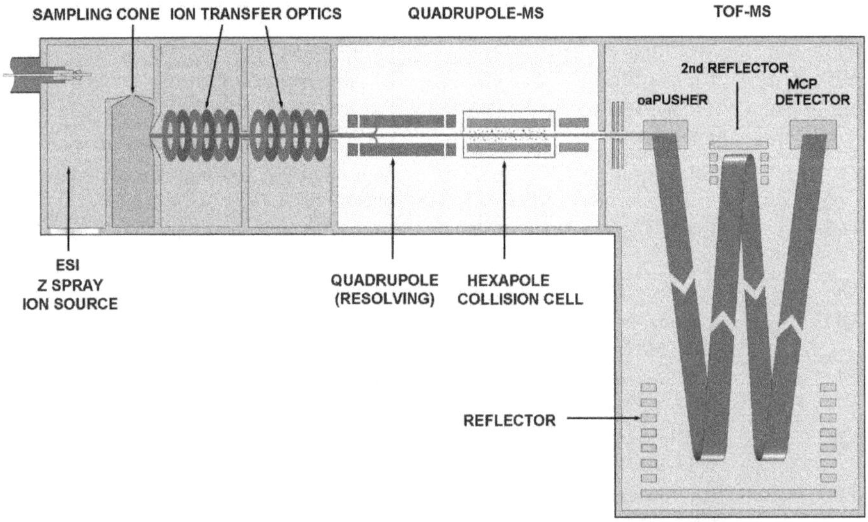

Fig. 4.84 The Q-TOF Ultima, Qh-oaTOF design, with ESI ion source in MS/MS mode. The TOF analyzer has a reflector that can either be operated using the large reflector alone (V-mode) or adding a second stage of ion reflection (W-mode) for higher resolving power (Courtesy of Waters Corporation, MS Technologies, Manchester, UK)

Widespread in use

Besides accommodating to their versatility, there is nothing new to understand with hybrid instruments. Exotic at a first glance, hybrids are governing today's market of mass spectrometers [133–135].

There is very strong competition between high-end QqTOF instruments, on the one side, and Qq-Orbitrap and LIT-Orbitrap hybrid instruments like the aforementioned LTQ-Orbitrap (Fig. 4.83), on the other. The Orbitrap instrument family shows remarkable flexibility in terms of how the Orbitrap analyzer is implemented as part of a complex hybrid system. The range not only includes Qq-Orbitrap and LIT-Orbitrap hybrids but recently even a Q-Orbitrap-tandemLIT configuration. The latter instrument, the Orbitrap Fusion is marketed as a *tribrid* because it incorporates three different types of mass analyzers (Fig. 4.85) [254, 255]. The purpose of the tandem LIT is to provide a higher-pressure LIT for precursor ion selection and ion fragmentation plus a lower-pressure LIT for effective mass analysis. The Orbitrap Fusion architecture permits a multitude of operational modes that allow tandem MS experiments to be run in parallel while a full range survey scan delivers accurate mass data of the next package of precursors to be interrogated or accurate mass of fragments.

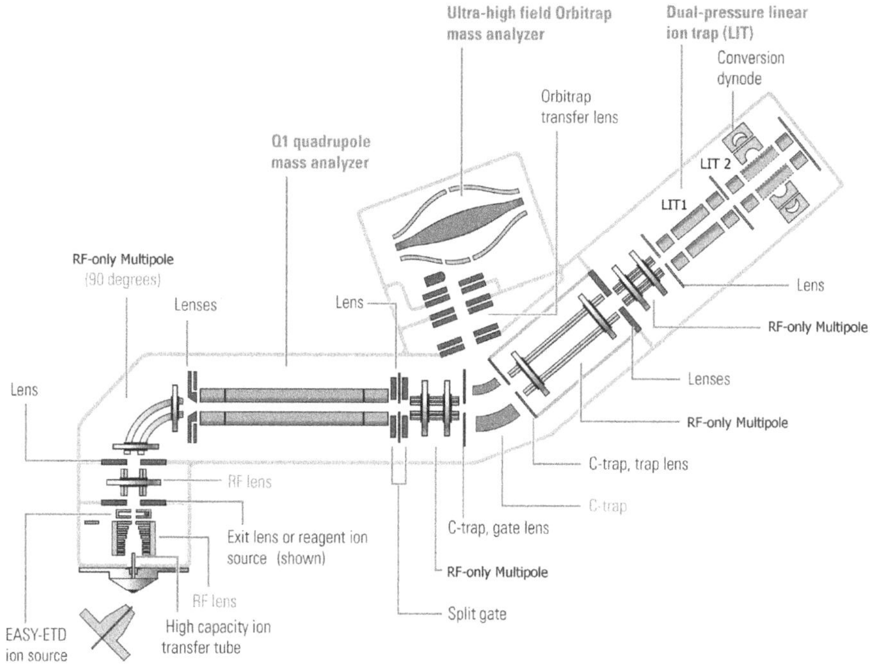

Fig. 4.85 The Orbitrap Fusion Lumos tribrid mass spectrometer. The first RF-only multipole is bent by 90° to get rid of neutrals before ions are entering the analyzer section comprising quadrupole (*orange*), Orbitrap (*blue*), and LIT/LIT (*green*) (Adapted from Thermo Fisher technical documentation with kind permission. © Thermo Fisher Scientific, Bremen, 2015)

The highest level of resolving power and mass accuracy can be achieved by replacing the oaTOF section with a FT-ICR analyzer. Those high-end hybrid instruments are either available as Qh-ICR by employing a quadrupole as first mass analyzer (Bruker Daltonik APEX-Q and Solarix instruments, Fig. 4.78) or as LIT-ICR, i.e., with a linear ion trap in front of the ICR cell (Thermo Scientific LTQ-FT series, Fig. 4.86).

4.10 Ion Mobility-Mass Spectrometry Systems

There is an increasing interest in *ion mobility spectrometry* (IMS) as it presents an effective means of separating gaseous ions [272, 273]. In IMS an electric field forces the ions to drift along a path through a countercurrent inert gas atmosphere whereby they are separated due to their collision cross sections. IMS does for gaseous ions what gas chromatography does for gaseous neutrals, and in fact, IMS was initially referred to as *plasma chromatography* (PC). IMS can separate isobaric ions of different charge state (size-to-charge ratio) resulting from their distinct speed of propagation along the electric field of the ion mobility tube or

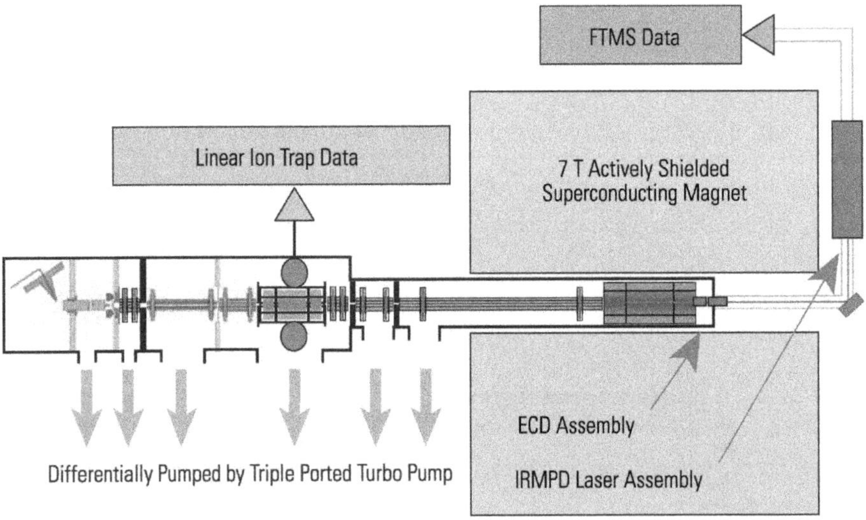

Fig. 4.86 Schematic of a LIT-FT-ICR hybrid instrument, the Thermo Scientific LTQ FT Ultra, incorporating a fully functional LTQ front end (as in LTQ Orbitrap) for highest versatility (Courtesy Thermo Fisher Scientific, Bremen)

distinguish isobars of the same charge state by their steric properties, i.e., it separates isomers and conformers alike by their shape. Thus, IMS is a valuable aid in biomolecular analysis [274–276].

Clearly, mass spectrometry is perfectly suited for the detection for gaseous ions eluting from an ion mobility device. Therefore, *ion mobility-mass spectrometry* (IM-MS) coupling has received considerable attention since the 1970s [277–279]. The IM-MS instrument provides the following functional features [272]:

- transfer of gaseous sample into the ion source,
- ion formation from neutral sample molecules at atmospheric pressure,
- accumulation of an ion package and injection into the drift region,
- measurement of drift velocities of the swarms of ions while passing the electric field of the drift region in a drift gas atmosphere, and
- detection of ions by a mass analyzer coupled to the IMS stage.

Hybrid, hyphenation, or something in between?
While a detailed treatment of ion mobility spectrometry is beyond the scope of this book, it is certainly useful to provide a brief description of the technique [272, 273]. In principle, IM-MS systems can be regarded as hyphenated instrumentation (for applications cf. Sect. 14.6) because the peculiarities of ion mobility demand an integrated instrumental approach.

(continued)

This distinguishes IM-MS from gas or liquid chromatography couplings to MS that may be coupled to and decoupled from a mass spectrometer as required [274, 280]. Therefore, IM-MS is dealt with here as a special case of hybridization.

4.10.1 Ion Mobility Separation

Ion mobility effects separation of ions based on their different velocities when accelerated by a constant electric field along a drift tube with a countercurrent inert gas, typically helium or nitrogen. The average velocity, v_D, of a drifting ion is then governed by the number of soft collisions it experiences within the drift tube. This number of collisions with the neutrals is directly proportional to the electric field strength, E, and the ion mobility constant K (in cm^2 V^{-1} s^{-1}).

$$v_D = K\,E \tag{4.50}$$

The value of K depends on the ion and the drift gas. Equation (4.50) is only valid up to field strengths of about 1000 V cm^{-1}, whereas above that electric field strength the proportionality between K and E is canceled [274].

The electric field needs to be weak enough so that collisions at given gas density dampen the ions to achieve an internal ion energy in equilibrium with the temperature of the bath gas [276]. Furthermore, gas discharges have strictly to be avoided. In the high-pressure regime (133–1013 mbar or 100–760 Torr) drift tubes are operated at 100–300 V cm^{-1} to deliver what in IMS is considered as high resolving power of 100–300. In the low-pressure regime, field strengths are limited to 10–30 V cm^{-1}. Unfortunately, lower pressure goes along with reduced resolving power of the device while coupling to mass analyzers is simplified due to reduced load on the vacuum system [276].

In the low-field regime, the value of K can be calculated from

$$K = \frac{3q}{16N}\sqrt{\frac{2\pi}{kT}}\sqrt{\left(\frac{m_g + m_i}{m_g m_i}\right)}\left(\frac{1}{\Omega}\right) \tag{4.51}$$

where q is the ionic charge, N the number density of the buffer gas, k is Boltzmann's constant, T is the absolute temperature, m_g is the mass of the buffer gas molecules, and m_i is the mass of the ions that have the collision cross section Ω [275, 280].

In the IM-MS experiment, q and Ω are a priori unknown, but m_i is derived from m/z as soon as the charge state z has been identified, which in turn delivers q from

$q = ze$. As hundreds of TOF mass spectra can be acquired during the tens of milliseconds required for one ion mobility run, the setup easily delivers high-quality MS data to identify the drift time-separated ions.

The reduced mobility, K_0, is calculated for comparing IMS data between runs obtained at different buffer gas temperature and pressure and also across different instruments. The reduced mobility, K_0, is obtained from:

$$K_0 = \frac{{l_D}^2}{t_D U_D} \frac{T_0}{T} \frac{p}{p_0} \tag{4.52}$$

where l_D is the length of the drift tube and U_D the voltage applied along it; the temperature is given in units of Kelvin ($T_0 = 273.2$ K) and the pressure in units of millibar ($p_0 = 1013$ mbar). K_0 has the physical dimension of cm^2 V^{-1} s^{-1}. Depending on the source, the equation for the reduced mobility may also be stated in the literature using the electric field strength instead of the voltage and the pressure in Torr:

$$K_0 = \frac{l_D}{t_D E_D} \frac{273.2\text{K}}{T} \frac{p}{760\,\text{Torr}} \tag{4.52a}$$

where l_D is the length of the drift tube and E_D the voltage applied divided by l_D [276].

For this classical approach to IMS, the theory of ion propagation is very well developed and allows to calculate the orientationally averaged collision cross sections with high confidence [275].

IM-TOF-MS The mass analyzer of an IM-MS instrument must be able to deliver a spectral acquisition rate that allows to collect mass spectra faster than the time span for elution of an IMS peak. As ion mobility separation proceeds in the order of tens of milliseconds, a typical IMS resolving power in the order of 100 implies that at least 100 mass spectra have to be acquired per IMS run. Only TOF analyzers are capable of delivering spectra at 100–1000 Hz, and thus, the IM-TOF-MS hybrid presents the natural combination for IM-MS (Fig. 4.87).

4.10.2 Stacked Ring Ion Guide

As an alternative to RF-only multipole ion guides, the *stacked ring ion guide* (SRIG) has been newly recognized since 2004. Ring electrodes (2–3 mm i.d.) are aligned with 1–2 mm insulating ceramics spacers in between them and supplied with an RF drive voltage ($U_{RF} \approx 100$ V at 1 MHz) that is reversed in phase between adjacent rings (Fig. 4.88) [118, 281]. Ions entering the SRIG experience a deep radial potential well with comparatively steep walls towards the inner ring surfaces when traveling though the apertures. The SRIG offers high transmission if operated with a thermalizing buffer gas at around 3 mbar. Interestingly, the SRIG not merely

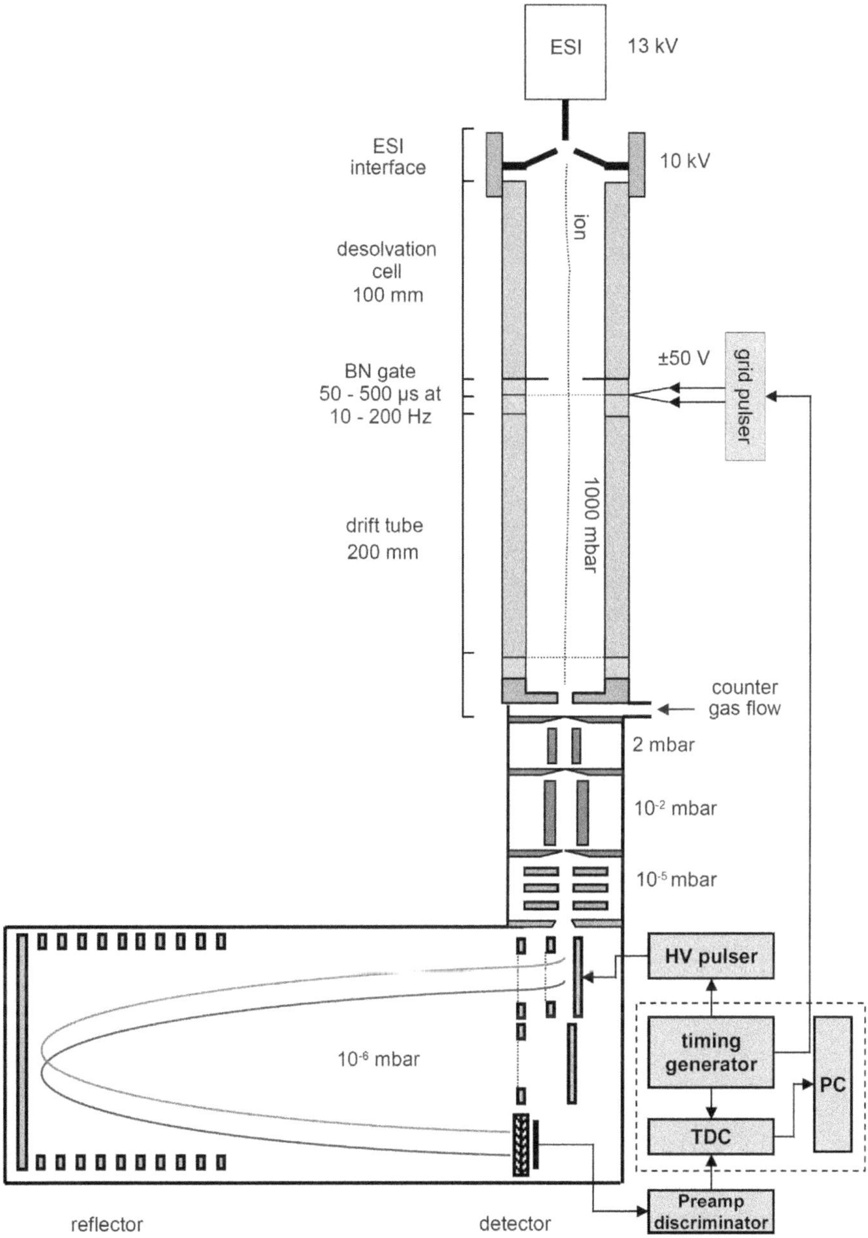

Fig. 4.87 Basic design of an ambient-pressure IMS-TOF mass spectrometer. Ions from an electrospray source are entering a desolvation chamber from where packets are pulsed into the ion mobility tube by means of a Bradbury-Nielsen (BN) ion gate. The ion path is shown uneven to indicate diffusion of ions. After ion mobility separation the ions are transferred into the reflector oaTOF analyzer via a differentially pumped interface (Courtesy of TofWerk AG, Thun, Switzerland)

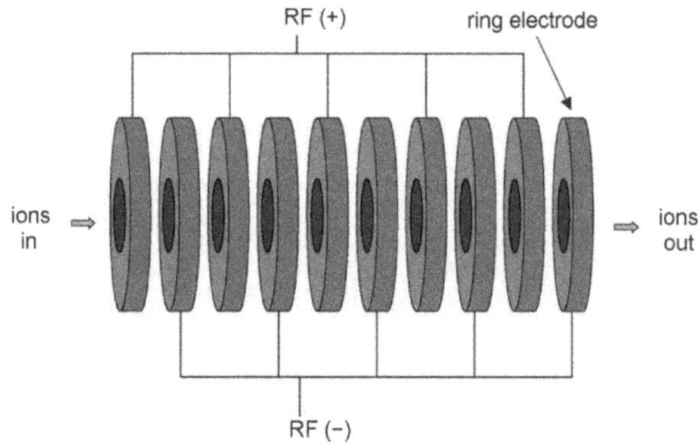

Fig. 4.88 A stacked ring ion guide. Rings are connected to an RF drive voltage in alteration of the phase. Normally tens of pairs are used to build one ion guide. Ions entering from the left experience a deep radial potential well with comparatively steep walls toward the inner ring surfaces when traveling though the apertures (Reproduced from Ref. [281] with permission. © Elsevier Science Publishers, 2007)

forms a kind of pipe for the ions, its effective potential more resembles a corrugated hose where the grooves act as low potential wells in axial direction, which are deep enough to restrain axial drift of thermalized ions by soft trapping.

To avoid stopping of the ions, a DC pulse can be delivered to a pair of rings causing the ions to move forth to the next potential groove. If the DC pulse makes a progression from pair to pair it creates a traveling wave (T-wave) that makes the ions "surf" along the SRIG (Fig. 4.89).

Such *traveling wave ion guides* (TWIGs) are incorporated in many Waters instruments to replace the more traditional RF-only multipoles as ion guides and collision cells, e.g., in the "triplequadrupoles" of the Xevo™ and Quattro Premier™ series that essentially are of Q-TWIG-Q design. The wave created by a potential of about 2 V is generally propagating at around 300 m s^{-1}. This provides an effective means of minimizing dwell times in the corresponding compartment.

4.10.3 Traveling Wave Ion Guides for IMS

When ions differing either in charge state or collision cross sections, or both, are entering the TWIG, the less mobile ones may occasionally transverse a wave in backward direction. Those ions lagging behind the traveling wave will exit later than those surfing on the wave. This makes the TWIG become an ion mobility separator.

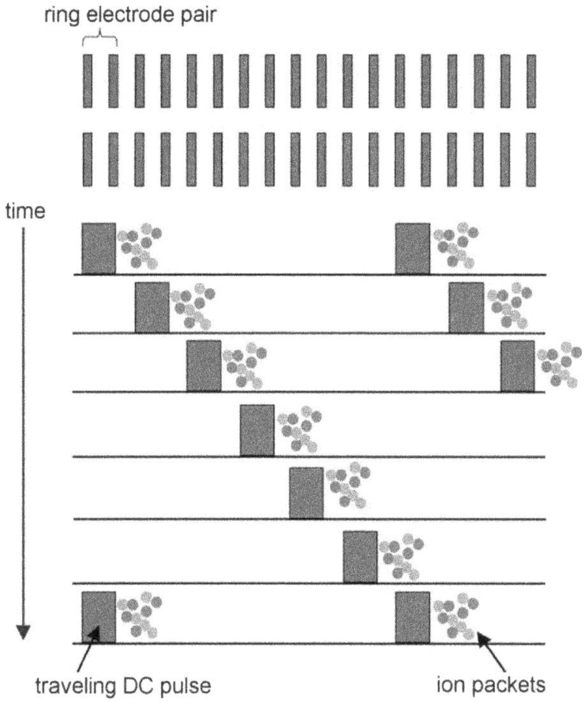

Fig. 4.89 Effect of a traveling wave DC pulse along a stacked ring ion guide. Ions in front of the DC pulse are moving along from stack to stack and are thus propulsed through the device (T-wave ion guide). A buffer gas is required to narrow down the thermal energy distribution (Reproduced from Ref. [281] with permission. © Elsevier Science Publishers, 2007)

Traveling wave
A specific type of IM-MS instrumentation using a *traveling-wave* (T-wave™) approach is available from Waters. In a T-wave ion mobility device ions are pushed by low-voltage waves established along a large stack of paired ring electrodes. However, the theory of ion mobility separation in the T-wave is not as fully understood as in traditional IMS devices [275, 280].

Obviously, multi-RF-ring electrode devices can be designed, optimized, and operated in numerous ways to

- guide ions on their transit from one instrument stage to another or across a pumping stage,
- keep ions on track while they are subjected to collisions with gas for excitation and fragmentation,

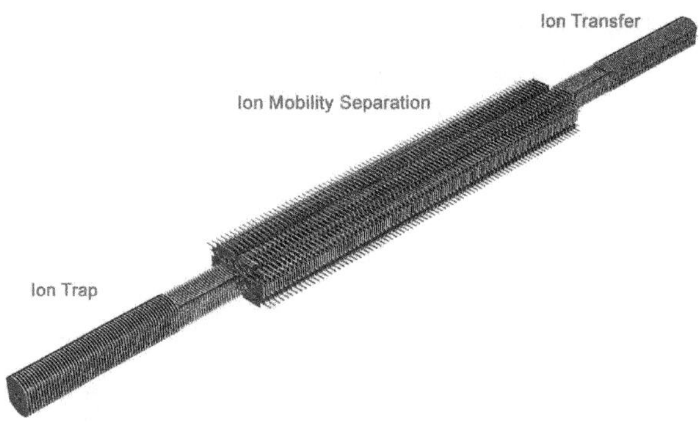

Fig. 4.90 Waters TriWave as incorporated in Synapt G2 instruments for ion mobility separation. Ions entering from the *left* are accumulated in the first section acting as the ion trap, then batch wise admitted into the ion mobility separation zone, and finally collected for transfer into the oaTOF analyzer (Adapted with permission. Courtesy of Waters MS Technologies)

- admit, stop, and collect ions to accumulate packets for subsequent IMS or mass analysis,
- provide ion mobility separation.

Compartments serving either purpose can be combined to form a linear operational unit as part of a more complex hybrid mass spectrometer (Fig. 4.90). With the exception of IMS, which is performed at 100–200 mbar of buffer gas countercurrent to the ion motion, multi-RF-ring electrode devices are typically operated in the 0.1–10 mbar pressure range. Thus, they are compatible with all sorts of applications of RF multipole ion guides.

4.10.4 Hybrid Instruments with IMS

A hybrid instrument comprising a mass-selecting quadrupole, a traveling wave ion mobility separator, and an oaTOF analyzer has been marketed by Waters as Synapt series of instruments (Fig. 4.91) [118, 281]. Additionally, this instrument incorporates a RF-ring electrode device in the interface region from ion source to the first mass-analyzing quadrupole. We will resume this topic in the context of interface design for electrospray ionization (Sect. 12.2).

Waters was the first company to offer IMS-tandem MS combinations and still seems to have the widest range of IM-MS instruments. More recently, Agilent (6560 Ion Mobility Q-TOF LC/MS) as well as Bruker with a new concept of *trapped ion mobility* (timsTOF) have also included this type of instrumentation in their portfolio. The designs are becoming more diverse as the technique receives more widespread use. Nonetheless, all IMS-tandem MS instruments rely on oaTOF as the final stage of mass analysis due to its unique combination of acquisition rate and resolving power.

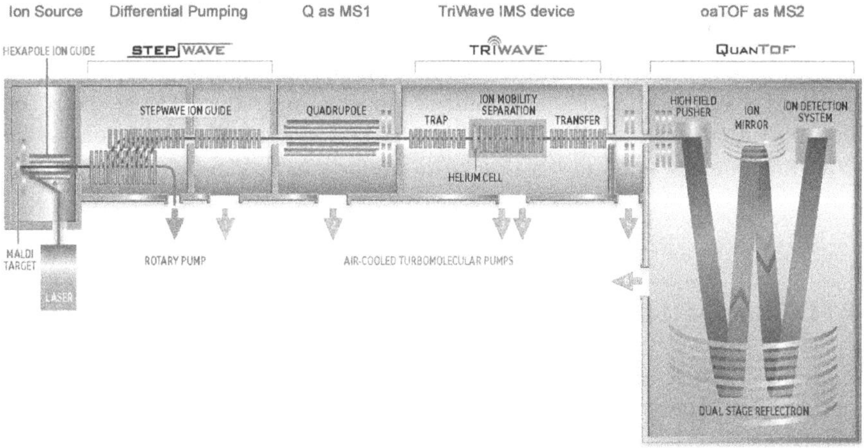

Fig. 4.91 The Waters Synapt G2-Si, a Q-IMS-oaTOF hybrid, here shown with MALDI source. The combination of three ring ion guide sections is used to build a complete IMS device comprising a trap at the entrance to supply ion packages, the IMS itself, and an ion guide for transfer to the mass analyzer (cf. TriWave in Fig. 4.89) (Adapted with permission. Courtesy of Waters MS Technologies)

4.10.5 Overview of Hybrid Instrumentation Including IM-MS

Classification

Mass spectrometers composed of different types of mass analyzers and ion-guiding devices are termed *hybrid instruments*. The components are combined in a way as to obtain mass spectrometers uniting the advantages of each subunit they are composed of. Thus, hybrids incorporate mass-analyzing, ion-guiding, ion-accumulating, ion separating, and ion-focusing elements in a way that ensures the most versatile and yet economic solution to obtaining a certain type of instrument.

Types of IMS

Drift tube ion mobility (DT-IMS) is the classical form of IMS. *Travelling-wave ion mobility* (TW-IMS) has been introduced and is marketed by Waters. In addition, there are *field asymmetric ion mobility* (FAIMS) and *differential ion mobility* (DMS) [282–284]. FAIMS devices are very compact and can externally be fitted to existing instruments with electrospray interface.

Relevant Representatives of Hybrid Instruments

Most newly introduced mass spectrometers are hybrid instruments in one way or another. Typically, they are designed as tandem mass spectrometers with a low-resolving first stage of *m/z* analysis (MS1) for precursor ion selection, e.g., Q, QIT, or LIT, and a high-resolving second stage for product ion analysis (MS2), e.g., oaTOF, Orbitrap, or FT-ICR.

Another family of hybrids includes ion mobility separation either in front of the mass spectrometer section or between MS1 and MS2. More widespread acceptance of IM-MS and instrument design by different manufacturers is leading to an increased diversity of instrumentation and modes of operation. Due to speed and sensitivity requirements, all dedicated IMS-tandem MS instruments rely on oaTOF as the final stage of mass analysis due to its unique combination of acquisition rate, duty cycle, and resolving power.

4.11 Ion Detection

The simplest detector is a *Faraday cup*, i.e., an electrode where the ions deposit their charge. The electric current flowing away from that electrode results in a voltage when passing through a resistor of high impedance. Faraday cups are still in use to measure abundance ratios with highest accuracy in *isotope ratio mass spectrometry* (IR-MS) [285]. Early in the era of Mattauch-Herzog-type instruments, the *photographic plate* has been the standard detection system (Sect. 4.3.5). With the advent of scanning mass spectrometers, *secondary electron multipliers* (SEM) became predominant [286]. These rely on the emission of secondary electrons from surfaces upon impact of energetic ions. Ion-counting detectors are not used in FT-ICR and Orbitrap instruments where *image current detection* is employed instead.

4.11.1 Analog-to-Digital Conversion

Ion packages of adjacent *m*/*z* values hit the detector very shortly after each other causing the signal to change at very high frequency. This requires the use of GHz-frequency digitizers for *analog-to-digital conversion.* Obviously, the final peak shape directly depends on the speed of the *analog-to-digital converter* (ADC) [45].

In case of an 8-bit ADC, for example, the intensity of the detector output is converted into a numerical value of 0–255 [287]. The *dynamic range* is the ratio obtained by dividing the intensity of the most intense signal by that of the weakest while both are correctly detected in the same spectrum. To improve the small dynamic range delivered by 8-bit ADCs (0–255), several tens to a few hundred single spectra are usually summed up. Most recent TOF and oaTOF instruments are therefore equipped with 8-bit or even 10-bit ADCs to provide a dynamic range of 10^4–10^5 after summation of several individual spectra.

Slower scanning instruments such as quadrupole, quadrupole ion trap, and magnetic sector instruments are typically equipped with 16–20-bit ADCs corresponding to intensity values of 0–65,535 (2^{16}–1) and 0–1,048,575 (2^{20}–1),

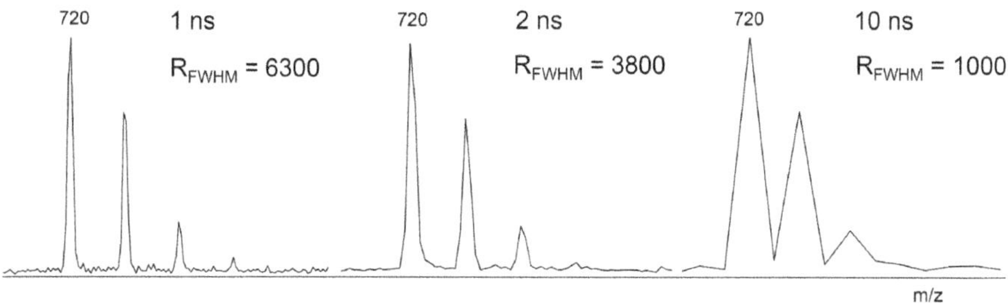

Fig. 4.92 The [60]fullerene molecular ion peak depicted at different settings of the dwell time per data point of the analog-to-digital converter obtained on the aforementioned instrument after PIE upgrade. At 1 ns per data point (1 GHz) the peaks are well resolved and resolution is limited by the analyzer. At 2 ns (500 MHz) some broadening occurs. At 10 ns (100 MHz) peak shapes are reduced to triangles because detection provides just about two points per *m/z*

respectively. This explains their advantage when a high linear dynamic range is required, e.g., for quantitation.

4.11.2 Digitization Rate

In particular, the resolving power of advanced TOF analyzers creates a need for high-speed ADCs. Modern TOF instruments incorporate 8-bit ADCs with a digitization rate of 4–5 GHz to suit their resolving power of up to $R = 45{,}000$. The *digitization rate* or *sampling rate* of an ADC may be reported as dwell time per data point, e.g., 1 ns, or as sampling frequency, e.g., 1 GHz (Fig. 4.92). Data points are also shown on a spectrum in Sect. 11.5.

General relevance
These considerations concerning the digitization rate are in no way restricted to TOF instruments but apply to any process of data acquisition. As a rule of thumb, good peak shapes require 6–10 data points per peak. This rule applies analogously to the number of single spectra per eluting chromatographic peak.

4.11.3 Time-to-Digital Conversion

Time-to-digital converters (TDC) had been employed in some early oaTOF instruments instead of analog-to-digital converters because of the much higher speed of TDCs. Speed in terms of sampling rate is needed to reach the high resolution of oaTOF analyzers, and speed in terms of data flow is a prerequisite to handle the enormous number of spectra per second. However, a TDC is a pulse-counting device that offers only 1 bit dynamic range (value 0 or 1) [287]. Detector–

TDC combinations easily suffer from saturation effects as they cannot distinguish the arrival of a single ion from that of several ions arriving simultaneously. The TDC response is therefore not proportional to ion flux. Thus, summation of many single spectra is also necessary to obtain a higher dynamic range via improved signal statistics. Nevertheless, the result is still unsatisfactory for quantitative analysis and for correct isotopic patterns. Furthermore, the dead time between subsequent counting events causes the second of a pair of ions having almost equal arrival times to remain undetected. Dead time effects within ion packages of a given *m*/*z* even cause *m*/*z* values to shift to the low-mass side (detection of early incoming ions only), which makes empirical dead-time corrections necessary for accurate mass measurements [287, 288].

4.11.4 Discrete Dynode Electron Multipliers

When an energetic particle impinges on the surface of a metal or a semiconductor, secondary electrons are emitted from that surface. The ease of such an emission is determined by the *electron(ic) work function* of the respective material, e.g., BeCu alloy oxide ($w_e \approx 2.4$ eV) [289]. The higher the velocity of the impacting particle [286, 290] and the lower the electron work function of the surface, the larger the number of secondary electrons. If an electrode opposite to the location of emission is held at more positive potential, all emitted electrons will be accelerated towards and hit that surface where they in turn cause the release of several electrons each. The avalanche of electrons produced over 12–18 discrete dynode stages held at about 100 V more positive potential each causes an electric current large enough to be detected by a sensitive preamplifier. Such a detector is called *secondary electron multiplier* (SEM, Fig. 4.93) [291]. The dynodes are normally cup-shaped, but stacks of Venetian blind-like dynodes have also been in use. Due to a certain air sensitivity of the emissive layer and in order to prevent arcing due to the high voltage, electron multipliers require operation in high vacuum.

The ion currents actually reaching the first dynode are chiefly in the picoampere range, but may span over a 10^{-18}–10^{-9} A range. Depending on the applied voltage, SEMs provide a gain of 10^6–10^8 [291]. The resulting current at the electron trap is the input of a nearby preamplifier providing another 10^6–10^9 gain. Its output current is then converted to a voltage signal which finally can be translated to an intensity value by means of an analog-to-digital converter (ADC).

How many ions per peak? A singly-charged ion corresponds to a charge of 1.6×10^{-19} C, and 1 A is equal to 1 C s^{-1}. Thus, an ion current of 10^{-15} A = 10^{-15} C s^{-1} is provided by about 6000 ions per second. If the detection of these ions during a scan in a GC-MS run taking 1 s over the *m*/*z* 40–400 range yields a mass spectrum consisting of some 30–60 peaks, this corresponds to 100–200 ions per peak. Such conditions define the detection limit of a scanning mass spectrometer.

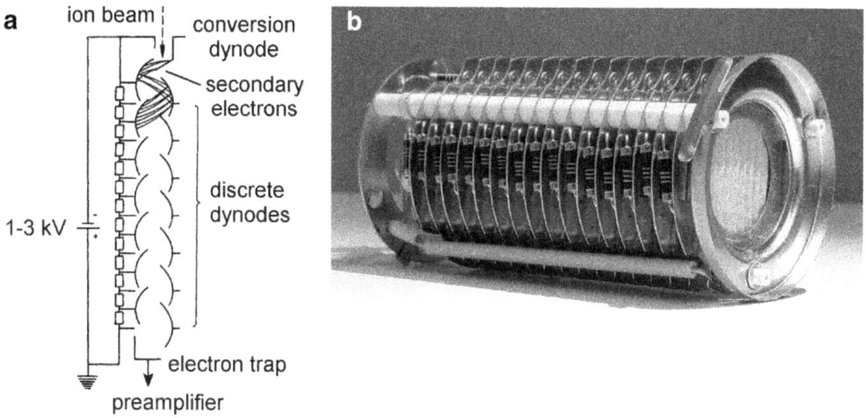

Fig. 4.93 Discrete dynode electron multipliers. (**a**) Schematic of a 14-stage SEM. (**b**) An old-fashioned 16-stage Venetian blind-type SEM clearly showing the resistors and ceramics insulators between the stacking dynodes at its side ((**a**) Adapted from Ref. [292] by permission. © Springer-Verlag Heidelberg, 1991)

> **Replacement may be on order**
> All types of secondary electron multipliers have limited life-time. They can deliver 0.1–10 C of extracted charge and are also limited by beam-induced destruction of the first dynode.

4.11.5 Channel Electron Multipliers

The cascade of secondary electrons can also be produced in a continuous tube. Such detectors, known as *channel electron multipliers* (CEM) or just *channeltrons*, are more compact and less expensive than discrete dynode SEMs. CEMs are preferably used in benchtop instruments. Their gain depends on the length-to-diameter ratio with an optimum ratio around 40–80 [293]. In a CEM, the high voltage drops continuously from the ion entrance to the electron exit of the tube requiring a sufficiently high resistance of the semiconducting material to withstand high voltage of about 2 kV. This is accomplished by an emissive layer of silicon dioxide overlying a conductive layer of lead oxide on the supporting heavily lead-doped glass tube [291, 294]. Straight CEMs are unstable at gains exceeding 10^4 because positive ions created inside by EI of residual gas are accelerated towards the input side of the tube where they randomly contribute to the signal causing spurious output pulses [294, 295]. A curved design shortens the free path for ion acceleration thereby suppressing noise from this so-called *ion-feedback*. Curved CEMs provide gains of up to 10^8 (Figs. 4.94 and 4.95).

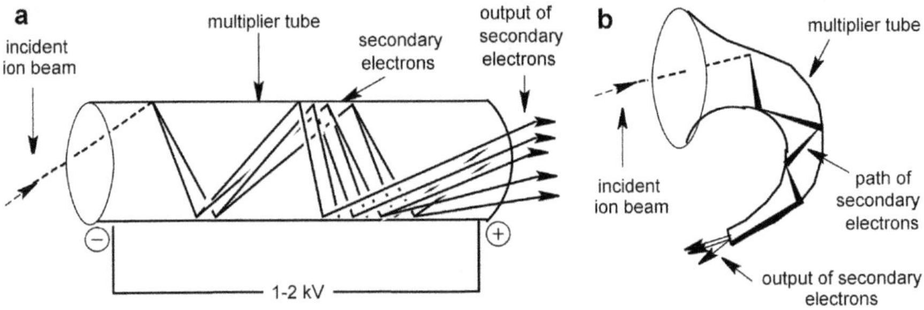

Fig. 4.94 Linear channel electron multiplier (**a**) and curved channel electron multiplier (**b**) (By courtesy of Waters Corporation, MS Technologies, Manchester, UK)

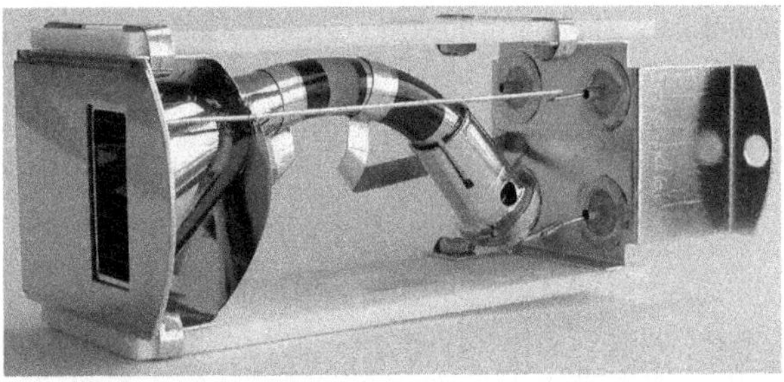

Fig. 4.95 Channeltron multiplier. Ions or electrons from a conversion dynode would enter from the left side. Amplification of secondary electrons occurs down the bent tube

Counting all sorts
Ion counting detectors also produce signals upon impact of energetic neutrals, electrons, or photons. Therefore, care has to be taken, not to allow other particles than the mass-analyzed ions to hit the detector.

4.11.6 Microchannel Plates

An extreme reduction of the size of a linear channeltron tube to some micrometers in diameter can be achieved. The cross section of such a single tube is by far too small to be of any use, however, millions of these tubes put together in a "bundle" yield a *channel electron multiplier array*; more common terms are *microchannel plate* or *multichannel plate* (MCP, Fig. 4.96). To avoid that the ions enter the microchannels parallel to their axis, these are inclined by some degrees from the perpendicular to the plate's surface. The gain of an MCP is 10^3–10^4, i.e., much lower than that of a SEM or CEM. Instead of a single MCP, two MCPs are often sandwiched together in such a way that the small angles oppose each other

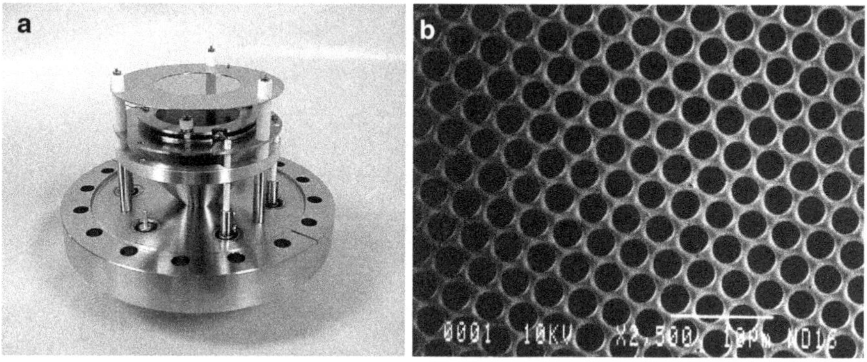

Fig. 4.96 MCP detector (top inner, glossy disk) mounted on top of a flange (**a**) and SEM micrograph of a high-resolving MCP showing channels of 2 μm diameter (**b**) (By courtesy of (**a**) R.M. Jordan Company, Grass Valley, CA and of (**b**) Burle Industries, Baesweiler)

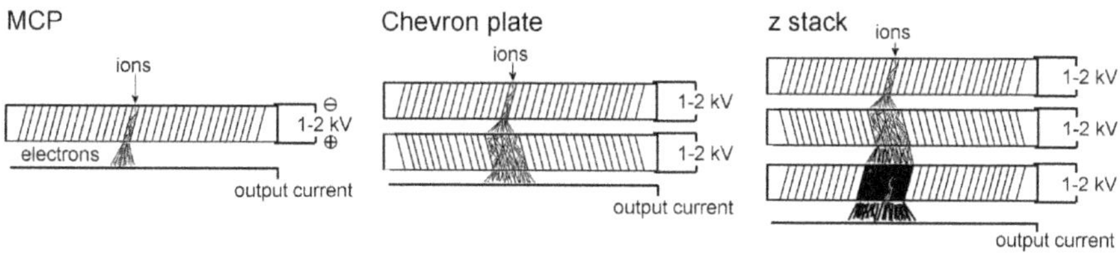

Fig. 4.97 Stacking of MCPs to increase gain. *From left*: single MCP, Chevron plate, and z-stack configuration. Note the loss of spatial resolution upon stacking

(*Chevron plate*, Fig. 4.97) to obtain gains of 10^6–10^7. Occasionally, even three MCPs are stacked analogously (*z-stack*, gain up to 10^8) [295, 296].

MCPs are produced as round plates of various sizes. Those of 2–5 cm in diameter are typically employed in mass spectrometers. An MCP may either be operated to give an integral output for all incident ions during a certain time interval, or the location of the impact may be conserved by connecting sectors of the MCP to individual registration channels. The first setup is more widespread, e.g., in TOF-MS to detect the electron current every nanosecond while the ions are arriving at the detector. The second setup can be used for imaging purposes, e.g., to construct an array detector (below).

4.11.7 Post-acceleration and Conversion Dynode

Discrimination of slower ions as compared to faster ions is observed with SEMs [297], CEMs, and MCPs as well [293, 298, 299]. This means a reduction in sensitivity upon reduction of the acceleration voltage of a mass spectrometer, and of course, with increasing ion mass. *Post-acceleration detectors* can reduce such effects and especially help to improve the sensitivity for high-mass ions [290, 299]. In post-

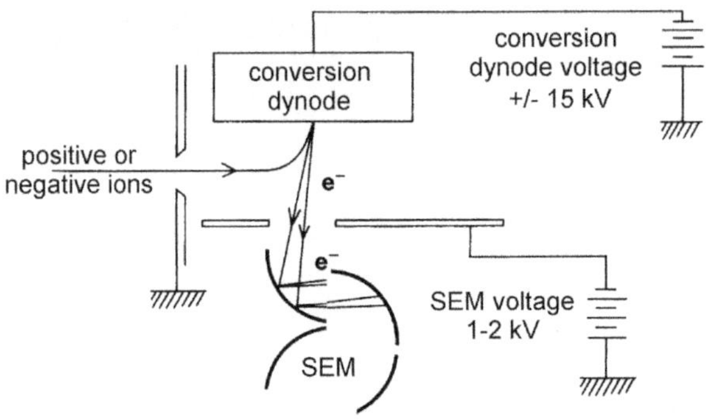

Fig. 4.98 Detector configuration with conversion dynode (By courtesy of JEOL, Tokyo)

acceleration detectors the ions are accelerated immediately in front of the detector by a voltage of 10–30 kV before they hit the first dynode or the first MCP.

The electron output of ion-counting detectors is usually measured with reference to ground potential, i.e., the first dynode is set to negative high voltage as to achieve acceleration of the electrons down the dynode assembly. In case of sector or TOF instruments, the deceleration of keV negative ions by the detector voltage is of comparatively minor importance. However, the slow ions exiting from quadrupole mass analyzers would stop before they reached the detector. Therefore, *conversion dynodes* are frequently placed in front of the SEM or CEM (Fig. 4.98) [291]. These are robust electrodes set to high potential (5–20 kV) of a polarity suitable to attract the ions actually exiting from the mass analyzer. Their impact on the conversion dynode creates secondary ions or electrons that can be used for subsequent detection. A conversion dynode detector also serves as a post-acceleration detector and gives almost equal sensitivity for positive and negative ion detection. In addition, neutrals and photons cannot reach the detector if the conversion dynode is placed out of the line of sight.

4.11.8 Focal Plane Detectors

Magnetic sector instruments are scanning devices usually focusing ions of one *m*/*z* value after the other onto a point detector. However, the mass-dispersive element of these instruments, i.e., the magnetic sector, is capable of producing an image of several neighboring *m*/*z* values simultaneously. *Focal plane detectors* (FPD) or *array detectors*, as they are often termed, can detect a small *m*/*z* range, i.e., ±2–5% of the center mass, at a time [293, 300, 301]. The ions impinging along the focal plane on the surface of an MCP (usually a Chevron plate) are converted to electrons. The electrons from the backside of the MCP stack are then converted into photons by a phosphor screen, and the light image is guided onto a photodiode array or a CCD detector by means of a fiber optical device. Such a multichannel electro-optical detection system typically improves sensitivity or signal-to-noise

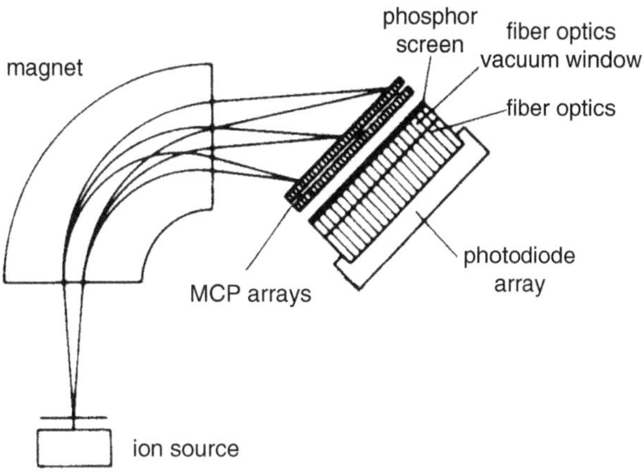

Fig. 4.99 Array detector in the focal plane of a magnetic sector to detect a small mass range simultaneously (By courtesy of Thermo Electron (Bremen) GmbH)

ratio, respectively, by a factor of 20–100, because less of the ion current is lost without being detected and fluctuations in the ion current are compensated [302, 303].

The resolution of an FPD is theoretically limited by the number of channels (512–2048). In practice, it is even less because the image suffers some broadening as it passes from the first MCP to the photodiode array (Fig. 4.99). Therefore, instruments with FPD can normally be switched from FPD to SEM detection, e.g., by vertical electrostatic deflection of the ion beam (Finnigan MAT900). Furthermore, quadrupole lenses or an inhomogeneous ESA behind the magnet are employed to achieve variable dispersion, i.e., to zoom the *m*/*z* range of simultaneous detection. Recent developments point towards fully integrated FPDs on a silicon chip [304].

4.12 Vacuum Technology

Vacuum systems are integral parts of any mass spectrometer, but vacuum technology definitely is a field of its own [305–309]. Thus the discussion of mass spectrometer vacuum systems will be restricted to the very basics.

4.12.1 Basic Mass Spectrometer Vacuum System

Generally, two pumping stages are employed to generate the high vacuum of a mass spectrometer. Usually, *rotary vane pumps* having *pumping speeds* of about 4–16 $m^3 h^{-1}$ are used to generate a medium vacuum of several Pascals. They are then connected to high-vacuum pumps in a way that their high-pressure side exhales into the medium vacuum of the rotary vane pumps, i.e., they are operated as *backing pumps*. This way, each pumping stage contributes a compression of some 10^4–10^5 to the total factor of 10^9–10^{10} between atmospheric pressure and the

Table 4.3 Pressure ranges in vacuum technology

Pressure range [Pa]	Pressure range [mbar]	Pressure range [mtorr]	Vacuum	Gas flow
10^5–10^2	1 bar–1 mbar	750 torr–750 mtorr	Rough vacuum (RV)	Viscous flow
10^2–10^{-1}	1–10^{-3}	750–0.75	Medium vacuum (MV)	Knudsen flow
10^{-1}–10^{-5}	10^{-3}–10^{-7}	0.75–7.5×10^{-5}	High vacuum (HV)	Molecular flow
$<10^{-5}$	$<10^{-7}$	$<7.5 \times 10^{-5}$	Ultrahigh vacuum (UHV)	Molecular flow

high vacuum of 10^{-4}–10^{-5} Pa (Table 4.3). The high-vacuum pumps can either be *turbomolecular pumps*, *oil diffusion pumps*, or *cryopumps* [310, 311].

Typical vacuum system The vacuum system of non-benchtop mass spectrometers consists of one to three rotary vane pumps and two or three turbo pumps. Rotary vane pumps are used for the inlet system(s) and as backing pumps for the turbo pumps. One turbo pump is mounted to the ion source housing, another one or two are operated at the analyzer. Thereby, a differentially pumped system is provided where local changes in pressure, e.g., from reagent gas in CI or collision gas in CID, do not notably influence the whole vacuum chamber.

4.12.2 High Vacuum Pumps

Turbomolecular pumps or *turbo pumps* having pumping speeds of 200–500 l s^{-1} are currently the standard high vacuum pumps in mass spectrometry. A high-speed rotor (50,000–60,000 rpm) is employed to transport the molecules out of the *vacuum manifold* (*vacuum chamber*). Turbo pumps can be switched on and off in minutes, have low power consumption (about 100 W), and thus can be operated either air- or water cooled. Furthermore, they provide clean, in particular oil-free, high vacuum, are compact, and can be mounted either vertically below or horizontally at the sides of the vacuum manifold. Their disadvantages are the risk of sudden damage (similar to hard disk drives) and potential high frequency noise. Fortunately, modern turbo pumps run for many years and their noise is negligible.

Special turbo pump designs provide more than one port to allow for their simultaneous connection to different pressure regions, e.g., ca. 10^{-5} mbar and ca. 10^{-3} mbar. Such multistage turbo pumps are very useful as one unit is able to support differential pumping of atmospheric pressure ionization interfaces.

Furthermore, newer turbo pumps are equipped with magnetic bearings rather than with oil-lubricated bearings. This cuts down on maintenance, as the yearly exchange of lubricant becomes needless and also guaranties oil-free high vacuum.

Recent turbo pump designs also accept higher pressure at their exhaust thereby allowing for replacement of rotary vane pumps by membrane pumps. This results in truly oil-free vacuum and offers more comfortable maintenance of the roughing pumps.

Oil diffusion pumps offer high pumping speeds (600–2000 l s^{-1}) at the cost of high power consumption (0.4–2 kW) and the need for a strong cooling water flow. The oil (perfluoropolypropylene glycols; Fomblin™, Santovac™) is thermally evaporated and the oil vapor supplies transport of gas molecules that enter it by diffusion. The gas-loaded oil vapor is condensed and the gas is removed from the liquid by the action of the backing pump. As diffusion pumps have no moving mechanical parts they are highly reliable and extremely silent. However, elongated use as well as sudden venting causes severe oil contaminations of the vacuum manifold. Diffusion pumps have almost been abandoned from modern mass spectrometers.

Cryopumps adsorb (freeze) residual gas to a surface cooled to the temperature of liquid nitrogen. They are highly efficient and provide clean vacuum, but cannot be operated without interruptions to recover the adsorber. Cryopumps are typically operated in combination with turbo pumps because they are only started after high-vacuum conditions are reached. Otherwise, the adsorber would soon be saturated.

4.13 Purchasing an Instrument

To some of us it can unexpectedly happen that we are faced with the task of having to buy a mass spectrometer, eventually for ourselves or on behalf of someone else. References to certain commercial instruments made in this chapter were in no way intended to preclude such a 100,000–1,000,000 € decision. The below guide may be useful in selecting an instrument that meets your requirements best.

Purpose
Define the tasks the mass spectrometer is going to be acquired for:

- Need for one dedicated or for several ionization methods?
- GC-MS, LC-MS, or ion mobility separation required?
- High resolution and accurate mass needed?
- Is tandem MS an issue or even a must?
- What sensitivity is needed?
- Is quantitative work important?
- Are you going to do mass spectral imaging?

Budget
Check your budget. A powerful and versatile second-hand machine from a proven company can be better than a toy-like single-purpose benchtop system.

Contact Sales
Get into contact with sales persons of all manufacturers offering suitable systems. Compare prices and modalities of customer training and support. Try to get information concerning longevity and product cycle (5, 10, 15 years?).

Demonstration
Make appointments for demonstration of those instruments that are likely to be acquired, e.g., for the top three of your ranking. Do not use completely unknown samples for this purpose. Otherwise, problems associated with your analyte might erroneously be regarded as a lack of instrumental performance.

Data System
Modern instruments form a unit with their data system. Does this offer the features you want? Does it allow for customization, "manual" settings, or corrections?

Analyzing Data
The software provided for analyzing the data is also of high relevance. Can you customize plots, lists, and reports, obtain molecular formulas, extract

Table 4.4 Rough estimates correlating instrumentation and factors affecting its cost

	Acquisition	Installation room requirements		Operation and long-term usage	
	Price of instrument	Footprint and weight	Power consumption, air conditioning load	Qualification of personnel	Maintenance
Time-of-flight	S–L	S–L	S–M	S–L	S–L
Magnetic sector	L–XL	L–XL	L–XL	L–XL	L
Linear quadrupole	S–M	S–M	S–M	S–M	S–M
Quadrupole ion trap	S–M	S – M	S–M	S–M	S–M
Linear quadrupole ion trap	M–L	S–M	S–M	M–L	M
Fourier transform-ion cyclotron resonance	XL–XXL	XL–XXL	XL–XXL	L–XL	XL–XXL
Orbitrap	L–XL	L	L	L–XL	L
Quadrupole-TOF hybrid	M–XL	M–L	L	M–L	L
Ion mobility-TOF hybrid	XL	L	L	L–XL	L–XL

Classified in the format of American dress sizes as S, M, L, XL, XXL chromatograms, get sophisticated output of data like Kendrick or van Krevelen plots?

Other Opinions

Use independent information from the published literature and ask current users of your top-choice mass spectrometers for the special strengths and shortcomings of those systems.

Investment and Cost of Ownership

Cost is not only affected by the price of acquisition of a mass spectrometer but also by operation in that it may have highly variable requirements of room, power, air conditioning, and operational skills (Table 4.4).

Avoid Buyer's Remorse

Keep in mind that any instrument acquisition inherently presents some compromise – none is perfect. Anyway, try to find the best for your needs and decide to be happy with your purchase afterwards.

References

1. Ligon WV Jr (1979) Molecular Analysis by Mass Spectrometry. Science 205:151–159. doi:10.1126/science.205.4402.151
2. Brunnée C (1987) The Ideal Mass Analyzer: Fact or Fiction? Int J Mass Spectrom Ion Proc 76:125–237. doi:10.1016/0168-1176(87)80030-7
3. Beynon JH (1960) Instruments. In: Beynon JH (ed) Mass Spectrometry and Its Applications to Organic Chemistry. Elsevier, Amsterdam
4. Habfast K, Aulinger F (1968) Massenspektrometrische Apparate. In: Kienitz H (ed) Massenspektrometrie. Weinheim, Verlag Chemie
5. Aulinger F (1968) Massenspektroskopische Geräte. In: Kienitz H (ed) Massenspektrometrie. Weinheim, Verlag Chemie
6. Brunnée C (1982) New Instrumentation in Mass Spectrometry. Int J Mass Spectrom Ion Phys 45:51–86. doi:10.1016/0020-7381(82)80100-9
7. Brunnée C (1997) 50 Years of MAT in Bremen. Rapid Commun Mass Spectrom 11:694–707. doi:10.1002/(SICI)1097-0231(199704)11:6<694::AID-RCM888>3.0.CO;2-K
8. Chapman JR, Errock GA, Race JA (1997) Science and Technology in Manchester: The Nurture of Mass Spectrometry. Rapid Commun Mass Spectrom 11:1575–1586. doi:10.1002/(SICI)1097-0231(199709)11:14<1575::AID-RCM22>3.0.CO;2-0
9. McLuckey SA (1998) Intrumentation for mass spectrometry. In: Hesso AE, Karjalainen UP, Jalonen JE, Karjalainen EJ (eds) Advances in Mass Spectrometry: Proc 14th Intl Mass Spectrometry Conf. Tampere, Finland, 1997. Elsevier, Amsterdam
10. Grayson MA (ed) (2002) Measuring Mass – From Positive Rays to Proteins. ASMS and CHF, Santa Fe and Philadelphia
11. Jennings KR (ed) (2012) A History of European Mass Spectrometry. IM Publications, Charlton Mill
12. Muenzenberg G (2013) Development of Mass Spectrometers from Thomson and Aston to Present. Int J Mass Spectrom 349–350:9–18
13. Doerr A, Finkelstein J, Jarchum I, Goodman C, Dekker B (2015) Nature Milestones: Mass Spectrometry. Nature Meth 12:1–21. www.nature.com/milestones/mass-spec

14. Badman ER, Cooks RG (2000) Miniature Mass Analyzers. J Mass Spectrom 35:659–671. doi:10.1002/1096-9888(200006)35:6<659::AID-JMS5>3.0.CO;2-V
15. Le Gac S, van den Berg A (eds) (2009) Miniaturization and Mass Spectrometry. The Royal Society of Chemistry, Cambridge
16. Baykut G, Franzen J (1994) Mobile Mass Spectrometry: A Decade of Field Applications. Trends Anal Chem 13:267–275. doi:10.1016/0165-9936(94)87063-2
17. Prieto MC, Kovtoun VV, Cotter RJ (2002) Miniaturized Linear Time-of-Flight Mass Spectrometer with Pulsed Extraction. J Mass Spectrom 37:1158–1162. doi:10.1002/jms.386
18. Arkin CR, Griffin TP, Ottens AK, Diaz JA, Follistein DW, Adams FW, Helms WR (2002) Evaluation of Small Mass Spectrometer Systems for Permanent Gas Analysis. J Am Soc Mass Spectrom 13:1004–1012. doi:10.1016/S1044-0305(02)00422-1
19. Fenselau C, Caprioli R (2003) Mass Spectrometry in the Exploration of Mars. J Mass Spectrom 38:1–10. doi:10.1002/jms.396
20. Hu Q, Noll RJ, Li H, Makarov A, Hardman M, Cooks RG (2005) The Orbitrap: A New Mass Spectrometer. J Mass Spectrom 40:430–443. doi:10.1002/jms.856
21. Wiley WC, McLaren IH (1955) Time-of-Flight Mass Spectrometer with Improved Resolution. Rev Sci Instrum 26:1150–1157. doi:10.1063/1.1715212
22. Stephens WE (1946) A Pulsed Mass Spectrometer with Time Dispersion. Phys Rev 69:691
23. Cameron AE, Eggers DF (1948) An Ion "Velocitron". Rev Sci Instrum 19:605–607. doi:10.1063/1.1741336
24. Wolff MM, Stephens WE (1953) A Pulsed Mass Spectrometer with Time Dispersion. Rev Sci Instrum 24:616–617. doi:10.1063/1.1770801
25. Wiley WC, McLaren IH (1997) Reprint of: Time-of-Flight Mass Spectrometer with Improved Resolution. J Mass Spectrom 32:4–11. doi:10.1002/(SICI)1096-9888(199701)32:1<1::AID-JMS467>3.0.CO;2-6
26. Harrington DB (1959) The time-of-flight mass spectrometer. In: Waldron JD (ed) Advances in Mass Spectrometry. Pergamon Press, Oxford
27. Gohlke RS, McLafferty FW (1993) Early Gas Chromatography/Mass Spectrometry. J Am Soc Mass Spectrom 4:367–371. doi:10.1016/1044-0305(93)85001-E
28. Guilhaus M (1995) The Return of Time-of-Flight to Analytical Mass Spectrometry. Adv Mass Spectrom 13:213–226
29. Guilhaus M, Mlynski V, Selby D (1997) Perfect Timing: Time-of-Flight Mass Spectrometry. Rapid Commun Mass Spectrom 11:951–962. doi:10.1002/(SICI)1097-0231(19970615)11:9<951::AID-RCM785>3.0.CO;2-H
30. Karas M, Hillenkamp F (1988) Laser Desorption Ionization of Proteins with Molecular Masses Exceeding 10000 Daltons. Anal Chem 60:2299–2301. doi:10.1021/ac00171a028
31. Weickhardt C, Moritz F, Grotemeyer J (1997) Time-of-Flight Mass Spectrometry: State-of-the-Art in Chemical Analysis and Molecular Science. Mass Spectrom Rev 15:139–162. doi:10.1002/(SICI)1098-2787(1996)15:3<139::AID-MAS1>3.0.CO;2-J
32. Cotter RJ (1997) Time-of-Flight Mass Spectrometry: Instrumentation and Applications in Biological Research. American Chemical Society, Washington, DC
33. Enke CG (1998) The Unique Capabilities of Time-of-Flight Mass Analyzers. Adv Mass Spectrom 14:197–219
34. Fuerstenau SD, Benner WH (1995) Molecular Weight Determination of Megadalton DNA Electrospray Ions Using Charge Detection Time-of-Flight Mass Spectrometry. Rapid Commun Mass Spectrom 9:1528–1538. doi:10.1002/rcm.1290091513
35. Fuerstenau SD, Benner WH, Thomas JJ, Brugidou C, Bothner B, Suizdak G (2001) Mass Spectrometry of an Intact Virus. Angew Chem Int Ed 40:541–544. doi:10.1002/1521-3773(20010202)40:3<541::AID-ANIE541>3.0.CO;2-K
36. Vestal ML (2009) Modern MALDI Time-of-Flight Mass Spectrometry. J Mass Spectrom 44:303–317. doi:10.1002/jms.1537

37. Guilhaus M (1995) Principles and Instrumentation in Time-of-Flight Mass Spectrometry. Physical and Instrumental Concepts. J Mass Spectrom 30:1519–1532. doi:10.1002/jms.1190301102
38. Ioanoviciu D (1995) Ion-Optical Solutions in Time-of-Flight Mass Spectrometry. Rapid Commun Mass Spectrom 9:985–997. doi:10.1002/rcm.1290091104
39. Cotter RJ (1992) Time-of-Flight Mass Spectrometry for the Analysis of Biological Molecules. Anal Chem 64:1027A–1039A. doi:10.1021/ac00045a726
40. Takach EJ, Hines WM, Patterson DH, Juhasz P, Falick AM, Vestal ML, Martin SA (1997) Accurate Mass Measurements Using MALDI-TOF with Delayed Extraction. J Protein Res 16:363–369. doi:10.1023/A:1026376403468
41. Vestal M, Juhasz P (1998) Resolution and Mass Accuracy in Matrix-Assisted Laser Desorption Ionization-Time-of-Flight. J Am Soc Mass Spectrom 9:892–911. doi:10.1016/S1044-0305(98)00069-5
42. Vestal M, Hayden K (2007) High Performance MALDI-TOF Mass Spectrometry for Proteomics. Int J Mass Spectrom 268:83–92. doi:10.1016/j.ijms.2007.06.21
43. Beavis RC, Chait BT (1989) Factors Affecting the Ultraviolet Laser Desorption of Proteins. Rapid Commun Mass Spectrom 3:233–237. doi:10.1002/rcm.1290030708
44. Toyoda M, Okumura D, Ishihara M, Katakuse I (2003) Multi-Turn Time-of-Flight Mass Spectrometers With Electrostatic Sectors. J Mass Spectrom 38:1125–1142. doi:10.1002/jms.546
45. Schuerch S, Schaer M, Boernsen KO, Schlunegger UP (1994) Enhanced Mass Resolution in Matrix-Assisted Laser Desorption/Ionization Linear Time-of-Flight Mass Spectrometry. Biol Mass Spectrom 23:695–700. doi:10.1002/bms.1200231108
46. Mamyrin BA (1994) Laser Assisted Reflectron Time-of-Flight Mass Spectrometry. Int J Mass Spectrom Ion Proc 131:1–19. doi:10.1016/0168-1176(93)03891-O
47. Brown RS, Lennon JJ (1995) Mass Resolution Improvement by Incorporation of Pulsed Ion Extraction in a Matrix-Assisted Laser Desorption/Ionization Linear Time-of-Flight Mass Spectrometer. Anal Chem 67:1998–2003. doi:10.1021/ac00109a015
48. Colby SM, King TB, Reilly JP (1994) Improving the Resolution of Matrix-Assisted Laser Desorption/Ionization Time-of-Flight Mass Spectrometry by Exploiting the Correlation Between Ion Position and Velocity. Rapid Commun Mass Spectrom 8:865–868. doi:10.1002/rcm.1290081102
49. Whittal RM, Li L (1995) High-Resolution Matrix Assisted Laser Desorption-Ionization in a Linear Time-of-Flight Mass Spectrometer. Anal Chem 67:1950–1954. doi:10.1021/ac00109a007
50. Vestal ML, Juhasz P, Martin SA (1995) Delayed Extraction Matrix-Assisted Laser Desorption Time-of-Flight Mass Spectrometry. Rapid Commun Mass Spectrom 9:1044–1050. doi:10.1002/rcm.1290091115
51. Dawson JHJ, Guilhaus M (1989) Orthogonal-Acceleration Time-of-Flight Mass Spectrometer. Rapid Commun Mass Spectrom 3:155–159. doi:10.1002/rcm.1290030511
52. Mirgorodskaya OA, Shevchenko AA, Chernushevich IV, Dodonov AF, Miroshnikov AI (1994) Electrospray-Ionization Time-of-Flight Mass Spectrometry in Protein Chemistry. Anal Chem 66:99–107. doi:10.1021/ac00073a018
53. Coles J, Guilhaus M (1993) Orthogonal Acceleration – A New Direction for Time-of-Flight Mass Spectrometry: Fast, Sensitive Mass Analysis for Continuous Ion Sources. Trends Anal Chem 12:203–213. doi:10.1016/0165-9936(93)80021-B
54. Selby DS, Mlynski V, Guilhaus M (2001) A 20 KV Orthogonal Acceleration Time-of-Flight Mass Spectrometer for Matrix-Assisted Laser Desorption/Ionization. Int J Mass Spectrom 210(211):89–100. doi:10.1016/S1387-3806(01)00438-9
55. Guilhaus M, Selby D, Mlynski V (2000) Orthogonal Acceleration Time-of-Flight Mass Spectrometry. Mass Spectrom Rev 19:65–107. doi:10.1002/(SICI)1098-2787(2000)19:2<65::AID-MAS1>3.0.CO;2-E

56. Selditz U, Nilsson S, Barnidge D, Markides KE (1999) ESI/TOF-MS Detection for Microseparation Techniques. Chimia 53:506–510
57. Charles L (2008) Influence of Internal Standard Charge State on the Accuracy of Mass Measurements in Orthogonal Acceleration Time-of-Flight Mass Spectrometers. Rapid Commun Mass Spectrom 22:151–155. doi:10.1002/rcm.3347
58. Guo C, Huang Z, Gao W, Nian H, Chen H, Dong J, Shen G, Fu J, Zhou Z (2008) A Homemade High-Resolution Orthogonal-Injection Time-of-Flight Mass Spectrometer with a Heated Capillary Inlet. Rev Sci Instrum 79:013109-1-013109/8. doi:10.1063/1.2832334
59. Prazen BJ, Bruckner CA, Synovec RE, Kowalski BR (1999) Enhanced Chemical Analysis Using Parallel Column Gas Chromatography with Single-Detector Time-of-Flight Mass Spectrometry and Chemometric Analysis. Analytical Chemistry 71:1093–1099. doi:10.1021/ac980814m
60. Hirsch R, Ternes TA, Bobeldijk I, Weck RA (2001) Determination of Environmentally Relevant Compounds Using Fast GC/TOF-MS. Chimia 55:19–22
61. Hsu CS, Green M (2001) Fragment-Free Accurate Mass Measurement of Complex Mixture Components by Gas Chromatography/Field Ionization-Orthogonal Acceleration Time-of-Flight Mass Spectrometry: An Unprecedented Capability for Mixture Analysis. Rapid Commun Mass Spectrom 15:236–239. doi:10.1002/1097-0231(20010215)15:3<236::AID-RCM197>3.0.CO;2-B
62. Chernushevich IV (2000) Duty Cycle Improvement for a Quadrupole-Time-of-Flight Mass Spectrometer and Its Use for Precursor Ion Scans. Eur J Mass Spectrom 6:471–479. doi:10.1255/ejms.377
63. Toyoda M (2010) Development of Multi-Turn Time-of-Flight Mass Spectrometers and Their Applications. Eur J Mass Spectrom 16:397–406. doi:10.1255/ejms.1076
64. Toyoda M, Shimma S, Aoki J, Ishihara M (2012) Multi-Turn Time-of-Flight Mass Spectrometers. J Mass Spectrom Soc Jpn 60:87–102. doi:10.5702/massspec.12-47
65. Ichihara T, Uchida S, Ishihara M, Katakuse I, Toyoda M (2007) Construction of a Palmtop Size Multi-Turn Time-of-Flight Mass Spectrometer "MULTUM-S". J Mass Spectrom Soc Jpn 55:363–368. doi:10.5702/massspec.55.363
66. Goesmann F, Rosenbauer H, Bredehoeft JH, Cabane M, Ehrenfreund P, Gautier T, Giri C, Krueger H, Le Roy L, MacDermott AJ, McKenna-Lawlor S, Meierhenrich UJ, Caro GMM, Raulin F, Roll R, Steele A, Steininger H, Sternberg R, Szopa C, Thiemann W, Ulamec S (2015) Organic Compounds on Comet 67P/Churyumov-Gerasimenko Revealed by COSAC Mass Spectrometry. Science 349:497–499. doi:10.1126/science.aab0689
67. Satoh T, Tsuno H, Iwanaga M, Kammei Y (2006) A New Spiral Time-of-Flight Mass Spectrometer for High Mass Analysis. J Mass Spectrom Soc Jpn 54:11–17. doi:10.5702/massspec.54.11
68. Satoh T, Sato T, Tamura J (2007) Development of a High-Performance MALDI-TOF Mass Spectrometer Utilizing a Spiral Ion Trajectory. J Am Soc Mass Spectrom 18:1318–1323. doi:10.1016/j.jasms.2007.04.010
69. Satoh T (2009) Development of a Time-of-Flight Mass Spectrometer Utilizing a Spiral Ion Trajectory. J Mass Spectrom Soc Jpn 57:363–369. doi:10.5702/massspec.57.363
70. Satoh T, Kubo A, Shimma S, Toyoda M (2012) Mass Spectrometry Imaging and Structural Analysis of Lipids Directly on Tissue Specimens by Using a Spiral Orbit Type Tandem Time-of-Flight Mass Spectrometer, SpiralTOF-TOF. Mass Spectrom 1:A0013. doi:10.5702/massspectrometry.A0013
71. Satoh T, Kubo A, Hazama H, Awazu K, Toyoda M (2014) Separation of Isobaric Compounds Using a Spiral Orbit Type Time-of-Flight Mass Spectrometer, MALDI-SpiralTOF. Mass Spectrom 3:S0027-1-S0027/5. doi:10.5702/massspectrometry.S0027
72. Sato H, Nakamura S, Teramoto K, Sato T (2014) Structural Characterization of Polymers by MALDI Spiral-TOF Mass Spectrometry Combined with Kendrick Mass Defect Analysis. J Am Soc Mass Spectrom 25:1346–1355. doi:10.1007/s13361-014-0915-y

73. Casares A, Kholomeev A, Wollnik H (2001) Multipass Time-of-Flight Mass Spectrometers with High Resolving Powers. Int J Mass Spectrom 206:267–273. doi:10.1016/S1387-3806(00)00391-2
74. Wollnik H, Casares A (2003) An Energy-Isochronous Multi-Pass Time-of-Flight Mass Spectrometer Consisting of Two Coaxial Electrostatic Mirrors. Int J Mass Spectrom 227:217–222. doi:10.1016/S1387-3806(03)00127-1
75. Yavor M, Verentchikov A, Hasin J, Kozlov B, Gavrik M, Trufanov A (2008) Planar Multi-Reflecting Time-of-Flight Mass Analyzer with a Jig-Saw Ion Path. Phys Procedia 1:391–400. doi:10.1016/j.phpro.2008.07.120
76. Klitzke CF, Corilo YE, Siek K, Binkley J, Patrick J, Eberlin MN (2012) Petroleomics by Ultrahigh-Resolution Time-of-Flight Mass Spectrometry. Energy & Fuels 26:5787–5794. doi:10.1021/ef300961c
77. Polyakova OV, Mazur DM, Artaev VB, Lebedev AT (2016) Rapid Liquid-Liquid Extraction for the Reliable GC/MS Analysis of Volatile Priority Pollutants. Environ Chem Lett 14:251–257. doi:10.1007/s10311-015-0544-0
78. Wolf RN, Wienholtz F, Atanasov D, Beck D, Blaum K, Borgmann C, Herfurth F, Kowalska M, Kreim S, Litvinov Y, Lunney D, Manea V, Neidherr D, Rosenbusch M, Schweikhard L, Stanja J, Zuber K (2013) ISOLTRAP's Multi-Reflection Time-of-Flight Mass Separator/Spectrometer. Int J Mass Spectrom 349–350:123–133. doi:10.1016/j.ijms.2013.03.020
79. Wolf RN, Eritt M, Marx G, Schweikhard L (2011) A Multi-Reflection Time-of-Flight Mass Separator for Isobaric Purification of Radioactive Ion Beams. Hyperfine Interact 199:115–122. doi:10.1007/s10751-011-0306-8
80. Wolf RN, Marx G, Rosenbusch M, Schweikhard L (2012) Static-Mirror Ion Capture and Time Focusing for Electrostatic Ion-Beam Traps and Multi-Reflection Time-of-Flight Mass Analyzers by Use of an In-Trap Potential Lift. Int J Mass Spectrom 313:8–14. doi:10.1016/j.ijms.2011.12.006
81. Nier AO (1991) The Development of a High Resolution Mass Spectrometer: A Reminiscence. J Am Soc Mass Spectrom 2:447–452. doi:10.1016/1044-0305(91)80029-7
82. Nier AO (1989) Some Reminiscences of Mass Spectrometry and the Manhattan Project. J Chem Educ 66:385–388. doi:10.1021/ed066p385
83. Nier AO (1990) Some Reflections on the Early Days of Mass Spectrometry at the University of Minnesota. Int J Mass Spectrom Ion Proc 100:1–13. doi:10.1016/0168-1176(90)85063-8
84. Duckworth HE, Barber RC, Venkatasubramanian VS (1986) Mass Spectroscopy. Cambridge University Press, Cambridge
85. Cooks RG, Beynon JH, Caprioli RM (1973) Instrumentation. In: Cooks RG, Beynon JH, Caprioli RM, Lester GR (eds) Metastable Ions. Elsevier, Amsterdam
86. Morrison JD (1986) Ion Focusing, Mass Analysis, and Detection. In: Futrell JH (ed) Gaseous Ion Chemistry and Mass Spectrometry. Wiley, New York
87. Dempster AJ (1918) A New Method of Positive Ray Analysis. Phys Rev 11:316–325. doi:10.1103/PhysRev.11.316
88. Cooks RG, Chen G, Wong P, Wollnik H (2014) Spectrometers Mass. In: Digital Encyclopedia of Applied Physics. Wiley-VCH, Weinheim. doi:10.1002/3527600434
89. Mattauch J, Herzog R (1934) Über Einen Neuen Massenspektrographen. Z Phys 89:786–795. doi:10.1007/BF01341392
90. Prohaska T, Irrgeher J, Zitek A, Jakubowski N (eds) (2015) Sector Field Mass Spectrometry for Elemental and Isotopic Analysis. Royal Society of Chemistry, Cambridge
91. Brunnée C, Voshage H (1964) Massenspektrometrie. Karl Thiemig Verlag KG, München
92. Bainbridge KT, Jordan EB (1936) Mass-Spectrum Analysis. 1. The Mass Spectrograph. 2. The Existence of Isobars of Adjacent Elements. Phys Rev 50:282–296. doi:10.1103/PhysRev.50.282
93. Johnson EG, Nier AO (1953) Angular Aberrations in Sector Shaped Electromagnetic Lenses for Focusing Beams of Charged Particles. Phys Rev 91:10–17. doi:10.1103/PhysRev.91.10

94. Todd JFJ (1995) Recommendations for Nomenclature and Symbolism for Mass Spectroscopy Including an Appendix of Terms Used in Vacuum Technology. Int J Mass Spectrom Ion Proc 142:211–240. doi:10.1016/0168-1176(95)93811-F
95. Morgan RP, Beynon JH, Bateman RH, Green BN (1978) The MM-ZAB-2F Double-Focussing Mass Spectrometer and MIKE Spectrometer. Int J Mass Spectrom Ion Phys 28:171–191. doi:10.1016/0020-7381(78)80124-7
96. Hintenberger H, König LA (1957) Über Massenspektrometer mit vollständiger Doppelfokussierung zweiter Ordnung. Z Naturforsch 12:773–785. doi:10.1515/zna-1957-1004
97. Guilhaus M, Boyd RK, Brenton AG, Beynon JH (1985) Advantages of a Second Electric Sector on a Double-Focusing Mass Spectrometer of Reversed Configuration. Int J Mass Spectrom Ion Proc 67:209–227. doi:10.1016/0168-1176(85)80020-3
98. Bill JC, Green BN, Lewis IAS (1983) A High Field Magnet with Fast Scanning Capabilities. Int J Mass Spectrom Ion Phys 46:147–150. doi:10.1016/0020-7381(83)80075-8
99. Matsuda H (1985) High-Resolution High-Transmission Mass Spectrometer. Int J Mass Spectrom Ion Proc 66:209–215. doi:10.1016/0168-1176(85)83010-X
100. Matsuda H (1989) Double-Focusing Mass Spectrometers of Short Path Length. Int J Mass Spectrom Ion Proc 93:315–321. doi:10.1016/0168-1176(89)80120-X
101. Paul W (1990) Electromagnetic Traps for Charged and Neutral Particles (Nobel Lecture). Angew Chem Int Ed 29:739–748. doi:10.1002/anie.199007391
102. Paul W (1993) Electromagnetic traps for charged and neutral particles. In: Nobel Prize Lectures in Physics. World Scientific Publishing, Singapore, pp 1981–1990
103. Paul W, Steinwedel H (1953) A New Mass Spectrometer Without Magnetic Field. Z Naturforsch 8A:448–450. doi:10.1515/zna-1953-0710
104. Paul W, Raether M (1955) Das elektrische Massenfilter. Z Phys 140:262–273. doi:10.1007/BF01328923
105. Lawson G, Todd JFJ (1972) Radio-Frequency Quadrupole Mass Spectrometers. Chem Brit 8:373–380
106. Dawson PH (1976) Quadrupole Mass Spectrometry and Its Applications. Elsevier, New York
107. Dawson PH (1986) Quadrupole Mass Analyzers: Performance, Design and Some Recent Applications. Mass Spectrom Rev 5:1–37. doi:10.1002/mas.1280050102
108. Douglas DJ (2009) Linear Quadrupoles in Mass Spectrometry. Mass Spectrom Rev 28:937–960. doi:10.1002/mas.20249
109. Blaum K, Geppert C, Müller P, Nörtershäuser W, Otten EW, Schmitt A, Trautmann N, Wendt K, Bushaw BA (1998) Properties and Performance of a Quadrupole Mass Filter Used for Resonance Ionization Mass Spectrometry. Int J Mass Spectrom 181:67–87. doi:10.1016/S1387-3806(98)14174-x
110. Amad MH, Houk RS (1998) High-Resolution Mass Spectrometry with a Multiple Pass Quadrupole Mass Analyzer. Anal Chem 70:4885–4889. doi:10.1021/ac980505w
111. Liyu Y, Amad MH, Winnik WM, Schoen AE, Schweingruber H, Mylchreest I, Rudewicz PJ (2002) Investigation of an Enhanced Resolution Triple Quadrupole Mass Spectrometer for High-Throughput Liquid Chromatography/Tandem Mass Spectrometry Assays. Rapid Commun Mass Spectrom 16:2060–2066. doi:10.1002/rcm.824
112. Denison DR (1971) Operating Parameters of a Quadrupole in a Grounded Cylindrical Housing. J Vac Sci Technol 8:266–269
113. Dawson PH, Whetten NR (1969) Nonlinear Resonances in Quadrupole Mass Spectrometers Due to Imperfect Fields. II. Quadrupole Mass Filter and the Monopole Mass Spectrometer. Int J Mass Spectrom Ion Phys 3:1–12. doi:10.1016/0020-7381(69)80054-9
114. Brubaker WM (1967) Comparison of Quadrupole Mass Spectrometers with Round and Hyperbolic Rods. J Vac Sci Technol 4:326
115. Gibson JR, Taylor S (2000) Prediction of Quadrupole Mass Filter Performance for Hyperbolic and Circular Cross Section Electrodes. Rapid Commun Mass Spectrom 14:1669–1673. doi:10.1002/1097-0231(20000930)14:18<1669::AID-RCM80>3.0.CO;2-%23

116. Chen W, Collings BA, Douglas DJ (2000) High-Resolution Mass Spectrometry with a Quadrupole Operated in the Fourth Stability Region. Anal Chem 72:540–545. doi:10.1021/ac990815u
117. Douglas DJ, Frank AJ, Mao D (2005) Linear Ion Traps in Mass Spectrometry. Mass Spectrom Rev 24:1–29. doi:10.1002/mas.20004
118. Giles K, Pringle SD, Worthington KR, Little D, Wildgoose JL, Bateman RH (2004) Applications of a Traveling Wave-Based Radio-Frequency-Only Stacked Ring Ion Guide. Rapid Commun Mass Spectrom 18:2401–2414. doi:10.1002/rcm.1641
119. Huang Y, Guan S, Kim HS, Marshall AG (1996) Ion Transport Through a Strong Magnetic Field Gradient by Radio Frequency-Only Octupole Ion Guides. Int J Mass Spectrom Ion Proc 152:121–133. doi:10.1016/0168-1176(95)04334-9
120. Douglas DJ, French JB (1992) Collisional Focusing Effects in Radiofrequency Quadrupoles. J Am Soc Mass Spectrom 3:398–408. doi:10.1016/1044-0305(92)87067-9
121. Tolmachev AV, Udseth HR, Smith RD (2000) Radial Stratification of Ions as a Function of Mass to Charge Ratio in Collisional Cooling Radio Frequency Multipoles Used as Ion Guides or Ion Traps. Rapid Commun Mass Spectrom 14:1907–1913. doi:10.1002/1097-0231(20001030)14:20<1907::AID-RCM111>3.0.CO;2-M
122. Collings BA, Campbell JM, Mao D, Douglas DJ (2001) A Combined Linear Ion Trap Time-of-Flight System with Improved Performance and MS^n Capabilities. Rapid Commun Mass Spectrom 15:1777–1795. doi:10.1002/rcm.440
123. Douglas DJ (1998) Applications of Collision Dynamics in Quadrupole Mass Spectrometry. J Am Soc Mass Spectrom 9:101–113. doi:10.1016/S1044-0305(97)00246-8
124. Thomson BA (1998) 1997 McBryde Medal Award Lecture Radio Frequency Quadrupole Ion Guides in Modern Mass Spectrometry. Can J Chem 76:499–505. doi:10.1139/v98-073
125. Lock CM, Dyer E (1999) Characterization of High Pressure Quadrupole Collision Cells Possessing Direct Current Axial Fields. Rapid Commun Mass Spectrom 13:432–448. doi:10.1002/(SICI)1097-0231(19990315)13:5<432::AID-RCM504>3.0.CO;2-I
126. Lock CM, Dyer E (1999) Simulation of Ion Trajectories Through a High Pressure Radio Frequency Only Quadrupole Collision Cell by SIMION 6.0. Rapid Commun Mass Spectrom 13:422–431. doi:10.1002/(SICI)1097-0231(19990315)13:5<422::AID-RCM503>3.0.CO;2-M
127. Adlhart C, Hinderling C, Baumann H, Chen P (2000) Mechanistic Studies of Olefin Metathesis by Ruthenium Carbene Complexes Using Electrospray Ionization Tandem Mass Spectrometry. J Am Chem Soc 122:8204–8214. doi:10.1021/ja9938231
128. Mao D, Douglas DJ (2003) H/D Exchange of Gas Phase Bradykinin Ions in a Linear Quadrupole Ion Trap. J Am Soc Mass Spectrom 14:85–94. doi:10.1016/S1044-0305(02)00818-8
129. Hager JW (2002) A New Linear Ion Trap Mass Spectrometer. Rapid Commun Mass Spectrom 16:512–526. doi:10.1002/rcm.607
130. Schwartz JC, Senko MW, Syka JEP (2002) A Two-Dimensional Quadrupole Ion Trap Mass Spectrometer. J Am Soc Mass Spectrom 13:659–669. doi:10.1016/S1044-0305(02)00384-7
131. Hofstadler SA, Sannes-Lowery KA, Griffey RH (2000) Enhanced Gas-Phase Hydrogen-Deuterium Exchange of Oligonucleotide and Protein Ions Stored in an External Multipole Ion Reservoir. J Mass Spectrom 35:62–70. doi:10.1002/(SICI)1096-9888(200001)35:1<62::AID-JMS913>3.0.CO;2-9
132. Collings BA, Scott WR, Londry FA (2003) Resonant Excitation in a Low-Pressure Linear Ion Trap. J Am Soc Mass Spectrom 14:622–634. doi:10.1016/S1044-0305(03)00202-2
133. Aebersold R, Mann M (2003) Mass Spectrometry-Based Proteomics. Nature 422:198–207. doi:10.1038/nature01511
134. Hopfgartner G, Husser C, Zell M (2003) Rapid Screening and Characterization of Drug Metabolites Using a New Quadrupole-Linear Ion Trap Mass Spectrometer. J Mass Spectrom 38:138–150. doi:10.1002/jms.420

135. Hager JW (2004) Recent Trends in Mass Spectrometer Development. Anal Bioanal Chem 378:845–850. doi:10.1007/s00216-003-2287-1
136. Koizumi H, Whitten WB, Reilly PTA (2008) Trapping of Intact, Singly-Charged, Bovine Serum Albumin Ions Injected from the Atmosphere with a 10-cm Diameter, Frequency-Adjusted Linear Quadrupole Ion Trap. J Am Soc Mass Spectrom 19:1942–1947. doi:10.1016/j.jasms.2008.08.007
137. Welling M, Schuessler HA, Thompson RI, Walther H (1998) Ion/Molecule Reactions, Mass Spectrometry and Optical Spectroscopy in a Linear Ion Trap. Int J Mass Spectrom Ion Proc 172:95–114. doi:10.1016/S0168-1176(97)00251-6
138. Londry FA, Hager JW (2003) Mass Selective Axial Ion Ejection from a Linear Quadrupole Ion Trap. J Am Soc Mass Spectrom 14:1130–1147. doi:10.1016/S1044-0305(03)00446-X
139. March RE, Todd JFJ (2005) Quadrupole Ion Trap Mass Spectrometry. Wiley, Hoboken
140. Blake TA, Ouyang Z, Wiseman JM, Takats Z, Guymon AJ, Kothari S, Cooks RG (2004) Preparative Linear Ion Trap Mass Spectrometer for Separation and Collection of Purified Proteins and Peptides in Arrays Using Ion Soft Landing. Anal Chem 76:6293–6305. doi:10.1021/ac048981b
141. Ramanathan R (ed) (2009) Mass Spectrometry in Drug Metabolism and Pharmacokinetics. Wiley, Hoboken
142. Dahl DA, Delmore JE, Appelhans AD (1990) SIMION PC/PS2 Electrostatic Lens Design Program. Rev Sci Instrum 61:607–609. doi:10.1063/1.1141932
143. Dahl DA (2000) SIMION for the Personal Computer in Reflection. Int J Mass Spectrom 200:3–25. doi:10.1016/S1387-3806(00)00305-5
144. Magparangalan DP, Garrett TJ, Drexler DM, Yost RA (2010) Analysis of Large Peptides by MALDI Using a Linear Quadrupole Ion Trap with Mass Range Extension. Anal Chem 82:930–934. doi:10.1021/ac9021488
145. March RE, Hughes RJ (1989) Quadrupole Storage Mass Spectrometry. Wiley, Chichester
146. March RE (1998) Quadrupole Ion Trap Mass Spectrometry: Theory, Simulation, Recent Developments and Applications. Rapid Commun Mass Spectrom 12:1543–1554. doi:10.1002/(SICI)1097-0231(19981030)12:20<1543::AID-RCM343>3.0.CO;2-T
147. March RE (2000) Quadrupole Ion Trap Mass Spectrometry. A View at the Turn of the Century. Int J Mass Spectrom 200:285–312. doi:10.1016/S1387-3806(00)00345-6
148. Stafford GC Jr (2002) Ion Trap Mass Spectrometry: A Personal Perspective. J Am Soc Mass Spectrom 13:589–596. doi:10.1016/S1044-0305(02)00385-9
149. March RE (2009) Quadrupole Ion Traps. Mass Spectrom Rev 28:961–989. doi:10.1002/mas.20250
150. March RE, Todd JFJ (eds) (1995) Practical Aspects of Ion Trap Mass Spectrometry Vol. 1 – Fundamentals of Ion Trap Mass Spectrometry. CRC Press, Boca Raton
151. March RE, Todd JFJ (eds) (1995) Practical Aspects of Ion Trap Mass Spectrometry Vol. 2 – Ion Trap Instrumentation. CRC Press, Boca Raton
152. March RE, Todd JFJ (eds) (1995) Practical Aspects of Ion Trap Mass Spectrometry Vol. 3 – Chemical, Environmental, and Biomedical Applications. CRC Press, Boca Raton
153. Yoshinari K (2000) Theoretical and Numerical Analysis of the Behavior of Ions Injected into a Quadrupole Ion Trap Mass Spectrometer. Rapid Commun Mass Spectrom 14:215–223. doi:10.1002/(SICI)1097-0231(20000229)14:4<215::AID-RCM867>3.0.CO;2-T
154. Alheit R, Kleinadam S, Vedel F, Vedel M, Werth G (1996) Higher Order Non-Linear Resonances in a Paul Trap. Int J Mass Spectrom Ion Proc 154:155–169. doi:10.1016/0168-1176(96)04380-7
155. Stafford GC Jr, Kelley PE, Syka JEP, Reynolds WE, Todd JFJ (1984) Recent Improvements in and Analytical Applications of Advanced Ion Trap Technology. Int J Mass Spectrom Ion Proc 60:85–98. doi:10.1016/0168-1176(84)80077-4
156. Wu HF, Brodbelt JS (1992) Effects of Collisional Cooling on Ion Detection in a Quadrupole Ion Trap Mass Spectrometer. Int J Mass Spectrom Ion Proc 115:67–81. doi:10.1016/0168-1176(92)85032-U

157. Plass WR, Li H, Cooks RG (2003) Theory, Simulation and Measurement of Chemical Mass Shifts in RF Quadrupole Ion Traps. Int J Mass Spectrom 228:237–267. doi:10.1016/S1387-3806(03)00216-1
158. Wuerker RF, Shelton H, Langmuir RV (1959) Electrodynamic Containment of Charged Particles. J Appl Phys 30:342–349. doi:10.1063/1.1735165
159. Ehlers M, Schmidt S, Lee BJ, Grotemeyer J (2000) Design and Set-Up of an External Ion Source Coupled to a Quadrupole-Ion-Trap Reflectron-Time-of-Flight Hybrid Instrument. Eur J Mass Spectrom 6:377–385. doi:10.1255/ejms.356
160. Forbes MW, Sharifi M, Croley T, Lausevic Z, March RE (1999) Simulation of Ion Trajectories in a Quadrupole Ion Trap: A Comparison of Three Simulation Programs. J Mass Spectrom 34:1219–1239. doi:10.1002/(SICI)1096-9888(199912)34:12<1219::AID-JMS897>3.0.CO;2-L
161. Coon JJ, Steele HA, Laipis P, Harrison WW (2002) Laser Desorption-Atmospheric Pressure Chemical Ionization: A Novel Ion Source for the Direct Coupling of Polyacrylamide Gel Electrophoresis to Mass Spectrometry. J Mass Spectrom 37:1163–1167. doi:10.1002/jms.385
162. Nappi M, Weil C, Cleven CD, Horn LA, Wollnik H, Cooks RG (1997) Visual Representations of Simulated Three-Dimensional Ion Trajectories in an Ion Trap Mass Spectrometer. Int J Mass Spectrom Ion Proc 161:77–85. doi:10.1016/S0168-1176(96)04416-3
163. Dawson PH, Hedman JW, Whetten NR (1969) Mass Spectrometer. Rev Sci Instrum 40:1444–1450. doi:10.1063/1.1683822
164. Dawson PH, Whetten NR (1970) A Miniature Mass Spectrometer. Anal Chem 42:103A–108A. doi:10.1021/ac60294a799
165. Griffiths IW, Heesterman PJL (1990) Quadrupole Ion Store (QUISTOR) Mass Spectrometry. Int J Mass Spectrom Ion Proc 99:79–98. doi:10.1016/0168-1176(90)85022-T
166. Griffiths IW (1990) Recent Advances in Ion-Trap Technology. Rapid Commun Mass Spectrom 4:69–73. doi:10.1002/rcm.1290040302
167. Kelley PE, Stafford GC Jr, Syka JEP, Reynolds WE, Louris JN, Todd JFJ (1986) New Advances in the Operation of the Ion Trap Mass Spectrometer. Adv Mass Spectrom 10B:869–870
168. Splendore M, Lausevic M, Lausevic Z, March RE (1997) Resonant Excitation and/or Ejection of Ions Subjected to DC and RF Fields in a Commercial Quadrupole Ion Trap. Rapid Commun Mass Spectrom 11:228–233. doi:10.1002/(SICI)1097-0231(19970131)11:2<228::AID-RCM735>3.0.CO;2-C
169. Creaser CS, Stygall JW (1999) A Comparison of Overtone and Fundamental Resonances for Mass Range Extension by Resonance Ejection in a Quadrupole Ion Trap Mass Spectrometer. Int J Mass Spectrom 190(191):145–151. doi:10.1016/S1387-3806(99)00022-6
170. Williams JD, Cox KA, Cooks RG, McLuckey SA, Hart KJ, Goeringer DE (1994) Resonance Ejection Ion Trap Mass Spectrometry and Nonlinear Field Contributions: The Effect of Scan Direction on Mass Resolution. Anal Chem 66:725–729. doi:10.1021/ac00077a023
171. Ding L, Sudakov M, Brancia FL, Giles R, Kumashiro S (2004) A Digital Ion Trap Mass Spectrometer Coupled with Atmospheric Pressure Ion Sources. J Mass Spectrom 39:471–484. doi:10.1002/jms.637
172. Cooks RG, Amy JW, Bier M, Schwartz JC, Schey K (1989) New Mass Spectrometers. Adv Mass Spectrom 11A:33–52
173. Kaiser RE Jr, Louris JN, Amy JW, Cooks RG (1989) Extending the Mass Range of the Quadrupole Ion Trap Using Axial Modulation. Rapid Commun Mass Spectrom 3:225–229. doi:10.1002/rcm.1290030706
174. Weber-Grabau M, Kelley P, Bradshaw S, Hoekman D, Evans S, Bishop P (1989) Recent Advances in Ion-Trap Technology. Adv Mass Spectrom 11A:152–153
175. Siethoff C, Wagner-Redeker W, Schäfer M, Linscheid M (1999) HPLC-MS with an Ion Trap Mass Spectrometer. Chimia 53:484–491

176. Eades DM, Johnson JV, Yost RA (1993) Nonlinear Resonance Effects During Ion Storage in a Quadrupole Ion Trap. J Am Soc Mass Spectrom 4:917–929. doi:10.1016/1044-0305(93)80017-S
177. Makarov AA (1996) Resonance Ejection from the Paul Trap: A Theoretical Treatment Incorporating a Weak Octapole Field. Anal Chem 68:4257–4263. doi:10.1021/ac960653r
178. Doroshenko VM, Cotter RJ (1997) Losses of Ions During Forward and Reverse Scans in a Quadrupole Ion Trap Mass Spectrometer and How to Reduce Them. J Am Soc Mass Spectrom 8:1141–1146. doi:10.1016/S1044-0305(97)00162-1
179. von Busch F, Paul W (1961) Nonlinear Resonances in Electric Mass-Filters as a Consequence of Field Irregularities. Z Phys 164:588–594. doi:10.1007/BF01378433
180. Dawson PH, Whetten NR (1969) Nonlinear Resonances in Quadrupole Mass Spectrometers Due to Imperfect Fields. I. Quadrupole Ion Trap. Int J Mass Spectrom Ion Phys 2:45–59. doi:10.1016/0020-7381(69)80005-7
181. Wang Y, Franzen J (1994) The Non-Linear Ion Trap. Part 3. Multipole Components in Three Types of Practical Ion Trap. Int J Mass Spectrom Ion Proc 132:155–172. doi:10.1016/0168-1176(93)03913-7
182. Franzen J (1994) The Non-Linear Ion Trap. Part 5. Nature of Non-Linear Resonances and Resonant Ion Ejection. Int J Mass Spectrom Ion Proc 130:15–40. doi:10.1016/0168-1176(93)03907-4
183. Snyder DT, Pulliam CJ, Ouyang Z, Cooks RG (2015) Miniature and Fieldable Mass Spectrometers: Recent Advances. Anal Chem 88:2–29. doi:10.1021/acs.analchem.5b03070
184. Pulliam CJ, Bain RM, Wiley JS, Ouyang Z, Cooks RG (2015) Mass Spectrometry in the Home and Garden. J Am Soc Mass Spectrom 26:224–230. doi:10.1007/s13361-014-1056-z
185. Ouyang Z, Wu G, Song Y, Li H, Plass WR, Cooks RG (2004) Rectilinear Ion Trap: Concepts, Calculations, and Analytical Performance of a New Mass Analyzer. Anal Chem 76:4595–4605. doi:10.1021/ac049420n
186. Peng WP, Goodwin MP, Nie Z, Volny M, Ouyang Z, Cooks RG (2008) Ion Soft Landing Using a Rectilinear Ion Trap Mass Spectrometer. Anal Chem 80:6640–6649. doi:10.1021/ac800929w
187. Berton A, Traldi P, Ding L, Brancia FL (2008) Mapping the Stability Diagram of a Digital Ion Trap (DIT) Mass Spectrometer Varying the Duty Cycle of the Trapping Rectangular Waveform. J Am Soc Mass Spectrom 19:620–625. doi:10.1016/j.jasms.2007.12.012
188. Ding L, Kumashiro S (2006) Ion Motion in the Rectangular Wave Quadrupole Field and Digital Operation Mode of a Quadrupole Ion Trap Mass Spectrometer. Rapid Commun Mass Spectrom 20:3–8. doi:10.1002/rcm.2253
189. Li X, Jiang G, Luo C, Xu F, Wang Y, Ding L, Ding C (2009) Ion Trap Array Mass Analyzer: Structure and Performance. Anal Chem 81:4840–4846. doi:10.1021/ac900478e
190. Brodbelt JS, Louris JN, Cooks RG (1987) Chemical Ionization in an Ion Trap Mass Spectrometer. Anal Chem 59:1278–1285. doi:10.1021/ac00136a007
191. Doroshenko VM, Cotter RJ (1997) Injection of Externally Generated Ions into an Increasing Trapping Field of a Quadrupole Ion Trap Mass Spectrometer. J Mass Spectrom 31:602–615. doi:10.1002/(SICI)1096-9888(199706)32:6<602::AID-JMS513>3.0.CO;2-G
192. Van Berkel GJ, Glish GL, McLuckey SA (1990) Electrospray Ionization Combined with Ion Trap Mass Spectrometry. Anal Chem 62:1284–1295. doi:10.1021/ac00212a016
193. Wang Y, Schubert M, Ingendoh A, Franzen J (2000) Analysis of Non-Covalent Protein Complexes Up to 290 KDa Using Electrospray Ionization and Ion Trap Mass Spectrometry. Rapid Commun Mass Spectrom 14:12–17. doi:10.1002/(SICI)1097-0231(20000115)14:1<12::AID-RCM825>3.0.CO;2-7
194. Lawrence EO, Livingston MS (1932) The Production of High-Speed Light Ions Without the Use of High Voltages. Phys Rev 40:19–35. doi:10.1103/PhysRev.40.19
195. Comisarow MB, Marshall AG (1996) The Early Development of Fourier Transform Ion Cyclotron Resonance (FT-ICR) Spectroscopy. J Mass Spectrom 31:581–585. doi:10.1002/(SICI)1096-9888(199606)31:6<581::AID-JMS369>3.0.CO;2-1

196. Smith LG (1951) New Magnetic Period Mass Spectrometer. Rev Sci Instrum 22:115–116. doi:10.1063/1.1745849
197. Sommer H, Thomas HA, Hipple JA (1951) Measurement of E/M by Cyclotron Resonance. Phys Rev 82:697–702. doi:10.1103/PhysRev.82.697
198. Baldeschwieler JD (1968) Ion Cyclotron Resonance Spectroscopy. Science 159:263–273. doi:10.1126/science.159.3812.263
199. Assamoto B (ed) (1991) Analytical Applications of Fourier Transform Ion Cyclotron Resonance Mass Spectrometry. Weinheim, VCH
200. Comisarow MB, Marshall AG (1974) Fourier Transform Ion Cyclotron Resonance Spectroscopy. Chem Phys Lett 25:282–283. doi:10.1016/0009-2614(74)89137-2
201. Comisarow MB, Marshall AG (1974) Frequency-Sweep Fourier Transform Ion Cyclotron Resonance Spectroscopy. Chem Phys Lett 26:489–490. doi:10.1016/0009-2614(74)80397-0
202. Wanczek K-P (1989) ICR Spectrometry – A Review of New Developments in Theory, Instrumentation and Applications. I. 1983–1986. Int J Mass Spectrom Ion Proc 95:1–38. doi:10.1016/0168-1176(89)83044-7
203. Marshall AG, Grosshans PB (1991) Fourier Transform Ion Cyclotron Resonance Mass Spectrometry: The Teenage Years. Anal Chem 63:215A–229A. doi:10.1021/ac00004a001
204. Amster IJ (1996) Fourier Transform Mass Spectrometry. J Mass Spectrom 31:1325–1337. doi:10.1002/(SICI)1096-9888(199612)31:12<1325::AID-JMS453>3.0.CO;2-W
205. Dienes T, Salvador JP, Schürch S, Scott JR, Yao J, Cui S, Wilkins CL (1996) Fourier Transform Mass Spectrometry-Advancing Years (1992-Mid 1996). Mass Spectrom Rev 15:163–211. doi:10.1002/(SICI)1098-2787(1996)15:3<163::AID-MAS2>3.0.CO;2-G
206. Marshall AG (2000) Milestones in Fourier Transform Ion Cyclotron Resonance Mass Spectrometry Technique Development. Int J Mass Spectrom 200:331–356. doi:10.1016/S1387-3806(00)00324-9
207. Smith RD (2000) Evolution of ESI-Mass Spectrometry and Fourier Transform Ion Cyclotron Resonance for Proteomics and Other Biological Applications. Int J Mass Spectrom 200:509–544. doi:10.1016/S1387-3806(00)00352-3
208. Marshall AG, Hendrickson CL, Shi SDH (2002) Scaling MS Plateaus with High-Resolution FT-ICR-MS. Anal Chem 74:252A–259A. doi:10.1021/ac022010j
209. Schaub TM, Hendrickson CL, Horning S, Quinn JP, Senko MW, Marshall AG (2008) High-Performance Mass Spectrometry: Fourier Transform Ion Cyclotron Resonance at 14.5 Tesla. Anal Chem 80:3985–3990. doi:10.1021/ac800386h
210. Boldin IA, Nikolaev EN (2011) Fourier Transform Ion Cyclotron Resonance Cell with Dynamic Harmonization of the Electric Field in the Whole Volume by Shaping of the Excitation and Detection Electrode Assembly. Rapid Commun Mass Spectrom 25:122–126. doi:10.1002/rcm.4838
211. Nikolaev EN (2015) Some Notes About FT ICR Mass Spectrometry. Int J Mass Spectrom 377:421–431. doi:10.1016/j.ijms.2014.07.051
212. Marshall AG, Chen T (2015) 40 Years of Fourier Transform Ion Cyclotron Resonance Mass Spectrometry. Int J Mass Spectrom 377:410–420. doi:10.1016/j.ijms.2014.06.034
213. Hendrickson CL, Quinn JP, Kaiser NK, Smith DF, Blakney GT, Chen T, Marshall AG, Weisbrod CR, Beu SC (2015) 21 Tesla Fourier Transform Ion Cyclotron Resonance Mass Spectrometer: A National Resource for Ultrahigh Resolution Mass Analysis. J Am Soc Mass Spectrom 26:1626–1632. doi:10.1007/s13361-015-1182-2
214. He F, Hendrickson CL, Marshall AG (2001) Baseline Mass Resolution of Peptide Isobars: A Record for Molecular Mass Resolution. Anal Chem 73:647–650. doi:10.1021/ac000973h
215. Bossio RE, Marshall AG (2002) Baseline Resolution of Isobaric Phosphorylated and Sulfated Peptides and Nucleotides by Electrospray Ionization FT-ICR-MS: Another Step Toward MS-Based Proteomics. Anal Chem 74:1674–1679. doi:10.1021/ac0108461
216. Nikolaev EN, Jertz R, Grigoryev A, Baykut G (2012) Fine Structure in Isotopic Peak Distributions Measured Using a Dynamically Harmonized Fourier Transform Ion Cyclotron Resonance Cell at 7 T. Anal Chem 84:2275–2283. doi:10.1021/ac202804f

217. Popov IA, Nagornov K, Vladimirov GN, Kostyukevich YI, Nikolaev EN (2014) Twelve Million Resolving Power on 4.7 T Fourier Transform Ion Cyclotron Resonance Instrument with Dynamically Harmonized Cell-Observation of Fine Structure in Peptide Mass Spectra. J Am Soc Mass Spectrom 25:790–799. doi:10.1007/s13361-014-0846-7
218. White FM, Marto JA, Marshall AG (1996) An External Source 7 T Fourier Transform Ion Cyclotron Resonance Mass Spectrometer with Electrostatic Ion Guide. Rapid Commun Mass Spectrom 10:1845–1849. doi:10.1002/(SICI)1097-0231(199611)10:14<1845::AID-RCM749>3.0.CO;2-%23
219. Marshall AG, Hendrickson CL (2002) Fourier Transform Ion Cyclotron Resonance Detection: Principles and Experimental Configurations. Int J Mass Spectrom 215:59–75. doi:10.1016/S1387-3806(01)00588-7
220. Marshall AG, Hendrickson CL, Jackson GS (1998) Fourier Transform Ion Cyclotron Resonance Mass Spectrometry: A Primer. Mass Spectrom Rev 17:1–35. doi:10.1002/(SICI)1098-2787(1998)17:1<1::AID-MAS1>3.0.CO;2-K
221. Shi SDH, Drader JJ, Freitas MA, Hendrickson CL, Marshall AG (2000) Comparison and Interconversion of the Two Most Common Frequency-to-Mass Calibration Functions for Fourier Transform Ion Cyclotron Resonance Mass Spectrometry. Int J Mass Spectrom 195 (196):591–598. doi:10.1016/S1387-3806(99)00226-2
222. Nikolaev EN, Gorshkov MV (1985) Dynamics of Ion Motion in an Elongated Cylindrical Cell of an ICR Spectrometer and the Shape of the Signal Registered. Int J Mass Spectrom Ion Proc 64:115–125. doi:10.1016/0168-1176(85)85003-5
223. Pan Y, Ridge DP, Wronka J, Rockwood AL (1987) Resolution Improvement by Using Harmonic Detection in an Ion Cyclotron Resonance Mass Spectrometer. Rapid Commun Mass Spectrom 1:120–121. doi:10.1002/rcm.1290010709
224. Nikolaev EN, Boldin IA, Jertz R, Baykut G (2011) Initial Experimental Characterization of a New Ultra-High Resolution FTICR Cell with Dynamic Harmonization. J Am Soc Mass Spectrom 22:1125–1133. doi:10.1007/s13361-011-0125-9
225. Derome AE (1987) Modern NMR Techniques for Chemistry Research. Pergamon Press, Oxford
226. Guan S, Marshall AG (1996) Stored Waveform Inverse Fourier Transform (SWIFT) Ion Excitation in Trapped-Ion Mass Spectrometry: Theory and Applications. Int J Mass Spectrom Ion Proc 157(158):5–37. doi:10.1016/S0168-1176(96)04461-8
227. Schweikhard L, Ziegler J, Bopp H, Luetzenkirchen K (1995) The Trapping Condition and a New Instability of the Ion Motion in the Ion Cyclotron Resonance Trap. Int J Mass Spectrom Ion Proc 141:77–90. doi:10.1016/0168-1176(94)04092-L
228. Comisarow MB, Marshall AG (1976) Theory of Fourier Transform Ion Cyclotron Resonance Mass Spectroscopy. I. Fundamental Equations and Low-Pressure Line Shape. J Chem Phys 64:110–119. doi:10.1063/1.431959
229. Comisarow MB (1978) Signal Modeling for Ion Cyclotron Resonance. J Chem Phys 69:4097–4104. doi:10.1063/1.437143
230. Hughey CA, Rodgers RP, Marshall AG (2002) Resolution of 11,000 Compositionally Distinct Components in a Single Electrospray Ionization FT-ICR Mass Spectrum of Crude Oil. Anal Chem 74:4145–4149. doi:10.1021/ac020146b
231. Huang Y, Li G-Z, Guan S, Marshall AG (1997) A Combined Linear Ion Trap for Mass Spectrometry. J Am Soc Mass Spectrom 8:962–969. doi:10.1016/S1044-0305(97)82945-5
232. Guan S, Marshall AG (1995) Ion Traps for Fourier Transform Ion Cyclotron Resonance Mass Spectrometry: Principles and Design of Geometric and Electric Configurations. Int J Mass Spectrom Ion Proc 146(147):261–296. doi:10.1016/0168-1176(95)04190-V
233. Caravatti P, Allemann M (1991) The Infinity Cell: A New Trapped-Ion Cell with Radiofrequency Covered Trapping Electrodes for FT-ICR-MS. Org Mass Spectrom 26:514–518. doi:10.1002/oms.1210260527
234. Kostyukevich YI, Vladimirov GN, Nikolaev EN (2012) Dynamically Harmonized FT-ICR Cell with Specially Shaped Electrodes for Compensation of Inhomogeneity of the Magnetic

Field. Computer Simulations of the Electric Field and Ion Motion Dynamics. J Am Soc Mass Spectrom 23:2198–2207. doi:10.1007/s13361-012-0480-1
235. Nicolardi S, Switzar L, Deelder AM, Palmblad M, van der Burgt YEM (2015) Top-Down MALDI-In-Source Decay-FTICR Mass Spectrometry of Isotopically Resolved Proteins. Anal Chem 87:3429–3437. doi:10.1021/ac504708y
236. Solouki T, Emmet MR, Guan S, Marshall AG (1997) Detection, Number, and Sequence Location of Sulfur-Containing Amino Acids and Disulfide Bridges in Peptides by Ultrahigh-Resolution MALDI FTICR Mass Spectrometry. Anal Chem 69:1163–1168. doi:10.1021/ac960885q
237. Wu Z, Hendrickson CL, Rodgers RP, Marshall AG (2002) Composition of Explosives by Electrospray Ionization Fourier Transform Ion Cyclotron Resonance Mass Spectrometry. Anal Chem 74:1879–1883. doi:10.1021/ac011071z
238. Senko MW, Hendrickson CL, Emmett MR, Shi SDH, Marshall AG (1997) External Accumulation of Ions for Enhanced Electrospray Ionization Fourier Transform Ion Cyclotron Resonance Mass Spectrometry. J Am Soc Mass Spectrom 8:970–976. doi:10.1016/S1044-0305(97)00126-8
239. Wang Y, Shi SDH, Hendrickson CL, Marshall AG (2000) Mass-Selective Ion Accumulation and Fragmentation in a Linear Octopole Ion Trap External to a Fourier Transform Ion Cyclotron Resonance Mass Spectrometer. Int J Mass Spectrom 198:113–120. doi:10.1016/S1387-3806(00)00177-9
240. Makarov A (2000) Electrostatic Axially Harmonic Orbital Trapping: A High-Performance Technique of Mass Analysis. Anal Chem 72:1156–1162. doi:10.1021/ac991131p
241. Scigelova M, Makarov A (2006) Orbitrap Mass Analyzer – Overview and Applications in Proteomics. Pract Proteomics 6:16–21. doi:10.1002/pmic.200600528
242. Makarov A, Denisov E, Lange O, Horning S (2006) Dynamic Range of Mass Accuracy in LTQ Orbitrap Hybrid Mass Spectrometer. J Am Soc Mass Spectrom 17:977–982. doi:10.1016/j.jasms.2006.03.006
243. Makarov A, Denisov E, Kholomeev A, Balschun W, Lange O, Strupat K, Horning S (2006) Performance Evaluation of a Hybrid Linear Ion Trap/Orbitrap Mass Spectrometer. Anal Chem 78:2113–2120. doi:10.1021/ac0518811
244. Macek B, Waanders LF, Olsen JV, Mann M (2006) Top-Down Protein Sequencing and MS^3 on a Hybrid Linear Quadrupole Ion Trap-Orbitrap Mass Spectrometer. Mol Cell Proteomics 5:949–958. doi:10.1074/mcp.T500042-MCP200
245. Perry RH, Cooks RG, Noll RJ (2008) Orbitrap Mass Spectrometry: Instrumentation, Ion Motion and Applications. Mass Spectrom Rev 27:661–699. doi:10.1002/mas.20186
246. Kingdon KH (1923) A Method for Neutralizing the Electron Space Charge by Positive Ionization at Very Low Pressures. Phys Rev 21:408–418. doi:10.1103/PhysRev.21.408
247. Knight RD (1981) Storage of Ions from Laser-Produced Plasmas. Appl Phys Lett 38:221–223. doi:10.1063/1.92315
248. Oksman P (1995) A Fourier Transform Time-of-Flight Mass Spectrometer. A SIMION Calculation Approach. Int J Mass Spectrom Ion Proc 141:67–76. doi:10.1016/0168-1176(94)04086-M
249. Hardman M, Makarov AA (2003) Interfacing the Orbitrap Mass Analyzer to an Electrospray Ion Source. Anal Chem 75:1699–1705. doi:10.1021/ac0258047
250. Olsen JV, de Godoy LMF, Li G, Macek B, Mortensen P, Pesch R, Makarov A, Lange O, Horning S, Mann M (2005) Parts Per Million Mass Accuracy on an Orbitrap Mass Spectrometer Via Lock Mass Injection into a C-Trap. Mol Cell Proteomics 4:2010–2021. doi:10.1074/mcp.T500030-MCP200
251. Perry RH, Hu Q, Salazar GA, Cooks RG, Noll RJ (2009) Rephasing Ion Packets in the Orbitrap Mass Analyzer to Improve Resolution and Peak Shape. J Am Soc Mass Spectrom 20:1397–1404. doi:10.1016/j.jasms.2009.02.011
252. Makarov A, Denisov E (2009) Dynamics of Ions of Intact Proteins in the Orbitrap Mass Analyzer. J Am Soc Mass Spectrom 20:1486–1495. doi:10.1016/j.jasms.2009.03.024

253. Makarov A, Denisov E, Lange O (2009) Performance Evaluation of a High-Field Orbitrap Mass Analyzer. J Am Soc Mass Spectrom 20:1391–1396. doi:10.1016/j.jasms.2009.01.005
254. Lebedev AT, Damoc E, Makarov AA, Samgina TY (2014) Discrimination of Leucine and Isoleucine in Peptides Sequencing with Orbitrap Fusion Mass Spectrometer. Anal Chem 86:7017–7022. doi:10.1021/ac501200h
255. Senko MW, Remes PM, Canterbury JD, Mathur R, Song Q, Eliuk SM, Mullen C, Earley L, Hardman M, Blethrow JD, Bui H, Specht A, Lange O, Denisov E, Makarov A, Horning S, Zabrouskov V (2013) Novel Parallelized Quadrupole/Linear Ion Trap/Orbitrap Tribrid Mass Spectrometer Improving Proteome Coverage and Peptide Identification Rates. Anal Chem 85:11710–11714. doi:10.1021/ac403115c
256. Amy JW, Baitinger WE, Cooks RG (1990) Building Mass Spectrometers and a Philosophy of Research. J Am Soc Mass Spectrom 1:119–128. doi:10.1016/1044-0305(90)85047-P
257. Futrell JH (2000) Development of Tandem Mass Spectrometry. One Perspective. Int J Mass Spectrom 200:495–508. doi:10.1016/S1387-3806(00)00353-5
258. McLuckey SA, Glish GL, Cooks RG (1981) Kinetic Energy Effects in Mass Spectrometry/ Mass Spectrometry Using a Sector/Quadrupole Tandem Instrument. Int J Mass Spectrom Ion Phys 39:219–230. doi:10.1016/0020-7381(81)80034-4
259. Glish GL, McLuckey SA, Ridley TY, Cooks RG (1982) A New "Hybrid" Sector/Quadrupole Mass Spectrometer for Mass Spectrometry/Mass Spectrometry. Int J Mass Spectrom Ion Phys 41:157–177. doi:10.1016/0020-7381(82)85032-8
260. Bradley CD, Curtis JM, Derrick PJ, Wright B (1992) Tandem Mass Spectrometry of Peptides Using a Magnetic Sector/Quadrupole Hybrid-the Case for Higher Collision Energy and Higher Radio-Frequency Power. Anal Chem 64:2628–2635. doi:10.1021/ac00045a028
261. Schoen AE, Amy JW, Ciupek JD, Cooks RG, Dobberstein P, Jung G (1985) A Hybrid BEQQ Mass Spectrometer. Int J Mass Spectrom Ion Proc 65:125–140. doi:10.1016/0168-1176(85) 85059-X
262. Ciupek JD, Amy JW, Cooks RG, Schoen AE (1985) Performance of a Hybrid Mass Spectrometer. Int J Mass Spectrom Ion Proc 65:141–157. doi:10.1016/0168-1176(85) 85060-6
263. Louris JN, Wright LG, Cooks RG, Schoen AE (1985) New Scan Modes Accessed with a Hybrid Mass Spectrometer. Anal Chem 57:2918–2924. doi:10.1021/ac00291a039
264. Loo JA, Münster H (1999) Magnetic Sector-Ion Trap Mass Spectrometry with Electrospray Ionization for High Sensitivity Peptide Sequencing. Rapid Commun Mass Spectrom 13:54–60. doi:10.1002/(SICI)1097-0231(19990115)13:1<54::AID-RCM450>3.0.CO;2-Y
265. Strobel FH, Solouki T, White MA, Russell DH (1991) Detection of Femtomole and Sub-Femtomole Levels of Peptides by Tandem Magnetic Sector/Reflectron Time-of-Flight Mass Spectrometry and Matrix-Assisted Laser Desorption Ionization. J Am Soc Mass Spectrom 2:91–94. doi:10.1016/1044-0305(91)80066-G
266. Bateman RH, Green MR, Scott G, Clayton E (1995) A Combined Magnetic Sector-Time-of-Flight Mass Spectrometer for Structural Determination Studies by Tandem Mass Spectrometry. Rapid Commun Mass Spectrom 9:1227–1233. doi:10.1002/rcm.1290091302
267. Aicher KP, Müller M, Wilhelm U, Grotemeyer J (1995) Design and Setup of an Ion Trap-Reflectron-Time-of-Flight Mass Spectrometer. Eur Mass Spectrom 1:331–340. doi:10.1255/ejms.117
268. Wilhelm U, Aicher KP, Grotemeyer J (1996) Ion Storage Combined with Reflectron Time-of-Flight Mass Spectrometry: Ion Cloud Motions As a Result of Jet-Cooled Molecules. Int J Mass Spectrom Ion Proc 152:111–120. doi:10.1016/0168-1176(95)04339-X
269. Morris HR, Paxton T, Dell A, Langhorne J, Berg M, Bordoli RS, Hoyes J, Bateman RH (1996) High Sensitivity Collisionally-Activated Decomposition Tandem Mass Spectrometry on a Novel Quadrupole/Orthogonal-Acceleration Time-of-Flight Mass Spectrometer. Rapid Commun Mass Spectrom 10:889–896. doi:10.1002/(SICI)1097-0231(19960610)10:8<889::AID-RCM615>3.0.CO;2-F

270. Shevchenko A, Chernushevich IV, Ens W, Standing KG, Thompson B, Wilm M, Mann M (1997) Rapid 'De Novo' Peptide Sequencing by a Combination of Nanoelectrospray, Isotopic Labeling and a Quadrupole/Time-of-Flight Mass Spectrometer. Rapid Commun Mass Spectrom 11:1015–1024. doi:10.1002/(SICI)1097-0231(19970615)11:9<1015::AID-RCM958>3.0.CO;2-H
271. Hopfgartner G, Chernushevich IV, Covey T, Plomley JB, Bonner R (1999) Exact Mass Measurement of Product Ions for the Structural Elucidation of Drug Metabolites with a Tandem Quadrupole Orthogonal-Acceleration Time-of-Flight Mass Spectrometer. J Am Soc Mass Spectrom 10:1305–1314. doi:10.1016/S1044-0305(99)00097-5
272. Borsdorf H, Eiceman GA (2006) Ion Mobility Spectrometry: Principles and Applications. Appl Spectrosc Rev 41:323–375. doi:10.1080/05704920600663469
273. Eiceman GA, Karpas Z, Hill HH Jr (2014) Ion Mobility Spectrometry. CRC Press, Boca Raton
274. Collins DC, Lee ML (2002) Developments in Ion Mobility Spectrometry-Mass Spectrometry. Anal Bioanal Chem 372:66–73. doi:10.1007/s00216-001-1195-5
275. Mukhopadhyay R (2008) IMS/MS: Its Time Has Come. Anal Chem 80:7918–7920. doi:10.1021/ac8018608
276. Bohrer BC, Merenbloom SI, Koeniger SL, Hilderbrand AE, Clemmer DE (2008) Biomolecule Analysis by Ion Mobility Spectrometry. Annu Rev Anal Chem 1:293–327. doi:10.1146/annurev.anchem.1.031207.113001
277. Karasek FW (1970) Drift-Mass Spectrometer. Res Developm 21:25–27
278. Karasek FW (1970) Plasma Chromatograph. Res Developm 21:34–37
279. Karasek FW, Cohen MJ, Carroll DI (1971) Trace Studies of Alcohols in the Plasma Chromatograph–Mass Spectrometer. J Chromatogr Sci 9:390–392. doi:10.1093/chromsci/9.7.390
280. Kanu AB, Dwivedi P, Tam M, Matz L, Hill HH Jr (2008) Ion Mobility-Mass Spectrometry. J Mass Spectrom 43:1–22. doi:10.1002/jms.1383
281. Pringle SD, Giles K, Wildgoose JL, Williams JP, Slade SE, Thalassinos K, Bateman RH, Bowers MT, Scrivens JH (2007) An Investigation of the Mobility Separation of Some Peptide and Protein Ions Using a New Hybrid Quadrupole/Travelling Wave IMS/Oa-ToF Instrument. Int J Mass Spectrom 261:1–12. doi:10.1016/j.ijms.2006.07.021
282. Guevremont R (2004) High-Field Asymmetric Waveform Ion Mobility Spectrometry: A New Tool for Mass Spectrometry. J Chromatogr A 1058:3–19. doi:10.1016/S0021-9673(04)01478-5
283. Kolakowski BM, Mester Z (2007) Review of Applications of High-Field Asymmetric Waveform Ion Mobility Spectrometry (FAIMS) and Differential Mobility Spectrometry (DMS). Analyst 132:842–864. doi:10.1039/B706039D
284. Harvey SR, Macphee CE, Barran PE (2011) Ion Mobility Mass Spectrometry for Peptide Analysis. Methods 54:454–461. doi:10.1016/j.ymeth.2011.05.004
285. Platzner IT, Habfast K, Walder AJ, Goetz A, Platzner IT (eds) (1997) Modern Isotope Ratio Mass Spectrometry. Wiley, Chichester
286. Stanton HE, Chupka WA, Inghram MG (1956) Electron Multipliers in Mass Spectrometry; Effect of Molecular Structure. Rev Sci Instrum 27:109. doi:10.1063/1.1715477
287. Weaver PJ, Laures AMF, Wolff JC (2007) Investigation of the Advanced Functionalities of a Hybrid Quadrupole Orthogonal Acceleration Time-of-Flight Mass Spectrometer. Rapid Commun Mass Spectrom 21:2415–2421. doi:10.1002/rcm.3052
288. Colombo M, Sirtori FR, Rizzo V (2004) A Fully Automated Method for Accurate Mass Determination Using High-Performance Liquid Chromatography with a Quadrupole/Orthogonal Acceleration Time-of-Flight Mass Spectrometer. Rapid Commun Mass Spectrom 18:511–517. doi:10.1002/rcm.1368
289. Allen JS (1947) An Improved Electron-Multiplier Particle Counter. Rev Sci Instrum 18:739–749. doi:10.1063/1.1740838

290. Wang GH, Aberth W, Falick AM (1986) Evidence Concerning the Identity of Secondary Particles in Post-Acceleration Detectors. Int J Mass Spectrom Ion Proc 69:233–237. doi:10.1016/0168-1176(86)87037-9
291. Busch KL (2000) The Electron Multiplier. Spectroscopy 15:28–33
292. Schröder E (1991) Massenspektrometrie – Begriffe und Definitionen. Springer, Heidelberg
293. Boerboom AJH (1991) Array Detection of Mass Spectra, a Comparison with Conventional Detection Methods. Org Mass Spectrom 26:929–935. doi:10.1002/oms.1210261103
294. Kurz EA (1979) Channel Electron Multipliers. Am Laboratory 11:67–82
295. Wiza JL (1979) Microchannel Plate Detectors. Nucl Instrum Methods 162:587–601. doi:10.1016/0029-554X(79)90734-1
296. Laprade BN, Labich RJ (1994) Microchannel Plate-Based Detectors in Mass Spectrometry. Spectroscopy 9:26–30
297. Alexandrov ML, Gall LN, Krasnov NV, Lokshin LR, Chuprikov AV (1990) Discrimination Effects in Inorganic Ion-Cluster Detection by Secondary-Electron Multiplier in Mass Spectrometry Experiments. Rapid Commun Mass Spectrom 4:9–12. doi:10.1002/rcm.1290040104
298. Geno PW, Macfarlane RD (1989) Secondary Electron Emission Induced by Impact of Low-Velocity Molecular Ions on a Microchannel Plate. Int J Mass Spectrom Ion Proc 92:195–210. doi:10.1016/0168-1176(89)83028-9
299. Hedin H, Håkansson K, Sundqvist BUR (1987) On the Detection of Large Organic Ions by Secondary Electron Production. Int J Mass Spectrom Ion Proc 75:275–289. doi:10.1016/0168-1176(87)83041-0
300. Hill JA, Biller JE, Martin SA, Biemann K, Yoshidome K, Sato K (1989) Design Considerations, Calibration and Applications of an Array Detector for a Four-Sector Tandem Mass Spectrometer. Int J Mass Spectrom Ion Proc 92:211–230. doi:10.1016/0168-1176(89)83029-0
301. Birkinshaw K (1997) Fundamentals of Focal Plane Detectors. J Mass Spectrom 32:795–806. doi:10.1002/(SICI)1096-9888(199708)32:8<795::AID-JMS540>3.0.CO;2-U
302. Cottrell JS, Evans S (1987) The Application of a Multichannel Electro-Optical Detection System to the Analysis of Large Molecules by FAB Mass Spectrometry. Rapid Commun Mass Spectrom 1:1–2. doi:10.1002/rcm.1290010103
303. Cottrell JS, Evans S (1987) Characteristics of a Multichannel Electrooptical Detection System and Its Application to the Analysis of Large Molecules by Fast Atom Bombardment Mass Spectrometry. Anal Chem 59:1990–1995. doi:10.1021/ac00142a021
304. Birkinshaw K, Langstaff DP (1996) The Ideal Detector. Rapid Commun Mass Spectrom 10:1675–1677. doi:10.1002/(SICI)1097-0231(199610)10:13<1675::AID-RCM712>3.0.CO;2-S
305. Hucknall DJ (1991) Vacuum Technology and Applications. Butterworth-Heinemann, Oxford
306. Pupp W, Hartmann HK (1991) Vakuum-Technik – Grundlagen und Anwendungen. Fachbuchverlag Leipzig, Leipzig
307. Wutz M, Adam H, Walcher W (1992) Theory and Practice of Vacuum Technology. Vieweg, Braunschweig/Wiesbaden
308. Lafferty JM (ed) (1998) Foundations of Vacuum Science and Technology. Wiley, New York
309. Umrath W (ed) (2001) Leybold Vacuum Products and Reference Book. Leybold Vacuum GmbH, Köln
310. Busch KL (2000) Vacuum in Mass Spectroscopy. Nothing Can Surprise You. Spectroscopy 15:22–25
311. Busch KL (2001) High-Vacuum Pumps in Mass Spectrometers. Spectroscopy 16:14–18

Practical Aspects of Electron Ionization

5

Learning Objectives

- Electron ionization ion sources – construction and operation
- Generating primary electrons for electron ionization
- Sample introduction into EI ion sources – methods and devices
- Databases of EI mass spectra

The use of *electron ionization* (EI) [1] dates back to the infancy of mass spectrometry in the early twentieth century. Before, only *spark source* (SS), *glow discharge* (GD), and *thermal ionization* (TI) had been in use [2]. In electron ionization, energetic electrons are shot onto gaseous neutrals to effect their ionization. EI definitely represents the classical approach to ionization in organic mass spectrometry. EI still remains an important technique for analyzing low- to medium-polarity, non-ionic organic compounds of molecular weights in the range of up to $M_r \approx$ 800 u. EI formerly has been referred to as *electron impact ionization* or simply *electron impact* (EI).

The physicochemical aspects of the ionization process in general, ion internal energy, and the principles determining the reaction pathways of excited ions have already been addressed (Chap. 2). Here, we will discuss practical aspects concerning the construction of EI ion sources and sample introduction systems. Finally, by considering EI mass spectral databases, this chapter directly leads over to the interpretation of EI mass spectra (Chap. 6).

J.H. Gross, *Mass Spectrometry*, DOI 10.1007/978-3-319-54398-7_5

5.1 Electron Ionization Ion Sources

5.1.1 Layout of an Electron Ionization Ion Source

The basic layout of any ion source has already been introduced (Sect. 4.1). The design is arranged so that an ion generated within an electric field as realized between two oppositely charged plates, will be accelerated towards the plate oppositely charged to itself. If the attracting plate has a hole or a slit, a beam of approximately monoenergetic ions is produced. For practical reasons, the attracting electrode is usually grounded and the location of ion generation is set to high potential. Doing so allows to keep the mass analyzer grounded, thereby contributing substantially to safety of operation (Fig. 5.1).

The beam of neutral gaseous analyte molecules enters the *ionization chamber* or *ion volume*, i.e., the actual region of ionization within the *ion source block*, in a line vertical to the paper plane and crosses the electron beam in the center. In order to reduce loss of ions by neutralizing collisions with the walls, the ions are pushed out immediately after generation by action of a low voltage applied to the *repeller* electrode [3, 4]. They are then accelerated and focused towards the mass analyzer. Efficient ionization and ion extraction are of key importance for the construction of ion sources producing focusable ion currents in the nanoampere range [5].

Modern ion sources are of compact design to simplify the handling during exchange and cleaning (Figs. 5.2 and 5.5). Magnetic sector instruments either come with *combination ion sources* switchable from EI to *chemical ionization* (CI), *fast atom bombardment* (FAB), or *field ionization/field desorption* (FI/FD). Particularly EI/CI/FAB and EI/FI/FD [7, 8] ion sources have been widespread in use.

Some instruments are equipped with ion sources having exchangeable ion volumes that can be accessed via a (separate) vacuum lock to allow for their exchange without breaking the high vacuum.

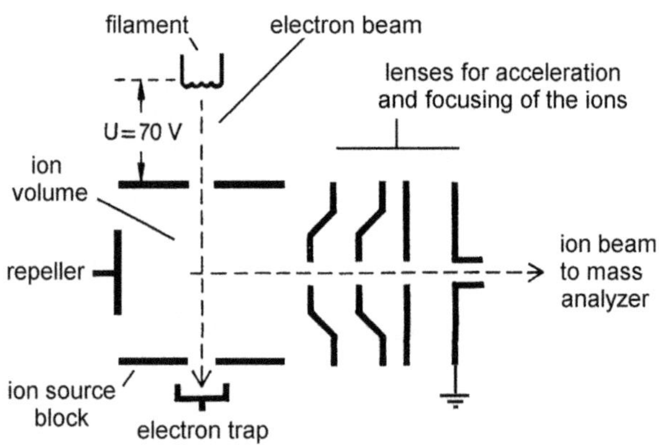

Fig. 5.1 Principle layout of an EI ion source (Adapted from Ref. [6] with permission. © Springer-Verlag Heidelberg, 1991)

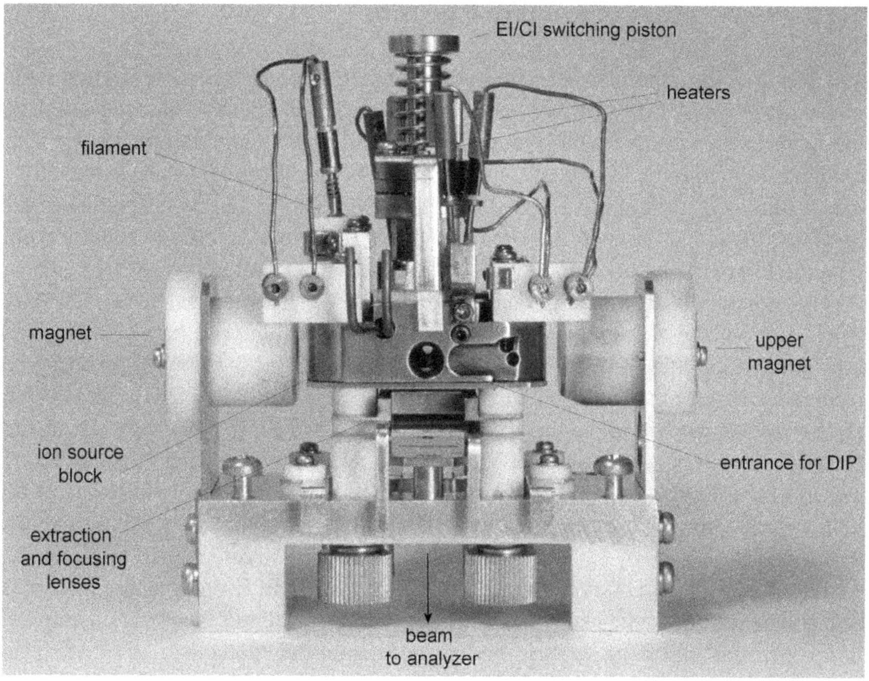

Fig. 5.2 EI/CI/FAB combination ion source of a JEOL JMS-700 sector instrument

More recently, there is a reverse trend to dedicated EI ion sources in order to achieve the utmost sensitivity. Dedicated sources – some even restricted to be used with *either* direct insertion probe *or* gas chromatograph – are optimized for trace level analyses. For covering a wide variety of samples, combination sources are hard to beat in versatility.

System contamination

High vacuum systems and ion sources, the more so, are almost inevitably prone to *contamination* in the process of *sample introduction*. Even though ion sources are operated at 150–250°C, decomposition products of low volatility cannot be removed by pumping. Instead, they form semiconducting layers on the surfaces which in turn cause defocusing due to badly defined potentials. Therefore, cleaning of an ion source is necessary on a regular basis. This includes disassembling, use of fine abrasives to polish the lenses, baking of the insulating ceramics, and thorough washing of the parts.

5.1.2 Generation of Primary Electrons

The beam of ionizing electrons is produced by *thermionic emission* from a resistively heated metal wire or *filament* typically made of rhenium or tungsten. The filament reaches up to 2000 °C during operation. Some reduction of the working temperature without loss of electron emission (1–10 mA mm^{-2}) can be achieved by use of thoriated iridium or thoriated rhenium filaments [9]. There is a wide variety of filaments available from different manufacturers working almost equally well, e.g., the filament can be a straight wire, a ribbon, or a small coil (Fig. 5.3).

The potential for acceleration of the primary electrons has to be carefully shielded from the acceleration voltage for the ions. Otherwise, badly defined ion kinetic energies cause substantial loss of resolution and mass accuracy. In addition, a pair of permanent magnets with their field aligned in parallel to the electron beam is attached above the filament and below the electron trap, thus preventing the electrons from spreading all over the ion volume (Fig. 5.2). This is achieved by action of the Lorentz force on divergent electrons which are forced to travel on helical paths; the resulting electron beam is about 1 mm in diameter. These features developed by Bleakney [10], and refined by Nier [11] were destined to direct the design of EI ion sources ever since [2, 4, 12] (the basic EI ion source is sometimes referred to as "Nier-type" ion source). Further improvements can be obtained by (*i*) more efficient shielding of the ion volume from the filament, a measure also reducing thermal decomposition of the analyte, and (*ii*) by use of stronger ion source magnets [3].

To achieve a more stable mode of operation, in modern instruments the heating current for the filament is *emission-controlled*, i.e., the current of the electron trap is used to keep emission comparatively independent from actual ion source conditions. Typical emission currents are in the range of 50–400 μA.

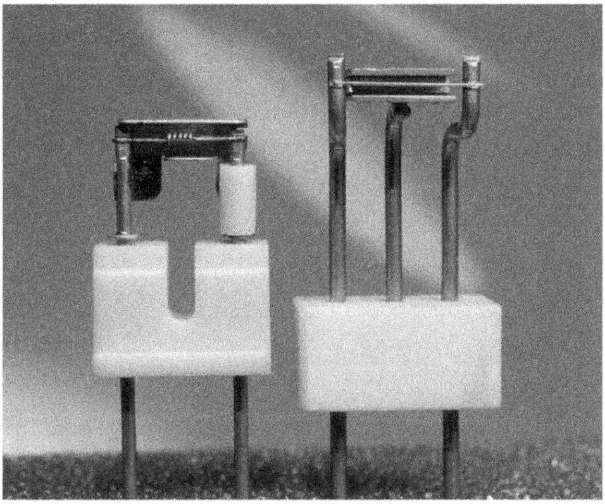

Fig. 5.3 Filaments for EI/CI ion sources. A coiled filament of the VG ZAB-2F (*left*) and a straight wire filament of the JEOL JMS-700 (*right*). The shields behind the filament are at the same potential as the wire itself and the white parts are made of ceramics for insulation

Filament lifetime
The lifetime of a filament is several weeks under proper operating conditions. However, this may become drastically shortened by the harsh conditions of aggressive analytes or reagent gases in chemical ionization, too high emission current, and in particular sudden breakdown of the high vacuum.

5.1.3 Overall Efficiency and Sensitivity of an EI Ion Source

The overall efficiency of an EI ion source depends on the intrinsic properties of the ionization process, the ion source design, and the actual operation parameters. The most astonishing fact is the extremely low ionization probability for a neutral entering the ion source. Only a minor fraction of the sample introduced becomes ionized, whereas the vast majority gets lost via the vacuum pumps. This is due to the disadvantageous combination of long mean free paths for ions and electrons and the low collision cross section of the electron itself. Remember, the path through the effective ionization volume is merely about 1 mm long. Nonetheless, EI provides high sensitivity as compared to other ionization methods.

In 70 eV EI mode, modern magnetic sector instruments are specified to have a sensitivity of about 4×10^{-7} C μg^{-1} for the molecular ion of methylstearate, *m/z* 298, at $R = 1000$. The charge of 4×10^{-7} C corresponds to 2.5×10^{12} electron charges. One microgram of methylstearate is equivalent to 3.4×10^{-9} mol or 2.0×10^{15} molecules. For a molecule entering the ionization volume one therefore calculates a chance of 1:800 to become ionized and to reach the detector as a molecular ion. The fraction of the neutrals that become ionized is definitely larger, maybe 1:100, because a significant fraction of them will dissociate to form fragment ions of other *m/z* values. Even then, a ratio of about 1:100 indicates an almost perfect ion source design as compared to $1{:}10^4$–10^5 in the 1970s. (For a comparison of EI to other ionization methods refer to Sect. 8.8.1.)

5.1.4 Optimization of Ion Beam Geometry

The extraction of ions and the shape of the ion beam can largely be improved if the acceleration voltage is applied in two or more successive stages instead of a single stage. In addition, by dividing the plates into an upper and a lower half or a left and a right one, the ion beam can be directed up and down or adjusted from right to left, respectively, by applying slightly different voltages to the corresponding halves (Figs. 5.1 and 5.2). This also allows for focusing of the ion beam.

In practice, the ion optical properties of an ion source are optimized by means of ion trajectory calculations. [13]. The standard tool for this task is the SIMION

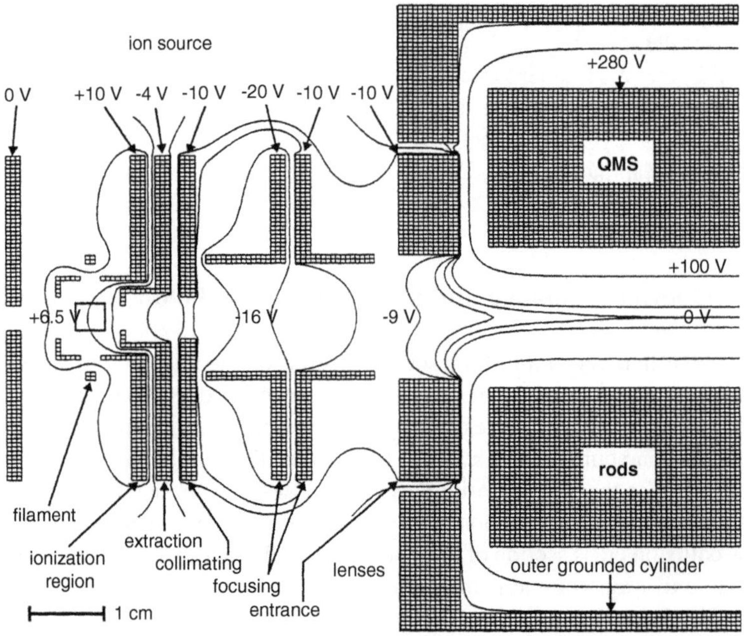

Fig. 5.4 The EI ion source of a quadrupole mass spectrometer with equipotentials as calculated by the computer simulation program SIMION three-dimensional version 6.0 (Reproduced from Ref. [15] with permission. © Elsevier Science, 1998)

software suite [14–17], while there are others, too [18]. Thus one can determine the optimum number, positions, voltages, and eventually shapes of the plates (Fig. 5.4). In order to compensate for slight mechanical deviations from theory and for effects exerted by contamination of the plates during elongated use, the voltages can be adjusted to yield optimum conditions.

Tuning the ion source

Usually, some *tuning* of the instrument is performed before actually starting measurements. Such a tuning procedure mainly means adjusting the voltages applied to the ion acceleration lenses of the ion source and eventually of some additional components of the ion optical system. Modern instruments may offer automatic tuning routines that are often faster and even more thorough than routine manual tuning would be. In any case, a reasonable mass spectrometer data system will also allow for manual corrections.

5.1.5 Mounting the Ion Source

While ion sources were rather fragile units in the past, modern ion sources are generally of compact design. Many manufacturers have understood that quick and reliable exchange of ion sources is as important in daily routine operations as the performance characteristics of the source. Thus, sources tend to be mounted via some sort of plugging mechanism that allows to insert or remove the ion source without touching any of the connection leads. Sometimes, a special probe-like tool is provided for exchange of the ion source. Some instruments require venting before and evacuation after exchanging ion sources (Fig. 5.5), others may even offer a vacuum lock that not only serves for the direct insertion probe but also allows for exchanging ion sources or at least ion volumes. Exchange of an ion source may thus require 15–60 min depending on whether the vacuum needs to be broken or not.

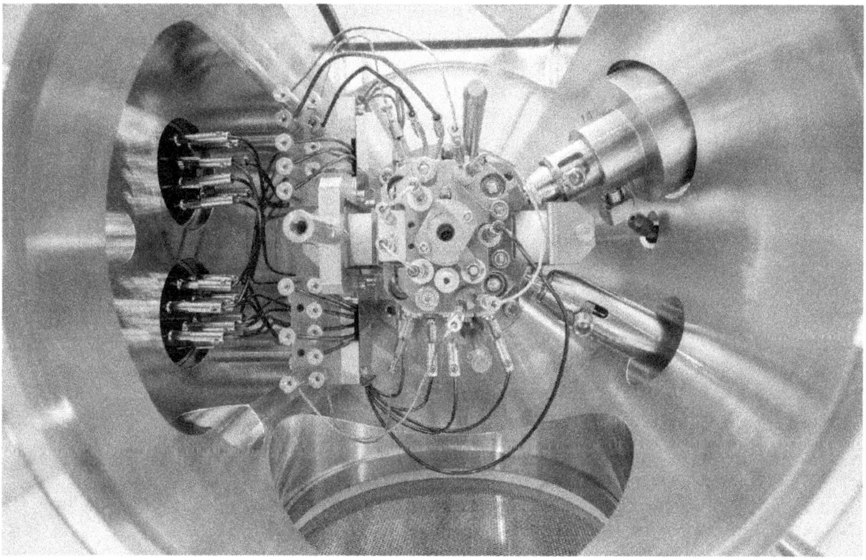

Fig. 5.5 An EI source mounted in the ion source housing of a JEOL AccuTOF GCx instrument. All voltages for operation are supplied via vacuum lead throughs from the left side. A connector to a gas chromatograph reaches down from the *upper right* while a connector to the reservoir inlet enters from the *lower right* side. Once the front cover plate bearing the vacuum lock has been mounted, a direct insertion probe can be introduced axially into the central notch of the ion source. The turbomolecular pump of the ion source housing is located directly below the protective wire mesh on the bottom

Nice to have
A window pane on top of the ion source housing allows to observe the probe during insertion, to locate an eventually lost sample vial, to roughly judge ion source contamination, and to check filament emission simply by observing whether it still shines brightly or remains dark.

5.2 Sample Introduction

For the purpose of sample introduction, any *sample introduction system* (also *sample inlet system* or *inlet*) can be employed that is suitable for the respective compound. Hence, *direct probes*, *reservoir inlets*, *gas chromatographs*, and even *liquid chromatographs* can be attached to an EI ion source. Which type of an inlet system is to be preferred depends on the type of sample to be analyzed. Whatever type the inlet system may be, it has to manage the same basic task, i.e., the transfer of the analyte from atmospheric conditions into the high vacuum of the EI ion source; Table 5.1 provides an overview.

Not for EI only
The below-mentioned sample introduction systems (reservoir inlets, various direct insertion probes, and chromatographs) are of equal importance to other ionization methods.

Table 5.1 Sample introduction systems for EI-MS

Inlet system	Principle	Analytes
Reservoir/ reference inlet	Heated reservoir with sample vapor	Low to medium boiling liquids
Direct insertion probe, DIP	Sample in heated/cooled glass/ metal vial as particles or film of analyte	Solids, waxes or high-boiling liquids
Direct exposure probe, DEP	Sample particles or film of analyte on resistively heated metal filament	Solids of extremely low volatility, especially if thermally labile
Gas chromatograph, GC	Elutes directly into ion source	Volatile components of mixtures
Liquid chromatograph, LC	Connected via particle beam interface	Analytes suitable for EI that cannot be separated by GC due to high polarity

5.2.1 Reservoir or Reference Inlet System

Highly volatile samples cannot be introduced into the ion source by means of a direct insertion probe even when cooling is applied. A *reference inlet system* or *reservoir inlet system* is better suited for that purpose [19]. The name of this type of inlet has been coined by the fact that reference inlets have been intended – and often are used for – the introduction of a mass calibrant (or *reference*) independent of the analyte in order to achieve internal mass calibration in accurate mass measurements (Sect. 3.6). Fluorocarbons such as *perfluorotributylamine* (PFTBA, aka FC43) or *perfluorokerosene* (PFK) can be admitted to the ion source via the reservoir inlet.

Reference/reservoir inlets serve equally well for the analysis of gases, solvents, and similar volatile samples. They are especially convenient when a continuous signal is desired for instrument tuning or long-lasting MS/MS experiments in ion chemistry. In addition, the components of a mixture are admitted to the ion source without fractionation, i.e., without affecting their partial pressures. Due to this property, reservoir inlets have extensively been used in the petroleum industry.

Typically, reference inlets are filled with a few microliters of liquid sample by means of a microliter syringe. Heating is applied to suppress adsorption of the analytes to the walls, and thus, to speed up the final removal of sample. As the analyte is exposed to prolonged heating, the application of reference inlet systems should be restricted to thermally stable analytes.

Basic components and features of a reference inlet system comprise (Fig. 5.6):

- Vessel of 30–100 ml that can be constantly heated to 80–200 °C.
- Access via a septum port or similar kind of injector.
- Connection to the ion source via a toggle valve (on/off) and a needle valve to adjust the partial pressure in the ion source housing.
- Roughing port to remove the sample after completion of the measurement by evacuation into a rotary or membrane pump.

Special reservoir types

To reduce the risks of catalytic degradation and selective adsorption of components of mixtures on the walls of the reservoir, an *all-glass heated inlet system* (AGHIS) [20, 21] and a teflon-coated reservoir inlet system have been commercially available as an alternative to stainless steel systems. To this end, *dynamic batch inlet systems* (DBIS) have been developed, where the analyte is transferred from the reservoir into the ion source by means of a capillary and where a carrier gas (H_2, He) can be used to reduce fractionation of mixtures having an extremely wide range of boiling points [21]. The *liquid introduction system* represents another variation of reservoir inlets where a few microliters of liquid are introduced by means of a kind of "micro DIP" [22].

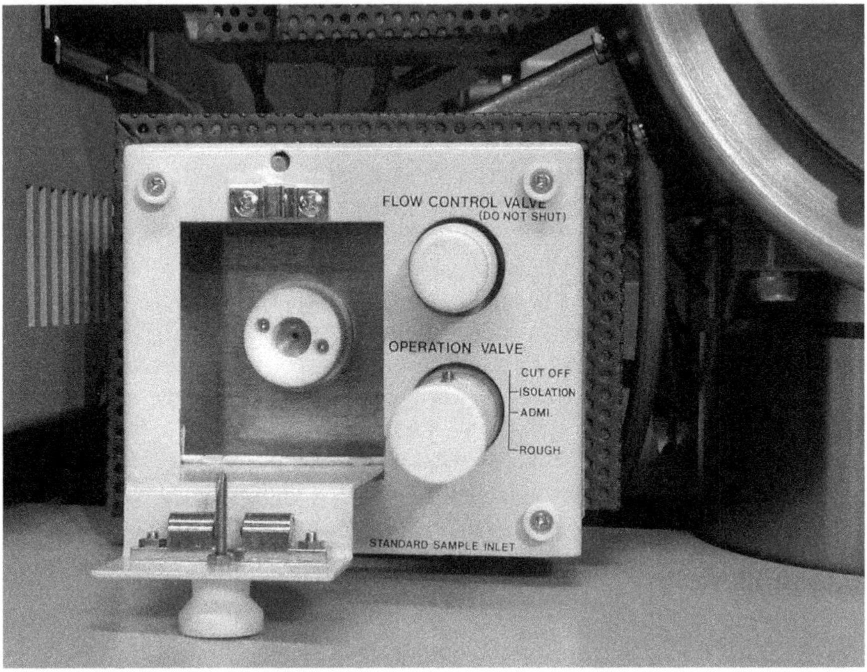

Fig. 5.6 Reservoir inlet of a JEOL JMS-700 sector instrument with the septum injection port opened. The "operation valve" switches between evacuation, isolation, and admission of the sample; a needle valve allows regulation of the sample flow. The GC transfer line crosses in the upper background from the GC (*left*) to the ion source housing (*upper right*)

5.2.2 Direct Insertion Probe

In early-day instrumentation, the introduction of solid samples into a mass spectrometer was performed by directly placing them inside the ion source, which was then mounted into the ion source housing, pumped down, and heated [23]. Obviously, exchanging the ion source for each run is laborious and too slow for routine work. A more convenient procedure is to use a micro *sample vial* or *crucible* containing some 0.1–2 µg of the analyte that can be directly applied close to the ion source by means of a *direct insertion probe* (DIP) or *direct inlet probe* (also DIP, Fig. 5.7). DIPs have been devised from the late 1950s and were in common use by the mid-1960s [24–26].

A DIP consists of a stainless steel shaft with a tip suitable to insert the sample vial. The shaft is polished to allow installation an effective vacuum seal against the O-rings of a vacuum lock. Being transferred into the high vacuum of the ion source housing through the *vacuum lock* [26], the probe is pushed in, eventually until it contacts the ion source block (Figs. 5.8 and 5.9). Spectra are then acquired while the analyte evaporates or sublimes from the vial directly into the ionization volume of

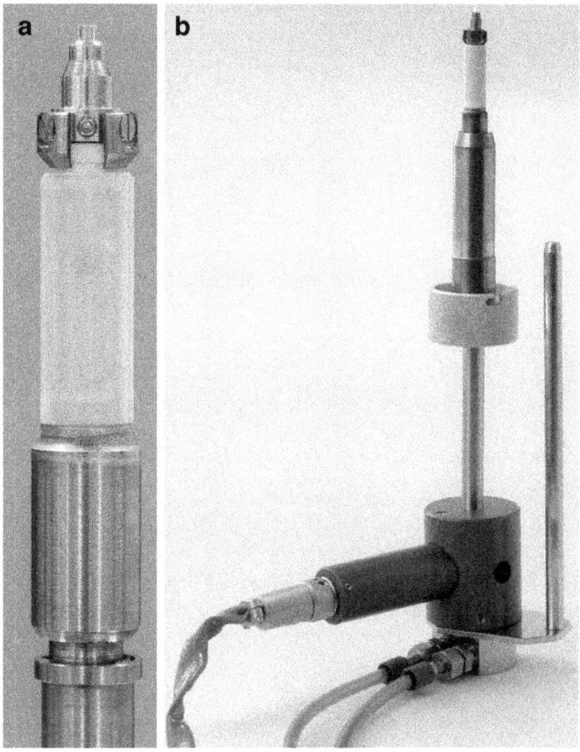

Fig. 5.7 Direct insertion probe (DIP) for use with EI, chemical ionization (CI), and field ionization (FI). (**a**) The copper probe tip holds the glass sample vial and is fitted to a temperature-controlled heater. The heater, a thermocouple, and cooling are provided inside. The (*white*) ceramics insulator protects the operator from the high voltage of the ion source. (**b**) Entire DIP of a JEOL JMS-700 equipped with water cooling

the ion source. Typically, the sample holder can be heated up to about 500 °C can be applied to enforce evaporation of the sample, which sometimes is accompanied by decomposition prior to evaporation. Special high-temperature probes reaching up to 1000 °C are also available. Modern direct probes have *temperature programed heaters* [27] allowing to set rates of 5–150 °C min^{-1} or are equipped with *ion current-controlled heaters* [28].

To prevent more volatile samples from suddenly evaporating a circulation watercooling is often incorporated in the DIP, and refrigerated probes for more volatile samples have also been developed [29]. Sometimes, glass wool is placed into the sample vial to increase the surface for adsorption, and thus to slow down evaporation of the sample; aluminum oxide and silica are also being used for this purpose [30]. Sudden evaporation causes distorted spectra and may even result in a temporary breakdown of the high vacuum.

5.2.3 Sample Vials for Use with Direct Insertion Probes

Sample vials for use with DIPs usually are about 2 mm in outer diameter and 10–20 mm in length. They are made from borosilicate glass or aluminum (Fig. 5.10). In general, the vials are disposed after use. However, although bearing

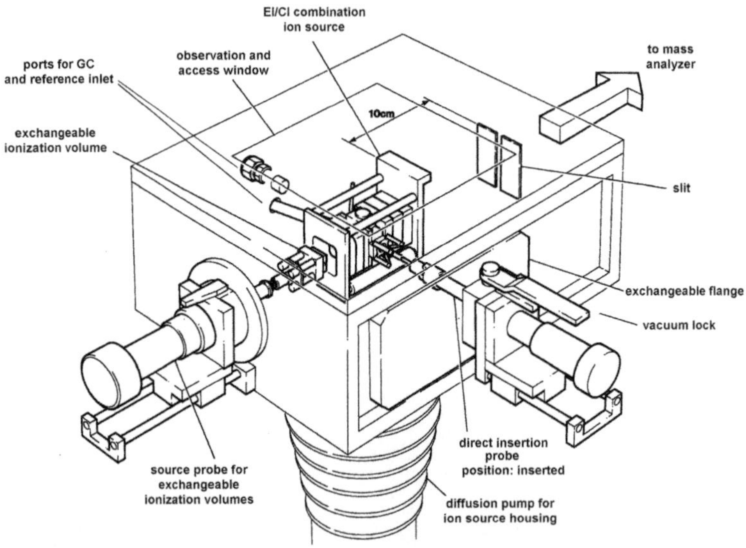

Fig. 5.8 Ion source housing of a Waters Micromass Autospec™ magnetic sector instrument. The ion source can be accessed from several directions to allow for simultaneous connection to DIP/DEP, GC and reference inlet system (By courtesy of Waters Corporation, MS Technologies, Manchester, UK)

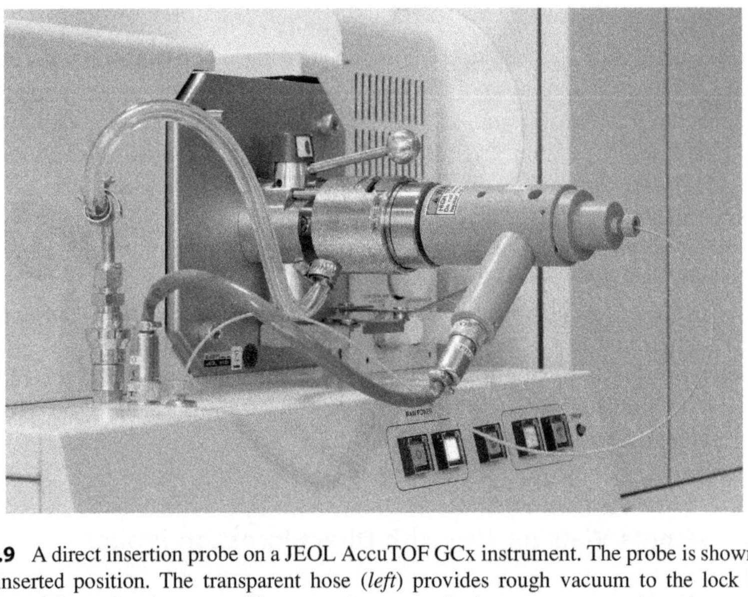

Fig. 5.9 A direct insertion probe on a JEOL AccuTOF GCx instrument. The probe is shown in its fully inserted position. The transparent hose (*left*) provides rough vacuum to the lock before insertion of the probe, the *gray* cable connection serves for heater power supply and temperature control, and the *light brown* capillary delivers pressurized gas for cooling the probe tip if required

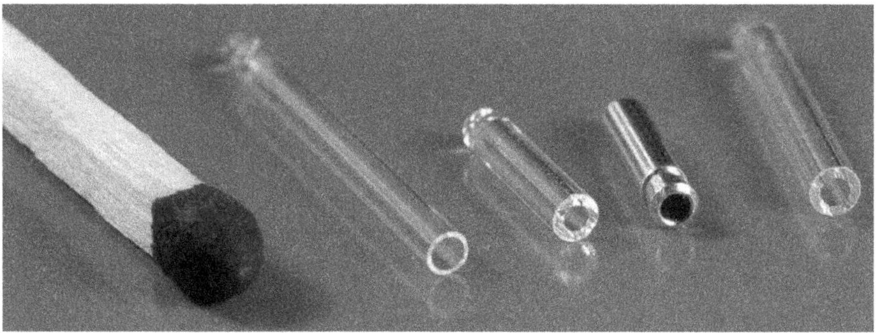

Fig. 5.10 Sample vials for different DIPs. From *left*: VG ZAB-2F, Finnigan TSQ700 glass and aluminum version, and JEOL JMS-700. The match illustrates the scale

the risk of memory effects or adsorption of analyte to residual pyrolysis products from previous samples, reusable quartz vials have also been employed in the past. The analyte may either be loaded in solution into the vial or as a tiny piece if solid or waxy (Fig. 5.11). Using solutions of known concentration allows for more reproducible loading of the vials which in other cases is not a prerequisite. The solvent should then be evaporated before insertion of the probe into the vacuum lock.

Disposable vials preferred
Disposable vials are devoid of memory effects. Glass vials bear the additional advantage of revealing the amount and position of sample within the vial. Afterwards, it is also possible that the analyte decomposes during the measurement yielding a black residue.

5.2.4 How to Run a Measurement with a Direct Insertion Probe

Direct insertion probes are suitable for use with electron ionization (EI), chemical ionization (CI, Chap. 7) and field ionization (FI, Sect. 8.5) as these methods require the introduction of gaseous sample into the ionization chamber of the respective ionization source.

The sample may either be loaded into the sample vial as a solid or from dilute solution. When a solid sample is provided, it is normally best to gently dip a fine needle or pin into the sample or to scratch some tiny crystals off the wall of the sample tube. An amount just visible with the bare eye is usually more than enough. The sample is then transferred into the sample vial, which is preferably fixed in a suitable holder. In case of a sample solution, one may either dip a pin into the solution to transfer a very small drop or one could use the smallest size of a microliter pipette, e.g., 0.5–10 μl tips. It is important to allow for the majority of

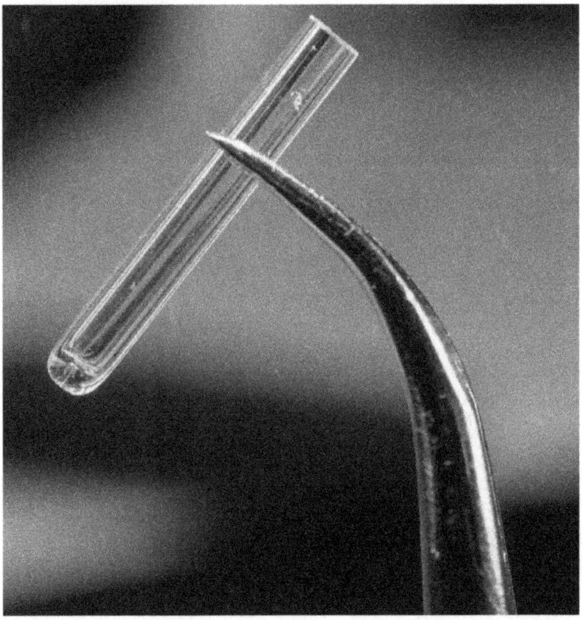

Fig. 5.11 Sample vial loaded with some analyte. The bright *yellow* speck halfway between the tip of the tweezers and upper rim of the vial is the solid material to be analyzed. Actually, this amount of sample is already in excess of what is ideally needed. The use of an additional amount of sample does not bear any advantage; rather, it may cause long-lasting ion source contamination

the solvent to evaporate leaving a film of the sample before inserting the probe. Otherwise, the drop will boil suddenly upon roughing, and thus, will spill the sample solution into the vacuum lock.

To start the measurement, the sample vial is mounted to the probe tip. Make sure that the tip has cooled down close to room temperature before placing the sample vial into the probe tip. The probe tip is generally equipped with some clipping or screwing mechanism to secure the vial in position. Losing the sample vial during transfer inside the vacuum lock can block the lock valve, result in air leaks from scratches or cause other damages. Dropping the vial inside the source housing may require venting and its removal prior to further operation or at least result in waiting time until the sample has evaporated to avoid superimposition of spectra. As any operator might use a vial once in a while, the rotor of the turbomolecular pump is protected from particle impact by a fine wire mesh cover (Fig. 5.5).

Preferably, the probe tip is cooled during insertion to prevent untimely evaporation of the analyte. Heating of the probe tip is only started when data acquisition is running. Typically, the probe tip is heated at a rate of 20–100 °C min^{-1} depending on sample volatility, and of course, on the scan speed of the mass spectrometer. Volatile sample will quickly evaporate during the first few seconds of a run, while "die-hards" can require heating to > 400 °C. After completion of the data acquisition, it is generally recommended to cool down the probe tip to < 100 °C before retracting it into the vacuum lock in order to avoid heat damages of the O-rings.

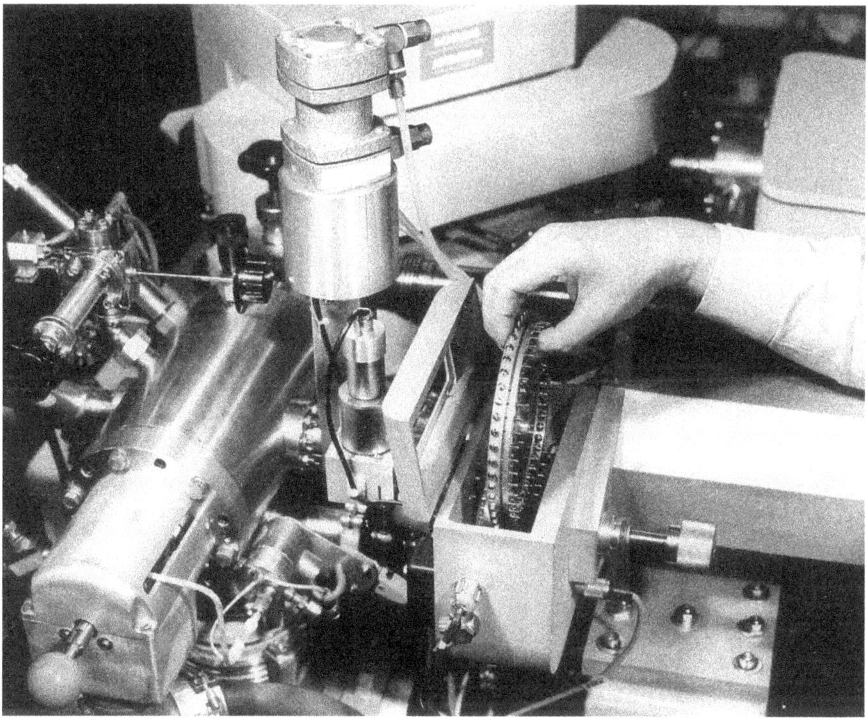

Fig. 5.12 Finnigan MAT AUDEVAP system where the turret wheel with 46 crucibles is being inserted into its housing. The probe mechanism is to the *right*, the vacuum lock and the ion source housing to the *left*. The mass spectrometer may either be a Finnigan MAT 212 or MAT 311 double-focusing sector instrument of BE geometry (Reproduced from Finnigan MAT technical documentation by courtesy of Thermo Fisher Scientific)

5.2.5 Automated Direct Insertion Probes

The first DIP for automated operation was presented in 1979 [31]. In 1982, with the Finnigan MAT AUDEVAP, a commercially available system appeared. It made use of a sample turret that could accommodate up to 46 aluminum crucibles. The probe would then pick up a crucible from the turret and move on through a vacuum lock (Fig. 5.12). Alternatively, the device could pick up DCI sample holders (Sect. 5.2.7) or even target tips for fast atom bombardment (FAB, Sect. 10.3). The AUDEVAP was designed to complete sample runs including data acquisition. Later, it was even possible to set up a system that performed internal mass calibration and formula assignment under data system control [32]. Worldwide, a few AUDEVAP systems are still in operation.

A modern and much more compact automated direct inlet probe is provided by Scientific Instruments Manufacturer (SIM). The SIM probe has a small diameter and is inserted into the ion source housing via a lock mechanism of very low dead

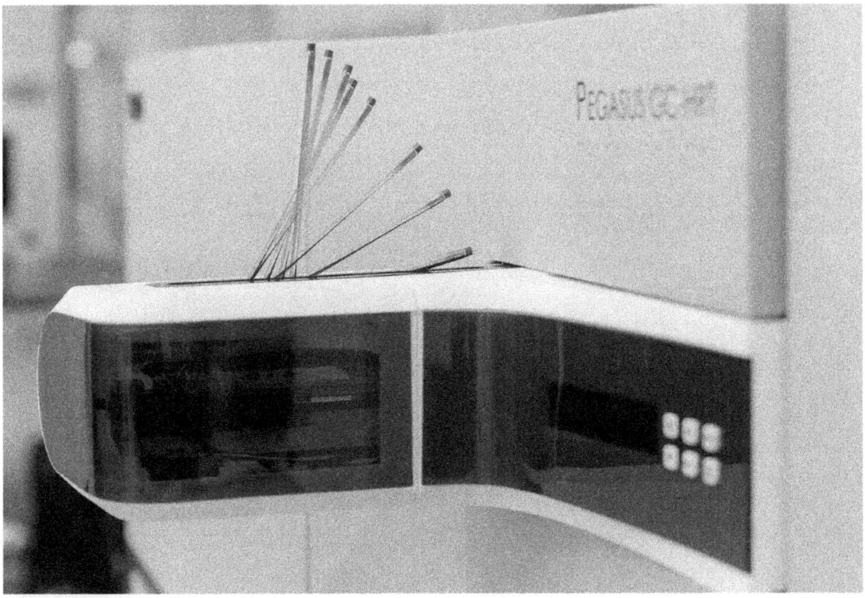

Fig. 5.13 Automated DIP in operation as visualized by multiple exposures. After having received the sample vial in vertical orientation, the rod is driven to the left and tilted downward for insertion through the lock. The photograph shows the SIM DIP mounted to a LECO Pegasus GC-HRT instrument

volume, thus permitting to quickly insert the probe even without prior evacuation of the vacuum lock (Fig. 5.13). The probes can either be loaded manually or be run in combination with an autosampler. The autosampler may either be employed to exchange filled sample vials on the DIP or pipette microliter volumes of liquid samples or solutions, respectively, into a vial at the probe tip. DIPs by SIM are custom-built for several instrument suppliers such as Agilent and LECO.

5.2.6 Fractionation When Using Direct Insertion Probes

The evaporation process out of the sample vial causes a certain degree of sample fractionation that can often be recognized from the *total ion chromatogram* (TIC) alone. Employing *reconstructed ion chromatograms* (RICs) in addition presents a valuable tool in identifying components of a simple mixture and in assigning their corresponding mass spectra. Generally, residual solvent is observed during the first few scans, while all other components appear more or less in order of increasing molecular weight as evaporation progresses.

Observing evaporation from a DIP The TIC of an EI measurement using a DIP already revealed ion formation during the first scans. After some period of relatively low TIC, heating of the DIP to about 200 °C finally led to evaporation of the

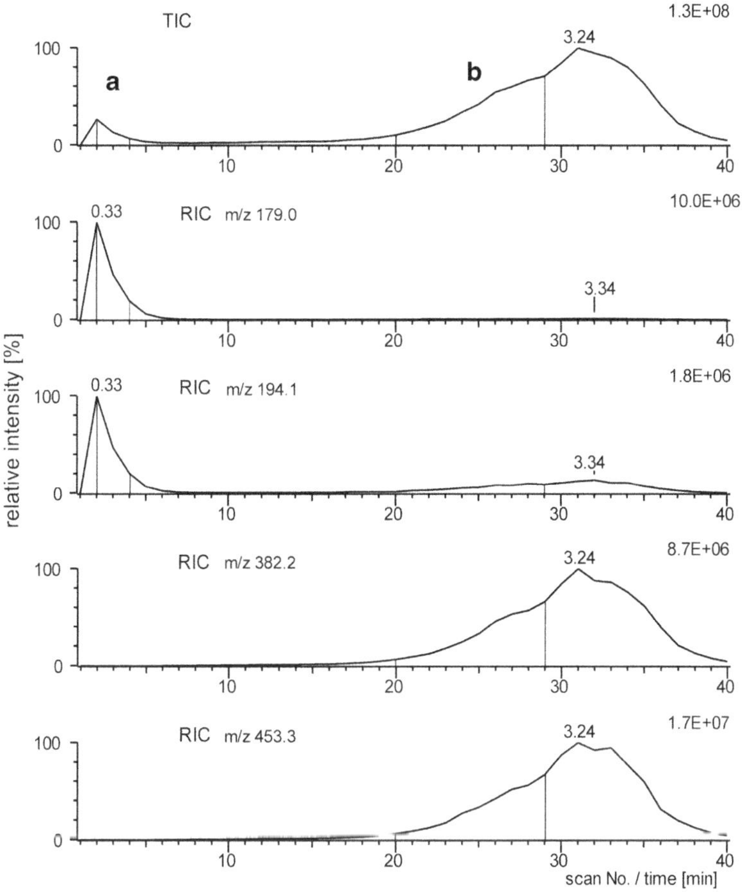

Fig. 5.14 Ion chromatograms from a DIP measurement. The TIC (*upper trace*) shows a bump during early scans that is also reflected in the RICs of *m/z* 179.0 and 194.1. Spectrum (**a**) corresponds to volatile impurities, whereas the RICs of *m/z* 382.2 and 453.3 are related to the target compound (**b**) that evaporates upon heating (cf. Fig. 5.15) (By courtesy of R. Gleiter, Organisch-Chemisches Institut, Universität Heidelberg)

major fraction of the sample, and thus produced a steeply rising TIC (Fig. 5.14). The TIC decreased again as all sample had evaporated. Thus, two different spectra were extracted from the data. The first was obtained by averaging scans 2–4, the second by averaging scans 20–29 (Fig. 5.15). Spectrum (**a**) corresponds to some impurities, whereas spectrum (**b**) represents the target compound, $C_{28}H_{47}NSi_2$.

Using RICs, the ions belonging to the same component can readily be identified from their parallel dependence in time (Fig. 5.14). The increase of the signal at *m/z* 194 in the chromatogram during late scans results from the presence of a minor signal at *m/z* 194 in the mass spectrum of the target compound. (More examples for the use of RICs are presented in Chap. 14.)

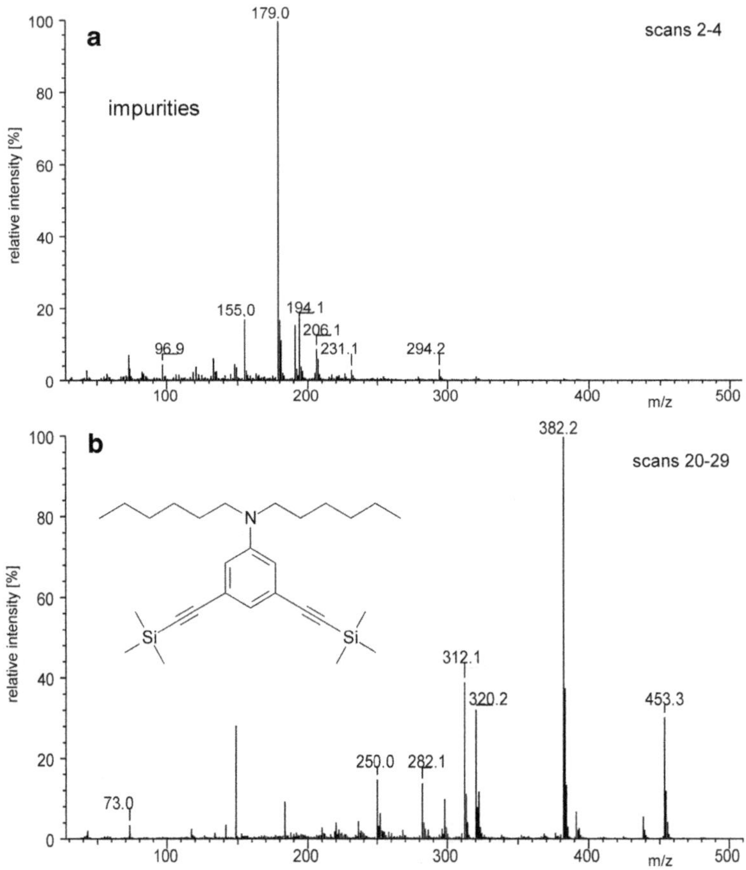

Fig. 5.15 Two EI mass spectra from the same sample. The spectrum obtained from scans 2–4 corresponds to some volatile impurities (**a**), the spectrum from scans 20–29 (**b**) represents the target compound (cf. TIC and RICs in Fig. 5.14) (By courtesy of R. Gleiter, Organisch-Chemisches Institut, Universität Heidelberg)

5.2.7 Direct Exposure Probe

Employing a *direct exposure probe* (DEP) may be helpful in case of analytes that cannot be evaporated from a sample vial without complete decomposition [33]. Here, the analyte is applied from solution or suspension to the outside of a thin wire loop or pin which is then directly exposed to the ionizing electron beam. This method has also been termed *in-beam* electron ionization. Early work describing the direct exposure of a sample to the electron beam came from Ohashi [34, 35], Constantin, [36] and Traldi [37, 38]. The idea behind the rapid heating of a DEP is to achieve evaporation faster than thermal degradation of the sample [39, 40]. This principle is realized in perfection with *energy-sudden* methods (Chaps. 10 and 11).

If the analyte is exposed to energetic electrons the method is called *direct electron ionization* (DEI) or *desorption electron ionization* (DEI), and accordingly it is termed *direct* or *desorption chemical ionization* (DCI) if the analyte is immersed in the reagent gas under conditions of chemical ionization (Chap. 7).

There are different types of DEPs in that some of them rely on the heated tip of a modified DIP [38], and others – widespread in use – that are capable of rapid resistive heating of a small loop made of chemically inert metal wire (rhenium). Resistively heated probes allow rates of several hundred °C s^{-1} and temperatures up to about 1500 °C (Fig. 5.16). As a consequence of rapid heating, fast scanning, e.g., 1 s per scan over the *m*/*z* range of interest, is required to follow the evaporation of the analyte. In either case, the use of a DEP allows to extend the temperature range for evaporation. In addition, it reduces thermal degradation as a result of heating the analyte faster than its thermal decomposition usually proceeds, and therefore expands the range of applications for EI and CI to some extent. In any case, employing direct exposure probes is by far no alternative to real desorption ionization methods [41, 42].

Application of DEI

The DEI technique has been applied to obtain mass spectra of four nonderivatized amino acids [38]. The method allowed for the observation of molecular ions and some primary fragment ions in contrast to conventional EI conditions which do not yield molecular ions. However, these additional signals are comparatively weak (Fig. 5.17).

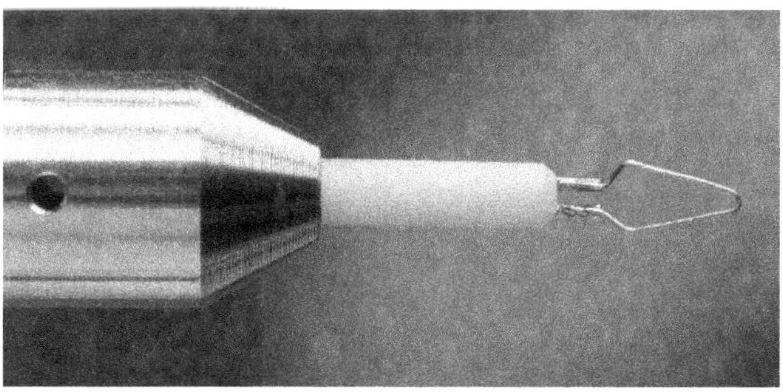

Fig. 5.16 Tip of a direct exposure probe of a GC-oaTOF mass spectrometer for EI and CI (By courtesy of Waters Corporation, MS Technologies, Manchester, UK)

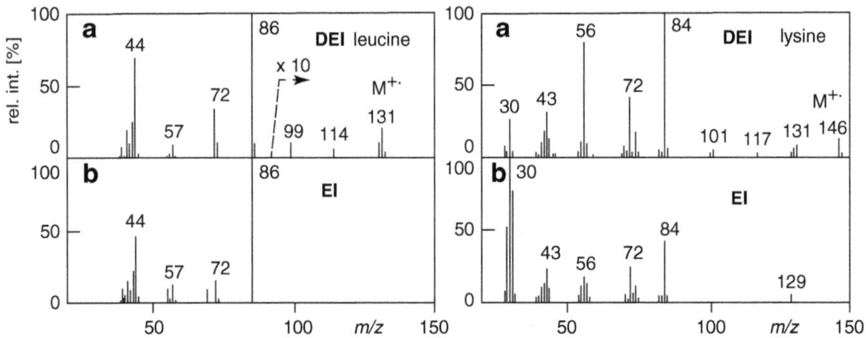

Fig. 5.17 Comparison of DEI (*upper*) and EI spectra (*lower*) of the amino acids leucine and lysine. In the leucine DEI spectrum the intensities above *m/z* 90 are shown in tenfold expansion (Adapted from Ref. [38] with permission. © John Wiley & Sons, 1982)

5.3 Pyrolysis Mass Spectrometry

The enormous temperatures attained on resistively heated sample holders can also be used to intentionally enforce the decomposition of nonvolatile samples, thereby yielding characteristic pyrolysis products. *Pyrolysis mass spectrometry* (Py-MS) can be applied to synthetic polymers [43], fossil biomaterial [44], food [45], and soil [46] analysis and even to characterize whole bacteria [47]. In polymer analysis, for example, Py-MS does of course not yield molecular weight distributions, though the type of polymer and the monomer units it is based on can usually be identified by Py-MS [43, 48]. Often, pyrolysis products are not directly introduced into the ion source but separated by GC beforehand. A detailed treatment of this branch of mass spectrometry is beyond the scope of the present book.

5.4 Gas Chromatograph

Gas chromatography (GC) provides the means for separation of volatile analytes in complex mixtures. GC eluting directly into the ion source of a mass spectrometer is called *GC-MS coupling* [49–51]. Capillary GC columns provide gas flow rates in the order of a few milliliters per minute, and therefore, their back end can be directly fitted into the entrance of the ion volume. In fact, the nano-LC-EI interface described in the next section is inspired by the standard direct coupling of capillary columns into EI ion sources.

EI is ideally suited as an ionization method for GC-MS applications. The specific properties of GC-MS are discussed later in more depth (Sect. 14.4). For the moment, it is sufficient to notice that proper coupling of a GC to an EI ion source neither exerts substantial effects on the EI process nor does it alter the fragmentation pathways of the ions.

5.5 Liquid Chromatograph

Chromatographic separation of polar analytes of low volatility can be performed by *liquid chromatography* (LC) prior to mass spectrometric analysis; such a setup is termed *LC-MS coupling*. Usually, atmospheric pressure ionization methods are employed when direct coupling of a liquid chromatograph to a mass spectrometer is required. However, it can be desirable to obtain EI spectra of LC-separated analytes or of dissolved analytes in general, e.g., when the analyte is only accessible by EI or when EI spectra are required for mass spectral database searches.

To this end, a simple and elegant solution makes use of very low flow rates as provided by nano-LC instrumentation [52, 53]. The flow from a fused silica column of 30 μm inner diameter is passed through a micro-nebulizer of just 5 μm inner diameter. The exit orifice of this nebulizer is slightly bent sideways into the ion source as to spray the droplets towards the opposite ion source wall (Fig. 5.18). A high ion source temperature of 200–300 °C serves to provide heat for solvent and analyte evaporation. An open source construction allows to keep the partial pressure of the solvent low inside the ionization volume, and thus, suppresses $[M+H]^+$ ion formation that would otherwise deteriorate the EI character of the spectra. As gas flow rates due to solvent vaporization are similar to flow rates of capillary GC,

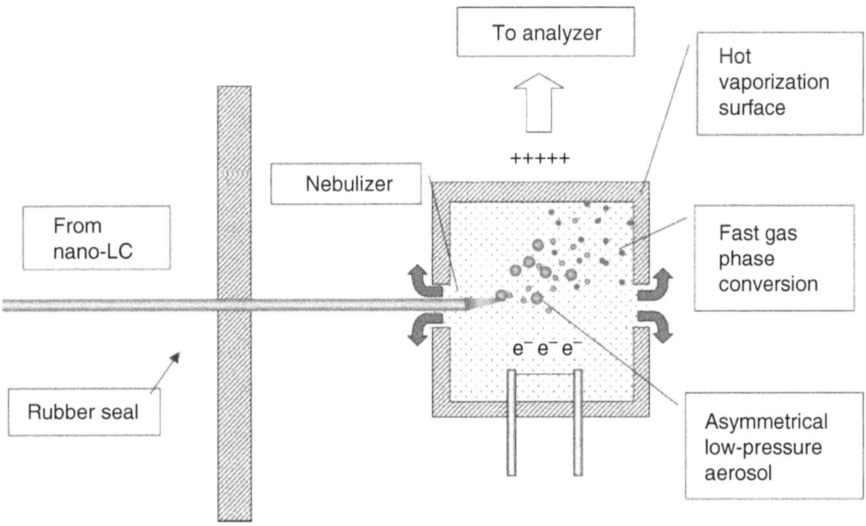

Fig. 5.18 Nano-LC-EI interface with direct connection of the LC capillary to a slightly modified EI ion source (Reproduced from Ref. [53] with permission. © Wiley Periodicals, Inc., 2005)

the nano-LC liquid flow of less than 1 μl min^{-1} can easily be accommodated by most ion source vacuum systems.

5.6 Low-Energy Electron Ionization Mass Spectra

Low-energy primary electrons limit the excess energy deposited onto a molecular ion. Using 12–15 eV instead of 70 eV electrons still ionizes most compounds while disadvantageous fragmentations are reduced. Superior EI mass spectra of large hydrocarbons can be obtained [54], even more so if the ion source is operated at 70 °C instead of 200 °C (Fig. 5.19). The concept of recording *low-energy, low-temperature EI mass spectra* has been postulated long ago [55] and has been extensively investigated since then [56–58]. Low-energy, low-temperature mass spectra are much easier to interpret than their conventional 70 eV counterparts for several reasons:

- The relative intensity of the molecular ion peak is enhanced, thus permitting this important peak to be identified more easily.
- Less fragmentation also means a simpler overall appearance of the spectrum.
- The fragmentation pattern is dominated by a few characteristic primary fragmentations carrying the largest portion of structural information.

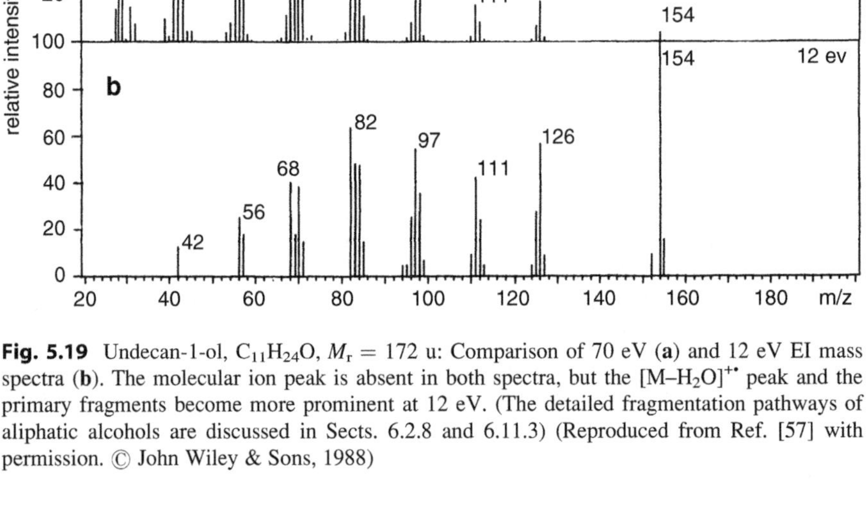

Fig. 5.19 Undecan-1-ol, $C_{11}H_{24}O$, M_r = 172 u: Comparison of 70 eV (**a**) and 12 eV EI mass spectra (**b**). The molecular ion peak is absent in both spectra, but the $[M–H_2O]^{+•}$ peak and the primary fragments become more prominent at 12 eV. (The detailed fragmentation pathways of aliphatic alcohols are discussed in Sects. 6.2.8 and 6.11.3) (Reproduced from Ref. [57] with permission. © John Wiley & Sons, 1988)

Unfortunately, there are also some disadvantages:

- The decreased ionization efficiency at 12–15 eV goes along with a significant loss of sensitivity (Sect. 2.3).
- Low ion source temperatures cause long-lasting "memory" of previous samples due to slow desorption from the surfaces that have been in contact with the sample vapor.
- A weak molecular ion peak may well be enhanced. However, a spectrum showing no molecular ion peak at 70 eV will not turn into a spectrum exhibiting a strong molecular ion peak at 12 eV.

Nonetheless, during the first decades of analytical mass spectrometry, low-energy EI spectra were the only way to minimize fragmentation, and thereby to increase the relative intensity of a weak molecular ion peak. Nowadays, EI mass spectra are preferably complemented with spectra obtained from so-called *soft ionization methods* (Chaps. 7, 8, 10, 11, 12, and 13).

Bad memories
Signals from previous samples in the mass spectrum of the actual analyte are usually termed *memory*. Memory is caused by contamination of ion source or sample introduction system. To reduce memory one should use the lowest amount of sample necessary to produce good spectra, keep the ion source around 200 °C, and allow some pumping between measurements.

5.7 Analytes for EI

Classical organic chemistry provides a wide variety of potential analytes for electron ionization, the only limitation being that the analyte should be able to evaporate or sublime without significant thermal decomposition. These requirements are usually met by saturated and unsaturated aliphatic and aromatic hydrocarbons and their derivatives such as halides, ethers, acids, esters, amines, amides etc. Heterocycles generally yield useful EI spectra, and flavones, steroids, terpenes and comparable compounds can successfully be analyzed by EI, too. Therefore, EI represents *the standard method* for such kinds of samples.

GC-EI-MS can be used for the direct analysis of mixtures, e.g., to analyze synthetic by-products; an advantage that made GC-EI-MS benchtop instruments become widespread in modern synthetic laboratories. The GC-EI-MS combination is especially successful in monitoring environmental pollutants such as polycyclic aromatic hydrocarbons (PAHs), polychlorinated biphenyls (PCBs), polychlorinated dibenzodioxins (PCDDs), polychlorinated dibenzofuranes (PCDFs), or other volatile organic compounds (VOCs).

While low- and medium-polarity analytes are usually well suited for EI, highly polar or even ionic compounds, e.g., diols or polyalcohols, amino acids, nucleosides, peptides, sugars, and organic salts should not be subjected to EI unless properly derivatized prior to EI-MS [59–64].

There is – as with any other ionization method – no strict upper limit for molecular mass, a range of up to 800 u being a realistic estimate. There are exceptions of up to 1300 u if the analyte is extremely nonpolar, like molecules having several fluoroalkyl or trialkylsilyl groups that significantly reduce polarity while increasing their mass.

5.8 Mass Analyzers for EI

In case of EI, there is no restriction as to the type of mass analyzer (Chap. 4). Magnetic sector instruments used to dominate EI applications in the early days of mass spectrometry. With the growing number of GC-MS applications, single quadrupole instruments became more popular because of significantly higher scan speeds and reduced cost. The demand for improved analytical selectivity via MS/MS approaches favored the use of triple quadrupole instruments and (linear) quadrupole ion traps. In recent years, accurate mass measurements have gained new interest thereby increasing the demand for magnetic sector analyzers and even more so for high-resolving oaTOF instruments. In principle, FT-ICR analyzers can be used in conjunction with EI, but rarely are because of their high cost. Recently, an Orbitrap-GC combination has also become commercially available.

5.9 Mass Spectral Databases for EI

EI mass spectra are excellently reproducible when measured under standard conditions (70 eV, ion source at 150–250 °C, pressure in the order of 10^{-4} Pa). This is not only the case for repeated measurements on the same instrument, but also between different types and brands of mass spectrometers. Large EI mass spectral libraries exist in either printed [65–67] or digitized form [68]. The most comprehensive EI mass spectral databases are the NIST/EPA/NIH Mass Spectral Database and the Wiley/NBS Mass Spectral Database [69–72].

Searching for a mass spectrum of an unknown substance in a mass spectral database often very quickly identifies the unknown, provided the corresponding spectrum is already available in the database. However, even if this is not case, the search might deliver similar spectra of closely related compounds, thus facilitating structure elucidation [73].

The obvious approach of comparing a mass spectrum of an unknown with a library spectrum is termed *forward library search* [74]. Normally, only a subset of the measured spectrum, i.e., a set of signals having intensities above a threshold value or a set of signals as defined by user input, is used to search the database. Database spectra closely matching that of the unknown are then displayed with a points score to judge the probability of the respective hit. In a so-called *reverse library search*, a library spectrum is compared to the mass spectra of unknowns in a way disregarding all peaks of the unknown's spectrum that are absent in the library spectrum. This prevents a misled search by background signals that might derive from column bleed, impurities, residual solvent, or memory.

5.9.1 NIST/EPA/NIH Mass Spectral Database

The 2014 version of the NIST/EPA/NIH Mass Spectral Database [69, 75] contains about 276,000 EI spectra of more than 242,000 compounds plus roughly 34,000 replicate spectra. For almost 83,000 compounds there is a compilation of 386,000 *Kovats retention index* (KRI) values as determined on nonpolar and polar columns. Since 2005, this database also offers CID spectra, which actually sum up to 193,000 spectra of 44,000 precursor ions generated from about 8,300 different compounds. The reason for the larger number of spectra over the number of ions is the inclusion of multiple spectra for a given ionic species as obtained by skimmer-CID, and CID on triplequadrupole and quadrupole ion trap instruments, respectively [76]. The NIST/EPA/NIH Mass Spectral Database is available as a stand-alone solution and also with – most probably – any commercial mass spectrometer that can be equipped with an EI ion source.

Searching the NIST/EPA/NIH mass spectral database The NIST/EPA/NIH mass spectral database (Vers. 2.0, 2011) was searched for spectra corresponding to the molecular formula $C_6H_{13}N$ and twenty-five compounds were found. Figure 5.20 shows the screenshot where the spectrum of *N*-(1-methylethylidene)-2-propanamine was selected for display. The structural formula is included in the spectral plot, while compound name, formula, molecular weight, CAS number, a tabular listing of the peaks, and a (here truncated) collection of synonyms are presented in the text window. To a certain extent it is possible to customize the information to be displayed in a specified window and to adjust the formatting.

Built-in or stand-alone

EI mass spectral databases can optionally be included in the software package of mass spectrometers. Thus, the EI spectra measured are directly searchable in the database by similarity search typically yielding a list of several hits. Alternatively, stand-alone solutions allow for sophisticated search algorithms and strategies (Table 5.2) [77–79].

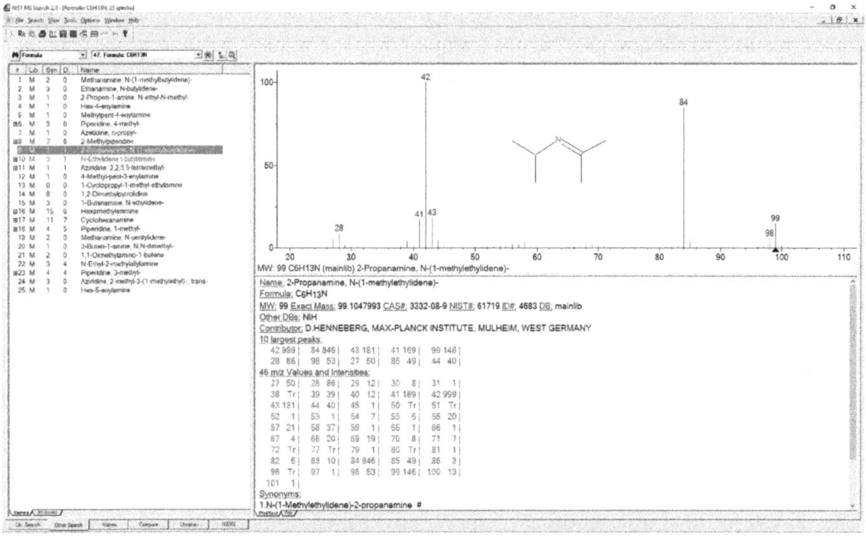

Fig. 5.20 Screenshot of NIST/EPA/NIH mass spectral database (V 2.0, 2011) after a formula search for spectra corresponding to $C_6H_{13}N$. Among 25 candidates, the spectrum of *N*-(1-methylethylidene)-2-propanamine has been selected for display. The database not only delivers the EI mass spectrum but also CAS number, contributor, listing, synonyms etc.

Table 5.2 Types of searches in the NIST/EPA/NIH Mass Spectral Database

Type of search	Explanation
Formula	Searches spectra corresponding to a chemical formula. Parentheses are resolved, e.g., $CH_3CH(C(CH_3)_3)_2$ is converted to $C_{10}H_{22}$. Constraints like name fragment or certain peaks can be selected
Molecular weight	Searches for spectra belonging to a defined molecular weight. Constraints like elements, required peaks etc. may be selected
Any peaks	A search based on a small number of peaks. Spectra can be searched using the largest peaks, or peaks in certain ranges of total intensity
Sequential search	Search through database for matches that satisfy the constraints selected by the user
CAS number	Search for compounds with specified CAS number
NIST number	The NIST number identifies a unique spectrum. Search used to retrieve such a spectrum for repeated examination
ID number	Each library spectrum has an additional identification number to correctly deal with user-edited spectra

5.9.2 Wiley Registry of Mass Spectral Data

The Wiley Registry of Mass Spectral Data dates back to the early 1960s when Stenhagen, Abrahamsson, and McLafferty started collecting mass spectra to be published in printed volumes of the Atlas of Mass Spectral Data in 1968 [65–67]. Different from the American Petroleum Institute's (API) spectral library, this project collected more spectra while applying lower restrictions to spectral quality. The reasoning behind that concept being that the probability to find a spectrum similar to that just measured in ones' own laboratory would be higher and that the spectrum of a similar compound may also provide useful guidance for the final elucidation of the unknown structure.

The Wiley Registry, 11th Edition as of 2014 contained more than 1.2 million spectra, about 943,000 chemical structures and EI spectra of 707,500 unique compounds. The Wiley Registry also provides tandem mass spectra of 45,298 ions. It may be obtained in a package combined with the NIST 2014 mass spectral data base and search software to provide the largest available general-purpose MS library.

In addition, specialty libraries for compound classes are available, e.g., the Mass Spectra of Pharmaceuticals and Agrochemicals by Kühnle, the Maurer/Pfleger/Weber Mass Spectral & GC Data of Drugs, Poisons, Pesticides, Pollutants, and their Metabolites or the Mass Spectra of Designer Drugs [80].

Searching for databases

There are several mass spectral databases available on the market today [80]. As collections and packages in the software world are subject to rapid changes, it is recommended to do a quick internet search for something like "EI mass spectral database" or "mass spectral library" to identify current options in this field.

5.9.3 Mass Spectral Databases: General Aspects

Although the coverage of these databases is enormous, and an easy-to-use interface is provided, one should be aware of potential pitfalls. The high score of a hit can be wrong, simply because the spectrum of the actual compound is still not included in database. A spectrum may be flawed by superimposition with some impurity peaks, which can in turn mislead the search. As a result, the unknown can generally not be perfectly identified by simple comparison with a library spectrum [75]. Nonetheless, mass spectral databases are highly useful, because even under unfavorable circumstances, they deliver spectra of similar compounds or isomers for comparison, or at least afford some characteristics of spectra of a compound class under investigation [73]. Ultimately, one should always cross check the hits from the database. Again: even the highest score hit can be wrong, so adequate interpretational skills are still indispensable (Chap. 6).

5.10 EI in a Nutshell

Basic Principle

Energetic electrons are capable of ionizing molecules in the (highly) dilute gas phase, i.e., in high vacuum. The process of *electron ionization* (EI) yields positive radical ions possessing rather high internal energy (Chap. 2). The initial molecular ion, $M^{+•}$, therefore tends to undergo numerous competing fragmentation reactions leading to fragment ions either by elimination of a radical or a molecule.

Hardness of Ionization

EI is generally considered a hard ionization method because it results in fragmentation of analyte molecular ions. The amount of fragmentation can be reduced by low-energy low-temperature techniques to some degree but it cannot be fully excluded. Soft ionization methods (Chaps. 7, 8, 10, 11, 12, and 13) are therefore recommended to complement EI mass spectral data.

Polarity

EI is a purely positive-ion method. The analyte can normally be detected by its molecular ions, $M^{+•}$, accompanied by numerous fragment ions thereof. Occasionally, $[M+H]^+$ ions can occur, in addition, by auto-protonation.

Analytes for EI

As EI requires gaseous samples for ionization, the analytes need to be volatile at least to some extent. EI can be employed for nonpolar to medium polar analytes. It is capable of analyzing molecules as small as hydrogen and up to about 800 u, in rare cases when low polarity and thermal stability are combined it may also work up to 1300 u. Nowadays, the use of EI is often restricted to smaller molecules of less than 600 u and to GC-MS applications.

Sample Introduction

Gases and liquids can directly be introduced by means of a reservoir inlet or after separation via a gas chromatograph. Solids are generally introduced using a direct insertion probe. Sufficient volatility provided, dilute solutions of solids can also be subjected to gas chromatography and analyzed by EI upon elution from the chromatographic column.

Instrumentation

Early on, EI-MS and MS in general employed magnetic sector analyzers. Later, upon commercial availability, linear quadrupole and quadrupole ion trap mass analyzers were frequently equipped with EI sources, especially for GC-MS applications due to their superior scan speed. During the last decade, oaTOF instruments, Q-TOF hybrids, and recently even Orbitrap analyzers have become available (mainly) for GC-MS as they combine fast spectral acquisition with the ability to deliver accurate mass data.

Accurate Mass

Due to stable and long-lasting ion currents, EI is well suited for high-resolution and accurate mass measurements. Internal mass calibration is generally required. The mass calibrant (PFTBA or PFK) is then admitted via the reservoir inlet. In GC-MS, background peaks from column bleed can also serve as internal mass calibrants.

Dissemination and Availability

EI paved the way for MS to become an analytical technique in organic chemistry. From the 1950s until the late 1970s, EI was the preferred ionization method for organic MS. As EI can be combined with a variety of mass analyzers, it has found widespread application – from past to present.

References

1. Field FH, Franklin JL (1957) Electron Impact Phenomena and the Properties of Gaseous Ions. Academic Press, New York
2. Nier AO (1990) Some Reflections on the Early Days of Mass Spectrometry at the University of Minnesota. Int J Mass Spectrom Ion Proc 100:1–13. doi:10.1016/0168-1176(90)85063-8
3. Schaeffer OA (1954) An Improved Mass Spectrometer Ion Source. Rev Sci Instrum 25:660–662. doi:10.1063/1.1771153
4. Fock W (1969) Design of a Mass Spectrometer Ion Source Based on Computed Ion Trajectories. Int J Mass Spectrom Ion Phys 3:285–291. doi:10.1016/0020-7381(69)85012-6
5. Koontz SL, Denton MB (1981) A Very High Yield Electron Impact Ion Source for Analytical Mass Spectrometry. Int J Mass Spectrom Ion Phys 37:227–239. doi:10.1016/0020-7381(81)80011-3
6. Schröder E (1991) Massenspektrometrie – Begriffe und Definitionen. Springer, Heidelberg
7. Hogg AM, Payzant JD (1978) Design of a Field Ionization/Field Desorption/Electron Impact Ion Source and Its Performance on a Modified AEIMS9 Mass Spectrometer. Int J Mass Spectrom Ion Phys 27:291–303. doi:10.1016/0020-7381(78)80116-8
8. Brunnée C (1967) A Combined Field Ionisation-Electron Impact Ion Source for High Molecular Weight Samples of Low Volatility. Z Naturforsch B 22:121–123. doi:10.1515/znb 1967-0203
9. Habfast K (1968) Massenspektrometrische Funktionselemente: Ionenquellen. In: Kienitz H (ed) Massenspektrometrie. Weinheim, Verlag Chemie
10. Bleakney W (1929) A New Method of Positive-Ray Analysis and Its Application to the Measurement of Ionization Potentials in Mercury Vapor. Phys Rev 34:157–160. doi:10.1103/PhysRev.34.157
11. Nier AO (1947) Mass Spectrometer for Isotope and Gas Analysis. Rev Sci Instrum 18:398–411. doi:10.1063/1.1740961
12. Nier AO (1991) The Development of a High Resolution Mass Spectrometer: A Reminiscence. J Am Soc Mass Spectrom 2:447–452. doi:10.1016/1044-0305(91)80029-7
13. Morrison JD (1986) Ion Focusing, Mass Analysis, and Detection. In: Futrell JH (ed) Gaseous Ion Chemistry and Mass Spectrometry. Wiley, New York
14. Dahl DA, Delmore JE, Appelhans AD (1990) SIMION PC/PS2 Electrostatic Lens Design Program. Rev Sci Instrum 61:607–609. doi:10.1063/1.1141932
15. Blaum K, Geppert C, Müller P, Nörtershäuser W, Otten EW, Schmitt A, Trautmann N, Wendt K, Bushaw BA (1998) Properties and Performance of a Quadrupole Mass Filter Used for Resonance Ionization Mass Spectrometry. Int J Mass Spectrom 181:67–87. doi:10.1016/S1387-3806(98)14174-x

16. Ehlers M, Schmidt S, Lee BJ, Grotemeyer J (2000) Design and Set-Up of an External Ion Source Coupled to a Quadrupole-Ion-Trap Reflectron-Time-of-Flight Hybrid Instrument. Eur J Mass Spectrom 6:377–385. doi:10.1255/ejms.356
17. Dahl DA (2000) SIMION for the Personal Computer in Reflection. Int J Mass Spectrom 200:3–25. doi:10.1016/S1387-3806(00)00305-5
18. Forbes MW, Sharifi M, Croley T, Lausevic Z, March RE (1999) Simulation of Ion Trajectories in a Quadrupole Ion Trap: A Comparison of Three Simulation Programs. J Mass Spectrom 34:1219–1239. doi:10.1002/(SICI)1096-9888(199912)34:12<1219::AID-JMS897>3.0.CO;2-L
19. Caldecourt VJ (1955) Heated Sample Inlet System for Mass Spectrometry. Anal Chem 27:1670. doi:10.1021/ac60106a058
20. Peterson L (1962) Mass Spectrometer All-Glass Heated Inlet. Anal Chem 34:1850–1851. doi:10.1021/ac60193a054
21. Roussis SG, Cameron AS (1997) Simplified Hydrocarbon Compound Type Analysis Using a Dynamic Batch Inlet System Coupled to a Mass Spectrometer. Energy Fuels 11:879–886. doi:10.1021/ef960221j
22. Pattillo AD, Young HA (1963) Liquid Sample Introduction System for a Mass Spectrometer. Anal Chem 35:1768. doi:10.1021/ac60204a075
23. Cameron AE (1954) Electron-Bombardment Ion Source for Mass Spectrometry of Solids. Rev Sci Instrum 25:1154–1156. doi:10.1063/1.1770970
24. Reed RI (1958) Electron Impact and Molecular Dissociation. Part I. Some Steroids and Triterpenoids. J Chem Soc:3432–3436. doi:10.1039/JR9580003432
25. Gohlke RS (1963) Obtaining the Mass Spectra of Non-Volatile or Thermally Unstable Compounds. Chem Industry:946–948
26. Junk GA, Svec HJ (1965) A Vacuum Lock for the Direct Insertion of Samples into a Mass Spectrometer. Anal Chem 37:1629–1630. doi:10.1021/ac60231a611
27. Kankare JJ (1974) Simple Temperature Programmer for a Mass Spectrometer Direct Insertion Probe. Anal Chem 46:966–967. doi:10.1021/ac60343a001
28. Franzen J, Küper H, Riepe W, Henneberg D (1973) Automatic Ion Current Control of a Direct Inlet System. Int J Mass Spectrom Ion Phys 10:353–357. doi:10.1016/0020-7381(73)83012-8
29. Sawdo RM, Blumer M (1976) Refrigerated Direct Insertion Probe for Mass Spectrometry. Anal Chem 48:790–791. doi:10.1021/ac60368a014
30. Li JJ (2011) Volatile Organic Compounds Analyzed by Direct Insertion Probe Mass Spectrometry. Can J Chem 89:1539–1541. doi:10.1139/v11-142
31. Hillig H, Kueper H, Riepe W, Ritter HP (1979) A Fully Automated Mass Spectrometer for the Analysis of Organic Solids. Anal Chim Acta 112:123–132. doi:10.1016/S0003-2670(01)83514-5
32. Huang N, Siegel MM, Muenster H, Weissenberg K (1999) On-Line Acquisition, Analysis, and E-Mailing of High-Resolution Exact-Mass Electron Impact/Chemical Ionization Mass Spectrometry Data Acquired Using an Automated Direct Probe. J Am Soc Mass Spectrom 10:1212–1216. doi:10.1016/S1044-0305(99)00112-9
33. Cotter RJ (1980) Mass Spectrometry of Nonvolatile Compounds by Desorption from Extended Probes. Anal Chem 52:1589A–1602A. doi:10.1021/ac50064a003
34. Ohashi M, Nakayama N (1978) In-Beam Electron Impact Mass Spectrometry of Aliphatic Alkohols. Org Mass Spectrom 13:642–645. doi:10.1002/oms.1210131106
35. Ohashi M, Tsujimoto K, Funakura S, Harada K, Suzuki M (1983) Detection of Pseudomolecular Ions of Tetra- and Pentasaccharides by In-Beam Electron Ionization Mass Spectrometry. Spectroscopy Int J 2:260–266
36. Constantin E, Nakatini Y, Ourisson G, Hueber R, Teller G (1980) Spectres de Masse de Phospholipides et Polypeptides Non Proteges. Une Méthode Simple d'Obtention du Spectre Complet. Tetrahedron Lett 21:4745–4746. doi:10.1016/0040-4039(80)88110-x
37. Traldi P, Vettori U, Dragoni F (1982) Instrument Parameterization for Optimum Use of Commercial Direct Inlet Systems. Org Mass Spectrom 17:587–592. doi:10.1002/oms.1210171112
38. Traldi P (1982) Direct Electron Impact – A New Ionization Technique? Org Mass Spectrom 17:245–246. doi:10.1002/oms.1210170510
39. Udseth HR, Friedman L (1981) Analysis of Styrene Polymers by Mass Spectrometry with Filament-Heated Evaporation. Anal Chem 53:29–33. doi:10.1021/ac00224a600

40. Daves GD Jr (1979) Mass Spectrometry of Involatile and Thermally Unstable Molecules. Acc Chem Res 12:359–365. doi:10.1021/ar50142a002
41. Peltier JM, MacLean DB, Szarek WA (1991) Determination of the Glycosidic Linkage in Peracetylated Disaccharides Comprised of D-Glucopyranose Units by Use of Desorption Electron-Ionization Mass Spectrometry. Rapid Commun Mass Spectrom 5:446–449. doi:10.1002/rcm.1290051005
42. Kurlansik L, Williams TJ, Strong JM, Anderson LW, Campana JE (1984) Desorption Ionization Mass Spectrometry of Synthetic Porphyrins. Biomed Mass Spectrom 11:475–481. doi:10.1002/bms.1200110908
43. Qian K, Killinger WE, Casey M, Nicol GR (1996) Rapid Polymer Identification by In-Source Direct Pyrolysis Mass Spectrometry and Library Searching Techniques. Anal Chem 68:1019–1027. doi:10.1021/ac951046r
44. Meuzelaar HLC, Haverkamp J, Hileman FD (1982) Pyrolysis Mass Spectrometry of Recent and Fossil Biomaterials. Elsevier, Amsterdam
45. Guillo C, Lipp M, Radovic B, Reniero F, Schmidt M, Anklam E (1999) Use of Pyrolysis-Mass Spectrometry in Food Analysis: Applications in the Food Analysis Laboratory of the European Commissions' Joint Research Center. J Anal Appl Pyrolysis 49:329–335
46. Schulten H-R, Leinweber P (1996) Characterization of Humic and Soil Particles by Analytical Pyrolysis and Computer Modeling. J Anal Appl Pyrolysis 38:1–53. doi:10.1016/S0165-2370(96)00954-0
47. Basile F, Beverly MB, Voorhees KJ (1998) Pathogenic Bacteria: Their Detection and Differentiation by Rapid Lipid Profiling with Pyrolysis Mass Spectrometry. Trends Anal Chem 17:95–109. doi:10.1016/S0165-9936(97)00103-9
48. Badawy SM (2004) Identification of Some Polymeric Materials by Low-Temperature Pyrolysis Mass Spectrometry. Eur J Mass Spectrom 10:613–617. doi:10.1255/ejms.668
49. Message GM (1984) Practical Aspects of Gas Chromatography/Mass Spectrometry. Wiley, New York
50. Budde WL (2001) Analytical Mass Spectrometry. ACS and Oxford University Press, Washington, DC and Oxford
51. Hübschmann H-J (2015) Handbook of GC-MS – Fundamentals and Applications. Wiley-VCH, Weinheim
52. Cappiello A, Famiglini G, Mangani F, Palma P (2002) A Simple Approach for Coupling Liquid Chromatography and Electron Ionization Mass Spectrometry. J Am Soc Mass Spectrom 13:265–273. doi:10.1016/S1044-0305(01)00363-4
53. Cappiello A, Famiglini G, Palma P, Siviero A (2005) Liquid Chromatography-Electron Ionization Mass Spectrometry: Fields of Application and Evaluation of the Performance of a Direct-EI Interface. Mass Spectrom Rev 24:978–989. doi:10.1002/mas.20054
54. Ludányi K, Dallos A, Kühn Z, Vékey D (1999) Mass Spectrometry of Very Large Saturated Hydrocarbons. J Mass Spectrom 34:264–267. doi:10.1002/(SICI)1096-9888(199904)34:4<264::AID-JMS749>3.0.CO;2-Q
55. Remberg G, Remberg E, Spiteller-Friedmann M, Spiteller G (1968) Massenspektren Schwach Angeregter Moleküle. 4. Mitteilung. Org Mass Spectrom 1:87–113. doi:10.1002/oms.1210010110
56. Bowen RD, Maccoll A (1983) Low-Energy, Low-Temperature Mass Spectra. I. Selected Derivatives of Octane. Org Mass Spectrom 18:576–581. doi:10.1002/oms.1210181216
57. Brophy JJ, Maccoll A (1988) Low-Energy, Low-Temperature Mass Spectra. 9. The Linear Undecanols. Org Mass Spectrom 23:659–662. doi:10.1002/oms.1210230906
58. Melaku A, Maccoll A, Bowen RD (1997) Low-Energy, Low-Temperature Mass Spectra. Part 17: Selected Aliphatic Amides. Eur Mass Spectrom 3:197–208. doi:10.1255/ejms.39
59. Blau G, King GS (eds) (1977) Handbook of Derivates for Chromatography. Heyden & Son, London
60. Poole CF (1977) Recent advances in the silylation of organic compounds for gas chromatography. In: Blau G, King GS (eds) Handbook of Derivates for Chromatography. Heyden & Son, London
61. Svendsen JS, Sydnes LK, Whist JE (1987) Mass Spectrometric Study of Dimethyl Esters of Trimethylsilyl Ether Derivatives of Some 3-Hydroxy Dicarboxylic Acids. Org Mass Spectrom 22:421–429. doi:10.1002/oms.1210220708

62. Svendsen JS, Whist JE, Sydnes LK (1987) A Mass Spectrometric Study of the Dimethyl Ester Trimethylsilyl Enol Ether Derivatives of Some 3-Oxodicarboxylic Acids. Org Mass Spectrom 22:486–492. doi:10.1002/oms.1210220803
63. Scribe P, Guezennec J, Dagaut J, Pepe C, Saliot A (1988) Identification of the Position and the Stereochemistry of the Double Bond in Monounsaturated Fatty Acid Methyl Esters by Gas Chromatography/Mass Spectrometry of Dimethyl Disulfide Derivatives. Anal Chem 60:928–931. doi:10.1021/ac00160a019
64. Pepe C, Sayer H, Dagaut J, Couffignal R (1997) Determination of Double Bond Positions in Triunsaturated Compounds by Means of Gas Chromatography/Mass Spectrometry of Dimethyl Disulfide Derivatives. Rapid Commun Mass Spectrom 11:919–921. doi:10.1002/(SICI)1097-0231(199705)11:8<919::AID-RCM924>3.0.CO;2-C
65. Abrahamsson S, Stenhagen E, McLafferty FW (1969) Atlas of Mass Spectral Data. Wiley, New York
66. Eight Peak Index of Mass Spectra (1983) Royal Society of Chemistry, London
67. McLafferty FW, Stauffer DB (1989) The Wiley/NBS Registry of Mass Spectral Data. Wiley-Interscience, New York
68. McLafferty FW, Gohlke RS (1959) Mass-Spectrometric Analysis: Spectral-Data File Utilizing Machine Filing and Manual Searching. Anal Chem 31:1160–1163. doi:10.1021/ac60151a025
69. Stein SE, Ausloos P, Lias SG (1991) Comparative Evaluations of Mass Spectral Databases. J Am Soc Mass Spectrom 2:441–443. doi:10.1016/1044-0305(91)85012-U
70. McLafferty FW, Stauffer DB, Twiss-Brooks AB, Loh SY (1991) An Enlarged Data Base of Electron-Ionization Mass Spectra. J Am Soc Mass Spectrom 2:432–437. doi:10.1016/1044-0305(91)85010-4
71. McLafferty FW, Stauffer DB, Loh SY (1991) Comparative Evaluations of Mass Spectral Data Bases. J Am Soc Mass Spectrom 2:438–440. doi:10.1016/1044-0305(91)85011-T
72. Henneberg D, Weimann B, Zalfen U (1993) Computer-Aided Interpretation of Mass Spectra Using Databases with Spectra and Structures. I. Structure Searches. Org Mass Spectrom 28:198–206. doi:10.1002/oms.1210280311
73. Zhu D, She J, Hong Q, Liu R, Lu P, Wang L (1988) ASES/MS: An Automatic Structure Elucidation System for Organic Compounds Using Mass Spectrometric Data. Analyst 113:1261–1265. doi:10.1039/AN9881301261
74. Kwiatkowski J, Riepe W (1979) A Combined Forward-Reverse Library Search System for the Identification of Low-Resolution Mass Spectra. Anal Chim Acta 112:219–231. doi:10.1016/S0003-2670(01)83551-0
75. Stein SE, Heller DN (2006) On the Risk of False Positive Identification Using Multiple Ion Monitoring in Qualitative Mass Spectrometry: Large-Scale Intercomparisons with a Comprehensive Mass Spectral Library. J Am Soc Mass Spectrom 17:823–835. doi:10.1016/j.jasms.2006.02.021
76. Milman BL (2005) Towards a Full Reference Library of MS^n Spectra. Testing of a Library Containing 3126 MS^2 Spectra of 1743 Compounds. Rapid Commun Mass Spectrom 19:2833–2839. doi:10.1002/rcm.2131
77. Stein S, Scott DR (1994) Optimization and Testing of Mass Spectral Library Search Algorithms for Compound Identification. J Am Soc Mass Spectrom 5:859–866. doi:10.1016/1044-0305(94)87009-8
78. Stein SE (1994) Estimating Probabilities of Correct Identification from Results of Mass Spectral Library Searches. J Am Soc Mass Spectrom 5:316–323. doi:10.1016/1044-0305(94)85022-4
79. Lebedev KS, Cabrol-Bass D (1998) New Computer Aided Methods for Revealing Structural Features of Unknown Compounds Using Low Resolution Mass Spectra. J Chem Inf Comput Sci 38:410–419
80. Halket JM, Waterman D, Przyborowska AM, Patel RKP, Fraser PD, Bramley PM (2005) Chemical Derivatization and Mass Spectral Libraries in Metabolic Profiling by GC/MS and LC/MS/MS. J Exp Bot 56:219–243. doi:10.1093/jxb/eri069

Fragmentation of Organic Ions and Interpretation of EI Mass Spectra

6

Learning Objectives

- Fragmentation reactions of organic ions
- Competing fragmentation pathways
- Bond cleavages of radical ions
- Bond cleavages of non-radical ions
- Rearrangement fragmentations
- Fragmentation reactions of important compound classes
- Characteristic ions and typical neutral losses
- Distonic ions and ion–neutral complexes
- Extracting structural information from mass spectra – tools and rules
- Interpreting mass spectra – systematic approaches

The following chapter introduces one of the key disciplines of organic mass spectrometry: the common fragmentation pathways of organic ions and the resulting methodology for the interpretation of *electron ionization* (EI) mass spectra. While being quite long, this chapter cannot be comprehensive, and thus, you even might want to look for further reading [1–3]. Of course, there is also a vast number of original publications dealing with compound classes and specific fragmentation pathways that should be consulted when trying to solve particular problems.

Intended as a systematic introduction to the topic this chapter emphasizes the most important fragmentation pathways rather than dwelling on countless compounds. Basic skills are provided as a guideline for further "learning by doing". Throughout the chapter we will keep an eye on the relationships between fragmentation patterns and gas phase ion chemistry. As a prerequisite for successfully working through these pages, some knowledge is needed on the general concept of mass spectrometry (Chap. 1) and of the basics of electron ionization (Chap. 5). In addition, you should

J.H. Gross, *Mass Spectrometry*, DOI 10.1007/978-3-319-54398-7_6

be familiar with the fundamentals of gas phase ion chemistry (Chap. 2) as well as with isotopic mass and isotopic distributions (Chap. 3).

Relevance beyond EI
Although the discussion of common fragmentation pathways of organic ions is embedded here in the context of EI mass spectrometry, their occurrence is not restricted to this technique. The reactions of isolated gaseous ions do not directly depend on the ionization method, but are almost exclusively governed by intrinsic properties of the respective ion and by its internal energy (Chap. 2).

6.1 Cleavage of a Sigma-Bond

6.1.1 Writing Conventions for Molecular Ions

Electron ionization mainly creates singly charged positive ions by ejection of one electron out of the neutral. If the precursor was a molecule, M, it will have an even number of electrons, i.e., be an *even-electron ion* (EE, also named *closed-shell ion*). The molecular ion formed upon EI must then be a positive *radical ion*, $M^{+\bullet}$, i.e., an *odd-electron ion* (OE, also named *open-shell ion*).

Definition
The *molecular ion*, $M^{+\bullet}$, has the same molecular formula as the corresponding neutral molecule. The neutral and its molecular ion only differ by one (or more) electron(s). A singly charged molecular ion can either be a positive radical ion, $M^{+\bullet}$, or a negative radical ion, $M^{-\bullet}$ (not in the case of EI, Table 6.1). The nominal mass of this ion corresponds to the sum of the nominal masses of the most abundant isotopes of the various atoms that make up the molecule [4, 5].

Note
The symbol $M^{+\bullet}$ does *not mean one added electron*. The radical ($^\bullet$) symbol is added to the molecular ion only to *indicate the remaining unpaired* electron after ionization. Addition of one electron (electron capture) to a neutral would make it a negative radical ion, $M^{-\bullet}$.

Table 6.1 Symbolism for charge and radical states

State of species	Symbol	Examples
Even-electron ion	+, –	CH_3^+, NH_4^+, EtO^-, CF_3^-
Odd-electron ion	+•, –•	$CH_4^{+\bullet}$, $C_{60}^{+\bullet}$, $C_{60}^{-\bullet}$, $CCl_4^{-\bullet}$
Radical, no charge	•	$CH_3^\bullet$, $OH^\bullet$, $H^\bullet$, $Br^\bullet$

When initially formulating the ionization process, we did not consider where the charge would reside (Sect. 2.1), e.g., for methane we simply wrote:

$$CH_4 + e^- \rightarrow CH_4^{+\bullet} + 2e^- \tag{6.1}$$

The tremendous changes in electronic structure and bonding that arise with the loss of an electron are by far better depicted by a formula representation including the σ-bonding electrons of the C–H bond. In small nonfunctionalized molecules such as methane, it is not possible to avoid the loss of a valence electron from a σ-bond upon electron ionization. The same is true for all other saturated hydrocarbons or a hydrogen molecule, for example. The resulting methane molecular ion may *formally* be represented either as a species resembling a combination of a methyl cation plus a hydrogen radical or a methyl radical plus a proton. Nevertheless, one may still assume that it resembles more the intact molecule than the evolving fragments – a statement being also in accordance with the basic assumptions of the QET (Sect. 2.5). Otherwise, fragmentation would proceed almost spontaneously, thereby excluding the detection of the molecular ion (Scheme 6.1).

Lone pairs or π-orbitals are the preferred sites of molecules where electrons become detached. The ease of doing so is directly reflected by their effect on ionization energy (Sect. 2.4) [6]. Therefore, it is common practice to write the charge of a molecular ion as if localized at the position of lowest ionization energy. This is of course not in full agreement with the real charge distributions in ions, but it has been established as a useful first step when writing down a fragmentation scheme. Appropriate formula representations of molecular ions of acetone, *N,N*-dimethyl-propylamine, tetrahydrothiophene, benzene, and 2-methyl-1-pentene are (Scheme 6.2).

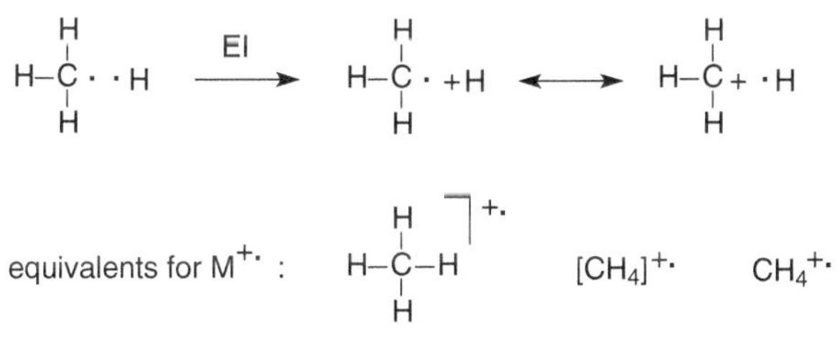

Scheme 6.1

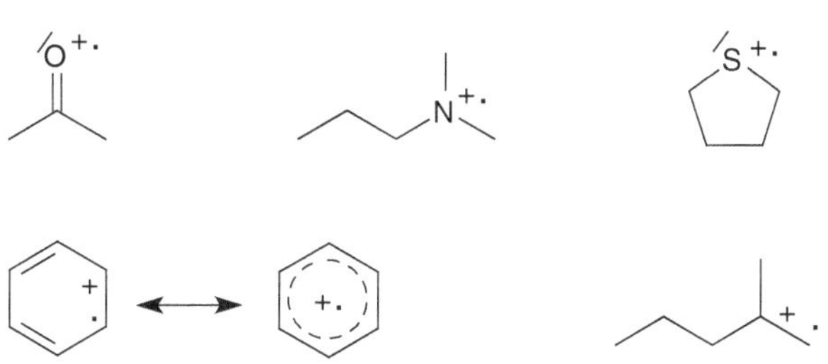

Scheme 6.2

6.1.2 σ-Bond Cleavage in Small Nonfunctionalized Molecules

The most intense peaks in the EI mass spectrum of methane are the molecular ion at *m/z* 16 and the fragment ion at *m/z* 15 (Fig. 6.1). Explicitly writing the electrons helps to understand the subsequent dissociations of $CH_4^{+\bullet}$ to yield CH_3^+, *m/z* 15, by $H^\bullet$ loss (σ_1) or H^+ by $CH_3^\bullet$ loss (σ_2), respectively (Scheme 6.3). In general, it is more convenient to write the molecular ion in one of the equivalent forms (Scheme 6.1). The charge and radical state are then attached to the brackets (often abbreviated as ⌉) enclosing the molecule. (It is advised to review the rules of Sect. 1.7 for terminology in the description of mass spectra).

The CH_3^+ fragment ion can also be seen in its relation to the molecular ion, i.e., it may be described as an $[M–H]^+$ ion. Accordingly, the proton could be written as

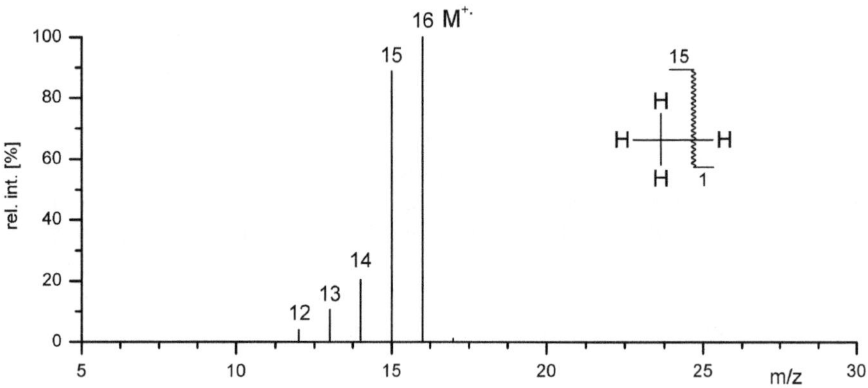

Fig. 6.1 EI mass spectrum of methane (Used by permission of NIST. © NIST 2002)

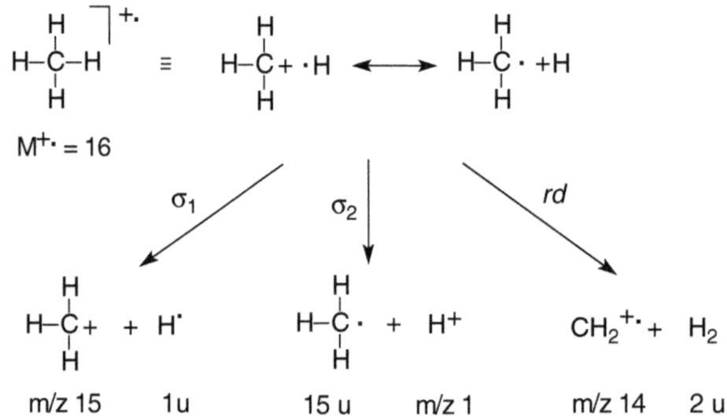

Scheme 6.3

$[M–CH_3]^+$. The $[M–H_2]^{+\bullet}$ ion at *m/z* 14, i.e., carbene molecular ion in this case, results from a rearrangement fragmentation (*rd*). Rearrangements are discussed later in this chapter.

The σ-bond cleavage represents a simple but very common type of fragmentation. Its occurrence does neither require particular functional groups nor heteroatoms in a molecular ion. The σ-bond cleavage proceeds via a loose transition state and therefore can become very rapid, provided that ions have sufficient internal energy (Sect. 2.5). Even if additional and perhaps energetically more favorable fragmentation pathways prevail, σ-bond cleavages will not vanish completely.

6.1.3 Even-Electron Rule

The *dissociation* or *fragmentation* of ions – as it is usually referred to in mass spectrometry – yields a fragment ion and a neutral. Depending on whether the fragmenting ion is an even-electron (EE) or an odd-electron (OE) species, certain fragmentation pathways may be allowed or forbidden. This has been generalized in the *even-electron rule* [7]. It serves as a reliable guideline rather than a strict rule for the fragmentation of ions, and thus for the interpretation of mass spectra. The even-electron rule is summarized in (Scheme 6.4).

Even-electron rule
Odd-electron ions (OE, such as molecular ions and fragment ions formed by rearrangements) may eliminate either a radical or an even-electron neutral species, but even-electron ions (EE, such as protonated molecules or fragment ions formed by a single bond cleavage) will not usually lose a radical to form an odd-electron cation. In other words, the successive loss of radicals is forbidden [8].

Scheme 6.4

$$[\text{odd}]^{+\bullet} \longrightarrow [\text{even}]^{+} + \text{R}^{\bullet}$$

$$[\text{odd}]^{+\bullet} \longrightarrow [\text{odd}]^{+\bullet} + \text{n}$$

$$[\text{even}]^{+} \longrightarrow [\text{even}]^{+} + \text{n}$$

$$[\text{even}]^{+} \not\longrightarrow [\text{odd}]^{+\bullet} + \text{R}^{\bullet}$$

Even-electron rule applied to methane According to the even-electron rule the molecular ion (OE) of methane should undergo the following dissociations:

$$CH_4^{+\bullet} \rightarrow CH_3^{+} + H^{\bullet} \quad (6.2)$$

$$CH_4^{+\bullet} \rightarrow CH_2^{+\bullet} + H_2 \quad (6.3)$$

Despite that it might initially be generated in a different electronic state and/or conformation, the $CH_2^{+\bullet}$ fragment ion (OE) can be expected to decompose further in a way identical to the molecular ion of carbene:

$$CH_2^{+\bullet} \rightarrow C^{+\bullet} + H_2 \quad (6.4)$$

$$CH_2^{+\bullet} \rightarrow CH^{+} + H^{\bullet} \quad (6.5)$$

Loss of a radical from a radical ion creates an even-electron fragment ion, CH_3^{+} (EE) in this case, which preferably may undergo subsequent loss of a molecule:

$$CH_3^{+} \rightarrow CH^{+} + H_2 \quad (6.6)$$

Loss of $H^{\bullet}$ from CH_3^{+} should not occur. It is noteworthy that even such a simple fragmentation scheme offers two independent pathways for the generation of CH^{+} (Eqs. 6.5 and 6.6).

Note

It is important to assign the correct charge and radical state to all species encountered and to carefully track them through a fragmentation scheme. Otherwise, "impossible" fragmentation pathways may be formulated, thereby misleading the assignment of elemental composition and molecular constitution.

Numerous exceptions to the even-electron rule have been described [8–10]. Violations tend to occur when the loss of a radical from an even-electron ion leads to the formation of an exceptionally stable ionic species or when highly excited ions are involved. Representatives of highly excited ions are small molecular ions having only a few degrees of freedom to randomize internal energy [9] or ions being subject to collision-induced dissociation (Sect. 9.3) [10, 11].

Hint

In chemistry, there usually is no strict "either ... or" – instead the ions behave like "more ... than ...".

6.1.4 σ-Bond Cleavage in Small Functionalized Molecules

The introduction of a charge-localizing heteroatom into a molecule is accompanied by obvious changes in the appearance of the mass spectrum. Withdrawal of an electron upon EI does not necessarily affect a σ-bond, because the lone pairs of the heteroatom may now provide an electron for ejection.

In the EI mass spectrum of iodomethane the molecular ion, $CH_3–I^{+\bullet}$, is detected as the base peak at *m/z* 142 (Fig. 6.2). An important new feature of the spectrum is the peak at *m/z* 127 due to an $[M–CH_3]^+$ ion. This signal is due to I^+ also formed by a process that can be classified as σ-bond cleavage. Here, a single electron shifts from the intact C–I bond to the radical site, thereby rupturing the bond. The peak is accompanied by a much less intense one at *m/z* 128 resulting from $HI^{+\bullet}$ by rearrangement (Scheme 6.5). Note that the peak at *m/z* 128 should not be interpreted as an isotopic peak of *m/z* 127, because iodine is monoisotopic! The remaining

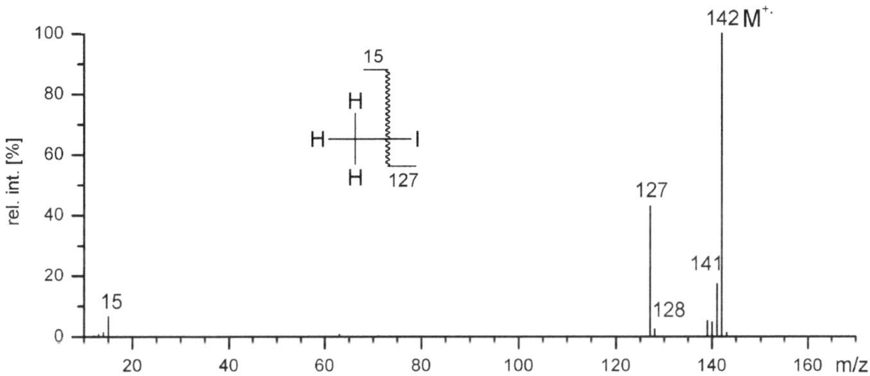

Fig. 6.2 EI mass spectrum of iodomethane. The molecular ion mainly decomposes to yield ionic fragments representing its major constituent groups, i.e., I^+, *m/z* 127 and CH_3^+, *m/z* 15 (Spectrum used by permission of NIST. © NIST 2002)

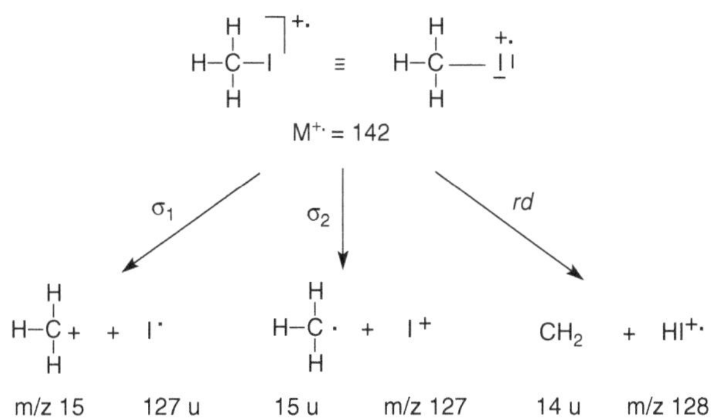

Scheme 6.5

peaks can be explained in the same manner as for methane, i.e., peaks can be assigned as $[M–H]^+$, *m/z* 141, $[M–H_2]^{+•}$, *m/z* 140, and $[M–H–H_2]^+$, *m/z* 139. Analogous to $H^•$ loss, $I^•$ loss, 127 u, also occurs generating the CH_3^+ ion, *m/z* 15.

Look for Hal$^+$
Halogenated compounds typically reveal the positive halogen ion and a less intense peak due to the hydrogen halogenide. In accordance with the incrementing electronegativities of the halogens their intensities follow the order $F^+ < Cl^+ < Br^+ < I^+$. In case of Br and Cl the isotopic patterns give additional evidence for their presence (Sect. 6.2.11) [12].

6.2 Alpha-Cleavage

6.2.1 α-Cleavage of Acetone Molecular Ion

The EI mass spectrum of acetone is rather simple: it shows three significant peaks at *m/z* 58, 43, and 15. According to the composition C_3H_6O, the peak at *m/z* 58 corresponds to the molecular ion. The base peak at *m/z* 43 is related to this signal by a difference of 15 u, a neutral loss that can almost certainly be assigned to loss of a methyl radical, $CH_3^•$. The peak at *m/z* 15 may then be expected to correspond to the ionic counterpart of the methyl radical, i.e., to the CH_3^+ carbenium ion (Fig. 6.3). In order to rationalize this mass spectrum in terms of ion chemistry, we consider the steps of electron ionization and subsequent fragmentation in detail.

The acetone molecule has two lone pairs at the oxygen that will at least formally be the preferred ones to remove an electron (Sect. 2.1). The excited molecular ion may then cleave off a methyl radical by simply shifting *one electron* (single-barbed arrow or "fishhook") from the CO–CH_3 bond to the radical site at the oxygen atom

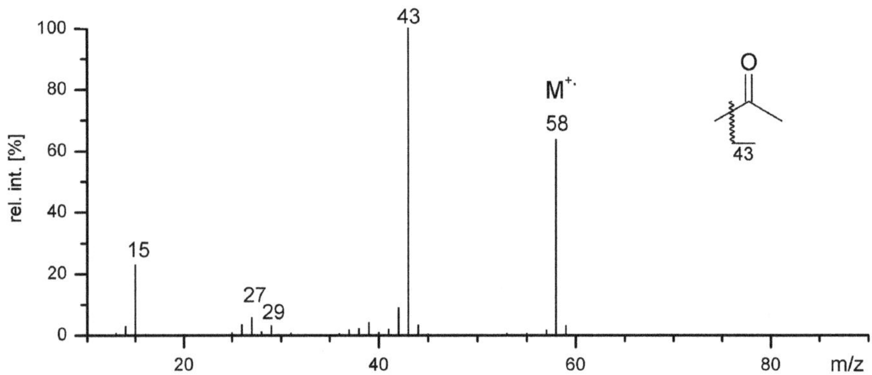

Fig. 6.3 EI mass spectrum of acetone (Used by permission of NIST. © NIST 2002)

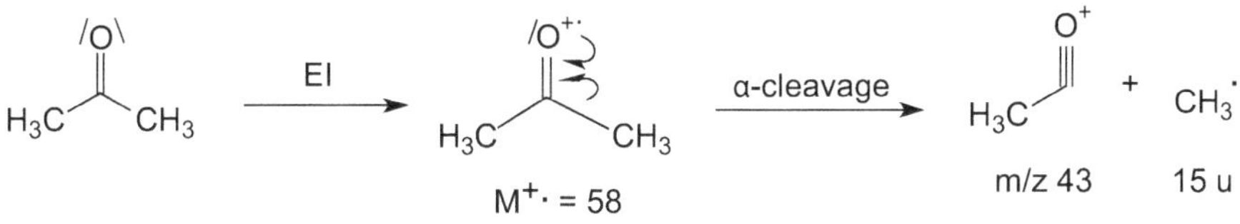

Scheme 6.6

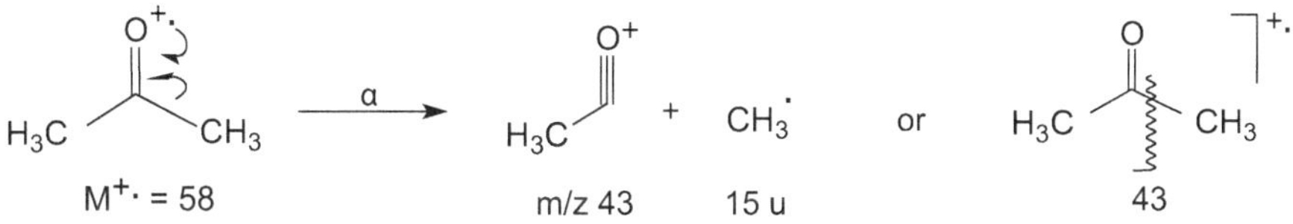

Scheme 6.7

allowing the products to drift apart (Scheme 6.6). This homolytic bond cleavage is a *radical-site initiated* process with *charge retention*, i.e., the ionic charge resides within the moiety where it was initially located. The process is also known as *α-cleavage*. The neutral fragment, $CH_3^{\bullet}$, is not detected by the mass spectrometer, while the charged fragment, $C_2H_3O^+$, leads to the base peak m/z 43.

Which bond is cleaved?

The term *α-cleavage* for this widespread *radical-site initiated process* with *charge retention* can be misleading, because the bond cleaved is not directly attached to the radical site, but to the next neighboring atom.

Including the ionization process, the lone pairs, and single-barbed arrows for each moving electron in the scheme is not necessary but presents a valuable aid. Alternatively, the α-cleavage may be indicated in a simplified manner (Scheme 6.7).

The first abbreviated form only shows the according electron shift, but it still explicitly gives the structures of the products. The second is useful to indicate which bond will be cleaved and what m/z the ionic product will have. Such a writing convention can of course be used for any other fragmentation pathway. The ionic product of the α-cleavage, an *acylium ion*, will not exactly have the angular structure as shown, however drawing it this way helps to identify the fragment as a part of the initial molecular ion. The charge in acylium ions can be substantially resonance-stabilized (Scheme 6.8).

6.2.2 Stevenson's Rule

The origin of the peak at m/z 43 in the EI mass spectrum of acetone should be quite clear now and we may examine the formation of the CH_3^+ ion, m/z 15, next. In

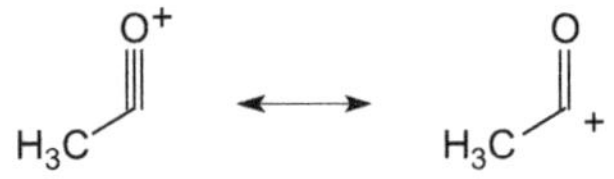

Scheme 6.8

principle, the ionic charge may reside on either fragment, the acyclium or the alkyl. In case of acetone, the formation of the acylium ion, CH_3CO^+, *m*/*z* 43, is preferred over the formation of the small carbenium ion, CH_3^+, *m*/*z* 15. The question which of the two incipient fragments will preferably retain the charge can be answered by means of Stevenson's Rule.

Stevenson's rule

When a fragmentation takes place, the positive charge remains on the fragment with the lowest ionization energy.

This criterion was originally established for the fragmentation of alkanes by Stevenson [13] and was later demonstrated to be generally valid [14, 15]. The rule can be rationalized on the basis of ion thermochemical considerations (Fig. 6.4). Assuming no reverse activation barrier, the difference in thermodynamic stability as expressed in terms of the difference of heats of formation of the respective products determines the preferred dissociation pathway:

$$\Delta H_{\mathrm{f(B+;A\bullet)}} - \Delta H_{\mathrm{f(A+;B\bullet)}} = \Delta\Delta H_{\mathrm{f(Prod)}} = \Delta E_0 \tag{6.7}$$

This can also be expressed in relation to the ionization energies of the radicals formed by both dissociations:

$$\Delta E_0 = IE_{\mathrm{B}\bullet} - IE_{\mathrm{A}\bullet} = E_{02} - E_{01} \tag{6.8}$$

Therefore, the radical having the lower ionization energy will dominate among the products [14, 16]. For example, in case of the α-cleavage of acetone, $CH_3C^{\bullet}{=}O$ has a by 2.8 eV lower *IE* than $^{\bullet}CH_3$ (Table 6.2). As ion internal energies are subject to a wide distribution, there is a substantial fraction of ions that may also dissociate to form the energetically more demanding pair of fragments. This is the reason for the "soft" character of the rule.

Both combinations occur

The homolytic dissociation of a bond generally proceeds to yield both product pairs, their relative abundances being basically governed by Stevenson's rule.

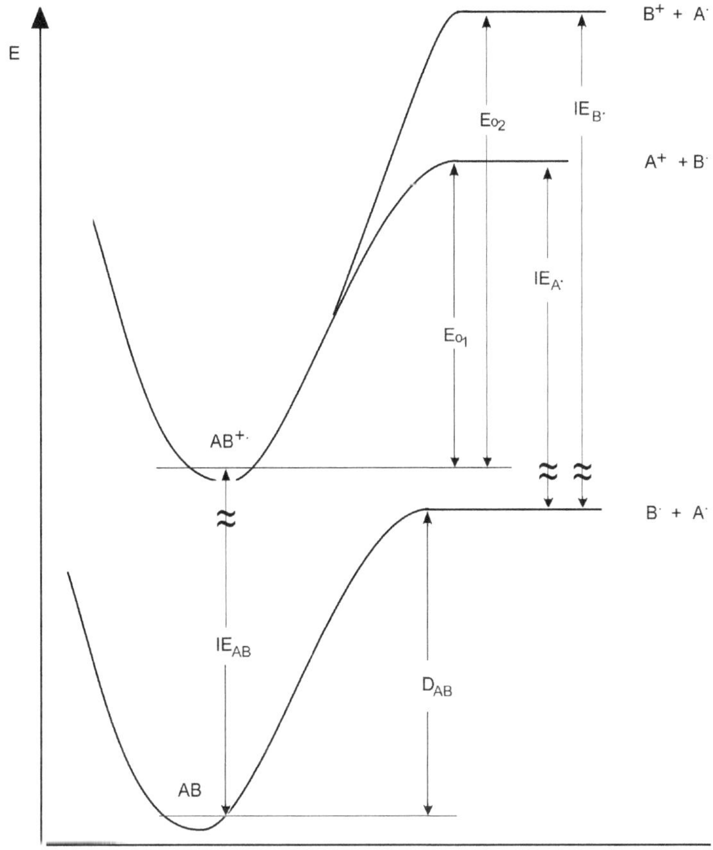

Fig. 6.4 Thermochemical description of Stevenson's rule (D_{AB} homolytic bond dissociation energy of bond A–B, *IE* ionization energy)

Without the thermochemical data, it is not easy to decide which pair of products will be preferred over the other. In general, the formation of the higher substituted and/or larger carbenium ion is preferred, because it can more easily stabilize a charge. However, the tendency is the same for the radicals and one may expect loss of ethyl to be favored over loss of methyl, for example. Thus, the formation of both the ionic and the radical fragments are of critical importance for the final distribution of products.

Reverse barrier needs consideration
The validity of Stevenson's rule requires no reverse activation energy barrier to exist for the fragmentation pathway. This requirement is usually fulfilled for simple bond cleavages, but not in case of rearrangement fragmentations.

Table 6.2 Ionization energies of some radicals[a]

Radical	IE^b [eV]	Radical	IE^b [eV]
$H^\bullet$	13.6	$CH_3O^\bullet$	10.7
$^\bullet CH_3$	9.8	$^\bullet CH_2OH$	7.6
$^\bullet C_2H_5$	8.4	$CH_3C^\bullet{=}O$	7.0
n-$^\bullet C_3H_7$	8.2	$C_2H_5C^\bullet{=}O$	5.7
i-$^\bullet C_3H_7$	7.6	$^\bullet CH_2Cl$	8.8
n-$^\bullet C_4H_9$	8.0	$^\bullet CCl_3$	8.1
i-$^\bullet C_4H_9$	7.9	$C_6H_5^\bullet$	8.3
s-$^\bullet C_4H_9$	7.3	$C_6H_5CH_2^\bullet$	7.2
t-$^\bullet C_4H_9$	6.8	$^\bullet CH_2NH_2$	6.3

[a] *IE* data extracted from Ref. [17] with permission © NIST 2002
[b] All values rounded to one decimal

6.2.3 α-Cleavage of Nonsymmetrical Aliphatic Ketones

Larger ketone molecules may have different alkyl groups at either side of the carbonyl group. Then, Stevenson's rule helps to decide which of them will mainly be detected as part of the acylium ion and which should preferably appear as carbenium ion. Overall, a nonsymmetrical ketone will yield four primary fragment ions in its EI mass spectrum.

The competing process of carbenium ion formation occurs as a companion of the α-cleavage and may be understood either as *charge site-induced cleavage* (also termed *inductive cleavage*, symbol *i*, or as σ-cleavage). In Scheme 6.9 the charge site-induced mechanism was chosen where the bonding electron pair is retained at the carbonyl fragment to yield an acyl radical and a carbenium ion. If the initial charge was directly assigned to the corresponding σ-bond, the very same products would also result from σ-cleavage.

EI mass spectrum of butanone At *m/z* 43, the EI mass spectrum of butanone shows a fragment due to ethyl loss from the molecular ion, which is largely preferred over methyl loss leading to a minor peak at *m/z* 57 (Fig. 6.5). Furthermore, the $C_2H_5^+$ ion, *m/z* 29, is more abundant than the less stable CH_3^+ ion, *m/z* 15. If the alkyl groups become larger than ethyl, an additional dissociation pathway will occur (Sect. 6.8).

In contrast to ketones [18] α-cleavage is less important as primary fragmentation for aliphatic aldehyde molecular ions [19, 20]. This is because α-cleavage of aldehyde molecular ions forms energetically unfavorable products, i.e., by loss of $H^\bullet$ or formation of the formyl ion, CHO^+, *m/z* 29. It was demonstrated by high-resolution mass spectrometry (Sect. 3.6) that only a fraction of the peak at *m/z* 29 originates from CHO^+ ions, while the majority is due to $C_2H_5^+$ ions from σ-cleavage or charge site-induced cleavage, respectively [21].

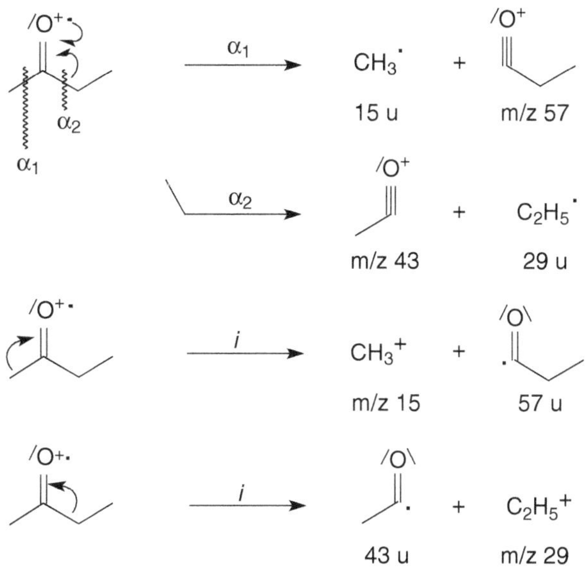

Scheme 6.9

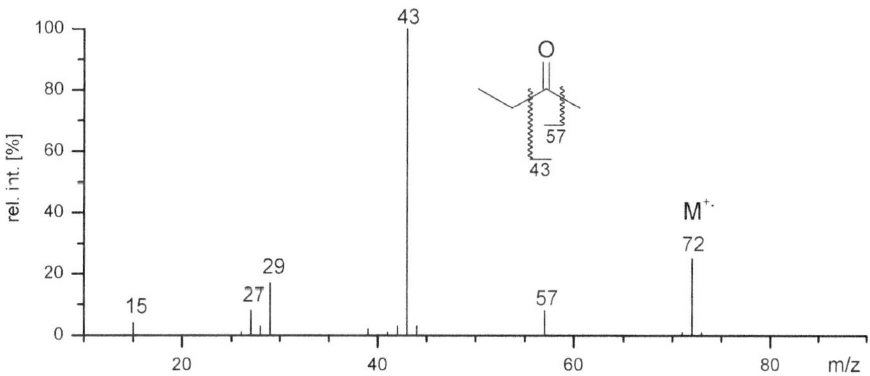

Fig. 6.5 EI mass spectrum of butanone (Used by permission of NIST. © NIST 2002)

6.2.4 Acylium Ions and Carbenium Ions

For larger ketones one can also expect larger acylium and alkyl fragments to occur. Such *series of homologous ions* are useful for deducing structural information from mass spectra. Ions such as those from the acylium ion series and the carbenium ion series are also known as *characteristic ions*. It is advisable to learn the nominal masses of the first members of each series by heart (Tables 6.3 and 6.4).

Isobaric ions
The acylium ions and the saturated carbenium ions are isobaric ions because they share the same nominal mass. However, their exact masses are different, i.e., CH_3CO^+, *m/z* 43.0178, and $C_3H_7^+$, *m/z* 43.0542.

Distinguishing carbenium ions from acylium ions Besides having different exact mass, carbenium ions and acylium ions fortunately exhibit different dissociation pathways thus allowing them to be distinguish by the peak pattern in the according mass spectra (Fig. 6.6).

Table 6.3 Carbenium ions

m/z (1 + 14*n*)	Carbenium ions $[C_nH_{2n+1}]^+$	Accurate mass [u][a]
15	CH_3^+	15.0229
29	$C_2H_5^+$	29.0386
43	*n*-$C_3H_7^+$, *i*-$C_3H_7^+$	43.0542
57	*n*-$C_4H_9^+$, *i*-$C_4H_9^+$, *sec*-$C_4H_9^+$, *tert*-$C_4H_9^+$	57.0699
71	$C_5H_{11}^+$ isomers	71.0855
85	$C_6H_{13}^+$ isomers	85.1011
99	$C_7H_{15}^+$ isomers	99.1168
113	$C_8H_{17}^+$ isomers	113.1325

[a]Values rounded to four decimals

Table 6.4 Acylium ions

m/z (15 + 14*n*)	Acylium ions $[C_nH_{2n-1}O]^+$	Accurate mass [u][a]
29	HCO^+	29.0022
43	CH_3CO^+	43.0178
57	$C_2H_5CO^+$	57.0335
71	$C_3H_7CO^+$	71.0491
85	$C_4H_9CO^+$	85.0648
99	$C_5H_{11}CO^+$ isomers	99.0804
113	$C_6H_{13}CO^+$ isomers	113.0961
127	$C_7H_{15}CO^+$ isomers	127.1117

[a]Values rounded to four decimals

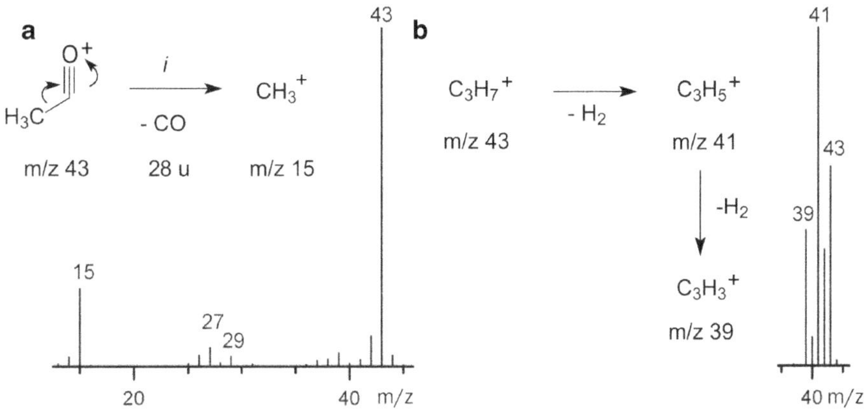

Fig. 6.6 Comparison of typical peak patterns and fragmentation pathways frequently found for (**a**) low-mass acylium ions and (**b**) low-mass carbenium ions

Acylium ions undergo charge-induced CO loss (–28 u), thereby forming carbenium ions, but they do not eliminate hydrogen molecules. This is exemplified by the dissociation $CH_3CO^+ \rightarrow CH_3^+ + CO$, which presents a second pathway for the generation of the peak at *m/z* 15 in the mass spectra of acetone and butanone.

Carbenium ions, especially from ethyl to butyl, show remarkable dehydrogenation, causing a characteristic pattern of peaks at *m/z*–2 and *m/z*–4, i.e., at the low-mass side of the corresponding peak.

While the mass spectra of both acetone (Fig. 6.3) and butanone (Fig. 6.5) show typical acylium ion peaks at *m/z* 43, the signals in the spectra of isopropyl ethyl thioether (Fig. 6.9), of 1-bromo-octane, (Fig. 6.10), and of isomeric decanes (Fig. 6.18) may serve as examples for carbenium ion signals.

The superimposition of both classes of ions causes signals representing an average pattern. The properties of larger carbenium ions are discussed in the section on alkanes (Sect. 6.6).

6.2.5 α-Cleavage When Heteroatoms Belong to the Aliphatic Chain

The charge-localizing heteroatom can also be part of the aliphatic chain as it is the case with amines, ethers, and alcohols. The mechanism of the α-cleavage remains unaffected by this change, i.e., still the bond second to the charge site is cleaved. Nevertheless, the structure of the charged fragments is quite changed, and consequently their further fragmentation pathways are also different.

In case of amine molecular ions the α-cleavage is clearly the dominating primary fragmentation pathway. The strong charge-stabilizing properties of the nitrogen atom keeps the fraction of charge migration fragments very low. The product ions are termed *immonium ions* (also *iminium ions*), because these can formally be obtained by electrophilic addition of a proton or carbenium ion to imines.

Scheme 6.10

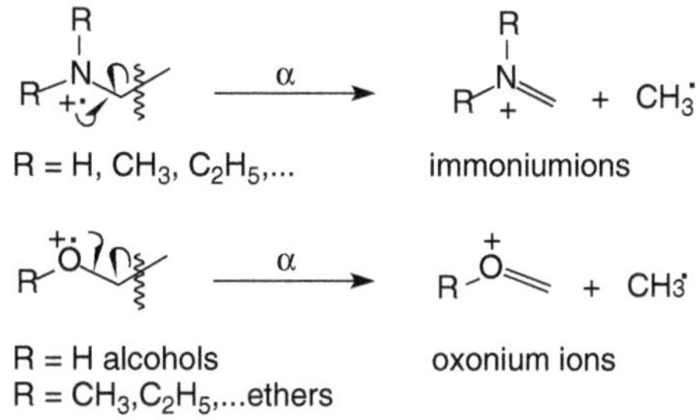

Table 6.5 Relative potential of functional groups to cause α-cleavage

Functional group	Relative value
–COOH	1
–Cl, –OH	8
–Br	13
–COOMe	20
–CO– (ketones)	43
–OMe	100
–I, –SMe	≈110
$–NHCOCH_3$	128
$–NH_2$	990
acetals	1600
$–NMe_2$	2100

From Ref. [30] with permission. © Georg Thieme Verlag, 2002

Immonium ions represent the most stable $[C_nH_{2n+2}N]^+$ isomers [22] and preferably undergo further decomposition on two widespread and thus highly important pathways for alkene loss [23, 24] (Sect. 6.12). *Oxonium ions* are the oxygen analogs of immonium ions. As oxygen is somewhat less charge-stabilizing than nitrogen, the competing formation of carbenium ions is more pronounced among the primary fragmentations of aliphatic ethers [25, 26] and alcohols [27], but still the α-cleavage represents the favored dissociation (Scheme 6.10).

6.2.6 α-Cleavage of Aliphatic Amines

The intensity of the molecular ion of aliphatic amines decreases with increasing molecular weight [28], the reason being their predisposition to α-cleavage. Analogous tendencies are observed for aliphatic ethers [26], hydrocarbons [29], aldehydes [19], and others.

A comparison of the relative strength of functional groups to cause α-cleavage is summarized in Table 6.5 [30]. This also corresponds to a rough measure of relative charge-stabilizing capability of the respective substituent, e.g., the ratio $H_2C{=}OH^+/H_2C{=}NH_2^+$ from 2-amino ethanol molecular ion is 2.3/100 and the ratio of $H_2C{=}OH^+/H_2C{=}SH^+$ from 2-thio ethanol molecular ion is 42/70 [15].

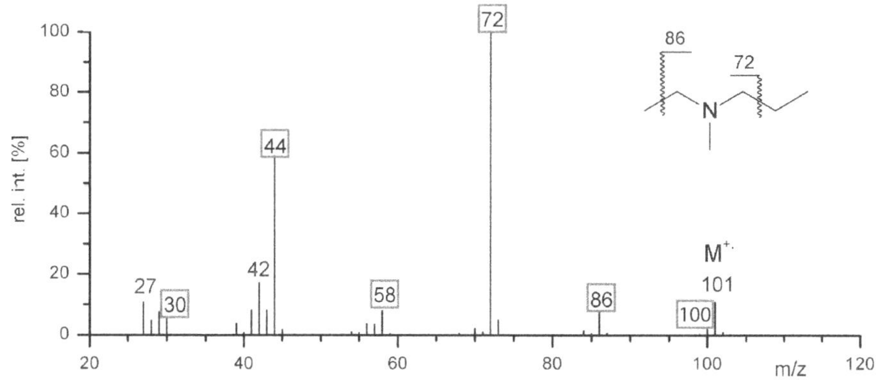

Fig. 6.7 EI mass spectrum of *N*-ethyl-*N*-methyl-propanamine. The molecular ion is detected at odd *m/z*, whereas the immonium fragment ions (marked with *green boxes*) all have even *m/z* values (Spectrum used by permission of NIST. © NIST 2002)

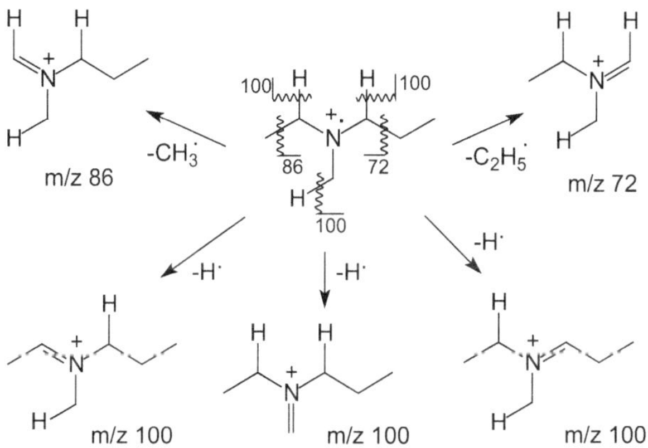

Scheme 6.11

The mass spectrum of *N*-ethyl-*N*-methyl-propanamine, $C_6H_{15}N$, shows the molecular ion peak at *m/z* 101 (Fig. 6.7). The primary fragmentations of the molecular ion are explained in terms of the α-cleavage and accordingly, the peaks at *m/z* 72 and 86 can be assigned as immonium fragment ions due to ethyl and methyl loss, respectively. There are three other pathways for α-cleavage! In order to identify those missing pathways, we have to write down the fragmentation scheme carefully checking every possibility. And of course, we have to examine the mass spectrum with sufficient care in order not to overlook an indicative peak. The peak at *m/z* 100 corresponds to $H^•$ loss and is also due to α-cleavage as can be easily recognized from Scheme 6.11. Three different positions to cleave off a $H^•$ as one of seven almost equivalent hydrogens are available. Despite these options, the peak at *m/z* 100 is still weak, the reason for this being the unfavorable thermodynamics of $H^•$ loss as compared to methyl loss (Table 2.2).

Table 6.6 Aliphatic immonium ions

m/z (16 + 14*n*)	Immonium ions $[C_nH_{2n+2}N]^+$	Accurate mass [u][a]
30	CH_4N^+	30.0338
44	$C_2H_6N^+$	44.0495
58	$C_3H_8N^+$	58.0651
72	$C_4H_{10}N^+$	72.0808
86	$C_5H_{12}N^+$	86.0964
100	$C_6H_{14}N^+$	100.1120
114	$C_7H_{16}N^+$	114.1277
128	$C_8H_{18}N^+$	128.1434

[a]Values rounded to four decimals

As with acylium ions and carbenium ions before, the series of homologous immonium ions is part of the mass spectrometrist's tool box. They can easily be recognized in the mass spectra and have even-numbered *m/z* values (Table 6.6). In the EI spectrum of *N*-ethyl-*N*-methyl-propanamine the series is completely present from *m/z* 30 up to *m/z* 100.

Recognizing primary amines
In the EI mass spectra of primary amines the methylene immonium ion, $CH_2{=}NH^+$, *m/z* 30, resulting from α-cleavage either represents the base peak or at least is the by far most abundant of the immonium ion series.

Even though α-cleavage seems to be a purely electronic process at first sight, the influence of ion internal energy and of the alkyl chain should not be neglected. Whereas $CH_2{=}NH^+$, *m/z* 30, is the predominating ionic product of fragmentations of highly excited primary amine molecular ions within the ion source, the metastable decompositions of such molecular ions yield $CH_3CH^+NH_2$ ($CH_3CH{=}NH_2{}^+$), *m/z* 44, and $CH_3CH_2CH^+NH_2$ ($CH_3CH_2H{=}NH_2{}^+$) *m/z* 58. This has been attributed to isomerization via $H^•$ shifts prior to dissociation [31].

6.2.7 Nitrogen Rule

When we restrict our selection to common elements in organic mass spectrometry (H, B, C, N, O, Si, S, P, F, Cl, Br, I, etc.) all but one of these elements having an odd number of valences also possess an odd mass number and those having an even number of valences also have even mass numbers. Nitrogen represents this only exception, which gives rise to the so-called *nitrogen rule* (Table 6.7).

Table 6.7 Examples illustrating the nitrogen rule

Number of nitrogens	Examples	$M^{+\bullet}$ at *m/z*
0	methane, CH_4	16
0	acetone, C_3H_6O	58
0	chloroform, $CHCl_3$	118
0	[60]fullerene, C_{60}	720
1	ammonia, NH_3	17
1	acetonitrile, C_2H_3N	41
1	pyridine, C_5H_5N	79
1	*N*-ethyl-*N*-methyl-propanamine, $C_6H_{15}N$	101
2	urea, CH_4N_2O	60
2	pyridazine, $C_4H_4N_2$	80
3	triazole, $C_2H_3N_3$	69
3	hexamethylphosphoric triamide, HMPTA, $C_6H_{18}N_3OP$	179

Nitrogen rule

If a compound contains an even number of nitrogen atoms (0, 2, 4, ...), its monoisotopic molecular ion will be detected at an even-numbered nominal *m/z* value. While, on the other hand, an odd number of nitrogen atoms (1, 3, 5, . . .) is indicated by an odd-numbered nominal *m/z*.

Warning

The concept of the nitrogen rule is often overly simplified in that it is assumed that an odd *m/z* value would always refer to one nitrogen and an even number would mean none. Again: the rule just states that odd *m/z* values imply an odd number of N and even *m/z* values an even number (including zero).

The rule may also be extended for use with fragment ions. This makes a practical tool to distinguish even-electron from odd-electron fragment ions and thus simple bond cleavages from rearrangements. However, some additional care has to be taken when applying the extended rule, because nitrogen might also be contained in the neutral, e.g., loss of NH_3, 17 u, or of $CONH_2^{\bullet}$, 44 u.

Rule

Cleaving off a radical (that contains no nitrogen) from any ion changes the nominal *m/z* value from odd to even or vice versa. Loss of a molecule (that contains no nitrogen) from an ion produces even nominal mass fragments from even mass ions and odd mass fragments from odd mass ions.

Nitrogen rule applied to methane To rationalize the mass spectrum of methane, reactions 6.2–6.6 were proposed. They all obey the rule. Just check the mass spectra and fragmentation schemes throughout this chapter for additional examples of the nitrogen rule:

$$CH_4{}^{+\bullet} \rightarrow CH_3{}^{+} + H^{\bullet}; m/z\ 16 \rightarrow m/z\ 15 \tag{6.2}$$

$$CH_4{}^{+\bullet} \rightarrow CH_2{}^{+\bullet} + H_2;\ m/z\ 16 \rightarrow m/z\ 14 \tag{6.3}$$

$$CH_2{}^{+\bullet} \rightarrow C^{+\bullet} + H_2;\ m/z\ 14 \rightarrow m/z\ 12 \tag{6.4}$$

$$CH_2{}^{+\bullet} \rightarrow CH^{+} + H^{\bullet};\ m/z\ 14 \rightarrow m/z\ 13 \tag{6.5}$$

$$CH_3{}^{+} \rightarrow CH^{+} + H_2;\ m/z\ 15 \rightarrow m/z\ 13 \tag{6.6}$$

6.2.8 α-Cleavage of Aliphatic Ethers and Alcohols

The molecular ions of aliphatic ethers do not behave much different from those of amines [25, 26]. However, oxygen is not directing their primary dissociations as strongly to the α-cleavage as nitrogen does in amines. Although α-cleavage is still dominant, there is a stronger tendency towards formation of carbenium ion fragments by charge migration. As can be expected, the structure of the alkyls also exerts a significant influence on the selection of a cleavage pathway.

EI mass spectra of aliphatic ethers The 70-eV EI mass spectra of two aliphatic ethers are compared in Fig. 6.8. Although being isomers, their spectra are clearly different. In case of methyl propyl ether, α-cleavage can occur by $H^{\bullet}$ loss, *m/z* 73, and preferably by $C_2H_5{}^{\bullet}$ loss resulting in the base peak at *m/z* 45. The thermodynamic advantage of $C_2H_5{}^{\bullet}$ loss over $CH_3{}^{\bullet}$ loss becomes evident from the diethyl ether spectrum. In accordance with Stevenson's rule, even two ethyl groups cleave off less $CH_3{}^{\bullet}$ than a single propyl loses $C_2H_5{}^{\bullet}$. It is tempting, although not trivial, to quantify the relative "ease" of fragmentation from the ratio of peak intensities. However, the primary fragment will undergo further fragmentation at an unknown rate, e.g., ethene loss from the oxonium ion at *m/z* 59 to yield the smaller one at *m/z* 31. Generally, oxonium ions are highly indicative of aliphatic ethers and alcohols. In the EI spectrum of diethyl ether the series from *m/z* 31 to *m/z* 73 is present (Table 6.8).

In case of alkanols, the methylene oxonium ion, $CH_2{=}OH^{+}$, *m/z* 31, deserves special attention. Resulting from α-cleavage, it undoubtedly marks spectra of primary alkanols, where it either represents the base peak or at least is the by far most abundant of the oxonium ion series (Fig. 6.9) [27]. The second important fragmentation route of aliphatic alcohols, loss of H_2O, is discussed in Sect. 6.11.

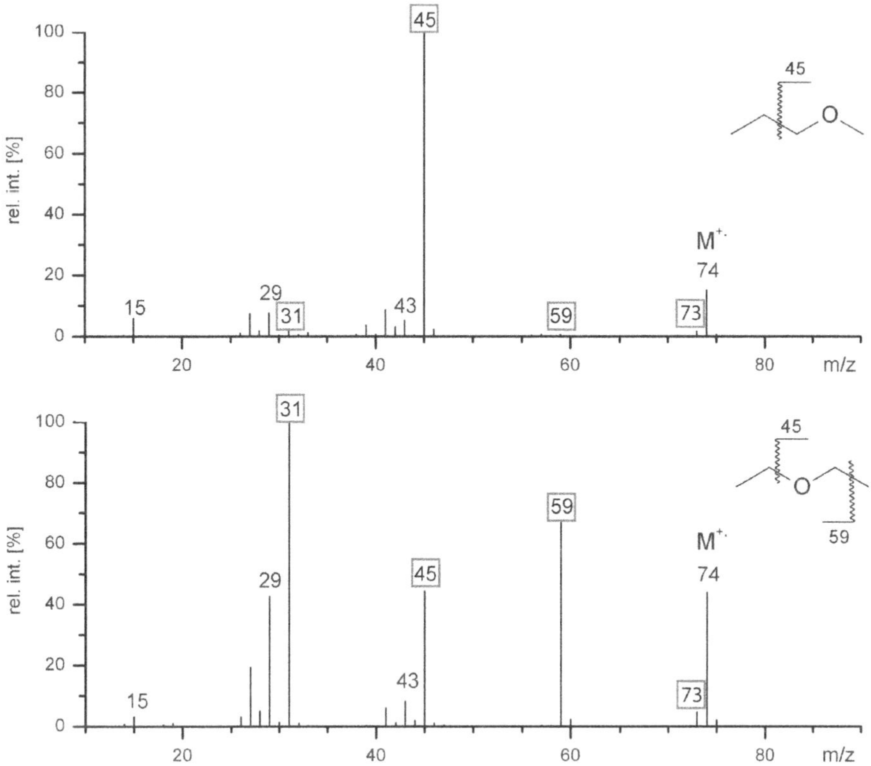

Fig. 6.8 EI mass spectra of methylpropylether and diethyl ether. Oxonium ion peaks are marked with *red boxes* (Spectra used by permission of NIST. © NIST 2002)

Table 6.8 Aliphatic oxonium ions

m/z (17 + 14*n*)	Oxonium ions $[C_nH_{2n+1}O]^+$	Accurate mass [u][a]
31	CH_3O^+	31.0178
45	$C_2H_5O^+$	45.0335
59	$C_3H_7O^+$	59.0491
73	$C_4H_9O^+$	73.0648
87	$C_5H_{11}O^+$	87.0804
101	$C_6H_{13}O^+$	101.0961
115	$C_7H_{15}O^+$	115.1117
129	$C_8H_{17}O^+$	129.1274

[a]Values rounded to four decimals

6.2.9 Charge Retention at the Heteroatom

The peak at *m/z* 45 in the spectrum of diethyl ether can neither be explained by α-cleavage nor by α-cleavage plus a subsequent cleavage, because the latter would demand carbene loss to occur, which is almost never observed (one of the rare

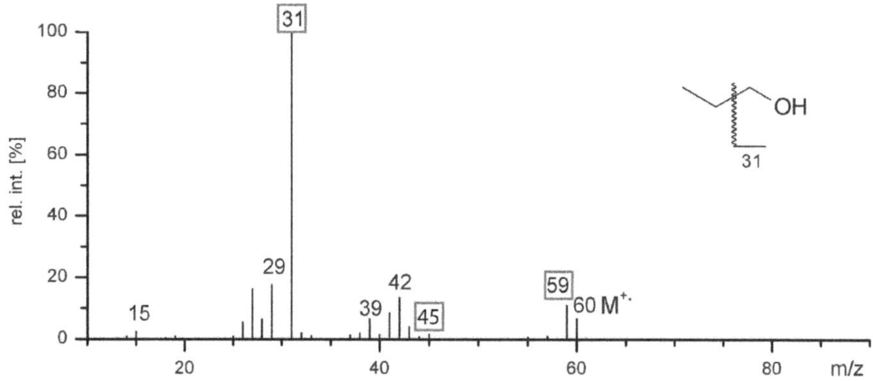

Fig. 6.9 EI mass spectrum of 1-propanol. Oxonium ion peaks are marked with *red boxes* (Used by permission of NIST. © NIST 2002)

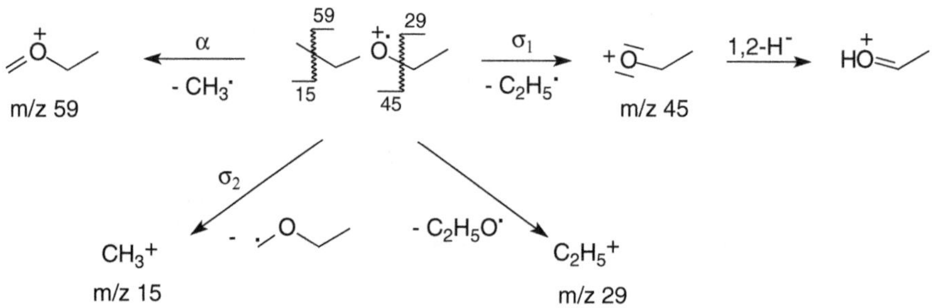

Scheme 6.12

examples is presented by formation of $HI^{+\bullet}$ from $CH_3I^{+\bullet}$). Obviously, the C–O bond can access a direct pathway for cleavage. Although some C–N bond cleavage can be observed in EI spectra of aliphatic amines, the cleavage of the C–O bond is gaining importance for the molecular ions of aliphatic ethers. It is a simple σ-bond cleavage as discussed for methane molecular ions, the only difference being the fact that one of the atoms connected by the σ-bond is not a carbon atom. As the heteroatom can stabilize the charge better than a primary carbon, the RX^+ fragment is preferably formed in such a case (σ_1). The product ion may then rearrange by 1,2-hydride shift to form an oxonium ion [32]. The formation of $C_2H_5^+$ fragment ions, *m*/*z* 29, directly competes with σ_1 (Scheme 6.12).

6.2.10 α-Cleavage of Thioethers

The EI mass spectra of thiols and thioethers also show a series of onium ions generated by α-cleavage of the molecular ion (Table 6.9). *Sulfonium ions* can easily

Table 6.9 Aliphatic sulfonium ions

m/z (33 + 14*n*)	Sulfonium ions $[C_nH_{2n+1}S]^+$	Accurate mass [u][a]
47	CH_3S^+	46.9950
61	$C_2H_5S^+$	61.0106
75	$C_3H_7S^+$	75.0263
89	$C_4H_9S^+$	89.0419
103	$C_5H_{11}S^+$	103.0576
117	$C_6H_{13}S^+$	117.0732
131	$C_7H_{15}S^+$	131.0889
145	$C_8H_{17}S^+$	145.1045

[a]Values rounded to four decimals

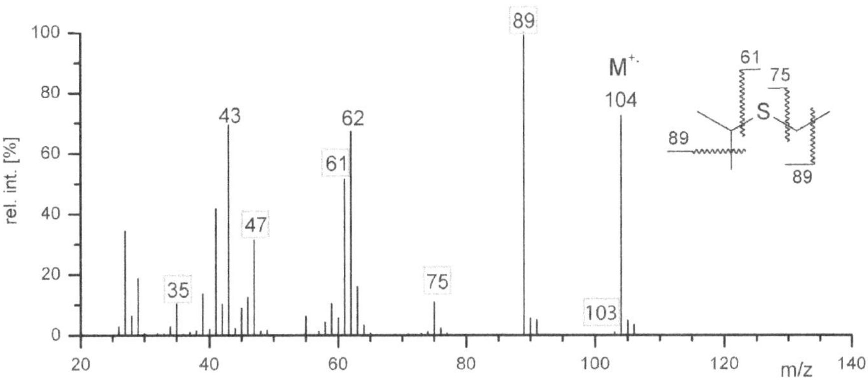

Fig. 6.10 EI mass spectrum of ethylisopropylthioether. Due to the isotopic composition of sulfur, the intensity of the $[M+2]^{+\bullet}$ ion is increased. The corresponding contributions can also be recognized for the sulfonium ions at *m/z* 47, 61, 75, and 89 (sulfonium ions are marked with *yellow boxes*). The peak at *m/z* 35 is due to H_3S^+ ions; also compare the spectrum of ethylpropylthioether (Fig. 6.46) (Spectrum used by permission of NIST. © NIST 2002)

be recognized from the isotopic pattern of sulfur (Fig. 6.10). The fragmentation patterns of thioethers will be discussed in greater detail later (Sects. 6.5.2 and 6.13.4).

6.2.11 α-Cleavage of Halogenated Hydrocarbons

Aliphatic halogenated hydrocarbons do not show abundant fragment ions due to α-cleavage [12]. As was found with aliphatic amines and ethers before, the molecular ion peak decreases in intensity as the molecular weight and branching of the alkyl chain increase. In general, the relative intensity of the molecular ion peak falls in the order I > Br > Cl > F (Sect. 6.1.4). For bromine the molecular ions are almost of the same relative intensity as for hydrogen, i.e., for the corresponding hydrocarbon. This corresponds to the inverse order of halogen electronegativities.

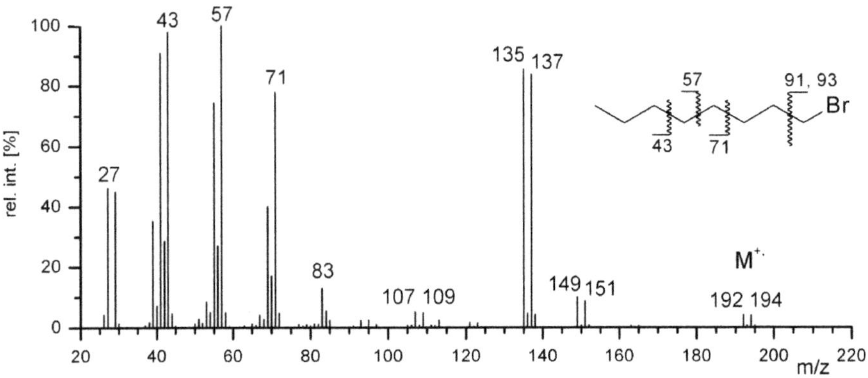

Fig. 6.11 EI mass spectrum of 1-bromo-octane. The product of the α-cleavage, *m/z* 91, 93 is of minor intensity, and the cyclic bromonium ion, *m/z* 135 and 137, dominates the spectrum (Spectrum used by permission of NIST. © NIST 2002)

Higher electronegativity of the halogen also causes a higher ionization energy of the RX molecule and an increase of α-cleavage products.

Fragmentation of 1-bromo-octane The 70-eV EI mass spectrum of 1-bromo-octane incorporates the characteristic fragmentations of aliphatic halogenated hydrocarbons (Fig. 6.11). All bromine-containing fragments are readily recognized from their bromine isotopic pattern (Sects. 3.1 and 3.2). The product of the α-cleavage, $[CH_2Br]^+$, *m/z* 91, 93, is of minor intensity, whereas a $[M–57]^+$ ion, *m/z* 135, 137, dominates the spectrum. The preference for the $[M–57]^+$ ion, $[C_4H_8Br]^+$, has been attributed to the possibility of forming a five-membered cyclic bromonium ion of low ring strain. This reaction differs from the preceding bond cleavages in that it is a displacement of an alkyl group, but it shares the common property of being a one-step process [33]. Analogous behavior is observed for the chlorohydrocarbons from hexyl through octadecyl that show the $[C_4H_8Cl]^+$ ion, *m/z* 91, 93. Fortunately, the isotopic patterns of Br and Cl are clearly different, thereby avoiding confusion of the isobaric $[C_4H_8Cl]^+$ and $[CH_2Br]^+$ ions. Iodo- and fluorohydrocarbons do not exhibit such cyclic halonium ions in their EI spectra. The remaining fragments can be explained by σ-cleavages leading to carbenium ions (Table 6.3, Scheme 6.13).

Beware of oversimplification

Early publications often oversimplified complex fragmentation processes. There are strong arguments that gas phase ionic reactions are generally stepwise processes. Thus, is more probable that complex fragmentations follow several discrete steps instead of single ones with simultaneous breaking and forming of several bonds [33].

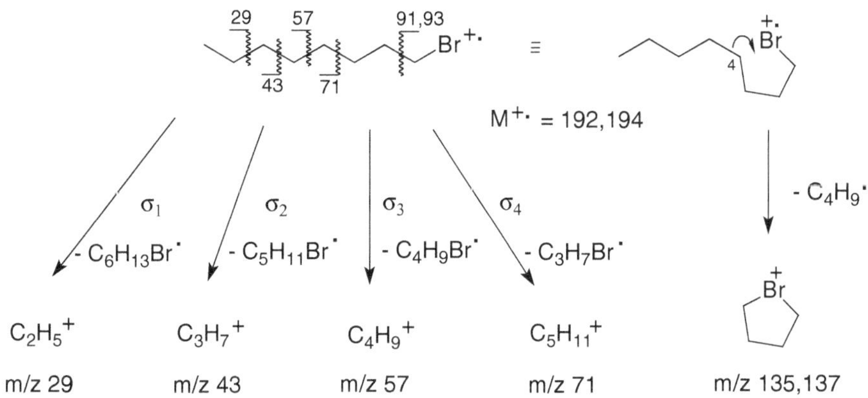

Scheme 6.13

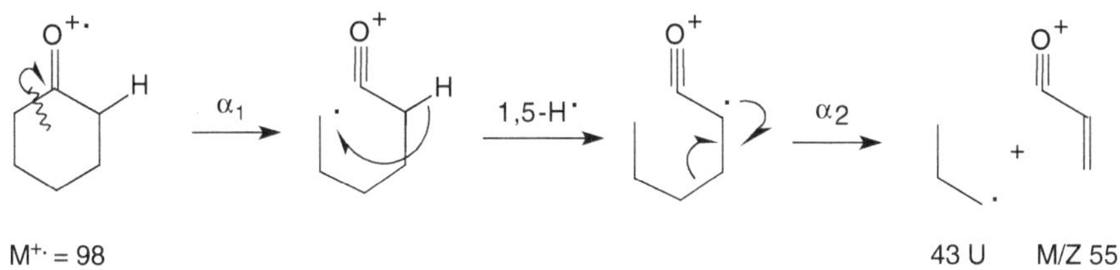

Scheme 6.14

6.2.12 Double α-Cleavage

Of course, α-cleavage can also occur in alicyclic ketones and other heteroatom-substituted alicyclic compounds. From a cycle, a single bond cleavage cannot release a neutral fragment, because this is still adhering to another valence of the functional group. To eliminate a propyl from cyclohexanone molecular ion, a three-step mechanism consisting of two α-cleavages and an intermediate 1,5-H$^{\bullet}$ shift is required (Scheme 6.14).

The mass spectrum of cyclohexanone has been examined by deuterium-labeling to reveal the mechanism effective for propyl loss, $[M-43]^+$, *m/z* 55, from the molecular ion, $M^{+\bullet} = 98$ [34, 35]. The corresponding signal represents the base peak of the spectrum (Fig. 6.12). Obviously, one deuterium atom is incorporated in the fragment ion that is shifted to *m/z* 56 in case of the [2,2,6,6-D_4]isotopolog. These findings are consistent with the above three-step mechanism.

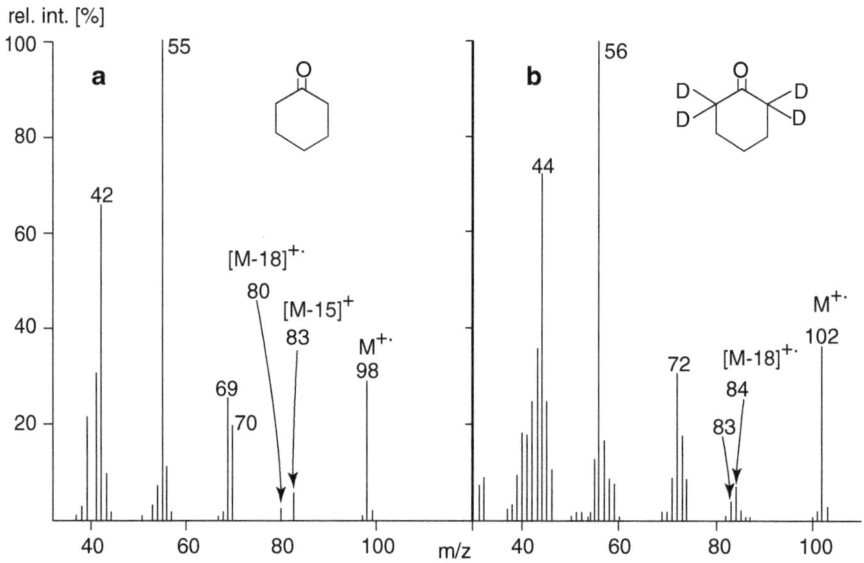

Fig. 6.12 70-eV EI mass spectra of cyclohexanone (**a**) and its deuterated isotopolog [2,2,6,6-D_4] (**b**) (Adapted from Ref. [34] with permission. © Springer-Verlag Wien, 1964)

6.2.13 Double α-Cleavage for the Identification of Regioisomers

Regioisomers of cyclohexanones, cyclohexylamines, cyclohexylalcohols and others can be identified by strict application of the mechanism of double α-cleavage. The method provides a valuable aid in structure elucidation even though there are some inherent limitations. While the double α-cleavage allows to distinguish substituents in positions 2 and/or 3 of the ring from those in position 4, it is, for example, impossible to distinguish a 2,3-dimethyl from a 2-ethyl or 3-ethyl derivative.

Structure elucidation of 2-ethyl-cyclohexylamine Propyl and pentyl losses from 2-ethyl-cyclohexylamine molecular ion, $M^{+\bullet} = 127$ (odd *m/z*) are competitive (Fig. 6.13). Pentyl loss, *m/z* 56 (even *m/z*), is favored over propyl loss, *m/z* 84 (even *m/z*), in accordance with Stevenson's rule. The peak at *m/z* 98 may be explained by ethyl loss due to a minor contribution of 1,4-$H^\bullet$ shift, i.e., from 3-position instead of the predominant 1,5-$H^\bullet$ shift from 2-position (Scheme 6.15). The $[M–CH_3]^+$ peak, *m/z* 112, is accompanied by a $[M–NH_3]^{+\bullet}$ signal, *m/z* 110, which is typical of primary (and to lower extent) secondary amines.

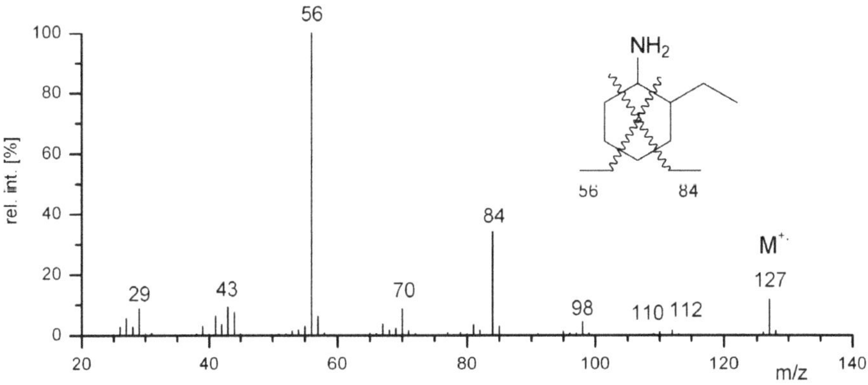

Fig. 6.13 EI mass spectrum of 2-ethyl-cyclohexylamine. Double α-cleavage allows to identify the substitution on one side of the ring (Spectrum used by permission of NIST. © NIST 2002)

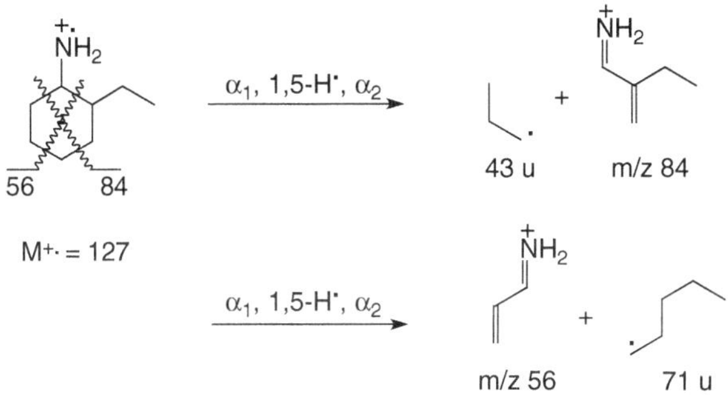

Scheme 6.15

6.3 Distonic Ions

6.3.1 Definition of Distonic Ions

For the case of the intermediate fragmentation products resulting from the first α-cleavage of cyclohexyl compounds the charge and the radical are not located at the same atom as is the case of molecular ions, but at distant positions. The term *distonic ion* was derived from the Greek word for 'separate' to describe such ionic species [36]. Distonic ions represent an ionic class of their own [36–38].

Definition
A *distonic ion* is a positive radical ion, which would formally arise by ionization of a zwitterion or a diradical, by isomerization or fragmentation

(continued)

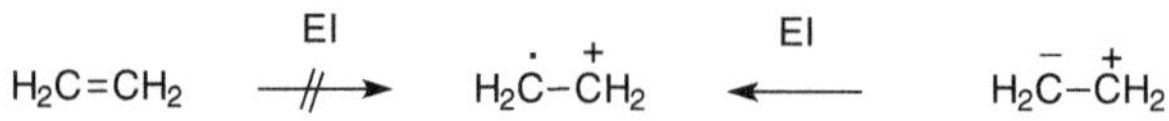

Scheme 6.16

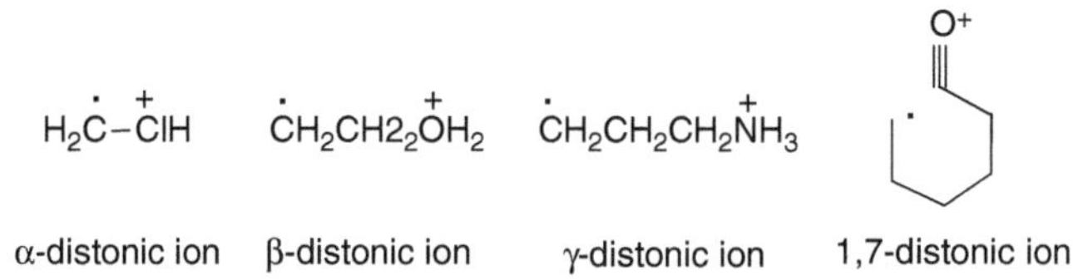

Scheme 6.17

of a 'classical' molecular ion, or by ion–molecule reactions. Consequently, distonic ions have charge and radical at different atoms in a conventional valence bond description [38, 39].

However, bearing charge and radical at separate sites is not a sufficient condition for an ion to be denoted distonic, e.g., the ethylene molecular ion may be written as such, but the corresponding neutral is *not* best represented as zwitterion and therefore the ethylene molecular ion by definition is *not* a distonic ion (Scheme 6.16).

The expressions *nonclassical* and *hypervalent* ion have also been used by some authors to describe distonic ions, but these are incorrect and thus should no longer be used. The term *ylidion* is limited to species where charge and radical are in adjacent positions. Thus, to describe the distance between charge and radical site, the terms α- (1,2-) *distonic ion*, β- (1,3-) *distonic* ion, γ- (1,4-) *distonic ion*, and so forth are now in use [38, 39] (Scheme 6.17).

6.3.2 Formation and Properties of Distonic Ions

Cleavage of a bond without immediate dissociation of the precursor radical ion is one way for generating distonic ions. Isomerization of molecular ions by hydrogen radical shift frequently leads to distonic ions prior to fragmentation and, moreover, the distonic isomers are often thermodynamically more stable than their "classical" counterparts [36] (Scheme 6.18).

The mutual interconversion of "classical" and distonic ions is not a fast process, because the isomers are separated by a comparatively high energy barrier. The activation energy for 1,2-$H^•$ shifts is substantially larger than for longer distance shifts such as 1,4- or 1,5-$H^•$ shifts. The activation energies and the heats of reaction have been determined for $H^•$ shifts in primary amine molecular ions (Fig. 6.14)

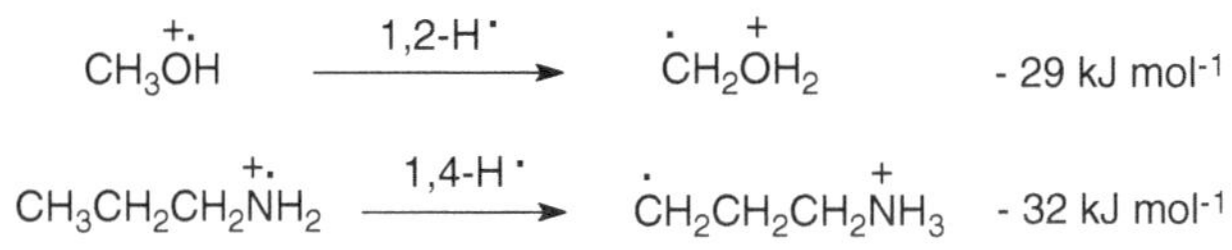

Scheme 6.18

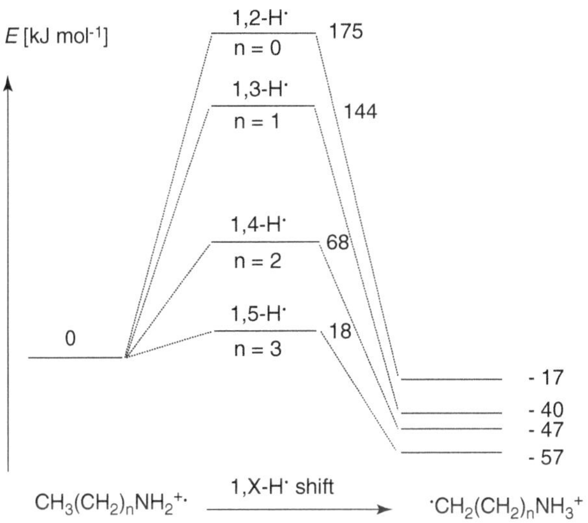

Fig. 6.14 Activation energies for isomerization of primary amine molecular ions to distonic isomers with the heats of formation of the precursor $M^{+\bullet}$ ions normalized to zero [41]

[31, 40, 41]. It has been argued that with increasing number of atoms between the positions, the ring strain in the respective C–H$^{\bullet}$–N transition states is reduced and that this is the reason for a significant decrease in activation energy [41]. In addition to the influence on transition states, the longer distance from charge to radical site also lowers the heats of formation of the distonic ions with respect to the "classical" ion precursors, i.e., any of these isomerizations is exothermic.

6.3.3 Distonic Ions as Intermediates

Distonic ions are of high relevance in the dissociation reactions of many ionized molecules as they play an important role as the central intermediates and products. It is likely that the long-lived molecular ions of many organic compounds exist in distonic form [39]. It has been shown, for example, that the long-lived radical ions of simple organophosphates spontaneously isomerize to distonic isomers [42] and that the ring-opening product of cyclopropane molecular ion is also distonic [43]. The next distonic ions we are going to learn about are the intermediates of the McLafferty rearrangement (Sect. 6.8).

6.4 Benzylic Bond Cleavage

The α-cleavage in molecular ions of ketones, amines, ethers, and similar functionalized compounds yields specific cleavage products of high importance for structure elucidation. Analogous behavior is observed in the mass spectra of phenylalkanes [44].

6.4.1 Cleavage of the Benzylic Bond in Phenylalkanes

Molecular ions of phenylalkanes are comparatively stable due to the good charge-stabilizing properties of the aromatic ring and thus, they normally give rise to intense peaks. Those molecular ions, possessing a benzylic bond preferably show cleavage of that bond as compared to the phenylic or homobenzylic position. As with the α-cleavage, the process is radical-initiated and follows the same basic scheme, i.e., dissociation of the bond second to the radical-site after transfer of a single electron towards the radical-site. The mass spectrum of *n*-propylbenzene is an example (Fig. 6.15 and Scheme 6.19).

The cleavages of the phenylic and homobenzylic bond are less important as can be seen from the minor peaks at *m*/*z* 77 and *m*/*z* 105 in the mass spectrum of *n*-

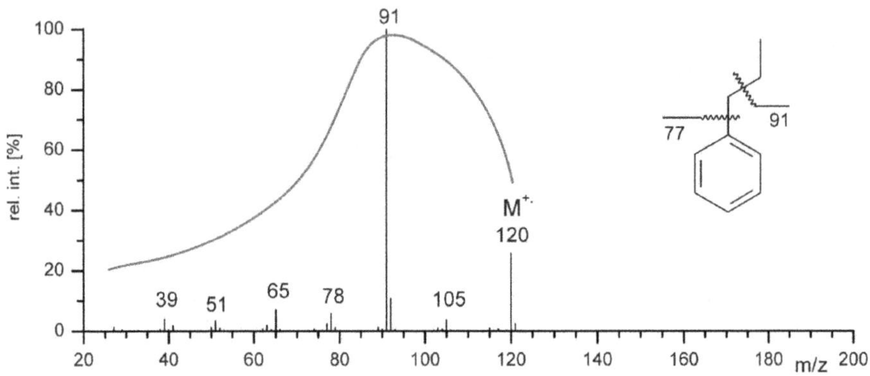

Fig. 6.15 EI mass spectrum of *n*-propylbenzene. The molecular ion peak and the primary fragment ion have significant intensity, whereas low-mass fragments are less abundant. The *red curve* illustrates the typical distribution of peak intensities versus *m*/*z* in EI spectra of aromatic compounds (Spectrum used by permission of NIST. © NIST 2002)

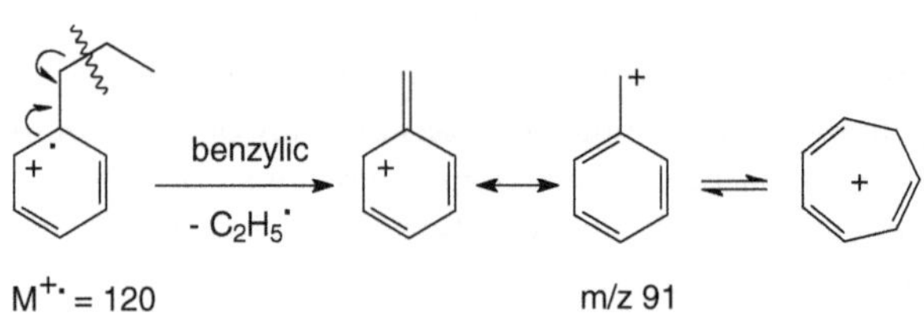

Scheme 6.19

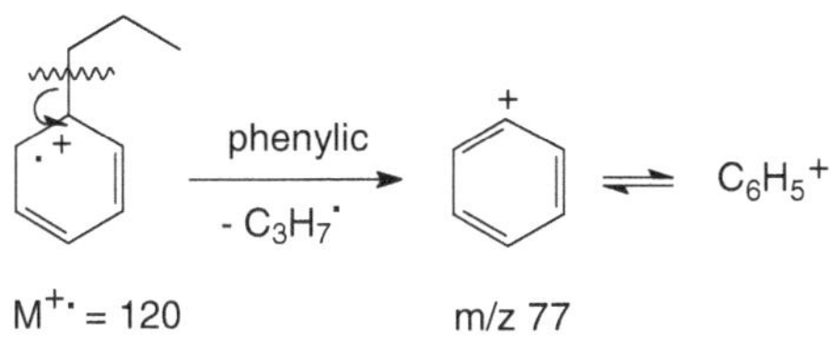

Scheme 6.20

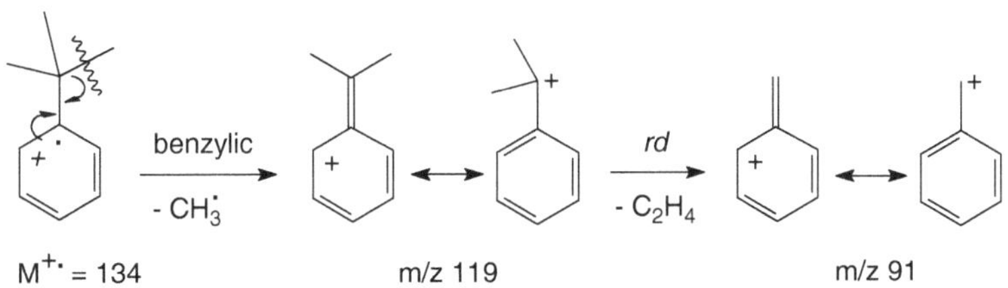

Scheme 6.21

propylbenzene. Nevertheless, phenylic bond cleavage does also occur and leads to further fragments. Due to its high thermodynamic stability, the $[C_7H_7]^+$ ion is not only formed by benzylic cleavage, but it is also obtained from many other fragmentation processes of phenylalkanes. The majority of mass spectra of such compounds clearly exhibit the corresponding peak at *m/z* 91 (Scheme 6.20).

Spectrum of *tert*-butylbenzene The first step of molecular ion dissociation of *tert*-butylbenzene, $C_{10}H_{14}$, proceeds via benzylic cleavage leading to $CH_3^{\bullet}$ and a primary fragment ion at *m/z* 119 (Scheme 6.21). In a second step, the $[C_7H_7]^+$ ion is formed from there by C_2H_4 loss even though this requires a complicated rearrangement that would not be expected at first sight (Fig. 6.16). Obviously, the driving force is the energetically favorable formation of $[C_7H_7]^+$ ions.

Many sources of $[C_7H_7]^+$ ions
The mere occurrence of the $[C_7H_7]^+$ ion – especially when it is of low intensity – is *not sufficient* to prove that the analyte belongs to the phenylalkanes. This ion and its characteristic fragments may also be observed *if there is any means of* generating a $[C_7H_7]^+$ fragment ion.

6.4.2 The Further Fate of $[C_6H_5]^+$ and $[C_7H_7]^+$

As already indicated in the preceding schemes, the resonance-stabilized benzyl ion, $[C_7H_7]^+$, initially formed by benzylic bond cleavage reversibly isomerizes to the tropylium and tolyl ion isomers (Scheme 6.22). The isomerization of $[C_7H_7]^+$ ions

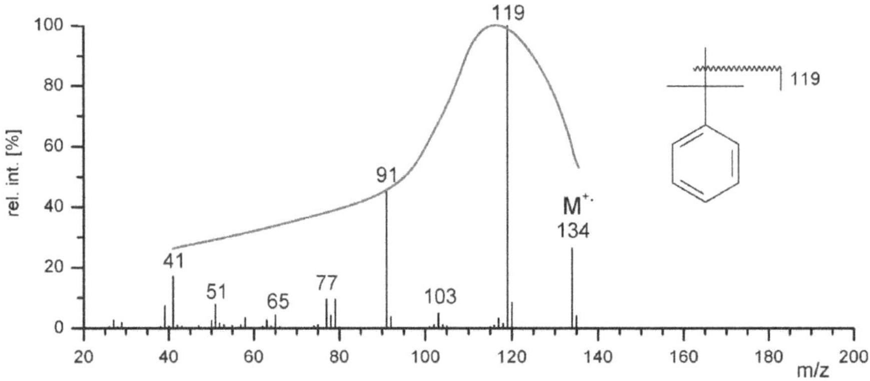

Fig. 6.16 EI spectrum of *tert*-butylbenzene. Again, molecular ion and primary fragment ion are dominating the spectrum and the *red curve* illustrates this typical distribution of peak intensities versus *m/z* in EI spectra of aromatic compounds (Spectrum used by permission of NIST. © NIST 2002)

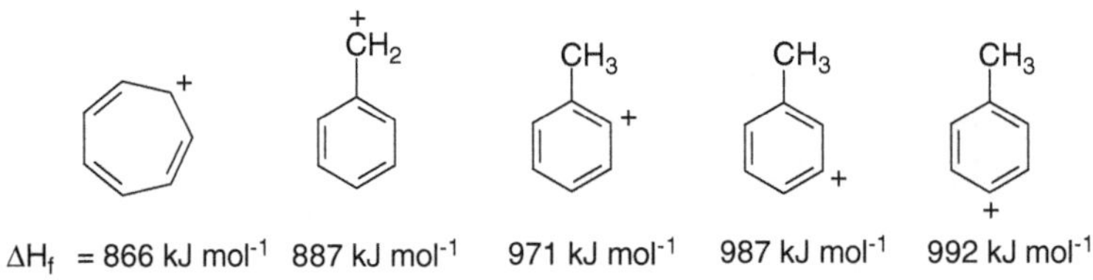

Scheme 6.22

has been the subject of numerous studies [45], revealing the tropylium ion as the thermodynamically most stable isomer [46, 47]. Provided sufficient lifetime, the process of benzyl/tropylium isomerization can be reversible ($E_0 = 167$ kJ mol^{-1} [45]), and then it necessarily goes along with a *scrambling* of hydrogens and of carbons as can be demonstrated by use of isotopically labeled compounds [48]. The degree of scrambling also depends on ion internal energy and on ion lifetime.

Scrambling

The illustrative term *scrambling* is used in mass spectrometry to describe rapid processes of (intramolecular) positional interchange of atoms. Scrambling may occur with hydrogens or may involve the complete carbon skeleton of an ion. Aryl radical ions and protonated aryl compounds are well known for their numerous scrambling processes [49].

Whatever the initial or preferred structure, the $[C_7H_7]^+$ ions dissociate by loss of ethyne, C_2H_2, to yield the cyclopentadienyl ion, $[C_5H_5]^+$, *m/z* 65, which fragments to yield $[C_3H_3]^+$, *m/z* 39, upon repeated ethyne loss (Scheme 6.23):

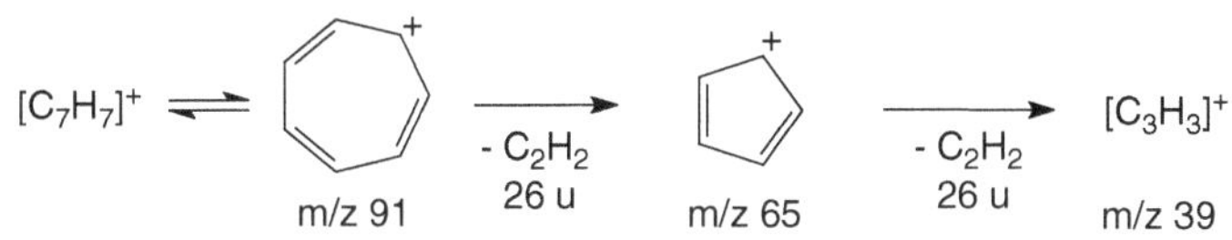

Scheme 6.23

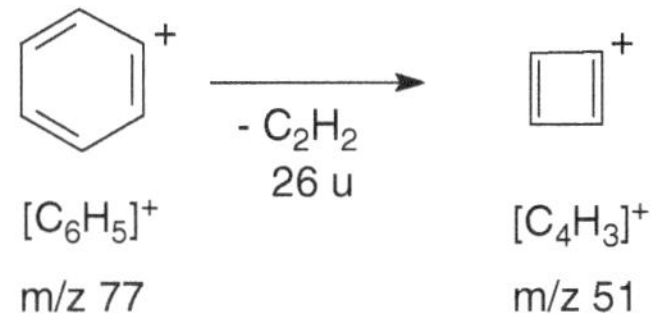

Scheme 6.24

The phenyl ion $[C_6H_5]^+$, *m/z* 77, also undergoes C_2H_2 loss, thereby generating the cyclobutadienyl ion, $[C_4H_3]^+$, *m/z* 51 (Scheme 6.24).

Characteristic ion series
Overall, the former two reactions lead to the typical appearance of the ion series *m/z* 39, 51, 65, 77, 91 in the EI mass spectra of phenylalkanes. However, one needs to be aware of the two competing reaction sequences leading to this series: (*i*) $M^{+\bullet} \rightarrow 91 \rightarrow 65 \rightarrow 39$ and (*ii*) $M^{+\bullet} \rightarrow 77 \rightarrow 51$; the latter usually being of lower intensity, which is in accordance with the preference for benzylic bond cleavage.

6.4.3 Isomerization of $[C_7H_8]^{+\bullet}$ and $[C_8H_8]^{+\bullet}$ Ions

The molecular ions of toluene and cycloheptatriene are capable of mutual isomerization prior to dissociation [44, 48, 50]. It has been known for long that hydrogen loss from toluene molecular ions takes place as if all eight positions within these ions were equivalent, and this has been interpreted in terms of complete hydrogen scrambling prior to dissociation (Scheme 6.25) [51]. The extent of isomerization becomes apparent from the close similarity of the toluene and cycloheptatriene EI mass spectra (Fig. 6.17). Loss of $H^\bullet$ from $[C_7H_8]^{+\bullet}$ leads to the formation of $[C_7H_7]^+$ ions, preferably of tropylium structure [49], and thus, to the typical fragment ion series described above.

Extensive isomerizations prior to dissociation are also observed for other ions having similar structural features. Deuterium labeling of some bicyclic aromatic systems has shown that complete or partial randomization of the aromatic hydrogens prior to dissociation can occur upon EI [52]. In detail, such observations were made in molecular ions of *i*) biphenyl prior to loss of $CH_3^\bullet$, C_2H_2, or $C_3H_3^\bullet$, *ii*) 1- and 2-cyanonaphthalenes before HCN expulsion, and *iii*) benzothiophene before

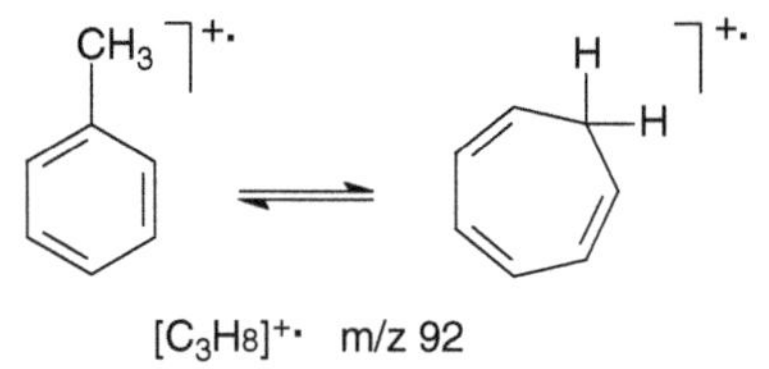

Scheme 6.25

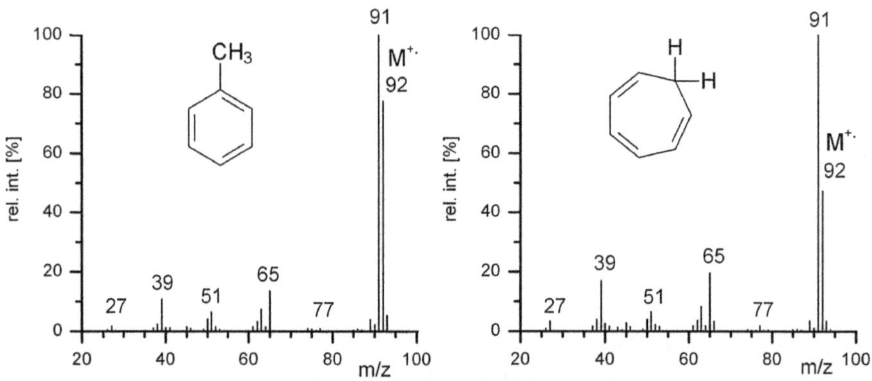

Fig. 6.17 Close similarity of the 70-eV EI mass spectra of toluene (*left*) and cycloheptatriene (*right*) (Spectra used by permission of NIST. © NIST 2002)

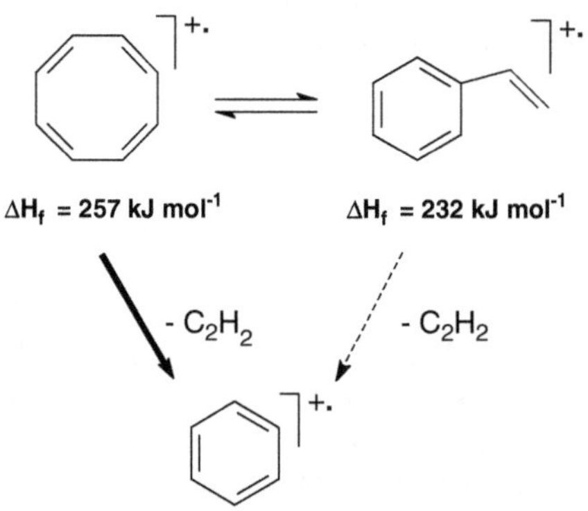

Scheme 6.26

C_2H_2 expulsion. Cyclooctatetraene and styrene molecular ions, $[C_8H_8]^{+\bullet}$, *m/z* 104, interconvert prior to loss of ethyne to yield benzene molecular ion, *m/z* 78. Because of the substantially lower overall activation energy, most of the $[C_6H_6]^{+\bullet}$ ions formed result from dissociation of cyclooctatetraene molecular ion (*bold arrow*) although this has the higher heat of formation [53] (Scheme 6.26).

6.4.4 Rings Plus Double Bonds

Based on valence rules, a general algorithm can be derived to distinguish between ions containing a different total number of double bonds and/or rings. As this algorithm does not allow to differentiate between a cyclic substructure and a double bond, the result is known as *double bond equivalents* (DBE) or simply *rings plus double bonds* ($r + d$). (The rarely used term *unsaturation* is not recommended because it does not imply cyclic structures.) The general equation for the determination of $r + d$ is:

$$r + d = 1 + 0.5 \times \sum_{i}^{i_{max}} N_i \ (V_i - 2) \tag{6.9}$$

where V_i represents the valence of an element and N_i is the number of atoms. For regular use, the expressions $0.5 \times (V_i - 2)$ should be calculated. For monovalent elements (H, F, Cl, Br, I) one obtains $0.5 \times (1 - 2) = -0.5$, for divalent elements (O, S, Se) $0.5 \times (2 - 2) = 0$ which is the reason why the contribution of divalent elements is cancelled. Proceeding with the higher valences yields:

$$r + d = 1 - 0.5\,N_{mono} + 0.5\,N_{tri} + N_{tetra} + 1.5N_{penta} + 2N_{hexa} + \dots \tag{6.10}$$

Restriction to formulas of the general type $C_cH_hN_nO_o$ reduces the expression to:

$$r + d = 1 + c - 0.5h + 0.5n \tag{6.11}$$

Here, other monovalent elements than hydrogen (F, Cl, Br, I) are counted "as hydrogens", other trivalent elements such as phosphorus are counted "as nitrogen" and tetravalent elements (Si, Ge) are handled the same way as carbons.

The $r + d$ algorithm produces integers for odd-electron ions and molecules, but nonintegers for even-electron ions that have to be rounded to the next lower integer, thereby allowing to distinguish even- from odd-electron species.

Care has to be taken when elements of changing valence are encountered, e.g., S in sulfoxides and sulfones or P in phosphates. In such a case, Eq. 6.9 or Eq. 6.10 have to be used, whereas Eq. 6.11 yields erroneous results (Table 6.10).

Table 6.10 Examples for the application of the $r + d$ algorithm according to Eq. 6.11

Name	Formula	$r + d$	Comment
Decane	$C_{10}H_{22}^{+\bullet}$	$1 + 10 - 11 = 0$	
Cyclohexanone	$C_6H_{10}O^{+\bullet}$	$1 + 6 - 5 = 2$	1 r + 1 d
Benzene	$C_6H_6^{+\bullet}$	$1 + 6 - 3 = 4$	1 r + 3 d
Benzonitrile	$C_7H_5N^{+\bullet}$	$1 + 7 - 2.5 + 0.5 = 6$	1 r + 5 d
Butyl ion	$C_4H_9^{+}$	$1 + 4 - 4.5 = 0.5$[a]	fragment[a]
Acetyl ion	CH_3CO^{+}	$1 + 2 - 1.5 = 1.5$[a]	1 d for C=O[b]
Dimethylsulfoxide	$C_2H_6SO^{+\bullet}$	$1 + 2 - 3 = 0$ $1 + 3 - 3 = 1$[c]	1 d expected[c] 1 d for tetravalent S

[a]Even-electron ions have 0.5 $r + d$ more than expected; round to next lower integer
[b]Values are correct for resonance structure with charge at carbon
[c]Attention! Sulfur is tetravalent in DMSO and should be treated like carbon

Apply the rules

Even-electron rule, Stevenson's rule, nitrogen rule, and $r + d$ algorithm belong to a collection of empirical rules and hints on how to systematically approach a mass spectrum of an unknown (Sect. 6.16). It is good practice to apply these during mass spectral interpretation, e.g., the $r + d$ algorithm as soon as the formula of a molecular ion or a fragment ion becomes apparent. This yields valuable information on possible substructures. Feel encouraged to practice their use while examining the numerous examples of spectra throughout this chapter!

6.5 Allylic Bond Cleavage

6.5.1 Cleavage of the Allylic Bond in Aliphatic Alkenes

The mass spectra of alkenes are governed by the alkyl moiety of the molecule and by the specific reactions characteristic for the double bond. Molecular ions are generally of low intensity – as is the case with all other purely aliphatic compounds discussed so far – and may even be fully absent [25, 54]. There is some preference for the cleavage of the allylic bond in the alkene molecular ions which can be treated analogously to α-cleavage and benzylic cleavage, but the double bond is the weakest cleavage-directing functional group (Scheme 6.27).

As hydrogen rearrangements prior to dissociation are prevalent in alkene molecular ions, the radical site migrates along the chain, thereby obscuring the original location of the double bond [55]. ^{2}H- and ^{13}C-labeling revealed that the molecular ions of 1-, 2-, 3-, and 4-octene completely interconvert within 10^{-9} s. The equilibration of double bond isomers by radical-site migration and concomitant hydrogen rearrangements do not involve the terminal hydrogens to a larger extent [56]. Generally, smaller unsaturated hydrocarbon ions undergo more extensive isomerization prior to decomposition than larger ones.

Isomerization first

Extensive isomerization prior to or between single steps of fragmentation makes the mass spectra of isomeric alkenes become very similar.

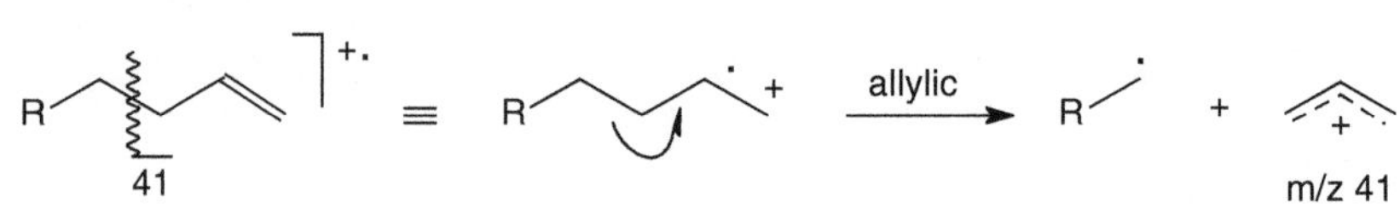

Scheme 6.27

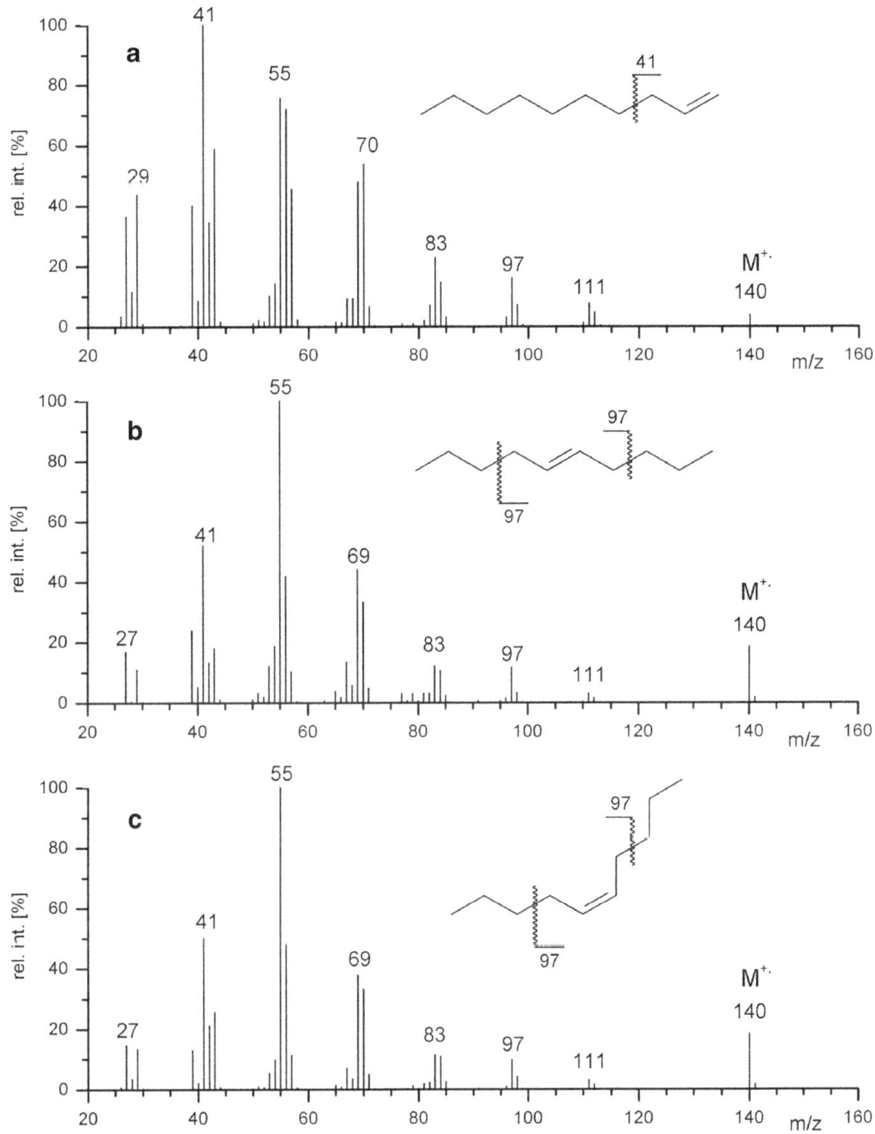

Fig. 6.18 EI mass spectra of isomeric decenes. The differences between 1-decene (**a**), (*E*)-5-decene (**b**), and (*Z*)-5-decene (**c**) are visible, but without reference spectra the isomers cannot be identified (Spectra used by permission of NIST. © NIST 2002)

Spectra of isomeric decenes compared The spectra of 1-decene, (*E*)-5-decene, and (*Z*)-5-decene are shown in Fig. 6.18. Whereas in the spectrum of 1-decene the basepeak at *m*/*z* 41 can easily be explained as a result of allylic cleavage, the base peak of both stereoisomeric 5-decenes is at *m*/*z* 55, and therefore, cannot result from direct allylic cleavage. It is impossible to find evidence for a certain isomer without reference spectra. At *m/z* 97, there is only a minor signal from allylic cleavage, and unfortunately such a peak is also observed in the spectrum of 1-decene. Consecutive fragmentations of the primary cleavage product give one reason for this close similarity, another being the influence of H• migrations prior to dissociation of the alkene molecular ions. Even comparison to reference spectra does not permit their proper identification as the differences between the stereoisomers are negligible.

6.5.2 Methods for the Localization of the Double Bond

The localization of a double bond is an important step in structure elucidation and therefore, it is not surprising that numerous approaches have been made to overcome the above limitations. The methods for immobilizing the double bond or for "freeze" isomerization include:

- epoxidation [57],
- iron and copper ion chemical ionization [58, 59],
- field ionization [60],
- collision-induced dissociation [55],
- formation of thioether derivatives [61, 62].

DMDS adducts The oxidative addition of dimethyl disulfide (DMDS) transforms the double bond to its 1,2-bis-thiomethyl derivative (Scheme 6.28a). Induced by charge localization at either sulfur atom, the molecular ions of DMDS adducts are prone to α-cleavage at the former double bond position (b). This yields sulfonium ions that are readily identified in the mass spectrum (Sect. 6.2.5). The method can be extended to dienes, trienes, and alkynes [63, 64].

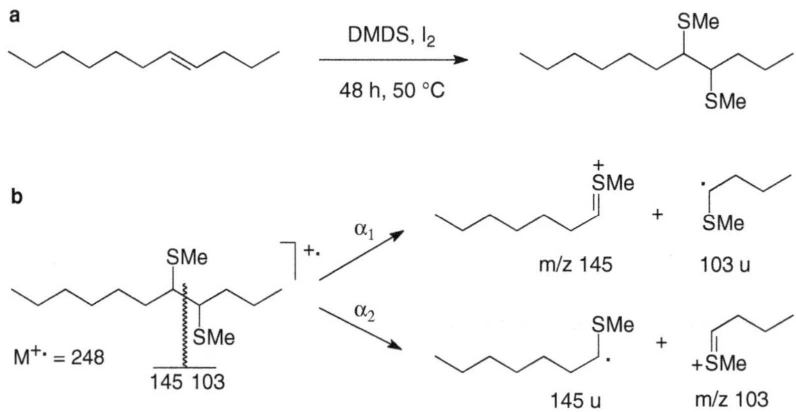

Scheme 6.28

6.6 Cleavage of Non-activated Bonds

6.6.1 Saturated Hydrocarbons

In a molecular ion of a straight-chain *n*-alkane there is no preferred position to localize the charge. Consequently, as in the case of methane, longer chain alkanes also suffer from substantial weakening of bonds upon electron ionization. The α-cleavage is not observed anymore. As expected, the primary step of dissociation is unspecific σ-bond cleavage at all but C_1–C_2 bonds, provided there are others. Methyl loss is negligible due to the unfavorable thermodynamics of this process. The resulting carbenium ions subsequently dissociate by loss of alkene molecules, preferably propene to pentene [65]. This process can occur repeatedly as long as the chain length of the fragment ion suffices [66]. As a result of these competing and consecutive ion dissociations, the base peak of aliphatic hydrocarbon spectra originates from low-mass carbenium ions, typically propyl, *m/z* 43, or butyl, *m/z* 57 (Table 6.3). Saturated carbenium ion fragments $[C_nH_{2n+1}]^+$ ($n = 3 - 7$) isomerize to common structures before decomposition, whereas the molecular ions retain their structure [67]. The molecular ion peak is usually apparent, but never as strong as in spectra of aromatic compounds [29]. For highly branched hydrocarbons it may even be absent (Scheme 6.29).

EI mass spectra of decane isomers The EI mass spectrum of *n*-decane is typical for linear saturated hydrocarbons (Fig. 6.19a). It shows smooth transitions of carbenium ion signal intensities from peak to peak, i.e., starting from *m/z* 29 the intensities steeply rise up to *m/z* 57, notably fall to about *m/z* 99, and then gradually diminish further up to the molecular ion peak that is somewhat stronger than the fragment peaks. Loss of $CH_3^•$ is not observed for energetic reasons. Branching of the aliphatic chain supports cleavage of the bonds adjacent to the branching point,

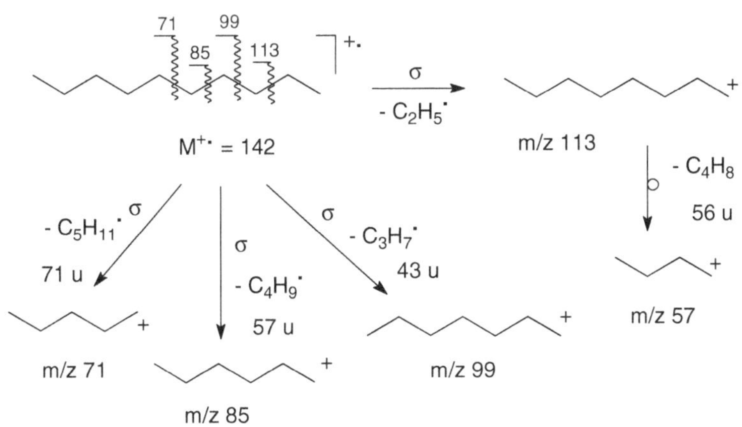

Scheme 6.29

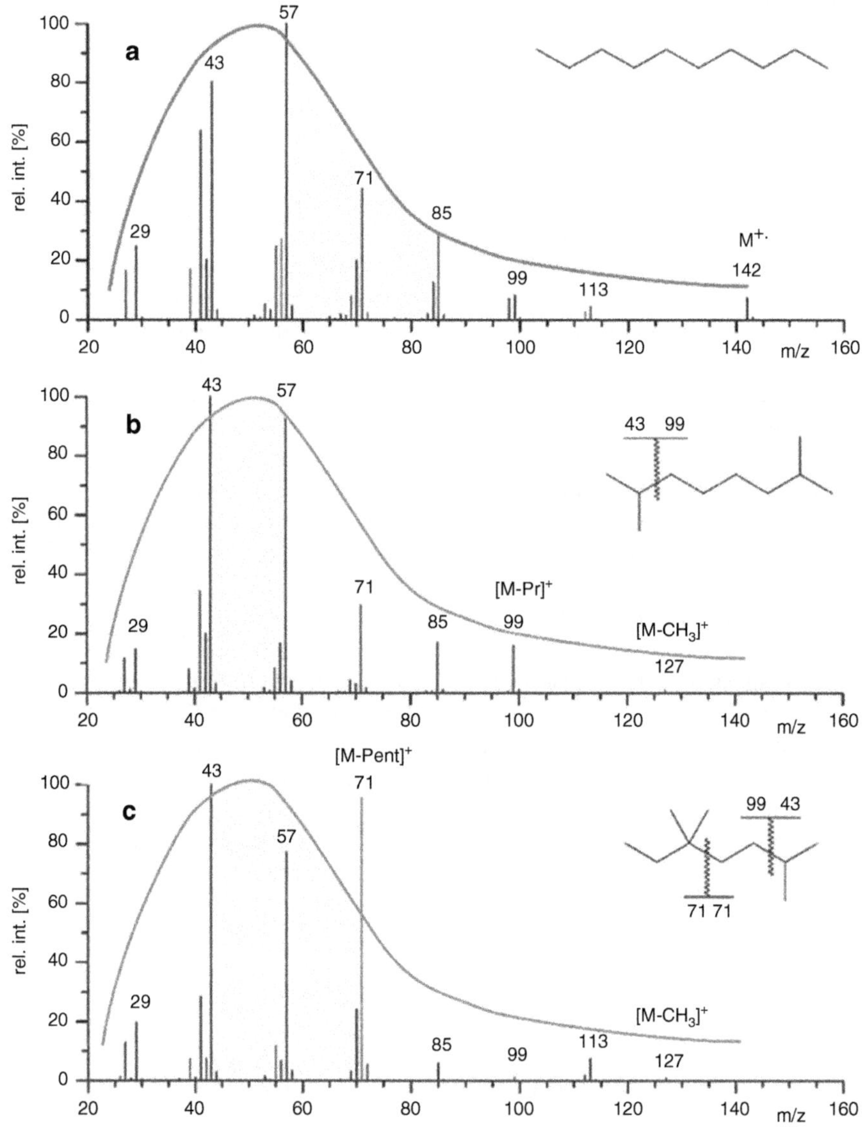

Fig. 6.19 EI mass spectra of *n*-decane (**a**), 2,7-dimethyloctane (**b**), and 2,5,5-trimethyl-heptane (**c**). The *red curve* in (**a**) has been fitted to smoothly follow the peak intensities along the *m/z* scale. Note how the same shape (*gray*) has different distances to the peak tops at *m/z* 71 and 99 in (**b**). The deviation from the smooth line becomes more obvious in (**c**) where $[M–Pent]^+$ really stands out while losses of Bu$^•$ and Pr$^•$ are notably reduced. Branched isomers also do not show the molecular ion peak anymore (Spectra used by permission of NIST. © NIST 2002)

because then secondary or tertiary carbenium ions and/or alkyl radicals are obtained (Fig. 6.19b, c). At least to some degree, this allows for the identification of isomers.

A closer look at the spectrum of *n*-decane also reveals fragment ions at *m/z* 84, 98, and 112, i.e., rearrangement ions at even mass number. The origin by loss of

Scheme 6.30

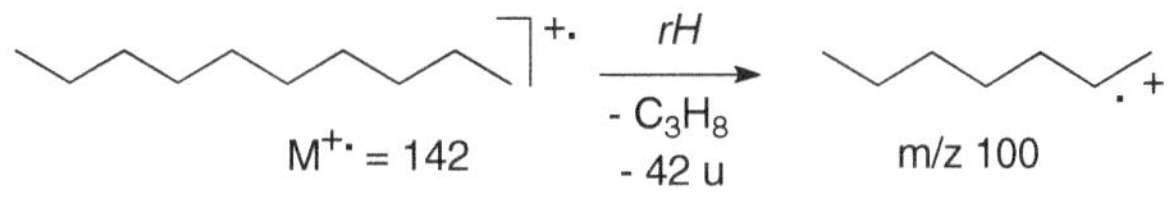

Scheme 6.31

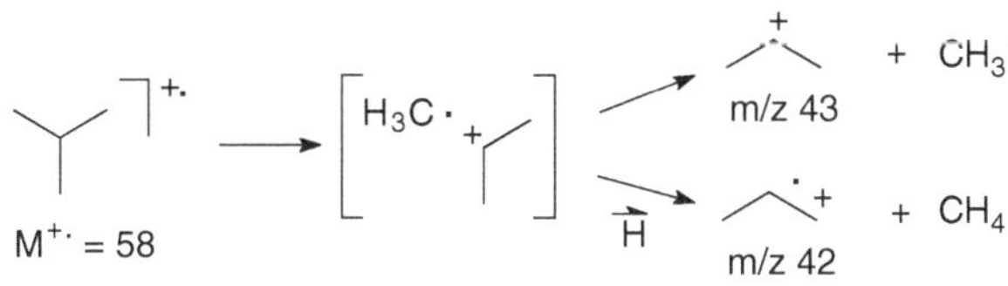

$H^{\bullet}$ from the accompanying carbenium ions at *m/z* 85, 99, and 113, respectively, can be excluded by application of the even-electron rule. Instead, alkane molecular ions may undergo alkane loss [68] (Scheme 6.30).

Theoretical and experimental studies revealed a common intermediate for the elimination of $CH_3^{\bullet}$ and CH_4 from isobutane and other alkanes of similar size. The additional hydrogen needed may originate from either one of the terminal positions of the propyl moiety [69, 70] (Scheme 6.31).

6.6.2 Carbenium Ions

Carbenium ions make up the largest portion of peaks in alkane mass spectra. They dissociate further by alkene loss with or without prior isomerization. Generally, such processes will yield a more stable isomer, e.g., the *tert*-butyl ion instead of other $[C_4H_9]^+$ isomers (Fig. 6.20).

Among the $[C_4H_9]^+$ isomers, only the *n*-butyl isomer can undergo fragmentations. It either yields an allyl ion, *m/z* 41, by loss of methane or an ethyl ion, *m/z* 29, by elimination of ethene. This is the reason why *tert*-butyl compounds exhibit strong *m/z* 41 and *m/z* 57 signals in their EI spectra (Figs. 6.21 and 6.24). In case of metastable $[C_4H_9]^+$ ions, methane loss is about 20-fold stronger than ethene loss because of the 1 eV higher activation energy in case of ethene loss [71].

Fragmentation of butyl ions In the EI mass spectrum of *tert*-butylchloride the molecular ion peak is absent and the signal of highest *m/z* is due to $[M\text{-}CH_3]^+$; note the Cl isotopic pattern of this signal (Fig. 6.21). The remaining portion of the spectrum is determined by the *tert*-butyl group, causing the base peak at *m/z* 57. The *tert*-butyl ion directly originates from σ-cleavage of the C–Cl bond. The ratio of the $[C_3H_5]^+$, *m/z* 41, and $[C_2H_5]^+$, *m/z* 29, fragments correlates well with the energetically favorable CH_4 loss from $[C_4H_9]^+$ ions (Fig. 6.20).

Besides alkene loss requiring sufficient chain length to occur, the smaller carbenium ions such as ethyl, propyl, or butyl ion exhibit remarkable dehydrogenation (Sect. 6.2.4). These single and even double H_2 eliminations lead to the

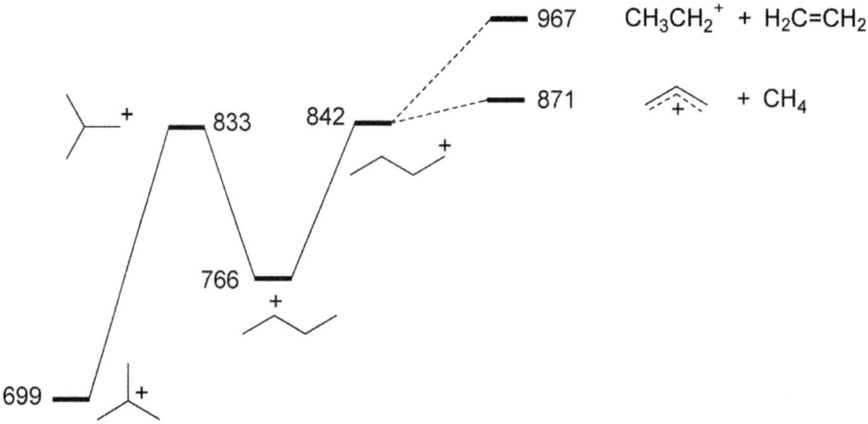

Fig. 6.20 Energetics of the isomerization and fragmentation pathways of $[C_4H_9]^+$ ions. Heat of formations are in kJ mol^{-1} (Redrawn from Ref. [71] with permission. © American Chemical Society, 1977)

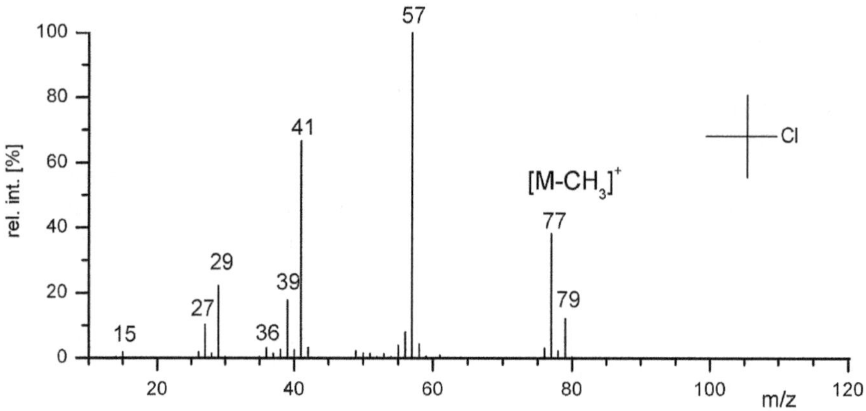

Fig. 6.21 EI mass spectrum of *tert*-butylchloride (Spectrum used by permission of NIST. © NIST 2002)

observation of characteristic accompanying peak patterns at *m*/*z*–2 and *m*/*z*–4, i.e., at the low-mass side of the corresponding carbenium ion peak.

Dirarylmethyl and triarylmethyl ions (trityl ions) are even more stable than the *tert*-butyl ion which is impressively demonstrated by the commercial availability of solid $[Ph_3C]^+[BF_4]^-$ and similar salts. Triphenylchloromethane dissociates in polar, inert solvents such as SO_2, and therefore, it is not surprising that EI spectra of triphenylmethyl compounds almost exclusively exhibit this ion together with some of its fragments, whereas the molecular ion peak is usually absent. Field desorption avoids this problem (Sect. 8.6).

6.6.3 Very Large Hydrocarbons

The mass spectra of very large hydrocarbons obey the same rules as their lower-mass counterparts. However, their peculiarities are worth mentioning. In case of linear chains, the EI spectrum shows an evenly expanding series of carbenium ion fragments of ever decreasing intensity. Given a clean background, the molecular ion (<1% rel. int.) can be well recognized at even *m/z* followed by the first fragment ion, $[M\text{-}29]^+$ (Fig. 6.22).

Limit of nominal mass

The first decimal of the *m/z* values of carbenium ions grows continuously with increasing *m/z* as a result of the negative mass defect of hydrogen (Sect. 3.5). Theoretically from $C_{32}H_{65}^+$ onwards (*m/z* 449.5081), rounding of the *m/z* value causes a shift to the next integer *m/z*, and thus would result in an assignment as *m/z* 450. This would also cause confusion due to the nitrogen rule. Therefore, nominal (integer) *m/z* values may not be used above *m/z* 400; instead inclusion of the first decimal is required also when dealing with LR mass spectra.

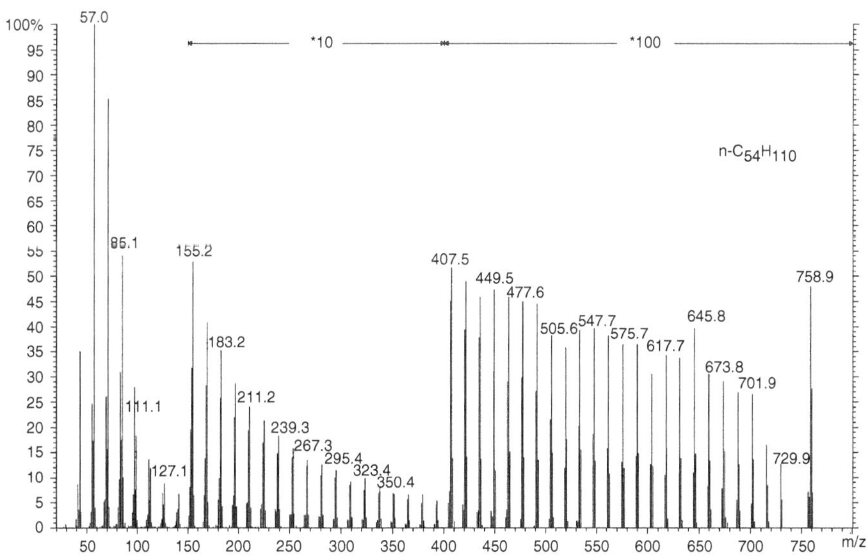

Fig. 6.22 DEI mass spectrum of tetrapentacontane, $n\text{-}C_{54}H_{110}$. The intensity scale is shown tenfold from *m/z* 150–400 and 100-fold above *m/z* 400. Note how the first decimal of the *m/z* values continuously rises with increasing *m/z* (By courtesy of W. Amrein, Labor für Organische Chemie, ETH Zürich)

Very large branched alkanes, such as 24,24-diethyl-19,29-dioctadecylheptatetracontane, $C_{87}H_{176}$, pose difficulties in obtaining useful mass spectra. Even 15-eV EI conditions are not sufficient for the detection of their molecular ions [72]. Beyond C_{40} alkanes, especially in case of mixtures such as hydrocarbon waxes or polyethylenes of low molecular weight, field desorption and matrix-assisted laser desorption/ionization are the ionization methods of choice (Chaps. 8 and 11).

6.7 Recognition of the Molecular Ion Peak

The molecular ion peak directly provides valuable information on the analyte. Provided the peak being of sufficient intensity, in addition to mere molecular mass, the accurate mass can reveal the molecular formula of the analyte, and the isotopic pattern may be used to derive limits of elemental composition (Sects. 3.5 and 3.6).

However, the peak of highest *m/z* in a mass spectrum must not necessarily represent the molecular ion of the analyte. This is often the case with EI spectra either as a result of rapidly fragmenting molecular ions or due to thermal decomposition of the sample (Sect. 6.11) In general, the stability of the molecular ion increases if π-bonding electrons for the delocalization of the charge are available and it decreases in the presence of preferred sites for bond cleavage.

In EI mass spectrometry, the molecular ion peak can be increased to a certain extent by measuring at low electron energy and ion source temperature (Sect. 5.1). Nonetheless, some compounds thermally decompose prior to evaporation or simply cannot form nondissociating molecular ions at all. The use of soft ionization methods is often the best way for coping with these problems. Unfortunately, even for the softest ionization method, there is no guarantee that the peak at highest *m/z* always corresponds to molecular mass.

Rule of thumb

The stability of molecular ions decreases roughly in the following order: aromatic compounds > conjugated alkenes > alkenes > alicyclic compounds > carbonyl compounds > linear alkanes > ethers > esters > amines > carboxylic acids > alcohols > branched alkanes [73].

6.7.1 Rules for Identifying the Molecular Ion Peak

In order to derive reliable analytical information, it is important to have some criteria at hand to identify the molecular ion peak (Fig. 6.23).

- The molecular ion must be the ion of highest *m/z* in the mass spectrum (besides the corresponding isotopic peaks).
- It has to be an odd-electron ion, $M^{+\bullet}$.

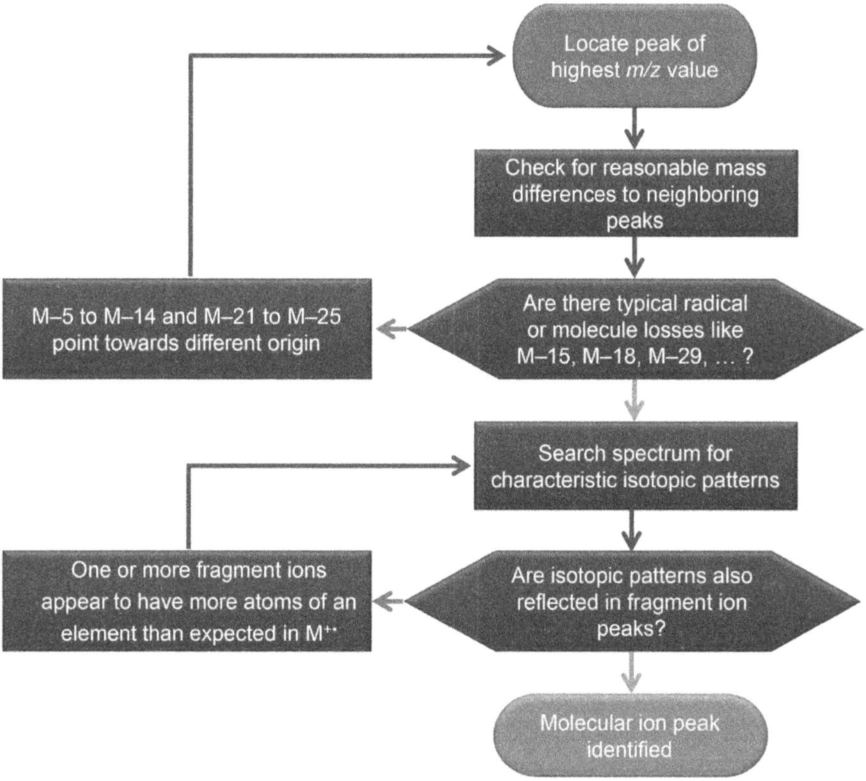

Fig. 6.23 Flow chart showing decisions and criteria for the identification of the molecular ion peak

- Peaks at the next lower *m*/*z* must be explainable in terms of reasonable losses, i.e., of common radicals or molecules. Signals at M–5 to M–14 and at M–21 to M–25 point towards a different origin of the presumed $M^{+•}$ (Table 6.11).
- Fragment ions may not show isotopic patterns due to elements that are not present in the presumed molecular ion.
- No fragment ion may contain a larger number of atoms of any particular element than the molecular ion does.

6.7.2 Common Neutral Losses

Neutral losses either proceed via elimination of radicals or intact molecules from the molecular ion. Some of these losses occur very frequently and it is thus useful to have a short compilation at hand before engaging in mass spectral interpretation (Table 6.11, for an extended version of this table cf. Appendix A.8).

Table 6.11 Commonly observed neutral losses from molecular ions

$[M–X]^+$	Radicals	$[M–XY]^{+\bullet}$	Molecules
−1	$H^\bullet$	−2	H_2
−15	$CH_3^\bullet$	−4	$2 \times H_2$
−16	$NH_2^\bullet$, $O^\bullet$	−17	NH_3
−17	$OH^\bullet$	−18	H_2O
−19	$F^\bullet$	−20	HF
−29	$C_2H_5^\bullet$	−27	HCN
−31	$OCH_3^\bullet$	−28	CO, C_2H_4, (N_2)
−33	$SH^\bullet$	−30	$H_2C{=}O$, NO
−35	$Cl^\bullet$	−32	CH_3OH, H_2S, (O_2)
−43	$C_3H_7^\bullet$, $CH_3CO^\bullet$	−34	H_2S
−45	$OC_2H_5^\bullet$, $COOH^\bullet$	−36	HCl
−57	$C_4H_9^\bullet$	−42	C_3H_6, $H_2C{=}C{=}O$
−79	$Br^\bullet$	−44	CO_2
−91	$C_7H_7^\bullet$	−46	C_2H_5OH, NO_2
−127	$I^\bullet$	−60	CH_3COOH

The case of 2,5,5-trimethylheptane The EI mass spectrum of 2,5,5-trimethylheptane (Fig. 6.19c) shows no molecular ion peak. The peak of highest *m/z* might be located either at *m/z* 113 or – upon closer inspection – at *m/z* 127. Whatever the right peak may be, this either would demand for 1, 3, 5, . . . nitrogen atoms or its interpretation as a fragment ion. However, the remaining mass spectrum does not reveal any hint for nitrogen-containing ions, e.g., immonium ions are absent. Instead, the spectrum suggests that there are carbenium ions and their accompanying fragments only. It is also awkward that $\Delta m/z = 14$ between *m/z* 113 and 127, which is a forbidden value for a pair of precursor and fragment ion. Thus, the peaks at *m/z* 113 and 127 both have to be fragment ions, most probably created by loss of $C_xH_y^\bullet$. Here, *m/z* 127 is explained as $[M–Et]^+$, while *m/z* 113 is assigned as $[M–Me]^+$.

6.8 McLafferty Rearrangement

Up to here, we have mainly discussed mass spectral fragmentations along the guideline of radical loss by simple cleavages, occasionally making some steps aside to learn about compound-specific reactions where appropriate. Next, we shall examine some pathways of alkene loss from molecular ions. Any loss of an intact molecule belongs to the rearrangement type of fragmentations. Among these, the *γ-H shift with β-cleavage*, commonly known as *McLafferty rearrangement* (McL), surely is the most prominent.

6.8.1 McL of Aldehydes and Ketones

The loss of alkenes from molecular ions of carbonyl compounds was noticed early on [18, 74]. Soon, a mechanism involving γ-H shift and β-cleavage was proposed and studied in detail [20, 21, 75, 76]. Strictly speaking, the term *McLafferty rearrangement* only describes an alkene loss from molecular ions of saturated aliphatic aldehydes, ketones, and carboxylic acids, the mechanism of which is analogous to the Norrish type-II photofragmentation in condensed-phase chemistry. However, a more generous use of the term to include all alkene losses essentially following this mechanism is useful for the recognition of analogies from a wide variety of molecular ions. Below, any fragmentation that can be described as a transfer of a γ-hydrogen to a double-bonded atom through a six-membered transition state causing alkene loss upon cleavage of the β-bond is regarded as a McLafferty rearrangement (Scheme 6.32) [77, 78].

The requirements for a McLafferty rearrangement in the broad sense are:

- Atoms A, B, and D can be carbons or heteroatoms.
- Atoms A and B must be connected by a double bond.
- At least one γ-hydrogen is available.
- The γ-H is selectively transferred to B via a six-membered transition state.
- The distance between the γ-H and the double-bonded atom must be less than 1.8×10^{-10} m [79, 80].
- The C_γ–H bond must be in plane with the acceptor group [81].

Ethene loss from butanal The EI mass spectrum of butanal, $M^{+\bullet}$ at *m/z* 72 (even-numbered *m/z* value), mainly shows carbenium fragment ions (Fig. 6.24). These simple bond cleavages can be easily recognized from the odd-numbered *m/z* values, i.e., *m/z* 15, 29, 43. As usual, the carbenium ions are accompanied by the products of their subsequent fragmentation by loss of H_2. Only the base peak at *m/z* 44 (also an even-numbered *m/z* value) stands out as it is represented by a loss of 28 u. Obviously, the $[M–28]^{+\bullet}$ ion is resulting from a rearrangement fragmentation, which corresponds to elimination of C_2H_4 via McL in this case.

Following the above general description of the McLafferty rearrangement, the peak at *m/z* 44 in the mass spectrum of butanal can be explained by C_2H_4 loss from the molecular ion. The process may either be formulated in a concerted manner (**a**) or as a stepwise process (**b**) (Scheme 6.33).

While the concerted pathway has been preferred in early publications on the subject, evidence for a stepwise mechanism involving distonic ion intermediates is presented in more recent work taking kinetic isotope effects into account [82]. This

Scheme 6.32

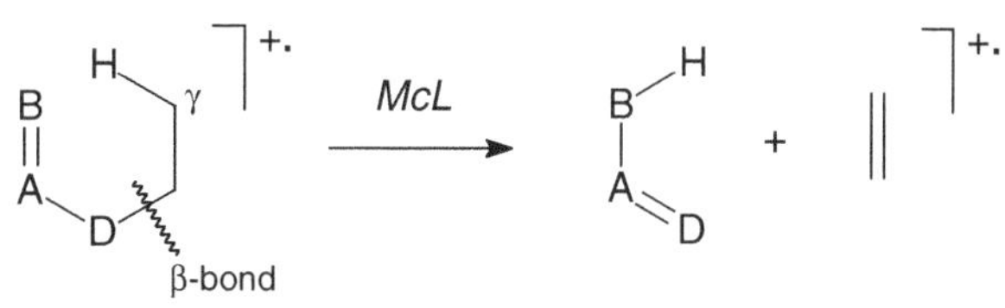

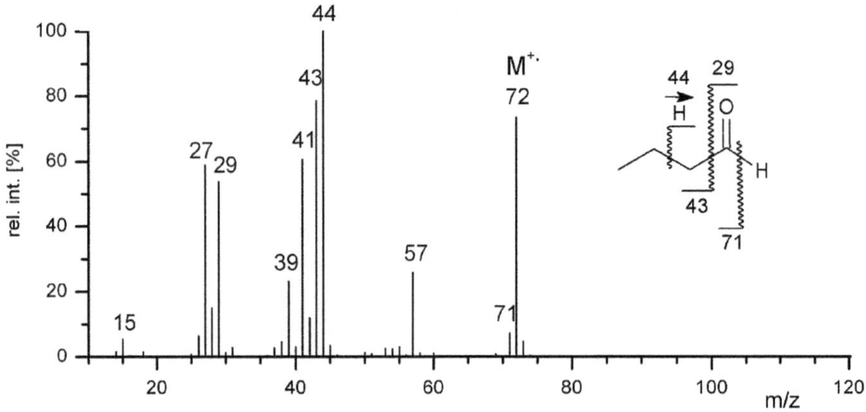

Fig. 6.24 EI mass spectrum of butanal. The base peak at *m/z* 44 is caused by the product of the McLafferty rearrangement. Note that here the peak at *m/z* 57 cannot result from $[C_4H_9]^+$, but is due to $[M–CH_3]^+$ (Spectrum used by permission of NIST. © NIST 2002)

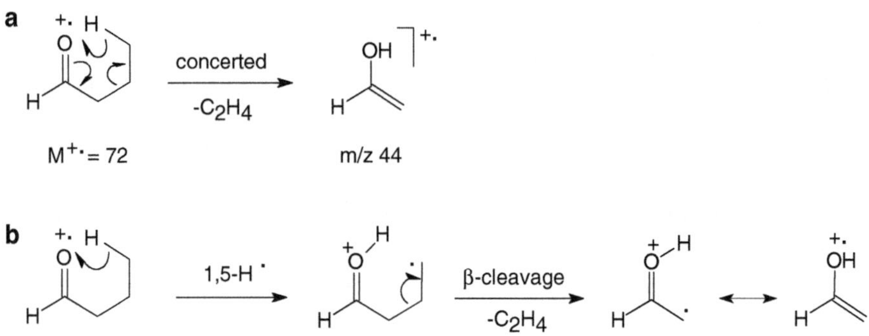

Scheme 6.33

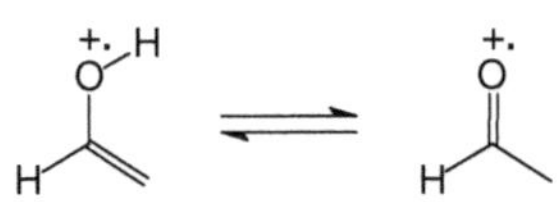

Scheme 6.34

is also in agreement with the postulation that reactions involving multiple bonds are generally stepwise processes [33, 83].

In principle, the enolic fragment ion may or may not tautomerize to the keto form before further fragmentation takes place (Scheme 6.34).

The gas-phase heats of formation of several enol positive ions of aliphatic aldehydes, ketones, acids, and esters were measured and compared with those of the corresponding keto ions. The enolic ions were found to be thermodynamically more stable by 58–129 kJ mol^{-1}. This is in marked contrast to the neutral tautomers, in which the keto forms are generally more stable [84]. The experimental findings also are in good agreement with MNDO calculations [85], and support the hypothesis that reketonization does not play a major role for further fragmentation. Anyway, it is helpful to consider tautomerization when seeking for subsequent decomposition pathways.

The McLafferty rearrangement itself proceeds via charge retention, i.e., as alkene loss from the molecular ion, but depending on the relative ionization energies of the respective enol and alkene products, the charge migration product, i.e., the corresponding alkene molecular ion is also observed, e.g., $C_2H_4^{+\bullet}$, *m*/*z* 28, in the EI spectrum of butanal.

The occurrence of the McLafferty rearrangement is strictly limited to molecular ions possessing at least one γ-hydrogen for transfer to the terminal atom at the double bond. Thus, blocking the γ-position, e.g., by introduction of alkyl or halogen substituents, effectively excludes this dissociation pathway.

No McL from 3,3-dimethyl-2-butanone In the EI mass spectrum of 3,3-dimethyl-2-butanone no fragment ion due to McLafferty rearrangement can be observed, because there is no γ-hydrogen available (Fig. 6.25). Instead, the products are exclusively formed by simple cleavages as evident from their odd-numbered *m*/*z* values. The highly stable *tert*-butyl ion, *m*/*z* 57, predominates over the acylium ion at *m*/*z* 43 (Sect. 6.6.2). The *tert*-butyl ion is also indicated by its characteristic fragment ions at *m*/*z* 29 and 41 (Sect. 6.6.2).

6.8.2 Fragmentation of Carboxylic Acids and Their Derivatives

The mass spectra of carboxylic acids and their derivatives are governed by both α-cleavage and McLafferty rearrangement. As expected, α-cleavage may occur at

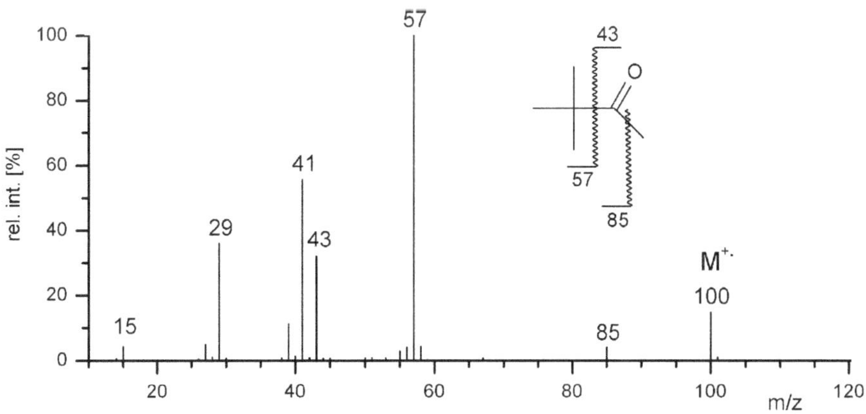

Fig. 6.25 EI spectrum of 3,3-dimethyl-2-butanone. The McLafferty rearrangement is suppressed, because there is no γ-hydrogen (Spectrum by permission of NIST. © NIST 2002)

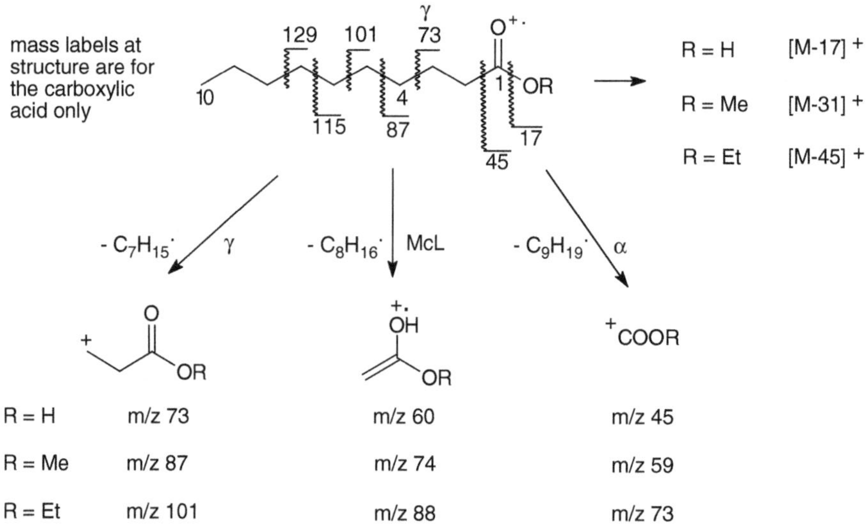

Scheme 6.35

either side of the carbonyl group causing $OH^{\bullet}$ loss, $[M–17]^+$, or alternatively alkyl loss. Whereas the α-cleavages can even be observed for formic acid where they are leading to $[M–OH]^+$, *m/z* 29, $[M–H]^+$, *m/z* 45, and the respective charge migration products, the McLafferty rearrangement can only occur from butanoic acid and its derivatives onwards (Scheme 6.35) [74]. Analogous to aliphatic aldehydes, the same fragment ions are obtained for a homologous series of carboxylic acids, provided they are not branched at the α-carbon. Thus, highly characteristic fragment ions make their recognition straightforward.

Typical alkanoic acid The molecular ion of decanoic acid, $C_{10}H_{20}O_2^{+\bullet}$, preferably eliminates octene via McLafferty rearrangement yielding $C_2H_4O_2^{+\bullet}$, *m/z* 60, as the base peak of the spectrum (Fig. 6.26). This process is accompanied by several σ-bond cleavages among which cleavage of the γ-bond is clearly favored. Resulting from α-cleavage, $OH^{\bullet}$ loss can be expected, but is often represented by a very minor peak in the spectra of carboxylic acids. The other product, $[M–R]^+$, $COOH^+$, *m/z* 45, is almost always observed together with the complementary $[M–45]^+$ ion, both of which normally belong to the ions of low abundance.

In aliphatic esters the fragments typical for carboxylic acids are shifted by 14 u to higher mass upon transition from the free acid to the methyl ester and by further 14 u for the ethyl ester [77, 78, 86, 87].

Esters of aliphatic carboxylic acids The mass spectrum of methyl heptanoate nicely meets the standard, and thus all peaks may be explained according to Scheme 6.36 (Fig. 6.27a). In principle, the same is true for the isomeric methyl 2-methylhexanoate, but here care has to be taken not to interpret the mass spectrum as belonging to an ethyl ester. This is because the 2-methyl substituent resides on

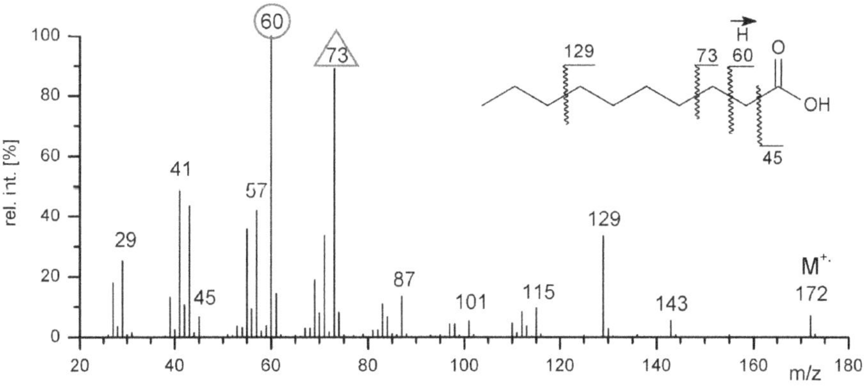

Fig. 6.26 EI mass spectrum of decanoic acid. The peak at *m/z* 60 due to McL is marked by a *blue circle*, the peak by γ-cleavage is marked by a *blue triangle* (Used by permission of NIST. © NIST 2002)

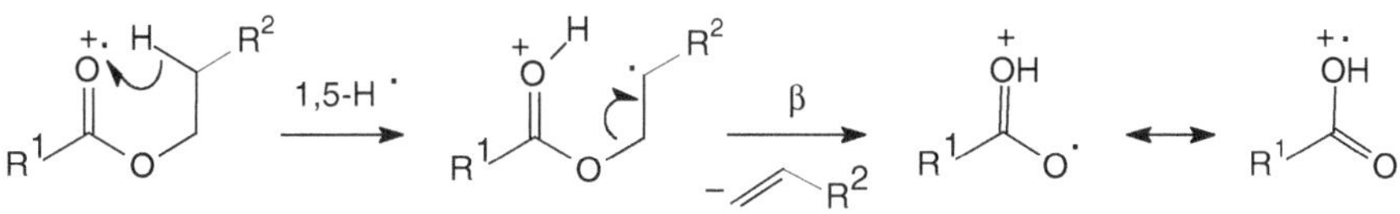

Scheme 6.36

the ionic products of McLafferty rearrangement and γ-cleavage, shifting both of them 14 u upwards. Nevertheless, a glance at the α-cleavage products, $[M–OMe]^+$ and $[COOMe]^+$, *m/z* 59, reveals the methyl ester.

For carboxylic acid ethyl and longer-chain aliphatic esters the McLafferty rearrangement can also occur on the alkoxy branch (R^2) of the molecular ion. It then competes as a second alkene loss with the reaction at R^1(Scheme 6.36). Independent of the alkyl chain, there are some frequently observed McL products (Table 6.12).

McL of the ester chain The base peak at *m/z* 88 in the mass spectrum of ethyl hexanoate results from butene loss from the molecular ion, $M^{+\bullet}$, *m/z* 144, via McLafferty rearrangement (Fig. 6.28). This product ion may then undergo ethene loss to yield the fragment ion at *m/z* 60. The remaining fragments can be rationalized by γ-cleavage, $[M–Pr]^+$, *m/z* 101, and α-cleavage products, $[M–OEt]^+$, *m/z* 99, respectively. The carbenium ions representing the alkyl portion of the molecule are formed by σ-bond cleavages. Note that the peaks pair at *m/z* 99, 101 and *m/z* 115, 117 do not reflect a chlorine isotopic pattern but just happen to show somewhat similar ratios of their intensities.

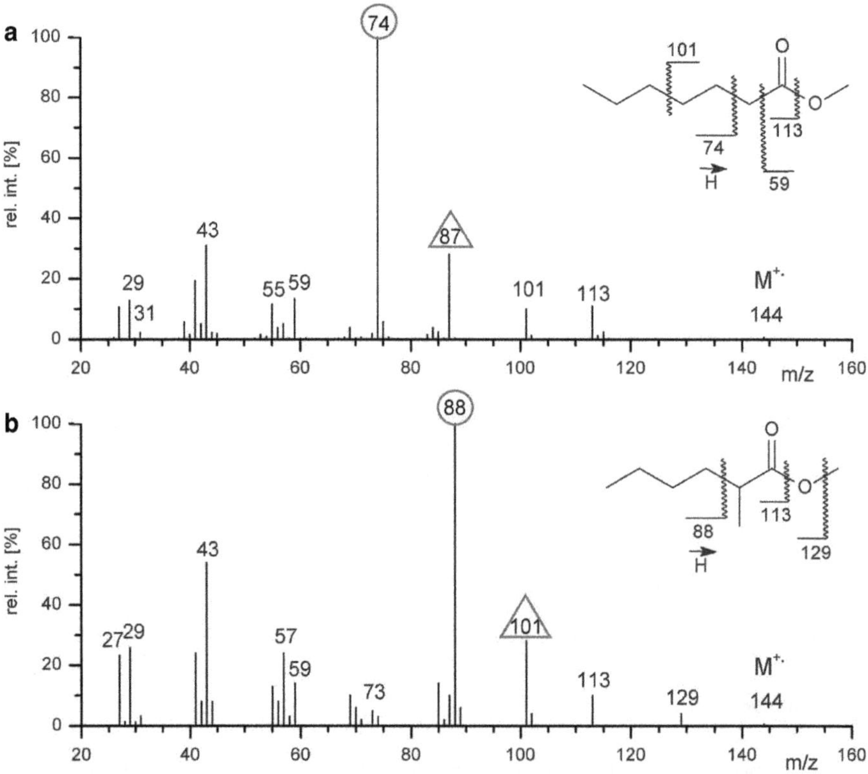

Fig. 6.27 EI mass spectra of methyl heptanoate (**a**) and methyl 2-methylhexanoate (**b**). The peaks due to McL at *m/z* 60 and 88, respectively, are marked by *blue circles*, the peaks by γ-cleavage at *m/z* 87 and 101, respectively, are marked by *blue triangles* (Spectra used by permission of NIST. © NIST 2002)

6.8.3 McL of Phenylalkanes

In addition to the previously described benzylic and phenylic cleavages (Sect. 6.4), phenylalkanes may undergo alkene loss by a mechanism that is perfectly analogous to the "true" McLafferty rearrangement, provided the alkyl substituent fulfills all requirements. The γ-hydrogen is transferred to the *ortho*-position where the aromatic ring serves as the accepting double bond (Scheme 6.37).

Independent of the alkyl substituent, $[C_7H_8]^{+\bullet}$, *m/z* 92, is obtained as the product ion, provided there are no other substituents at the ring. The product is an isomer of toluene molecular ion, and as such it readily stabilizes by $H^\bullet$ loss to yield the even-electron $[C_7H_7]^+$ species, *m/z* 91, which then produces the well-known characteristic fragments (*m/z* 65, 39). Provided that there is no prior isomerization of the molecular ion, this dissociation is prohibited if both *ortho*-positions are substituted and/or if there is no γ-hydrogen in the alkyl group.

Table 6.12 Frequent product ions of the McLafferty rearrangement

Precursor	Product structure	Formula	Accurate mass [u][a]
Aldehyde	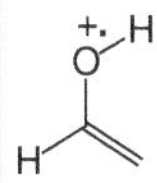	$C_2H_4O^{+\bullet}$	44.0257
Alkyl methyl ketone	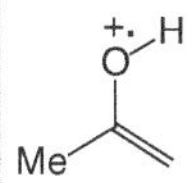	$C_3H_6O^{+\bullet}$	58.0413
Carboxylic acid	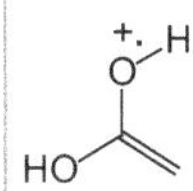	$C_2H_4O_2^{+\bullet}$	60.0206
Carboxylic acid amide	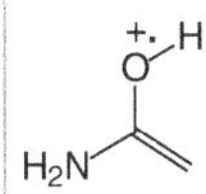	$C_2H_5NO^{+\bullet}$	59.0366
Methyl carboxylates	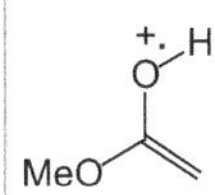	$C_3H_6O_2^{+\bullet}$	74.0362
Ethyl carboxylates	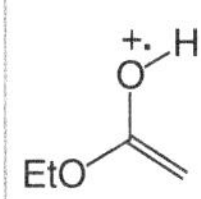	$C_4H_8O_2^{+\bullet}$	88.0519

[a]Values rounded to four decimals

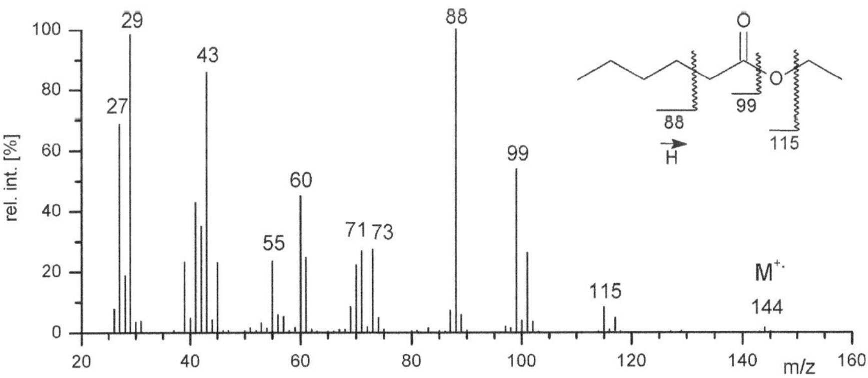

Fig. 6.28 EI spectrum of ethyl hexanoate (Used by permission of NIST. © NIST 2002)

In case of alkyl benzylethers, aldehyde loss can occur following the same reaction pathway. For example, acetaldehyde is eliminated from the molecular ions of benzylethylether, thus producing $[C_7H_8]^{+\bullet}$ fragment ions. Again, evidence has been presented for a stepwise mechanism involving a distonic intermediate [88].

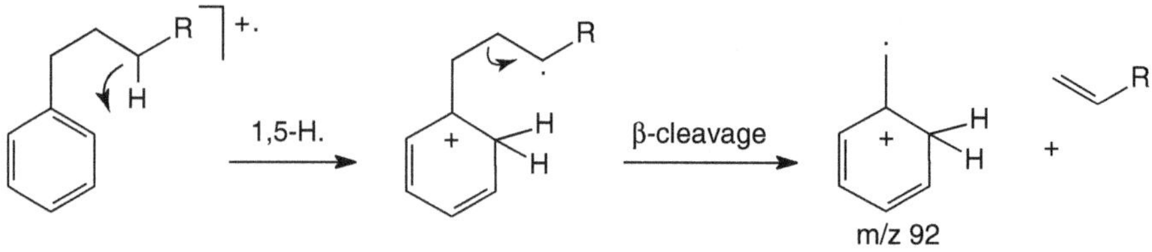

Scheme 6.37

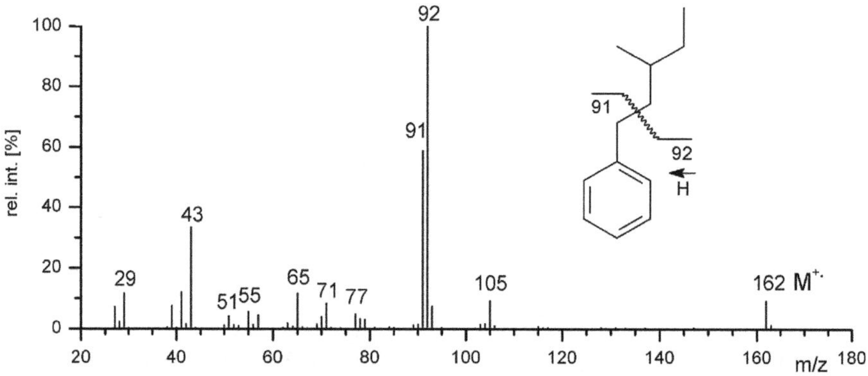

Fig. 6.29 EI mass spectrum of (3-methylpentyl)-benzene. McLafferty rearrangement and benzylic cleavage are clearly dominating. In the low-mass range carbenium ions and the "aromatic fragments" are present (Spectrum used by permission of NIST. © NIST 2002)

Pentene loss by McL The base peak in the EI mass spectrum of (3-methylpentyl)-benzene, *m/z* 92 (even-numbered *m/z* value), results from McLafferty rearrangement of the molecular ion at *m/z* 162 (even-numbered *m/z* value, Fig. 6.29). The difference of 70 u indicates pentene loss. As long as pentene loss may occur, there is not much difference to spectra of benzene isomers bearing 2-methylpentyl-, 4-methylpentyl, or *n*-hexyl. Reference spectra are needed for distinguishing between those isomers, because the spectra only differ in relative peak intensities. Also note the product of benzylic cleavage at *m/z* 91 and the related series of fragment ions at *m/z* 39, 51, 65, and 77. The additional peaks correspond to carbenium ions from the alkyl chain, i.e., *m/z* 29, 43, 57, 71.

Superimposition of series

In the lower *m/z* range, the EI spectrum of (3-methylpentyl)-benzene (Fig. 6.29) shows the superimposition of two series of ions, namely those

(continued)

belonging to $[C_7H_7]^+$, *m/z* 91, and related fragments at *m/z* 39, 51, 65, 77 as well as carbenium ions at *m/z* 29, 43, 57, 71. Thus, the characteristics of both parts of the molecule can quickly be read from this portion of the spectrum. From there, it would be a short way to an unknown structure.

"Luck is what happens when preparation meets opportunity" (Seneca): Admittedly, to discover this treasure of information in the low-mass range you have to be familiar with the *m/z* values of typical ion series. Learn them by heart or at least compile a sheet with your own collection.

6.8.4 McL with Double Hydrogen Transfer

Alkene loss via McLafferty rearrangement at the alkoxy group of aliphatic and aromatic carboxylic acid esters competes with yet another reaction path, where two hydrogens instead of one as in the "normal McLafferty product" are transferred to the charge site. This second pathway leading to alkenyl loss has early been noticed [86] and has become known as *McLafferty rearrangement with double hydrogen transfer* (*r2H*) (Scheme 6.38).

Labeling studies indicate that this process is by far not as site-specific as its better known counterpart [89, 90]. Based on thermochemical data, evidence has been presented for a two-step mechanism that finally yields a carbonyl-protonated carboxylic acid and the unsaturated radical. While the final products are well described, the second step has not fully been elucidated [91, 92] (Scheme 6.39).

Competition of McL and r2H The competition of alkene and alkenyl loss is demonstrated by the presence of peaks at *m/z* 122 (McL) and *m/z* 123 (r2H) in the EI mass spectrum of isopropyl benzoate (Fig. 6.30) [92]. Of course, both primary fragmentations are competing with the predominating α-cleavage at the carbonyl group yielding the highly characteristic *benzoyl ion*, $[C_7H_5O]^+$, *m/z* 105 (Scheme 6.40) [93]. The benzoyl ion, essentially an aromatic acylium ion, dissociates by CO

$$[R^1COOR^2]^{+\bullet} \xrightarrow{r2H} [R^1C(OH)_2]^+ + [R^2\text{-}2H]^\bullet$$

Scheme 6.38

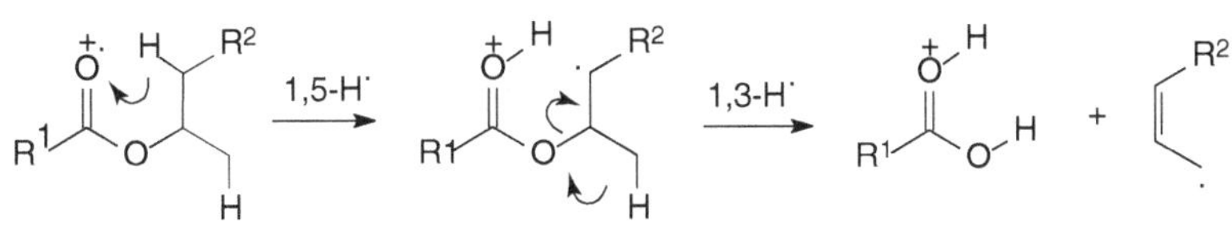

Scheme 6.39

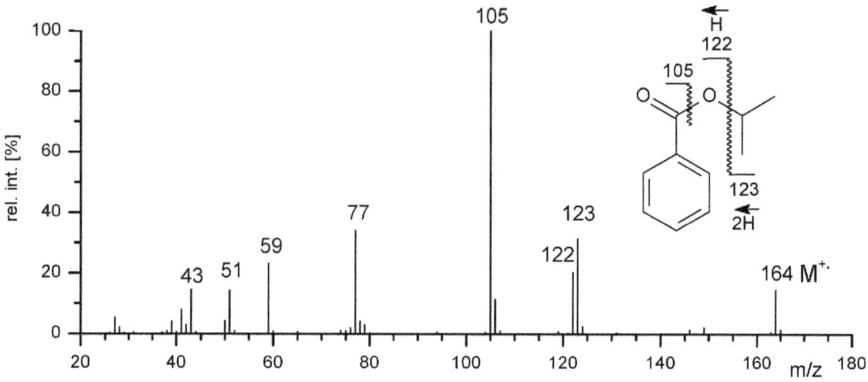

Fig. 6.30 EI spectrum of isopropyl benzoate (Used by permission of NIST. © NIST 2002)

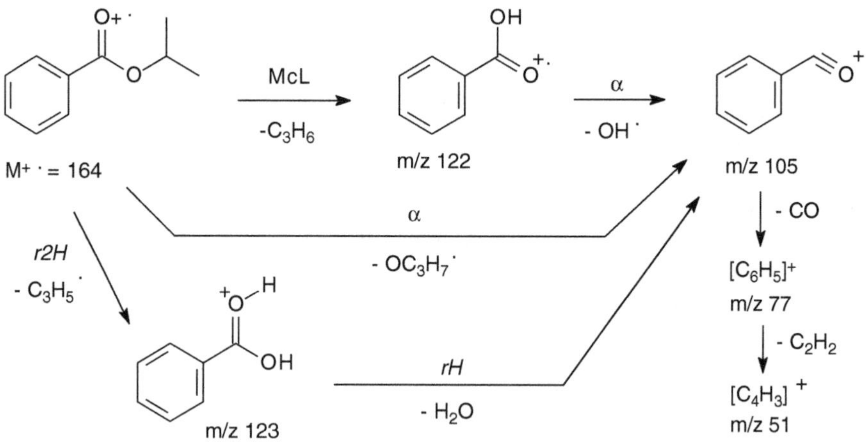

Scheme 6.40

loss to yield the phenyl ion, *m/z* 77, and finally by C_2H_2 loss the cyclobutadienyl ion, *m/z* 51 (Sect. 6.4.2).

6.8.5 Benzyl Versus Benzoyl

The ion series *m/z* 51, 77, 105 is a reliable indicator for benzoyl substructures, e.g., from benzaldehyde, benzoic acid, and its derivatives as well as from acetophenone, benzophenone, etc. In contrast to benzylic compounds, the peaks at *m/z* 39, 65, and 91 are almost absent (Fig. 6.31). If a peak at *m/z* 105 and the complete series *m/z* 39, 51, 65, 77, 91 are present, this strongly points towards the composition $[C_7H_7]^+$, and thus to phenylalkanes.

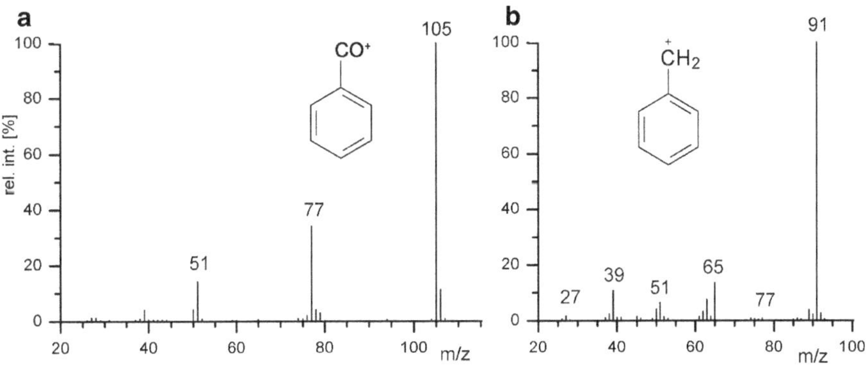

Fig. 6.31 Typical appearance of peak series as caused by (**a**) benzoyl or (**b**) benzyl as part of a molecule's structure

6.8.6 Ubiquitous Plasticizers

Phthalates, especially di-2-ethylhexyl phthalate (also known as di-octyl phthalate, DOP), are commonly used plasticizers in synthetic polymers. Unfortunately, they are extracted from the polymers upon exposure to solvents such as dichloromethane, chloroform, or toluene, e.g., from syringes, tubing, vials etc. Therefore, they are often detected as impurities. They are easily recognized from their peaks at *m/z* 149 (often base peak), *m/z* 167, and $[M-(R-2H)]^+$ (*m/z* 279 in case of DOP). The molecular ion is often absent in their EI spectra.

The fragment ions at *m/z* 149, $[C_8H_5O_3]^+$, and 167, $[C_8H_7O_4]^+$, are especially prominent in the EI spectra of phthalates. The formation of the $[C_8H_5O_3]^+$ ion was initially attributed to a McLafferty rearrangement followed by loss of an alkoxy radical and final stabilization to a cyclic oxonium ion [94]. However, it has been shown that four other pathways in total lead to its formation excluding the above one [95, 96]. The most prominent fragmentation pathways are (Scheme 6.41).

6.9 Retro-Diels-Alder Reaction

6.9.1 Mechanism of the Retro-Diels-Alder Reaction

Molecular ions containing a cyclohexene unit may fragment to form conjugated di-olefinic (*diene*) and mono-olefinic (*ene*) products. This fragmentation pathway was first recognized by Biemann as formally analogous to the retro-Diels-Alder (RDA) reaction of neutrals in the condensed phase [73]. The fragmentation can in principle proceed in a concerted manner (**a**) or stepwise, as if it proceeds as a double α-cleavage with the first being an allylic cleavage (**b**) (Scheme 6.42).

As most ion dissociation processes, the RDA reaction is endothermic, e.g., by 185 kJ mol^{-1} in case of ethene loss from cyclohexene molecular ion [97]. The

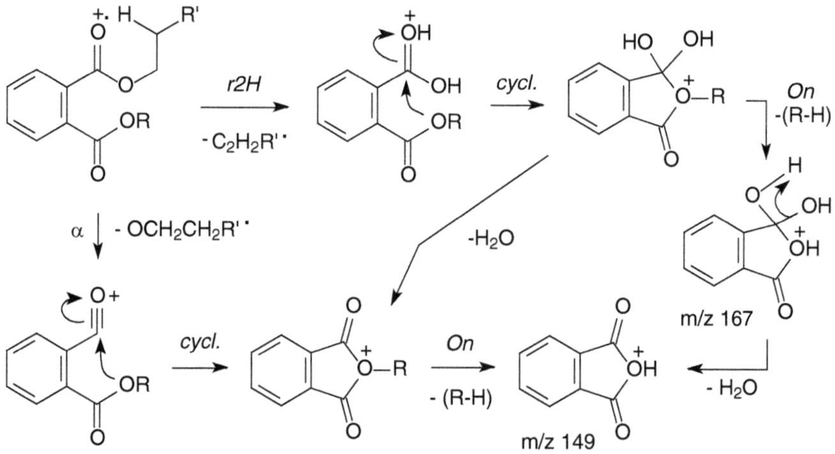

Scheme 6.41

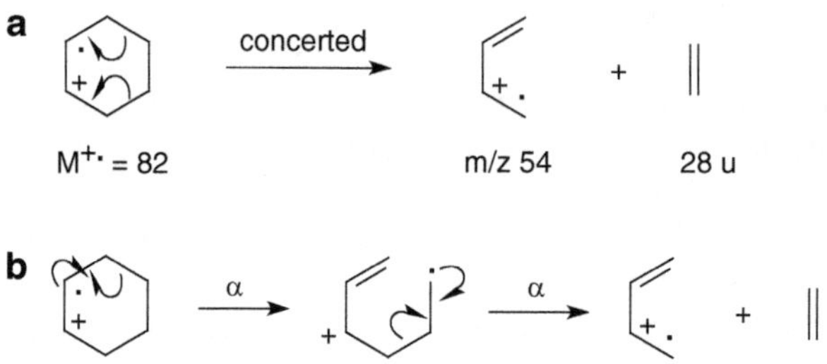

Scheme 6.42

charge usually resides at the diene fragment, but the ene fragment is also frequently observed in mass spectra. The fraction of charge retention and charge migration products has been studied [98]. As may be expected, competition for the charge is greatly influenced by the substitution pattern of the cyclohexene derivative and by the presence or absence of heteroatoms in the respective fragments.

In case of 3,5,5-trimethylcyclohexene, for example, the molecular ion $[C_9H_{16}]^{+\bullet}$, *m/z* 124, undergoes isobutene loss, C_4H_8, 56 u, via RDA reaction resulting in a $[C_5H_8]^{+\bullet}$ fragment, that causes the base peak at *m/z* 68, which is also the only significant peak at even-numbered *m/z* (Scheme 6.43). The peak due to the charge migration product $[C_4H_8]^{+\bullet}$, *m/z* 56, is of rather low intensity (Fig. 6.32).

The McLafferty rearrangement and the RDA reaction have several features in common:

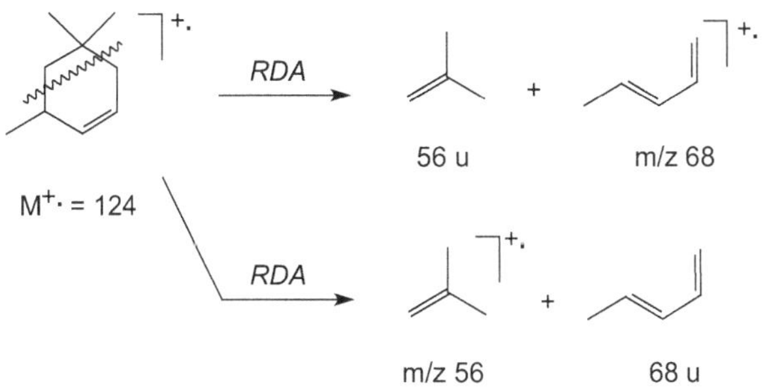

Scheme 6.43

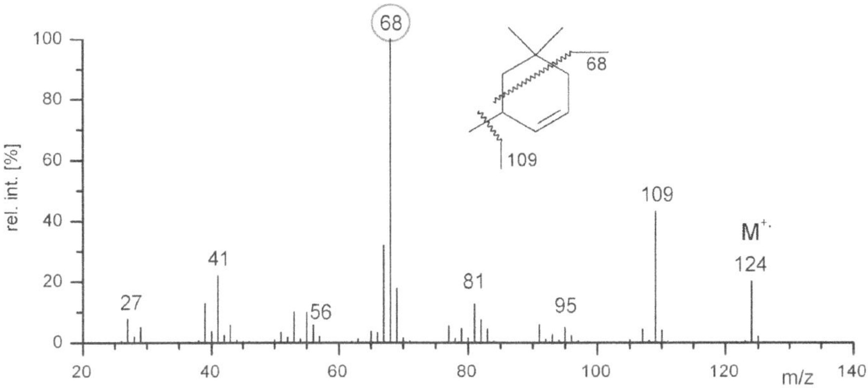

Fig. 6.32 EI mass spectrum of 3,5,5-trimethylcyclohexene. The molecular ion undergoes isobutene loss, 56 u, via RDA reaction yielding the base peak at *m/z* 68, which is also the only significant peak at even-numbered *m/z* (*orange circle*). The charge migration product at *m/z* 56 is of low intensity (Spectrum used by permission of NIST. © NIST 2002)

- McL and RDA belong to the rearrangement type of fragmentations, although the name conceals this fact in case of the latter.
- Both represent pathways for alkene loss from molecular ions.
- McL and RD are highly versatile in structure elucidation.

Provided the double bond does not migrate prior to RDA reaction, the alkene loss is perfectly regiospecific, and it does not really suffer from extensive substitution at the cyclohexene unit. Thus, substitution patterns can be revealed from the mass spectrum (**a**). The RDA reaction also proceeds independent of whether the six-membered ring contains heteroatoms or not (**b**) (Scheme 6.44).

6.9.2 Widespread Occurrence of the RDA Reaction

Obviously, the RDA reaction has the potential needed for a widespread mass spectral fragmentation [97, 99, 100]. Any molecule that can at least formally be

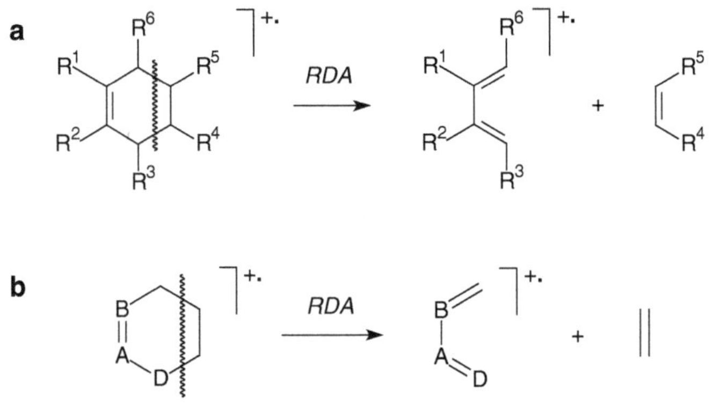

Scheme 6.44

synthesized by a Diels-Alder reaction is a potential candidate for the mass spectral RDA reaction. In addition, the RDA reaction is not restricted to positive radical ions, but it may also occur from even-electron ions as well as from negative radical ions, $M^{-\bullet}$. These findings remind us of the fact that ionic reactions are determined by the intrinsic properties and the internal energy of the ions, and thus only indirectly by the ionization technique used for their creation.

Few restrictions apply for RDA
In fact, almost any molecular ion having a six-membered ring that contains one double bond can undergo the RDA reaction to eliminate a (substituted) alkene or a corresponding heteroanalog.

6.9.3 RDA Reaction in Natural Products

The RDA reaction is often observed from steroid molecular ions, and it can be very indicative of steroidal structure [97, 100–102]. The extent of the RDA reaction depends on whether the central ring junction is *cis* or *trans*. The mass spectra of Δ^7-steroidal olefins, for example, show a marked dependence on the stereochemistry of the A/B ring juncture, in accordance with orbital symmetry rules for a thermal concerted process.

The RDA reaction is also a typical process of flavones, naphthoflavones, and methoxynaphthoflavones [103]. In many cases it provides intact A- and B-ring fragments, and therefore, it is of high relevance for structure elucidation. The intensity ratio of A- to B-ring fragments was found to be strongly influenced by the substituent position, i.e., to be very sensitive to the charge distribution within the molecular ion [104]. The pentacyclic triterpene molecular ion below also shows RDA (Scheme 6.45).

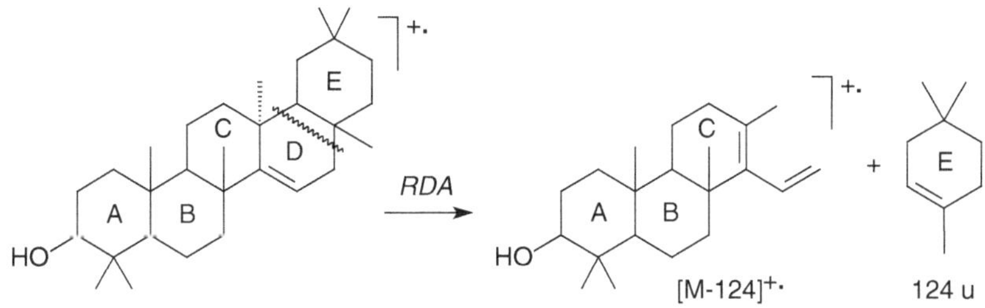

Scheme 6.45

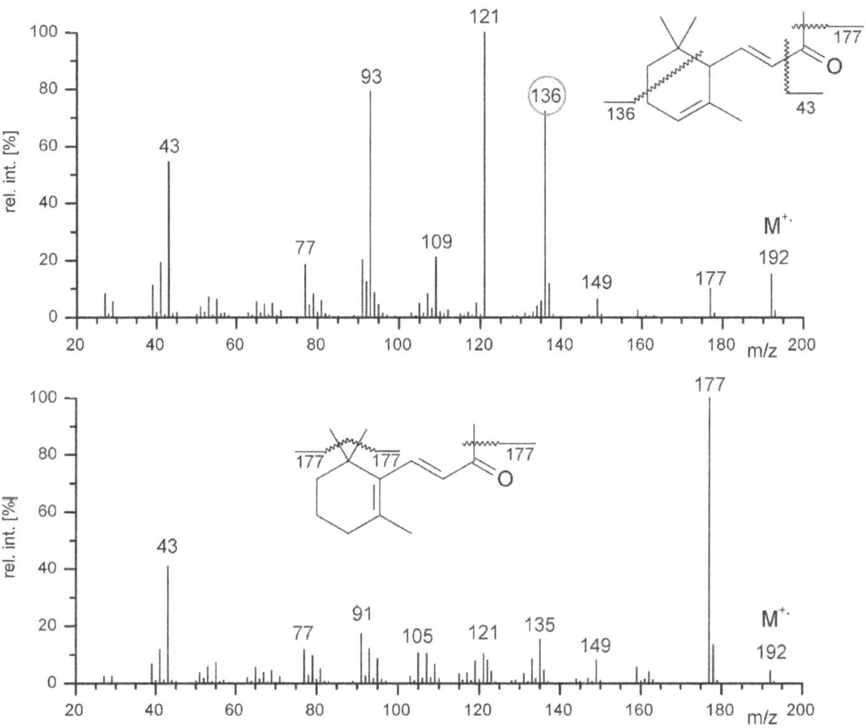

Fig. 6.33 EI mass spectra of α- (**a**) and β-ionone (**b**). RDA reaction proceeds via loss of isobutene, causing the peak at *m/z* 136 in case of α-ionone, whereas ethene loss is almost absent in the β-ionone spectrum. In (**a**) the product ion peak of the RDA reaction stands out due to its even-numbered *m/z* (*orange circle*) (Spectra used by permission of NIST. © NIST 2002)

Influence of Positional Isomerism on the RDA Reaction As often observed in mass spectrometry, seemingly small changes in ion structure may cause significant changes in the mass spectra of the respective analytes. Let us compare the mass spectra of α- and β-ionone (Fig. 6.33). While α-ionone significantly dissociates to yield the fragment ion at *m/z* 136 upon isobutene loss via RDA reaction, its isomer β-ionone mainly exhibits an intense $[M{-}CH_3]^+$ signal [73]. This is because the geminal methyl substituents are in allylic position to the ring double bond in the latter, and moreover, in this case methyl loss by allylic bond cleavage yields a thermodynamically favorable tertiary allyl ion.

6.10 Elimination of Carbon Monoxide

As we know by now, the elimination of small stable molecules represents a frequent fragmentation route of odd- and even-electron ions. Second to alkene loss, we will consider some of the numerous pathways for loss of carbon monoxide, CO. In contrast to the preceding reactions, CO loss does not follow a single mechanism. Instead, a wide range of molecular and fragment ions can undergo loss of CO. Therefore, this is rather a compound-specific view in the context of CO loss than a collection of compounds exhibiting a certain reaction mechanism. In retrospect, we actually already have encountered some CO losses (Sects. 6.2.4 and 6.8.4).

6.10.1 CO Loss from Phenols

Phenols exhibit a strong molecular ion peak often representing the base peak in their spectra. The most characteristic fragment ions of phenols are caused by loss of CO from the molecular ion [105], and subsequent $H^{\bullet}$ loss, thereby forming $[M–28]^{+\bullet}$ and $[M–29]^{+}$ ions, respectively (Scheme 6.46 and Fig. 6.34), the identity of which have been ascertained by HR-MS as $[M–CO]^{+\bullet}$ and $[M–CHO]^{+}$ [106]. This initially unexpected fragmentation proceeds via ketonization of the molecular ion prior to elimination of CO. The mechanism has been verified by D-labeling. These experiments also revealed that only about one third of the $H^{\bullet}$ cleaved off from the cyclopentadiene ion, *m/z* 66, originates from the former OH group, whereas the majority is derived from the ring [107].

Similar pathways
The above mechanism of CO loss from phenols is perfectly analogous to HCN loss from aniline and other aminoarenes (Sect. 6.15.2).

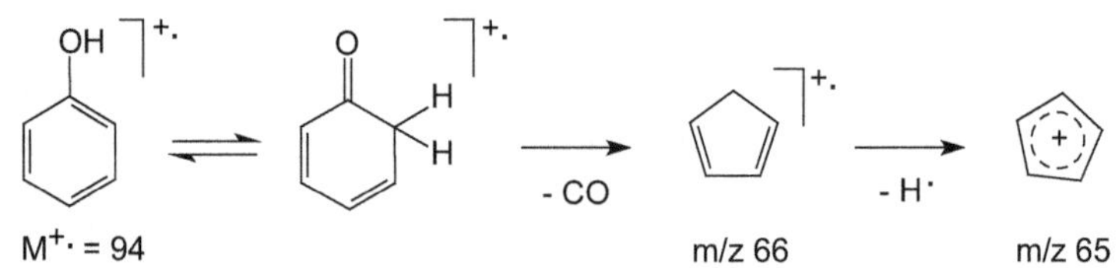

Scheme 6.46

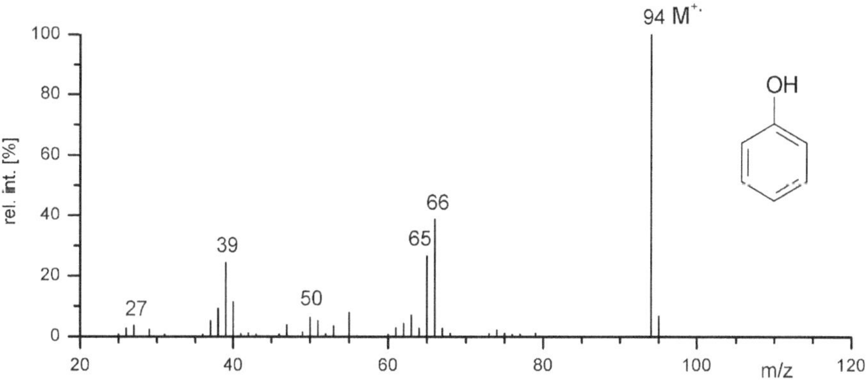

Fig. 6.34 EI mass spectrum of phenol showing an intense peak due to CO loss at *m/z* 66. Note that the $M^{+•}$ ion peak, *m/z* 94, and the product of CO loss, *m/z* 66, both are at even-numbered *m/z* (Spectrum used by permission of NIST. © NIST 2002)

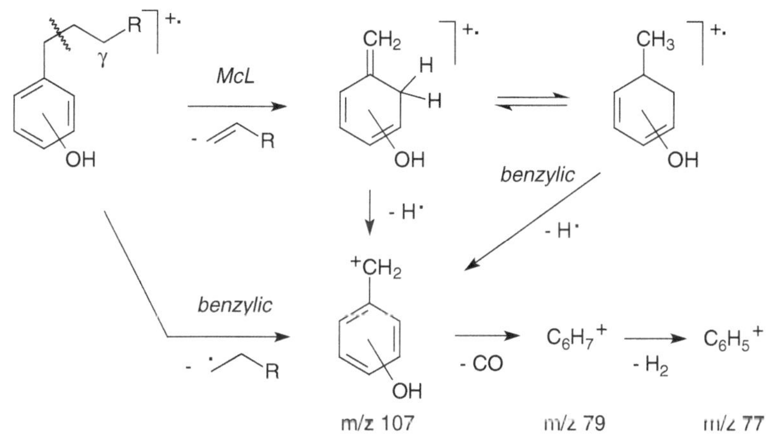

Scheme 6.47

Alkylphenol molecular ions preferably dissociate by benzylic bond cleavage, e.g., $[M–H]^+$ ions are observed in case of methylphenols. Provided a γ-hydrogen is available in alkyl substituents of sufficient chain length, the benzylic bond cleavage competes with the McLafferty rearrangement [108], the product ion of this being an isomer of methylphenol molecular ion. Loss of $H^•$ from the latter yields a $[C_7H_7O]^+$ ion, *m/z* 107, that may dissociate further by CO loss, thus forming a protonated benzene ion, $[C_6H_7]^+$, *m/z* 79. This tells us that CO loss occurs equally well from even-electron phenolic ions (Scheme 6.47).

Accurate mass identifies fragmentation pathways Ethyl loss clearly predominates over methyl loss in the EI mass spectrum of 2-(1-methylpropyl)

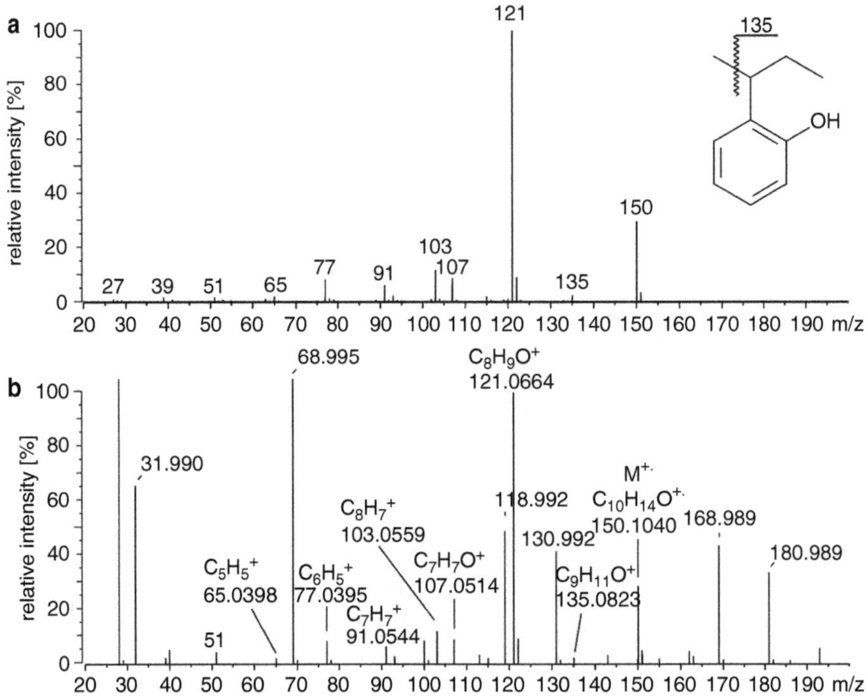

Fig. 6.35 LR- (**a**) and HR-EI (**b**) mass spectra of 2-(1-methylpropyl)phenol. The elemental compositions as obtained from accurate mass measurement are directly attached to the corresponding peaks. Peaks bearing labels in *small font size* (e.g., 31.990) are due to PFK and residual air used for internal mass calibration (Sect. 3.6)

phenol. It proceeds via benzylic bond cleavage, the products of which are detected as the base peak at *m*/*z* 121 and *m*/*z* 135 (3%), respectively (Fig. 6.35a). The McLafferty rearrangement does not play a role, as the peak at *m*/*z* 122 (8.8%) is completely due to the ^{13}C isotopic contribution to the peak at *m*/*z* 121. From the HR-EI spectrum (Fig. 6.35b) the alternative pathway for the formation of a $[M–29]^+$ peak, i.e., $[M–CO–H]^+$, can be excluded, because the measured accurate mass of this singlet peak indicates $C_8H_9O^+$. HR-MS data also reveal that the peak at *m*/*z* 107 corresponds to $[M–CH_3–CO]^+$ and that the one at *m*/*z* 103 corresponds to $[M–C_2H_5–H_2O]^+$. Although perhaps unexpected, the loss of H_2O from phenolic fragment ions is not unusual.

6.10.2 CO and C_2H_2 Loss from Quinones

Quinones [109] and aromatic ketones such as flavones [104], fluorenone, anthraquinone, and similar compounds [110] dissociate by competing and consecutive losses of CO and C_2H_2. Multiple CO losses may also occur subsequent to the RDA reaction of flavones [104]. As these molecules all have large π-electron systems to stabilize the charge, they show intense molecular ion peaks that often represent the base peak in those spectra. Typically any available carbonyl group is expelled as CO in the course of complete dissociation of the molecular ion; sometimes CO first, sometimes alternating with C_2H_2 loss.

Elimination of molecules from benzoquinone 1,4-Benzoquinone represents the perfect prototype of this fragmentation pattern. The subsequent eliminations of intact molecules of CO (28 u) and/or C_2H_2 (26 u) causes a series exclusively comprising odd-electron fragment ions (Scheme 6.48 and Fig. 6.36). This results

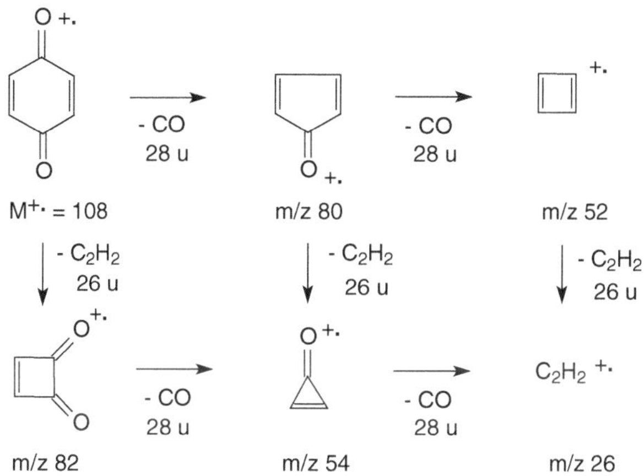

Scheme 6.48

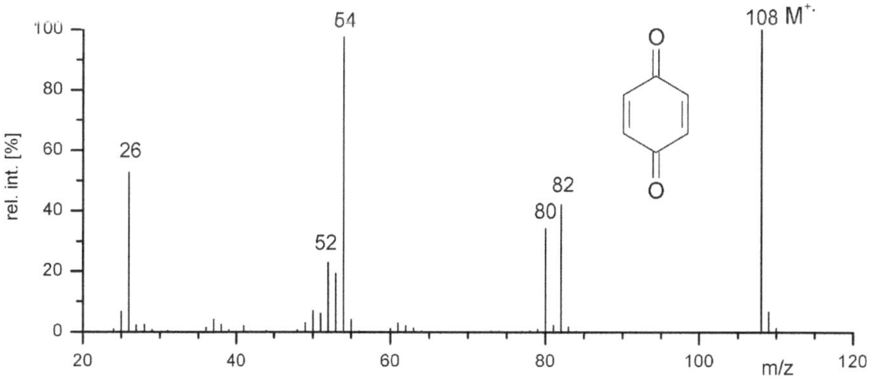

Fig. 6.36 EI mass spectrum of 1,4-benzoquinone. All peaks bearing a *m/z* label correspond to OE ions as the molecular ion exclusively eliminates intact molecules, in other words, the series starts with $M^{+\bullet}$ at even-numbered *m/z* and never switches to odd-numbered *m/z* values (Spectrum used by permission of NIST. © NIST 2002)

in characteristic fragment ions as a result of sequences such as $[M–28–26–28]^{+•}$ or $[M–28–26–26]^{+•}$.

6.10.3 Fragmentation of Arylalkylethers

The molecular ions of arylmethylethers preferably dissociate by loss of a formaldehyde molecule or by loss of the alkyl group via C–O bond cleavage [88, 111]. The latter process yields an even-electron phenolic ion, $C_6H_5O^+$, *m/z* 93, that readily expels CO (Scheme 6.48 and Fig. 6.37) [112, 113] (Scheme 6.49).

Astonishingly, the study of the mechanism of formaldehyde loss from anisole revealed two different pathways for this process, one involving a four- and one a five-membered cyclic transition state (Fig. 6.38) [114]. The four-membered transition state conserves aromaticity in the ionic product, which therefore has the lower

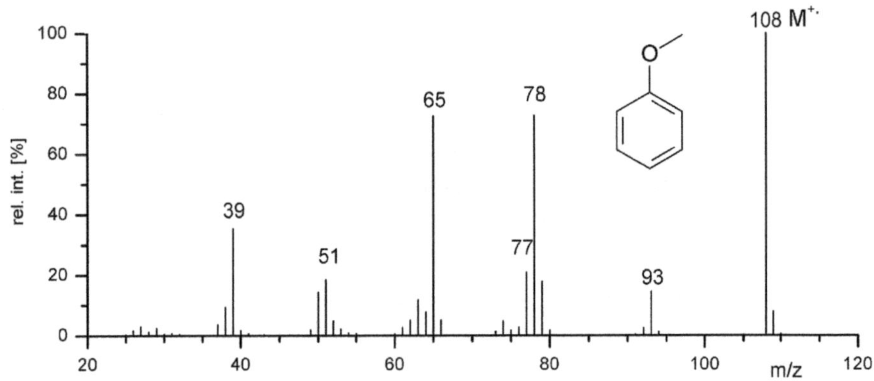

Fig. 6.37 EI mass spectrum of anisole exhibiting a strong $[M–H_2CO]^{+•}$ peak at *m/z* 78 (Spectrum used by permission of NIST. © NIST 2002)

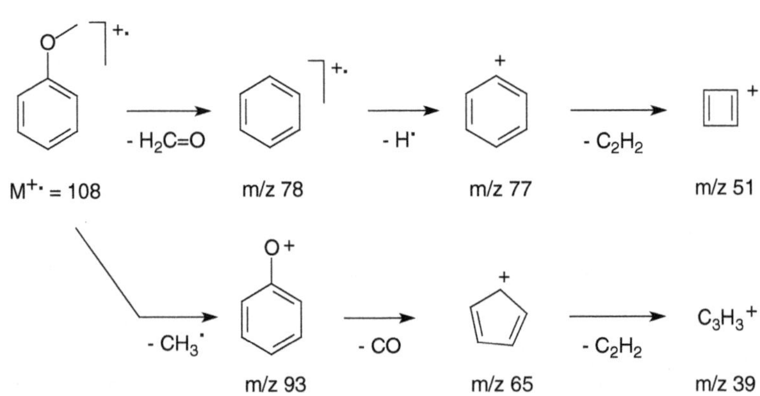

Scheme 6.49

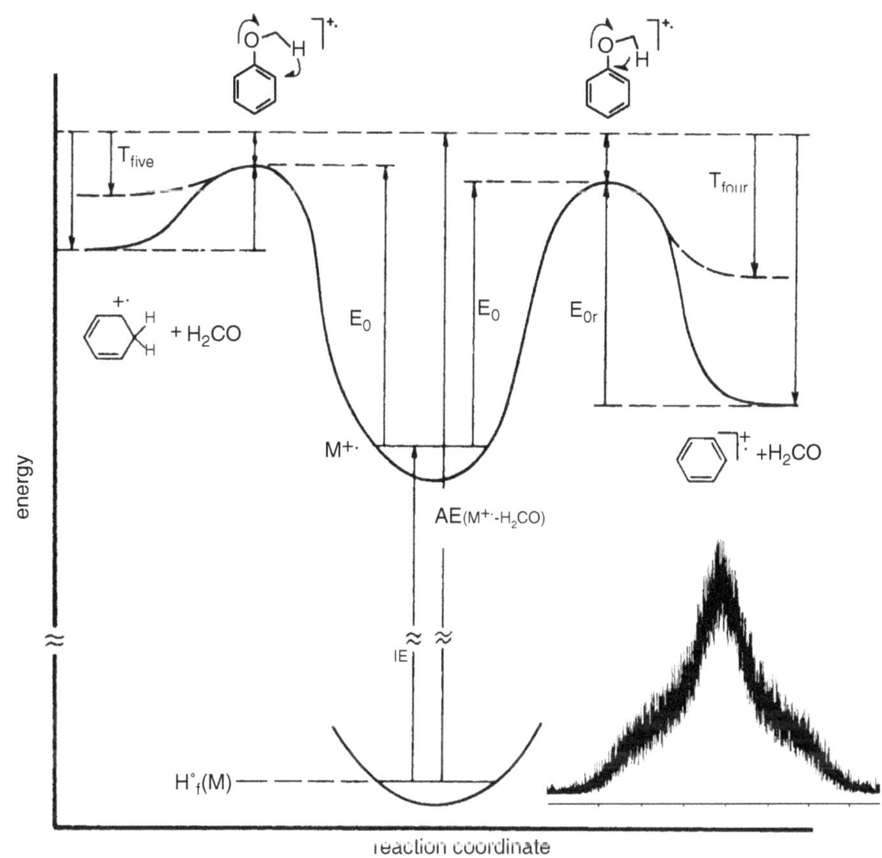

Fig. 6.38 Energetics of formaldehyde loss from anisole. The *inset* shows the composite metastable peak due to two different amounts of kinetic energy release (Adapted from Ref. [114] with permission. © American Chemical Society, 1973)

heat of formation. Prompted by the observation of a composite metastable peak, this rather unusual behavior could be uncovered by deconvolution of two different values of kinetic energy release with the help of metastable peak shape analysis (Sect. 2.8).

In case of longer-chain alkyl substituents, alkene loss can compete with the McLafferty rearrangement as is observed from suitably substituted phenylalkanes (Sect. 6.8.3), e.g., ethene loss from phenetole and its derivatives [111].

Approach for of structure elucidation The EI spectrum of an "unknown" compound is shown in Fig. 6.39. The molecular ion (OE) appears at *m/z* 156, the base peak at *m/z* 128, the difference of 28 u may be attributed to CO, C_2H_4, or N_2 (Sect. 6.10.6), and thus, we have to think of a rearrangement fragmentation to explain this. Further, the spectrum exhibits peaks showing a chlorine isotopic pattern, that of Cl_1 to be exact. The Cl_1 pattern is obvious at *m/z* 156, 158, *m/z* 128, 130 and assumably could also occur at *m/z* 111, 113 and *m/z* 100, 102. The combination of an intense $M^{+\bullet}$

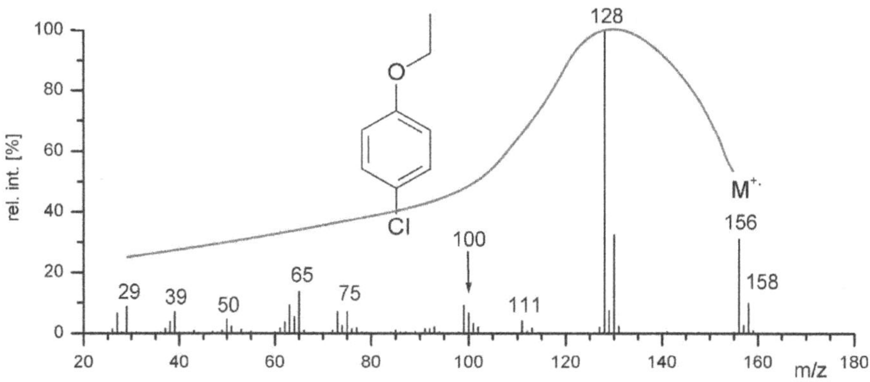

Fig. 6.39 EI mass spectrum of 4-chlorophenetole. The chlorine isotopic pattern is found in the signals corresponding to $M^{+\bullet}$, m/z 156, $[M–C_2H_4]^{+\bullet}$, m/z 128, $[M–OEt]^+$, m/z 111, and $[M–C_2H_4–CO]^{+\bullet}$, m/z 100. Also note the distribution of peak intensities (*red curve*) typical for an EI spectrum of an aromatic compound (Spectrum used by permission of NIST. © NIST 2002)

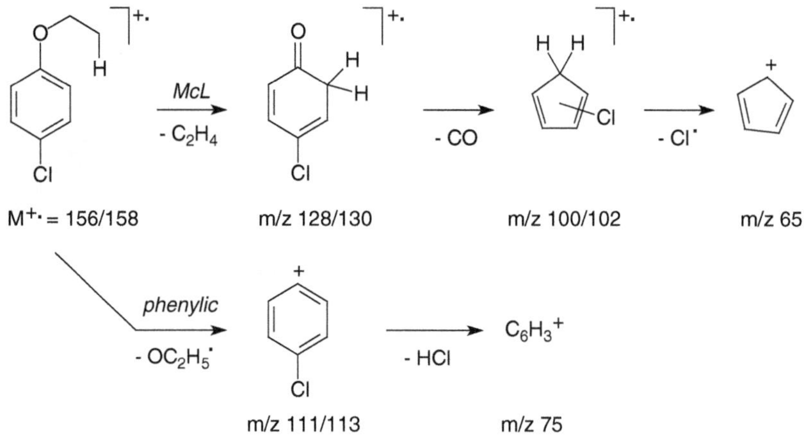

Scheme 6.50

peak and primary fragment plus low-intensity fragments at m/z 39, 50, 65, 75 reveal an aromatic compound. The fact that the series expected for a benzyl substituent is slightly different from our observation here points towards double substitution at the phenyl ring, i.e., H is missing as it has been substituted by something else. Assuming Cl, C_6H_5, and eventually C_2H_4 as constituents of the unknown, this sums up to a molecular mass of 140 u. The missing 16 u might be added by one O atom. Thus, we try to build a structure based on the composition C_8H_9ClO. Calculating r+d yields $8 - 5 + 1 = 4$, which fits to the aromatic system. After gathering such basic information, one may try to find out the structure by iteratively assuming a structure and trying to correlate this to the fragment ions observed. In this particular case, accurate mass data to verify the molecular formula and the neutral loss(es) would be very helpful. The most important fragmentation pathways are summarized in Scheme 6.50.

6.10.4 CO Loss from Transition Metal Carbonyl Complexes

Transition metal carbonyl complexes successively eliminate all CO ligands upon electron ionization until the bare metal remains. Pure carbonyl complexes as well as many other complexes with carbonyl ligands can therefore be readily identified from their characteristic CO losses which are – dependent on the metal – often observed in combination with the eye-catching isotopic pattern of the respective metal (Fig. 6.40). According to ^{13}C-labeling experiments, extensive isomerization may precede the dissociation of the carbonyl complexes [115]. Furthermore, the different bond strength of the M–CO bond in heterometallic transition-metal dimers can be deduced from the mass spectral fragmentation pattern of the carbonyl complexes, e.g., selective ^{12}CO loss from Mn in $[Mn(CO)_5Re(^{13}CO)_5]$ has been interpreted in terms of stronger Re–CO bonds [116].

6.10.5 CO Loss from Carbonyl Compounds

A molecule of CO may also be eliminated from malonates [117], β-keto esters [118], phenoxyacetates [119], and many other compounds containing similar structural features. Whatever the mechanism of CO loss might be, in none of the above cases does CO loss proceed by a simple bond cleavage. Instead, multistep rearrangements are necessary to "cut" the CO moiety out of the precursor ion.

Sources for CO loss

The detection of CO loss from molecular or fragment ions usually indicates the presence of carbonyl groups. However, it is less indicative of molecular structure than the highly specific reactions discussed before, because a multitude of rearrangement processes can be effective. These might even lead to CO loss in cases where no carbonyl group exists, e.g., from phenols.

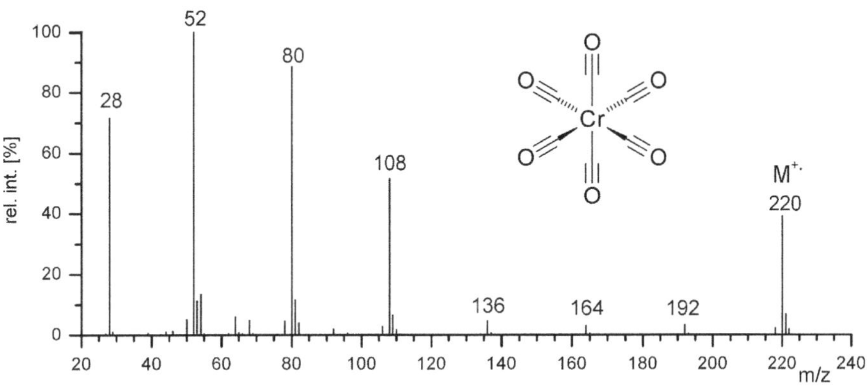

Fig. 6.40 EI mass spectrum of hexacarbonylchromium. All six CO ligands are eliminated until the bare metal ion, *m/z* 52, remains. The isotopic pattern of chromium can well be recognized from the more intense signals (Used by permission by NIST. © NIST 2002)

Table 6.13 Example of the differentiation of isobaric neutral losses

Generation of fragment	Type of peak	Sequence (a) and *m/z*	Sequence (b) and *m/z*
0th	Singlet	$M^{+\bullet} = 182.0798$	
		$\downarrow - N_2$	
1st	Singlet	154.0737	
		$\downarrow - N_2$	$\downarrow - C_2H_4$
2nd	Doublet	126.0675 (10%)	126.0424 (90%)
		$\downarrow - C_2H_4$	$\downarrow - CO$
3rd	Doublet	98.0362 (61%)	98.0475 (39%)

6.10.6 Differentiation Between Loss of CO, N_2, and C_2H_4

Carbon monoxide, CO, 27.9949 u, is a nominal isobar of ethene, C_2H_4, 28.0313 u, and nitrogen, N_2, 28.0061 u, and the separation of these gases themselves by means of HR-MS has already been described (Sect. 3.6). Accordingly, the difference in accurate mass for a given pair of peaks can be used to decide which of these neutrals has been eliminated, e.g., we employed HR-MS to uniquely identify the $[M–29]^+$ peak from 2-(1-methylpropyl)phenol as $[M–C_2H_5]^+$ (Sect. 6.9.1). The elimination of N_2, CO, and/or C_2H_4 can even occur on consecutive and competing fragmentation pathways from the very same analyte [120].

High resolution distinguishes losses of CO, N_2, and C_2H_4 The molecular ion of ethyl-*trans*-3-methyltetrazole-5-acrylate, $[C_7H_{10}O_2N_4]^{+\bullet}$, *m/z* 182.0798, exhibits two fragmentation sequences involving loss of N_2, C_2H_4, and/or CO, in different order. This way, isobaric fragment ions at *m/z* 98 and 126 are formed that cannot be distinguished by LR-MS. HR-MS resolves both signals as doublets and thus deconvolutes the competing pathways (Table 6.13) [120].

Hint

In case of doubt which neutral loss(es) are effective, it is highly recommended to obtain HR-MS data to avoid ambiguities. Moreover, the differences in accurate mass for a given pair of peaks can be used to identify the neutral loss even though the composition of the ions themselves might still be unknown.

6.11 Thermal Degradation Versus Ion Fragmentation

Heating of the sample, a common procedure enforcing evaporation from the crucible placed onto a direct insertion probe, may cause unwanted reactions prior to ionization. Thus, non-mass spectral but thermal reactions can effect that the mass spectrum does not represent the analyte itself, but its decomposition product(s). Sometimes, those thermal reactions are difficult to recognize, because the same neutral loss may also occur by a true mass spectral fragmentation of the corresponding molecular ion. In even more disadvantageous circumstances, the thermal decomposition does not yield a single defined derivative, but a complex mixture of pyrolysis products. This is the case with highly polar natural products such as saccharides, nucleotides, and peptides or when ionic compounds such as organic salts or metal complexes are to be measured.

6.11.1 Decarbonylation and Decarboxylation

Thermal degradation prior to ionization can cause decarbonylation or decarboxylation of the analyte. Decarbonylation, is observed for α-ketocarboxylic acids and α-ketocarboxylic acid esters, while decarboxylation is typical for β-oxo-carboxylic acids such as malonic acid and its derivatives and di-, tri-, or polycarboxylic acids.

6.11.2 Retro-Diels-Alder Reaction

The Diels-Alder reaction is reversible at elevated temperatures, and therefore its products can decompose prior to evaporation by RDA reaction of the neutral in the condensed phase. The mass spectral RDA reaction has already been discussed in detail (Sect. 6.9).

6.11.3 Loss of H_2O from Alkanols

Aliphatic alcohols show a strong tendency to thermally eliminate water. This is of special relevance if volatile alkanols are introduced via the reference inlet system or by means of a gas chromatograph. Then, the mass spectra correspond to the respective alkenes rather than to the alkanols that were intended to be analyzed. Water is often not detected, simply because mass spectra are frequently acquired starting from m/z 40 to omit background from residual air.

Interestingly, the molecular ions of alkanols also strongly tend to lose H_2O [27, 121, 122], which is their second important fragmentation route in addition to α-cleavage (Sect. 6.2.5). It has been demonstrated that the large majority of H_2O loss from the molecular ion proceeds by 1,4-elimination, whereas only some minor percentage of H_2O loss is due to other 1,x-eliminations. Following the labeling results, a cyclic intermediate can be assumed that decomposes further by loss of ethene [122]. These findings are not only supported by deuterium labeling studies but also by the fact that H_2O loss does play a less important role in the mass spectra of methanol, ethanol, and the propanols (Scheme 6.51).

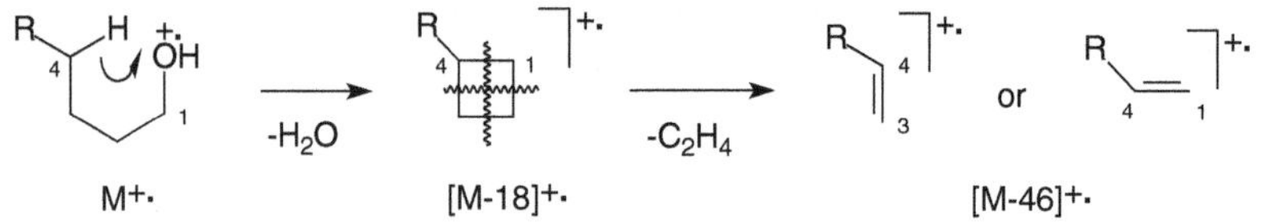

Scheme 6.51

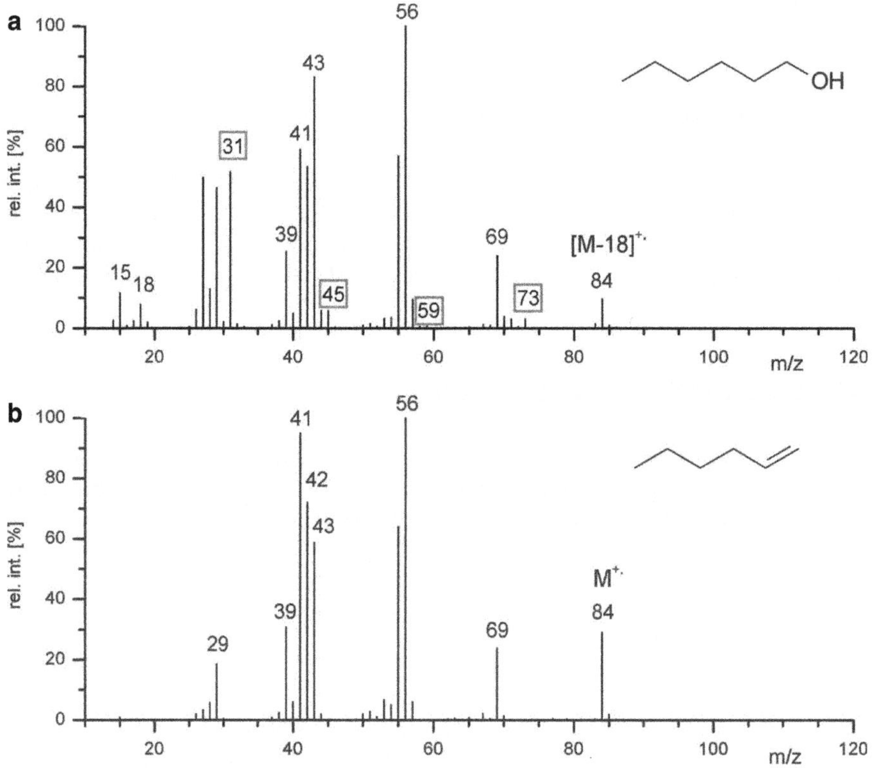

Fig. 6.41 Comparison of the EI mass spectra of 1-hexanol, $M_r = 102$ u (**a**) and 1-hexene, $M_r = 84$ u (**b**). Watch for similarities as well as for differences. Would you have noted the oxonium ion series in (**a**) if these ions had not been marked by *red boxes*? Also note that the peak at *m*/*z* 31 is the most intensive oxonium ion signal because this spectrum belongs to a primary alcohol (Spectra used with permission by NIST. © NIST 2002)

Similarity of alcohol and alkene spectra The EI mass spectra of 1-hexanol, $M_r = 102$ u, and 1-hexene, $M_r = 84$ u, are similar because the molecular ion peak is absent in the mass spectrum of hexanol (Fig. 6.41). However, a more careful examination of the hexanol spectrum reveals peaks at *m*/*z* 18, 19, 31, 45, and 59 that are absent in the hexene spectrum. These are due to $H_2O^{+\bullet}$, H_3O^+, and to oxonium ions ($H_2C{=}OH^+$, $H_3CCH{=}OH^+$ etc.) which are reliable indicators of aliphatic alcohols and ethers (Table 6.8).

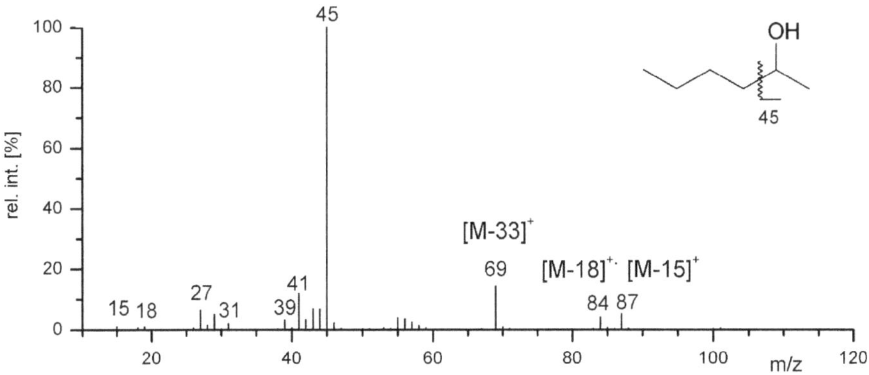

Fig. 6.42 EI mass spectrum of 2-hexanol, $M_r = 102$ u (Spectrum used with permission by NIST. © NIST 2002)

In addition to the observation of oxonium ions, alkanols may occasionally be identified from the occurrence of a seemingly [M–3] peak while the molecular ion is absent (Fig. 6.42). The unusual difference of 3 u results from neighboring $[M-CH_3]^+$ and $[M-H_2O]^{+\bullet}$ peaks. In these cases, a [M–33] peak indicates consecutive losses of $CH_3^{\bullet}$ and H_2O in either order, i.e., $[M-H_2O-CH_3]^+$ and $[M-CH_3-H_2O]^+$. (Sect. 6.6.4). Alternatively, the sequence of $[M-H_2O]^{+\bullet}$ and $[M-H_2O-C_2H_4]^{+\bullet}$ may occur (Scheme 6.51).

Indication of alkanols

EI spectra of aliphatic alcohols rarely show molecular ion peaks and, in any case, these are weak signals. Instead $[M-15]^+$, $[M-18]^{+\bullet}$, $[M-33]^+$ (losses of $CH_3^{\bullet}$ and H_2O in either sequence) and occasionally $[M-46]^+$ (loss of H_2O and then C_2H_4) are observed.

6.11.4 EI Mass Spectra of Organic Salts

Ammonium, phosphonium, oxonium salts and the like cannot be evaporated without substantial or complete decomposition, and thus EI-MS does not serve well for their characterization. Nevertheless, if a sample that happens to be an organic salt has incidentally been analyzed by EI-MS, it is helpful to know about their recognition. The EI mass spectra usually appear to result from the corresponding amines, phosphines, or ethers, but fortunately, the anion cannot 'hide'.

Ammonium salts in EI The EI mass spectrum of tetrabutylammonium iodide shows a peak of low intensity (0.6%) for the $[Bu_4N]^+$ ion, *m/z* 242. A 'molecular

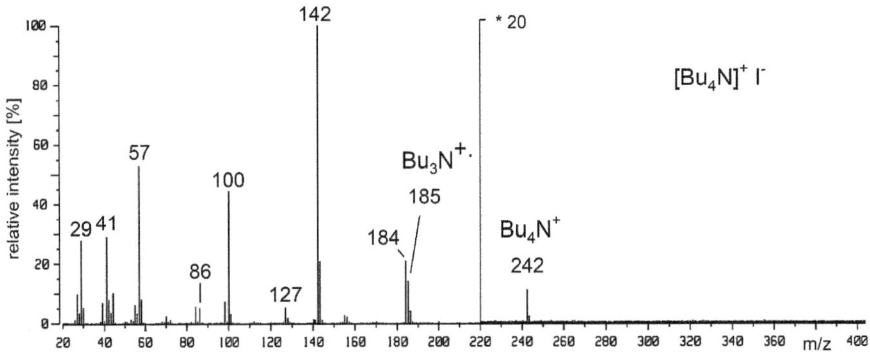

Fig. 6.43 EI mass spectrum of tetrabutylammonium iodide. The intensity scale is 20-fold above *m/z* 220, i.e., disregarding the peaks at *m/z* 127 and 128 this spectrum is very similar to the mass spectrum of pure tributylamine (Fig. 6.44b; for the field desorption mass spectrum cf. Sect. 8.6)

ion' of the salt that would occur at *m/z* 369 is not observed. The majority of the sample decomposes and the spectrum closely resembles that of pure tributylamine showing its molecular ion peak at *m/z* 185 (the fragmentation of which is explained in Sect. 6.12.1). Closer inspection, however, reveals the existence of peaks at *m/z* 127 and 128 corresponding to I^+ and $HI^{+\bullet}$, respectively (Fig. 6.43).

6.12 Alkene Loss from Onium Ions

Up to this point, aliphatic *onium ions* such as *immonium*, *oxonium*, and *sulfonium ions* have only been referred to as even-electron ionic products of the α-cleavage occurring from molecular ions of amines, alcohols, ethers, thiols, and thioethers (Sect. 6.2.5). All these and analogous onium ions are capable of further fragmentation reactions, the majority of which are alkene losses [123] yielding fragments of high relevance for structure elucidation.

The first of these reactions requires a γ-hydrogen, and thus at least one C_3-alkyl substitutent. It may either be regarded as the *even-electron analogy of the McLafferty rearrangement* (*McL*, Sect. 6.8) as it will be treated here [77, 78, 124], or alternatively, as a *retro-ene reaction* [125, 126].

The second alkene loss can occur from any onium ion bearing at least one C_2-alkyl moiety, which obviously is the least demanding prerequisite for an alkene loss (ethene) to proceed. By this process, the whole substituent is cleaved off the heteroatom with concomitant nonspecific hydrogen transfer from the leaving group to the heteroatom [25, 28]. In accordance with its occurrence from onium ions, this alkene loss is sometimes termed *onium reaction* (*On*) [30, 54, 127–130]. Thus, we obtain the following general fragmentation scheme for alkene losses from suitably substituted onium ions (Scheme 6.52).

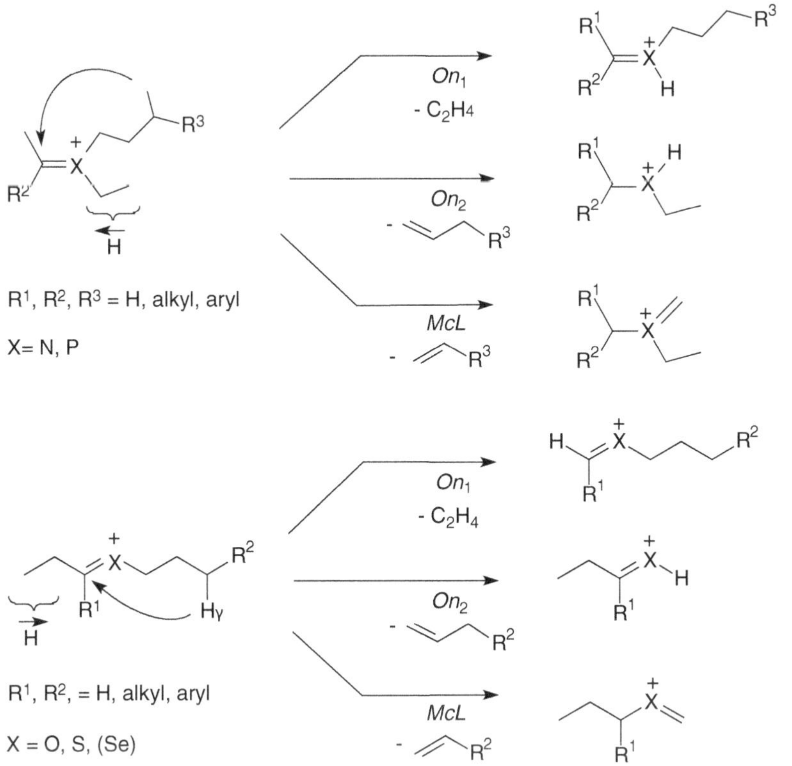

Scheme 6.52

6.12.1 McL of Onium Ions

The McLafferty rearrangement of onium ions is accompanied by the same 100% regioselectivity for γ-H transfer as is observed for odd-electron ions. This has repeatedly been demonstrated by deuterium labeling experiments [124, 127, 129, 131]. This γ-selectivity also supports the general findings that immonium ions neither undergo random hydrogen nor carbon skeleton rearrangements prior to fragmentation [22, 124, 132]. The generally observed inertness of onium ions towards isomerization which is in contrast to $[C_nH_{2n+1}]^+$ (Sect. 6.6.1) and $[C_2H_{2n-1}]^+$ ions (Sect. 6.5.1) can be attributed to the preferred charge localization at the heteroatom [133].

The origin of the moving hydrogen and the structures of the product ions of the McLafferty rearrangement are well known. A large amount of experimental data is in perfect agreement with a heterolytic stepwise mechanism, initiated by a 1,5-hydride shift [124, 127, 131, 134–136] (Scheme 6.53).

The carbenium ion intermediate then eliminates the alkene by charge-induced cleavage of a C–C bond. The most striking argument for a carbenium ion intermediate is presented by the influence of the γ-substituent R on the competition of

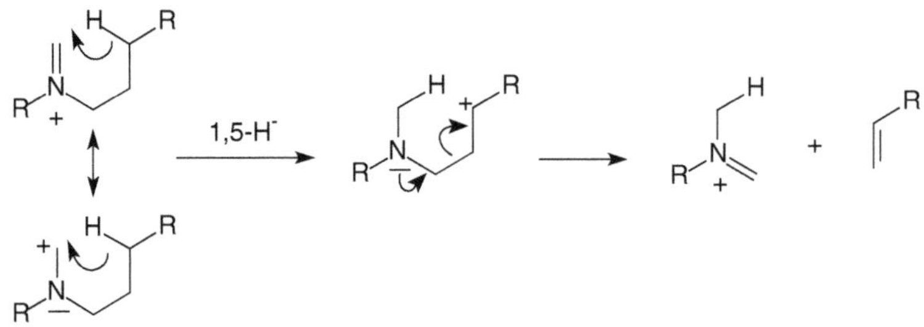

Scheme 6.53

onium reaction and McL. If R = H, i.e., for propyl-substituted immonium ions, the products of both reactions exhibit similar abundance. If R = Me or larger or if even two alkyls are present, the McLafferty rearrangement becomes extremely dominant, because then its intermediate is a secondary or tertiary carbenium ion, respectively, in contrast to a primary carbenium ion intermediate in case of R = H. The importance of relative carbenium ion stability for onium ion fragmentations (Sect. 6.12.2) will become more apparent when dealing with the mechanism of the onium reaction.

McL always useful
Regardless of the exact mechanism and regardless of whatever the correct name, the McLafferty rearrangement of onium ions is one of those processes allowing to reliably track ionic structures through a mass spectrum.

Fragmentation of aliphatic amines Comparing the EI mass spectra of tripropylamine (Fig. 6.44a) and tributylamine [128] (Fig. 6.44b) shows that the latter basically can be explained by two reactions: α-cleavage of the molecular ion at *m*/*z* 185 forming a dibutylmethyleneimmonium ion, *m*/*z* 142, undergoing double propene loss (42 u) via consecutive McLafferty rearrangements (Scheme 6.54). The propyl substitutents of the primary iminum ion fragment from tripropylamine, *m*/*z* 114, on the other side, allow for both fragmentations equally well, i.e., ethene loss via McL and propene loss via onium reaction, yielding peaks at *m*/*z* 86 and 72, respectively.

McL of oxonium ions The McLafferty rearrangement of onium ions is not necessarily as obvious as in the case of the immonium ions from aliphatic amines above. Especially, when other dissociation pathways are effectively competing, the corresponding signals can be of comparatively low intensity. The EI mass spectrum of butylisopropylether represents such a case: only the primary fragment ion at *m*/*z* 101 is able to undergo McL to form the oxonium ion at *m*/*z* 59 (Fig. 6.45 and Scheme 6.56). The peak at *m*/*z* 56 is due to $[C_4H_8]^{+\bullet}$ ions by loss of isopropanol

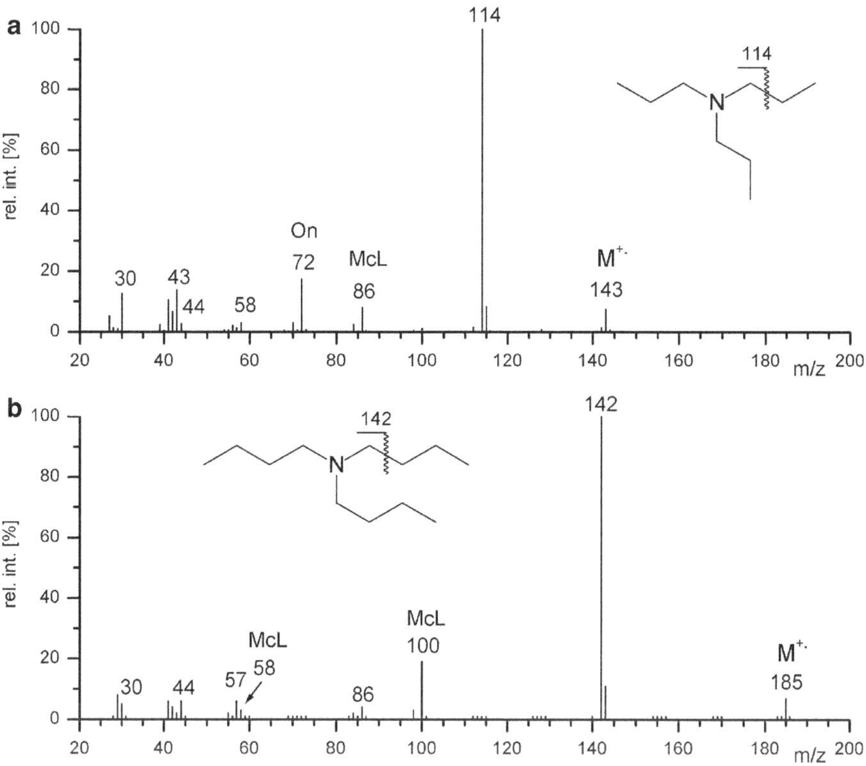

Fig. 6.44 EI mass spectra of tripropylamine (**a**) and tributylamine (**b**). For both compounds, the immonium ion series are completely present from *m/z* 30 onwards (Spectra used by permission of NIST. © NIST 2002)

from the molecular ion [137, 138]. Eliminations of ROH from ionized ethers are usually of low abundance, but can gain importance in case of branching at the α-carbon.

How to approach spectra By now, you should have gotten used to approach spectra in this way:

- Identify molecular ion peak (Sect. 6.7).
- Carefully look for isotopic patterns of Cl, Br, Si, and S; use a ^{13}C peak to estimate the number of carbon atoms (Chap. 3).
- Check for even- versus odd-numbered *m/z* values, changes from even to odd, and vice versa. Apply even-electron rule.
- Apply nitrogen rule.
- Judge from the intensity distribution as to whether the compound should rather be aliphatic or aromatic.
- Look for characteristic ion series (also when boxes and circles are missing!).

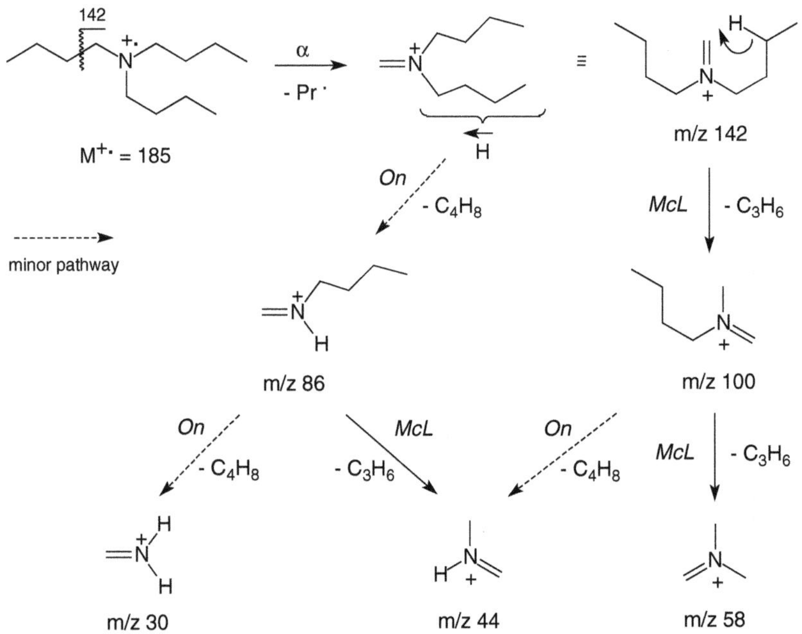

Scheme 6.54

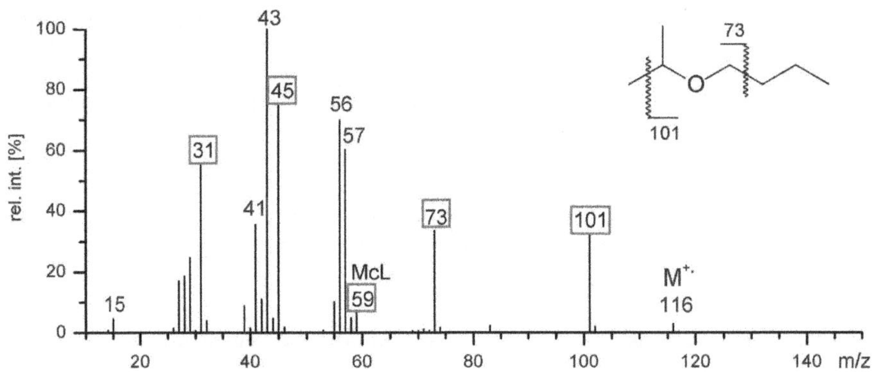

Fig. 6.45 EI mass spectrum of butylisopropylether. The intense oxonium ion peaks (*red boxes*) clearly indicate that this spectrum must belong to an aliphatic ether or alcohol. Here, the primary oxonium fragment $[M–CH_3]^{+\bullet}$, *m/z* 101, undergoes McL to yield the oxonium ion at *m/z* 59 via loss of C_3H_8 (Spectrum used by permission of NIST. © NIST 2002)

6.12.2 Onium Reaction

The loss of alkenes from aliphatic onium ions via onium reaction comprises scission of the C–X bond and concomitant transfer of a hydrogen from the leaving alkyl moiety to the heteroatom. This seemingly simple reaction has to be regarded as a multistep process that involves *ion–neutral complex* (INC) intermediates. The properties of ion–neutral complexes are discussed in detail below (Sect. 6.13). Here, we restrict ourselves to the application of this concept to achieve a consistent explanation of the behavior of onium ions.

The onium reaction of immonium ions [127, 129, 130, 136, 139, 140] and oxonium ions [32, 125, 141, 142] has been studied exhaustively. Imagine an isopropyl-propylmethyleneimmonium ion, *m/z* 114, where the reaction is initiated by heterolytic elongation of the C–N bond (Scheme 6.55). Having passed the transition state, the reaction would normally be expected to proceed by direct dissociation to yield a $C_3H_7^+$ ion, *m/z* 43 (imine loss). Alternatively, the incipient propyl ion might stay with the imine, thus forming an ion–neutral complex INC_1. The decision which of these channels will be followed depends on the ion internal energy, i.e., the less energetic ions will prefer INC formation, whereas the highly

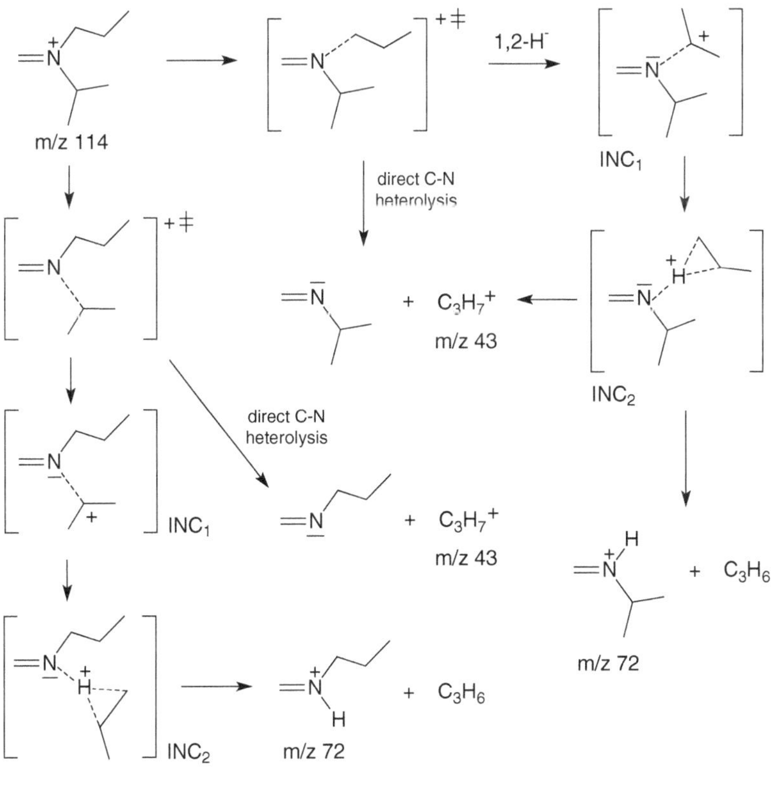

Scheme 6.55

excited ones are prone to dissociation. An INC can be regarded as the gas phase analog to solvation of ions in the condensed phase. Here, the lone pair of the imine acts as a donor for the carbenium ion. As ion and neutral are mutually free and mainly held together by Coulombic attraction, isomerization of the incipient 1-propyl ion to a 2-propyl ion via 1,2-hydride shift can take place. This goes along with a stabilization of about 60 kJ mol^{-1} (Table 2.3). The stabilization energy must of course be stored in internal degrees of freedom, thereby contributing to some further excitation of INC_1. Direct dissociation of INC_1 is also detected as imine loss. By considering the propyl ion as a protonated propene molecule it becomes reasonable that within the INC a proton may be attracted by the imine having a by 100–140 kJ mol^{-1} higher proton affinity (*PA*, Sect. 2.12) than the leaving alkene [124, 143–145]. Therefore, the proton is almost quantitatively transferred to the imine, and the heat of reaction of 140 kJ mol^{-1} causes additional excitation. Thus, INC_2, also called *proton-bridged complex* (PBC), finally decomposes to give an immonium ion, *m/z* 72, and propene, 42 u.

More examples for onium reactions The spectra of *N*-ethyl-*N*-methyl-propylamine (Fig. 6.6), tripropylamine, and tributylamine (Fig. 6.44) also exemplify alkene loss from immonium ions via an onium reaction. Oxonium ions are involved in the fragmentation of diethylether and methylpropylether (Fig. 6.7) and many others have been published [125, 141, 142, 146]. Below, the fragmentation of butyl-isopropylether is shown (Scheme 6.56).

The onium reaction and the McLafferty rearrangement of onium ions are closely related to each other in so far as that they often occur from the very same ion. However, the knowledge of the above mechanisms reveals significant differences in the way they proceed and it sheds light on the competition of onium reaction and McL: During the onium reaction alkyl substituents with no branch at C_α (adjacent to the heteroatom) have to be cleaved off via a transition state resembling a primary carbenium ion. Branching at C_α will effect dramatic change on the ease of bond heterolysis. As pointed out, analogous effects are observed for the McL in case of substitution at C_γ (Sect. 6.12.1 and Fig. 6.44). It becomes clear that the reaction

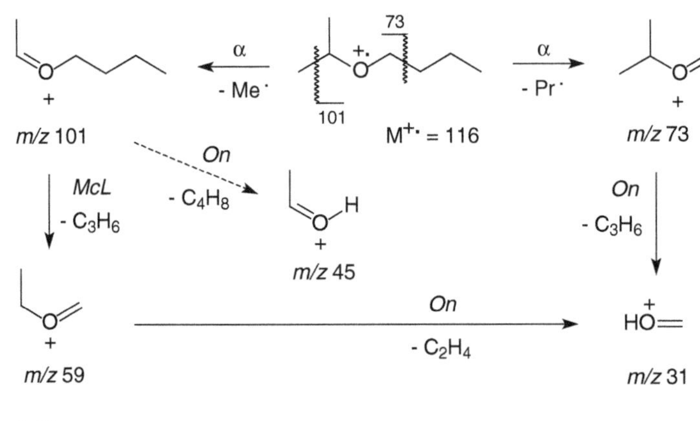

Scheme 6.56

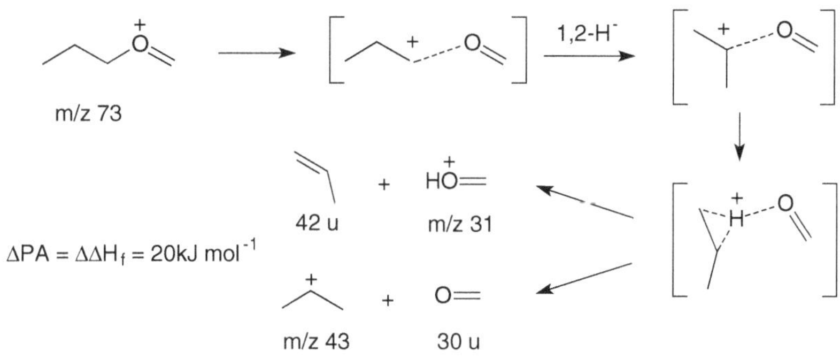

Scheme 6.57

pathway passing through the higher branched carbenium ion intermediate will be observed as the predominating process.

In case of immonium ion fragmentations, the large difference of proton affinities, Δ*PA*, between imine and alkene clearly favors the formation of immonium ion plus neutral alkene, whereas imine loss is restricted to highly energetic precursors.

In decomposing oxonium ions the situation is quite different, i.e., the preference for alkene loss is much less emphasized and aldehyde (ketone) loss is gaining importance. The observed changes are in good agreement with the postulated mechanism of the onium reaction [125, 147]. The alternative pairs of oxonium ion plus alkene and aldehyde plus carbenium ion may be formed with a preference for the first one, because Δ*PA* is comparatively small (20–60 kJ mol^{-1}) or even zero, e.g., for the acetone/isobutene pair [125, 145, 147] (Scheme 6.57).

6.13 Ion–Neutral Complexes

During the above discussion of the mechanism of the onium reaction we encountered another type of reactive intermediates of unimolecular ion fragmentations: *ion–neutral complexes* (INC) [24, 37, 148–151]. In contrast to *distonic ions* (Sect. 6.3) ion–neutral complex intermediates add some bimolecular reaction characteristics to fragmentation pathways of isolated ions. This is effected by allowing an incipient neutral fragment to remain some time with the ionic part, both derived from the same precursor ion, thus enabling processes that otherwise could only occur from bimolecular ion-molecule reactions. The final products of such fragmentations are governed by the properties of the species involved, e.g., by the relative proton affinities of the partners as was the case with the onium reaction.

6.13.1 Evidence for the Existence of Ion–Neutral Complexes

INCs were first referred to by Rylander and Meyerson [152, 153]. Soon, the concept that the decomposition of oxonium and immonium ions involve INCs (Sect. 6.12.2) was put forth by Bowen and Williams [125, 139, 140, 147], and the analogies to solvolysis were described by Morton [148]. Still, mass spectrometrists were too much used to strictly unimolecular reactions as to assimilate this concept without stringent proof.

Conclusive evidence for INCs was first presented by Longevialle and Botter [154, 155] who demonstrated the transfer of a proton from an imine fragment to an amino group located on the opposite side of the rigid skeleton of bifunctional steroidal amines [155]. Such a proton transfer cannot proceed without the intermediacy of an INC; otherwise, a conventional hydrogen shift would have bridged the distance of about 10^{-9} m between the respective groups which is about five times too far.

The occurrence of this unexpected reaction chiefly depends on the ion's internal energy: energetic molecular ions undergo α-cleavage leading to an immonium ion, $[C_2H_6N]^+$, *m/z* 44, while less energetic ions and especially metastable ions show imine loss. Obviously, mutual rotation of the reacting partners has to precede the final acid-base reaction preferably causing imine loss, i.e., an $[M–C_2H_5N]^{+\bullet}$ fragment, $[M–43]^{+\bullet}$. This is possible because the attractive forces between the radical and the ion are strong enough to prevent spontaneous dissociation by forming an INC. Now, mutual rotation of the reacting partners allows additional dissociation channels to be explored. Finally, the proton transfer to the amine is thermodynamically favorable, because the proton affinity of ethylideneimine, 891 kJ mol^{-1}, is presumably lower than that of the steroidal amine radical (as estimated from the proton affinity of cyclohexylamine [143], this is about 920 kJ mol^{-1}, i.e., $\Delta PA \approx$ 29 kJ mol^{-1}).

Proton transfer will be prevented when the initial fragments separate too rapidly for the partners to rotate into a suitable configuration. Here, the lower limit for the intermediate's lifetime can be estimated as 10^{-11} s (Scheme 6.58). The competition between the α-cleavage and the INC-mediated reaction is therefore governed by the amount of ion internal energy.

6.13.2 Attractive Forces in Ion–Neutral Complexes

The term ion–neutral complex is applied to species in which an ion and a neutral are held together mainly by electrostatic attraction [151]. The INC must be held together by attracting positive and negative charges and an electron-donating or -accepting group, respectively, rather than by the action of covalent bonds. This can accomplished by ion-dipole and ion-induced dipole interactions. The formation of an INC can be compared to solvolysis reactions in the condensed phase with subsequent mutual solvation of the partners [148]. Typically, the stabilization energy V_r is in the range of 20–50 kJ mol^{-1}.

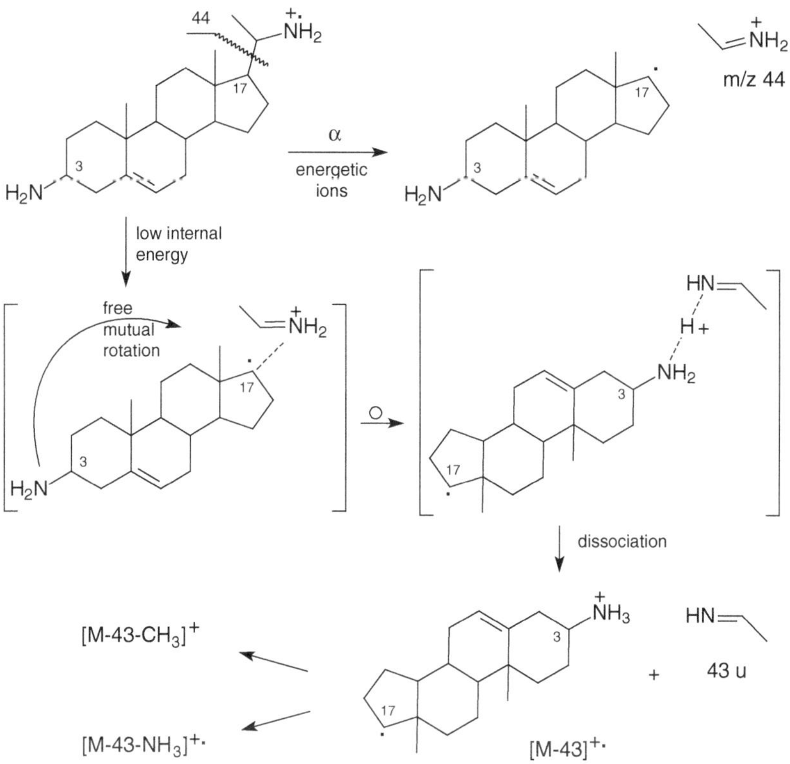

Scheme 6.58

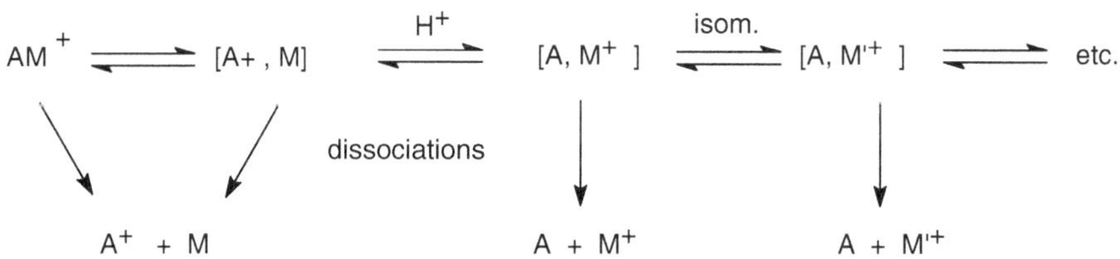

Scheme 6.59

Consider the dissociation of an ion AM^+ that may either dissociate to form the fragments A^+ and M or the INC [A^+, M] allowing free mutual rotation and thus reorientation of the constituents. Within the INC, A^+ and M can recombine only if they attain a well-defined mutual orientation, i.e., the system has to freeze rotational degrees of freedom. Such a configuration allowing covalent bonds to be formed is termed *locked-rotor critical configuration* [149–151, 156] and any reaction channel, e.g., proton transfer or recombination, has to pass this *entropic bottleneck*. The INC [A^+, M] can in principle undergo multiple isomerizations and may dissociate at any of these isomeric states (Scheme 6.59).

INCs mean slow reactions

Any reaction depending on a certain configuration to be attained, i.e., "classical" rearrangement fragmentations and especially INC-mediated processes, exhibit comparatively low rate constants that are in part due to entropic bottlenecks that need to be passed (cf. *tight transition states*, Sect. 2.5). Therefore, high ion internal energies tend to discriminate between INC-mediated reactions, but favor direct bond cleavages.

6.13.3 Criteria for Ion–Neutral Complexes

A species can be considered as an INC if its lifetime is long enough to allow for other chemical reactions than the mere dissociation of the incipient particles. This is the minimum criterion that has to be fulfilled to term a reactive intermediate an ion–neutral complex, because otherwise any transition state would also represent an INC [151, 157]. In addition, the *reorientation criterion* [24, 149] should be met, i.e., free reorientation of the particles involved must be possible. Although still regarded provisional by the authors, McAdoo and Hudson have provided a useful collection of additional characteristics of ion–neutral complex-mediated dissociations [158, 159]:

- Complete dissociation by the bond cleavage that forms the INC will be observed and will increase in importance relative to the INC-mediated pathway as internal energy increases.
- INC-mediated processes will be among the lowest energy reactions of an ion.
- Reactions within and between partners may occur below the dissociation thresholds for simple dissociations.
- Alternative mechanisms consistent with the observations would require much higher energy transition states – transition states in which multiple bond breakings and makings occur simultaneously, or even transition states of impossible geometries.
- The observed kinetic isotope effects are usually large (because of low excess energy in the transition states).
- The kinetic energy released in corresponding metastable decompositions may be very small.

6.13.4 Ion–Neutral Complexes of Radical Ions

The intermediacy of ion–neutral complexes is neither restricted to even-electron fragmentations nor to complexes that consist of a neutral molecule and an ion. In

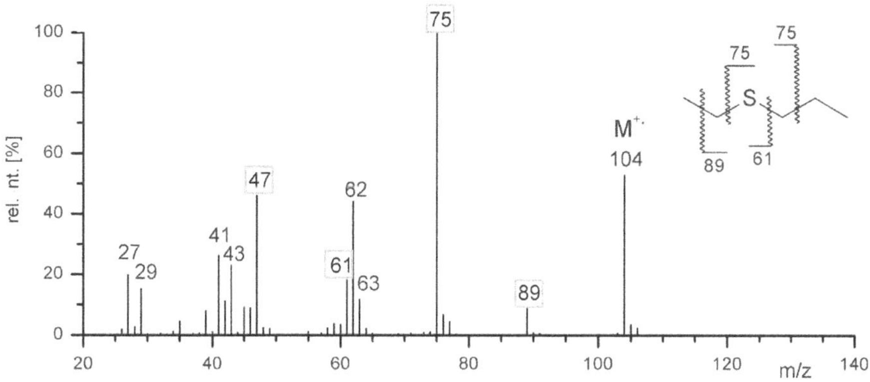

Fig. 6.46 EI mass spectrum of ethylpropylthioether. (Also compare to the spectrum of ethylisopropylthioether, Fig. 6.10. The isotopic pattern is discussed in Sect. 3.2). Sulfonium ions are marked with *yellow boxes* (Spectrum used by permission of NIST. © NIST 2002)

addition, radical-ion complexes and radical ion–neutral complexes occur that may dissociate to yield the respective fragments or can even *reversibly interconvert* by hydride, proton, or hydrogen radical shifts. Many examples are known from aliphatic alcohols [160, 161], alkylphenylethers [162–164], and thioethers [165].

The tricky fragmentations of a thioether The unimolecular reactions of the molecular ion of ethyl-propylthioether (Fig. 6.46, Scheme 6.60) [165] chiefly are (*i*) loss of a methyl from the ethyl or the propyl group, (*ii*) loss of an ethyl from the propyl group, both leading to *sulfonium ions* [166] (Sect. 6.2.5), and (*iii*) elimination of propene or an allyl radical by transfer of one or two hydrogen atoms, respectively, from the propyl group to the sulfur. On the microsecond time scale, the loss of $CH_3^{\bullet}$ involves only the propyl entity and is preceded by an isomerization of this group. Partial loss of the positional identity of the hydrogen atoms of the propyl group occurs, but incorporation of hydrogen or carbon atoms from the ethyl group into the formed neutral species does not occur. Cleavage of a C–S bond assisted by a 1,2-hydride shift in the incipient carbenium ion leads to an INC of a thioethoxy radical and a 2-propyl ion. The INC may recombine to form the molecular ion of ethylisopropylthioether (cf. Fig. 6.9) prior to $CH_3^{\bullet}$ loss, or react by proton transfer to give another INC, which may dissociate or undergo hydrogen atom transfer, followed by elimination of an allyl radical. The partial loss of positional identity of the hydrogen atoms during the decomposition of the metastable ions is mainly a result of reversible proton transfer between the constituents, which competes favorably with 1,2-hydride shifts within the carbenium ion entity of the complex.

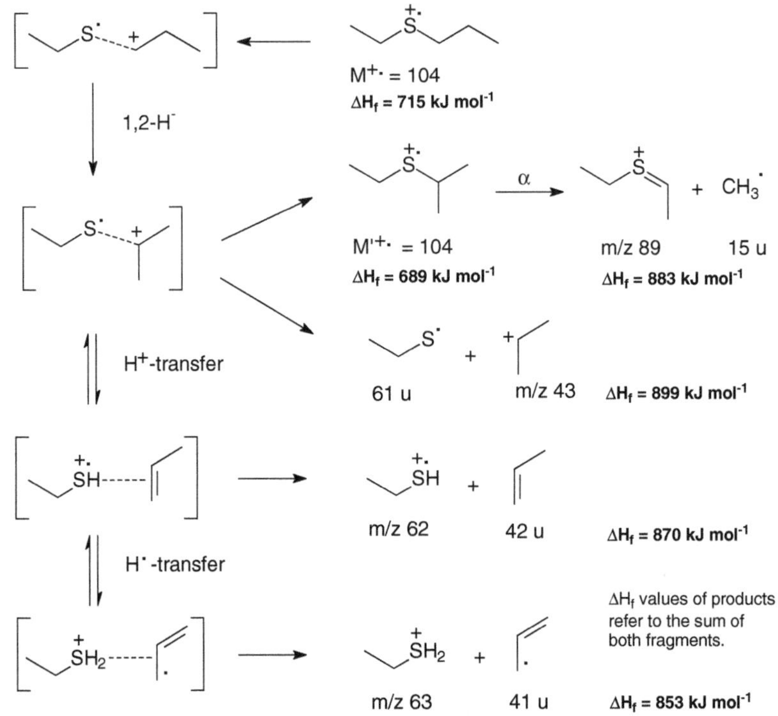

Scheme 6.60

6.14 *Ortho* Elimination (*Ortho* Effect)

The *ortho elimination* (*ortho effect*) has been stated to belong to the diagnostically most important mass spectral fragmentations [167]. Indeed, from the first report on this process [94] until the present, there is a continuing interest in this topic concerning a wide range of compounds [168–173]. The driving force for these research activities stems from a strict relation of this process to the substitution pattern of aryl compounds. The existence of a suitably 1,2-disubstituted *cis*-double bond presents an essential structural requirement for this rearrangement-type fragmentation, and this double bond is usually part of an aromatic system, hence the name.

Effect or elimination?

Although not being the correct term to describe a reaction, the term *ortho effect* is well established, and another occasionally used term, *retro-1,4-addition*, is redundant; *1,4-elimination* would describe the same.

(continued)

Scheme 6.61

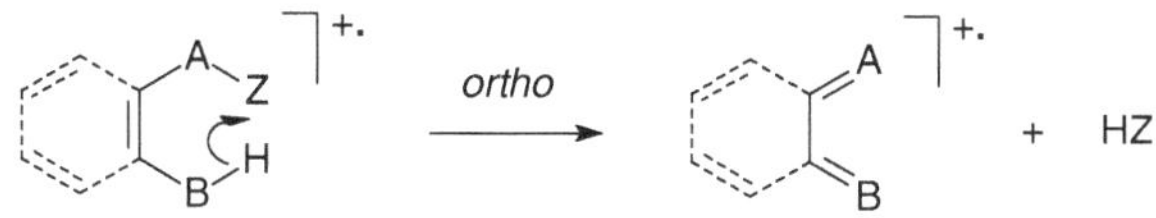

Unfortunately, this might be confused with 1,4-H_2O-eliminations from aliphatic alcohols, for example. Therefore, the term *ortho elimination* is suggested and used here.

6.14.1 *Ortho* Elimination from Molecular Ions

Commonly, *ortho* elimination refers to a hydrogen transfer via a six-membered transition state at *ortho*-disubstituted aromatic compounds. In practice, the reacting entities are almost in position to form this six-membered transition state. The general mechanism of the *ortho* elimination is as follows (Scheme 6.61).

The charge can reside on either product, but charge retention at the diene product is generally predominant. As the 1,2-disubstituted *cis*-double bond must not necessarily belong to an aryl group, the optional part of the molecule has been drawn in dashed style in the above scheme. In addition to the substitution pattern, the *ortho* elimination requires substituent A to bear a hydrogen-accepting leaving group, Z, and substituent B to be a hydrogen donor, e.g., hydroxyl, amino, thiol, or even alkyl [174].

Structural requirements for *ortho* elimination The leaving methyl of 2-hydroxyacetophenone (Fig. 6.47a) is not a suitable hydrogen acceptor, and therefore homolytic cleavages predominate. Here, these are loss of a methyl by α-cleavage, $[M–CH_3]^+$, *m/z* 121, and loss of an acyl by phenylic cleavage, $[M–COCH_3]^+$, *m/z* 93. On the other hand, all requirements for the *ortho* elimination are met in the 2-methylbenzoic acid molecular ion (Fig. 6.47b) [94]. As usual, homolytic cleavages are still competing with the *ortho* elimination [175], but the additional fragments due to loss of intact molecules containing one hydrogen from the donor site cannot be overlooked. Thus, α-cleavage, $[M–OH]^+$, *m/z* 119, is overrun by loss of water, $[M–H_2O]^{+\bullet}$, *m/z* 118, and phenylic cleavage, $[M–COOH]^+$, *m/z* 91, has to compete with formal loss of formic acid, $[M–HCOOH]^{+\bullet}$, *m/z* 90 (Scheme 6.62). Consequently, such neutral losses are absent in the mass spectra of the *meta* and *para* isomers.

As indicated by metastable ion studies of isopropylbenzoic acids [176], the formation of the ion at *m/z* 90 should be described as a two-step process, i.e., the product rather is $[M–OH–CHO]^{+\bullet}$ than $[M–HCOOH]^{+\bullet}$; yet another example to the list of violations of the even-electron rule (Sect. 6.1.3).

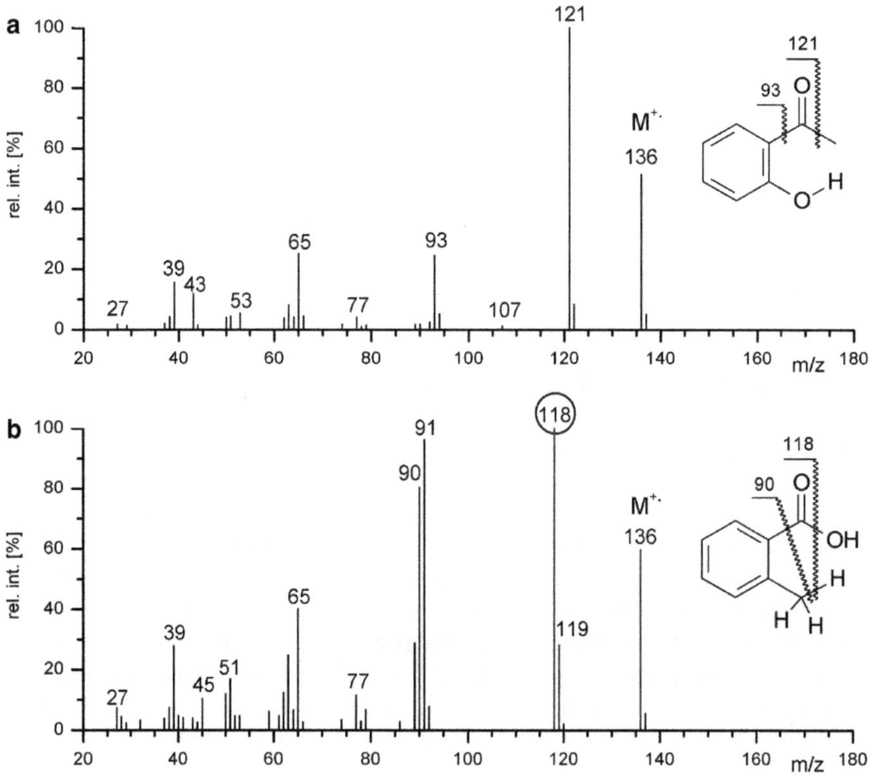

Fig. 6.47 EI mass spectra of (**a**) 2-hydroxyacetophenone and (**b**) 2-methylbenzoic acid. In (**a**) methyl is not an effective H acceptor and therefore 2-hydroxyacetophenone eliminates $CH_3^{\bullet}$ while in (**b**) OH in 2-methylbenzoic acid readily takes the $H^{\bullet}$ to form H_2O (*purple circle*) (Spectra used by permission of NIST. © NIST 2002)

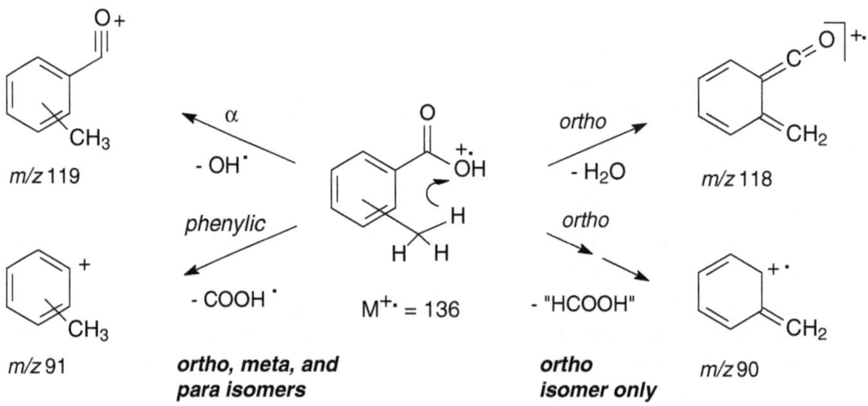

Scheme 6.62

6.14.2 *Ortho* Elimination from Even-Electron Ions

As with the McLafferty rearrangement and the retro-Diels-Alder reaction before, the occurrence of the *ortho* elimination is not restricted to molecular ions. It may equally well proceed in even-electron species.

***Ortho* eliminations from OE and EE ions** Examination of the mass spectrum of isopropylbenzoic acid reveals that the molecular ion, *m/z* 164, as well as the [M–CH_3]$^+$ ion, *m/z* 149, eliminate H_2O via *ortho* elimination yielding fragment ions at *m/z* 146 and 131, respectively (Fig. 6.48) [176]. The [M–CH_3–H_2O]$^+$ ion, a homolog of the benzoyl ion, decomposes further by loss of CO, thereby creating a fragment that overall corresponds to [M–CH_3–HCOOH]$^+$, *m/z* 103 (Scheme 6.63).

Fragmentation of 1,2-bis(trimethylsiloxy)benzene The molecular ion of 1,2-bis (trimethylsiloxy)benzene, *m/z* 254, undergoes methyl loss by Si–C bond cleavage as typically observed for silanes (Fig. 6.49). Rearrangement of the [M–CH_3]$^+$ ion then yields [Si(Me)$_3$]$^+$, *m/z* 73 (base peak). This is not an *ortho* elimination with concomitant $H^•$ transfer as defined in the strict sense, but the observed reaction is still specific for the *ortho*-isomer [167, 177]. In the spectra of the *meta*- and *para*-isomers the [Si(Me)$_3$]$^+$ ion is of lower abundance, the [M–CH_3]$^+$ ion representing the base peak in their spectra. Moreover, the *m/z* 73 ion is then generated directly from the molecular ion which is clearly different from the two-step pathway of the *ortho*-isomer (Scheme 6.64).

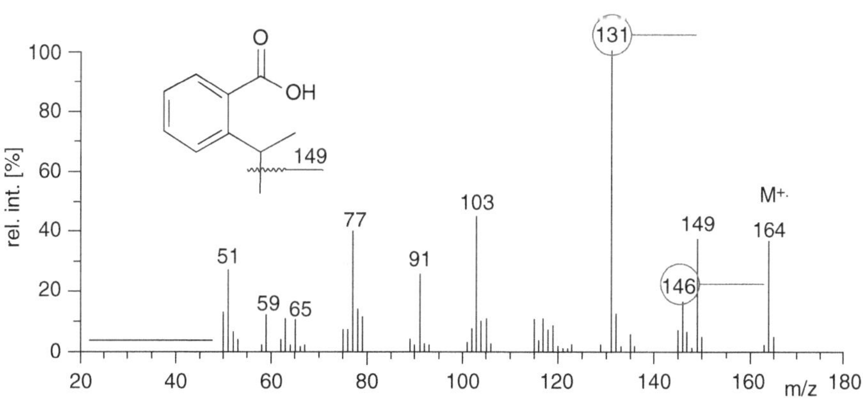

Fig. 6.48 EI mass spectrum of isopropylbenzoic acid. Both $M^{+•}$ (OE) and [M–CH_3]$^+$ (EE) ions undergo H_2O loss by *ortho* elimination (indicated by *purple lines* and *circles*). The horizontal line in the *m/z* 20–50 range indicates that there was no data available, which does not necessarily imply that there would be no ions if the range had been included during the acquisition of the spectrum (Spectrum used by permission of NIST. © NIST 2002)

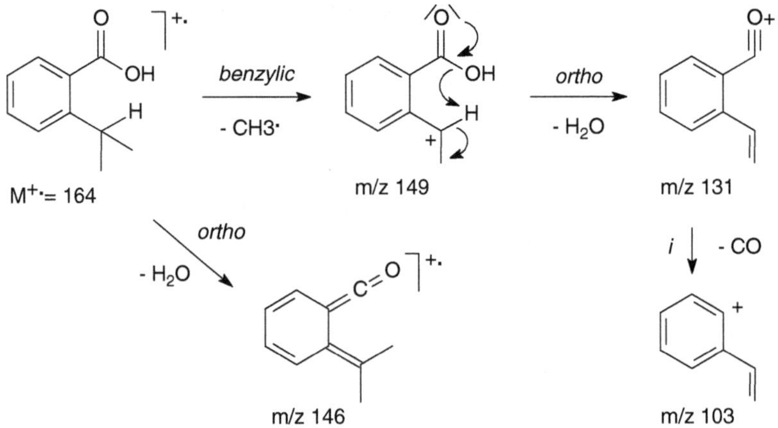

Scheme 6.63

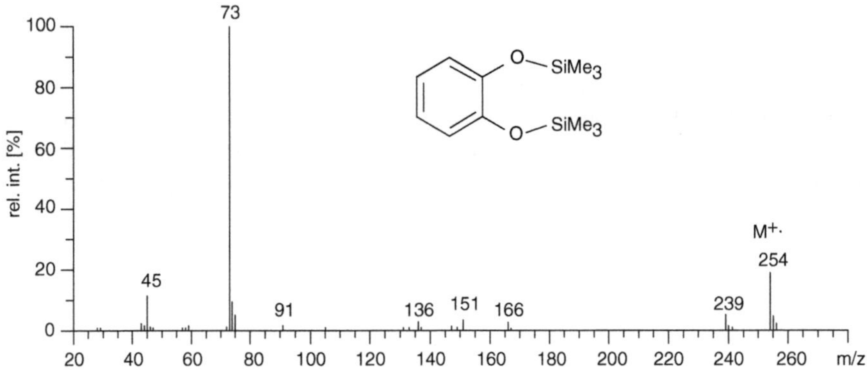

Fig. 6.49 EI mass spectrum of 1,2-bis(trimethylsiloxy)benzene. The isotopic pattern of silicon is clearly visible in the signals at *m/z* 73, 239, and 254 (Sect. 3.2) (Spectrum used by permission of NIST. © NIST 2002)

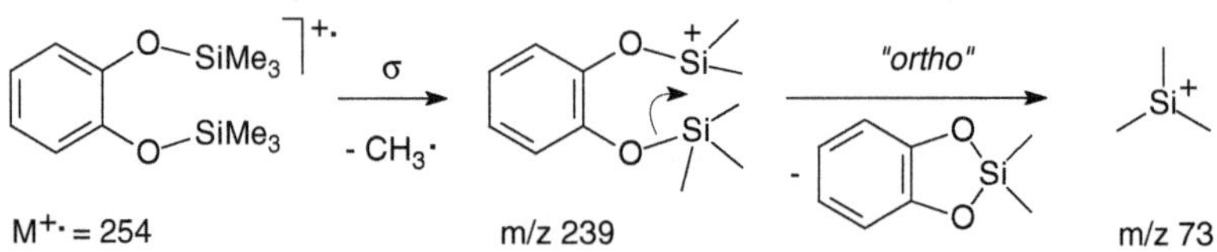

Scheme 6.64

Silylation
Trimethylsilyl (TMS) derivatives are frequently employed to volatize alcohols [177, 178], carboxylic acids [179, 180], and other compounds [181] for mass spectrometry, and for GC-MS applications in particular. The EI mass spectra of TMS derivatives exhibit weak molecular ion peaks, clearly visible $[M\text{–}CH_3]^+$ signals and often $[Si(Me)_3]^+$, *m/z* 73, as the base peak.

6.14.3 *Ortho* Elimination the Fragmentation of Nitroarenes

Nitroarenes are recognized from their characteristic neutral losses due to the NO_2 substituent. Normally, all theoretically possible fragment ions, the plausible $[M\text{–}NO_2]^+$ and $[M\text{–}O]^{+\bullet}$ ions as well as the unexpected $[M\text{–}NO]^+$ ion, are observed. It is worth noting that molecular ions are 1,2-distonic by definition, because nitro-arene molecules are best represented as zwitterion (Sect. 6.3). The molecular ion may either dissociate directly by loss of an oxygen atom or a NO_2 molecule or it may rearrange prior to loss of $NO^\bullet$. For the latter process, two reaction pathways have been suggested, one of them involving intermediate formation of a nitrite, and the other proceeding via a three-membered cyclic intermediate (Scheme 6.65) [182]. Thus, the characteristic series of $[M\text{–}16]^{+\bullet}$ (generally weak signal), $[M\text{–}30]^+$, and $[M\text{–}46]^+$ ions is obtained, e.g., for nitrobenzene:

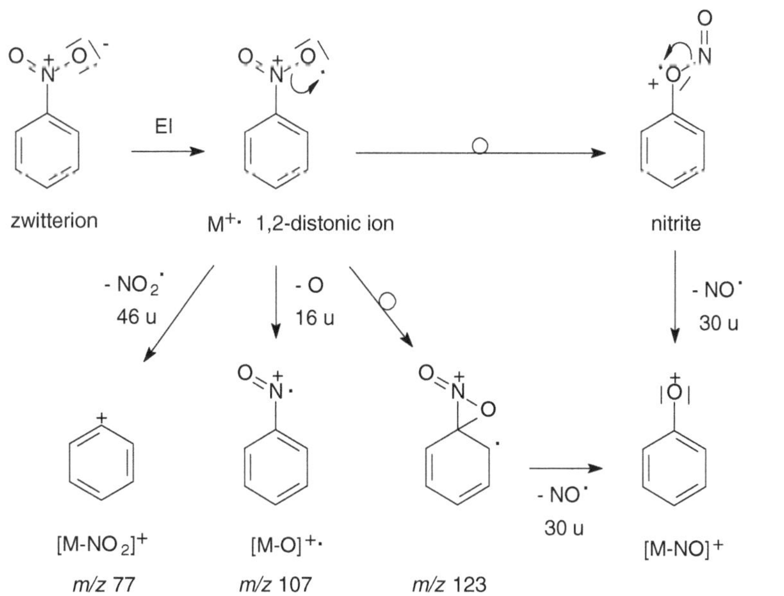

Scheme 6.65

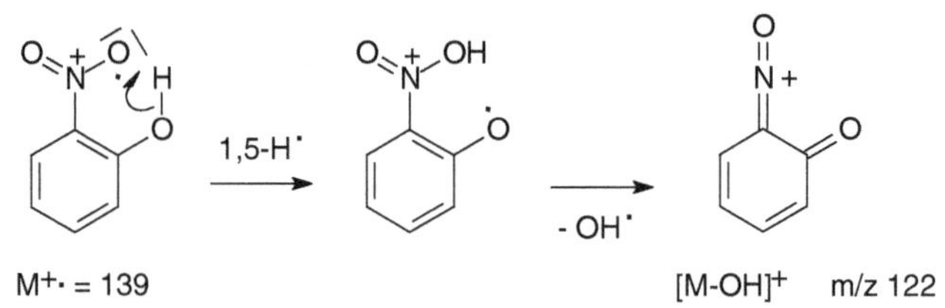

Scheme 6.66

Differentiation of isomeric nitrophenols *Ortho*-substituted nitroarenes can be distinguished from *meta*- or *para*-substituted isomers due to a characteristic change in their mass spectra. In the presence of a hydrogen-donating *ortho* substituent, $[M–OH]^+$ replaces the $[M–O]^{+•}$ fragment ion. In case of nitrophenols, the ion at *m/z* 122 appears in place of the one at *m/z* 123 (Scheme 6.66 and Fig. 6.50c). Here, the mechanism which resembles the previously discussed *ortho* eliminations is shown [183]:

6.15 Heterocyclic Compounds

As mentioned in the beginning of this chapter, it is not possible in this book to deliver a comprehensive treatment of the fragmentations of organic ions. Nevertheless, a short reference to MS of heterocyclic compounds should be made here, while being aware that this topic could easily fill an entire book of its own [184].

6.15.1 Saturated Heterocyclic Compounds

The molecular ions of small saturated heterocyclic compounds exhibit a strong tendency for *transannular cleavages* that often give rise to the base peak. These transannular cleavages can formally be regarded as clean cuts across the ring. Other fragmentation pathways including ring-opening bond scissions followed by consecutive cleavages and α-cleavage also play a role and start to compete effectively with the characteristic ring cleavage as the number of substituents at the ring increases [185–187] (Scheme 6.67).

The methyloxirane molecular ion, *m/z* 58, easily fragments by α-cleavage preferably yielding a $[M–CH_3]^+$ ion, *m/z* 43, and a $[M–H]^+$ ion, *m/z* 57 (Fig. 6.51). The more characteristic transannular ring cleavage leads to loss of formaldehyde, thus explaining the base peak at *m/z* 28 as a $C_2H_4^{+•}$ ion. Ring opening and consecutive fragmentation leads to fragment ions such as $[CH_2OH]^+$, *m/z* 31, $[CHO]^+$, *m/z* 29, and $[CH_3]^+$, *m/z* 15 (Scheme 6.68).

Four-membered rings Comparing the spectra of methyloxirane and its isomer oxetane reveals a clear difference in that the $[M–CH_3]^+$ ion, *m/z* 43, is almost absent because of the missing methyl group, whereas the $[M–H]^+$ ion, *m/z* 57, remains

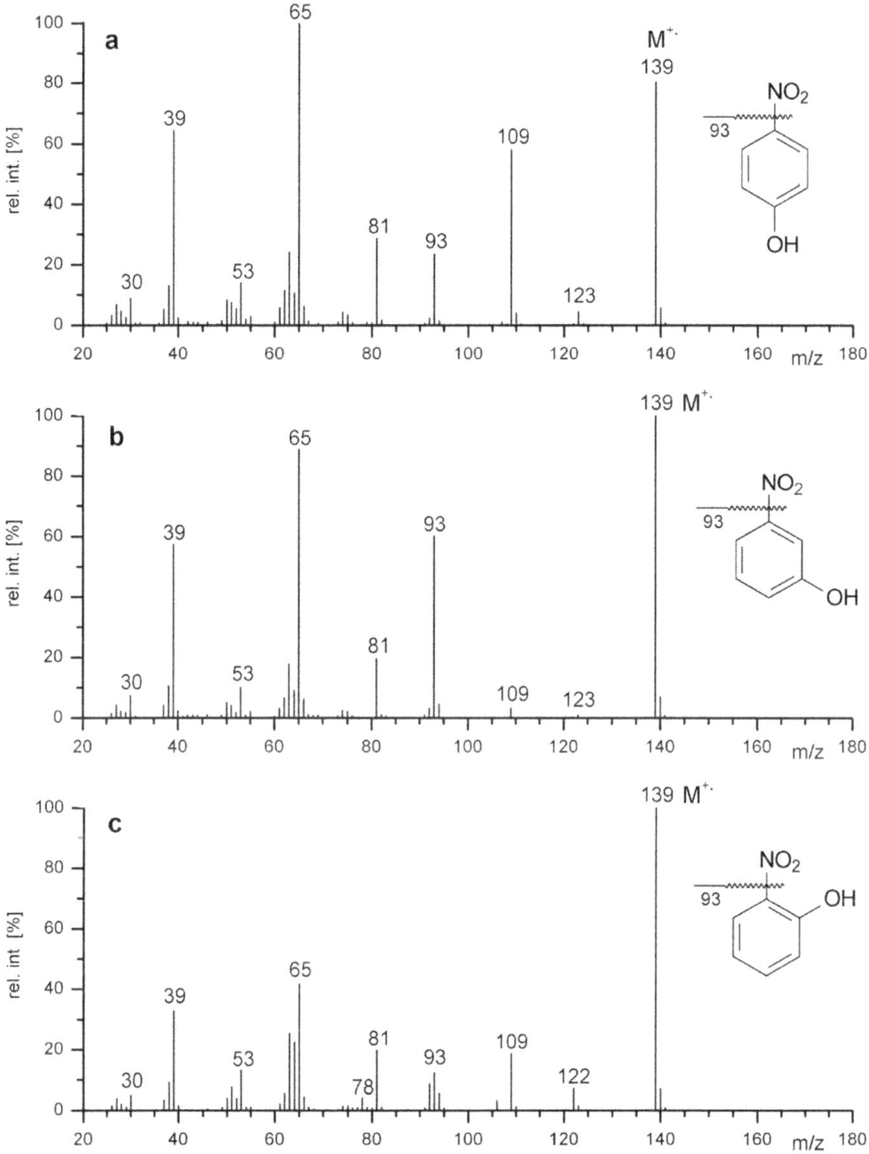

Fig. 6.50 EI mass spectra of isomeric nitrophenols: (**a**) *para*-, (**b**) *meta*-, (**c**) *ortho*-nitrophenol. The fragment ions by loss of NO_2 at *m/z* 93 and NO at *m/z* 109 are observed in all spectra, whereas only for the *ortho* isomer, the fragment ion $[M–OH]^+$, *m/z* 122, replaces $[M–O]^{+\bullet}$, *m/z* 123 (Spectra used by permission of NIST. © NIST 2002)

unaffected (Fig. 6.52a). The transannular ring cleavage, however, benefits from this reduced number of competing routes and thus, the $[M–H_2CO]^{+\bullet}$ ion, *m/z* 28, is definitely dominant. The better charge-localizing capability of nitrogen as in

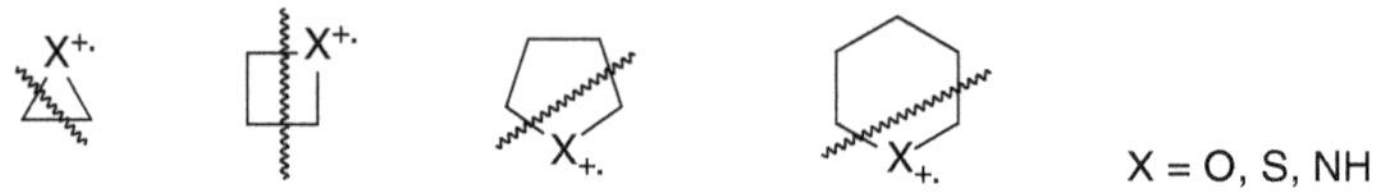

Scheme 6.67

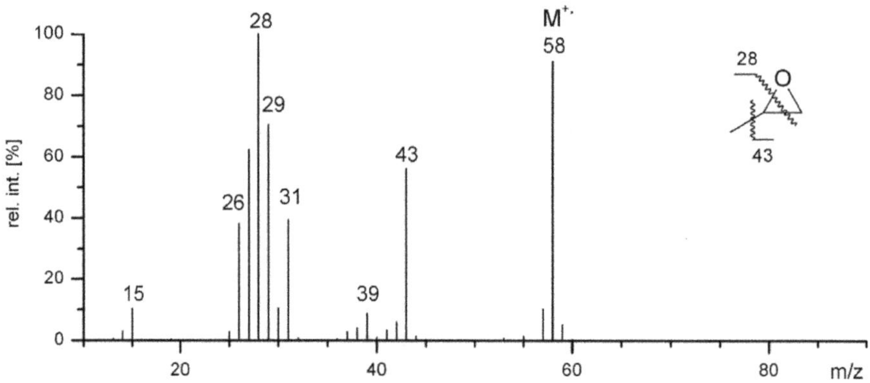

Fig. 6.51 EI mass spectrum of methyloxirane (Spectrum used by permission of NIST)

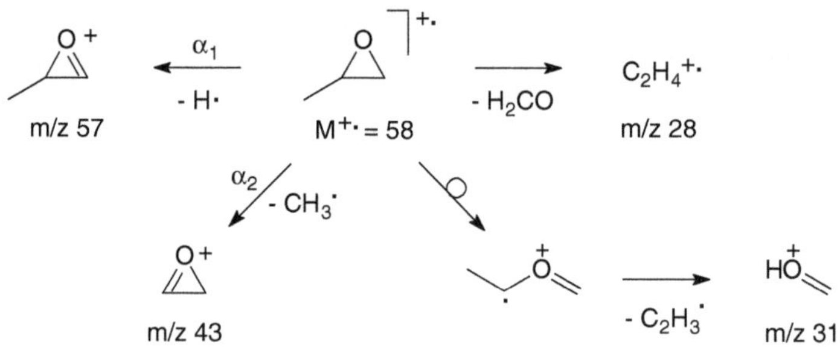

Scheme 6.68

azetidine pronounces radical-induced cleavages as compared to the oxetane spectrum, i.e., a $[M{-}CH_3]^+$ ion, *m*/*z* 42, is observed due to ring opening and the $[M{-}H]^+$ ion, *m*/*z* 56, from α-cleavage (Sect. 6.2) is also more prominent (Fig. 6.52b). Here, transannular ring cleavage of the *N*-heterocycle effects loss of methyleneimine, and the $[M{-}H_2CNH]^{+\bullet}$ ion forms the base peak (Scheme 6.69).

Think of isomers

Methyloxirane and oxetane are C_3H_6O isomers, but acetone, propanal, methyl vinylether, and 2-propenol also belong to this group. This reminds us to be careful when assigning structures to empirical formulas and when deducing structural information from $r + d$ values (Sect. 6.4.4).

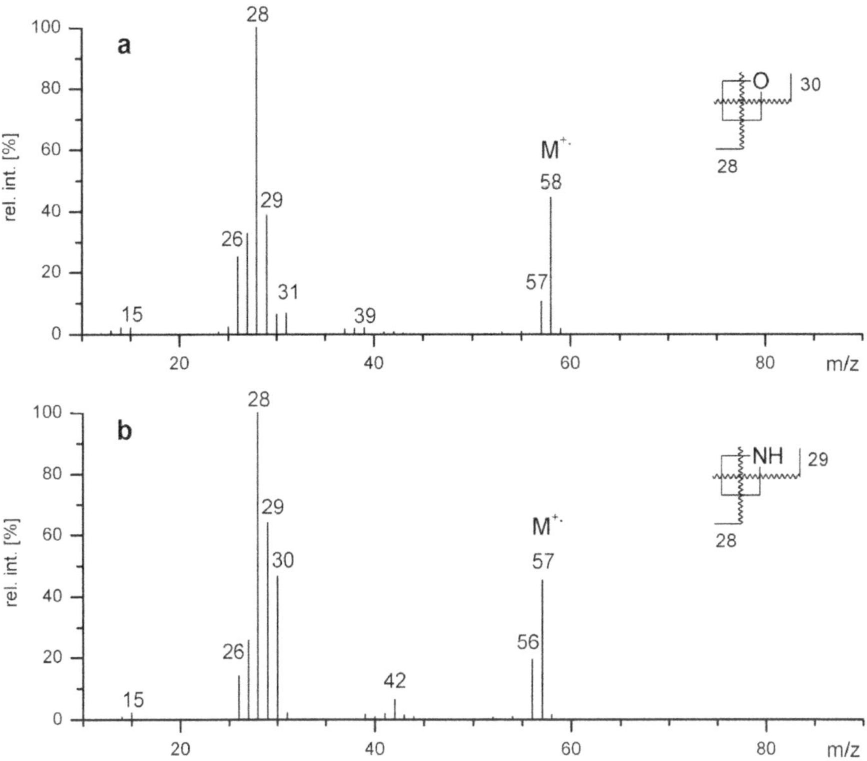

Fig. 6.52 EI mass spectra of oxetane (**a**) and azetidine (**b**) (Spectra used by permission of NIST. © NIST 2002)

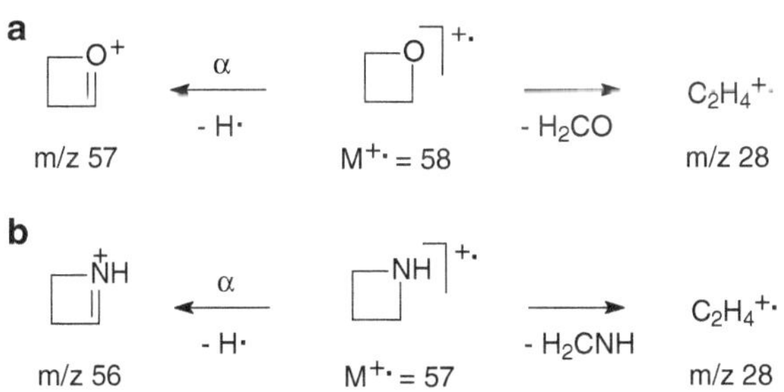

Scheme 6.69

Loss of formaldehyde is not only among the processes of low activation energy for oxirane and oxetane molecular ions, but also in case of larger cyclic ether molecular ions such as those of tetrahydrofurane and tetrahydropyran [188]. Again, imine loss from *N*-heterocycles [189] behaves analogously. The mass spectra of tetrahydrofuran, pyrrolidine, tetrahydropyran, and piperidine are compared below (Fig. 6.53). The strong $[M–H]^+$ peaks in all of those four spectra are due to α-cleavage.

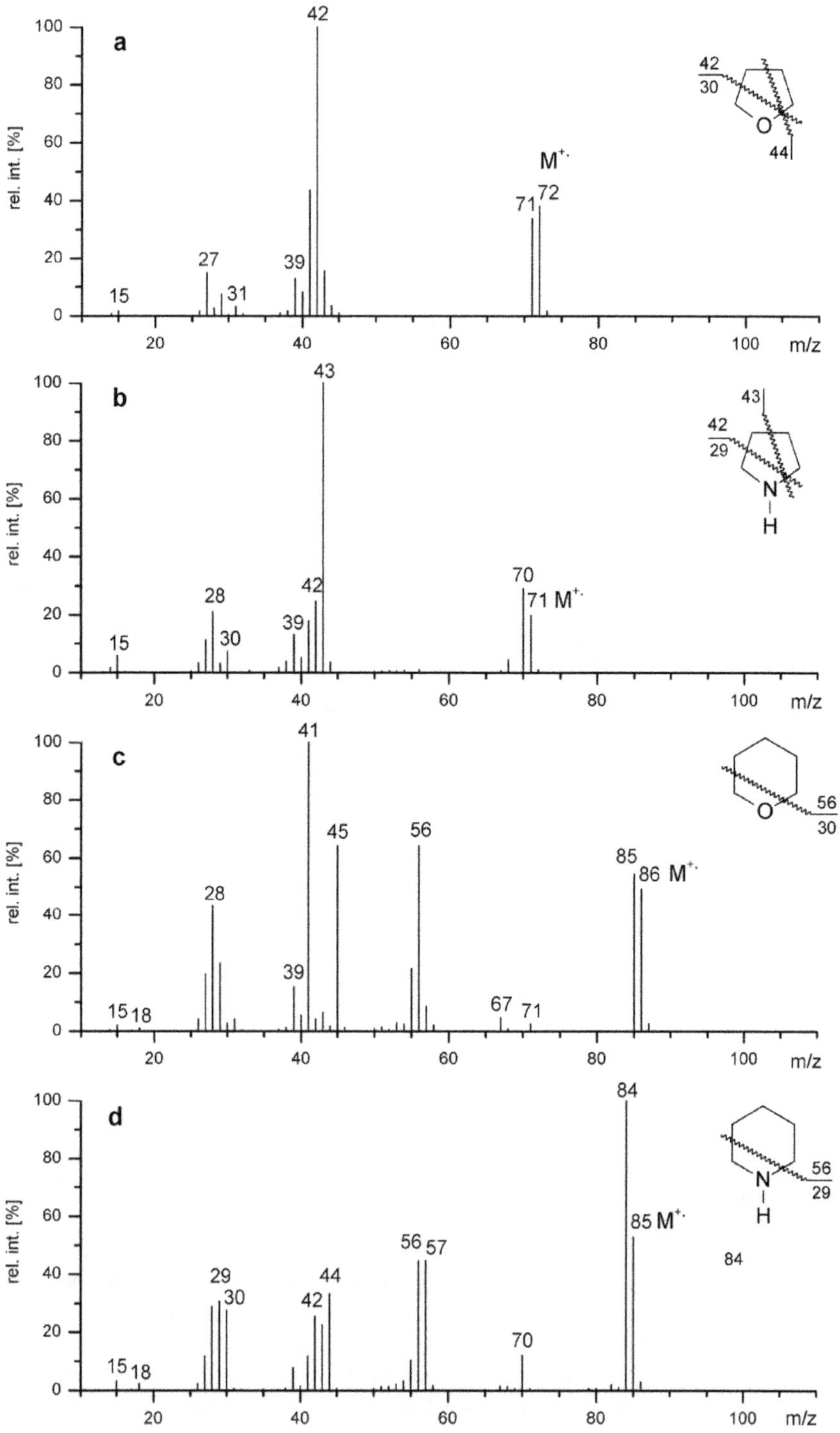

Fig. 6.53 EI mass spectra of tetrahydrofuran (**a**), pyrrolidine (**b**), tetrahydropyran (**c**), and piperidine (**d**) (Spectra used by permission of NIST. © NIST 2002)

6.15.2 Aromatic Heterocyclic Compounds

Pyridine and numerous other aromatic *N*-heterocycles eliminate a molecule of hydrogen cyanide, HCN, 27 u, from their molecular ions. It has been demonstrated that the molecule eliminated from pyridine molecular ions, *m/z* 79, definitely is HCN and not its isomer hydrogen isocyanide, HNC [190, 191]. The fragmentation of pyridine molecular ions to form $[C_4H_4]^{+\bullet}$, *m/z* 52, and HCN was reported to proceed via a tight transition state [192], which is in some disagreement with the small kinetic energy release of 43 meV [193]. The fragmentation threshold of 12.1 eV for this process is well beyond the ionization energy of 9.3 eV [17], thus demonstrating comparatively high energy requirements [192]. HCN loss from aromatic *N*-heterocycles is the equivalent to C_2H_2 loss from aromatic hydrocarbons. As anticipated, the peak at *m/z* 53 in the spectrum of pyridine reveals that (after subtraction of the isotopic contribution of ^{13}C) a minor fraction of the pyridine molecular ions eliminates C_2H_2, 26 u (Fig. 6.54).

Indole fragmentations Indole molecular ions, *m/z* 117, preferably dissociate by loss of HCN (Fig. 6.55) [194]. The $[C_7H_6]^{+\bullet}$ fragment ion, *m/z* 90, then stabilizes by $H^\bullet$ loss to form an even-electron species, $[C_7H_5]^+$, *m/z* 89, which decomposes further by loss of ethyne (Scheme 6.70).

Indole derivatives are widespread natural compounds, and mass spectrometry of indoles [194, 195], especially of indole alkaloids, has been of special interest ever since [196–198].

In case of the pyrrole molecular ion, HCN loss is somewhat less important than with indole, i.e., the $[M–C_2H_2]^{+\bullet}$ ion at *m/z* 41 is more abundant than the $[M–HCN]^{+\bullet}$ ion at *m/z* 40. This may in part be due to the twofold chance of C_2H_2 elimination (Fig. 6.56). The introduction of *N*-substituents has similar effects as observed for the saturated heterocycles mentioned earlier, i.e., rearrangement fragmentations and α-cleavage of the substituent take control [199] (Scheme 6.71).

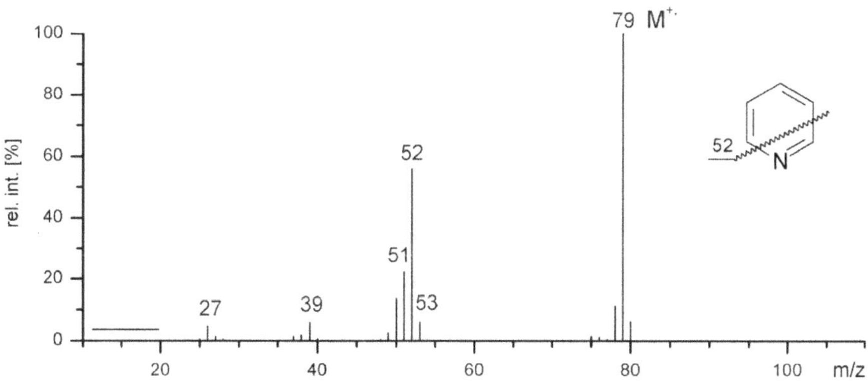

Fig. 6.54 EI mass spectrum of pyridine. Loss of HCN, 27 u, from the molecular ion, *m/z* 79 (OE ion, odd-numbered *m/z*), represents the most important primary fragmentation to yield the product at *m/z* 52 (OE ion, even-numbered *m/z*; cf. nitrogen rule) (Spectrum used by permission of NIST. © NIST 2002)

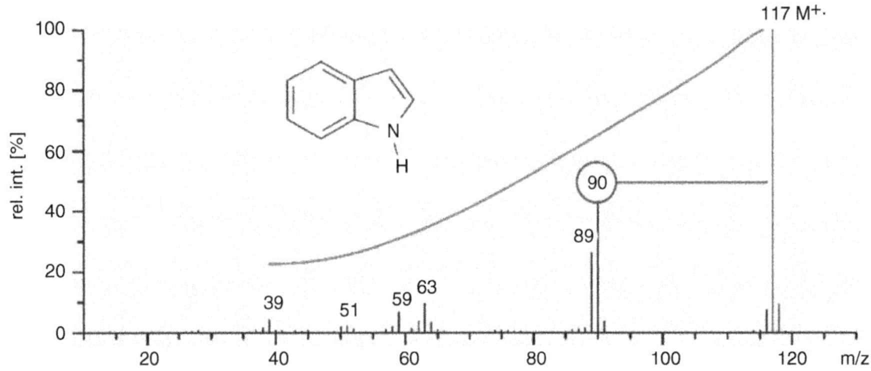

Fig. 6.55 EI mass spectrum of indole. The loss of HCN from $M^{+•}$ ion (OE ion, odd-numbered *m/z*) is marked by a *dark green line* and the resulting fragment at *m/z* 90 (OE ion, even-numbered *m/z*) is marked by a *dark green circle*. Note the diminishing peak intensities towards lower *m/z* (*red line*), which are indicative of aromatic heterocyclic compounds (Used by permission of NIST. © NIST 2002)

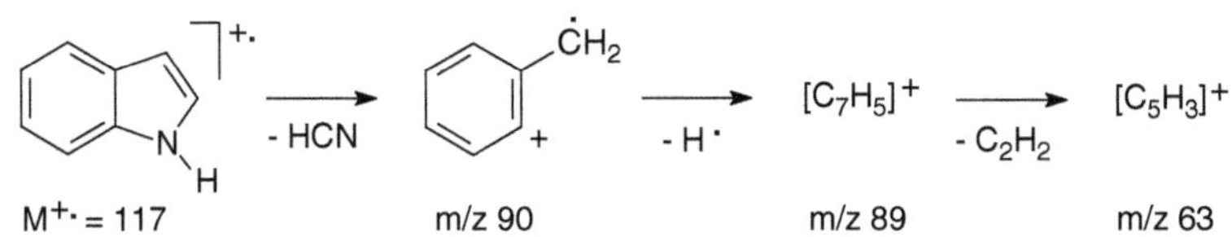

Scheme 6.70

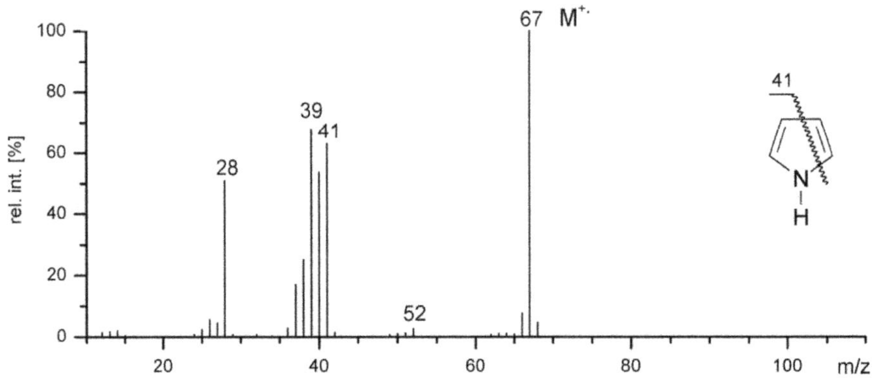

Fig. 6.56 EI mass spectrum of pyrrole. Elimination of C_2H_2 slightly predominates over loss of HCN (Spectrum used by permission of NIST. © NIST 2002)

The mass spectrum of aniline has been known since the early days of mass spectrometry [107]. Initially, the observed $[M–27]^{+•}$ ion was interpreted in terms of HCN loss (Fig. 6.57a). The mechanism for loss of the elements of H, N, and C from aminoarenes is perfectly analogous to CO loss from phenols (Sect. 6.10.1)

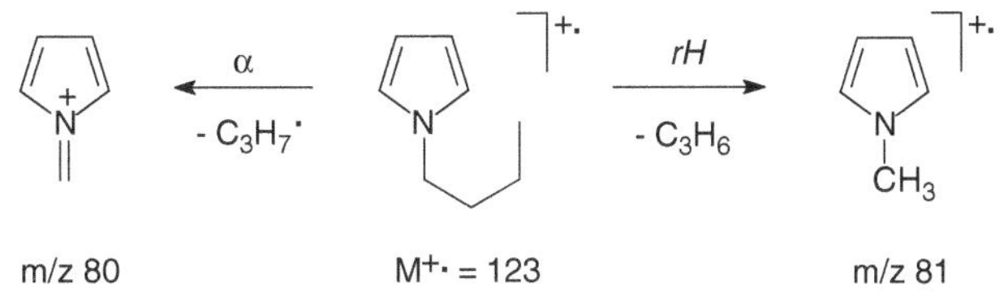

Scheme 6.71

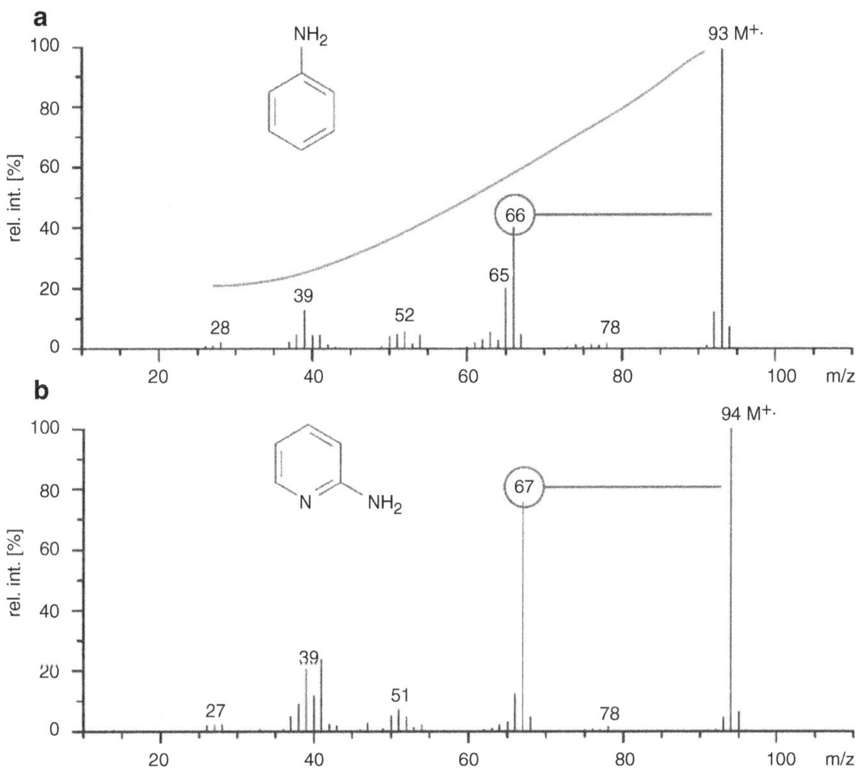

Fig. 6.57 EI mass spectra of aniline (**a**) and 2-aminopyridine (**b**). Different in mechanism from the *N*-heterocycles, but very similar in appearance: the aromatic amine molecular ions eliminate HNC (marked by *dark green lines* and *circles*). Note that the loss of HNC from $M^{+\bullet}$ in (**a**) causes a switch from odd-numbered *m/z* to even-numbered *m/z* while in (**b**) the same difference of 27 u results in a switch from even-numbered *m/z* to odd-numbered *m/z* (cf. nitrogen rule in Sect. 6.2.5). Again, intensive $M^{+\bullet}$ ions and diminishing peak intensities (*red line* in (**a**)) towards lower *m/z* indicate aromatic heterocyclic compounds. (Spectra used by permission of NIST. © NIST 2002)

[200]. More recently, it could be demonstrated that loss of hydrogen isocyanide, HNC, occurs rather than losing the more stable neutral species HCN, a behavior typical of ionized pyridine [191].

Interestingly, the three isomeric aminopyridine molecular ions display ion chemistry similar to aniline molecular ions, i.e., metastable HNC loss [191], instead

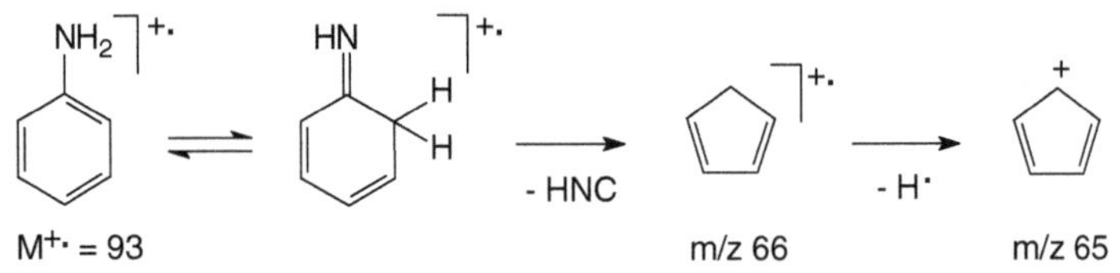

Scheme 6.72

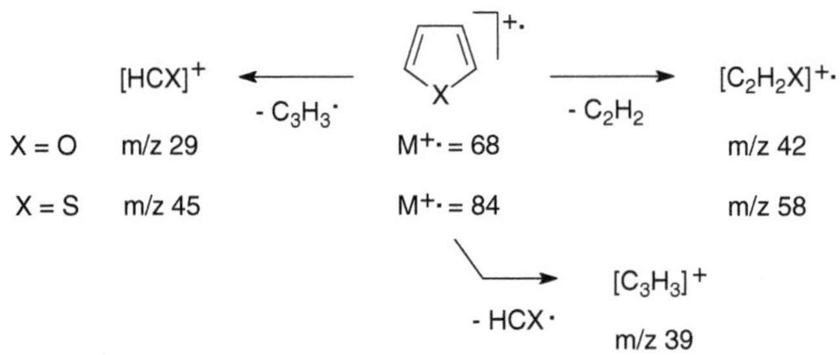

Scheme 6.73

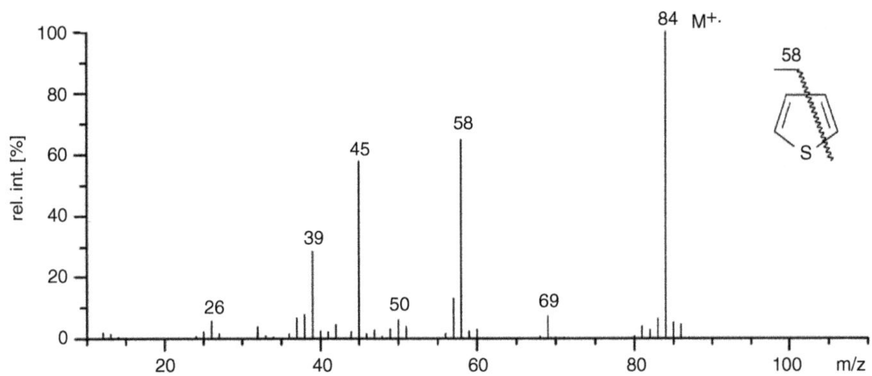

Fig. 6.58 EI mass spectrum of thiophene. The isotopic pattern of sulfur directly reveals its presence in the ions detected at *m/z* 45, 58, (69), and 84 (Spectrum used by permission of NIST. © NIST 2002)

of HCN loss which should also be possible due to the pyridine core of the molecule (Fig. 6.57b) (Scheme 6.72).

The mass spectra of furanes are governed by a strong $[M{-}HCO]^+$ signal and the corresponding, but weaker peak at *m/z* 29 belonging to the formyl ion [201]. Analogous behavior is observed for thiophene, i.e., the spectrum shows a $[M{-}HCS]^+$ peak, *m/z* 39, and the thioformyl ion, $[HCS]^+$, at *m/z* 45 (Scheme 6.73 and Fig. 6.58). Mass spectra of [2-^{13}C]thiophene and of [2-D]thiophene showed that the thioformyl ion is generated after carbon skeleton rearrangement, whereas hydrogen scrambling seemed to be absent [202]. In addition to this marked fragmentation route, the molecular ions of furanes and thiophenes preferably decompose by C_2H_2 loss [203], a behavior resembling that of pyrroles and quinones (Sect. 6.10.2). Mass spectra of substituted furanes and thiophenes are discussed in the literature [201, 204, 205].

6.16 Guide to the Interpretation of Mass Spectra

6.16.1 Summary of Rules

1. Identify the molecular ion! This is an important initial step, because it is needed to derive the molecular composition (Sect. 6.7). If the EI spectrum does not allow for the identification of the molecular ion, soft ionization methods should be employed in addition.
2. The mass differences between the presumed molecular ion and primary fragments must correspond to realistic chemical compositions (Sect. 6.7, Table 6.11).
3. The calculated and experimental isotopic patterns have to agree with the molecular formula postulated (Sect. 3.6).
4. The derived molecular formula must obey the nitrogen rule (Sect. 6.2.5). An odd-numbered m/z value of the molecular ion requires 1, 3, 5, ... nitrogen atoms to be contained, whereas an even m/z value belongs to 0, 2, 4, ... nitrogen atoms.
5. Homolytic cleavages cause odd-numbered mass differences between fragment and molecular ion (Sect. 6.2.5). Rearrangement fragmentations cause even-numbered mass differences. This rule toggles if odd numbers of nitrogen are contained in the neutral loss.
6. In general, fragmentations obey the even-electron rule (Sect. 6.1.3). Odd-electron fragments from rearrangement fragmentations behave as if they were molecular ions of the respective smaller molecule.
7. The competition of homolytic cleavages is governed by Stevenson's rule (Sect. 6.2.2). Thermodynamic stability of the pairs of products formed is decisive in selecting the preferred fragmentation route.
8. Calculate $r + d$ to check formula proposals and to derive some structural characteristics (Sect. 6.4.4).
9. Write down a fragmentation scheme, thereby carefully tracking the origin of primary fragment ions and of characteristic ions used for structure assignment. From the purely analytical point of view this is very useful. However, one should keep in mind that any proposed fragmentation scheme remains a working hypothesis unless experimental confirmation is available.
10. Employ additional techniques, such as measurement of accurate mass (Sect. 3.6), tandem mass spectrometry, or other spectroscopic methods to crosscheck and to refine your assignments.

6.16.2 Systematic Approach to Mass Spectra

1. Collect background information such as origin of the sample, presumed compound class, solubility, thermal stability, or other spectroscopic information.
2. Write *m/z* labels for all relevant peaks and calculate mass differences between prominent peaks. Do you recognize characteristic ion series or mass differences that point to common neutral losses?
3. Check which ionization method was used and examine the general appearance of the mass spectrum. Is the molecular ion peak intense (as with aromatic, heterocyclic, polycyclic compounds) or weak (as with aliphatic and multifunctional compounds, cf. Fig. 6.23)? Are there typical impurities (solvent, grease, plasticizers) or background signals (residual air, column bleed in GC-MS)?
4. Is accurate mass data available for some of the peaks?
5. Now, follow the above rules to proceed.
6. Derive information on the presence/absence of functional groups.
7. Be careful when using collections of common neutral losses and *m/z*-to-structure relationship tables – they're never comprehensive. Even worse, one tends to get stuck on the first assumption.

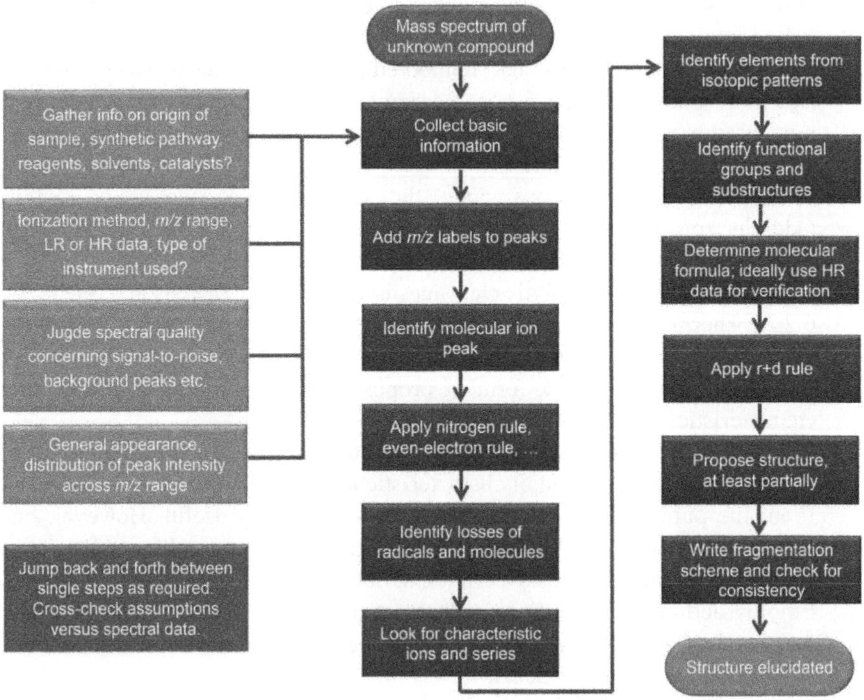

Fig. 6.59 Guide to systematic interpretation of EI mass spectra

8. Put together the known structural features and try to assign the structure to the unknown sample. Sometimes, only partial structures of the analyte can be derived or isomers cannot be distinguished.
9. Crosscheck proposed molecular structure and mass spectral data. This is also recommended between the single steps of mass spectral interpretation.
10. Are there reference spectra available (at least of similar compounds) either from the literature or from mass spectral databases (Sect. 5.9)?
11. Never rigidly follow this scheme! Sometimes, a step back or forth may accelerate the process or help to avoid pitfalls (Fig. 6.59).
12. Good luck!

References

1. Budzikiewicz H, Djerassi C, Williams DH (1967) Mass Spectrometry of Organic Compounds. Holden-Day, San Francisco
2. McLafferty FW, Turecek F (1993) Interpretation of Mass Spectra. University Science Books, Mill Valley
3. Splitter JS, Turecek F (eds) (1994) Applications of Mass Spectrometry to Organic Stereochemistry. Weinheim, Verlag Chemie
4. Price P (1991) Standard Definitions of Terms Relating to Mass Spectrometry. A Report from the Committee on Measurements and Standards of the Amercian Society for Mass Spectrometry. J Am Soc Mass Spectrom 2:336–348. doi:10.1016/1044-0305(91)80025-3
5. Todd JFJ (1995) Recommendations for Nomenclature and Symbolism for Mass Spectroscopy Including an Appendix of Terms Used in Vacuum Technology. Int J Mass Spectrom Ion Proc 142:211–240
6. Svec HJ, Junk GA (1967) Electron-Impact Studies of Substituted Alkanes. J Am Chem Soc 89:790–796. doi:10.1021/ja00980a010
7. Friedman L, Long FA (1953) Mass Spectra of Six Lactones. J Am Chem Soc 75:2832–2836. doi:10.1021/ja01108a013
8. Karni M, Mandelbaum A (1980) The 'Even-Electron Rule'. Org Mass Spectrom 15:53–64. doi:10.1002/oms.1210150202
9. Bowen RD, Harrison AG (1981) Loss of Methyl Radical from Some Small Immonium Ions: Unusual Violation of the Even-Electron Rule. Org Mass Spectrom 16:180–182. doi:10.1002/oms.1210160408
10. Nizigiyimana L, Rajan PK, Haemers A, Claeys M, Derrick PJ (1997) Mechanistic Aspects of High-Energy Collision-Induced Dissociation Proximate to the Charge in Saturated Fatty Acid *n*-Butyl Esters Cationized With Lithium. Evidence for Hydrogen Radical Removal. Rapid Commun Mass Spectrom 11:1808–1812. doi:10.1002/(SICI)1097-0231(19971030)11:16<1808::AID-RCM43>3.0.CO;2-R
11. Veith HJ, Gross JH (1991) Alkane Loss from Collisionally Activated Alkylmethyleneimmonium Ions. Org Mass Spectrom 26:1061–1064. doi:10.1002/oms.1210261206
12. McLafferty FW (1962) Mass Spectrometric Analysis. I. Aliphatic Halogenated Compounds. Anal Chem 34:2–15. doi:10.1021/ac60181a003
13. Stevenson DP (1951) Ionization and Dissociation by Electronic Impact. Ionization Potentials and Energies of Formation of *sec*-Propyl and *tert*-Butyl Radicals. Some Limitations on the Method. Discuss Faraday Soc 10:35–45. doi:10.1039/df9511000035

14. Audier HE (1969) Ionisation et Fragmentation en Spectrometrie de Masse I. Sur la Répartition de la Charge Positive Entre Fragment Provenant des Mêmes Ruptures. Org Mass Spectrom 2:283–298. doi:10.1002/oms.1210020307
15. Harrison AG, Finney CD, Sherk JA (1971) Factors Determining Relative Ionic Abundances in Competing Fragmentation Reactions. Org Mass Spectrom 5:1313–1320. doi:10.1002/oms.1210051109
16. Levsen K (1978) Reaction Mechanisms. In: Fundamental Aspects of Organic Mass Spectrometry. Verlag Chemie, Weinheim
17. http://webbook.nist.gov/
18. Sharkey AG Jr, Shultz JL, Friedel RA (1956) Mass Spectra of Ketones. Anal Chem 28:934–940. doi:10.1021/ac60114a003
19. Gilpin JA, McLafferty FW (1957) Mass Spectrometric Analysis: Aliphatic Aldehydes. Anal Chem 29:990–994. doi:10.1021/ac60127a001
20. Liedtke RJ, Djerassi C (1969) Mass Spectrometry in Structural and Stereochemical Problems. CLXXXIII. A Study of the Electron Impact Induced Fragmentation of Aliphatic Aldehydes. J Am Chem Soc 91:6814–6821. doi:10.1021/ja01052a046
21. Harrison AG (1970) The High-Resolution Mass Spectra of Aliphatic Aldehydes. Org Mass Spectrom 3:549–555. doi:10.1002/oms.1210030504
22. Levsen K, McLafferty FW (1974) Metastable Ion Characteristics. XXVII. Structure and Unimolecular Reactions of $[C_2H_6N]^+$ and $[C_3H_8N]^+$ Ions. J Am Chem Soc 96:139–144. doi:10.1021/ja00808a023
23. Bowen RD (1991) The Chemistry of $[C_nH_{2n+2}N]^+$ Ions. Mass Spectrom Rev 10:225–279. doi:10.1002/mas.1280100304
24. Bowen RD (1991) Ion-Neutral Complexes. Acc Chem Res 24:364–371. doi:10.1021/ar00012a002
25. Djerassi C, Fenselau C (1965) Mass Spectrometry in Structural and Stereochemical Problems. LXXXIV. The Nature of the Cyclic Transition State in Hydrogen Rearrangements of Aliphatic Ethers. J Am Chem Soc 87:5747–5762. doi:10.1021/ja00952a039
26. McLafferty FW (1957) Mass Spectrometric Analysis of Aliphatic Ethers. Anal Chem 29:1782–1789. doi:10.1021/ac60132a036
27. Friedel RA, Shultz JL, Sharkey AG Jr (1956) Mass Spectra of Alcohols. Anal Chem 28:927–934. doi:10.1021/ac60114a002
28. Gohlke RS, McLafferty FW (1962) Mass Spectrometric Analysis of Aliphatic Amines. Anal Chem 34:1281–1287. doi:10.1021/ac60190a025
29. O'Niel MJ Jr, Wier TP Jr (1951) Mass Spectrometry of Heavy Hydrocarbons. Anal Chem 23:830–843. doi:10.1021/ac60054a004
30. Hesse M, Meier H, Zeeh B (2002) Massenspektren. In: Spektroskopische Methoden in der Organischen Chemie, 6te Aufl. Georg Thieme Verlag, Stuttgart
31. Audier HE, Milliet A, Sozzi G, Denhez JP (1984) The Isomerization Mechanisms of Alkylamines: Structure of $[C_2H_6N]^+$ and $[C_3H_8N]^+$ Fragment Ions. Org Mass Spectrom 19:79–81. doi:10.1002/oms.1210190206
32. Phillips GR, Russell ME, Solka BH (1975) Structure of the $[C_2H_5O]^+$ Ion in the Mass Spectrum of Diethyl Ether. Org Mass Spectrom 10:819–823. doi:10.1002/oms.1210101002
33. McAdoo DJ, Hudson CE (1984) Gas Phase Ionic Reactions Are Generally Stepwise Processes. Int J Mass Spectrom Ion Proc 62:269–276. doi:10.1016/0168-1176(84)87113-X
34. Williams DH, Budzikiewicz H, Pelah Z, Djerassi C (1964) Mass Spectroscopy and Its Application to Structural and Stereochemical Problems. XLIV. Fragmentation Behavior of Monocyclic Ketones. Monatsh Chem 95:166–177
35. Seibl J, Gäumann T (1963) Massenspektren Organischer Verbindungen. 2. Mitteilung: Cyclohexanone. Helv Chim Acta 46:2857–2872. doi:10.1002/hlca.19630460743
36. Yates BF, Bouma WJ, Radom L (1984) Detection of the Prototype Phosphonium (CH_2PH_3), Sulfonium (CH_2SH_2), and Chloronium (CH_2ClH) Ylides by Neutralization-Reionization

Mass Spectrometry: A Theoretical Prediction. J Am Chem Soc 106:5805–5808. doi:10.1021/ja00332a008
37. Grützmacher H-F (1992) Unimolecular Reaction Mechanisms: The Role of Reactive Intermediates. Int J Mass Spectrom Ion Proc 118(119):825–855. doi:10.1016/0168-1176(92)85087-G
38. Hammerum S (1988) Distonic Radical Cations in the Gaseous and Condensed Phase. Mass Spectrom Rev 7:123–202. doi:10.1002/mas.1280070202
39. Stirk KM, Kiminkinen MLK, Kenttämaa HI (1992) Ion-Molecule Reactions of Distonic Radical Cations. Chem Rev 92:1649–1665. doi:10.1021/cr00015a008
40. Hammerum S, Derrick PJ (1986) Thermodynamics of Intermediate Ion-Molecule Complexes or Kinetics of Competing Reactions? The Reactions of Low-Energy Isobutylamine and Neopentylamine Molecular Ions. J Chem Soc, Perkin Trans 2:1577–1580. doi:10.1039/P29860001577
41. Yates BF, Radom L (1987) Intramolecular Hydrogen Migration in Ionized Amines: A Theoretical Study of the Gas-Phase Analogues of the Hofmann-Löffler and Related Rearrangements. J Am Chem Soc 109:2910–2915. doi:10.1021/ja00244a009
42. Zeller L, Farrell J Jr, Vainiotalo P, Kenttämaa HI (1992) Long-Lived Radical Cations of Simple Organophosphates Isomerize Spontaneously to Distonic Structures in the Gas Phase. J Am Chem Soc 114:1205–1214. doi:10.1021/ja00030a013
43. Sack TM, Miller DL, Gross ML (1985) The Ring Opening of Gas-Phase Cyclopropane Radical Cations. J Am Chem Soc 107:6795–6800. doi:10.1021/ja00310a008
44. Grubb HM, Meyerson S (1963) Mass spectra of alkylbenzenes. In: McLafferty FW (ed) Mass Spectrometry of Organic Ions. Academic Press, New York
45. McLafferty FW, Bockhoff FM (1979) Collisional Activation and Metastable Ion Characteristics. 67. Formation and Stability of Gaseous Tolyl Ions. Org Mass Spectrom 14:181–184. doi:10.1002/oms.1210140402
46. Cone C, Dewar MJS, Landman D (1977) Gaseous Ions. 1. MINDO/3 Study of the Rearrangement of Benzyl Cation to Tropylium. J Am Chem Soc 99:372–376. doi:10.1021/ja00444a011
47. Traeger JC, McLoughlin RG (1977) Threshold Photoionization and Dissociation of Toluene and Cycloheptatriene. J Am Chem Soc 99:7351–7352. doi:10.1021/ja00464a041
48. Howe I, McLafferty FW (1971) Unimolecular Decomposition of Toluene and Cycloheptatriene Molecular Ions. Variation of the Degree of Scrambling and Isotope Effect With Internal Energy. J Am Chem Soc 93:99–105. doi:10.1021/ja00730a019
49. Kuck D (2002) Half a Century of Scrambling in Organic Ions: Complete, Incomplete, Progressive and Composite Atom Interchange. Int J Mass Spectrom 213:101–144. doi:10.1016/S1387-3806(01)00533-4
50. Mormann M, Kuck D (1999) Protonated 1,3,5-Cycloheptatriene and 7-Alkyl-1,3,5-Cycloheptatrienes in the Gas Phase: Ring Contraction to the Isomeric Alkylbenzenium Ions. J Mass Spectrom 34:384–394. doi:10.1002/(SICI)1096-9888(199904)34:4<384::AID-JMS770>3.0.CO;2-8
51. Rylander PN, Meyerson S, Grubb HM (1957) Organic Ions in the Gas Phase. II. The Tropylium Ion. J Am Chem Soc 79:842–846. doi:10.1021/ja01561a016
52. Cooks RG, Howe I, Tam SW, Williams DH (1968) Studies in Mass Spectrometry. XXIX. Hydrogen Scrambling in Some Bicyclic Aromatic Systems. Randomization Over Two Rings. J Am Chem Soc 90:4064–4069. doi:10.1021/ja01017a025
53. Borchers F, Levsen K (1975) Isomerization of Hydrocarbon Ions. III. $[C_8H_8]^+$, $[C_8H_8]^{2+}$, $[C_6H_6]^+$, and $[C_6H_5]^+$ Ions. Org Mass Spectrom 10:584–594. doi:10.1002/oms.1210100804
54. Budzikiewicz H (1998) Massenspektrometrie – Eine Einführung. Wiley-VCH, Weinheim
55. Nishishita T, McLafferty FW (1977) Metastable Ion Characteristics. XXXXVII. Collisional Activation Mass Spectra of Pentene and Hexene Molecular Ions. Org Mass Spectrom 12:75–77. doi:10.1002/oms.1210120206

56. Borchers F, Levsen K, Schwarz H, Wesdemiotis C, Winkler HU (1977) Isomerization of Linear Octene Cations in the Gas Phase. J Am Chem Soc 99:6359–6365. doi:10.1021/ja00461a031
57. Schneider B, Budzikiewicz H (1990) A Facile Method for the Localization of a Double Bond in Aliphatic Compounds. Rapid Commun Mass Spectrom 4:550–551. doi:10.1002/rcm.1290041217
58. Peake DA, Gross ML (1985) Iron(I) Chemical Ionization and Tandem Mass Spectrometry for Locating Double Bonds. Anal Chem 57:115–120. doi:10.1021/ac00279a031
59. Fordham PJ, Chamot-Rooke J, Guidice E, Tortajada J, Morizur J-P (1999) Analysis of Alkenes by Copper Ion Chemical Ionization Gas Chromatography/Mass Spectrometry and Gas Chromatography/Tandem Mass Spectrometry. J Mass Spectrom 34:1007–1017. doi:10.1002/(SICI)1096-9888(199910)34:10<1007::AID-JMS854>3.0.CO;2-E
60. Levsen K, Weber R, Borchers F, Heimbach H, Beckey HD (1978) Determination of Double Bonds in Alkenes by Field Ionization Mass Spectrometry. Anal Chem 50:1655–1658. doi:10.1021/ac50034a022
61. Buser H-R, Arn H, Guerin P, Rauscher S (1983) Determination of Double Bond Position in Mono-Unsaturated Acetates by Mass Spectrometry of Dimethyl Disulfide Adducts. Anal Chem 55:818–822. doi:10.1021/ac00257a003
62. Scribe P, Guezennec J, Dagaut J, Pepe C, Saliot A (1988) Identification of the Position and the Stereochemistry of the Double Bond in Monounsaturated Fatty Acid Methyl Esters by Gas Chromatography/Mass Spectrometry of Dimethyl Disulfide Derivatives. Anal Chem 60:928–931. doi:10.1021/ac00160a019
63. Pepe C, Dif K (2001) The Use of Ethanethiol to Locate the Triple Bond in Alkynes and the Double Bond in Substituted Alkenes by Gas Chromatography/Mass Spectrometry. Rapid Commun Mass Spectrom 15:97–103. doi:10.1002/1097-0231(20010130)15:2<97::AID-RCM196>3.0.CO;2-3
64. Pepe C, Sayer H, Dagaut J, Couffignal R (1997) Determination of Double Bond Positions in Triunsaturated Compounds by Means of Gas Chromatography/Mass Spectrometry of Dimethyl Disulfide Derivatives. Rapid Commun Mass Spectrom 11:919–921. doi:10.1002/(SICI)1097-0231(199705)11:8<919::AID-RCM924>3.0.CO;2-C
65. Levsen K, Heimbach H, Shaw GJ, Milne GWA (1977) Isomerization of Hydrocarbon Ions. VIII. The Electron Impact Induced Decomposition of *N*-Dodecane. Org Mass Spectrom 12:663–670. doi:10.1002/oms.1210121103
66. Lavanchy A, Houriet R, Gäumann T (1979) The Mass Spectrometric Fragmentation of *n*-Alkanes. Org Mass Spectrom 14:79–85. doi:10.1002/oms.1210140205
67. Levsen K (1975) Isomerization of Hydrocarbon Ions. I. Isomeric Octanes. Collisional Activation Study. Org Mass Spectrom 10:43–54. doi:10.1002/oms.1210100108
68. Traeger JC, McAdoo DJ, Hudson CE, Giam CS (1998) Why Are Alkane Eliminations from Ionized Alkanes so Abundant? J Am Soc Mass Spectrom 9:21–28. doi:10.1016/S1044-0305(97)00225-0
69. Olivella S, Solé A, McAdoo DJ, Griffin LL (1994) Unimolecular Reactions of Ionized Alkanes: Theoretical Study of the Potential Energy Surface for $CH_3^{\bullet}$ and CH_4 Losses from Ionized Butane and Isobutane. J Am Chem Soc 116:11078–11088. doi:10.1021/ja00103a025
70. McAdoo DJ, Bowen RD (1999) Alkane Eliminations from Ions in the Gas Phase. Eur Mass Spectrom 5:389–409. doi:10.1255/ejms.303
71. Williams DH (1977) A Transition State Probe. Acc Chem Res 10:280–286. doi:10.1021/ar50116a002
72. Ludányi K, Dallos A, Kühn Z, Vékey D (1999) Mass Spectrometry of Very Large Saturated Hydrocarbons. J Mass Spectrom 34:264–267. doi:10.1002/(SICI)1096-9888(199904)34:4<264::AID-JMS749>3.0.CO;2-Q
73. Biemann K (1962) Application of Mass Spectrometry in Organic Chemistry, Especially for Structure Determination of Natural Products. Angew Chem Int Ed 1:98–111. doi:10.1002/anie.196200981

74. Happ GP, Stewart DW (1952) Rearrangement Peaks in the Mass Spectra of Certain Aliphatic Acids. J Am Chem Soc 74:4404–4408. doi:10.1021/ja01137a050
75. McLafferty FW (1956) Mass Spectrometric Analysis. Broad Applicability to Chemical Research. Anal Chem 28:306–316. doi:10.1021/ac60111a005
76. McLafferty FW (1965) Mass Spectrometric Analysis: Molecular Rearrangements. Anal Chem 31:82–87. doi:10.1021/ac60145a015
77. Kingston DGI, Bursey JT, Bursey MM (1974) Intramolecular Hydrogen Transfer in Mass Spectra. II. McLafferty Rearrangement and Related Reactions. Chem Rev 74:215–245. doi:10.1021/cr60288a004
78. Zollinger M, Seibl J (1985) McLafferty Reactions in Even-Electron Ions? Org Mass Spectrom 20:649–661. doi:10.1002/oms.1210201102
79. Djerassi C, Tökés L (1966) Mass Spectrometry in Structural and Stereochemical Problems. XCIII. Further Observations on the Importance of Interatomic Distance in the McLafferty Rearrangement. Synthesis and Fragmentation Behavior of Deuterium-Labeled 12-Oxo Steroids. J Am Chem Soc 88:536–544. doi:10.1021/ja00955a027
80. Djerassi C, von Mutzenbecher G, Fajkos J, Williams DH, Budzikiewicz H (1965) Mass Spectrometry in Structural and Stereochemical Problems. LXV. Synthesis and Fragmentation Behavior of 15-Oxo Steroids. The Importance of Inter-Atomic Distance in the McLafferty Rearrangement. J Am Chem Soc 87:817–826. doi:10.1021/ja01082a022
81. Henion JD, Kingston DGI (1974) Mass Spectrometry of Organic Compounds. IX. McLafferty Rearrangements in Some Bicyclic Ketones. J Am Chem Soc 96:2532–2536. doi:10.1021/ja00815a035
82. Stringer MB, Underwood DJ, Bowie JH, Allison CE, Donchi KF, Derrick PJ (1992) Is the McLafferty Rearrangement of Ketones Concerted or Stepwise? The Application of Kinetic Isotope Effects. Org Mass Spectrom 27:270–276. doi:10.1002/oms.1210270319
83. Dewar MJS (1984) Multibond Reactions Cannot Normally Be Synchronous. J Am Chem Soc 106:209–219. doi:10.1021/ja00313a042
84. Holmes JL, Lossing FP (1980) Gas-Phase Heats of Formation of Keto and Enol Ions of Carbonyl Compounds. J Am Chem Soc 102:1591–1595. doi:10.1021/ja00525a021
85. Hrušák J (1991) MNDO Calculations on the Neutral and Cationic [CH_3-CO-R] Systems in Relation to Mass Spectrometric Fragmentations. Z Phys Chem 172:217–226
86. Beynon JH, Saunders RA, Williams AE (1961) The High Resolution Mass Spectra of Aliphatic Esters. Anal Chem 33:221–225. doi:10.1021/ac60170a017
87. Harrison AG, Jones EG (1965) Rearrangement Reactions Following Electron Impact on Ethyl and Isopropyl Esters. Can J Chem 43:960–968. doi:10.1139/v65-124
88. Wesdemiotis C, Feng R, McLafferty FW (1985) Distonic Radical Ions. Stepwise Elimination of Acetaldehyde from Ionized Benzyl Ethyl Ether. J Am Chem Soc 107:715–716. doi:10.1021/ja00289a040
89. Benoit FM, Harrison AG (1976) Hydrogen Migrations in Mass Spectrometry. II. Single and Double Hydrogen Migrations in the Electron Impact Fragmentation of Propyl Benzoate. Org Mass Spectrom 11:1056–1062. doi:10.1002/oms.1210111006
90. Müller J, Krebs G, Lüdemann F, Baumgartner E (1981) Wasserstoff-Umlagerungen beim Elektronenstoß-Induzierten Zerfall von H^6-Benzoesäure-*n*-Propylester-Tricarbonylchrom. J Organomet Chem 218:61–68. doi:10.1016/S0022-328X(00)80987-0
91. Benoit FM, Harrison AG, Lossing FP (1977) Hydrogen Migrations in Mass Spectrometry. III. Energetics of Formation of $[R'CO_2H_2]^+$ in the Mass Spectra of $R'CO_2R$. Org Mass Spectrom 12:78–82. doi:10.1002/oms.1210120207
92. Tajima S, Azami T, Shizuka H, Tsuchiya T (1979) An Investigation of the Mechanism of Single and Double Hydrogen Atom Transfer Reactions in Alkyl Benzoates by the Ortho Effect. Org Mass Spectrom 14:499–502. doi:10.1002/oms.1210140908
93. Elder JF Jr, Beynon JH, Cooks RG (1976) The Benzoyl Ion. Thermochemistry and Kinetic Energy Release. Org Mass Spectrom 11:415–422. doi:10.1002/oms.1210110414

94. McLafferty FW, Gohlke RS (1959) Mass Spectrometric Analysis-Aromatic Acids and Esters. Anal Chem 31:2076–2082. doi:10.1021/ac60156a062
95. Djerassi C, Fenselau C (1965) Mass Spectrometry in Structural and Stereochemical Problems. LXXXVI. The Hydrogen-Transfer Reactions in Butyl Propionate, Benzoate, and Phthalate. J Am Chem Soc 87:5756–5762. doi:10.1021/ja00952a041
96. Yinon J (1988) Mass Spectral Fragmentation Pathways in Phthalate Esters. A Tandem Mass Spectrometric Collision-Induced Dissociation Study. Org Mass Spectrom 23:755–759. doi:10.1002/oms.1210231104
97. Turecek F, Hanus V (1984) Retro-Diels-Alder Reaction in Mass Spectrometry. Mass Spectrom Rev 3:85–152. doi:10.1002/mas.1280030104
98. Turecek F, Hanuš V (1980) Charge Distribution Between Formally Identical Fragments: the Retro-Diels-Alder Cleavage. Org Mass Spectrom 15:4–7. doi:10.1002/oms.1210150104
99. Kühne H, Hesse M (1982) The Mass Spectral Retro-Diels-Alder Reaction of 1,2,3,4-Tetrahydronaphthalene, Its Derivatives and Related Heterocyclic Compounds. Mass Spectrom Rev 1:15–28. doi:10.1002/mas.1280010104
100. Budzikiewicz H, Brauman JI, Djerassi C (1965) Mass Spectrometry and Its Application to Structural and Stereochemical Problems. LXVII. Retro-Diels-Alder Fragmentation of Organic Molecules Under Electron Impact. Tetrahedron 21:1855–1879. doi:10.1016/S0040-4020(01)98656-9
101. Dixon JS, Midgley I, Djerassi C (1977) Mass Spectrometry in Structural and Stereochemical Problems. 248. Stereochemical Effects in Electron Impact Induced Retro-Diels-Alder Fragmentations. J Am Chem Soc 99:3432–3441. doi:10.1021/ja00452a041
102. Djerassi C (1992) Steroids Made It Possible: Organic Mass Spectrometry. Org Mass Spectrom 27:1341–1347. doi:10.1002/oms.1210271203
103. Barnes CS, Occolowitz JL (1964) Mass Spectra of Some Naturally Occurring Oxygen Heterocycles and Related Compounds. Aust J Chem 17:975–986. doi:10.1071/CH9640975
104. Ardanaz CE, Guidugli FH, Catalán CAN, Joseph-Nathan P (1999) Mass Spectral Studies of Methoxynaphthoflavones. Rapid Commun Mass Spectrom 13:2071–2079. doi:10.1002/(SICI)1097-0231(19991115)13:21<2071::AID-RCM746>3.0.CO;2-K
105. Aczel T, Lumpkin HE (1960) Correlation of Mass Spectra with Structure in Aromatic Oxygenated Compounds. Aromatic Alcohols and Phenols. Anal Chem 32:1819–1822. doi:10.1021/ac50153a035
106. Beynon JH (1960) Correlation of molecular structure and mass spectra. In: Beynon JH (ed) Mass Spectrometry and Its Applications to Organic Chemistry. Elsevier, Amsterdam
107. Momigny J (1953) The Mass Spectra of Monosubstituted Benzene Derivatives. Phenol, Monodeuteriophenol, Thiophenol, and Aniline. Bull Soc Royal Sci Liège 22:541–560
108. Occolowitz JL (1964) Mass Spectrometry of Naturally Occurring Alkenyl Phenols and Their Derivatives. Anal Chem 36:2177–2181. doi:10.1021/ac60217a043
109. Stensen WG, Jensen E (1995) Structural Determination of 1,4-Naphthoquinones by Mass Spectrometry/Mass Spectrometry. J Mass Spectrom 30:1126–1132. doi:10.1002/jms.1190300809
110. Beynon JH, Lester GR, Williams AE (1959) Specific Molecular Rearrangements in the Mass Spectra of Organic Compounds. J Phys Chem 63:1861–1869. doi:10.1021/j150581a018
111. Pelah Z, Wilson JM, Ohashi M, Budzikiewicz H, Djerassi C (1963) Mass Spectrometry in Structural and Stereochemical Problems. XXXIV. Aromatic Methyl and Ethyl Ethers. Tetrahedron 19:2233–2240. doi:10.1016/0040-4020(63)85038-3
112. Molenaar-Langeveld TA, Ingemann S, Nibbering NMM (1993) Skeletal Rearrangements Preceding Carbon Monoxide Loss from Metastable Phenoxymethylene Ions Derived from Phenoxyacetic Acid and Anisole. Org Mass Spectrom 28:1167–1178. doi:10.1002/oms.1210281031
113. Zagorevskii DV, Régimbal J-M, Holmes JL (1997) The Heat of Formation of the $[C_6,H_5,O]^+$ Isomeric Ions. Int J Mass Spectrom Ion Proc 160:211–222. doi:10.1016/S0168-1176(96)04497-7

114. Cooks RG, Bertrand M, Beynon JH, Rennekamp ME, Setser DW (1973) Energy Partitioning Data as an Ion Structure Probe. Substituted Anisoles. J Am Chem Soc 95:1732–1739. doi:10.1021/ja00787a006
115. Alexander JJ (1975) Mechanism of Photochemical Decarbonylation of Acetyldicarbonyl-H^5-Cyclopentadienyliron. J Am Chem Soc 97:1729–1732. doi:10.1021/ja00840a018
116. Coville NJ, Johnston P (1989) A Mass-Spectral Investigation of Site-Selective Carbon Monoxide Loss from Isotopically Labeled $[MnRe(CO)_{10}]^+$. J Organomet Chem 363:343–350. doi:10.1016/0022-328X(89)87121-9
117. Tobita S, Ogino K, Ino S, Tajima S (1988) On the Mechanism of Carbon Monoxide Loss from the Metastable Molecular Ion of Dimethyl Malonate. Int J Mass Spectrom Ion Proc 85:31–42. doi:10.1016/0168-1176(88)83003-9
118. Moldovan Z, Palibroda N, Mercea V, Mihailescu G, Chiriac M, Vlasa M (1981) Mass Spectra of Some β-Keto Esters. A High Resolution Study. Org Mass Spectrom 16:195–198. doi:10.1002/oms.1210160503
119. Vairamani M, Mirza UA (1987) Mass Spectra of Phenoxyacetyl Derivatives. Mechanism of Loss of CO from Phenyl Phenoxyacetates. Org Mass Spectrom 22:406–409. doi:10.1002/oms.1210220705
120. Tou JC (1974) Competitive and Consecutive Eliminations of Molecular Nitrogen and Carbon Monoxide (or Ethene) from Heterocyclics Under Electron Impact. J Heterocycl Chem 11:707–711. doi:10.1002/jhet.5570110508
121. Meyerson S, Leitch LC (1964) Organic Ions in the Gas Phase. XIV. Loss of Water from Primary Alcohols Under Electron Impact. J Am Chem Soc 86:2555–2558. doi:10.1021/ja01067a005
122. Bukovits GJ, Budzikiewicz H (1983) Mass Spectroscopic Fragmentation Reactions. XXVIII. The Loss of Water from *n*-Alkan-1-ols. Org Mass Spectrom 18:219–220. doi:10.1002/oms.1210180509
123. Bowen RD (1993) The Role of Ion-Neutral Complexes in the Reactions of Onium Ions and Related Species. Org Mass Spectrom 28:1577–1595. doi:10.1002/oms.1210281234
124. Bowen RD (1980) Potential Energy Profiles for Unimolecular Reactions of Isolated Organic Ions: Some Isomers of $[C_4H_{10}N]^+$ and $[C_5H_{12}N]^+$. J Chem Soc, Perkin Trans 2:1219–1227. doi:10.1039/P29800001219
125. Bowen RD, Derrick PJ (1993) Unimolecular Reactions of Isolated Organic Ions: The Chemistry of the Oxonium Ions $[CH_3CH_2CH_2CH_2O{=}CH_2]^+$ and $[CH_3CH_2CH_2CH{=}OCH_3]^+$. Org Mass Spectrom 28:1197–1209. doi:10.1002/oms.1210281035
126. Solling TI, Hammerum S (2001) The Retro-Ene Reaction of Gaseous Immonium Ions Revisited. J Chem Soc Perkin Trans 2:2324–2428. doi:10.1039/B105386H
127. Veith HJ, Gross JH (1991) Alkene Loss from Metastable Methyleneimmonium Ions: Unusual Inverse Secondary Isotope Effect in Ion-Neutral Complex Intermediate Fragmentations. Org Mass Spectrom 26:1097–1105. doi:10.1002/oms.1210261214
128. Budzikiewicz H, Bold P (1991) A McLafferty Rearrangement in an Even-Electron System: C_3H_6 Elimination from the α-Cleavage Product of Tributylamine. Org Mass Spectrom 26:709–712. doi:10.1002/oms.1210260808
129. Bowen RD, Colburn AW, Derrick PJ (1993) Unimolecular Reactions of Isolated Organic Ions: Reactions of the Immonium Ions $[CH_2{=}N(CH_3)CH(CH_3)_2]^+$, $[CH_2{=}N(CH_3)CH_2CH_2CH_3]^+$ and $[CH_2{=}N(CH_2CH_2CH_3)_2]^+$. J Chem Soc Perkin Trans 2:2363–2372. doi:10.1039/P29930002363
130. Gross JH, Veith HJ (1994) Propene Loss from Phenylpropylmethyleneiminium Ions. Org Mass Spectrom 29:153–154. doi:10.1002/oms.1210290307
131. Gross JH, Veith HJ (1993) Unimolecular Fragmentations of Long-Chain Aliphatic Iminium Ions. Org Mass Spectrom 28:867–872. doi:10.1002/oms.1210280808
132. Uccella NA, Howe I, Williams DH (1971) Structure and Isomerization of Gaseous $[C_3H_8N]^+$ Metastable Ions. J Chem Soc B:1933–1939. doi:10.1039/J29710001933

133. Levsen K, Schwarz H (1975) Influence of Charge Localization on the Isomerization of Organic Ions. Tetrahedron 31:2431–2433. doi:10.1016/0040-4020(75)80249-3
134. Bowen RD (1982) Unimolecular Reactions of Isolated Organic Ions: Olefin Elimination from Immonium Ions $[R^1R^2N{=}CH_2]^+$. J Chem Soc Perkin Trans 2:409–413. doi:10.1039/P29820000409
135. Bowen RD (1989) Reactions of Isolated Organic Ions. Alkene Loss from the Immonium Ions $[CH_3CH{=}NHC_2H_5]^+$ and $[CH_3CH{=}NHC_3H_7]^+$. J Chem Soc Perkin Trans 2:913–918. doi:10.1039/P29890000913
136. Bowen RD, Colburn AW, Derrick PJ (1990) Unimolecular Reactions of the Isolated Immonium Ions $[CH_3CH{=}NHC_4H_9]^+$, $[CH_3CH_2CH{=}NHC_4H_9]^+$ and $[(CH_3)_2C{=}NHC_4H_9]^+$. Org Mass Spectrom 25:509–516. doi:10.1002/oms.1210251005
137. Bowen RD, Maccoll A (1990) Unimolecular Reactions of Ionized Ethers. J Chem Soc Perkin Trans 2:147–155. doi:10.1039/P29900000147
138. Traeger JC, Hudson CE, McAdoo DJ (1990) Energy Dependence of Ion-Induced Dipole Complex-Mediated Alkane Eliminations from Ionized Ethers. J Phys Chem 94:5714–5717. doi:10.1021/j100378a021
139. Bowen RD, Williams DH (1979) Non-Concerted Unimolecular Reactions of Ions in the Gas-Phase: The Importance of Ion-Dipole Interactions in Carbonium Ion Isomerizations. Int J Mass Spectrom Ion Phys 29:47–55. doi:10.1016/0020-7381(79)80017-0
140. Bowen RD, Williams DH (1980) Unimolecular Reactions of Isolated Organic Ions. The Importance of Ion-Dipole Interactions. J Am Chem Soc 102:2752–2756. doi:10.1021/ja00528a038
141. Bowen RD, Derrick PJ (1992) The Mechanism of Ethylene Elimination from the Oxonium Ions $[CH_3CH_2CH{=}OCH_2CH_3]^+$ and $[(CH_3)_2C{=}OCH_2CH_3]^+$. J Chem Soc Perkin Trans 2:1033–1039. doi:10.1039/P29920001033
142. Nguyen MT, Vanquickenborne LG, Bouchoux G (1993) On the Energy Barrier for 1,2-Elimination of Methane from Dimethyloxonium Cation. Int J Mass Spectrom Ion Proc 124:R11–R14. doi:10.1016/0168-1176(93)80099-Z
143. Lias SG, Liebman JF, Levin RD (1984) Evaluated Gas Phase Basicities and Proton Affinities of Molecules; Heats of Formation of Protonated Molecules. J Phys Chem Ref Data 13:695–808. doi:10.1063/1.555719
144. Lias SG, Bartmess JE, Liebman JF, Holmes JL, Levin RD, Mallard WG (1988) Gas-Phase Ion and Neutral Thermochemistry. J Phys Chem Ref Data 17(Supplement 1):861 pp.
145. Hunter EPL, Lias SG (1998) Evaluated Gas Phase Basicities and Proton Affinities of Molecules: An Update. J Phys Chem Ref Data 27:413–656. doi:10.1063/1.556018
146. Bowen RD, Colburn AW, Derrick PJ (1992) Unimolecular Reactions of Isolated Organic Ions: The Chemistry of the Unsaturated Oxonium Ion $[CH_2{=}CHCH{=}OCH_3]^+$. Org Mass Spectrom 27:625–632. doi:10.1002/oms.1210270517
147. Bowen RD, Stapleton BJ, Williams DH (1978) Nonconcerted Unimolecular Reactions of Ions in the Gas Phase: Isomerization of Weakly Coordinated Carbonium Ions. J Chem Soc Chem Commun:24–26. doi:10.1039/C39780000024
148. Morton TH (1982) Gas Phase Analogues of Solvolysis Reactions. Tetrahedron 38:3195–3243. doi:10.1016/0040-4020(82)80101-4
149. Morton TH (1992) The Reorientation Criterion and Positive Ion-Neutral Complexes. Org Mass Spectrom 27:353–368. doi:10.1002/oms.1210270404
150. Longevialle P (1992) Ion-Neutral Complexes in the Unimolecular Reactivity of Organic Cations in the Gas Phase. Mass Spectrom Rev 11:157–192. doi:10.1002/mas.1280110302
151. McAdoo DJ (1988) Ion-Neutral Complexes in Unimolecular Decompositions. Mass Spectrom Rev 7:363–393. doi:10.1002/mas.1280070402
152. Rylander PN, Meyerson S (1956) Organic Ions in the Gas Phase. I. The Cationated Cyclopropane Ring. J Am Chem Soc 78:5799–5802. doi:10.1021/ja01603a021

153. Meyerson S (1989) Cationated Cyclopropanes as Reaction Intermediates in Mass Spectra: an Earlier Incarnation of Ion-Neutral Complexes. Org Mass Spectrom 24:267–270. doi:10.1002/oms.1210240412
154. Longevialle P, Botter R (1983) Electron Impact Mass Spectra of Bifunctional Steroids. The Interaction Between Ionic and Neutral Fragments Derived from the Same Parent Ion. Org Mass Spectrom 18:1–8. doi:10.1002/oms.1210180102
155. Longevialle P, Botter R (1983) The Interaction Between Ionic and Neutral Fragments from the Same Parent Ion in the Mass Spectrometer. Int J Mass Spectrom Ion Phys 47:179–182. doi:10.1016/0020-7381(83)87165-4
156. Redman EW, Morton TH (1986) Product-Determining Steps in Gas-Phase Broensted Acid-Base Reactions. Deprotonation of 1-Methylcyclopentyl Cation by Amine Bases. J Am Chem Soc 108:5701–5708. doi:10.1021/ja00279a007
157. Filges U, Grützmacher H-F (1986) Fragmentations of Protonated Benzaldehydes via Intermediate Ion/Molecule Complexes. Org Mass Spectrom 21:673–680. doi:10.1002/oms.1210211012
158. Hudson CE, McAdoo DJ (1984) Alkane Eliminations from Radical Cations Through Ion-Radical Complexes. Int J Mass Spectrom Ion Proc 59:325–332. doi:10.1016/0168-1176(84)85106-X
159. McAdoo DJ, Hudson CE (1987) Ion-Neutral Complex-Mediated Hydrogen Exchange in Ionized Butanol: A Mechanism for Nonspecific Hydrogen Migration. Org Mass Spectrom 22:615–621. doi:10.1002/oms.1210220908
160. Hammerum S, Audier HE (1988) Experimental Verification of the Intermediacy and Interconversion of Ion-Neutral Complexes as Radical Cations Dissociate. J Chem Soc Chem Commun:860–861. doi:10.1039/C39880000860
161. Traeger JC, Hudson CE, McAdoo DJ (1991) Isomeric Ion-Neutral Complexes Generated from Ionized 2-Methylpropanol and *n*-Butanol: The Effect of the Polarity of the Neutral Partner on Complex-Mediated Reactions. J Am Soc Mass Spectrom 3:409–416. doi:10.1016/1044-0305(92)87068-A
162. Sozzi G, Audier HE, Mourgues P, Milliet A (1987) Alkyl Phenyl Ether Radical Cations in the Gas Phase: A Reaction Model. Org Mass Spectrom 22:746–747. doi:10.1002/oms.1210221111
163. Blanchette MC, Holmes JL, Lossing FP (1989) The Fragmentation of Ionized Alkyl Phenyl Ethers. Org Mass Spectrom 24:673–678. doi:10.1002/oms.1210240826
164. Harnish D, Holmes JL (1991) Ion-Radical Complexes in the Gas Phase: Structure and Mechanism in the Fragmentation of Ionized Alkyl Phenyl Ethers. J Am Chem Soc 113:9729–9734. doi:10.1021/ja00026a003
165. Zappey HW, Ingemann S, Nibbering NMM (1991) Isomerization and Fragmentation of Aliphatic Thioether Radical Cations in the Gas Phase: Ion-Neutral Complexes in the Reactions of Metastable Ethyl Propyl Thioether Ions. J Chem Soc Perkin Trans 2:1887–1892. doi:10.1039/P29910001887
166. Broer WJ, Weringa WD (1980) Potential Energy Profiles for the Unimolecular Reactions of $[C_3H_7S]^+$ Ions. Org Mass Spectrom 15:229–234. doi:10.1002/oms.1210150504
167. Schwarz H (1978) Some Newer Aspects of Mass Spectrometric Ortho Effects. Top Curr Chem 73:231–263. doi:10.1007/BFb0050140
168. Meyerson S, Drews H, Field EK (1964) Mass Spectra of Ortho-Substituted Diarylmethanes. J Am Chem Soc 86:4964–4967. doi:10.1021/ja01076a044
169. Grützmacher H-F (1981) Mechanisms of Mass Spectrometric Fragmentation Reactions. XXXII. The Loss of *Ortho* Halo Substituents from Substituted Thiobenzamide Ions. Org Mass Spectrom 16:448–450. doi:10.1002/oms.1210161006
170. Ramana DV, Sundaram N, George N (1987) Ortho Effects in Organic Molecules on Electron Impact. 14. Concerted and Stepwise Ejections of SO_2 and N_2 from *N*-Arylidene-2-Nitrobenzenesulfenamides. Org Mass Spectrom 22:140–144. doi:10.1002/oms.1210220305

171. Sekiguchi O, Noguchi T, Ogino K, Tajima S (1994) Fragmentation of Metastable Molecular Ions of Acetylanisoles. Int J Mass Spectrom Ion Proc 132:172–179. doi:10.1016/0168-1176(93)03937-H
172. Barkow A, Pilotek S, Grützmacher H-F (1995) *Ortho* Effects: A Mechanistic Study. Eur Mass Spectrom 1:525–537. doi:10.1255/ejms.88
173. Danikiewicz W (1998) Electron Ionization-Induced Fragmentation of *N*-Alkyl-*o*-Nitroanilines: Observation of New Types of *Ortho* Effects. Eur Mass Spectrom 4:167–179. doi:10.1255/ejms.206
174. Spiteller G (1961) The *Ortho* Effect in the Mass Spectra of Aromatic Compounds. Monatsh Chem 92:1147–1154
175. Martens J, Praefcke K, Schwarz H (1975) Spectroscopic Investigations. IX. Analytical Importance of the *Ortho* Effect in Mass Spectrometry. Benzoic and Thiobenzoic Acid Derivatives. Z Naturforsch B 30:259–262. doi:10.1515/znb-1975-3-426
176. Smith JG, Wilson GL, Miller JM (1975) Mass Spectra of Isopropyl Benzene Derivatives. A Study of the *Ortho* Effect. Org Mass Spectrom 10:5–17. doi:10.1002/oms.1210100103
177. Schwarz H, Köppel C, Bohlmann F (1974) Electron Impact-Induced Fragmentation of Acetylene Compounds. XII. Rearrangement of Bis(Trimethylsilyl) Ethers of Unsaturated α,ω-Diols and Mass Spectrometric Identification of Isomeric Phenols. Tetrahedron 30:689–693. doi:10.1016/S0040-4020(01)97065-6
178. Krauss D, Mainx HG, Tauscher B, Bischof P (1985) Fragmentation of Trimethylsilyl Derivatives of 2-Alkoxyphenols: a Further Violation of the 'Even-Electron Rule'. Org Mass Spectrom 20:614–618. doi:10.1002/oms.1210201005
179. Svendsen JS, Sydnes LK, Whist JE (1987) Mass Spectrometric Study of Dimethyl Esters of Trimethylsilyl Ether Derivatives of Some 3-Hydroxy Dicarboxylic Acids. Org Mass Spectrom 22:421–429. doi:10.1002/oms.1210220708
180. Svendsen JS, Whist JE, Sydnes LK (1987) A Mass Spectrometric Study of the Dimethyl Ester Trimethylsilyl Enol Ether Derivatives of Some 3-Oxodicarboxylic Acids. Org Mass Spectrom 22:486–492. doi:10.1002/oms.1210220803
181. Halket HM, Zaikin VG (2003) Derivatization in Mass Spectrometry – 1. Silylation. Eur J Mass Spectrom 9:1–21. doi:10.1255/ejms.527
182. Beynon JH, Bertrand M, Cooks RG (1973) Metastable Loss of Nitrosyl Radical from Aromatic Nitro Compounds. J Am Chem Soc 95:1739–1745. doi:10.1021/ja00787a007
183. Meyerson S, Puskas I, Fields EK (1966) Organic Ions in the Gas Phase. XVIII. Mass Spectra of Nitroarenes. J Am Chem Soc 88:4974–4908. doi:10.1021/ja00973a036
184. Porter QN, Baldas J (1971) Mass Spectrometry of Heterocyclic Compounds. Wiley Interscience, New York
185. Schwarz H, Bohlmann F (1973) Mass Spectrometric Investigation of Amides. II. Electron-Impact Induced Fragmentation of (Phenylacetyl)Aziridine, -Pyrrolidine, and -Piperidine. Tetrahedron Lett 38:3703–3706. doi:10.1016/S0040-4039(01)87012-X
186. Nakano T, Martin A (1981) Mass Spectrometric Fragmentation of the Oxetanes of 3,5-Dimethylisoxazole, 2,4-Dimethylthiazole, and 1-Acetylimidazole. Org Mass Spectrom 16:55–61. doi:10.1002/oms.1210160202
187. Grützmacher H-F, Pankoke D (1989) Rearrangement Reactions of the Molecular Ions of Some Substituted Aliphatic Oxiranes. Org Mass Spectrom 24:647–652. doi:10.1002/oms.1210240822
188. Collin JE, Conde-Caprace G (1968) Ionization and Dissociation of Cyclic Ethers by Electron Impact. Int J Mass Spectrom Ion Phys 1:213–225. doi:10.1016/0020-7381(68)85001-6
189. Duffield AM, Budzikiewicz H, Williams DH, Djerassi C (1965) Mass Spectrometry in Structural and Stereochemical Problems. LXIV. A Study of the Fragmentation Processes of Some Cyclic Amines. J Am Chem Soc 87:810–816. doi:10.1021/ja01082a021
190. Burgers PC, Holmes JL, Mommers AA, Terlouw JK (1983) Neutral Products of Ion Fragmentations: Hydrogen Cyanide and Hydrogen Isocyanide (HNC) Identified by Collisionally Induced Dissociative Ionization. Chem Phys Lett 102:1–3. doi:10.1016/0009-2614(83)80645-9

191. Hop CECA, Dakubu M, Holmes JL (1988) Do the Aminopyridine Molecular Ions Display Aniline- or Pyridine-Type Behavior? Org Mass Spectrom 23:609–612. doi:10.1002/oms.1210230811
192. Rosenstock HM, Stockbauer R, Parr AC (1981) Unimolecular Kinetics of Pyridine Ion Fragmentation. Int J Mass Spectrom Ion Phys 38:323–331. doi:10.1016/0020-7381(81)80077-0
193. Burgers PC, Holmes JL (1989) Kinetic Energy Release in Metastable-Ion Fragmentations. Rapid Commun Mass Spectrom 3:279–280. doi:10.1002/rcm.1290030809
194. Cardoso AM, Ferrer AJ (1999) Fragmentation Reactions of Molecular Ions and Dications of Indoleamines. Eur Mass Spectrom 5:11–18. doi:10.1255/ejms.244
195. Rodríguez JG, Urrutia A, Canoira L (1996) Electron Impact Mass Spectrometry of Indole Derivatives. Int J Mass Spectrom Ion Proc 152:97–110. doi:10.1016/0168-1176(95)04344-6
196. Hesse M (1974) Indolalkaloide, Teil 2: Spektren. Weinheim, VCH
197. Hesse M (1974) Indolalkaloide, Teil 1: Text. Weinheim, VCH
198. Biemann K (2002) Four Decades of Structure Determination by Mass Spectrometry: From Alkaloids to Heparin. J Am Soc Mass Spectrom 13:1254–1272. doi:10.1016/S1044-0305(02)00441-5
199. Duffield AM, Beugelmans R, Budzikiewicz H, Lightner DA, Williams DH, Djerassi C (1965) Mass Spectrometry in Structural and Stereochemical Problems. LXIII. Hydrogen Rearrangements Induced by Electron Impact on N-n-Butyl- and N-n-Pentylpyrroles. J Am Chem Soc 87:805–810. doi:10.1021/ja01082a020
200. Aubagnac JL, Campion P (1979) Mass Spectrometry of Nitrogen Heterocycles. X. Contribution to the Behavior of the Aniline Ion and Aminopyridine Ions Prior to Fragmentation by Loss of Hydrogen Cyanide. Org Mass Spectrom 14:425–429. doi:10.1002/oms.1210140806
201. Heyns K, Stute R, Scharmann H (1966) Mass Spectrometric Investigations. XII. Mass Spectra of Furans. Tetrahedron 22:2223–2235. doi:10.1016/S0040-4020(01)82143-8
202. De Jong F, Sinnige HJM, Janssen MJ (1970) Carbon Scrambling in Thiophene Under Electron Impact. Rec Trav Chim Pays-Bas 89:225–226. doi:10.1002/recl.19700890214
203. Williams DH, Cooks RG, Ronayne J, Tam SW (1968) Studies in Mass Spectrometry. XXVII. The Decomposition of Furan, Thiophene, and Deuterated Analogs Under Electron Impact. Tetrahedron Lett 9:1777–1780. doi:10.1016/S0040-4039(01)99049-5
204. Riepe W, Zander M (1979) The Mass Spectrometric Fragmentation Behavior of Thiophene Benzologs. Org Mass Spectrom 14:455–456. doi:10.1002/oms.1210140812
205. Rothwell AP, Wood KV, Gupta AK, Prasad JVNV (1987) Mass Spectra of Some 2- and 3 Cycloalkenylfurans and Cycloalkenylthiophenes and Their Oxy Derivatives. Org Mass Spectrom 22:790–795. doi:10.1002/oms.1210221206

7 Chemical Ionization

Learning Objectives

- Ion formation by ion–molecule reactions
- Processes of positive-ion formation other than electron ionization
- Pathways of negative-ion formation
- Softness of chemical ionization techniques
- Applications of chemical ionization mass spectrometry
- Chemical ionization processes at atmospheric pressure
- Atmospheric pressure chemical ionization
- Atmospheric pressure photoionization
- Overview of chemical ionization techniques

Mass spectrometrists have ever been searching for ionization methods softer than EI, because molecular weight determination is key for structure elucidation. *Chemical ionization* (CI) is the first of the so-called *soft ionization methods* we are going to discuss (cf. Fig. 1.4). Historically, *field ionization* (FI, Sect. 8.5) is the elder technique, and thus CI can be regarded as the second soft ionization method introduced to organic mass spectrometry. Nonetheless, CI shares some similarities with EI making its discussion next to EI convenient. CI goes back to experiments of Talrose in the early 1950s [1] and was developed to an analytically useful technique by Munson and Field in the mid-1960s [2–5]. Since then, the basic concept of CI has been extended and applied in numerous different ways, meanwhile providing experimental conditions for a wide diversity of analytical tasks [5–7].

J.H. Gross, *Mass Spectrometry*, DOI 10.1007/978-3-319-54398-7_7

7.1 Basics of Chemical Ionization

7.1.1 Formation of Ions in Positive-Ion Chemical Ionization

In chemical ionization, new ionized species are formed when gaseous molecules interact with ions, i.e., chemical ionization is based on *ion–molecule reactions* (Sect. 2.13). Chemical ionization may involve the transfer of an electron, proton, or other ions between the reactants [8], that is, between the neutral analyte M and the *reagent ions* generated from the *reagent gas* [9, 10].

CI differs from what we have encountered in mass spectrometry so far because *bimolecular processes* are used to generate analyte ions. The occurrence of bimolecular reactions requires a sufficiently large number of ion–molecule collisions during the dwell time of the reactants in the ion source. This is achieved by significantly increasing the partial pressure of the reagent gas. Assuming reasonable collision cross sections and an ion source residence time of microseconds [11], a molecule will undergo 30–70 collisions at an ion source pressure of about 2.5×10^2 Pa (2.5 mbar) [12]. The 10^3–10^4-fold excess of reagent gas also effectively shields the analyte molecules from direct ionization by primary electrons, a prerequisite to suppress competing EI of the analyte.

Let us first consider *positive-ion chemical ionization* (PICI). In PICI, there are four fundamental pathways of positive-ion formation from a neutral analyte molecule M. First, there is *proton transfer*:

$$M + [BH]^+ \rightarrow [M + H]^+ + B \tag{7.1}$$

For proton transfer, the reagent ion $[BH]^+$ has to act as Brønsted acid. Proton transfer yields protonated analyte molecules, $[M+H]^+$, i.e., even-electron ions that are detected at [M+1]. Although proton transfer is generally considered to yield protonated analyte molecules, $[M+H]^+$, acidic analytes themselves may form both $[M+H]^+$ and $[M–H]^-$ ions by mutual proton exchange, a behavior exploited for *negative-ion chemical ionization* (NICI, Sect. 7.5).

Second, an analyte molecule may receive a charge by adduct formation via *electrophilic addition*:

$$M + X^+ \rightarrow [M + X]^+ \tag{7.2}$$

Electrophilic addition of X^+ occurs by attachment of the entire reagent ion to an analyte molecule if protonation of M is not feasible. For example, $[M+NH_4]^+$ ions are often formed when ammonia reagent gas is used. Thus, even-electron ions are detected at an *m/z* value above M, the exact position of which depends on the adduct actually formed.

Third, *anion abstraction* can occur:

$$M + X^+ \rightarrow [M - A]^+ + AX \tag{7.3}$$

Hydride abstraction is a commonly occurring case of *anion abstraction*, e.g., aliphatic alcohols rather yield $[M{-}H]^+$ ions, $[M{-}1]^+$, than $[M{+}H]^+$ ions [13, 14]. Strong leaving groups like mesylate or tosylate may also lead to even-electron cation formation via loss of an anionic group.

The fourth pathway is *charge transfer* (CT):

$$M + X^{+\bullet} \rightarrow M^{+\bullet} + X \tag{7.4}$$

Charge transfer, also known as *charge exchange* (CE), differs from the previous three processes in that it yields molecular ions, $M^{+\bullet}$, i.e., odd-electron species. Although being positive radical ions, the products of charge transfer tend to provide notably less fragmentation than those formed upon electron ionization, because the average ion internal energy from CT is much lower than after EI. CT thus yields radical ions behaving similar to molecular ions in low-energy electron ionization (Sect. 5.6).

A sort of molecular ion?
It has been common to denote $[M{+}H]^+$ and $[M{-}H]^+$ ions as *quasi-molecular ions* because they comprise the otherwise intact analyte molecule and are detected in place of a "true" molecular ion, $M^{+\bullet}$, when soft ionization methods are employed. The term was also applied to $[M{+}alkali]^+$ ions created by soft ionization methods other than CI. Recent recommendations are to avoid the term *quasi-molecular ion* [9, 10]. Now, ions are addressed more specifically, e.g., $[M{+}H]^+$ as *protonated molecules*, $[M{-}H]^-$ as *deprotonated molecules*, $[M{+}Na]^+$ ions as *sodiated molecules*, and in general $[M{+}X]^+$ as *cationized molecules*.

7.1.2 Chemical Ionization Ion Sources

CI ion sources exhibit close similarity to EI ion sources (Sect. 5.1). In fact, some EI ion sources can actually be switched to CI operation in seconds, i.e., they are constructed as *EI/CI combination ion sources*. Such a change requires the EI ion source to be modified according to the needs of holding a comparatively high pressure of reagent gas (some 10^2 Pa) without allowing too much leakage into the ion source housing [15]. This is accomplished by axially inserting some inner wall, e.g., a small cylinder, into the ion volume leaving only narrow entrances and exits of the ionizing primary electrons, the sample inlets, and the exiting ion beam. The ports for the reference inlet, the gas chromatograph (GC) and the direct insertion probe (DIP) need to be tightly connected to the respective inlet system during operation, e.g., the empty DIP is inserted even when another inlet actually provides the sample flow into the ion volume. The reagent gas is introduced directly into the

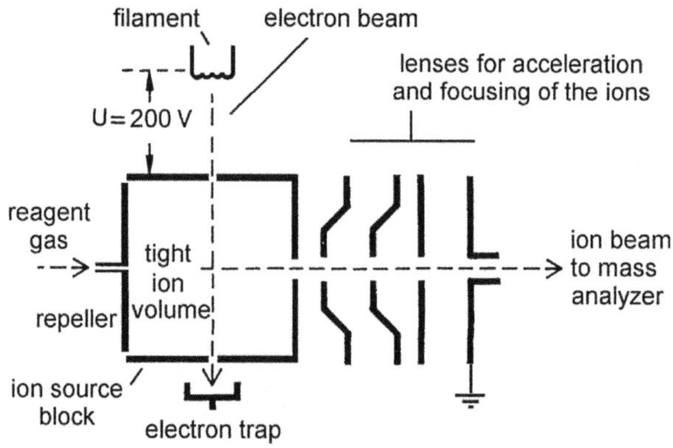

Fig. 7.1 Layout of a chemical ionization ion source (Adapted from Ref. [16] by permission. © Springer-Verlag Heidelberg, 1991)

ion volume to ensure maximum pressure inside at minimum losses to the ion source housing (Fig. 7.1). During CI operation, the pressure in the ion source housing typically rises by a factor of 20–50 (5×10^{-4}–10^{-3} Pa) as compared to the background pressure of the instrument. Thus, a sufficient pumping speed of $200\ l\ s^{-1}$ or more is necessary to maintain stable operation in CI mode. The energy of the primary electrons is preferably adjusted to some 200 eV, because electrons of lower energy experience difficulties in penetrating the reagent gas.

7.1.3 Chemical Ionization Techniques and Terms

In its original implementation, chemical ionization delivered positive ions [2–5], and therefore, for many practitioners the acronym CI used without further specifications still stands for *positive-ion chemical ionization* (PICI) where the latter term should clearly be preferred. For negative ions, the term *negative-ion chemical ionization* (NICI) should be used [8]. Table 7.1 provides an overview of CI terms and acronyms. The last technique listed there, *electron capture* (EC) or *electron capture negative ionization* (ECNI) does not represent chemical ionization in the strict sense, as will be outlined later (Sect. 7.6).

7.1.4 Sensitivity of Chemical Ionization

Ionization in CI is the result of one or several competing chemical reactions. Therefore, the sensitivity (Sect. 1.6) in CI strongly depends on the conditions of the experiment. For comparison of sensitivity data, the reagent gas, its pressure, and the ion source temperature have to be stated in addition to primary electron energy and electron current. Specifications of magnetic sector instruments, for example, state a sensitivity of about $4 \times 10^{-8}\ C\ \mu g^{-1}$ for the $[M+H]^+$ ion of methylstearate,

Table 7.1 Terms and acronyms related to chemical ionization

Polarity	Method	Acronym	Explication
Positive	Positive-ion chemical ionization (or positive chemical ionization)	PICI (or PCI)	Strictly speaking, any CI technique delivering even-electron positive analyte ions. (Sometimes used in the restricted sense of ion formation by protonation.)
	Charge transfer (or charge exchange)	CT (or CE)	Positive radical ions are formed by exchange/transfer of an electron.
Negative	Negative-ion chemical ionization (or negative chemical ionization)	NICI (or NCI)	Any CI technique delivering even-electron negative analyte ions
	Electron capture	EC (or ECNI)	Not a CI technique in the strict sense. However, ion source operation is equal to NICI

m/z 299, at $R = 1000$ in positive-ion CI mode with methane reagent gas. This is approximately one order of magnitude less than for EI. While the ion current that can be generated from a sample by CI tends to be lower than in EI, it is worth considering that most of this ion current is delivered by ions like $[M+H]^+$ or $[M+NH_4]^+$ that are directly related to intact molecules. Assigning the correct molecular mass is therefore easier to accomplish even in the presence of impurities.

7.2 Protonation in Chemical Ionization

7.2.1 Source of Protons

The formation of $[M+H]^+$ ions due to bimolecular processes between ions and their neutral molecular counterparts is called *autoprotonation*, a special form of *self-chemical ionization* (self-CI). Self-CI is a chemical ionization process, where the reagent ions are formed by an ionized species of the analyte itself [17]. In EI-MS, autoprotonation is an unwanted phenomenon. $[M+H]^+$ ions from autoprotonation are promoted by increasing the ion source pressure and lowering the temperature. Furthermore, the formation of $[M+H]^+$ ions is favored if the analyte is highly volatile and/or has acidic hydrogens. Thus, self-CI can cause a misinterpretation of mass spectra either by an overestimation of the number of carbon atoms from the ^{13}C isotopic peak due to exaggerated [M+1] ion abundance (Sect. 3.2) or by indicating a molecular mass which seems to be higher by 1 u than it really is (Fig. 7.6 and cf. *nitrogen rule* Sect. 6.2.7). In CI-MS with methane or ammonia reagent gas, however, the process of autoprotonation is intentionally exploited to generate the reagent ions.

Chemi-ionization
Chemi-ionization means ionization of internally excited molecules upon interaction with other neutrals by *electron detachment*. This corresponds to $M^* + X \rightarrow MX^{+\bullet} + e^-$. Chemi-ionization is different from CI in that there is no ion–molecule reaction involved (cf. Penning ionization, Sect. 2.1.3) [8, 18].

Transition from $M^{+\bullet}$ to $[M+H]^+$ The contribution of some autoprotonation causes an increase in [M+1] peak intensity that may be hard to recognize, and thus, can erroneously be interpreted as a larger number of carbon atoms than actually present (Fig. 7.2, Sect. 3.2). The appearance of the signal shifts upon transition from pure molecular ion formation to pure protonation. Conditions resulting in an intermediate situation are therefore to be avoided. Clean EI spectra require low partial pressure of the sample in the ion source while clean CI spectra demand for a correct adjustment of the reagent gas pressure in order to avoid residual EI.

7.2.2 Methane Reagent Gas Plasma

The EI mass spectrum of methane has already been discussed (Sect. 6.1). It shows peaks from all ionic species listed in Eq. 7.5. Raising the partial pressure of methane from the EI standard value of about 10^{-4} Pa to 10^2 Pa significantly alters the ion

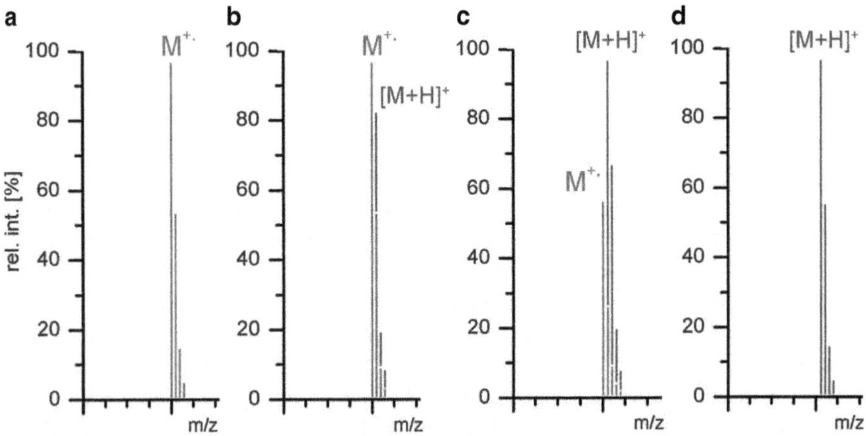

Fig. 7.2 Stepwise change of signal appearance upon transition from pure molecular ion formation (*red peak portions*) to protonated molecules (*blue peak portions*). (**a**) Pure molecular ion peak with correct isotope pattern, (**b**) some contribution of $[M+H]^+$ causes an excessively intensive [M+1] peak, (**c**) mostly $[M+H]^+$, and (**d**) pure $[M+H]^+$ ion signal with correct isotope pattern. Only pure $M^{+\bullet}$ and pure $[M+H]^+$ result in undistorted isotope patterns

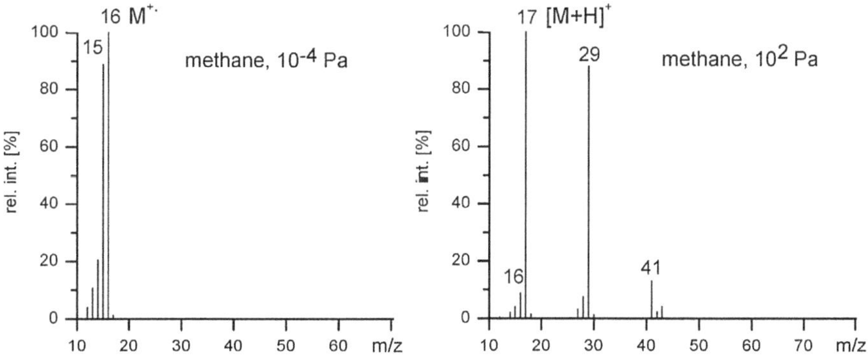

Fig. 7.3 Comparison of the methane spectrum upon electron ionization at different ion source pressures: (**a**) approx. 10^{-4} Pa, (**b**) approx. 10^{2} Pa. The latter represents the typical methane reagent gas spectrum in positive-ion CI

population [1]. The molecular ion, $CH_4^{+\bullet}$, *m/z* 16, almost vanishes and a new species, CH_5^+, *m/z* 17, is detected instead [19]. Some additional ions occur at higher mass, the most prominent being $C_2H_5^+$, *m/z* 29, and $C_3H_5^+$, *m/z* 41 (Fig. 7.3) [20, 21]. Clearly, the positive-ion CI spectrum of methane is governed by competing and consecutive bimolecular reactions in the ion source [4, 6, 12]:

$$CH_4 + e^- \rightarrow CH_4^{+\bullet},\ CH_3^+,\ CH_2^{+\bullet},\ CH^+,\ C^{+\bullet},\ H_2^{+\bullet},\ H^+ \quad (7.5)$$

$$CH_4^{+\bullet} + CH_4 \rightarrow CH_5^+ + CH_3^\bullet \quad (7.6)$$

$$CH_3^+ + CH_4 \rightarrow C_2H_7^+ \rightarrow C_2H_5^+ + H_2 \quad (7.7)$$

$$CH_2^{+\bullet} + CH_4 \rightarrow C_2H_4^{+\bullet} + H_2 \quad (7.8)$$

$$CH_2^{+\bullet} + CH_4 \rightarrow C_2H_3^+ + H_2 + H^\bullet \quad (7.9)$$

$$C_2H_3^+ + CH_4 \rightarrow C_3H_5^+ + H_2 \quad (7.10)$$

$$C_2H_5^+ + CH_4 \rightarrow C_3H_7^+ + H_2 \quad (7.11)$$

The relative abundances of the product ions change dramatically as the ion source pressure increases from EI conditions to 25 Pa. Above 100 Pa, the relative concentrations become stabilized at levels represented by the CI spectrum of methane reagent gas [4, 22]. Fortunately, in CI the ion source pressure is usually in this range of 10^2 Pa and thus in this plateau region of relative ion abundances, thereby ensuring reproducible CI conditions. The influence of the ion source temperature is more pronounced than in EI because the high collision rate rapidly effects a thermal equilibrium.

Reagent gas plasma
The simultaneous presence of free electrons, protons, and numerous ionic and radical species in the ionized reagent gas has led to its description as a *reagent gas plasma*.

7.2.3 CH_5^+ and Related Ions

The protonated methane ion, CH_5^+, represents a reactive as well as fascinating species in the methane reagent gas plasma. In 1991, its structure had been calculated as shown in Scheme 7.1 [19] and the chemical behavior of the CH_5^+ ion indeed appears to be compatible with a stable structure, involving a three-center two-electron bond associating two hydrogens and the carbon atom.

Rearrangement of this structure due to exchange between one of these hydrogens and one of the three remaining hydrogens seemingly is a fast process induced by interactions with the chemical ionization gas. Recent work indicates that all five C–H bonds are rendered equal by extremely rapid zero-point motion thereby precluding the assignment of a unique CH_5^+ ion structure [23]. For the $C_2H_7^+$ intermediate during $C_2H_5^+$ ion formation several isomerizing structures are discussed [20, 21]. In protonated fluoromethane, the conditions are quite different, promoting a weak C–F and a strong F–H bond [24].

7.2.4 Energetics of Protonation

The tendency of a (basic) molecule B to accept a proton is quantitatively described by its *proton affinity* (*PA*, Sect. 2.12). For the process of protonation we have to consider the gas phase reaction of a base, B_g, with a proton [3]:

$$B_g + H_g^+ \rightarrow [BH]_g^+ \tag{7.12}$$

Now, the proton affinity of B is defined as the negative of the corresponding heat of reaction upon formation of $[BH]_g^+$:

Scheme 7.1

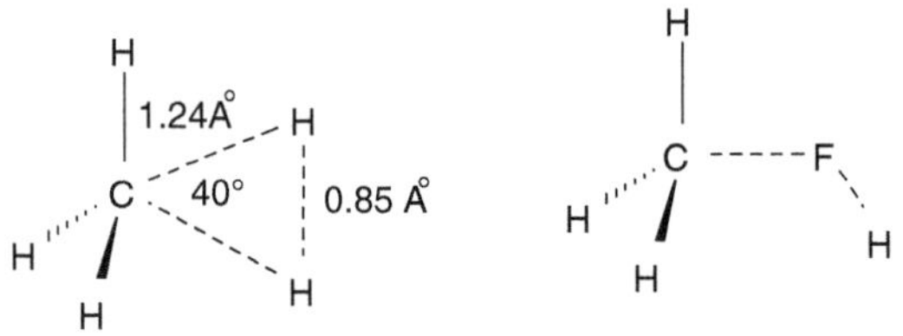

$$PA_{(B)} = -\Delta H_r^{\ 0} \tag{7.13}$$

The inversion of the algebraic sign of $\Delta H_r^{\ 0}$ serves to express a more exothermal protonation in terms of a larger proton affinity of B.

To judge the chances of protonation under CI conditions, one has to compare the *PA* of the neutral analyte M with that of the complementary base B of the proton-donating reagent ion $[BH]^+$ (Brønsted acid). Protonation will occur as long as the process is exothermic, i.e., if $PA_{(B)} < PA_{(M)}$. The heat of reaction has basically to be distributed among the degrees of freedom of the $[M+H]^+$ analyte ion [14, 25]. Accordingly, the minimum internal energy of the $[M+H]^+$ ions is well approximated by:

$$E_{\text{int}(M+H)} \approx \Delta PA = PA_{(M)} - PA_{(B)} \tag{7.14}$$

Some additional thermal energy will also be contained in the $[M+H]^+$ ions. Having *PA* data at hand (Table 2.6), one can easily judge whether a reagent ion will be able to protonate the analyte of interest and how much energy will be put into the $[M+H]^+$ ion.

Influence of the substrate The CH_5^+ reagent ion is able to protonate C_2H_6 because Eq. 7.14 gives $\Delta PA = PA_{(C2H6)} - PA_{(CH4)} = 601 - 552 = 49$ kJ mol^{-1}. The product, protonated ethane, $C_2H_7^+$, is immediately stabilized by H_2 loss to yield $C_2H_5^+$ [20, 21]. In case of tetrahydrofuran, protonation to yield $[C_4H_8O+H]^+$ is more exothermic: $\Delta PA = PA_{(C4H8O)} - PA_{(CH4)} = 831 - 552 = 279$ kJ mol^{-1}, and thus, results in some more fragmentation of the $[M+H]^+$ ions.

7.2.5 Impurities of Higher *PA* than the Reagent Gas

Due to the above energetic considerations, impurities of the reagent gas having a higher *PA* than the neutral reagent gas are protonated by the reagent ion [3]. Residual water is a frequent source of contamination. Higher concentrations of water in the reagent gas may even alter its properties completely, i.e., H_3O^+ becomes the predominant species in a CH_4/H_2O mixture under CI conditions (Fig. 7.4) [26].

Impurities change reagent gas
Any analyte of suitable *PA* may be regarded as a basic impurity of the reagent gas, and thus becomes protonated in excellent yield. Heteroatoms and π-electron systems are the preferred sites of protonation. Nevertheless, the additional proton is often mobile within the ion, sometimes even accompanied by its exchange with otherwise fixed hydrogens [27, 28].

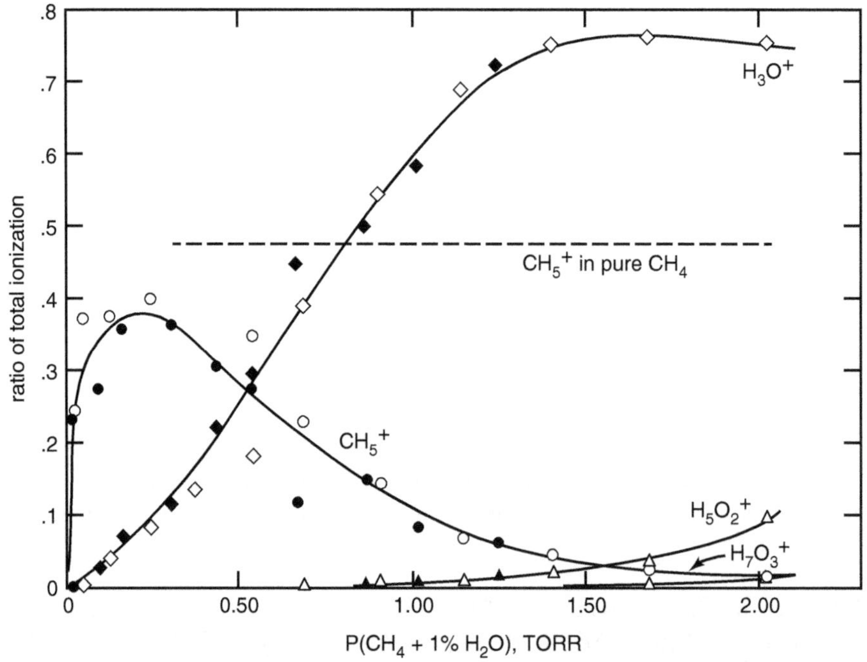

Fig. 7.4 Relative concentrations of CH_5^+ and H_3O^+ ions vs. pressure of a mixture of CH_4 (99%) and H_2O (1%). 1 Torr = 133 Pa (Reproduced from Ref. [26] by permission. © American Chemical Society, 1965)

7.2.6 Methane Reagent Gas PICI Spectra

The $[M+H]^+$ ion peak in methane reagent gas PICI spectra – generally denoted *methane-CI spectra* – is usually intense and often represents the base peak [29–31]. Although protonation in CI is generally exothermic by 1–4 eV, the degree of fragmentation of $[M+H]^+$ ions is much lower than that observed for the same analytes under 70-eV EI conditions. This is because $[M+H]^+$ ions have (*i*) a narrow internal energy distribution, and (*ii*) fast radical-induced bond cleavages are prohibited, because solely intact molecules are eliminated from these even-electron ions. Electrophilic addition fairly often gives rise to $[M+C_2H_5]^+$ and $[M+C_3H_5]^+$ adduct ions. Thus, [M+29] and [M+41] peaks are sometimes observed in addition to the expected – usually clearly dominating – [M+1] peak. Occasionally, hydride abstraction may occur instead of protonation.

Obscured hydride abstractions
Hydride abstractions are difficult to recognize. To identify a $[M–H]^+$ peak occurring instead of a $[M+H]^+$ peak it is useful to examine the mass differences between the signal in question and the products of electrophilic addition. In that case, [M+29] and [M+41] appear as if they were [M+31] and [M+43] peaks, respectively. An apparent loss of 16 u can be indicative of an $[M+H–H_2O]^+$ ion instead of an $[M+H–CH_4]^+$ ion.

PICI of methionine There is a greatly reduced fragmentation in the methane reagent gas PICI spectrum of methionine as compared to the according EI spectrum (Fig. 7.5). Only small stable molecules such as NH_3, HCOOH, and MeSH are eliminated from the $[M+H]^+$ ion, *m*/*z* 150, which yields the base peak. In addition, the PICI spectrum perfectly reveals the isotopic pattern that indicates the presence of sulfur. The horizontal line (Fig. 7.5b) means that this range was not acquired in the PICI spectrum as to keep the spectrum free from reagent ion signals. The spectra were, however, plotted on the same *m*/*z* scales to simplify the comparison.

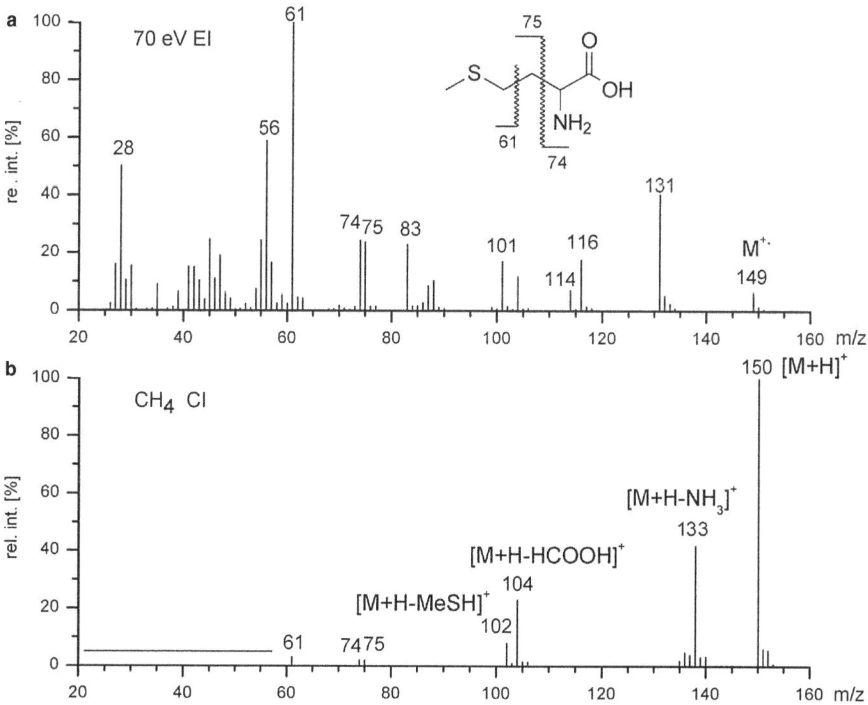

Fig. 7.5 Comparison of (**a**) 70-eV EI spectrum and (**b**) methane reagent gas PICI spectrum of the amino acid methionine

Low-mass range in CI

Resulting from the large excess of reagent gas, its spectrum often is of higher intensity than that of the analyte. Therefore, CI spectra are usually acquired starting above the *m/z* range occupied by reagent ions, e.g., above *m/z* 50 for methane or above *m/z* 70 for isobutane. Background subtraction can alternatively be applied to remove these peaks, but this approach suffers from variations in the reagent ion abundances upon admission of the analyte.

7.2.7 Other Reagent Gases in PICI

As pointed out, the value of ΔPA determines whether a particular analyte can be protonated by a certain reactant ion and how exothermic the protonation will be. Considering other reagent gases than methane therefore allows some tuning of the PICI conditions. The employed reagent gases and ions are chiefly:

- hydrogen and hydrogen-containing mixtures [14, 25, 32],
- isobutane [33–37],
- ammonia [34, 38–44],
- dimethylether [45],
- diisopropylether [46],
- acetone [13],
- acetaldehyde [13],
- benzene [47],
- iodomethane [48],
- nitrous oxide [39, 49, 50], and
- transition metal ions like Cu^+ [51] and Fe^+ [52].

Among these, methane, isobutane, and ammonia are the by far most common reagent gases in PICI (Table 7.2). Nitrous oxide and transition metal ions are

Table 7.2 Common PICI reagent gases (chiefly protonating)

Reagent gas	Reagent ions	Neutral from reagent ions	*PA* of neutral product [kJ mol^{-1}]	Analyte ions and relative analyte ion masses
H_2	H_3^+	H_2	424	$[M+H]^+$, $[M-H]^+$ [M+1], [M–1]
CH_4	CH_5^+ ($C_2H_5^+$ and $C_3H_5^+$)	CH_4	552	$[M+H]^+$, also $[M+C_2H_5]^+$ and $[M+C_3H_5]^+$ [M+1], [M+29], [M+41]
i-C_4H_{10}	*t*-$C_4H_9^+$	*i*-C_4H_8	820	$[M+H]^+$, also $[M+C_4H_9]^+$, (eventually $[M+C_3H_3]^+$, $[M+C_3H_5]^+$ and $[M+C_3H_7]^+$), [M+1], [M+57]
NH_3	NH_4^+	NH_3	854	$[M+H]^+$, $[M+NH_4]^+$, [M+1], [M+18]

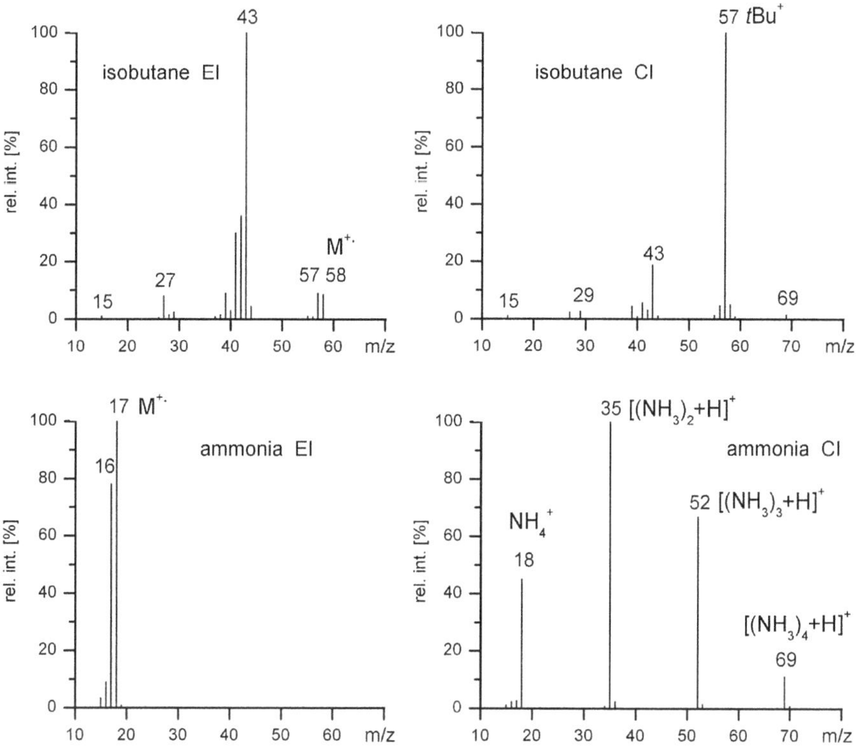

Fig. 7.6 Standard EI vs. positive-ion CI spectra of isobutane (*upper*) and ammonia (*lower part*). Ammonia forms abundant $[(NH_3)_n+H]^+$ cluster ions upon CI

particularly useful in locating double bonds. The EI and CI spectra of ammonia and isobutane reagent gas are compared in Fig. 7.6.

Isobutane is an especially versatile reagent gas, because (*i*) it provides low-fragmentation PICI spectra of all but the most nonpolar analytes, (*ii*) gives almost exclusively one well-defined adduct ($[M+C_4H_9]^+$, [M+57]) if any (Fig. 7.7), and (*iii*) can also be employed for electron capture negative ionization (Sect. 7.4).

Cluster ions

Cluster ions are formed by the agglomeration of polar species, mostly molecules, around an ion as a common center of charge, thereby essentially creating a solvent sphere around that ion. Cluster ions occur when a sufficiently large number of ion–neutral collisions provides the occasion. Cluster ions are therefore frequently formed in CI with polar reagent gases, from liquid matrices (Chap. 10), and generally when analytes at high concentration are subjected to soft ionization. Typical examples of cluster ions are $[(H_2O)_n+H]^+$, $[(NH_3)_n+H]^+$, [*n*M+H]+, etc. Cluster ions may also be generated by ionization of neutral clusters.

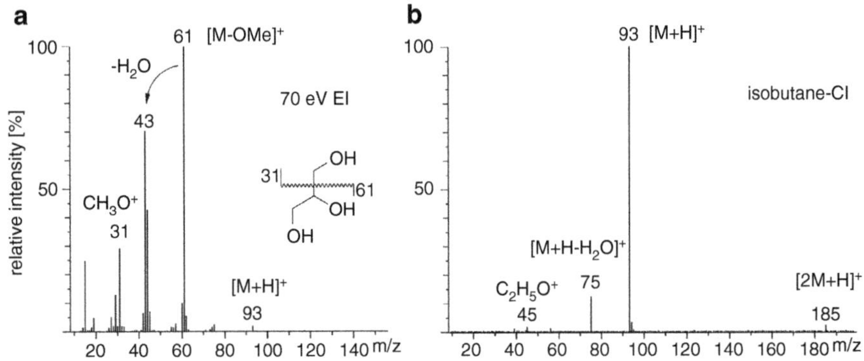

Fig. 7.7 70-eV EI (**a**) vs. isobutane-PICI spectrum of glycerol (**b**). Even in EI mode, an $[M+H]^+$ ion by autoprotonation is observed rather than $M^{+\bullet}$. Besides $[M+H]^+$, the PICI spectrum shows only few fragment ions and a weak $[2M+H]^+$ cluster ion signal

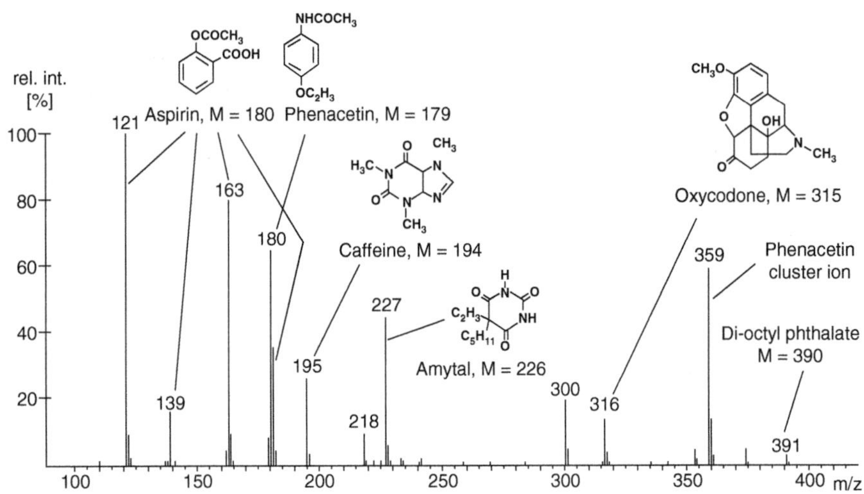

Fig. 7.8 Isobutane PICI mass spectrum of gastric contents in an overdose case (Reproduced from Ref. [33] by permission. © American Chemical Society, 1970)

Quick clinical diagnosis In a drug overdose case evidence was available of ingestion of Percodan (a mixture of several common drugs). The isobutane-PICI spectrum of the gastric extract was obtained (Fig. 7.8) [33]. All drugs formed an $[M+H]^+$ ion. Due to the low exothermicity of protonation by the *tert*-$C_4H_9^+$ ion, most $[M+H]^+$ ions did not fragment, solely that of aspirin showed intense fragment ion peaks that can be assigned as $[M+H–H_2O]^+$, *m*/*z* 163; $[M+H–H_2C{=}CO]^+$, *m*/*z* 139; and $[M+H–CH_3COOH]^+$, *m*/*z* 121. Phenacetine, in addition to the $[M+H]^+$ ion at *m*/*z* 180, formed a $[2M+H]^+$ cluster ion, *m*/*z* 359.

The spectra in both Figs. 7.7 and 7.8 tell us some important facts:

- Cluster ions like $[2M+H]^+$ are frequently formed in CI-MS and this needs to be considered when interpreting CI spectra of unknown samples.
- Today, in an overdose case one would perform the analysis by LC-MS in combination with other soft ionization techniques, but this example from 1970 demonstrates the softness of PICI.
- In addition, Fig. 7.8 may serve as an eye-opener for what can be achieved in mixture analysis when fragmentation is virtually absent and most or preferably all ions correspond to intact molecular species contained in a mixture (Sects. 14.7 and 14.8).

7.3 Proton Transfer Reaction-Mass Spectrometry

By combining the principles of PICI with an apparatus derived from *selected-ion flow tube* (SIFT) experiments, the technique of *proton transfer reaction-mass spectrometry* (PTR-MS) has been developed as a dedicated tool for the analysis of *volatile organic compounds* (VOCs) at parts-per-trillion by volume (pptv) level in air [53, 54]. PTR-MS is highly useful as a fast and quantitative method for the determination of VOCs as proven by numerous applications in food control, environmental and atmospheric research, as well as in medicine, e.g., to analyze the exhaled breath of patients [53–57]. Recent instrumental developments in PTR-MS result in even higher sensitivity for trace component analysis [58, 59].

7.3.1 Reagent ion Formation in PTR-MS

When water vapor is passed through the discharge of a hollow-cathode ion source it is ionized by primary electrons, basically by EI. Due to ion–molecule reaction sequences the product ion mixture forms H_3O^+ ions with high selectivity of up to 99.5% (Sect. 7.2.5) [53, 54]. Even $N_2^{+\bullet}$ or N^+ ions from nitrogen rapidly react with water molecules in the source region to result in more H_3O^+ ions. Thus, a high (typical count rates of $\approx 10^6$ counts s^{-1}) and almost pure flux of hydronium primary ions is provided that may then serve as reagent ions in a PICI process:

$$M + H_3O^+ \rightarrow [MH]^+ + H_2O \tag{7.15}$$

Fortunately this proton transfer reaction can generally occur for all VOCs as their *PA*s exceed that of water ($PA_{water} = 697$ kJ mol^{-1}) allowing for their exothermic protonation.

7.3.2 Analyte Ion Formation in PTR-MS

Different from classical CI sources, PTR-MS separates reagent ion generation from the stage of analyte ion formation. For the latter step, PTR-MS makes use of an ion flow tube

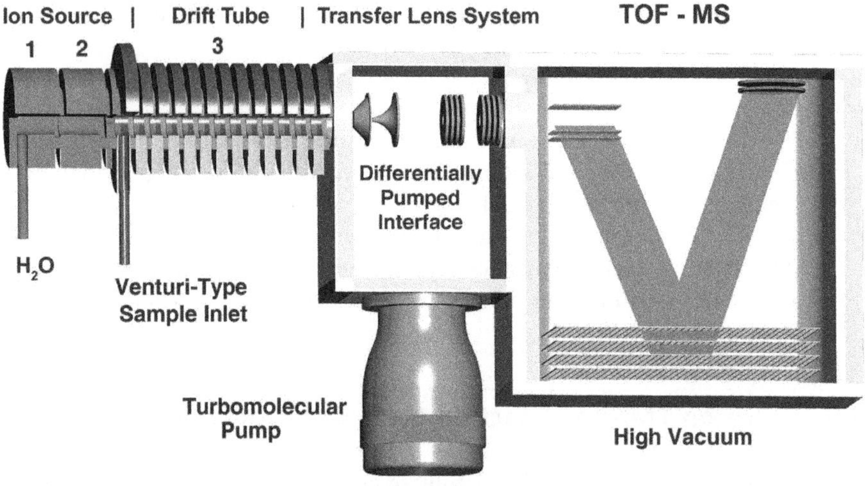

Fig. 7.9 PTR mass spectrometer. The ion source of the Ionicon PTR-TOF 2000™ is divided into a compartment for reagent ion generation from H_2O by (*1*) a hollow cathode and (*2*) a source drift region in front of the sample inlet, and (*3*) the drift tube for analyte ion formation. The TOF analyzer has its own turbomolecular pump to maintain high vacuum (*not shown*) (By courtesy of Ionicon Analytik GmbH, Innsbruck, Austria)

similar to a device used in IMS (Sect. 4.10), which provides sufficient time for effective reactions according to Eq. 7.14. Thus, ions are extracted from the hollow-cathode source, passed through a short drift region, and delivered to the extended reaction region, at the entrance of which the sample air containing the VOCs is continuously admitted (Fig. 7.9). Due to the purity of the H_3O^+ reagent ions delivered, there is no need for an ion flux-limiting quadrupole system to preselect reagent ions [53, 54].

On its way from the Venturi-type inlet to the downstream end of the drift section, H_3O^+ ions undergo nonreactive and reactive collisions with any one of the components of air [53, 54]. The water reagent gas PICI process causes the analyzed VOCs to be converted into $[M+H]^+$ ions.

The flow tube, which is about 20 cm long, acts as a reaction region that is maintained at about 1 mbar by action of a vacuum pump attached to its exit. These conditions afford thermalization and effective proton transfer as the hydronium ions drift along together with the VOC-loaded air. As PTR-MS does not necessitate an additional buffer gas, the analyte air is not diluted any further, a feature that contributes to the high sensitivity of the method. Furthermore, the original mole fraction of the analytes in the air is maintained.

VOCs in the Manaus area VOCs in air originate from natural (emission by plants and animals) and anthropogenic sources (usage of fossil fuels, evaporation of solvents, gases from landfill sites). Even without anthropogenic contributions, the Earth's atmosphere would consist of a complex mixture of VOCs [55]. Methane (2 pptv) is by far the most common organic compound in the Earth's atmosphere,

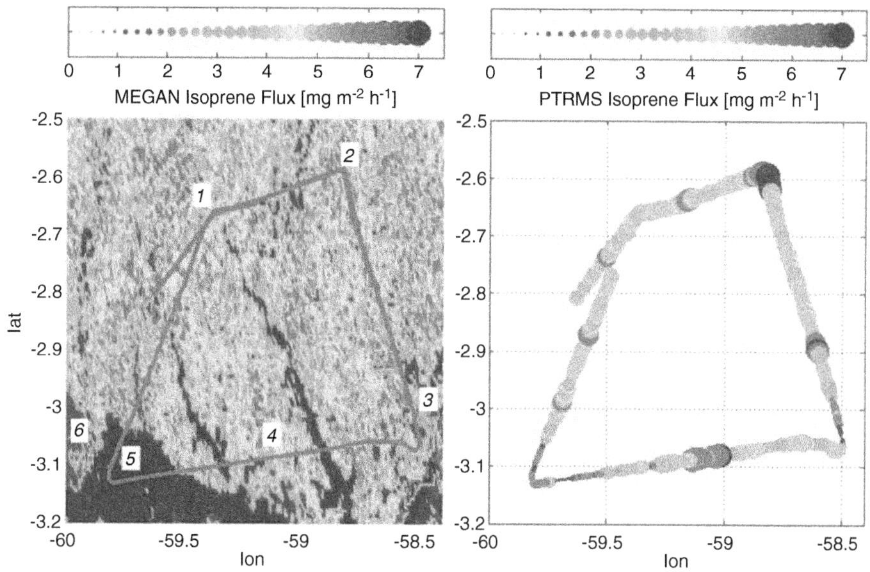

Fig. 7.10 Isoprene emission map generated for flight conditions from MEGAN (*left*) compared to airborne PTR-MS measurements (*right*). The *gray line* on the *left panel* depicts the flight track. Numbers *1–6* on the *left side* mark different land cover types: (*1*) mixed forest/plantation, (*2*) primary tropical forest, (*3*) soybean plantations, (*4*) mixed forest/plantation, (*5*) water, (*6*) Manaus urban region (Reproduced from Ref. [60] by permission. © The American Geophysical Union, 2007)

while other VOCs are in the ppbv range [55]. Isoprene, C_5H_8, and monoterpenes are important VOCs for modeling atmospheric chemistry in Amazonia [60]. The model of *emissions of gases and aerosols from nature* (MEGAN), estimates VOC fluxes and can describe the large observed variations associated with land-use change in the region of Manaus (Brasil). Airborne PTR-MS measurements of isoprene, detected as $[C_5H_9]^+$, *m/z* 69, were conducted by flying a racetrack pattern north-east of Manaus at constant altitude of 675 m above sea level. The racetrack of 320 km covered various landscapes such as primary forest, mixed water/forest, soybean plantations, and agricultural areas. In Fig. 7.9, the left panel depicts the isoprene emission map calculated from MEGAN, with the flight track plotted in gray. The right panel shows the surface flux calculated from airborne PRT-MS (Fig. 7.10) [60].

7.4 Charge Transfer Chemical Ionization

Charge transfer (CT) or *charge exchange* (CE) ionization occurs when an ion–neutral reaction takes place in which the ionic charge is transferred to the neutral [8]. In principle, any of the reagent systems discussed so far is capable of effecting

CT because the respective reagent molecular ions $X^{+\bullet}$ are also present in the plasma:

$$X^{+\bullet} + M \rightarrow M^{+\bullet} + X \tag{7.16}$$

With methane, isobutane, or ammonia, however, proton transfer is still prevailing. Therefore, reagent gases suitable for CT should exhibit abundant molecular ions even under the conditions of CI, whereas potentially protonating species have to be absent or at least of minor abundance.

CE or CE?
The acronym CE is also used for *capillary electrophoresis*, a separation method. CE may be coupled to a mass spectrometer via an electrospray interface (Chaps. 12 and 14), and thus CE-CI and CE-ESI-MS must not be confused. The term charge transfer (CT) avoids these ambiguities.

7.4.1 Energetics of CT

The energetics of CT is determined by the *ionization energy* of the neutral analyte, $IE_{(M)}$, and the *recombination energy* of the reagent ion, $RE_{(X+\bullet)}$. Recombination of an atomic or molecular ion with a free electron is the inverse of its ionization. $RE_{(X+\bullet)}$ is defined as the exothermicity of the gas phase reaction [7]:

$$X^{+\bullet} + e^{-} \rightarrow X \tag{7.17}$$

The recombination energy of the reagent ion $X^{+\bullet}$ is defined as the negative value of the corresponding heat of neutralization:

$$RE_{(X+\bullet)} = -\Delta H_r^{\,0} \tag{7.18}$$

For monoatomic ions, the *RE* has the same numeric value as the *IE* of the neutral; for diatomic or polyatomic species differences may occur due to storage of energy in internal modes or electronic excitation. Ionization of the analyte via CT is effected if [61]:

$$RE_{(X+\bullet)} - IE_{(M)} > 0 \tag{7.19}$$

Now, the heat of reaction, and thus the minimum internal energy of the analyte molecular ion, is given by [62]:

$$E_{int(M+\bullet)} \geq RE_{(X+\bullet)} - IE_{(M)} \tag{7.20}$$

(The $\geq$ sign indicates the additional contribution of thermal energy.) In summary, no CT is expected if $RE_{(X+\bullet)}$ is less than $IE_{(M)}$; $M^{+\bullet}$ ions are predominantly expected if

$RE_{(X+\bullet)}$ is slightly above $IE_{(M)}$; extensive fragmentation occurs if $RE_{(X+\bullet)}$ is notably greater than $IE_{(M)}$ [62]. Accordingly, the "softness" of CTCI can be adjusted by choosing a reagent gas of suitable *RE*. Fortunately, the differences between *RE*s and *IE*s are small, and unless highest accuracy is required, *IE* data may be used to estimate the effect of a CT reagent gas (Table 2.1).

CTCI mass spectra closely resemble low-energy EI spectra (Sect. 5.6) because molecular ions are formed upon CT. As the sensitivity of CTCI is superior to low-energy EI [61], CTCI may be preferred over low-energy EI. The degree of fragmentation in CTCI is generally reduced as compared to EI because:

- The ion internal energy of the molecular ions is lower according to Eq. 7.20.
- The energy distribution is narrower, i.e., the high energy tail of the ion internal energy distribution as present in EI is cut off in CTCI.
- Some collisional cooling of the incipient molecular ions can occur that is not available in the strictly unimolecular regime of EI.

7.4.2 Reagent Gases for CTCI

Numerous gases are employed for CTCI. Reagent gases such as hydrogen [25] or methane can also affect CT. Typically, pure compounds are employed as CT reagent gases, but occasionally they are diluted with nitrogen to act as an inert or sometimes reactive buffer gas (Table 7.3). Compared to protonating CI conditions,

Table 7.3 CTCI reagent gases [7, 62, 65–68, 72]

Reagent gas	Reagent ion	*RE* or *RE* range [eV]
$C_6H_5NH_2$	$C_6H_5NH_2^{+\bullet}$	7.7
C_6H_5Cl	$C_6H_5Cl^{+\bullet}$	9.0
C_6H_6	$C_6H_6^{+\bullet}$	9.2
$NO^\bullet : N_2 = 1 : 9$	NO^+	9.3
$C_6F_6 : CO_2 = 1 : 9$	$C_6F_6^{+\bullet}$	10.0
$CS_2 : N_2 = 1 : 9$	$CS_2^{+\bullet}$	9.5–10.2
H_2S	$H_2S^{+\bullet}$	10.5
$COS : CO = 1 : 9$	$COS^{+\bullet}$	11.2
Xe	$Xe^{+\bullet}$	12.1, 13.4
N_2O ($: N_2 = 1 : 9$)	$N_2O^{+\bullet}$	12.9
CO_2	$CO_2^{+\bullet}$	13.8
CO	$CO^{+\bullet}$	14.0
Kr	$Kr^{+\bullet}$	14.0, 14.7
N_2	$N_2^{+\bullet}$	15.3
H_2	$H_2^{+\bullet}$	15.4
Ar	$Ar^{+\bullet}$	15.8, 15.9
Ne	$Ne^{+\bullet}$	21.6, 21.7
He	$He^{+\bullet}$	24.6

the reagent gas is typically admitted at somewhat lower pressure (15–80 Pa). Primary electron energies are reported in the 100–600 eV range.

The major reagent gases for CTCI are:

- benzene [47, 63, 64],
- chlorobenzene [65],
- carbon disulfide [66, 67],
- carbon oxysulfide [66–70],
- carbon monoxide [62, 66, 68],
- nitrogen [66],
- nitrogen oxide [62, 71],
- dinitrogen oxide [67, 71],
- argon [66], and
- xenon [66, 68].

CTCI of cyclohexene We want to compare the CTCI spectra of cyclohexene with the according 70-eV EI spectrum. Different CT reagent gases show different degrees of fragmentation (Fig. 7.11) [73]. The relative intensity of the molecular ion increases as the RE of the reagent gas decreases. As the sensitivity of CTCI is superior to low-energy EI [61], CTCI may be preferred over low-energy EI.

7.4.3 Compound Class-Selective CTCI

The energy distribution upon CT largely differs from that obtained upon EI in that the CT process delivers an energetically well-defined ionization of the neutral. Choosing the appropriate reagent gas allows for the selective ionization of a targeted compound class contained in a complex mixture [61, 64, 65, 74]. The differentiation is possible due to the characteristic range of *IE*s for each compound class. This property of CE-CI can also be applied to construct breakdown graphs (Sect. 2.11) from a set of CE-CI mass spectra by using reagent ions of stepwise increasing $RE_{(X^{+\bullet})}$, e.g., $C_6F_6^{+\bullet}$, $CS_2^{+\bullet}$, $COS^{+\bullet}$, $Xe^{+\bullet}$, $N_2O^{+\bullet}$, $CO^{+\bullet}$, $N_2^{+\bullet}$ [68, 72].

CTCI of fuels CTCI allows for the direct determination of the molecular weight distributions of the major aromatic components in liquid fuels and other petroleum products [61, 65, 74]. The approach involves selective CT between $C_6H_5Cl^{+\bullet}$ and the substituted benzenes and naphthalenes in the sample. In this application, chlorobenzene also serves as the solvent for the fuel to avoid interferences with residual solvent. Thus, the paraffinic components present in the fuel can be suppressed in the resulting CE-CI mass spectra (Fig. 7.12) [65].

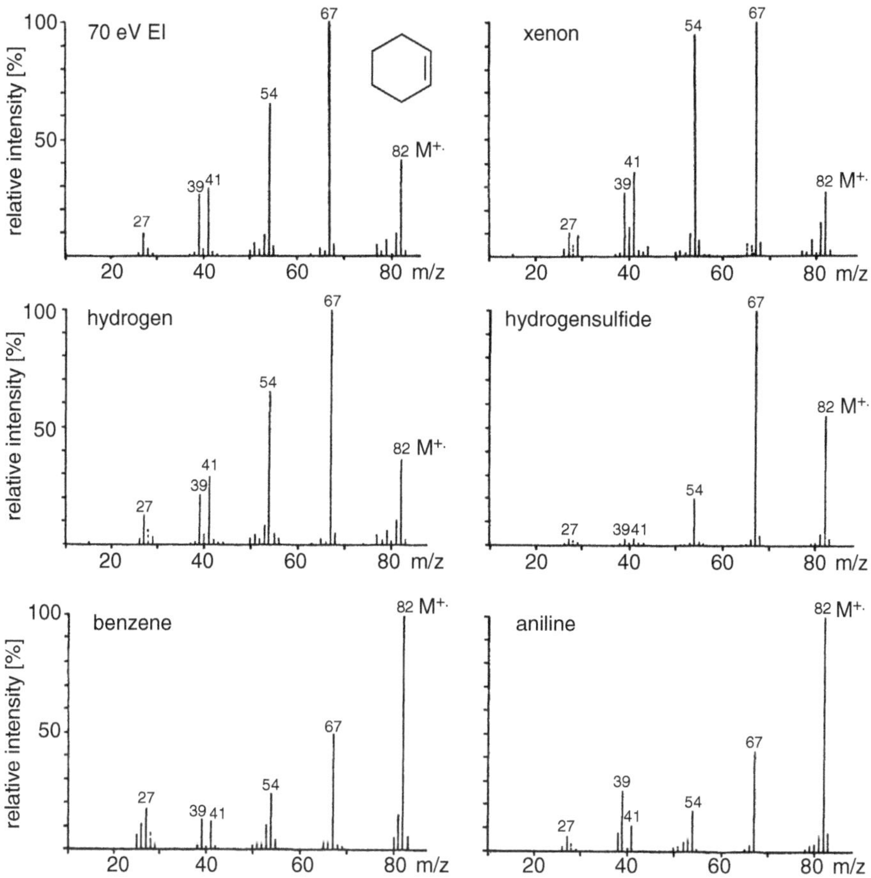

Fig. 7.11 Comparison of CTCI spectra of cyclohexene with that of the according 70-eV EI spectrum recorded with different reagent gases (Adapted from Ref. [73] by permission. © John Wiley & Sons, 1976)

7.4.4 Regio- and Stereoselectivity in CTCI

Small differences in activation energy, E_0, that exist between analogous fragmentations of regioisomers [66, 67, 69, 70] or stereoisomers do not cause significant differences in their 70-eV EI spectra. Pathways leading to a pair of different fragment ions cannot be distinguished, because minor differences in the respective *appearance energies* (*AE*s) are overridden by the excess energy of the fragmenting ions (Sect. 2.5). The situation changes if an energy-tunable ionization method is applied, which in addition offers a narrow internal energy distribution of the ions. Then, a significant alteration of relative intensities of a pair of fragments

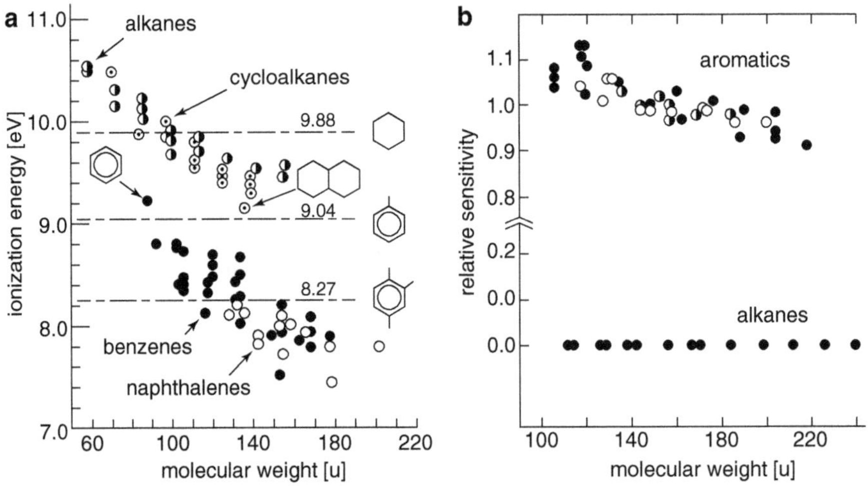

Fig. 7.12 (**a**) Ionization energies of certain classes of organic molecules as a function of their molecular weight, and (**b**) relative sensitivities for (○) alkylbenzenes, (●) polyolefines, and (◑) substituted naphthalenes in chlorobenzene CTCI (Adapted from Ref. [65] by permission. © American Chemical Society, 1983)

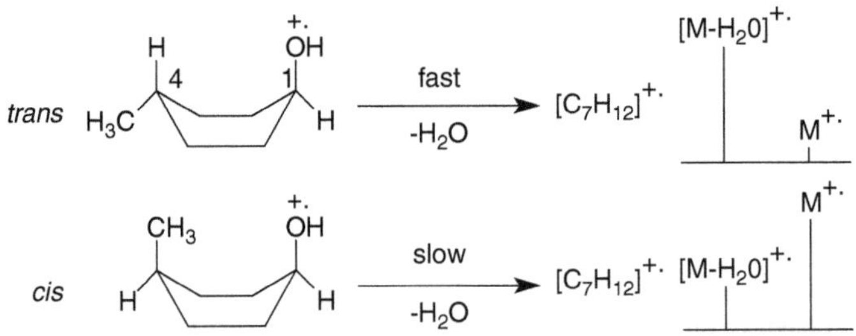

Scheme 7.2

could be effected if the appearance energies $AE_{(F1)}$ and $AE_{(F1')}$ of these fragments from isomeric precursors were just below $RE_{(x+\bullet)}$.

Distinguishing epimers In epimeric 4-methylcyclohexanols the methyl and the hydroxyl group can either both reside in axial position (*cis*) or one is equatorial and the other axial (*trans*). In the *trans* isomer, stereospecific 1,4–H_2O elimination should proceed easily (Sect. 6.11), while H_2O loss from the *cis* isomer is more demanding. CE-CI using $C_6F_6^{+\bullet}$ reagent ions clearly reveals the difference between these stereoisomers from the according $M^{+\bullet}/[M–H_2O]^{+\bullet}$ ratio determined as *trans* : *cis* = 0.09: 2.0 = 23) [72] (Scheme 7.2).

7.5 Negative-Ion Chemical Ionization

In any CI plasma, ions of both polarities, positive *and* negative, are formed simultaneously, e.g., $[M+H]^+$ and $[M–H]^-$ ions, and it is just a matter of the polarity of the acceleration voltage which ions are going to be extracted from the ion source [75]. Thus, from a technical point of view, *negative-ion chemical ionization* (NICI) [76] mass spectra can readily be obtained.

As in PICI, there are also several pathways in NICI leading to the formation of negative ions [77–80]. First, in case of acidic molecules, such as carboxylic acids [81], diimides, or phenols, there is dissociation leading to *deprotonation*:

$$M \rightarrow [M-H]^- + H^+ \tag{7.21}$$

While deprotonation can occur spontaneously, the presence of a proton-accepting base, B, either delivered by some species of the reagent gas or by the excess of other analyte neutrals (cf. autoprotonation, Sect. 7.2.1) accelerates the process:

$$M + B \rightarrow [M-H]^- + [BH]^+ \tag{7.21a}$$

Second, *nucleophilic addition*, i.e., anion attachment, can occur:

$$M + A^- \rightarrow [M+A]^- \tag{7.22}$$

Third, *ion-pair formation*, induced by direct interaction with an energetic electron (Sect. 2.1), can also play a role:

$$M + e^- \rightarrow [M-B]^- + B^+ + e^- \tag{7.23}$$

Nonetheless, ion-pair formation is generally the energetically least favorable process. Each of these processes delivers even-electron analyte anions.

Nucleophilic addition The NICI mass spectrum of tetraiodoethene, $I_2C=CI_2$, has been obtained using isobutane reagent gas (Fig. 7.13). The negative molecular ion, $M^{-\bullet}$, at *m/z* 531.6 has a relative intensity of just 0.15%, while the product of nucleophilic addition, $[M+I]^-$, *m/z* 658.5, yields the base peak [82]. Losses of $I^\bullet$ and I_2 from $M^{-\bullet}$ are also observed. The series of peaks at *m/z* 126.9, 253.8, and 380.7 corresponds to traces of iodine present as impurity of tetraiodoethene. The iodine is also ionized by both electron capture (EC, next paragraph) and iodide addition. The spectrum nicely exemplifies the superimposition of mass spectra of two components of a mixture. It is not always simple to tell the corresponding peaks apart; accurate mass measurements or tandem mass spectrometry may be required. It is worth noting the mass defect introduced by the iodine and the ^{13}C isotopic peak of merely 2% due to only two carbon atoms present.

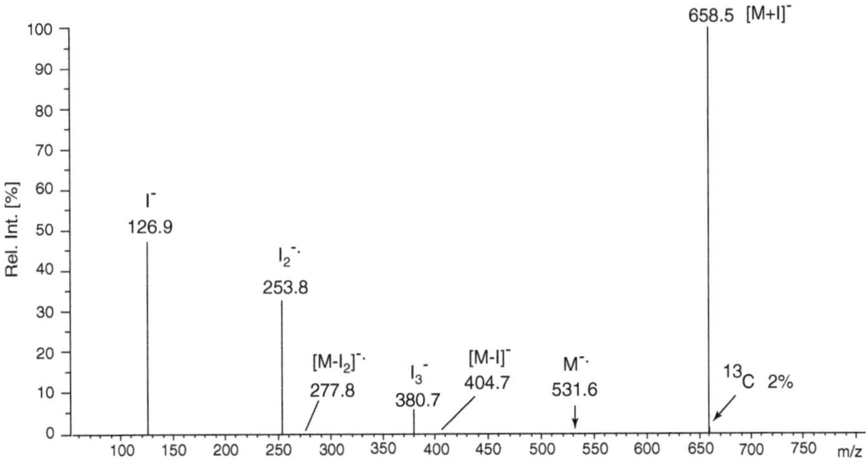

Fig. 7.13 NICI mass spectrum of tetraiodoethene (isobutane reagent gas, electron emission 300 μA at 200 eV, and ion source temperature of 200 °C) (Adapted from Ref. [82] with permission. © Wiley-VCH, Weinheim, 2007)

Competitors to classical NICI
Over the last decade, NICI applications have diminished because these analyses have mostly been carried out by negative-ion *atmospheric pressure chemical ionization* (APCI, Sect. 7.8). APCI is compatible with liquid chromatography (Chap. 14) and can readily be implemented on instruments with electrospray ionization interface (ESI, Chap. 12). Such instruments have an enormous market share, and thus, it is often more convenient and economic to switch between ESI and APCI as required. APCI will be dealt with a the end of this chapter.

7.6 Electron Capture Negative Ionization

There is one further process of negative-ion formation: *electron capture* (EC) or *electron attachment* [76]. EC is a resonance process whereby an electron of low kinetic energy is incorporated into an orbital of an atom or molecule [8]. The method employing this process is termed *electron capture negative ionization* (ECNI). Electron capture negative ionization is of special interest, because it provides superior sensitivity towards many toxic and/or environmentally relevant substances [83–87].

Strictly speaking, ECNI is not a subtype of NICI because the electrons are not provided by a reagent ion. In ECNI, the reagent gas solely serves as a moderator to decelerate the energetic electrons injected from the filament to close to thermal energy. Nonetheless, the ion source conditions to achieve ECNI are the same as for NICI. In fact, the processes discussed in Eqs. 7.21, 7.22, and 7.23 often compete with EC, and thus, characteristics of NICI and ECNI can simultaneously appear in mass spectra [88].

7.6.1 Ion Formation by Electron Capture

When a neutral molecule interacts with an electron of high kinetic energy, the positive radical ion is generated by EI. If the electrons have less energy than the *IE* of the respective neutral, EI is prohibited. As the electrons approach thermal energy, EC can occur instead. Under EC conditions, there are three different processes of ion formation [78, 89–92].

First, *resonance electron capture* yields the negative molecular ion, $M^{-\bullet}$:

$$M + e^{-} \rightarrow M^{-\bullet} \tag{7.24}$$

Second, *dissociative electron capture* can result in fragment ion formation by immediate loss of a radical from the incipient molecular radical anion:

$$M + e^{-} \rightarrow [M - A]^{-} + A^{\bullet} \tag{7.25}$$

Third, *ion-pair formation* can also occur:

$$M + e^{-} \rightarrow [M - B]^{-} + B^{+} + e^{-} \tag{7.26}$$

Molecular radical anions, $M^{-\bullet}$, are generated by capture of electrons with 0–2 eV kinetic energy, whereas fragment ions are generated by capture of electrons from 0 to 15 eV. Ion pair formation tends to occur when electron energies exceed 10 eV [91]. Odd-electron molecular anions are exclusively formed by resonance electron capture, whereas even-electron fragment ions are formed by dissociative electron capture and ion-pair formation.

7.6.2 Energetics of Electron Capture

The potential energy curves of a neutral molecule AB and the potential ionic products from Eqs. 7.24, 7.25, and 7.26 are compared below (Fig. 7.14). These graphs reveal that the formation of negative molecular ions, $AB^{-\bullet}$, is energetically more favorable than homolytic bond dissociation of AB and that the $AB^{-\bullet}$ ions have internal energies close to the activation energy for dissociation [76, 78, 89]. The negative molecular ions from EC are therefore definitely less excited than their positive counterparts from 70-eV EI.

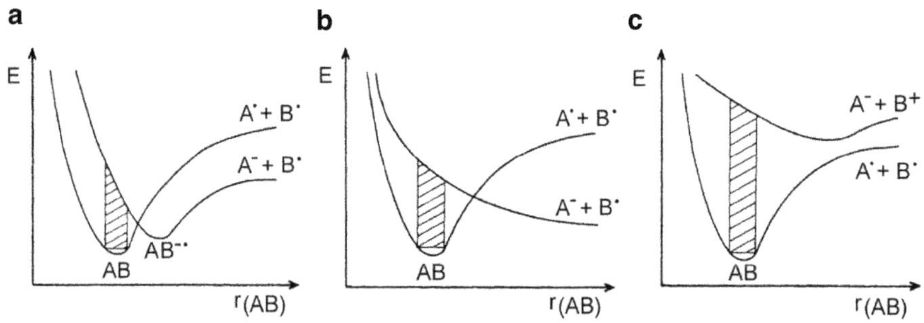

Fig. 7.14 Energetics of (**a**) resonance electron capture, (**b**) dissociative electron capture, and (**c**) ion-pair formation (Adapted from Ref. [89] by permission. © John Wiley & Sons, 1981)

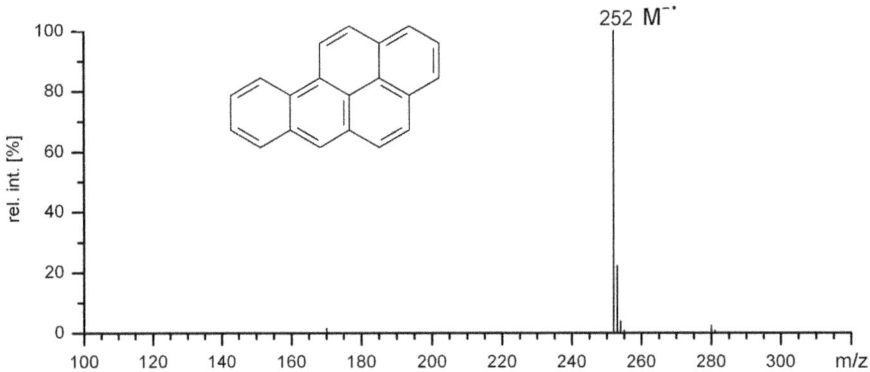

Fig. 7.15 EC spectrum of benzo[a]pyrene (isobutane buffer gas, ion source 200 °C). The two additional minor signals correspond to impurities of the sample

EC of benzo[a]pyrene The EC mass spectrum of benzo[a]pyrene, $C_{20}H_{12}$, shows the negative molecular ion exclusively at *m/z* 252 (Fig. 7.15). This spectrum is representative for EC spectra of *polycyclic aromatic hydrocarbons* (PAHs) [93, 94]. One particular PAH, fluoranthene, has recently received much attention as its $M^{-\bullet}$ ion serves as electron donating reagent ion in *electron transfer dissociation* (ETD, Sect. 9.15).

The energetics of the EC process $M + e^- \rightarrow M^{-\bullet}$ (Eq. 7.24) are determined by the *electron affinity* (*EA*) of the neutral. The electron affinity is the negative of the enthalpy of the attachment of a zero kinetic energy electron to a neutral molecule or atom:

$$-\Delta H_r = EA_{(M)} \tag{7.27}$$

Just like the *IE* of a molecule is governed by the atom of lowest *IE* within that neutral (Sect. 2.1), the *EA* of a molecule is basically determined by the atom of

Table 7.4 Selected electron affinities [97]

Compound	*EA* [eV]	Compound	*EA* [eV]
Carbon dioxide	–0.600	Pentachlorobenzene	0.729
Naphthalene	–0.200	Tetrachloromethane	0.805
Acetone	0.002	Biphenylene	0.890
1,2-Dichlorobenzene	0.094	Nitrobenzene	1.006
Benzonitrile	0.256	Octafluorocyclobutane	1.049
Molecular oxygen	0.451	Pentafluorobenzonitrile	1.084
Carbon disulfide	0.512	2-Nitronaphthalene	1.184
Benzo[e]pyrene	0.534	1-Bromo-4-nitrobenzene	1.292
Tetrachloroethylene	0.640	Antimony pentafluoride	1.300

highest electronegativity. This is why analytes with halogens, in particular fluorine and chlorine, as well as with nitro groups make attractive candidates for EC (Table 7.4) [95]. If EC occurs with a neutral of negative *EA*, the electron–molecule complex will have a short lifetime (*autodetachment*), but in case of positive *EA* a negative molecular ion can persist.

Dissociative EC Consider the dissociative EC process $CF_2Cl_2 + e^- \rightarrow F^- + CFCl_2^{\bullet}$ and let the potential energy of CF_2Cl_2 be zero. The homolytic bond dissociation energy $D_{(F\text{–}CFCl2)}$ has been calculated as 4.93 eV. Now, the potential energy of the products is 4.93 eV less the electron affinity of a fluorine atom ($EA_{(F\bullet)} = 3.45$ eV), i.e., the process is endothermic by 1.48 eV. The experimental *AE* of the fragments is 1.80 eV. This yields a minimum excess energy of 0.32 eV (Fig. 7.16) [96].

7.6.3 Creating Thermal Electrons

Thermionic emission from a heated metal filament is the standard source of free electrons. However, after acceleration into the ion source, those electrons usually carry 10–200 eV rather than thermal energy (0.1–1 eV) and need to be decelerated for EC. Buffer gases such as methane, isobutane, or carbon dioxide serve well for that purpose, but others have also been used [77, 88, 98]. These gases do not form negative ions themselves while effectively moderating the energetic electrons to thermal energy [84]. Despite inverse polarity of the extraction voltage, the same conditions as for PICI in terms of buffer gas pressure, ion source temperature, and energy of primary electrons can usually be applied. Lowering the ion source temperature provides lower-energy electrons, e.g., assuming a Maxwell-Boltzmann energy distribution the mean electron energy is 0.068 eV at 250 °C and 0.048 eV at 100 °C [84].

Alternatively to direct supply from a heated filament, electrons of well-defined low energy can be delivered into the ion volume by an electron monochromator [92, 96, 99–101].

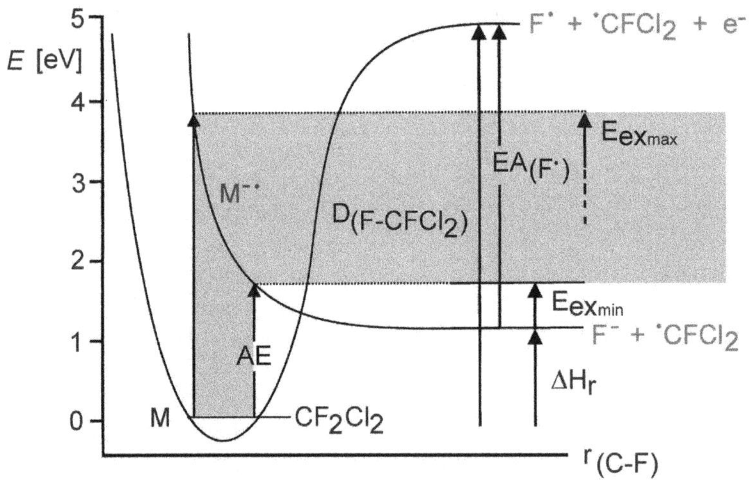

Fig. 7.16 Potential energy diagram of the dissociative EC process of dichloro-difluoromethane. The molecular radical anion (*blue*) does not possess a minimum on the energy surface but immediately dissociates via $CF_2Cl_2 + e^- \rightarrow F^- + CFCl_2^{\bullet}$ (*green products*), whereas the competing formation of two radicals is outside the energy window (*red products*)

NICI and ECNI in practice

Both NICI and ECNI are comparatively sensitive to ion source conditions [80, 100]. The actual ion source temperature, the buffer gas, the amount of sample introduced, and ion source contaminations each play important roles. Regular cleaning of the ion source is important [85]. It much depends on the actual analyte and instrument setting which of the competing processes outlined in Eqs. 7.21, 7.22, 7.23, 7.24, 7.25, and 7.26 finally prevails. Interlaboratory comparisons of NICI and ECNI spectra are therefore not as reliable as in case of 70-eV EI spectra.

7.6.4 Appearance of ECNI Spectra

ECNI spectra generally exhibit strong molecular ions and no primary fragment ions (Fig. 7.15) or in some cases just a few (Fig. 7.17). As $M^{-\bullet}$ is an odd-electron species, homolytic bond cleavages as well as rearrangement fragmentations may occur. Apart from the opposite charge, there are close similarities to the fragmentation pathways of positive molecular ions (Chap. 6) [80, 90, 91].

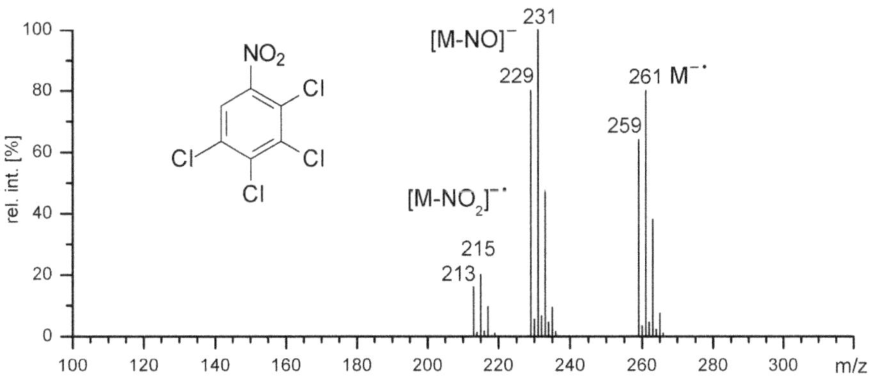

Fig. 7.17 Methane EC spectrum of 2,3,4,5-tetrachloronitrobenzene (Redrawn from Ref. [91] by permission. © John Wiley & Sons, 1988)

ECNI spectrum of PFK Perfluorokerosine (PFK), a mixture of numerous perfluorinated compounds, is frequently employed as mass calibrant in EI where it delivers spectra that almost exclusively represent $[C_nF_{2n-1}]^+$ fragment ions like $[C_5F_9]^+$, *m/z* 231 (Sect. 3.6.2). In ECNI, the situation changes because low-energy molecular anions are formed, a large fraction of which does not undergo fragmentation (Fig. 7.18). Roughly the upper half of the ECNI spectrum of PFK is thus made up by peaks at even *m/z* values while the lower half shows $[C_nF_{2n-1}]^-$ fragment ions fragment ion peaks of similar intensity at odd *m/z* values, e.g., $[C_5F_9]^-$, *m/z* 231, or $[C_6F_{11}]^-$, *m/z* 281 (cf. nitrogen rule, Sect. 6.2.7). The peak at *m/z* 153.1 is caused by residual nitrobenzyl alcohol that had been used the previous day as a matrix in fast atom bombardment (Chap. 10) on this instrument.

7.6.5 Applications of ECNI

ECNI, especially when combined with GC-MS (Sects. 14.2, 14.3, and 14.4), is commonly used in the monitoring of halogenated compounds and nitrocompounds as often represented in environmental pollutants such as dioxins [96, 100, 101], pesticides [96], halogenated metabolites [86], food contaminants [102, 103], DNA adducts [95], explosives [79, 104, 105], and others [83, 84, 106–108].

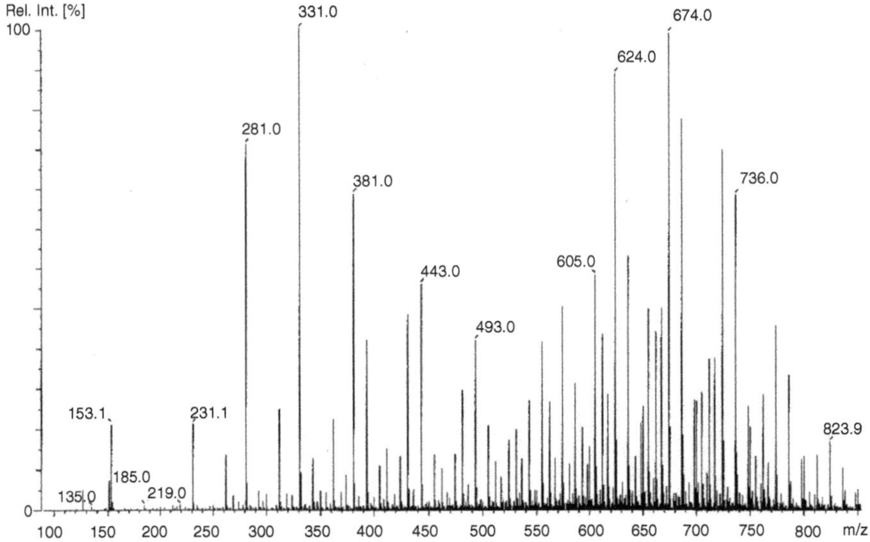

Fig. 7.18 ECNI spectrum of perfluorokerosene (PFK) as obtained with isobutane buffer gas. While fragment ions prevail in the lower half of the *m/z* range, molecular ions of the numerous constituents are characteristic of the upper half

7.7 Desorption Chemical Ionization

In CI, the analyte is generally introduced into the ion source via *direct insertion probe* (DIP), *gas chromatograph* (GC), or *reservoir inlet* (Sect. 5.2). However, CI can also be used in conjunction with sample introduction by a *direct exposure probe* (DEP). This is known as *desorption chemical ionization* (DCI) [34, 109, 110]. In DCI, the analyte is applied from solution or suspension to the outside of a thin resistively heated wire loop or coil. Then, the analyte is directly exposed to the reagent gas plasma while being rapidly heated at rates of several hundred °C s^{-1} and to temperatures up to about 1500 °C (Sect. 5.2). The analytical result depends on the actual shape of the wire, the sample application method, and the heating rate [111, 112]. The rapid heating of the sample plays an important role in promoting molecular species rather than pyrolysis products [113]. In contrast to *desorption electron ionization* (DEI), DCI is more frequently applied [112, 114–116]. An appropriate experimental setup provided, accurate mass measurements can be achieved in DCI mode [117].

Pyrolysis DCI of cellulose The pyrolysis (Py) DCI mass spectrum of cellulose, H$(C_6H_{10}O_5)_n$OH, as acquired using NH_3 reagent gas, 100 eV of electron energy, and scanning *m/z* 140–700 at 2 s per cycle shows a series of distinct signals. The peaks are separated by 162 u, i.e., by $C_6H_{10}O_5$ saccharide units. The main signals are due

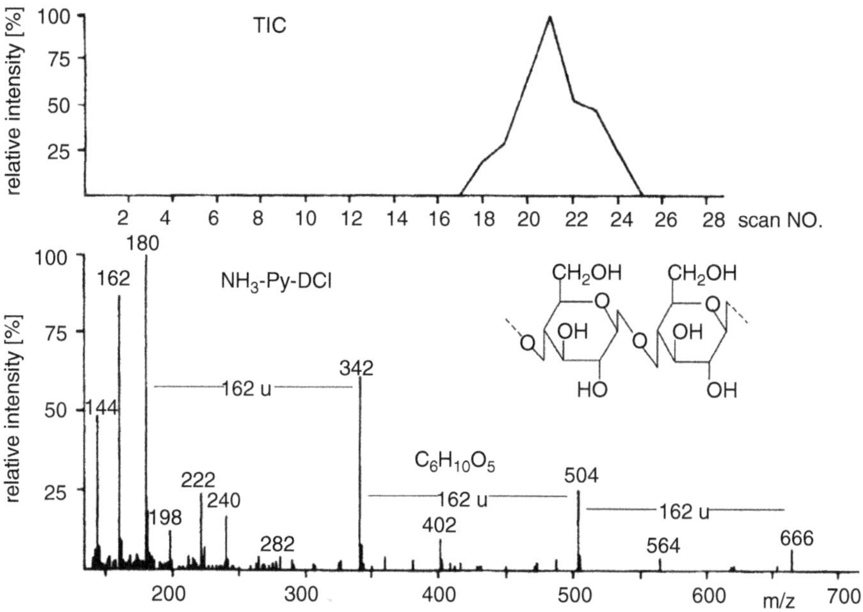

Fig. 7.19 Ammonia-Py-DCI mass spectrum of cellulose and total ion current (Adapted from Ref. [111] by permission. © Research Council of Canada, 1994)

to ions from anhydro-oligosaccharides, $[(C_6H_{10}O_5)_n+NH_4]^+$, formed upon heating of the cellulose in the ammonia CI plasma (Fig. 7.19) [111].

Other terms

Although *desorption chemical ionization* being the correct term [112], DCI is sometimes referred to as *direct CI*, *direct exposure CI*, *in-beam CI*, or even *surface ionization*. Nowadays, DCI is rarely used, because in most instances one of the various desorption/ionization methods serves the purpose much better (Chaps. 8, 10, 11, 12 and 13).

7.8 Atmospheric Pressure Chemical Ionization

Up to this point, we have exclusively dealt with ionization in (high) vacuum. The attempt for online mass spectrometric detection for liquid chromatographic separations (Sects. 14.1 and 14.5) initiated the development of a wealth of ionization methods and interfaces permitting ionization at atmospheric pressure to be directly and continuously attached to high vacuum mass analyzers.

7.8.1 Atmospheric Pressure Ionization

Atmospheric pressure ionization (API) was the first technique to directly connect solution phase analyte supply with a mass analyzer [118]. In API, a dilute solution of the analyte is injected at atmospheric pressure into a stream of hot nitrogen (≈200 °C) to rapidly evaporate the solvent. The vapor passes through a tube bearing radioactive ^{63}Ni, a β emitter (Fig. 7.20). The electrons emitted by ^{63}Ni induce a complex sequence of reactions finally delivering reagent ions for chemical ionization. Thus, starting with the ionization of N_2, consecutive ion–molecule reactions eventually lead to the formation of $[(H_2O)_n+H]^+$ cluster ions:

$$N_2 + e^- \rightarrow N_2^{+\bullet} + 2e^- \tag{7.28}$$

$$N_2^{+\bullet} + N_2 + N_{2(3rd\ body)} \rightarrow N_4^{+\bullet} + N_{2(3rd\ body)} \tag{7.29}$$

$$N_4^{+\bullet} + H_2O \rightarrow H_2O^{+\bullet} + 2N_2 \tag{7.30}$$

$$H_2O^{+\bullet} + H_2O \rightarrow H_3O^+ + OH^\bullet \tag{7.31}$$

$$H_3O^+ + H_2O \rightarrow \left[(H_2O)_2 + H\right]^+ \tag{7.32}$$

Here, only the first step of $[(H_2O)_n+H]^+$ cluster ion formation is explicitly formulated. As the *PA* of H_2O (697 kJ mol^{-1}) is essentially below that of any

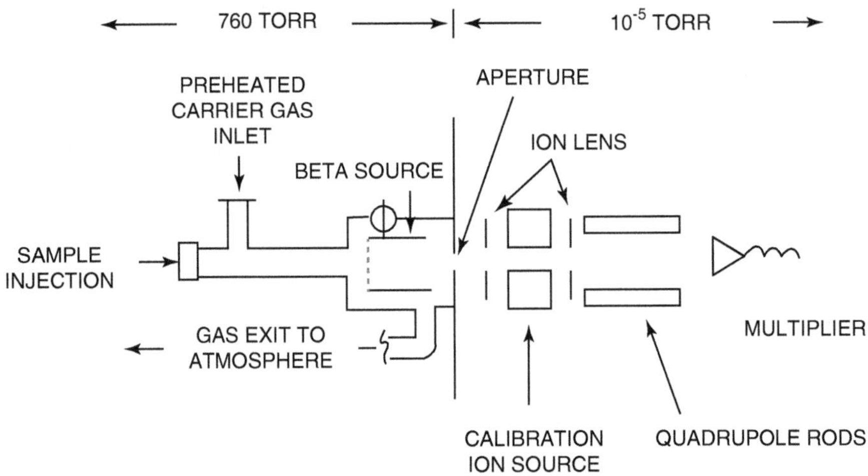

Fig. 7.20 The original implementation of API. Here, primary electrons are delivered by a ^{63}Ni foil. For API, the filament of the EI calibration source was switched off and only the electrostatic lenses where used to pass the ions into the quadrupole mass analyzer chosen for its tolerance to moderate vacuum conditions (Reproduced from Ref. [118] with permission. © The American Chemical Society, 1973)

organic molecule that could be of interest as potential analyte (Table 2.6), water cluster ions protonate the analyte molecules by a chemical ionization process at atmospheric pressure [118–120]:

$$[H_2O)_n + H]^+ + M \rightarrow [M + H]^+ + nH_2O \tag{7.33}$$

Always the same reaction
Did you notice that the reaction $H_2O^{+\bullet} + H_2O \rightarrow H_3O^+ + OH^\bullet$ (Eq. 7.31) follows the same pattern as does the reaction $CH_4^{+\bullet} + CH_4 \rightarrow CH_5^+ + CH_3^\bullet$ (Eq. 7.6) that is relevant for PICI using methane reagent gas? In fact, this general reaction, $M^{+\bullet} + M \rightarrow [M+H]^+ + [M-H]^\bullet$, is observed whenever a molecular ion is formed in an excess of neutral molecules of the same species, provided the number of collisions during its lifetime permits ion–molecule reactions to occur.

7.8.2 Atmospheric Pressure Chemical Ionization

Ion sources using a radioactive ^{63}Ni foil are not ideally suitable for the common laboratory as the occasional need for abrasive cleaning of the source inevitably leads to radioactive contamination. The Horning group thus refined API by replacing ^{63}Ni, the primary source of ionization, with a corona discharge [121, 122]. The reagent ion plasma is now maintained by a corona discharge between the sharp tip of a needle and the spray chamber walls serving as the counter electrode. The improved technique providing enhanced primary ion formation was termed *atmospheric pressure chemical ionization* (APCI). Basically, APCI represents an atmospheric-pressure variant of "classical" vacuum chemical ionization. In contrast to CI, ion–molecule reactions occurring at atmospheric pressure are employed for analyte ion production.

Nebulization of the analyte solution is effected by action of the pneumatic nebulizer. The transformation of the aerosol into a vapor composed of solvent and highly diluted sample is then performed in a heater cartridge set to about 500 °C (Fig. 7.21).

In APCI, the ions are transferred into the mass analyzer by use of the same atmosphere-to-vacuum interface as employed in electrospray ionization (ESI), the design of which will be pointed out along with the development of ESI (Sect. 12.2). As a benefit, ESI sources can easily be switched to APCI operation. To do so, the ESI spray head is exchanged for a unit comprising a pneumatic nebulizer and a heated spray chamber with a needle electrode mounted in front of the sampling orifice, while the atmosphere-to-vacuum interface stays in place [123–125].

Older APCI sources require a liquid flow of 200–1000 μl min^{-1} for effective vaporization and ionization. While this is fine for liquid chromatography coupling,

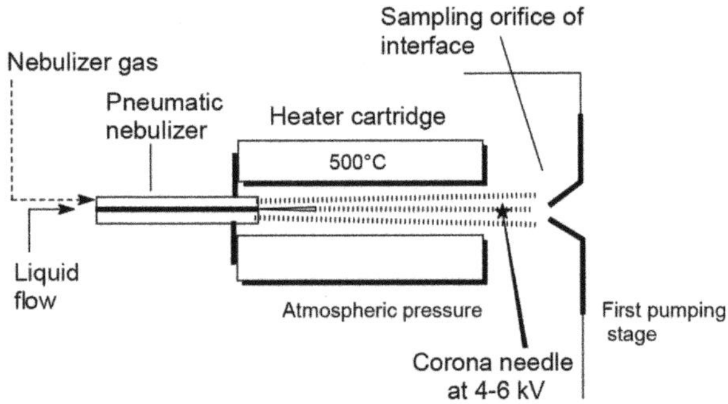

Fig. 7.21 APCI source. The liquid flow is pneumatically sprayed into a heated vaporizer where ionization is initiated by a corona discharge at atmospheric pressure. The atmospheric pressure-to-vacuum interface serves appropriately for all types of API techniques without any alterations

direct injection using a syringe pump is hampered by such a high flow. More recent APCI source designs also permit stable operation using a liquid flow of just 5–20 μl min^{-1}. Typical corona discharge currents are in the order of 10 μA, and thus, the blueish discharge is only visible in virtual darkness (Fig. 7.22).

API techniques
Atmospheric pressure ionization as originally devised in 1973 has never been widely applied as it was almost immediately replaced by atmospheric pressure chemical ionization. Nonetheless, *atmospheric pressure ionization* has survived as a collective term to encompass the manifold ionization methods employing analyte ion formation at atmospheric pressure.

7.8.3 Positive Ion Formation in APCI

Apart from initiation by a corona discharge, the pathway of reagent ion formation in APCI follows the route just discussed in API:

$$\text{corona discharge} + N_2 \rightarrow N_2^{+\bullet} + e^- \tag{7.34}$$

$$N_2^{+\bullet} + N_2 + N_{2(\text{3rd body})} \rightarrow N_4^{+\bullet} + N_{2(\text{3rd body})} \tag{7.35}$$

$$N_4^{+\bullet} + H_2O \rightarrow 2N_2 + H_2O^{+\bullet} \tag{7.36}$$

Ion–molecule reactions are fast at atmospheric pressure because collision rates are in the order of $10^9\ \text{s}^{-1}$. Seemingly bimolecular reactions can in fact be termolecular, because a neutral collision partner like N_2 in Eq. 7.35 is required for immediate removal of excess energy (Table 7.5) [126–128].

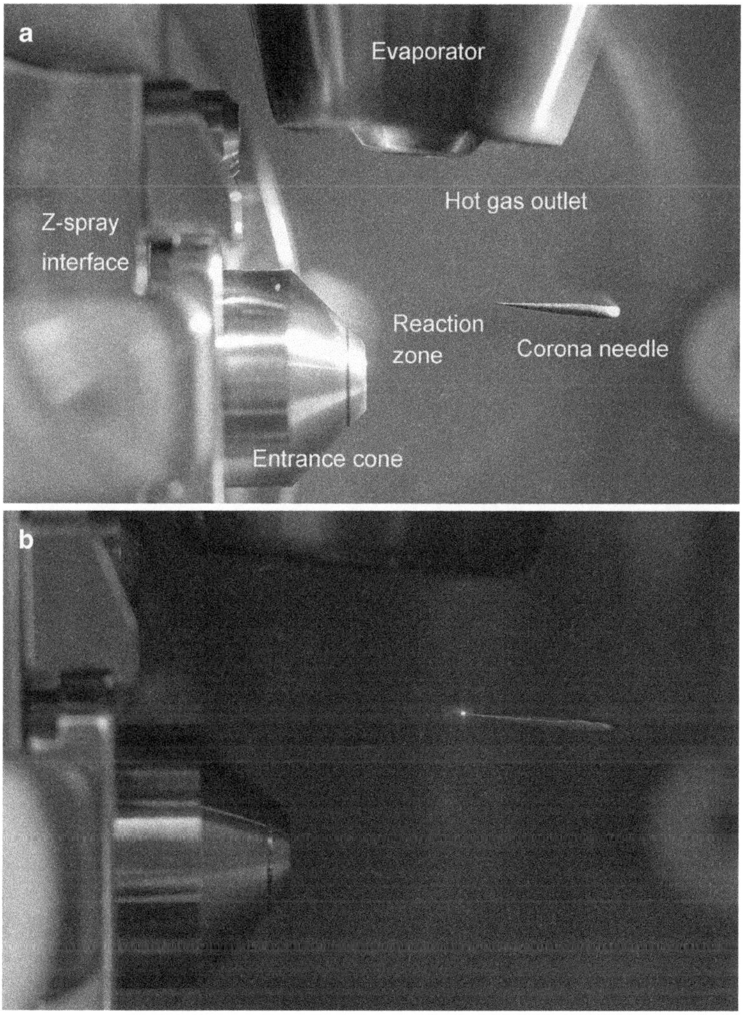

Fig. 7.22 APCI source of a Waters SQD2 instrument attached to a Z-spray interface. (**a**) APCI source as seen in daylight, (**b**) shaded source in operation. The blueish corona discharge corresponding to about 10 μA discharge current at the tip of the needle is only visible in virtual darkness

Table 7.5 Comparison of typical conditions and occurrence of elementary processes in atmospheric pressure ionization and vacuum ionization techniques

Parameter or reaction	API methods	Vacuum ionization
Pressure	1000 mbar	10^{-6} mbar
Mean free molecular path	100 nm	100 m
Hard sphere collision number	10^9 s^{-1}	1 s^{-1}
Number density of O_2	10^{14}–10^{18} molecules cm^{-3}	10^4–10^7 molecules cm^{-3}
Number density of H_2O	10^{13}–10^{16} molecules cm^{-3}	10^3–10^6 molecules cm^{-3}
Source residence time of ions	10 ms to 1 s	1 µs
Unimolecular decay of ions	None to rarely	Yes
Bimolecular reactions	Yes	No
Termolecular reactions	Yes	No

Next, the $H_2O^{+\bullet}$ ions rapidly form cluster ions:

$$H_2O^{+\bullet} + H_2O \rightarrow H_3O^+ + OH^\bullet \tag{7.37}$$

$$H_3O^+ + nH_2O \rightarrow \left[(H_2O)_n + H\right]^+ \tag{7.38}$$

The $[(H_2O)_n + H]^+$ ions then act as reagent ions [127]:

$$M + \left[(H_2O)_n + H\right]^+ \rightarrow [M + H]^+ + nH_2O \tag{7.39}$$

The concentration of water in the actual atmosphere of the reaction zone as well as the dwell time exert a strong influence on the $[(H_2O)_n + H]^+$ cluster ion distribution (Fig. 7.23) [128]. The relative contribution of the individual $[(H_2O)_n + H]^+$ cluster ions on the process of analyte ion formation may thus be subject to wide variation.

Ammonium adducts are frequent in APCI of medium polar compounds. $[M+NH_4]^+$ ions are observed, for example, with oxygen-rich molecules, in particular in absence of basic functional groups, e.g., polyethylene glycols, ketones, di-or triacylglycerols, and polysiloxanes:

$$M + [NH_4]^+ \rightarrow [M + NH_4]^+ \tag{7.40}$$

Ammonium ions may be delivered along with the sample or can be formed from trace amounts of ammonia in the atmosphere.

Common reaction scheme

The same sequence of reactions, although initiated by different sources of primary ionization, is observed not only in APCI but also in *atmospheric pressure photoionization* (APPI, Sect. 7.9) and *direct analysis in real time* (Sect. 13.8) [127, 129].

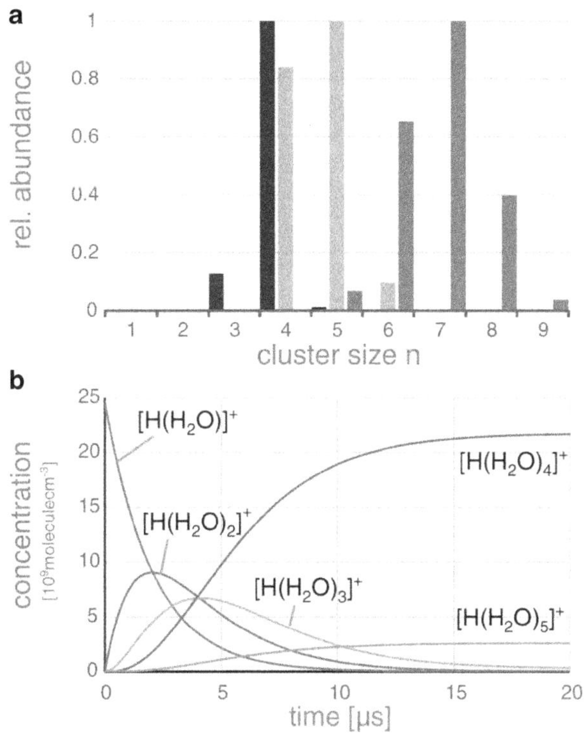

Fig. 7.23 (**a**) Bar graph representing the relative $[(H_2O)_n + H]^+$ cluster ion distribution for $n = 1–9$ in the presence of 1 ppm (v/v, *black*), 100 ppm (v/v, *light grey*), and 1 ‰ (v/v, *dark grey*) H_2O mixing ratio at 1000 mbar. (**b**) Temporal evolution of the concentrations of $[(H_2O)_n + H]^+$ cluster ions when starting H_3O^+ at a mixing ratio of 1 ppt as the only initial charged species present. Water background mixing ratio 10 ppm, $p =$ 1000 mbar. Clusters with $n =$ 6–9 are not discernible on this scale (Reproduced from Ref. [128] with permission. © Springer, 2014)

7.8.4 Negative-Ion Formation in APCI

All ionization processes known of NICI may occur in negative-ion formation in APCI, depending on the analyte. Oxygen is an important player as it easily forms $O_2^{-\bullet}$ reagent ions by electron capture [126, 127]:

$$O_2 + e^- \rightarrow O_2^{-\bullet} \tag{7.41}$$

These $O_2^{-\bullet}$ ions form adducts by association with the analyte M:

$$O_2^{-\bullet} + M \rightarrow [M + O_2]^{-\bullet} \tag{7.42}$$

Alternatively, negative molecular ions directly formed by electron capture can attach to molecular oxygen, thereby yielding the same product:

$$M^{-\bullet} + O_2 \rightarrow [M + O_2]^{-\bullet} \tag{7.43}$$

$[M + O_2]^{-\bullet}$ may either be detected as such or may dissociate to yield radical anions:

$$[M + O_2]^{-\bullet} \rightarrow M^{-\bullet} + O_2 \tag{7.44}$$

The latter dissociation requires $EA_M > EA_{O2}$, as oxygen would otherwise retain the electron.

The loss of a hydroperoxyl radical may lead to $[M - H]^-$ ions, i.e., proton abstraction, if the gas phase acidity of $[M - H]^-$ exceeds that of $HOO^{\bullet}$:

$$[M + O_2]^{-\bullet} \rightarrow [M - H]^- + HOO^{\bullet} \tag{7.45}$$

Halogenide ions can also play a role in analyte ion formation:

$$M + Hal^- \rightarrow [M + Hal]^- \tag{7.46}$$

Halogenide adducts can be observed when the analyte and/or a solvent are halogenated. Finally, adduct ion formation can occur with less abundant anions such as CO_3^-, NO_2^-, or OH^-.

7.8.5 APCI Spectra

The nature of the APCI plasma varies widely as both solvent and nebulizing gas contribute to the composition of the CI plasma, and thus, APCI spectra can resemble PICI, CTCI, NICI, or ECNI spectra depending on the actual conditions and ion polarity. The influence of solvent components, temperature, and other parameters explains why APCI conditions suffer from comparatively low reproducibility as compared to other ionization methods.

The heater cartridge typically operated at around 500 °C may lead to the impression of APCI as being a harsh ionization technique. However, the opposite is true. The softness of APCI even exceeds that of "classical" CI in the vacuum environment. The reasons for this apparent softness of APCI are numerous:

- The temperature of the aerosol droplets stays at the boiling temperature of the solvent until evaporation is complete. Thus, the temperature essentially remains below 70–100 °C and only rises to about 150–200 °C towards the exit of the heater cartridge.
- All excess energy of freshly formed analyte ions is effectively dissipated into the surrounding gas, because at atmospheric pressure, 10^6 ion–neutral collisions per millisecond guarantee immediate thermalization (Table 7.5) [128].
- Thermal energy at 150–200 °C is only about 0.1–0.2 eV, while bond breaking normally requires 2–3 eV.

- Decomposition rates at low internal energy are far too slow to permit a high amount of fragmentation within the few milliseconds between nebulization and entry into the interface.

APCI spectra are therefore characterized by no or at least a very moderate level of fragmentation.

The greatest advantage of APCI over ESI is that it actively generates ions from neutrals. Thus, APCI provides mass spectrometry with the means of applying low- to medium-polarity analytes eluting from a liquid chromatograph [130]. The use of APCI rapidly expanded in the mid-1990, perhaps because by then elaborate vacuum interfaces had become available from ESI technology. Nowadays, APCI is used where LC separation is required, but ESI is not applicable to the compound class of interest [130–133]. A set of typical APCI spectra is provided below.

Positive-ion APCI of triacylglycerols Liquid chromatographic separation of triacylglycerols from soybean oil delivered dozens of fats differing in type and combination of fatty acids. The positive-ion APCI mass spectra of two selected triacylglycerols, triolein (OOO) and 1(3)-palmitoyl-2-stearoyl-3(1)-linoleoyl glycerol (PSL), are shown in Fig. 7.24 [131]. The APCI spectra exhibit $[M+H]^+$ ions and fragment ions characteristic of fatty acid composition and – to a certain degree – of isomers. While triolein can only form one distinctive diacyl fragment $[OO]^+$, the other fat yields $[PS]^+$, $[PL]^+$, and $[LS]^+$ as primary fragment ions. The fatty acids themselves are also revealed by their acylium ions in the low-mass range.

Negative-ion APCI of chloro-nitrobenzofurazan derivatives Negative-ion APCI spectra of alkylamino derivatives of 4-chloro-7-nitrobenzofurazan (NBDCl) were measured from acetonitrile/methanol solution. While the *N,N*-dimethylamino derivative preferably forms the radical anion, $M^{-\bullet}$, *m/z* 208, the *N*-ethyl isomer prefers the $[M-H]^-$ ion, *m/z* 207. This major change in spectral appearance is due to the missing slightly acidic hydrogen in the NBDCl isomer with the tertiary amino group. This demonstrates the strong influence of analyte structure on negative-ion (AP)CI spectra (Fig. 7.25) [134, 135].

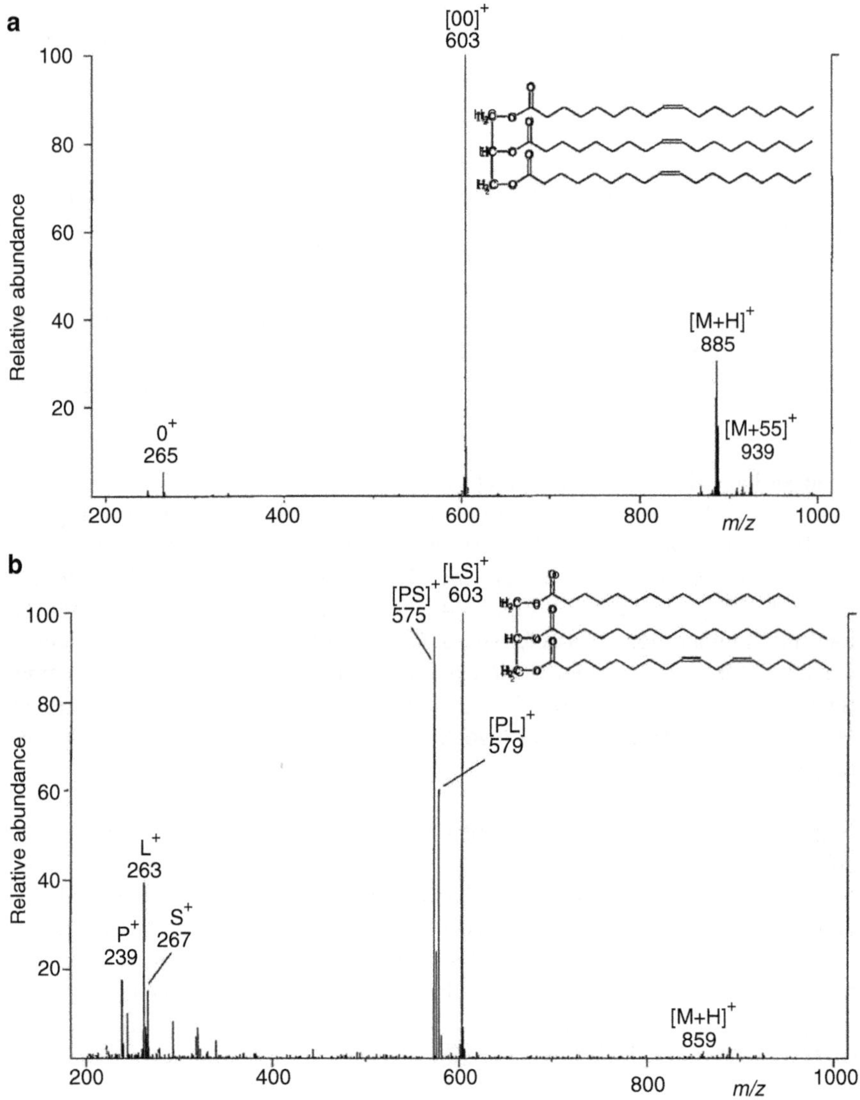

Fig. 7.24 Positive-ion APCI mass spectra of (**a**) triolein (OOO) and (**b**) 1(3)-palmitoyl-2-stearoyl-3 (1)-linoleoyl glycerol (PSL) from soybean oil. The $[M+55]^+$ ion in (**a**) is a solvent (proprionitrile) adduct (Reproduced from Ref. [131] with permission. © John Wiley & Sons, Ltd, 1997)

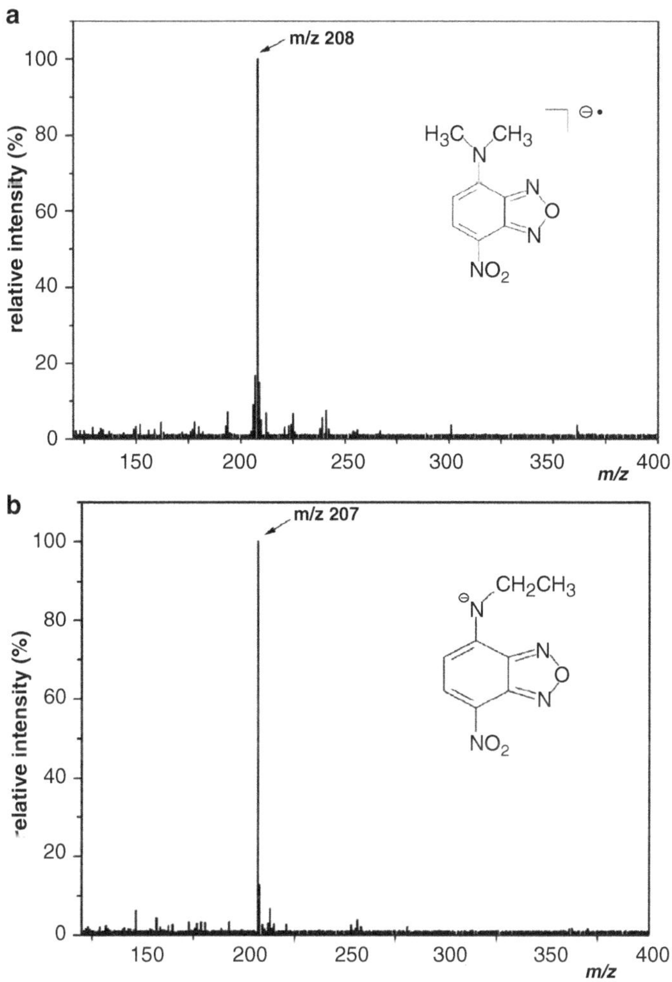

Fig. 7.25 Negative-ion APCI spectra of alkylamino derivatives of 4-chloro-7-nitrobenzofurazan (NBDCl). (**a**) The *N,N*-dimethylamino derivative preferably forms the radical anion, $M^{-\bullet}$, while (**b**) the *N*-ethyl form prefers the $[M-H]^-$ ion (Adapted from Ref. [135] with permission. © The Royal Society of Chemistry, 2002)

7.9 Atmospheric Pressure Photoionization

Atmospheric pressure photoionization (APPI) was introduced in 2000 [136] as a complement or alternative to APCI [130, 137, 138]. In APPI, a UV light source replaces the corona discharge-powered plasma, while the pneumatic sprayer and the heated vaporizer remain almost unaffected (Fig. 7.26) [139–141]. Apart from

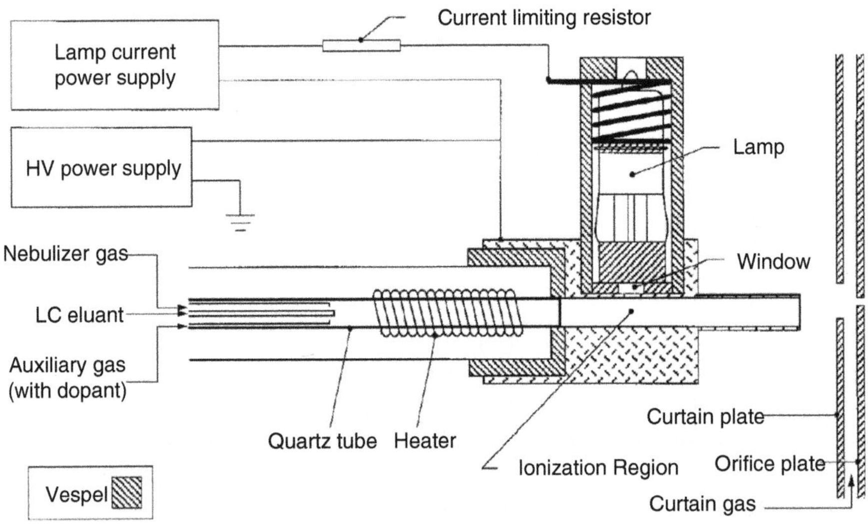

Fig. 7.26 APPI source comprising the heated nebulizer probe, photoionization UV lamp and mounting bracket (Reproduced from Ref. [136] by permission. © American Chemical Society, 2000)

the UV light, the most relevant modification is the use of a quartz tube to guide the hot vapor toward the sampling orifice. Quartz is required to transmit the UV light emitted by a noble gas discharge lamp.

Quick method switching
Modern instruments with atmospheric pressure ion sources are all constructed as to permit easy exchange of spray heads for rapid switching between ESI, APCI, and APPI [139, 142]. There is no interruption of instrument vacuum and mounting of spray heads takes just a minute, but there is a 10–15-min delay for APCI or APPI vaporizers to fully heat up for operation or to sufficiently cool down before removal is possible without risk of injury from hot parts.

7.9.1 Ion Formation in APPI

Statistically, the light emitted by the UV lamp will be absorbed by solvent molecules or eventually by nitrogen used for spraying, rather than by the analyte molecules. Therefore, the energy of the UV photons and the ionization energies of the compounds are decisive for the initiation of the APPI process (Fig. 7.27) [141]. In APPI, krypton lamps are commonly used as UV light source. In addition to the main emission of photons bearing 10.0 eV of energy there is a smaller fraction of photons of 10.6 eV. According to this energy level, krypton achieves ionization of most analytically relevant compounds while it blanks ionization of

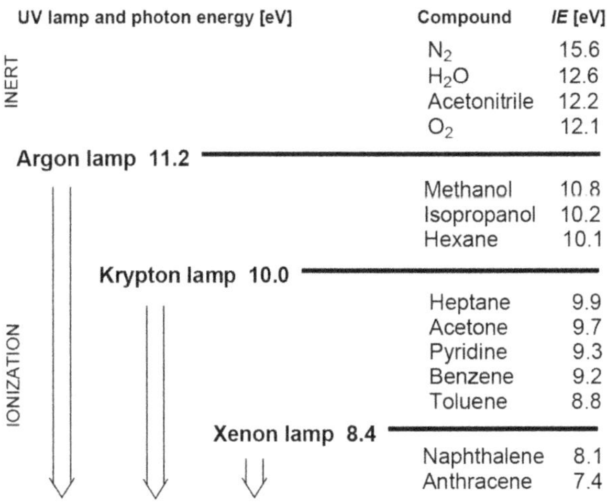

Fig. 7.27 Relationship between UV lamps and their photon energies used for APPI and ionization energies of typical compounds

some frequently used solvents and atmospheric gases [142]. APPI therefore has a higher compound class selectivity than APCI.

Provided the analyte, AB, has a UV chromophore, it can absorb the light to undergo *photoexcitation*, which merely delivers excited neutrals:

$$AB + h\nu \rightarrow AB^* \tag{7.47}$$

These electronically excited molecules AB* can either undergo radiative decay

$$AB^* \rightarrow AB + h\nu \tag{7.48}$$

or radiationless decay processes such as *photodissociation* to yield radicals

$$AB^* \rightarrow A^\bullet + B^\bullet \tag{7.49}$$

or *collisional quenching* with neutrals (N):

$$AB^* + N \rightarrow AB + N^* \tag{7.50}$$

More advantageous from the application point of view is *photoionization* (PI) of the analyte where AB* essentially represents a transition state:

$$AB + h\nu \rightarrow AB^* \rightarrow AB^{+\bullet} + e^- \tag{7.51}$$

However, photoionization of analyte molecules is neither energetically nor statistically a favored process [141]. Even if ions $AB^{+\bullet}$ have formed, they can be lost by neutralization via *recombination* with free electrons present in the plasma, eventually along with moderating ion–neutral collisions:

$$AB^{+\bullet} + e^- \rightarrow AB^* \tag{7.52}$$

$$AB^{+\bullet} + e^- + N \rightarrow AB + e^- + N \tag{7.52a}$$

Instead of relying on direct photoionization to occur, one normally would prefer a chemical ionization process where the reagent ions are formed by photoionization of a reagent gas. If the solvent (S) cannot be photoionized to play this role, a UV-absorbing dopant (D) may be added [136, 140, 143–146]. The dopant ions may then react with the analyte by *charge transfer*:

$$D^{+\bullet} + AB \rightarrow AB^{+\bullet} + D \tag{7.53}$$

Alternatively, dopant ions can lead to the formation of solvent reagent ions:

$$D^{+\bullet} + S \rightarrow [D - H]^{\bullet} + [S + H]^+ \tag{7.54}$$

These $[S+H]^+$ ions can finally protonate the analyte molecules [141, 142]:

$$[S + H]^+ + AB \rightarrow S + [AB + H]^+ \tag{7.55}$$

Methanol, for example, cannot be ionized by use of a krypton lamp, but addition of some acetone as dopant will allow the processes described in Eqs. 7.53, 7.54, and 7.55 to occur. Obviously, rich chemistry is involved until the neutral analyte has been transformed into $AB^{+\bullet}$ or $[AB+H]^+$ ions with sufficient efficiency [145, 146].

Negative-ion formation in APPI can occur by mechanisms analogous to APCI where electron capture by molecular oxygen initiates the cascade of reactions (Sect. 7.8.5).

More of CI than expected
Overall and in general, much of what happens in APPI bears close resemblance to APCI and CI, while the role of direct photoionization for analyte ion formation is less pronounced than suggested by its name.

7.9.2 APPI Spectra

The appearance of APPI spectra strongly depends on the actual combination of UV lamp, solvent, analyte, and eventually dopant. It is not always straightforward to predict whether protonation or molecular ion formation will dominate a positive-ion APPI spectrum, and analogously, whether deprotonation or radical anion formation will be observed in negative-ion mode. As a rule of thumb, molecules of higher

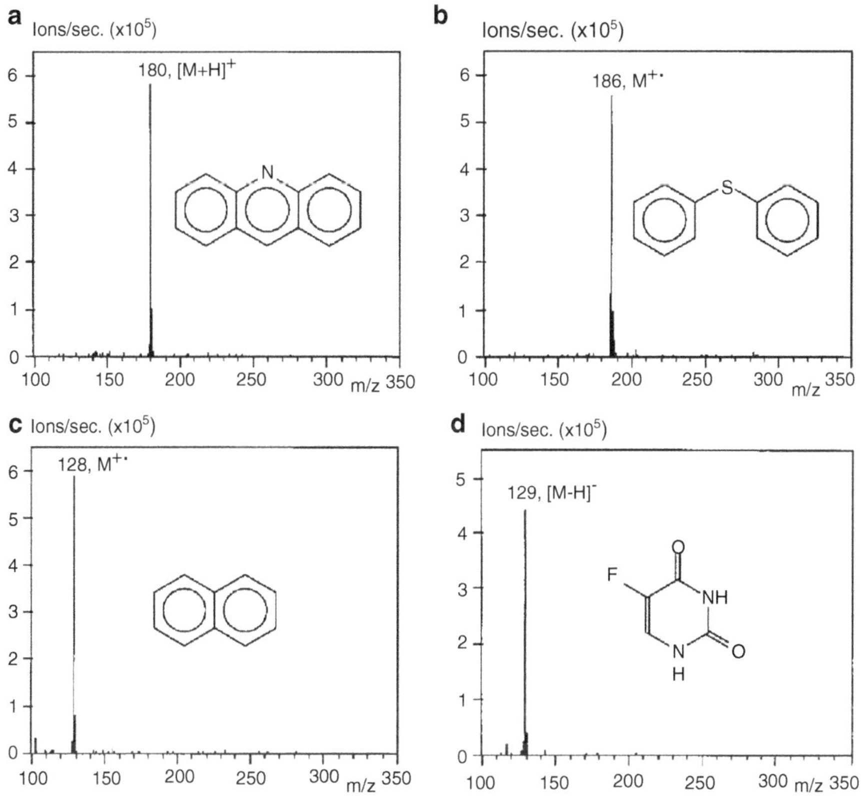

Fig. 7.28 Positive-ion APPI spectra of (**a**) acridine, (**b**) diphenyl sulfide, and (**c**) naphthalene showing how *PA* and *IE* of a compound affect ion formation. (**d**) Negative-ion APPI spectrum of 5-fluorouracil where the acidity of the imide is sufficient to form $[M–H]^-$ ions (Adapted from Ref. [136] with permission. © American Chemical Society, 2000)

proton affinity (*PA*) tend to form $[M+H]^+$ ions while nonpolar analytes, in particular those of low ionization energy (*IE*), preferably form $M^{+\bullet}$ ions [145]. In negative-ion mode, acidic molecules easily deliver $[M–H]^-$ ions, while those of high electron affinity (*EA*) undergo electron capture to yield $M^{-\bullet}$ ions. Unfortunately, APPI tends towards mixed ion formation, e.g., $M^{+\bullet}$ beside $[M+H]^+$ ions, the ratio of which is strongly influenced by the actual dopant [140, 143, 147, 148]. Like APCI, APPI often provides spectra showing almost exclusively ions representing the intact molecule. Some typical APPI spectra are compiled below (Fig. 7.28) [136].

One compound ionized by three methods Often, different soft ionization methods can be employed for the same compound with comparable success [149]. This does, however, not imply that each method is delivering the same type of analyte ion of a given compound. A comparison of positive-ion electrospray

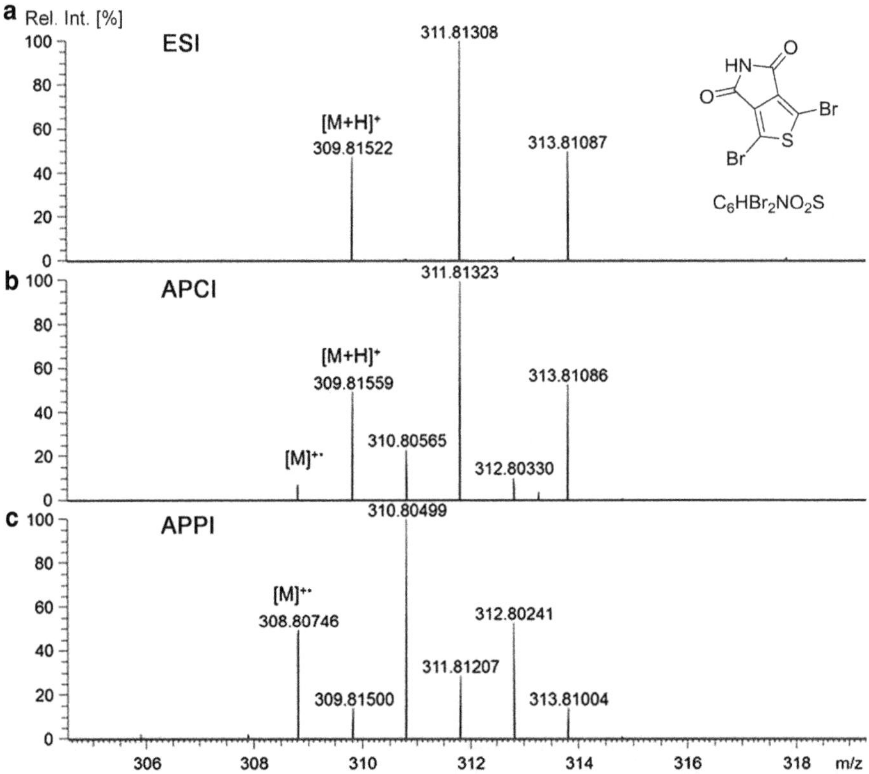

Fig. 7.29 Comparison of positive-ion (**a**) ESI, (**b**) APCI, and (**c**) APPI spectra of dibromothieno [3,4-*c*]pyrrole-4,6-dione. Note that there is also a small contribution of $M^{+\bullet}$ in APCI (Adapted from Ref. [148] by permission. © Wiley, 2014)

ionization (ESI, Chap. 12), APCI, and APPI spectra of dibromothieno[3,4-*c*]pyrrole-4,6-dione demonstrates this fact (Fig. 7.29) [148]. While ESI will exclusively deliver even-electron ions, both APCI and APPI may either result in formation of $[M+H]^+$ or $M^{+\bullet}$ ions depending on parameters such as ionization energy of the analyte and of the solvent as well as on their relative proton affinities.

Effect of different dopants In APPI, the formation of molecular ions, $M^{+\bullet}$, versus protonated molecules, $[M+H]^+$, also strongly depends on the type of dopant used [145, 146, 148]. A comparison of positive-ion APPI spectra of dibromothieno [3,4-*c*]pyrrole-4,6-dione as obtained using either chlorobenzene, bromobenzene, toluene, or no dopant exemplifies this effect (Fig. 7.30) [148].

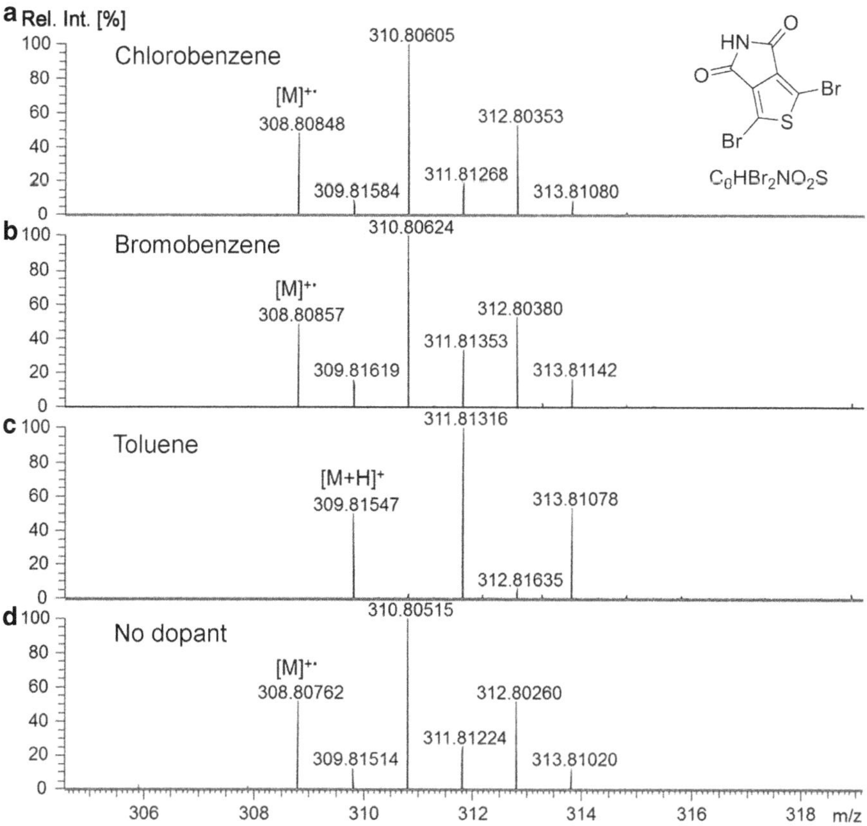

Fig. 7.30 Influence of dopants on positive-ion APPI spectra of dibromothieno[3,4-*c*]pyrrole-4,6-dione. The formation of $M^{+\bullet}$ versus $[M+H]^+$ ions depends on the actual dopant: (**a**) chlorobenzene, (**b**) bromobenzene, (**c**) toluene, and (**d**) no dopant (Adapted from Ref. [148] by permission. © Wiley, 2014)

Analyte supply from solution
Both APCI and APPI differ from vacuum CI in that the analyte is supplied from dilute solutions rather than by direct evaporation of liquids or solids from a probe or reservoir inlet. This does not only ensure the compatibility of APCI and APPI with liquid chromatography (Sect. 14.5) but also results in a softer transition from condensed phase to gas phase. Nonetheless, all CI methods involve gas phase ionization, and thus, require some evaporation to be performed prior to ionization as an integral part of the technique. All CI techniques are therefore perfectly compatible with gas chromatography (Sect. 14.4).

7.10 Overview of CI, APCI, and APPI

Common Features of Chemical Ionization Techniques

The term *chemical ionization* (CI) usually applies to all ionization processes that proceed via ion–molecule reactions. In CI, analyte molecules, M, are ionized by reacting with *reagent ions* generated in a foregoing process from a *reagent gas*. Classically, chemical ionization was performed on the microsecond-time scale in medium vacuum, typically at about 1 mbar (1 collision μs^{-1}). The occurrence of ion–molecule reactions is not restricted to the vacuum environment – on the contrary, rates of bimolecular reactions increase along with rising pressure. Performing chemical ionization on the millisecond-time scale and at atmospheric pressure (10^6 collisions ms^{-1}) thus improves ionization efficiency. Additionally, immediate thermalization of the freshly formed ions reduces fragmentation.

Fundamental Ionization Pathways

Chemical ionization proceeds either by transfer of an electron, proton, or other ions between the reactants. Positive-ion chemical ionization (PICI) comprises four fundamental pathways of ion formation from neutrals: proton transfer, electrophilic addition, anion abstraction, and charge transfer (CT). Negative-ion chemical ionization (NICI) either involves deprotonation, nucleophilic addition, or ion-pair formation. A fourth process observed along with NICI is electron capture (EC). However, electron capture negative ionization (ECNI) is not a chemical ionization process in the strict sense. These fundamental ionization pathways apply whether CI is performed in vacuum or at atmospheric pressure and independent of whether the primary step of reagent ion formation is initiated by energetic electrons (vacuum CI), a corona discharge (APCI), UV photons (APPI), or any other source.

Analytes

Whether an analyte is suitable to be analyzed by a CI technique depends on the type of particular CI process to be applied. Obviously, protonating PICI will be beneficial for other compounds than CTCI or ECNI. In general, most analytes accessible to electron ionization (EI, Sect. 5.6) can be analyzed by protonating PICI. PICI spectra are particularly useful as a complement to EI spectra when molecular ion peaks are absent or very weak in EI. CTCI and ECNI play a role where selectivity and/or very high sensitivity for a certain compound class is desired (Table 7.6). The typical mass range for vacuum CI reaches from 60 u (above reagent ions) to 1200 u. APCI and APPI are softer due to immediate thermalization of the ions, and thus, extend the upper range of ions representing the intact molecule to about 2000 u. APPI can deliver ions of less polar analytes than APCI.

Today, desorption chemical ionization (DCI) and particularly pyrolysis-DCI are rarely used because APCI, APPI, and many other soft ionization methods, especially those combining desorption and ionization (Chaps. 8, 10, 11, 12, and 13) offer more promising and more convenient ways of mass spectral analysis. Nonetheless, there are exceptions when materials such as resins, varnishes, rubbers, and others of similar complexity are to be studied.

Table 7.6 Chemical ionization for different groups of analytes

Analyte	Thermodynamic properties[a]	Example	Suggested CI pathway
Low polarity, no heteroatoms	Low to high *IE*, low *PA*, low *EA*	Alkanes, alkenes, aromatic hydrocarbons	CTCI
Low to medium polarity, one or two heteroatoms	Low to medium *IE*, medium to high *PA*, low *EA*	Alcohols, amines, esters, heterocyclic compounds	PICI, CTCI
Medium to high polarity, some heteroatoms	Low to medium *IE*, high *PA* and low *EA*	Diols, triols, amino acids, disaccharides, substituted aromatic or heterocyclic compounds	PICI
Low to high polarity, halogens (especially F or Cl)	Medium *IE*, low *PA*, medium to high *EA*	Halogenated and nitrocompounds, derivatives, e.g., trifluoroacetate, pentafluorobenzyl	ECNI
High polarity, medium to high molecular mass	Low to medium *IE*, high *PA* and low *EA*	Mono- to tetrasaccharides, other polar oligomers, complex materials	DCI
High polarity, very high molecular mass	Decomposition products of low to medium *IE*, high *PA* and low *EA*	humic compounds, synthetic polymers, complex materials	Py-DCI

[a]*IE* ionization energy, *PA* proton affinity, *EA* electron affinity

Table 7.7 Ions formed by chemical ionization techniques

Analytes	Positive ions	Negative ions
Nonpolar	$M^{+\bullet}$	$M^{-\bullet}$
Medium polarity	$M^{+\bullet}$ and/or $[M+H]^+$, $[M+cat]^{+a}$,{*clusters* $[2M]^{+\bullet}$ and/or $[2M+H]^+$, $[2M+cat]^{+a}$}[b]	$M^{-\bullet}$ and/or $[M–H]^-$, $[M+an]^{-a}${*clusters* $[2M]^{-\bullet}$ and/or $[2M–H]^-$, $[2M+an]^{-a}$}[b]
Polar	$[M+H]^+$, $[M+cat]^{+a}$,{*clusters* $[2M+H]^+$, $[2M+cat]^{+a}$ }[b]	$[M–H]^-$, $[M+an]^{-a}${*clusters* $[2M–H]^-$, $[2M+an]^{-a}$}[b]

[a]Cation cat^+ and anion an^-
[b]Braces denote occasionally accompanying species

Ions Formed

The various options for selecting pathways of ion formation and the variety of available CI methods result in a comparatively large number of different types of analyte ions that can occur. The chiefly occurring type of analyte ions strongly depends on such general parameters as mass, polarity, volatility, and intrinsic properties like ionization energy, proton affinity, or electron affinity. And then, the selection of either positive-ion or negative-ion mode creates a different set of analyte ions. Table 7.7 provides a basic classification.

Relationship to Other Ionization Techniques
Reaction sequences analogous to *atmospheric pressure chemical ionization* (APCI) do occur whenever ionization is performed in an atmosphere with traces of water, e.g., *direct analysis in real time* (DART, Sect. 13.8).

References

1. Talrose VL, Ljubimova AK (1998) Secondary Processes in the Ion Source of a Mass Spectrometer (Presented by Academician N.N. Semenov 27 Viii 1952) – Reprinted from Report of the Soviet Academy of Sciences, Vol LXXXVI, -N5 (1952). J Mass Spectrom 33:502–504
2. Munson MSB, Field FH (1965) Reactions of Gaseous Ions. XV. Methane + 1% Ethane and Methane + 1% Propane. J Am Chem Soc 87:3294–3299. doi:10.1021/ja01093a002
3. Munson MSB (1965) Proton Affinities and the Methyl Inductive Effect. J Am Chem Soc 87:2332–2336. doi:10.1021/ja01089a005
4. Munson MSB, Field FH (1966) Chemical Ionization Mass Spectrometry. I General Introduction. J Am Chem Soc 88:2621–2630. doi:10.1021/ja00964a001
5. Munson MSB (2000) Development of Chemical Ionization Mass Spectrometry. Int J Mass Spectrom 200:243–251. doi:10.1016/S1387-3806(00)00301-8
6. Richter WJ, Schwarz H (1978) Chemical Ionization – A Highly Important Productive Mass Spectrometric Analysis Method. Angew Chem 90:449–469. doi:10.1002/anie.197804241
7. Harrison AG (1992) Chemical Ionization Mass Spectrometry. CRC Press, Boca Raton
8. Todd JFJ (1995) Recommendations for Nomenclature and Symbolism for Mass Spectroscopy Including an Appendix of Terms Used in Vacuum Technology. Int J Mass Spectrom Ion Proc 142:211–240. doi:10.1016/0168-1176(95)93811-F
9. Sparkman OD (2006) Mass Spectrometry Desk Reference. Global View Publishing, Pittsburgh
10. Murray KK, Boyd RK, Eberlin MN, Langley GJ, Li L, Naito Y (2013) Definitions of Terms Relating to Mass Spectrometry (IUPAC Recommendations 2013). Pure Appl Chem 85:1515–1609. doi:10.1351/PAC-REC-06-04-06
11. Griffith KS, Gellene GI (1993) A Simple Method for Estimating Effective Ion Source Residence Time. J Am Soc Mass Spectrom 4:787–791. doi:10.1016/1044-0305(93)80036-X
12. Field FH, Munson MSB (1965) Reactions of Gaseous Ions. XIV. Mass Spectrometric Studies of Methane at Pressures to 2 Torr. J Am Chem Soc 87:3289–3294. doi:10.1021/ja01093a001
13. Hunt DF, Ryan JFI (1971) Chemical Ionization Mass Spectrometry Studies. I. Identification of Alcohols. Tetrahedron Lett 12:4535–4538. doi:10.1016/S0040-4039(01)97523-9
14. Herman JA, Harrison AG (1981) Effect of Reaction Exothermicity on the Proton Transfer Chemical Ionization Mass Spectra of Isomeric C_5 and C_6 Alkanols. Can J Chem 59:2125–2132. doi:10.1139/v81-307
15. Beggs D, Vestal ML, Fales HM, Milne GWA (1971) Chemical Ionization Mass Spectrometer Source. Rev Sci Inst 42:1578–1584. doi:10.1063/1.1684943
16. Schröder E (1991) Massenspektrometrie – Begriffe und Definitionen. Springer-Verlag, Heidelberg
17. Ghaderi S, Kulkarni PS, Ledford EB Jr, Wilkins CL, Gross ML (1981) Chemical Ionization in Fourier Transform Mass Spectrometry. Anal Chem 53:428–437. doi:10.1021/ac00226a011
18. Price P (1991) Standard Definitions of Terms Relating to Mass Spectrometry. A Report from the Committee on Measurements and Standards of the Amercian Society for Mass Spectrometry. J Am Soc Mass Spectrom 2:336–348. doi:10.1016/1044-0305(91)80025-3
19. Heck AJR, de Koning LJ, Nibbering NMM (1991) Structure of Protonated Methane. J Am Soc Mass Spectrom 2:454–458. doi:10.1016/1044-0305(91)80030-B

20. Mackay GI, Schiff HI, Bohme KD (1981) A Room-Temperature Study of the Kinetics and Energetics for the Protonation of Ethane. Can J Chem 59:1771–1778. doi:10.1139/v81-265
21. Fisher JJ, Koyanagi GK, McMahon TB (2000) The $C_2H_7^+$ Potential Energy Surface: A Fourier Transform Ion Cyclotron Resonance Investigation of the Reaction of Methyl Cation with Methane. Int J Mass Spectrom 195(196):491–505. doi:10.1016/S1387-3806(99)00231-6
22. Drabner G, Poppe A, Budzikiewicz H (1990) The Composition of the Methane Plasma. Int J Mass Spectrom Ion Proc 97:1–33. doi:10.1016/0168-1176(90)85037-3
23. Thompson KC, Crittenden DL, Jordan MJT (2005) $CH_5^{+\bullet}$: Chemistry's Chameleon Unmasked. J Am Chem Soc 127:4954–4958. doi:10.1021/ja0482280
24. Heck AJR, de Koning LJ, Nibbering NMM (1991) On the Structure and Unimolecular Chemistry of Protonated Halomethanes. Int J Mass Spectrom Ion Proc 109:209–225. doi:10.1016/0168-1176(91)85105-U
25. Herman JA, Harrison AG (1981) Effect of Protonation Exothermicity on the Chemical Ionization Mass Spectra of Some Alkylbenzenes. Org Mass Spectrom 16:423–427. doi:10.1002/oms.1210161002
26. Munson MSB, Field FH (1965) Reactions of Gaseous Ions. XVI Effects of Additives on Ionic Reactions in Methane. J Am Chem Soc 87:4242–4247. doi:10.1021/ja00947a005
27. Kuck D, Petersen A, Fastabend U (1998) Mobile Protons in Large Gaseous Alkylbenzenium Ions. The 21-Proton Equilibration in Protonated Tetrabenzylmethane and Related "Proton Dances". Int J Mass Spectrom 179(180):129–146. doi:10.1016/S1387-3806(98)14168-4
28. Kuck D (2002) Half a Century of Scrambling in Organic Ions: Complete, Incomplete, Progressive and Composite Atom Interchange. Int J Mass Spectrom 213:101–144. doi:10.1016/S1387-3806(01)00533-4
29. Fales HM, Milne GWA, Axenrod T (1970) Identification of Barbiturates by Chemical Ionization Mass Spectrometry. Anal Chem 42:1432–1435. doi:10.1021/ac60294a040
30. Milne GWA, Axenrod T, Fales HM (1970) Chemical Ionization Mass Spectrometry of Complex Molecules. IV Amino Acids. J Am Chem Soc 92:5170–5175. doi:10.1021/ja00720a029
31. Fales HM, Milne GWA (1970) Chemical Ionization Mass Spectrometry of Complex Molecules. II Alkaloids. J Am Chem Soc 92:1590–1597. doi:10.1021/ja00709a028
32. Herman JA, Harrison AG (1981) Energetics and Structural Effects in the Fragmentation of Protonated Esters in the Gas Phase. Can J Chem 59:2133–2145. doi:10.1139/v81-308
33. Milne GWA, Fales HM, Axenrod T (1970) Identification of Dangerous Drugs by Isobutane Chemical Ionization Mass Spectrometry. Anal Chem 42:1815–1820. doi:10.1021/ac60307a048
34. Takeda N, Harada KI, Suzuki M, Tatematsu A, Kubodera T (1982) Application of Emitter Chemical Ionization Mass Spectrometry to Structural Characterization of Aminoglycoside Antibiotics. Org Mass Spectrom 17:247–252. doi:10.1002/oms.1210170602
35. McGuire JM, Munson B (1985) Comparison of Isopentane and Isobutane as Chemical Ionization Reagent Gases. Anal Chem 57:680–683. doi:10.1021/ac00280a024
36. McCamish M, Allan AR, Roboz J (1987) Poly(dimethylsiloxane) as Mass Reference for Accurate Mass Determination in Isobutane Chemical Ionization Mass Spectrometry. Rapid Commun Mass Spectrom 1:124–125. doi:10.1002/rcm.1290010711
37. Maeder H, Gunzelmann KH (1988) Straight-Chain Alkanes As Reference Compounds for Accurate Mass Determination in Isobutane Chemical Ionization Mass Spectrometry. Rapid Commun Mass Spectrom 2:199–200. doi:10.1002/rcm.1290021003
38. Hunt DF, McEwen CN, Upham RA (1971) Chemical Ionization Mass Spectrometry. II. Differentiation of Primary, Secondary, and Tertiary Amines. Tetrahedron Lett 12:4539–4542. doi:10.1016/S0040-4039(01)97524-0
39. Busker E, Budzikiewicz H (1979) Studies in Chemical Ionization Mass Spectrometry. 2. Isobutane and Nitric Oxide Spectra of Alkynes. Org Mass Spectrom 14:222–226. doi:10.1002/oms.1210140412

40. Keough T, DeStefano AJ (1981) Factors Affecting Reactivity in Ammonia Chemical-Ionization Spectrometry. Org Mass Spectrom 16:527–533. doi:10.1002/oms.1210161205
41. Hancock RA, Hodges MG (1983) A Simple Kinetic Method for Determining Ion-Source Pressures for Ammonia CIMS. Int J Mass Spectrom Ion Phys 46:329–332. doi:10.1016/0020-7381(83)80119-3
42. Rudewicz P, Munson B (1986) Effect of Ammonia Partial Pressure on the Sensitivities for Oxygenated Compounds in Ammonia Chemical Ionization Mass Spectrometry. Anal Chem 58:2903–2907. doi:10.1021/ac00127a003
43. Lawrence DL (1990) Accurate Mass Measurement of Positive Ions Produced by Ammonia Chemical Ionization. Rapid Commun Mass Spectrom 4:546–549. doi:10.1002/rcm.1290041216
44. Brinded KA, Tiller PR, Lane SJ (1993) Triton X-100 As a Reference Compound for Ammonia High-Resolution Chemical Ionization Mass Spectrometry and as a Tuning and Calibration Compound for Thermospray. Rapid Commun Mass Spectrom 7:1059–1061. doi:10.1002/rcm.1290071119
45. Wu HF, Lin YP (1999) Determination of the Sensitivity of an External Source Ion Trap Tandem Mass Spectrometer Using Dimethyl Ether Chemical Ionization. J Mass Spectrom 34:1283–1285. doi:10.1002/(SICI)1096-9888(199912)34:12<1283::AID-JMS900>3.0.CO;2-M
46. Barry R, Munson B (1987) Selective Reagents in Chemical Ionization Mass Spectrometry: Diisopropyl Ether. Anal Chem 59:466–471. doi:10.1021/ac00130a019
47. Allgood C, Lin Y, Ma YC, Munson B (1990) Benzene as a Selective Chemical Ionization Reagent Gas. Org Mass Spectrom 25:497–502. doi:10.1002/oms.1210251003
48. Srinivas R, Vairamani M, Mathews CK (1993) Gase-Phase Halo Alkylation of C_{60}-Fullerene by Ion-Molecule Reaction Under Chemical Ionization. J Am Soc Mass Spectrom 4:894–897. doi:10.1016/1044-0305(93)87007-Y
49. Budzikiewicz H, Blech S, Schneider B (1991) Studies in Chemical Ionization. XXVI. Investigation of Aliphatic Dienes by Chemical Ionization with Nitric Oxide. Org Mass Spectrom 26:1057–1060. doi:10.1002/oms.1210261205
50. Schneider B, Budzikiewicz H (1990) A Facile Method for the Localization of a Double Bond in Aliphatic Compounds. Rapid Commun Mass Spectrom 4:550–551. doi:10.1002/rcm.1290041217
51. Fordham PJ, Chamot-Rooke J, Guidice E, Tortajada J, Morizur JP (1999) Analysis of Alkenes by Copper Ion Chemical Ionization Gas Chromatography/Mass Spectrometry and Gas Chromatography/Tandem Mass Spectrometry. J Mass Spectrom 34:1007–1017. doi:10.1002/(SICI)1096-9888(199910)34:10<1007::AID-JMS854>3.0.CO;2-E
52. Peake DA, Gross ML (1985) Iron(I) Chemical Ionization and Tandem Mass Spectrometry for Locating Double Bonds. Anal Chem 57:115–120. doi:10.1021/ac00279a031
53. Lindinger W, Jordan A (1998) Proton-Transfer-Reaction Mass Spectrometry (PTR-MS): Online Monitoring of Volatile Organic Compounds at pptv Levels. Chem Soc Rev 27:347–354. doi:10.1039/a827347z
54. Lindinger W, Hansel A, Jordan A (1998) Online Monitoring of Volatile Organic Compounds at pptv Levels by Means of Proton-Transfer-Reaction Mass Spectrometry (PTR-MS). Medical Applications, Food Control and Environmental Research. Int J Mass Spectrom Ion Proc 173:191–241. doi:10.1016/S0168-1176(97)00281-4
55. Blake RS, Monks PS, Ellis AM (2009) Proton-Transfer Reaction Mass Spectrometry. Chem Rev 109:861–896. doi:10.1021/cr800364q
56. de Gouw J, Warneke C (2007) Measurements of Volatile Organic Compounds in the Earth's Atmosphere Using Proton-Transfer-Reaction Mass Spectrometry. Mass Spectrom Rev 26:223–257. doi:10.1002/mas.20119
57. Fay LB, Yeretzian C, Blank I (2001) Novel Mass Spectrometry Methods in Flavour Analysis. Chimia 55:429–434

58. Sulzer P, Hartungen E, Hanel G, Feil S, Winkler K, Mutschlechner P, Haidacher S, Schottkowsky R, Gunsch D, Seehauser H, Striednig M, Juerschik S, Breiev K, Lanza M, Herbig J, Maerk L, Maerk TD, Jordan A (2014) A Proton Transfer Reaction-Quadrupole Interface Time-of-Flight Mass Spectrometer (PTR-QiTOF): High Speed Due to Extreme Sensitivity. Int J Mass Spectrom 368:1–5. doi:10.1016/j.ijms.2014.05.004
59. Edtbauer A, Hartungen E, Jordan A, Hanel G, Herbig J, Juerschik S, Lanza M, Breiev K, Maerk L, Sulzer P (2014) Theory and Practical Examples of the Quantification of CH_4, CO, O_2, and CO_2 with an Advanced Proton-Transfer-Reaction/Selective-Reagent-Ionization Instrument (PTR/SRI-MS). Int J Mass Spectrom 365-366:10–14. doi:10.1016/j.ijms.2013.11.014
60. Karl T, Guenther A, Yokelson RJ, Greenberg J, Potosnak M, Blake DR, Artaxo P (2007) The Tropical Forest and Fire Emissions Experiment: Emission, Chemistry, and Transport of Biogenic Volatile Organic Compounds in the Lower Atmosphere Over Amazonia. J Geophys Res Atmos 112:D18302-1–D18302/17. doi: 10.1029/2007JD008539
61. Hsu CS, Qian K (1993) Carbon Disulfide Charge Exchange as a Low-Energy Ionization Technique for Hydrocarbon Characterization. Anal Chem 65:767–771. doi:10.1021/ac00054a020
62. Einolf N, Munson B (1972) High-Pressure Charge Exchange Mass Spectrometry. Int J Mass Spectrom Ion Phys 9:141–160. doi:10.1016/0020-7381(72)80040-8
63. Allgood C, Ma YC, Munson B (1991) Quantitation Using Benzene in Gas Chromatography/Chemical Ionization Mass Spectrometry. Anal Chem 63:721–725. doi:10.1021/ac00007a014
64. Subba Rao SC, Fenselau C (1978) Evaluation of Benzene as a Charge Exchange Reagent. Anal Chem 50:511–515. doi:10.1021/ac50025a036
65. Sieck LW (1983) Determination of Molecular Weight Distribution of Aromatic Components in Petroleum Products by Chemical Ionization Mass Spectrometry with Chlorobenzene as Reagent Gas. Anal Chem 55:38–41. doi:10.1021/ac00252a013
66. Li YH, Herman JA, Harrison AG (1981) Charge Exchange Mass Spectra of Some C_5H_{10} Isomers. Can J Chem 59:1753–1759. doi:10.1139/v81-263
67. Abbatt JA, Harrison AG (1986) Low-Energy Mass Spectra of Some Aliphatic Ketones. Org Mass Spectrom 21:557–563. doi:10.1002/oms.1210210906
68. Herman JA, Li YH, Harrison AG (1982) Energy Dependence of the Fragmentation of Some Isomeric $C_6H_{12}^{+\cdot}$ Ions. Org Mass Spectrom 17:143–150. doi:10.1002/oms.1210170309
69. Chai R, Harrison AG (1981) Location of Double Bonds by Chemical Ionization Mass Spectrometry. Anal Chem 53:34–37. doi:10.1021/ac00224a010
70. Keough T, Mihelich ED, Eickhoff DJ (1984) Differentiation of Monoepoxide Isomers of Polyunsaturated Fatty Acids and Fatty Acid Esters by Low-Energy Charge Exchange Mass Spectrometry. Anal Chem 56:1849–1852. doi:10.1021/ac00275a021
71. Polley CW Jr, Munson B (1983) Nitrous Oxide As Reagent Gas for Positive Ion Chemical Ionization Mass Spectrometry. Anal Chem 55:754–757. doi:10.1021/ac00255a037
72. Harrison AG, Lin MS (1984) Stereochemical Applications of Mass Spectrometry. 3. Energy Dependence of the Fragmentation of Stereoisomeric Methylcyclohexanols. Org Mass Spectrom 19:67–71. doi:10.1002/oms.1210190204
73. Hsu CS, Cooks RG (1976) Charge Exchange Mass Spectrometry at High Energy. Org Mass Spectrom 11:975–983. doi:10.1002/oms.1210110909
74. Roussis S (1999) Exhaustive Determination of Hydrocarbon Compound Type Distributions by High Resolution Mass Spectrometry. Rapid Commun Mass Spectrom 13:1031–1051. doi:10.1002/(SICI)1097-0231(19990615)13:11<1031::AID-RCM602>3.0.CO;2-8
75. Hunt DF, Stafford GC Jr, Crow FW (1976) Pulsed Positive- and Negative-Ion Chemical Ionization Mass Spectrometry. Anal Chem 48:2098–2104. doi:10.1021/ac50008a014
76. von Ardenne M, Steinfelder K, Tümmler R (1971) Elektronenanlagerungs-Massenspektrographie Organischer Substanzen. Springer, Heidelberg

77. Dougherty RC, Weisenberger CR (1968) Negative Ion Mass Spectra of Benzene, Naphthalene, and Anthracene. A New Technique for Obtaining Relatively Intense and Reproducible Negative Ion Mass Spectra. J Am Chem Soc 90:6570–6571. doi:10.1021/ja01025a090
78. Dillard JG (1973) Negative Ion Mass Spectrometry. Chem Rev 73:589–644. doi:10.1021/cr60286a002
79. Bouma WJ, Jennings KR (1981) Negative Chemical Ionization Mass Spectrometry of Explosives. Org Mass Spectrom 16:330–335. doi:10.1002/oms.1210160802
80. Budzikiewicz H (1986) Studies in Negative Ion Mass Spectrometry. XI. Negative Chemical Ionization (NCI) of Organic Compounds. Mass Spectrom Rev 5:345–380. doi:10.1002/mas.1280050402
81. Kurvinen JP, Mu H, Kallio H, Xu X, Hoy CE (2001) Regioisomers of Octanoic Acid-Containing Structured Triacylglycerols Analyzed by Tandem Mass Spectrometry Using Ammonia Negative Ion Chemical Ionization. Lipids 36:1377–1382. doi:10.1007/s11745-001-0855-9
82. Gross JH (2009) Mass Spectrometry. In: Andrews DL (ed) Encyclopedia of Applied Spectroscopy. Wiley-VCH, Weinheim
83. Hunt DF, Crow FW (1978) Electron Capture Negative Ion Chemical Ionization Mass Spectrometry. Anal Chem 50:1781–1784. doi:10.1021/ac50035a017
84. Ong VS, Hites RA (1994) Electron Capture Mass Spectrometry of Organic Environmental Contaminants. Mass Spectrom Rev 13:259–283. doi:10.1002/mas.1280130305
85. Oehme M (1994) Quantification of Fg-Pg Amounts by Electron Capture Negative Ion Mass Spectrometry – Parameter Optimization and Practical Advice. Fresenius J Anal Chem 350:544–554. doi:10.1007/BF00321803
86. Bartels MJ (1994) Quantitation of the Tetrachloroethylene Metabolite *N*-Acetyl-*S*-(Trichlorovinyl)Cysteine in Rat Urine Via Negative Ion Chemical Ionization Gas Chromatography/Tandem Mass Spectrometry. Biol Mass Spectrom 23:689–694. doi:10.1002/bms.1200231107
87. Fowler B (2000) The Determination of Toxaphene in Environmental Samples by Negative Ion Electron Capture High Resolution Mass Spectrometry. Chemosphere 41:487–492. doi:10.1016/S0045-6535(99)00476-2
88. Laramée JA, Arbogast BC, Deinzer ML (1986) Electron Capture Negative Ion Chemical Ionization Mass Spectrometry of 1,2,3,4-Tetrachlorodibenzo-*p*-dioxin. Anal Chem 58:2907–2912. doi:10.1021/ac00127a004
89. Budzikiewicz H (1981) Mass Spectrometry of Negative Ions. 3. Mass Spectrometry of Negative Organic Ions. Angew Chem 93:635–649. doi:10.1002/anie.198106241
90. Bowie JH (1984) The Formation and Fragmentation of Negative Ions Derived from Organic Molecules. Mass Spectrom Rev 3:161–207. doi:10.1002/mas.1280030202
91. Stemmler EA, Hites RA (1988) The Fragmentation of Negative Ions Generated by Electron Capture Negative Ion Mass Spectrometry: A Review with New Data. Biomed Environ Mass Spectrom 17:311–328. doi:10.1002/bms.1200170415
92. Jensen KR, Voorhees KJ (2015) Analytical Applications of Electron Monochromator-Mass Spectrometry. Mass Spectrom Rev 34:24–42. doi:10.1002/mas.21395
93. Buchanan MV, Olerich G (1984) Differentiation of Polycyclic Aromatic Hydrocarbons Using Electron Capture Negative Chemical Ionization. Org Mass Spectrom 19:486–489. doi:10.1002/oms.1210191005
94. Oehme M (1983) Determination of Isomeric Polycyclic Aromatic Hydrocarbons in Air Particulate Matter by High-Resolution Gas Chromatography/Negative Ion Chemical Ionization Mass Spectrometry. Anal Chem 55:2290–2295. doi:10.1021/ac00264a021
95. Giese RW (1997) Detection of DNA Adducts by Electron Capture Mass Spectrometry. Chem Res Toxicol 10:255–270. doi:10.1021/tx9601263
96. Laramée JA, Mazurkiewicz P, Berkout V, Deinzer ML (1996) Electron Monochromator-Mass Spectrometer Instrument for Negative Ion Analysis of Electronegative Compounds.

Mass Spectrom Rev 15:15–42. doi:10.1002/(SICI)1098-2787(1996)15:1<15::AID-MAS2>3.0.CO;2-E
97. NIST webbook. http://webbook.nist.gov/
98. Williamson DH, Knighton WB, Grimsrud EP (2000) Effect of Buffer Gas Alterations on the Thermal Electron Attachment and Detachment Reactions of Azulene by Pulsed High Pressure Mass Spectrometry. Int J Mass Spectrom 195(196):481–489. doi:10.1016/S1387-3806(99)00142-6
99. Wei J, Liu S, Fedoreyev SA, Vionov VG (2000) A Study of Resonance Electron Capture Ionization on a Quadrupole Tandem Mass Spectrometer. Rapid Commun Mass Spectrom 14:1689–1694. doi:10.1002/1097-0231(20000930)14:18<1689::AID-RCM75>3.0.CO;2-G
100. Carette M, Zerega Y, Perrier P, Andre J, March RE (2000) Rydberg Electron-Capture Mass Spectrometry of 1,2,3,4-Tetrachlorodibenzo-*p*-Dioxin. Eur Mass Spectrom 6:405–408. doi:10.1255/ejms.362
101. Zerega Y, Carette M, Perrier P, Andre J (2002) Rydberg Electron Capture Mass Spectrometry of Organic Pollutants. Organohal Comp 55:151–154
102. Bendig P, Maier L, Lehnert K, Knapp H, Vetter W (2013) Mass Spectra of Methyl Esters of Brominated Fatty Acids and Their Presence in Soft Drinks and Cocktail Syrups. Rapid Commun Mass Spectrom 27:1083–1089. doi:10.1002/rcm.6543
103. Jenske R, Vetter W (2008) Gas Chromatography/Electron-Capture Negative Ion Mass Spectrometry for the Quantitative Determination of 2- and 3-Hydroxy Fatty Acids in Bovine Milk Fat. J Agric Food Chem 56:5500–5505. doi:10.1021/jf800647w
104. Yinon J (1982) Mass Spectrometry of Explosives: Nitro Compounds, Nitrate Esters, and Nitramines. Mass Spectrom Rev 1:257–307. doi:10.1002/mas.1280010304
105. Cappiello A, Famiglini G, Lombardozzi A, Massari A, Vadalà GG (1996) Electron Capture Ionization of Explosives with a Microflow Rate Particle Beam Interface. J Am Soc Mass Spectrom 7:753–758. doi:10.1016/1044-0305(96)00015-3
106. Knighton WB, Grimsrud EP (1995) High-Pressure Electron Capture Mass Spectrometry. Mass Spectrom Rev 14:327–343. doi:10.1002/mas.1280140406
107. Aubert C, Rontani J-F (2000) Perfluoroalkyl Ketones: Novel Derivatization Products for the Sensitive Determination of Fatty Acids by Gas Chromatography/Mass Spectrometry in Electron Impact and Negative Chemical Ionization Modes. Rapid Commun Mass Spectrom 14:960–966. doi:10.1002/(SICI)1097-0231(20000615)14:11<960::AID-RCM972>3.3.CO;2-R
108. Kato Y, Okada S, Atobe K, Endo T, Haraguchi K (2012) Selective Determination of Mono- and Dihydroxylated Analogs of Polybrominated Diphenyl Ethers in Marine Sponges by Liquid Chromatography Tandem Mass Spectrometry. Anal Bioanal Chem 404:197–206. doi:10.1007/s00216-012-6132-2
109. Cotter RJ (1980) Mass Spectrometry of Nonvolatile Compounds by Desorption from Extended Probes. Anal Chem 52:1589A–1602A. doi:10.1021/ac50064a003
110. Kurlansik L, Williams TJ, Strong JM, Anderson LW, Campana JE (1984) Desorption Ionization Mass Spectrometry of Synthetic Porphyrins. Biomed Mass Spectrom 11:475–481. doi:10.1002/bms.1200110908
111. Helleur RJ, Thibault P (1994) Optimization of Pyrolysis-Desorption Chemical Ionization Mass Spectrometry and Tandem Mass Spectrometry of Polysaccharides. Can J Chem 72:345–351. doi:10.1139/v94-053
112. Vincenti M (2001) The Renaissance of Desorption Chemical Ionization Mass Spectrometry: Characterization of Large Involatile Molecules and Nonpolar Polymers. Int J Mass Spectrom 212:505–518. doi:10.1016/S1387-3806(01)00492-4
113. Beuhler RJ, Flanigan E, Greene LJ, Friedman L (1974) Proton Transfer Mass Spectrometry of Peptides. Rapid Heating Technique for Underivatized Peptides Containing Arginine. J Am Chem Soc 96:3990–3999. doi:10.1021/ja00819a043

114. Cullen WR, Eigendorf GK, Pergantis SA (1993) Desorption Chemical Ionization Mass Spectrometry of Arsenic Compounds Present in the Marine and Terrestrial Environment. Rapid Commun Mass Spectrom 7:33–36. doi:10.1002/rcm.1290070108
115. Juo CG, Chen SW, Her GR (1995) Mass Spectrometric Analysis of Additives in Polymer Extracts by Desorption Chemical Ionization and Collisional Induced Dissociation with B/E Linked Scanning. Anal Chim Acta 311:153–164. doi:10.1016/0003-2670(95)00183-Z
116. Chen G, Cooks RG, Jha SK, Green MM (1997) Microstructure of Alkoxy and Alkyl Substituted Isocyanate Copolymers Determined by Desorption Chemical Ionization Mass Spectrometry. Anal Chim Acta 356:149–154. doi:10.1016/S0003-2670(97)00504-7
117. Pergantis SA, Emond CA, Madilao LL, Eigendorf GK (1994) Accurate Mass Measurements of Positive Ions in the Desorption Chemical Ionization Mode. Org Mass Spectrom 29:439–444. doi:10.1002/oms.1210290808
118. Horning EC, Horning MG, Carroll DI, Dzidic I, Stillwell RN (1973) New Picogram Detection System Based on a Mass Spectrometer with an External Ionization Source at Atmospheric Pressure. Anal Chem 45:936–943. doi:10.1021/ac60328a035
119. Horning EC, Carroll DI, Dzidic I, Haegele KD, Horning MG, Stillwell RN (1974) Atmospheric Pressure Ionization (API) Mass Spectrometry. Solvent-Mediated Ionization of Samples Introduced in Solution and in a Liquid Chromatograph Effluent Stream. J Chromatogr Sci 12:725–729. doi:10.1093/chromsci/12.11.725
120. Carroll DI, Dzidic I, Stillwell RN, Horning MG, Horning EC (1974) Subpicogram Detection System for Gas Phase Analysis Based Upon Atmospheric Pressure Ionization (API) Mass Spectrometry. Anal Chem 46:706–704. doi:10.1021/ac60342a009
121. Carroll DI, Dzidic I, Stillwell RN, Haegele KD, Horning EC (1975) Atmospheric Pressure Ionization Mass Spectrometry. Corona Discharge Ion Source for Use in a Liquid Chromatograph-Mass Spectrometer-Computer Analytical System. Anal Chem 47:2369–2373. doi:10.1021/ac60364a031
122. Dzidic I, Stillwell RN, Carroll DI, Horning EC (1976) Comparison of Positive Ions Formed in Nickel-63 and Corona Discharge Ion Sources Using Nitrogen, Argon, Isobutane, Ammonia and Nitric Oxide as Reagents in Atmospheric Pressure Ionization Mass Spectrometry. Anal Chem 48:1763–1768. doi:10.1021/ac50006a035
123. Bruins AP (1991) Mass Spectrometry with Ion Sources Operating at Atmospheric Pressure. Mass Spectrom Rev 10:53–77. doi:10.1002/mas.1280100104
124. Tsuchiya M (1995) Atmospheric Pressure Ion Sources, Physico-Chemical and Analytical Applications. Adv Mass Spectrom 13:333–346
125. Schiewek R, Lorenz M, Giese R, Brockmann K, Benter T, Gaeb S, Schmitz OJ (2008) Development of a Multipurpose Ion Source for LC-MS and GC-API-MS. Anal Bioanal Chem 392:87–96. doi:10.1007/s00216-008-2255-x
126. Warscheid B, Hoffmann T (2001) Structural Elucidation of Monoterpene Oxidation Products by Ion Trap Fragmentation Using on-Line Atmospheric Pressure Chemical Ionization Mass Spectrometry in the Negative Ion Mode. Rapid Commun Mass Spectrom 15:2259–2272. doi:10.1002/rcm.504
127. Derpmann V, Albrecht S, Benter T (2012) The Role of Ion-Bound Cluster Formation in Negative Ion Mass Spectrometry. Rapid Commun Mass Spectrom 26:1923–1933. doi:10.1002/rcm.6303
128. Klee S, Derpmann V, Wissdorf W, Klopotowski S, Kersten H, Brockmann KJ, Benter T, Albrecht S, Bruins AP, Dousty F, Kauppila TJ, Kostiainen R, O'Brien R, Robb DB, Syage JA (2014) Are Clusters Important in Understanding the Mechanisms in Atmospheric Pressure Ionization? Part 1: Reagent Ion Generation and Chemical Control of Ion Populations. J Am Soc Mass Spectrom 25:1310–1321. doi:10.1007/s13361-014-0891-2
129. McEwen CN, Larsen BS (2009) Ionization Mechanisms Related to Negative Ion APPI, APCI, and DART. J Am Soc Mass Spectrom 20:1518–1521. doi:10.1016/j.jasms.2009.04.010

130. Hayen H, Karst U (2003) Strategies for the Liquid Chromatographic-Mass Spectrometric Analysis of Non-Polar Compounds. J Chromatogr A 1000:549–565. doi:10.1016/S0021-9673(03)00505-3
131. Mottram H, Woodbury SE, Evershed RP (1997) Identification of Triacylglycerol Positional Isomers Present in Vegetable Oils by High Performance Liquid Chromatography/Atmospheric Pressure Chemical Ionization Mass Spectrometry. Rapid Commun Mass Spectrom 11:1240–1252. doi:10.1002/(SICI)1097-0231(199708)11:12<1240::AID-RCM990>3.0.CO;2-5
132. Reemtsma T (2003) Liquid Chromatography-Mass Spectrometry and Strategies for Trace-Level Analysis of Polar Organic Pollutants. J Chromatogr A 1000:477–501. doi:10.1016/S0021-9673(03)00507-7
133. Covey TR, Thomson BA, Schneider BB (2009) Atmospheric Pressure Ion Sources. Mass Spectrom Rev 28:870–897. doi:10.1002/mas.20246
134. Hayen H, Jachmann N, Vogel M, Karst U (2003) LC-Electron Capture-APCI(-)-MS Determination of Nitrobenzoxadiazole Derivatives. Analyst 128:1365–1372. doi:10.1039/B308752B
135. Hayen H, Jachmann N, Vogel M, Karst U (2002) LC-Electron Capture APCI-MS for the Determination of Nitroaromatic Compounds. Analyst 127:1027–1030. doi:10.1039/B205477A
136. Robb DB, Covey TR, Bruins AP (2000) Atmospheric Pressure Photoionization: an Ionization Method for Liquid Chromatography-Mass Spectrometry. Anal Chem 72:3653–3659. doi:10.1021/ac0001636
137. Keski-Hynnilä H, Kurkela M, Elovaara E, Antonio L, Magdalou J, Luukkanen L, Taskinen J, Koistiainen R (2002) Comparison of Electrospray, Atmospheric Pressure Chemical Ionization, and Atmospheric Pressure Photoionization in the Identification of Apomorphine, Dobutamine, and Entacapone Phase II Metabolites in Biological Samples. Anal Chem 74:3449–3457. doi:10.1021/ac011239g
138. Syage JA, Hanold KA, Lynn TC, Horner JA, Thakur RA (2004) Atmospheric Pressure Photoionization. II Dual Source Ionization. J Chromatogr A 1050:137–149. doi:10.1016/j.chroma.2004.08.033
139. Yang C, Henion JD (2002) Atmospheric Pressure Photoionization Liquid Chromatographic-Mass Spectrometric Determination of Idoxifene and Its Metabolites in Human Plasma. J Chromatogr A 970:155–165. doi:10.1016/S0021-9673(02)00882-8
140. Kauppila TJ, Kuuranne T, Meurer EC, Eberlin MN, Kotiaho T, Koistiainen R (2002) Atmospheric Pressure Photoionization Mass Spectrometry. Ionization Mechanism and the Effect of Solvent on the Ionization of Naphthalenes. Anal Chem 74:5470–5479. doi:10.1021/ac025659x
141. Raffaeli A, Saba A (2003) Atmospheric Pressure Photoionization Mass Spectrometry. Mass Spectrom Rev 22:318–331. doi:10.1002/mas.10060
142. Kauppila TJ, Syage JA, Benter T (2015) Recent Developments in Atmospheric Pressure Photoionization-Mass Spectrometry. Mass Spectrom Rev XX:1–27. doi:10.1002/mas.21477
143. Kauppila TJ, Kostiainen R, Bruins AP (2004) Anisole, a New Dopant for Atmospheric Pressure Photoionization Mass Spectrometry of Low Proton Affinity, Low Ionization Energy Compounds. Rapid Commun Mass Spectrom 18:808–815. doi:10.1002/rcm.1408
144. Robb DB, Covey TR, Bruins AP (2001) Atmospheric Pressure Photoionization (APPI): A New Ionization Technique for LC/MS. Adv Mass Spectrom 15:391–392
145. Kauppila TJ, Kersten H, Benter T (2014) The Ionization Mechanisms in Direct and Dopant-Assisted Atmospheric Pressure Photoionization and Atmospheric Pressure Laser Ionization. J Am Soc Mass Spectrom 25:1870–1881. doi:10.1007/s13361-014-0988-7
146. Ahmed A, Choi CH, Kim S (2015) Mechanistic Study on Lowering the Sensitivity of Positive Atmospheric Pressure Photoionization Mass Spectrometric Analyses: Size-Dependent Reactivity of Solvent Clusters. Rapid Commun Mass Spectrom 29:2095–2101. doi:10.1002/rcm.7373

147. Kauppila TJ, Kotiaho T, Kostiainen R, Bruins AP (2004) Negative Ion-Atmospheric Pressure Photoionization-Mass Spectrometry. J Am Soc Mass Spectrom 15:203–211. doi:10.1016/j.jasms.2003.10.012
148. Sioud S, Kharbatia N, Amad MH, Zhu Z, Cabanetos C, Lesimple A, Beaujuge P (2014) The Formation of [M-H]+ Ions in *n*-Alkyl-Substituted Thieno[3,4-*c*]-Pyrrole-4,6-Dione Derivatives During Atmospheric Pressure Photoionization Mass Spectrometry. Rapid Commun Mass Spectrom 28:2389–2397. doi:10.1002/rcm.7031
149. Fredenhagen A, Kuehnoel J (2014) Evaluation of the Optimization Space for Atmospheric Pressure Photoionization (APPI) in Comparison with APCI. J Mass Spectrom 49:727–736. doi:10.1002/jms.3401

Field Ionization and Field Desorption

8

Learning Objectives

- Ion formation by action of very strong electric fields
- Desorption of ions into the gas phase by strong electric fields
- Softness of field ionization and field desorption
- Methods of sample introduction for field ionization and field desorption
- General properties and fields of application of the title methods
- Applications to air- and moisture-sensitive samples
- Complex mixture analysis by combining gas chromatography and high-resolution mass spectrometry with field ionization and field desorption

8.1 Evolution of Field Ionization and Field Desorption

The first observation of the desorption of positive ions from surfaces by high electrostatic fields was made by means of a field ion microscope [1, 2]. The mass spectrometric analysis of some field-ionized gases followed soon [2–4]. In 1959, H. D. Beckey presented the first focusing field ionization ion source [5]. In these early experiments electric field strengths of about 10^8 V cm^{-1} (1 V$Å^{-1}$) were generated at sharp tungsten tips [2, 4, 5]. The method of *field ionization* (FI) was soon extended to analyzing volatile liquids [6–10] and solids introduced by evaporation from a sample vial in close proximity to the ionizing tip or wire electrode [11]. FI, still embryonic in the mid-1960s, had soon to compete with chemical ionization (CI, Chap. 7) [12]. The major breakthrough came from its further development to *field desorption* (FD), because FD circumvents the evaporation of the analyte prior to ionization [13, 14]. Instead, the processes of ionization *and* subsequent desorption of the formed ions are centered on the surface of the *field*

J.H. Gross, *Mass Spectrometry*, DOI 10.1007/978-3-319-54398-7_8

emitter. The specific charm of FI-MS and especially of FD-MS arises from their extraordinary softness of ionization, in many cases yielding solely intact molecular ions, and from the capability of FD to handle neutral as well as ionic analytes [15–24]. FD-MS initially flourished from the mid-1970s to the mid-1980s, but soon suffered from the advent of fast-atom bombardment (FAB) and later electrospray ionization (ESI) mass spectrometry [23]. Then, however, the unique capabilities of FD-MS were rediscovered [25–27], even more so with the advent of advanced sample introduction [28, 29] and the adaptation of FI and FD ion sources to oaTOF and FT-ICR mass analyzers [30–35].

8.2 Field Ionization Process

Inghram and Gomer described and explained the process of *field ionization* of a single hydrogen atom [3, 4, 36]: If a hydrogen atom resides on a metal surface, its proton-electron potential is only slightly distorted. However, in the presence of an electric field in the order of 2 $VÅ^{-1}$ (1 Å = 10^{-10} m) with the metal at positive polarity, this distortion becomes remarkable (Fig. 8.1). As a result, the electron can become detached from the proton by tunneling into the bulk metal through a potential barrier that is only a few angstroms wide and some electronvolts high [19, 37]. Thereby, the hydrogen atom becomes ionized, and the resulting proton is immediately driven away by action of the electric field. Interestingly, the situation is quite similar for an isolated hydrogen atom. Here, the electric field causes analogous distortion of the potential, and with sufficient field strength, the atom is field ionized, too. This means that atoms or molecules can be ionized by the mere action of a strong electric field independent of whether they have been adsorbed to the anodic surface or whether they are moving freely through the space between the electrodes.

Field ionization essentially is a autoionization-type process, i.e., an internally supra-excited atom or molecular moiety loses an electron spontaneously without further interaction with an energy source [38]. Different from electron ionization, there is no excess energy transferred onto the incipient ion, and thus, dissociation of the ions is reduced to a minimum.

$$M \rightarrow M^{+\bullet} + e^- \tag{8.1}$$

Electric fields sufficient to effect field ionization are only obtained in close proximity to sharp tips, edges, or thin wires. The smaller the radius of the curvature of the anode, the further away (1–10 nm) the field sufficing to cause ionization (Fig. 8.1). The importance of sufficient electric field strength is reflected by the extreme decrease in half-life calculated for a hydrogen atom: it is in the order of 0.1 s at 0.5 $VÅ^{-1}$, 0.1 ns at 1.0 $VÅ^{-1}$, and 0.1 f. at 2.5 $VÅ^{-1}$ [19].

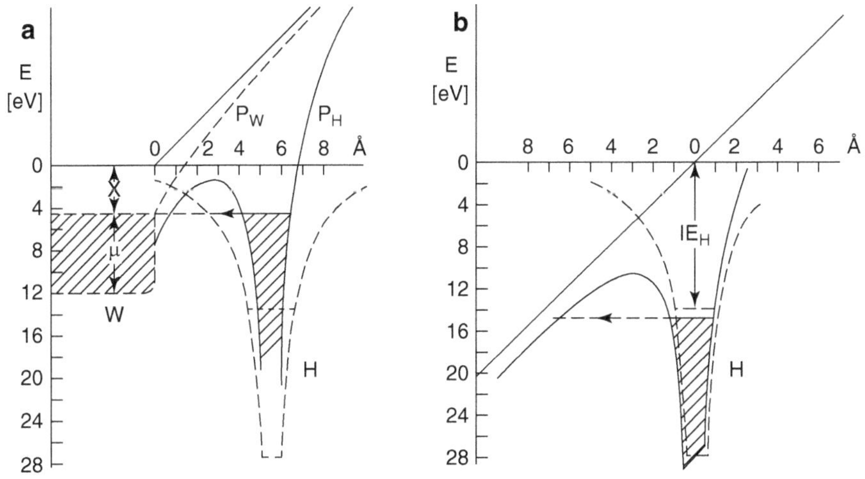

Fig. 8.1 Field ionization of a hydrogen atom (H) (**a**) close to a tungsten surface (*W*), (**b**) isolated. Conditions and symbols: electric field 2 $VÅ^{-1}$, P_W image potential of W distorted by the field, P_H potential of the hydrogen atom distorted by the field, X work function, μ Fermi level. *Dashed lines* represent potentials in absence of the electric field (Adapted from Ref. [4] by permission. © Verlag der Zeitschrift für Naturforschung, 1955)

Naming the parts

The field anode is usually referred to as *field emitter*, *FI emitter*, or *FD emitter*. The properties of the field emitter are of key importance for FI- and FD-MS. The electrode opposed to the emitter is called *field cathode* or simply *counter electrode*.

8.3 FI and FD Ion Sources

In FI- and FD-MS, a voltage of 8–12 kV is applied between *field emitter* (field anode) and *counter electrode* (field cathode) usually located 2–3 mm in front of the emitter. Thus, the desorbing ions are accelerated to 8–12 keV kinetic energy, clearly exceeding the amount which can be handled by a double-focusing magnetic sector instrument (typically used in conjunction with FI/FD ion sources). These contradictory requirements can be met by setting the counter electrode to negative potential to establish the high field gradient for ion generation while adjusting the difference between emitter and ground potential to the actual acceleration voltage (Fig. 8.2) [39]. With the emitter grounded and the counter electrode at high negative potential even slow ion beams can be delivered for mounting FD ion sources to FT-ICR or oaTOF instruments [30, 40].

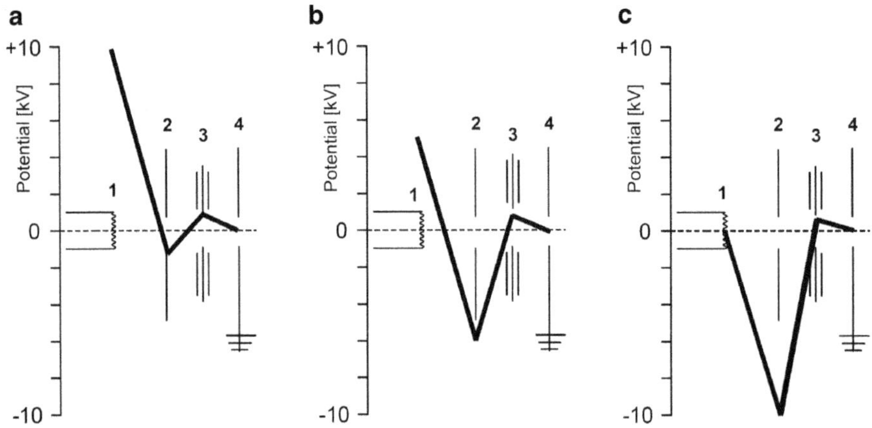

Fig. 8.2 Potentials (*bold lines*) along different FI/FD ion sources to realize full extraction voltage while delivering ions of defined kinetic energy to the analyzer. The part numbers correspond to: (*1*) emitter, (*2*) counter electrode, (*3*) optional electrostatic lenses, (*4*) analyzer entrance slit. (**a**) Instruments with high acceleration voltage, (**b**) instruments with medium acceleration voltage as is often the case in magnetic sector instruments, and (**c**) instruments requiring slow ions, e.g., FT-ICR or oaTOF instruments

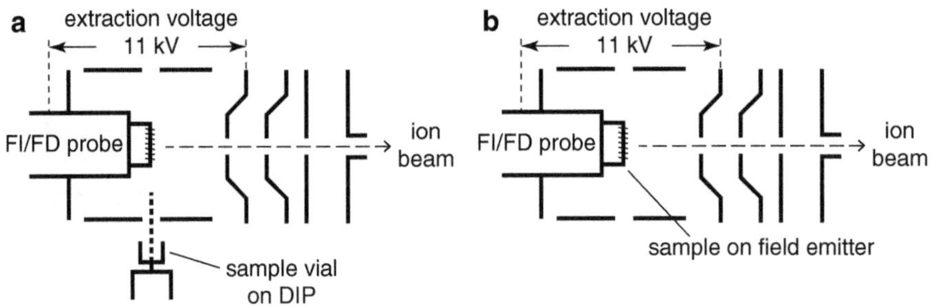

Fig. 8.3 Schematic of an FI/FD ion source (**a**) in FI mode, (**b**) in FD mode. The distance between emitter and counter electrode is exaggerated for clarity (Adapted from Ref. [41] by permission. © Springer-Verlag, Heidelberg, 1991)

In FI mode, the analyte is introduced via external inlet systems such as a direct probe, a reservoir inlet, or a gas chromatograph (Sects. 5.2 and 5.4). In FD mode, the analyte is supplied directly on the surface of the field emitter. Doing so not only guarantees a more efficient usage of the sample, it also combines the steps of ionization and desorption, thereby minimizing the risk of thermal decomposition prior to ionization (Figs. 8.3 and 8.4). This is especially important in case of highly polar or ionic analytes that cannot be evaporated without thermal degradation.

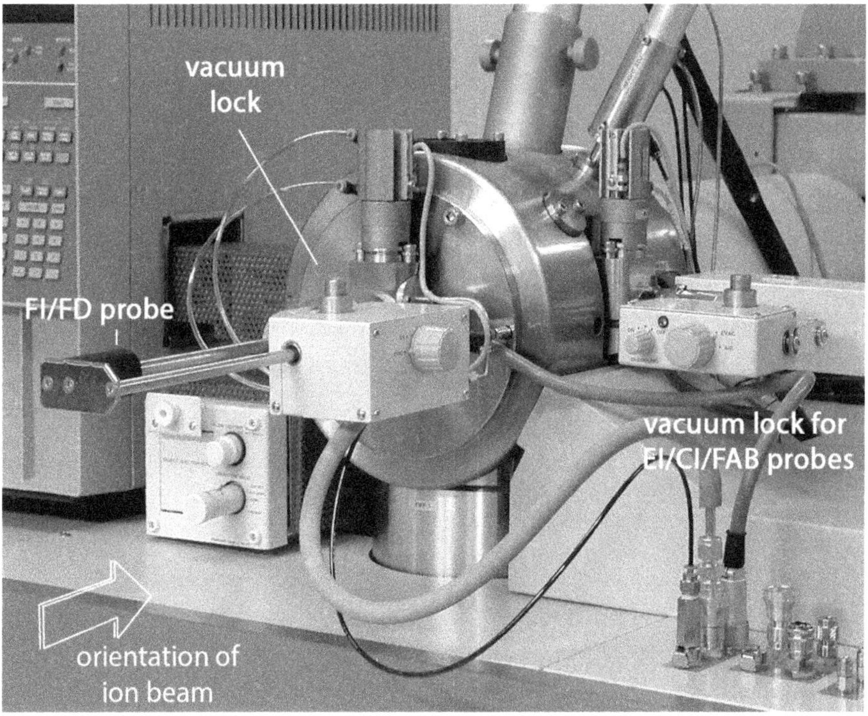

Fig. 8.4 FD probe inserted into the vacuum lock. FD probes are generally inserted in axial position to free the vacuum lock of the DIP for FI use. The emitter wire is now oriented vertically to comply with the beam geometry of the magnetic sector analyzer

8.4 Field Emitters

8.4.1 Blank Metal Wires as Emitters

In the first FI experiments, the high electric field strength was obtained at sharply pointed tungsten tips [2, 4, 5]. Later, edges of sharp blades [42] and wires of a few micrometers in diameter were used. Wires are advantageous because the emitting surface of a smooth blade is approximately two orders of magnitude smaller than that of a smooth wire at the same field strength under normal working conditions (Fig. 8.5). Simple wire emitters can be used for field desorption of nonpolar [43] or electrolytic analytes [44]. As thin wires are fragile and can break during electric discharges, sharp edges should be avoided in their vicinity, e.g., by polishing the counter electrode [45].

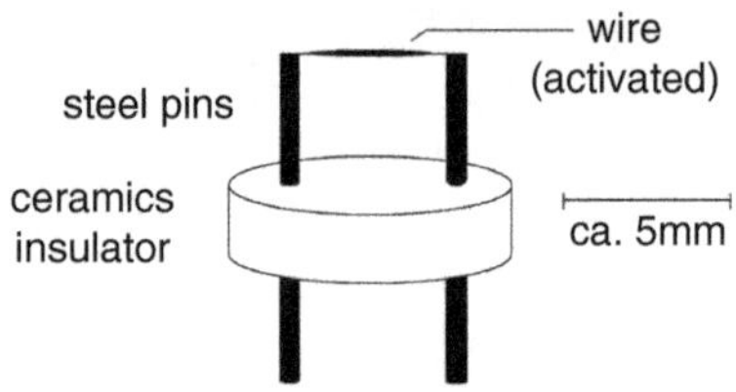

Fig. 8.5 A wire emitter: high voltage is supplied via the emitter-holding pins. These also serve to pass a current for resistive heating through the (activated) wire

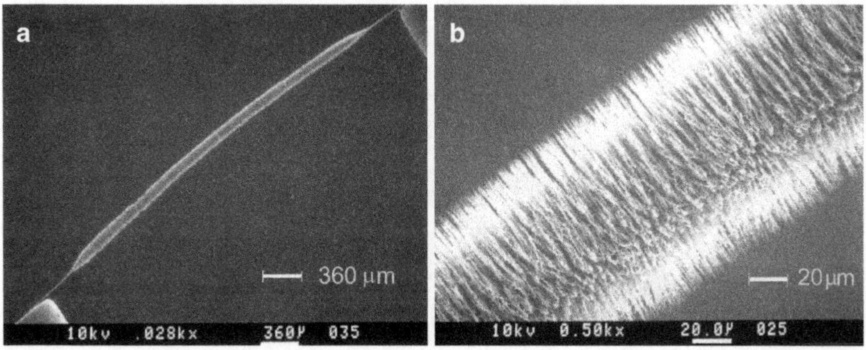

Fig. 8.6 SEM pictures of activated tungsten wire emitters; (**a**) overview showing the thin tungsten wire close to the holders and the whisker-bearing middle section, (**b**) detail of the central part revealing whiskers (By courtesy of Carbotec, Bergisch Gladbach, Germany)

8.4.2 Activated Emitters

The electric field strength on the emitter can greatly be enhanced by creating dendritic microneedles (*whiskers*) on its surface, by a process known as *emitter activation*. FI- and FD-MS require emitters of reproducible high quality, and therefore the activation procedure has received much attention. The high-temperature activation of 10 μm tungsten wires with pure benzonitrile vapor takes 3–7 h [46], but it may be accelerated by reversal of the polarity of the high voltage during activation [47], or by using indane, indene, indole, or naphthalene as the activating agent [48]. The activation procedures with benzonitrile or indene are employed commercially to produce carbon whiskers on emitters (Fig. 8.6). Microneedle growth is also achieved by decomposition of hexacarbonyltungsten, $W(CO)_6$, on a cathode producing an electric discharge [49]. A self-controlling mechanism which draws ions preferably to the top of the growing tungsten needles has been suggested [49]. SEM pictures of activated emitter surfaces and single whiskers have an aesthetic appeal [47–52].

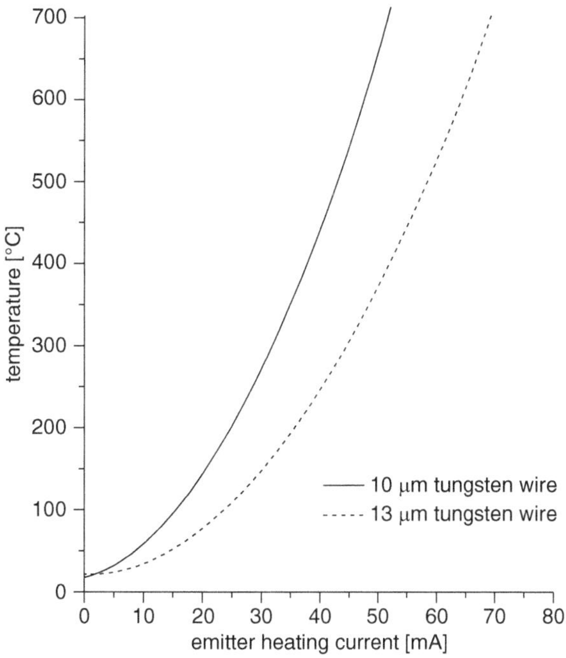

Fig. 8.7 Calibration of EHC vs. temperature for emitters activated with carbon needles on 10-μm and 13-μm tungsten wire (By courtesy of Carbotec, Bergisch Gladbach, Germany)

8.4.3 Emitter Temperature

Emitters can be heated by applying an electric current via the emitter holders. It is somewhat difficult to establish a precise calibration of emitter temperature versus *emitter heating current* (EHC) [53, 54]. The actual temperature not only depends on the emitter material, but also on diameter and length of the emitter as well as on length and area density of the whiskers. A useful estimate for tungsten emitters with carbon whiskers is given below (Fig. 8.7).

In practice, moderate heating of the emitter at constant current serves to reduce adsorption to its surface during FI measurements. Heating at a constant rate (1–20 mA min^{-1}) is frequently employed to enforce desorption of analytes from the emitter in FD-MS. Electric discharges resulting from too massive ion desorption can be avoided by emission-controlled emitter heating [55–57]. Where the EHC is regulated as to achieve a constant ion emission current, typically in the range of 1–100 nA. At the end, the emitter is cleaned for subsequent measurements by baking for 2–5 s at 800–1000 °C at 50–60 mA (activated tungsten emitters of 10 μm diameter) or at 80–100 mA (emitters of 13 μm).

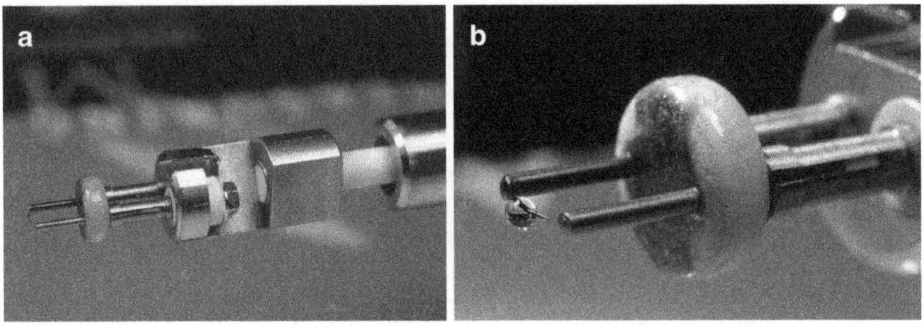

Fig. 8.8 FD probe. (**a**) Emitter holder of a JEOL FD probe tip, (**b**) a drop formed of 1–2 μl of analyte solution placed onto the activated emitter by means of a microliter syringe

8.4.4 Handling of Activated Emitters

Activated wire emitters are extremely fragile, because after activation the material behaves more like ceramics than like a metal wire. The slightest touch with a syringe needle as well as electric discharges during operation cause immediate destruction of the emissive wire. Delicate handling of the emitter is therefore a prerequisite [23]. Follow these guidelines for longer emitter lifespans:

- Use tweezers for emitter manipulation. Grasp the emitter either at the robust ceramics socket or at both steel pins simultaneously.
- Bake the emitter before first use in order to outgas and clean the emitter.
- When applying analyte solutions onto the emitter, only the emerging drop should come in contact with the emitter wire, but not the syringe needle (Fig. 8.8).
- Avoid excessive loading, as analyte solution may spread even onto the steel pins. From there, it can be washed back during loading of the subsequent sample.
- Allow complete evaporation of the solvent before insertion into the vacuum lock (Fig. 8.4).
- Switch on the high voltage only after the high vacuum has fully recovered.
- Switch off the high voltage after completion of the measurement.
- Finally, repeatedly bake the emitter to remove sample residues.

Adequate handling provided, an emitter can last for up to 20 measurements.

Better don't dip it

To apply a solution of the analyte, the emitter can either be *dipped into*, or alternatively, a drop of 1–2 μl can be *transferred onto* the emitter by means of a microliter syringe [52]. The latter method exhibits better reproducibility and avoids contamination of the emitter pins. Special micromanipulators are available to handle the syringe [14], but with some exercise a skilled operator can accomplish it manually.

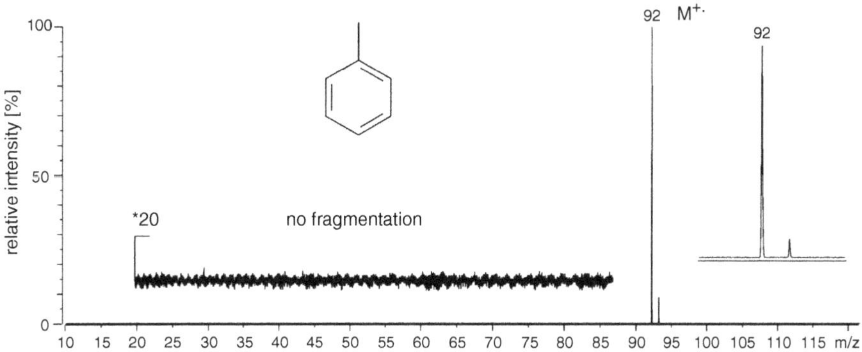

Fig. 8.9 FI spectrum of toluene. The molecular ion and its isotopolog are the only observed entities. (The CID spectrum of field-ionized toluene is shown in Sect. 9.3, the EI spectrum is discussed in Sect. 6.4)

8.5 Field Ionization Mass Spectrometry

FI mass spectra are normally characterized by intense molecular ion peaks accompanied by no or in some cases just a few fragment ions [9, 11, 58]. Especially in case of nonpolar low-mass analytes, FI-MS can serve for molecular ion mass spectrometry (Fig. 8.9) [59]. This property made FI-MS a standard tool for hydrocarbon analysis in the petroleum industry [6, 7, 10, 12, 25, 59–61]. FI performs nicely for samples that can reasonably be evaporized, but it exhibits poor sensitivity for polyhalogenated compounds such as $CHCl_3$ or PFK. FI usually fails with highly polar or even ionic compounds due to thermal decomposition. Nonetheless, there is no rule without exceptions: FI can, for example, create low-abundant "molecular ions", more appropriately described as cation-radical pairs $[C{+}A]^{+\bullet}$, of ionic liquids [62].

Although convenient at first sight, the lack of fragment ion peaks in FI spectra also means a lack of structural information. If data beyond a mere estimate of the elemental composition based on the isotopic pattern are asked for, then tandem MS employing collision-induced dissociation (CID, Chap. 9) is the preferred standard of structure elucidation. Fortunately, the fragmentation pathways of $M^{+\bullet}$ ions in CID are the same as in EI-MS (Chap. 6).

Low ion currents by FI

In FI-MS, the ionization efficiency is very low, because of the low probability for a neutral effusing from any inlet system towards the field emitter to come close enough to the whiskers. Consequently, FI-MS produces very low ion currents. The application of FI-MS is therefore restricted to samples that are too volatile for FD-MS or require prior gas chromatographic separation.

Table 8.1 Ions formed by FI

Analytes	Ions formed
Nonpolar	$M^{+\bullet}$, M^{2+}, occasionally $M^{3+\bullet}$, rarely $[M+H]^+$
Medium polarity	$M^{+\bullet}$, M^{2+} and/or $[M+H]^+$
Polar	$[M+H]^+$
Ionic	Generally thermal decomposition

8.5.1 Origin of $[M+H]^+$ Ions in FI-MS

FI mass spectra can show signals due to reactions of the analyte with the emitter surface or between molecules adsorbed to that surface. In case of acetone, it was demonstrated that $[M+H]^+$ ions are produced mainly by a *field-induced proton-transfer* reaction in the physically adsorbed layer [63]. The mechanism of this field-induced reaction depends on the existence of tautomeric structures of the neutral molecule. Besides the $[M+H]^+$ ions, $[M–H]^\bullet$ radicals are formed in an overall reaction analogous to CH_5^+ formation in CI:

$$M^{+\bullet} + M \rightarrow [M + H]^+ + [M - H]^\bullet \tag{8.2}$$

Furthermore, the radicals formed upon field-induced hydrogen abstraction can lead to polymerization products on the emitter surface [63]. Criteria to distinguish $M^{+\bullet}$ from $[M+H]^+$ ions have been published [64]. Besides analyte polarity and acidity of the solvent used for sample deposition onto the emitter, lower electric field strength and lower emitter temperature are likely to cause stronger $[M+H]^+$ ion contributions [64]. Analytes possessing exchangeable hydrogens strongly tend to form $[M+H]^+$ ions in FI-MS. Occasionally, the protonated molecule occurs in favor of the molecular ion that even may be hardly present (cf. Table 8.1).

8.5.2 Multiply-Charged Ions in FI-MS

Multiply charged ions of minor abundance are frequently observed in FI and FD mass spectra. Their increased abundance as compared to EI spectra can be rationalized by either of the following two-step processes: (*i*) *Post-ionization* of gaseous $M^{+\bullet}$ ions can occur due to the probability for an $M^{+\bullet}$ ion to suffer a second or even third ionization while drifting away from the emitter surface [65, 66]. Especially ions generated in locations not in close vicinity of the counter electrode pass numerous whiskers on their first 10–100 μm of flight:

$$M \rightarrow M^{+\bullet} + e^- \tag{8.3}$$

$$M^{+\bullet} \rightarrow M^{2+} + e^- \tag{8.4}$$

(*ii*) Alternatively, a surface-bound ion, $M^{+\bullet}{}_{(surf)}$, is formed and ionized for a second time before leaving the surface [67–69]:

$$M \rightarrow M^{+\bullet}{}_{(surf)} + e^- \quad (8.5)$$

$$M^{+\bullet}{}_{(surf)} \rightarrow M^{2+} + e^- \quad (8.6)$$

The most commonly formed types of ions in FI are summarized in Table 8.1.

Multiple charges compress *m/z* scale
For recognizing multiply charged ions, it is important to keep in mind that the *m/z* scale is compressed by a factor equal to the number of charges *z* (Sects. 3.8 and 4.2).

8.5.3 Field-Induced Dissociation

In certain cases, the advantageous property of the strong electric field to effect soft ionization can be accompanied by *field-induced dissociation*, another type of field-induced reactions [58, 70, 71]. For example, the fragment ions in the FI spectra of low-mass aliphatic amines, ketones, and hydrocarbons are formed by field-induced dissociation [58, 63]. Field-induced dehydrogenation [72, 73] presents a severe problem to the FI and FD analysis of saturated hydrocarbon mixtures reaching beyond C_{40}, because signals from unsaturated compounds at low levels are superimposed by $[M–H_2]^{+\bullet}$ peaks [74–77]. A reduction of the emitter potential can reduce field-induced dehydrogenation to some degree.

8.5.4 Accurate Mass FI Spectra

Accurate mass complements FI with other valuable information. Unfortunately, FI delivers very low ion currents, which on scanning sector instruments make it difficult to achieve accurate mass measurements. This is because (*i*) high resolution requires narrow slits, and thus, goes along with low transmission, and (*ii*) internal reference masses have to be distributed over the entire range making interferences more likely. While HR-FI-MS on sector instruments is neither new nor impossible [78–81], it is generally outside routine operation [62]. The attachment of FI/FD ion sources to oaTOF instruments has made it quite a bit easier, because a single point of reference, a so-called *lock mass*, is normally sufficient [30, 31].

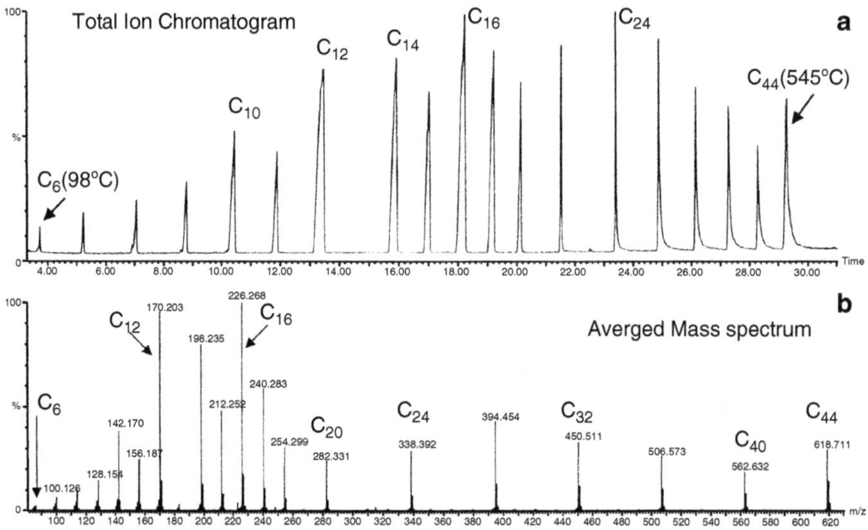

Fig. 8.10 GC-FI-oaTOF-MS total ion chromatogram and averaged mass spectrum of C_6–C_{44} *n*-paraffins. The masses of the paraffin molecular ions are all accurate (Reproduced from Ref. [31] with permission. © American Chemical Society, 2002)

8.5.5 Coupling Gas Chromatography to FI-MS

The coupling of gas chromatography to FI-MS was first attempted in the early 1970s [82, 83], but suffered from poor instrument capabilities of that time. Recent advances with oaTOF instrumentation allow for fast acquisition of spectra, comparatively high resolution, and more importantly, straightforward accurate mass measurements in GC-FI-MS. Thus, GC-FI-MS has become a trusted tool in several laboratories, especially in the petroleum community [30, 31, 84, 85]. To maintain full ionization efficiency, it is common that an accumulation period of 1 s per spectrum is followed by flash-heating the emitter for 0.1–0.2 s [30, 31]. These applications have also been driving the development of EI/FI/FD [40] and EI/CI/FI combination sources for GC-oaTOF instruments [86].

GC-FI-MS of paraffins GC-FI-oaTOF-MS measurements were performed on paraffins from C_6 to C_{44}, covering the wide boiling range from 98 to 545 °C, delivering GC separation and accurate mass information in one run. Main components such as the C_{12}, C_{14}, and C_{16} alkanes caused some broadening of their gas chromatographic peaks, eventually due to adsorption/desorption from the emitter surface resulting in a temporal spread [31]. Figure 8.10 shows the gas chromatogram as represented by the total ion chromatogram and the averaged mass spectrum over the complete acquisition period. Although FI of the entire mixture would have yielded a similar mass spectrum, this approach avoids mutual interference during ionization, and additionally, delivers isomer recognition from retention times.

8.6 FD Spectra

FD can be regarded the softest ionization method in mass spectrometry, even though electrospray ionization and matrix-assisted laser desorption ionization can transfer much larger ions into the gas phase [26, 87]. This is mainly because the ionization process itself does not transfer any extra energy to the incipient ions. Problems normally arise above molecular weights of 3000 u where the heated emitter causes thermal decomposition of the sample.

FD delivers $M^{+\bullet}$ of chlorotriphenylmethane The extraordinarily stable trityl ion, Ph_3C^+, *m/z* 243, tends to dominate mass spectra (Sect. 6.6.2). Thus, neither the EI spectrum of chlorotriphenylmethane nor that of its impurity triphenylmethanol show molecular ions (Fig. 8.11). An isobutane PICI spectrum also shows the trityl ion almost exclusively, although some hint is obtained from the Ph_2COH^+ ion, *m/z* 183, that cannot be explained as a fragment of a chlorotriphenylmethane ion. Only FD reveals the presence of the alcohol by its molecular ion at *m/z* 260, while that of the chloride is detected at *m/z* 278. Both molecular ions undergo some $OH^\bullet$ or $Cl^\bullet$ loss, respectively, to yield the Ph_3C^+ fragment ion of minor intensity.

8.6.1 Ion Formation by Field Ionization in FD-MS

In *field ionization* (as an experimental configuration) *field ionization* (the process) is the major pathway of ion generation. In *field desorption* from activated emitters, the analyte may also undergo *field ionization*. Presuming that the molecules are deposited in layers on the shanks of the whiskers or between them, this requires that (*i*) analytes of low polarity are polarized by action of the electric field, (*ii*) become mobile upon heating, and (*iii*) finally reach the locations of ionizing electric field strength at the tips of the whiskers (Fig. 8.12). The requirement of mobility of the polarized molecules can either be fulfilled via gas phase transport or surface diffusion [52]. As the level of mobility to travel some ten micrometers along a whisker is clearly below that for evaporation from a separate inlet system, thermal decomposition of the field-ionized analyte in FD-MS is much reduced as compared to FI-MS.

The relevance of the FI mechanism of ionization decreases as the polarity of the analyte increases. In certain cases such as sucrose, for example, it is not easy to decide whether gas phase mobility of the neutral and molecular ions jointly formed by FI still play a role [88, 89] or not [90].

EI, FI and FD mass spectra of D-Glucose D-Glucose evaporates into the ion source without complete decomposition as demonstrated by its FI spectrum (Fig. 8.13). FD yields a spectrum with a very low degree of fragmentation that is most probably due to the required slight heating of the emitter. The occurrence of $M^{+\bullet}$ ions, *m/z* 180, and $[M+H]^+$ ions, *m/z* 181, in the FD spectrum suggests that ion formation occurs via field ionization and field-induced proton transfer, respectively.

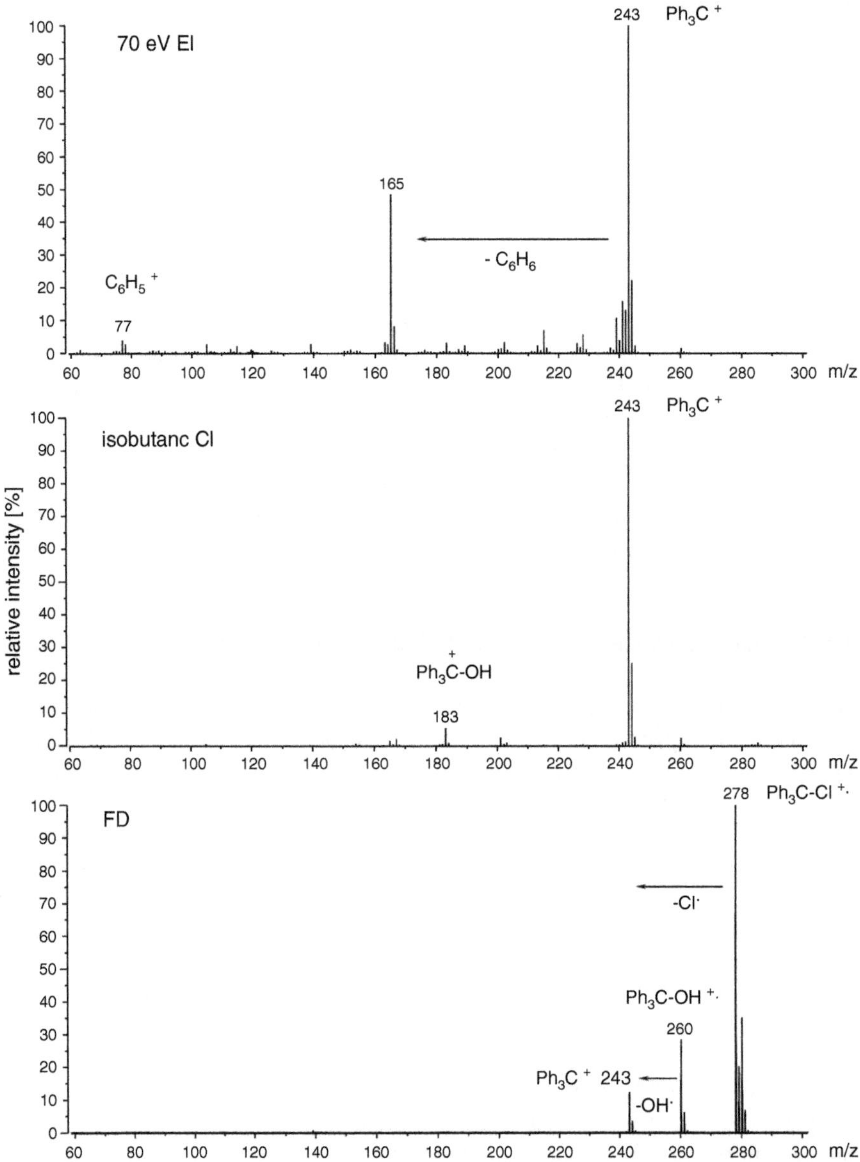

Fig. 8.11 Comparison of EI, PICI, and FD mass spectra of chlorotriphenylmethane containing some triphenylmethanol (By courtesy of C. Limberg, Humboldt University, Berlin)

However, thermal energy plus a hard ionization method (as EI) effect extreme fragmentation. By comparing the EI and FI spectra, the effects of thermal energy may roughly be distinguished from those of EI itself.

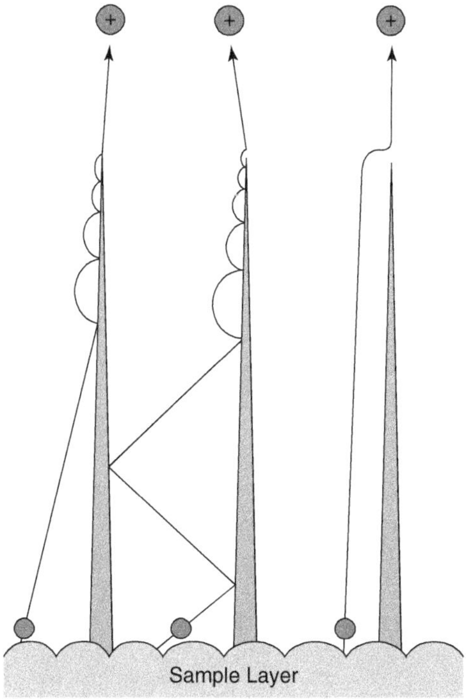

Fig. 8.12 The transport of neutrals to the tips of the field-enhancing whiskers (Reproduced from Ref. [52] by permission. © Elsevier Science, 1981)

8.6.2 Desorption of Preformed Ions in FD-MS

Analytes of very high polarity are not further ionized by field ionization. Here, the prevailing pathways are *protonation* or *cationization*, i.e., the attachment of alkali ions to molecules [91]. The subsequent desorption of the ions from the surface is effected by the action of the electric field. As $[M+Na]^+$ and $[M+K]^+$ ions are already present in the condensed phase, the field strength required for their desorption is lower than that for field ionization or field-induced $[M+H]^+$ ion formation [44, 92]. The desorption of ions is also effective in case of ionic analytes.

Bare wire emitters in FD-MS FD from untreated wire emitters to which alkali metal salts were added was used to obtain mass spectra of tartaric acid, arginine, pentobarbital, and other compounds [91, 93]. Besides $[M+H]^+$ ions, m/z 175, the FD mass spectrum of arginine exhibits $[M+Na]^+$, m/z 197, and $[M+K]^+$, m/z 213, ions due to alkali metal cationization as well as $[2M+H]^+$, m/z 349, cluster ions (Fig. 8.14) [44].

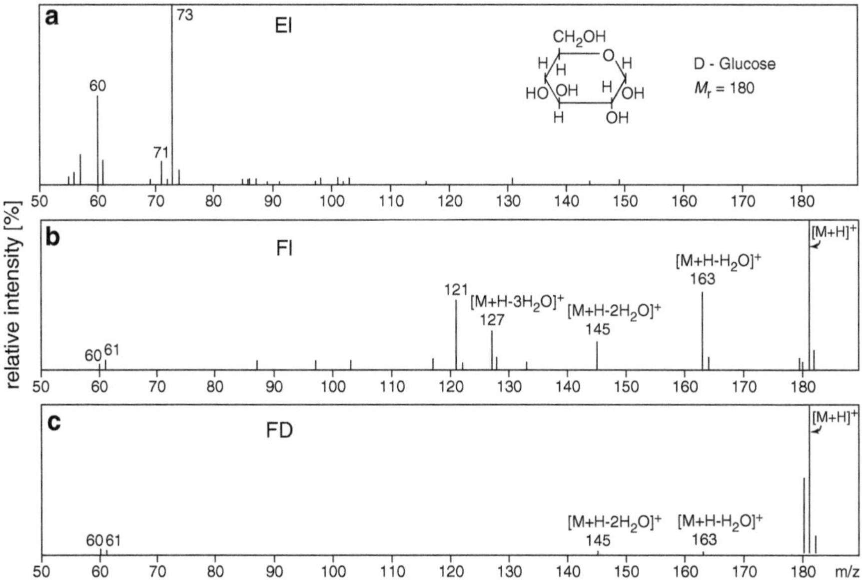

Fig. 8.13 D-Glucose mass spectra: (**a**) EI only yields ions that are due to decomposition and fragmentation, (**b**) FI still produces several fragments, and (**c**) FD almost exclusively gives ions related to the intact molecule (Adapted from Ref. [13] by permission. © Elsevier Science, 1969)

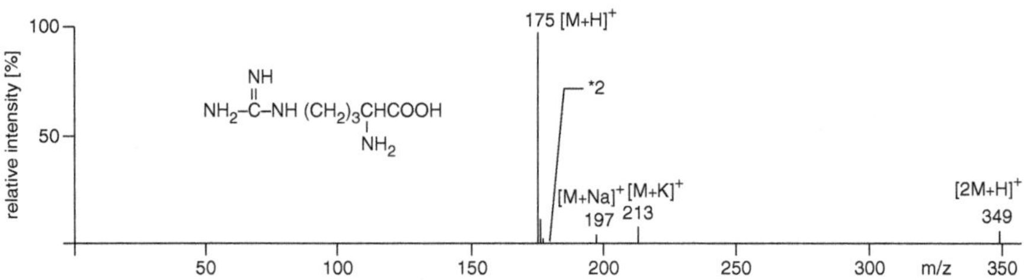

Fig. 8.14 The FD mass spectrum of arginine, $M_r = 174$, desorbed from an untreated metal wire emitter in the presence of alkali ions (Adapted from Ref. [44] by permission. © John Wiley & Sons, 1977)

Two major concepts of ion formation and desorption have been suggested, but it has remained a matter of debate whether the concept of *field-induced desolvation* [94–96] or that of *ion evaporation* [97, 98] more appropriately describes the event. Although different in several aspects, the models are coherent in that ions are created in the condensed phase and subsequently desorbed into the gas phase. Both recognize the electric field as the driving force to effect extraction of ionic species after charge separation within the layer adsorbed onto the emitter surface.

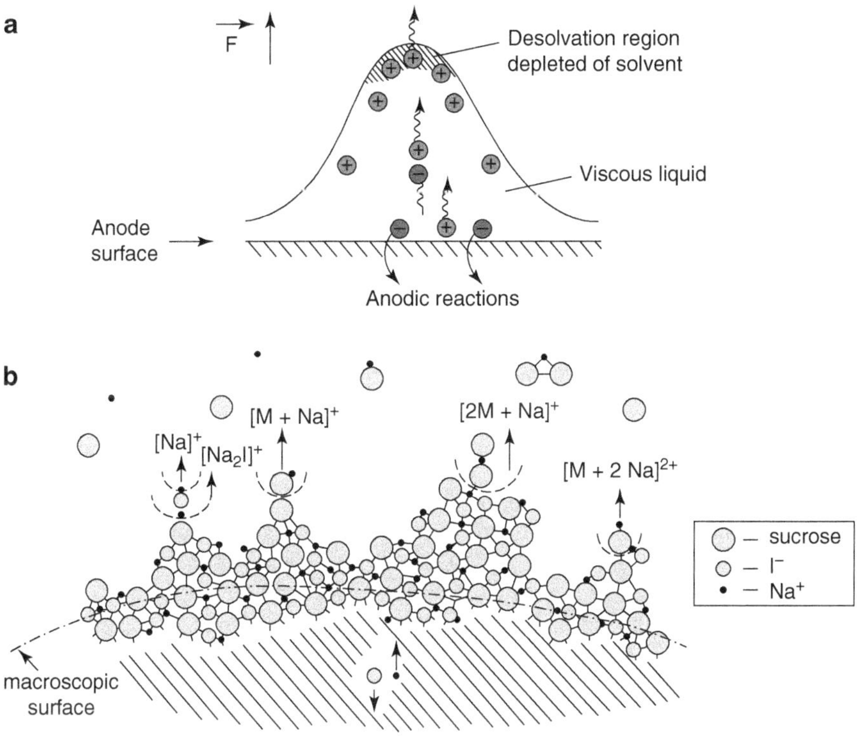

Fig. 8.15 The desolvation of ions. (**a**) Charge separation inside a protuberance, (**b**) continuous reconstruction of the surface allows for successive rupture of intermolecular bonds and stepwise desolvation of the ions (Reproduced from Ref. [96] by permission. © Elsevier Science, 1984)

Protuberances are assumed to develop from where ions can escape into the gas phase as a result of the field-enhancing effect of these protrusions. The differences of the models may in part be attributed to the different experimental and theoretical approaches. The model of the Röllgen group is much based on microscopic observation of protuberances from glassy sample layers (Fig. 8.15) [94, 95], whereas the Derrick group assumes their size to be a thousand-fold smaller (Fig. 8.16) [97]. Thus, the latter emphasizes the role of mobility of molecules instead of microscopic viscous flow of the surface layer.

8.6.3 Cluster Ion Formation in FD-MS

Highly polar analytes which strongly tend towards cationization, frequently form cluster ions such as $[n\mathrm{M+H}]^+$ and $[n\mathrm{M+alkali}]^+$ in addition to $[\mathrm{M+H}]^+$ and $[\mathrm{M+alkali}]^+$ ions. A priori, there is no reason why these cluster ions should not be interpreted as resulting from "impurities". However, the sequence of events can serve as a reliable criterion to distinguish components of higher molecular weight

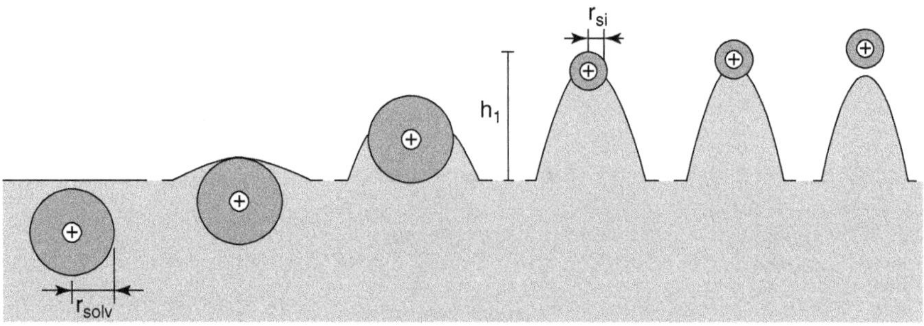

Fig. 8.16 Schematic model for ion evaporation. r_{solv} is the radius of the solvation sphere, r_{si} the radius of the separating ion, and h_1 the height of the protuberance when the radius of its parabolic tip equals r_{si} (Reproduced from Ref. [98] by permission. © Elsevier Science, 1987)

from cluster ions. Cluster ions are preferably formed when the coverage of the emitter surface is still high, i.e., in the beginning of desorption. As desorption proceeds, the probability for cluster ion formation decreases, because the surface layer is diminished. In addition, a continuously rising emitter heating current leads to further thermal decomposition of clusters. Whereas cluster ions decrease in abundance, true higher-mass components require higher emitter temperature to become mobile and ionized thereafter (cf. Sect. 8.4.1). Doubly charged cluster ions, e.g., $[M+2Na]^{2+}$, may also occur. Such doubly or even multiply charged ions can serve to extend the mass range accessible by FD-MS [26].

Cluster ion formation of polar molecules During the acquisition of an FD mass spectrum of a putatively clean disaccharide, a series of ions at higher *m/z* was observed in addition to $[M+H]^+$, *m/z* 341 and $[M+Na]^+$, *m/z* 363. Those ions could be interpreted either in terms of cluster ions or of higher oligosaccharides, respectively. The high-mass ions were only observed soon after the onset of desorption, while their abundance decreased remarkably at somewhat higher emitter current. Thereby, these signals could be assigned to cluster ions such as $[2M+Na]^+$, *m/z* 703, and $[3M+Na]^+$, *m/z* 1043 (Fig. 8.17).

Cluster ions or real high-mass component?
Cluster ions of the general formula $[nM+X]^+$, less frequently also $[nM]^{+\bullet}$, mainly appear at the onset of desorption and then decrease in abundance along with the diminishing amount of sample on the emitter. Finally, cluster ions disappear towards the end of desorption. Whether or not the observed peaks at higher *m/z* correspond to cluster ions can thus be answered by watching the intensity of cluster ion peaks along the period of desorption/ionization.

(continued)

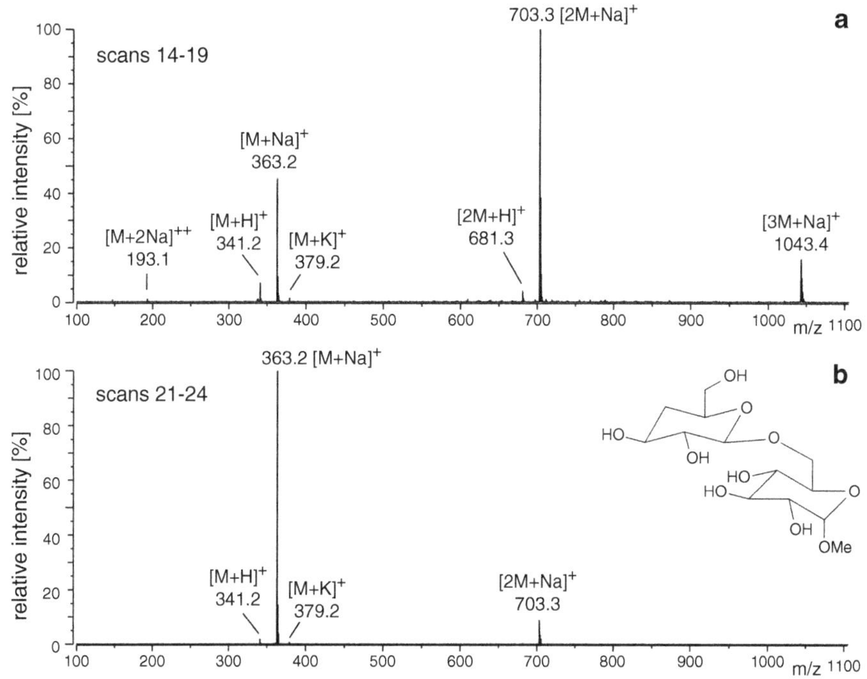

Fig. 8.17 FD mass spectra of a disaccharide (**a**) at the beginning of desorption, (**b**) towards end of desorption [99] (By courtesy of H. Friebolin, Heidelberg University)

Generally, the amount of cluster ion production increases (*i*) at high sample load on the emitter and (*ii*) with higher polarity of the analyte (cf. Sect. 8.6.4).

The value of $\Delta m/z$ between adjacent cluster ion peaks directly reflects the mass of the neutral analyte M. This can also be exploited to identify whether M is detected as $M^{+\bullet}$, $[M+H]^+$, or $[M+Na]^+$.

8.6.4 FD-MS of Ionic Analytes

The intact cation C^+ of an ionic analyte of the general composition $[C^+A^-]$ always causes the base peak in positive-ion FD mass spectra. In addition, singly charged cluster ions of the $[C_nA_{n-1}]^+$ type are observed [100, 101]. Their abundance and the maximum of n varies depending on the ionic species encountered as well as on the actual experimental parameters such as temperature and sample load of the emitter (Figs. 8.18 and 8.19). The advantage of these cluster ions is that the mass difference between the members of the series corresponds to $[C^+A^-]$. Thus, the counterion A^-

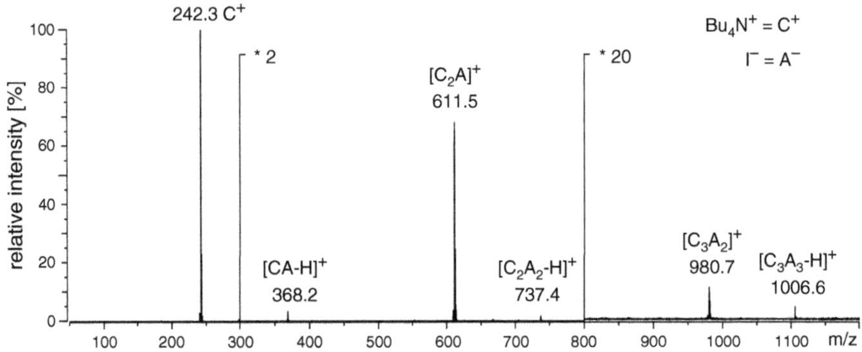

Fig. 8.18 FD mass spectrum of $[(n\text{-}C_4H_9)_4N]^+\ I^-$. The intact ammonium ion is detected at *m/z* 242; additional signals are due to cluster ions. (For the EI spectrum cf. Sect. 6.11.4)

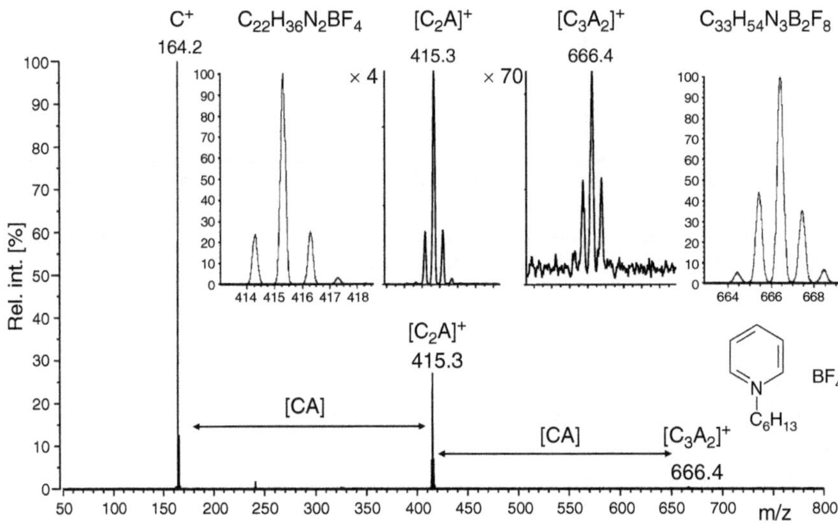

Fig. 8.19 LIFDI mass spectrum of *N*-hexylpyridinium tetrafluoroborate in methanol at a concentration of 0.1 μl ml^{-1} scanned over the *m/z* 50–800 range. The *insets* show the $[C_2A]^+$ and $[C_3A_2]^+$ cluster ions for comparison of the experimental and calculated isotopic patterns that are characteristic of one and two boron atoms, respectively. The mass of [CA] is obtained from $\Delta(m/z)$ between adjacent cluster ion peaks (Reproduced from Ref. [110] with permission. © Elsevier Science Publishers, 2007)

can be determined by subtraction of the mass of C^+. Moreover, the isotopic pattern of the anion is reflected in the cluster ion signals, facilitating the identification of chloride and bromide, for example. Interestingly, ionic species corresponding to some sort of "molecular ion of the salt" can also be formed. Usually, such ions are of much lower intensity than the even-electron cluster ions. Applications of FD-MS to detect cations are manifold and include organic cations [16, 20, 100–104] as well as inorganic ones [105, 106] even down to the trace level [107], e.g., for trace-metal analysis in physiological fluids of patients suffering from multiple sclerosis [108].

Zwitterions are generally not easy to analyze by MS. Depending on the acidity of the proton-donating site and on the basicity of the proton-accepting site either the cationic or the anionic species can be formed preferentially. Adding acids to the solution of the analyte prior to loading of the emitter can significantly enhance the signal resulting from the protonated species [109].

Cluster ions reveal cation and anion of salts Ionic liquids (ILs) are perfect representatives of ionic analytes. LIFDI (essentially FD, cf. Sect. 8.6) spectra of ILs such as *N*-hexylpyridinium tetrafluoroborate (Fig. 8.19) are dominated by the cation peak, C^+ here at *m*/*z* 164, that is accompanied by a strong first cluster ion signal, $[(C^+)_2+BF_4^-]^+$ at *m*/*z* 415, and by a weak second cluster ion signal. The corresponding boron isotopic patterns (B_1 and B_2) are clearly visible. Furthermore, the softness of the FD process is demonstrated by the fact that even the weakly bound cluster ions exhibit almost no fragmentation in metastable ion spectra, but require collisions to induce dissociation [110].

8.6.5 Temporal Evolution of FD Spectral Acquisition

During an FD run, the FD emitter heating current is generally ramped from 0 to 2 mA to several tens of milliamperes to effect mobilization and desorption/ionization of the analyte on the emitter surface. Thus, a typical total ion chromatogram (TIC) shows a section of very low intensity up to the onset of desorption. There, the TIC rises steeply to the maximum of ion production and then falls quickly after the complete sample has been consumed. The final FD spectrum is best obtained by addition of those scans exhibiting good signal intensity.

FD analysis of an organic solid compound The FD spectrum of α-cyano-4-hydroxycinnamic acid, $C_{10}H_7NO_3$, (CHCA, a matrix compound in MALDI-MS) depicts the typical process of mass spectral acquisition in FD-MS (Fig. 8.20). During the first 35 scans there is almost no desorption, then the analyte is desorbed and ionized during scans 35–46 (EHC ca. 25–30 mA), and finally, the TIC drops after consumption of the sample. To achieve good signal-to-noise ratio, scans 37–44 where accumulated. The resulting FD spectrum mainly shows the $M^{+\bullet}$ ion at *m*/*z* 189.1, which is accompanied by a $[2M]^{+\bullet}$ cluster ion at *m*/*z* 378.1. Both ionic species are also accompanied by fragment ion peaks of very low intensity corresponding to some loss of $OH^\bullet$ and H_2O from $M^{+\bullet}$ and $[2M]^{+\bullet}$ ions, respectively.

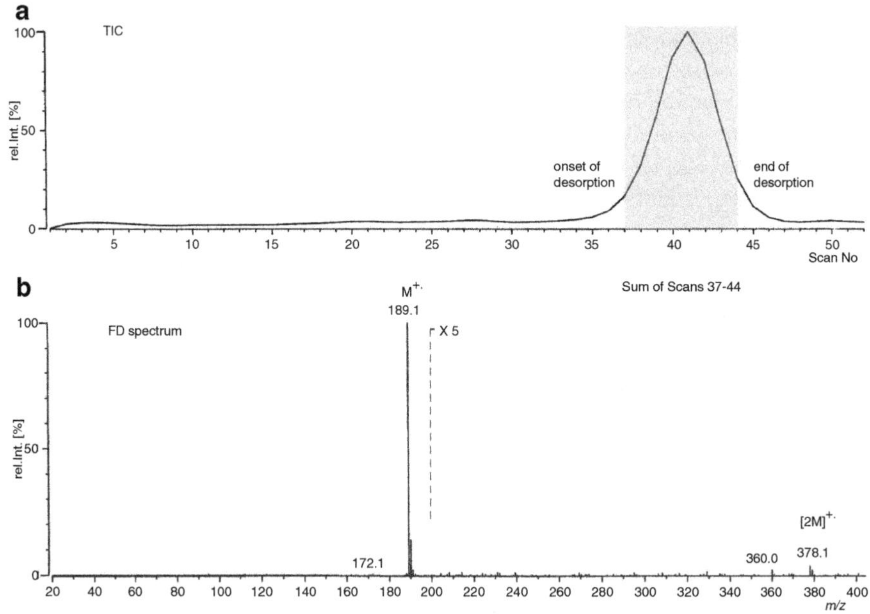

Fig. 8.20 Acquisition of an FD mass spectrum of CHCA. (**a**) TIC, (**b**) resulting FD spectrum. Desorption/ionization occurs during scans No. 35–46. Scans 37–44 where accumulated to provide the final FD spectrum, which mainly shows the $M^{+\bullet}$ ion at *m/z* 189.1 and a $[2M]^{+\bullet}$ cluster ion at *m/z* 378.1

Shape of the TIC

Pure analytes often show a comparatively sharp onset of desorption. Desorption then lasts for several scans until the sample is consumed. Finally, the intensity of the signals rapidly drops to zero again. In case of mixtures, some fractionation by molecular weight of the components is observed (Fig. 8.21).

8.6.6 Best Anode Temperature and Thermal Decomposition

The onset of desorption of an analyte depends not solely on its intrinsic properties, but also on the extraction voltage and the applied emitter heating current. FD spectra are typically acquired while the *emitter heating current* (EHC) is increased at a constant rate (1–8 mA min^{-1}). Alternatively, the heating can be regulated in a emission-controlled manner [55–57]. The desorption usually begins before the competing thermal decomposition of the analytes becomes severe. Nevertheless, increasing temperature of the emitter transfers additional thermal energy onto the desorbing ions, thereby effecting some fragmentation. The optimum temperature of

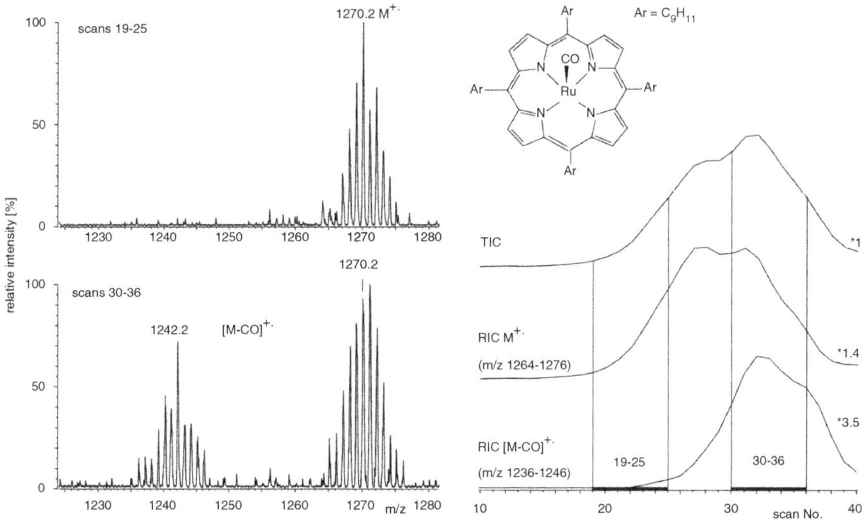

Fig. 8.21 Thermal CO loss during FD measurement of a ruthenium-carbonyl-porphyrin complex (Adapted from Ref. [111] by permission. © IM Publications, 1997)

the emitter where a sufficiently intense signal at the lowest level of fragmentation is obtained has been termed *best anode temperature* (BAT) [19, 37].

FD spectrum of a ruthenium-carbonyl-porphyrin complex The FD spectrum of a ruthenium-carbonyl-porphyrin complex shows an isotopic pattern very close to the theoretical distribution (Sect. 3.2). The loss of the carbonyl ligand chiefly results from thermal decomposition. A spectrum accumulated close to BAT (scans 19–25, EHC 25–30 mA) is nearly devoid of CO loss, while a spectrum accumulated of scans 30–36 (35–40 mA) shows significant CO loss (Fig. 8.21). This is demonstrated by comparison of the total ion chromatogram (TIC) with the reconstructed ion chromatogram (RIC) of $M^{+\bullet}$ and $[M–CO]^{+\bullet}$. The FD spectrum of a lower-mass complex was essentially devoid of signals of CO loss because lower emitter currents were sufficient to effect desorption [111].

8.6.7 FD-MS of Polymers

FD-MS is well suited for the analysis of low- to medium-polarity synthetic oligomers and polymers [26, 27, 70, 74, 75, 77, 112–114]. In advantageous cases, polymer molecules beyond molecular weights of 10,000 u can be measured [115]. Besides the mass analyzer used, limiting factors for the mass range are thermal decomposition of polymer and presence or absence of charge-stabilizing groups. Polystyrene, for example, with its combination of aromatic rings and low polarity is close to an ideal case for FD-MS. Heteroatoms are also useful because of

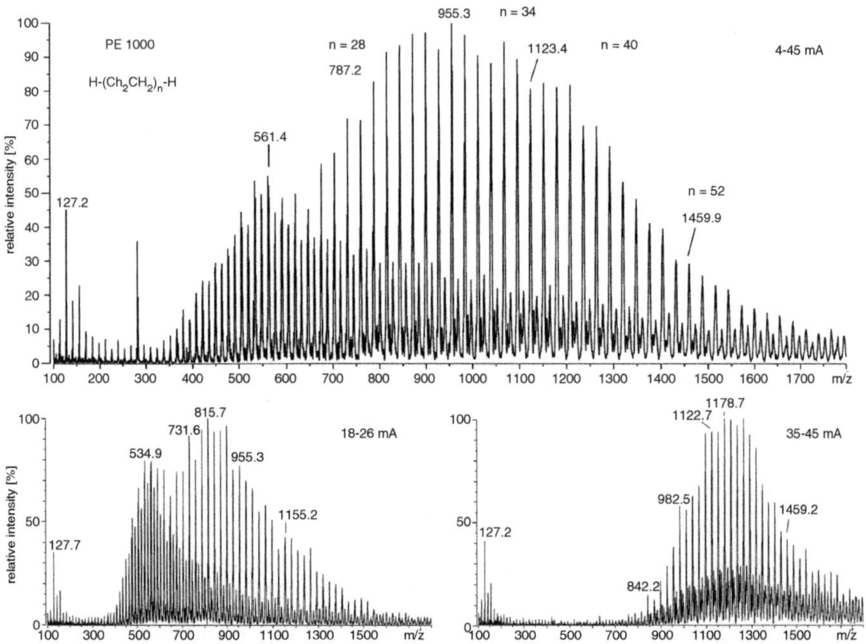

Fig. 8.22 FD spectra of PE 1000 (emitter potential 10 kV, EHC 4–45 mA). *Insets* show selected ranges corresponding to different EHCs (Adapted from Ref. [77] by permission. © IM Publications, 2000)

their general capability to serve as proton- or metal ion-accepting sites. The worst case for MS is that of polyethylene (PE) [74, 75, 77]: the FD mass spectra of PE oligomers can be obtained up to *m*/*z* 3500; however, starting at around C_{40} hydrocarbons, field-induced and thermally induced dehydrogenation can no longer be suppressed and thermal decomposition of the hydrocarbon chains start playing a role above 2000 u.

FD mass spectrum of polyethylene The FD mass spectrum of polyethylene of nominal average molecular weight 1000 u (PE 1000) was obtained by summing of all scans where desorption occurred, i.e., over the 4–45 mA EHC range (Fig. 8.22) [77]. The result represents the molecular weight distribution of the polymer. The according experimental average molecular weight can be calculated by means of Eq. 3.2 (Sect. 3.1). The fractionating effect of emitter heating and the significant changes in spectral appearance are demonstrated by the spectra in the lower part of the figure showing two selected portions of the total ion desorption.

8.6.8 Negative-Ion Field Desorption – An Exotic Exception

Negative-ion FD-MS for the direct detection of the anion A^- and cluster ions of the general composition $[C_{n-1}A_n]^-$ can, in principle, be performed [116, 117]. Nonetheless, negative-ion FD-MS has remained an exception. This is due to the fact that electrons are easily emitted from activated emitters well before negative ions start to desorb. Then, the strong emission of electrons causes a spark discharge that ends up in the destruction of the emitter. Low emitter voltages and larger emitter–counter electrode distance can help to avoid such problems [118]. Neutral analytes can give rise to $[M–H]^-$ ions or products of nucleophilic addition, e.g., $[M+Cl]^-$ ions [119]. Thus, if anions are of interest, they are generally analyzed indirectly by FD-MS via the formation of cluster ions with their positive counterion.

With the advent of fast atom bombardment (FAB, Chap. 10), the interest in negative-ion FD-MS vanished. Nowadays, matrix-assisted laser desorption/ionization (MALDI, Chap. 11), or electrospray ionization (ESI, Chap. 12) are by far preferred for analyzing anions.

8.6.9 Types of Ions in FD-MS

At first sight, FD produces a disadvantageous variety of ions depending on the polarity of the analyte and on the presence or absence of impurities such as alkali metal ions. However, with some knowledge of the ions formed, the signals can be deconvoluted without difficulty (Table 8.2).

Never one adduct alone

One type of alkali adduct ion almost never occurs exclusively, i.e., $[M+H]^+$, $[M+Na]^+$ and $[M+K]^+$ (M+1, M+23 and M+39) are observed with varying relative intensities at 22 u and 16 u distance, respectively. This facilitates the recognition of those peaks and effectively allows for the assignment of the molecular weight.

Table 8.2 Ions formed by FD

Method	Analytes	Ions formed
FD	Nonpolar	$M^{+\bullet}$, M^{2+}, occasionally $M^{3+\bullet}$
FD	Medium polarity	$M^{+\bullet}$, M^{2+} and/or $[M+H]^+$, $[M+alkali]^+$, occasionally $[2M]^{+\bullet}$ and/or $[2M+H]^+$, $[2M+alkali]^+$, rarely $[M+2H]^{2+}$, $[M+2\ alkali]^{2+}$
FD	Polar	$[M+H]^+$, $[M+alkali]^+$, often $[2M+H]^+$, $[2M+alkali]^+$, occasionally $[nM+H]^+$, $[nM+alkali]^+$, rarely $[M+2H]^{2+}$, $[M+2\ alkali]^{2+}$
FD	Ionic[a]	C^+, $[C_n+A_{n-1}]^+$, rarely $[CA]^{+\bullet}$

[a]Comprising cation C^+ and anion A^-

8.7 Liquid Injection Field Desorption Ionization

Numerous analytes could be good candidates for FD-MS, but undergo immediate decomposition by reacting with ambient air and/or water during conventional emitter loading. Emitter loading under inert conditions such as in a glove box does not really avoid the problem, because the emitter still needs to be mounted to the probe before insertion into the vacuum lock.

Liquid injection field desorption ionization (LIFDI) presents a major breakthrough for FD-MS of reactive analytes [29, 120]. The risk of decomposition before starting the measurement is greatly reduced because the analyte, dissolved at about 0.1–0.2 mg ml^{-1}, can be handled under inert conditions. It is transported through a fused silica capillary by the sucking action of the ion source vacuum and then spreads out over the entire emitter driven by capillary forces and adsorption. Careful alignment of the sample transfer capillary with respect to the emitter axis is crucial for reliable wetting. The small volume of solvent transferred (ca. 40 nl) evaporates within seconds. As the sample is supplied from the "backside" to the emitter, there neither is a need to remove the capillary during the measurement, nor to change the adjustment of the emitter inside the ion source (Fig. 8.23). Instead, the emitter interrupts the contact to the capillary as it slightly bends toward the counter electrode as soon as the high voltage is switched on. Thus, LIFDI simplifies the delicate procedure of emitter loading and allows for its repeated loading without breaking the vacuum between successive measurements. This also avoids frequent focusing of the ion source [29, 110, 121]. Together with faster ramping of the EHC, up to 30 mA min^{-1} as enabled by lower sample load, this causes up to tenfold reduced measurement times in LIFDI as compared to conventional FD-MS. In any other respect, FD and LIFDI spectra are equivalent.

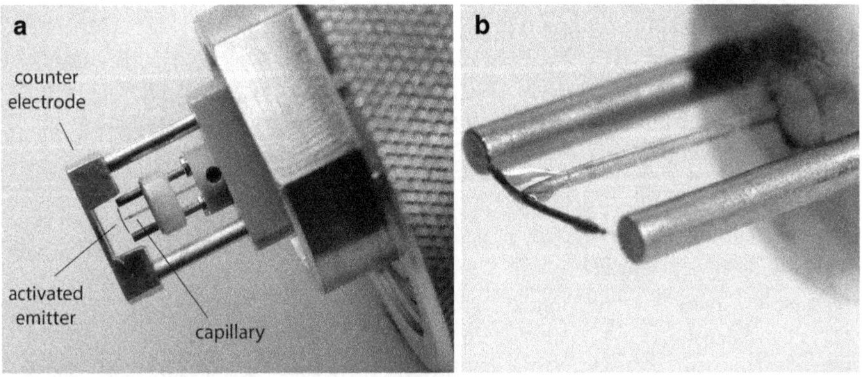

Fig. 8.23 (**a**) LIFDI probe tip with the fused silica capillary that delivers the sample to the "backside" of the activated emitter; here, the counter electrode is part of the probe, and (**b**) wetting of the emitter with solvent spreading out over the activated zone. The 13-μm tungsten wire connecting this section to the posts is barely visible (By courtesy of Linden CMS, Leeste, Germany)

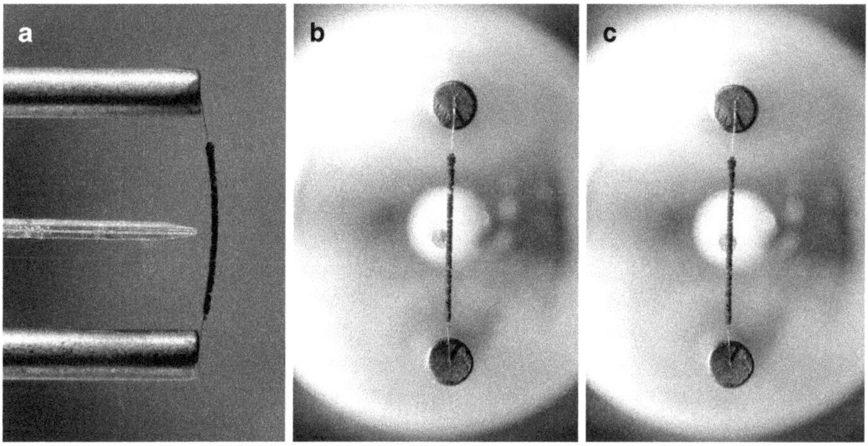

Fig. 8.24 Alignment of the fused silica capillary on the emitter axis; the photographs are similar to what would be observed using a 8× magnifying glass. (**a**) Side view to show the distance between the tip of the capillary and the activated emitter, (**b**, **c**) on axis views. In (**b**) the capillary is left side off-axis while in (**c**) it is well aligned

The majority of LIFDI applications either deals with sensitive compounds such as transition metal complexes [29, 121, 122] or belongs to the group of petroleomics applications [32, 123–125]. Using an extremely low liquid flow rate even allows to continuously deliver sample solution to an emitter at high voltage, permiting continuous-flow (CF-)LIFDI experiments [33, 126]. More recently, an automated LIFDI system has been introduced [127].

8.7.1 Positioning of the Capillary

Accurate positioning of the silica capillary that delivers the analyte solution to the emitter inside the ion source is crucial for LIFDI operation. The tip of the capillary has to approach as closely as possible without ever touching the emitter. Furthermore, it needs to be aligned in order to allow the emerging drop to bridge the gap between the capillary exit and the activated emitter. The simplest way to accomplish this seemingly tricky task is to align the capillary before insertion of the probe. To do so, a magnifying glass (8–10 fold) is recommended. Also, it is important to observe the adjustment on-axis of the capillary, as looking at the assembly in a slightly sideways manner would cause erroneous alignment due to parallax error (Fig. 8.24). The capillary is then positioned by turning a small screw located in the base of the emitter holder.

LIFDI-MS of sensitive compounds Transition metal complexes are readily analyzed by LIFDI-MS. A dichloro nickel carbene complex dissolved in acetonitrile not only forms the expected $[M–Cl]^+$ ion, *m/z* 375.3, but also a molecular ion,

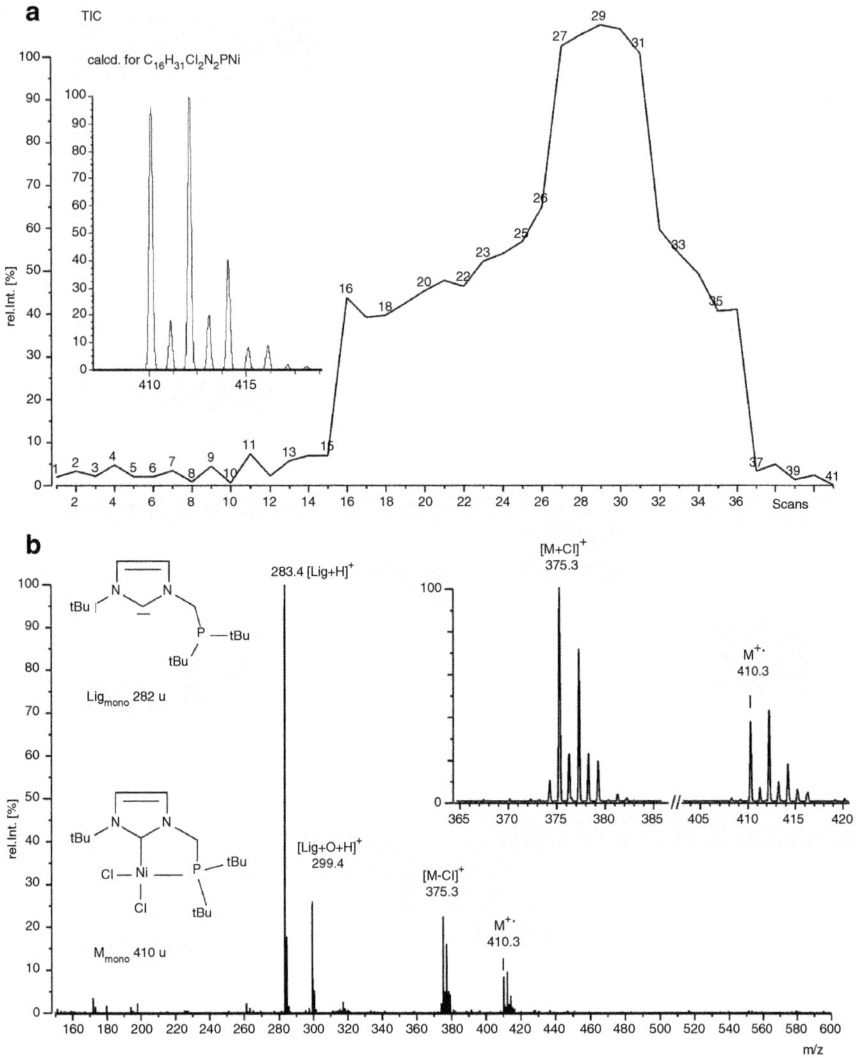

Fig. 8.25 (**a**) TIC and (**b**) LIFDI mass spectrum obtained from a nickel carbene complex in acetonitrile solution shows peaks due to excess free ligand $[Lig+H]^+$, *m/z* 283.4, and its oxide $[Lig+O+H]^+$, *m/z* 299.4, plus those corresponding to the complex. Note the intense $M^{+\bullet}$ ion at *m/z* 410.3 accompanying the $[M–Cl]^+$ ion at *m/z* 375.3. The isotopic pattern of the molecular ion is in good agreement with the calculated isotopic distribution (cf. inserts) (Reproduced from Ref. [121] with permission. © Springer-Verlag, Heidelberg, 2006)

m/z 410.3, of somewhat lower abundance. The isotopic patterns of the signals are in very good agreement with the calculated isotopic distributions (Fig. 8.25). Peaks due to the free ligand and its oxide are also observed. The corresponding TIC is

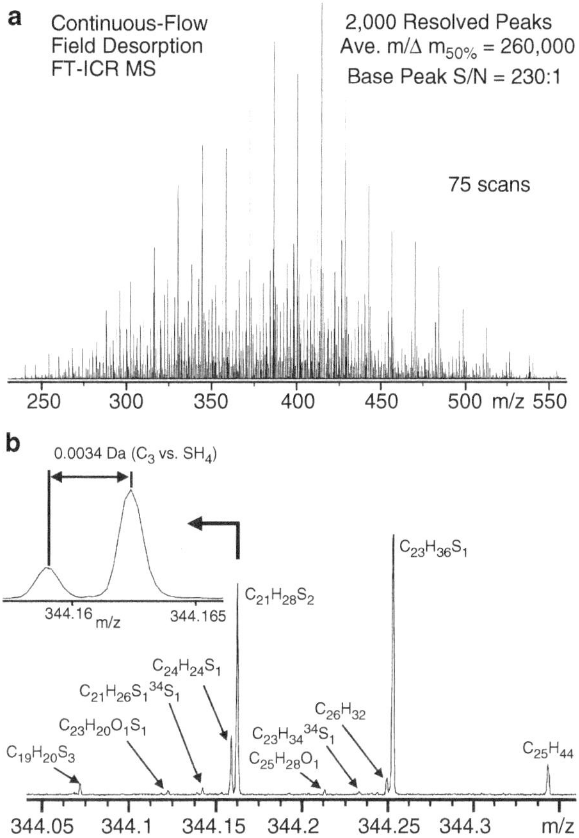

Fig. 8.26 CF-LIFDI-FT-ICR mass spectral analysis of a refinery process stream sample. (**a**) Spectrum as obtained from 75 single spectra accumulated during 1 h. (**b**) Extreme mass scale expansion at nominal *m/z* 344 from the broadband mass spectrum reveals the complexity of the sample. The resolution of the 3.4×10^{-3} u distant C_3 vs. SH_4 doublet can be observed at *m/z* 344.25 and separately in the inset at *m/z* 344.16 (Adapted from Ref. [33] with permission. © John Wiley & Sons Ltd, 2004)

typical for FD experiments and clearly reveals the onset of desorption/ionization at medium EHC and the completion of the measurement when the sample is consumed [121].

Continuous-flow LIFDI-FT-ICR-MS Extremely complex crude oil fractions with each component at a very low concentration can be analyzed by continuous-flow LIFDI-FT-ICR-MS. CF-LIFDI delivers improved spectral quality as a stable FD-generated ion current can be sustained to allow for measurement times totaling up to 1 h. With the ionizing high voltage switched on, the sample solution (0.1 mg ml^{-1}) is delivered at 75 nl min^{-1} through a 10 μm i.d. capillary onto the emitter which is moderately heated using an EHC of 15 mA. The example shows the CF-LIFDI-FT-ICR spectrum of a refinery process stream sample (Fig. 8.26) [33].

8.8 General Properties of FI-MS and FD-MS

8.8.1 Sensitivity of FI-MS and FD-MS

In FD mode, the sensitivity (Sect. 1.6) of magnetic sector instruments is about 4×10^{-11} C μg^{-1} for the $[M+H]^+$ ion of cholesterol, *m/z* 387, at $R = 1000$. This is 10^4 times less than specified for those instruments in EI mode and 10^3 times less than for CI mode.

In FI mode, the sensitivity of such instruments is about 4×10^{-9} A Pa^{-1} for the molecular ion of acetone, *m/z* 58, at $R = 1000$. This corresponds to an ion current of 4×10^{-13} A at a realized ion source pressure of 10^{-4} Pa.

Although the ion currents produced by FI/FD ion sources are by orders of magnitude smaller than those from EI or CI ion sources, the detection limits are quite good. In general, about 0.1 ng of sample yield a sufficient signal-to-noise ratio (S/N $\geq$ 10) in FD-MS. This is because most of the ion current is collected in a single ionic species (including the isotopologs). Furthermore, the background of FI/FD ion sources is very clean, providing a good signal-to-background ratio.

Comparison of sensitivity data The comparison of 70-eV EI, CI, NICI and FI on the average reveals a 200-fold lower total ion current from FI as compared to EI. If only molecular ion peak intensities are compared, the FI spectra become much more appealing (Fig. 8.27) [86]. The concentration of the ion current on the molecular ions and the concomitant clarity of FI spectra are certainly the most attractive features of FI-MS.

8.8.2 Analytes and Practical Considerations for FI, FD, and LIFDI

Analytes for FI have to be evaporated prior to ionization, and thus any sample suitable for EI (Sect. 5.10) or CI (Sect. 7.10) yields low-fragmentation FI mass spectra. For FD and LIFDI, the analyte should be soluble to at least 0.01 mg ml^{-1} in some solvent. Concentrations of 0.1–2 mg ml^{-1} are ideal for FD and about 0.1–0.2 mg ml^{-1} should be used for LIFDI. Significantly higher sample loads result in overloading the emitter, and in turn cause its destruction due to electric discharge. In case of extremely low solubility, repeated application of solution to the emitter is also possible. For FD, fine suspensions or dispersions are acceptable, whereas these will block the capillary in LIFDI. Pure water tends not to wet the emitter surface – a problem that can be circumvented by addition of some methanol before transferring the solution to the emitter. Whatever the solvent for FD, it should be volatile enough to evaporate prior to introduction of the probe into the vacuum lock, while small volumes of dimethylformamide or dimethylsulfoxide, for example, can also be evaporated in the rough vacuum of the vacuum lock. The analyte may be neutral or ionic. However, anions are usually detected solely in an indirect manner, i.e., from corresponding cluster ions. Solutions containing metal salts, e.g., from buffers or excess of noncomplexed metals, are to be avoided,

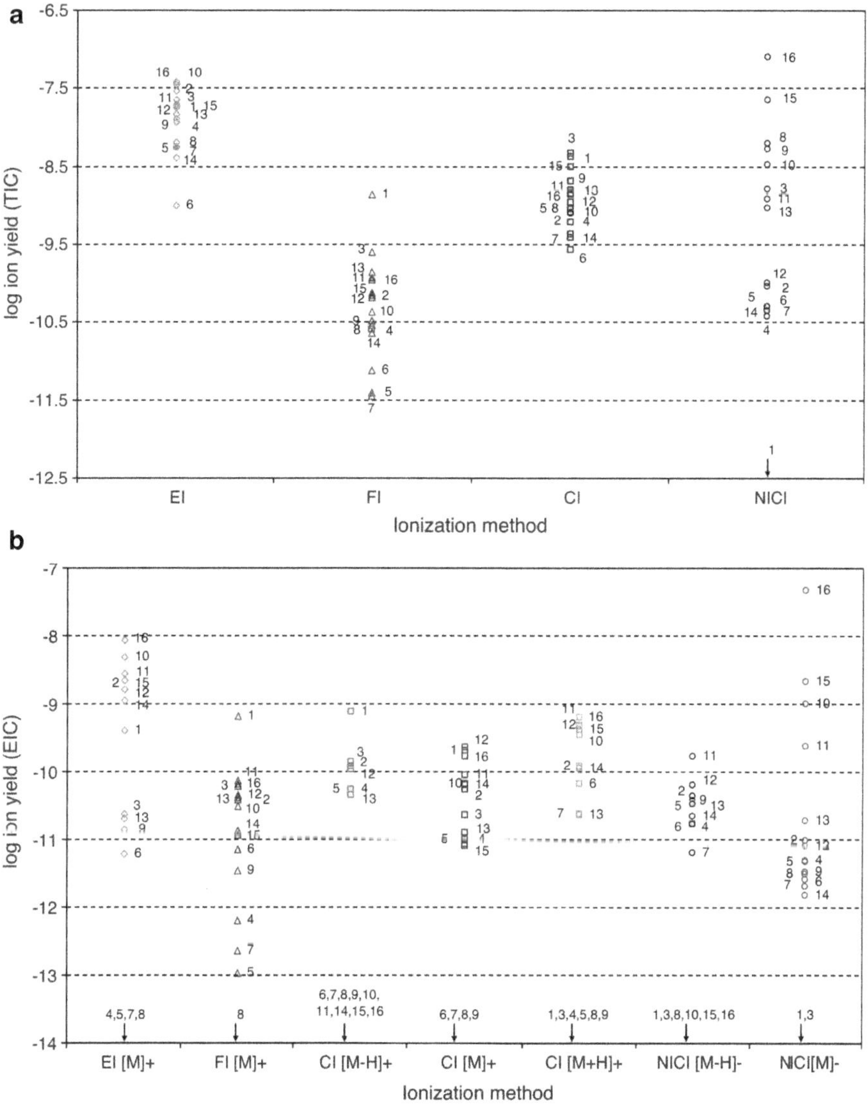

Fig. 8.27 Comparison of (**a**) total ion currents and (**b**) ion currents due to molecular ions or otherwise ionized intact molecules typical for GC-MS as obtained by 70-eV EI, FI, positive-ion CI and negative-ion CI both using methane reagent gas (Reproduced from Ref. [86] with permission. © John Wiley & Sons, Ltd., 2009)

because sudden desorption of the metal ions at higher emitter current often leads to rupture of the emitter. A mass range up to 3000 u is easily covered by FD, and cases reaching up to 10,000 u have been reported.

8.8.3 Mass Analyzers for FI and FD

In FI and FD, ions of 10–12 keV kinetic energy are generated as a continuous ion current. Compared to EI or CI the ion current is weak and tends to fluctuate. The voltage drop across the whiskers (roughly proportional to the whisker length) causes an energy spread of the ions which results in poor resolution with single-focusing magnetic sector instruments [45]. Therefore, double-focusing magnetic sector instruments were the standard in FD-MS for decades. Although linear quadrupoles have been adapted to FI/FD ion sources rather successfully [128, 129], they never became widespread with FI/FD. More recently, oaTOF and FT-ICR analyzers have been equipped with FD/LIFDI sources [34, 35, 123, 126, 127, 130, 131].

Most promising in terms of performance per instrument cost and size is the approach to attach LIFDI to Orbitrap analyzers, in particular to the Thermo Fisher Exactive and Exactive-Q series of instruments. With these particular instruments, the LIFDI source is mounted "at the rear" end, i.e., via the HCD cell (Sect. 9.10). In case of the Exactive-Q type, this unconventional way of mounting the LIFDI source sacrifices the ability to use the instrument's tandem MS capabilities in LIFDI mode, while, on the other hand, it permits to keep the atmospheric pressure source ready while switching back and forth between ESI or APCI and LIFDI operation.

LIFDI of Grubb's catalyst Olefin metathesis by use of Grubbs catalyst, $C_{46}H_{65}Cl_2N_2PRu$ (Grubbs type II), is a common process in preparative organic chemistry. The air- and moisture-sensitive catalyst has been analyzed by using an Exactive Orbitrap instrument with a prototype LIFDI source attached via the HCD cell. The molecular ion signal in this spectrum exhibits about $R = 40.000$. The mass errors of all major peaks are below 1 mu when compared to the calculated isotopic pattern for $[C_{46}H_{65}Cl_2N_2PRu]^{+\bullet}$ (Fig. 8.28).

8.9 FI, FD, and LIFDI at a Glance

Basic Principle

Field ionization (FI) and field desorption (FD) rely on the ionization of neutrals by action of very strong electric fields in the order of 10 V nm^{-1}. The electric field enables the detachment of an electron from the neutral via a tunneling mechanism. While the electron moves into the field anode (aka field emitter) the resulting molecular ion gets ejected from the surface. Field ionization as a mechanism of ion formation can occur in both the gas phase or in the condensed phase at the emitter surface. The technique is also termed *field ionization* when the analyte is supplied via the gas phase to effect ionization of gaseous neutrals. It is termed *field desorption* when the analyte is deposited onto the field emitter prior to exposure to the electric field. Liquid injection field desorption/ionization is a special variant of sample supply for FD-MS. LIFDI allows for sample deposition under inert conditions and enables quicker and smoother operation of FD.

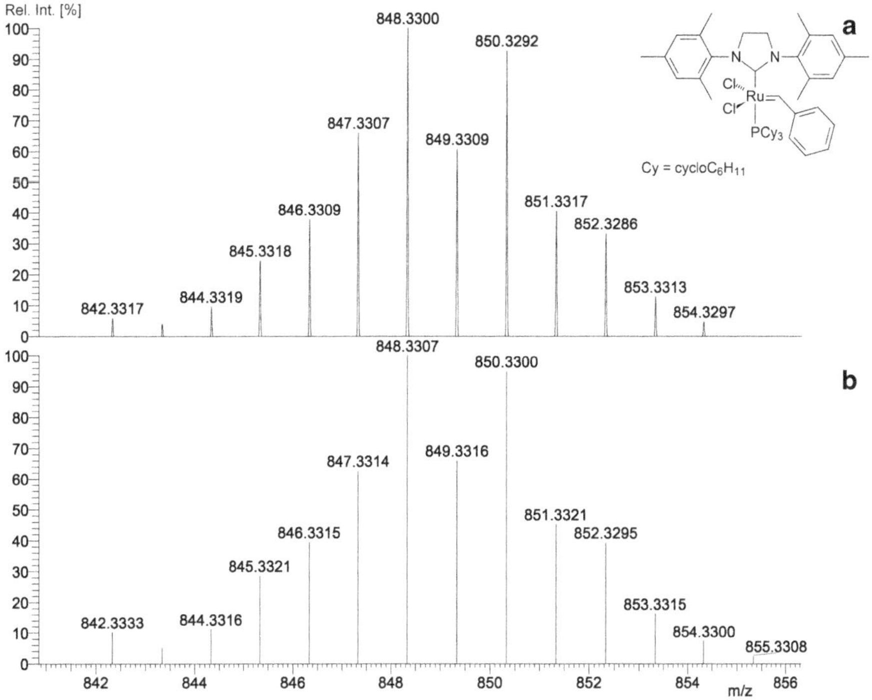

Fig. 8.28 Partial LIFDI spectrum of Grubbs catalyst as obtained by using an Exactive Orbitrap instrument with a prototype source attached via the HCD cell. (**a**) Molecular ion signal, (**b**) calculated isotopic pattern for $[C_{46}H_{65}Cl_2N_2PRu]^{+\bullet}$ (Reproduced with kind permission of Linden CMS, Leeste)

Analytes for FI-MS

Analytes need to be vaporized prior to ionization. Thus, sample supply can be performed from a reservoir inlet, from a sample vial attached to a direct insertion probe, or via a gas chromatograph. The analyte may have low to medium polarity. Normally, FI can be employed for analytes up to about 1000 u.

Analytes for FD-MS

Analytes should preferably be soluble in standard solvents (DMF and DMSO should be avoided due to insufficient volatility). Solutions of 0.1–2.0 mg ml^{-1} are suitable for deposition on the emitter. If necessary, even fine suspensions or emulsions may be transferred onto the emitter. The analyte may have low to high polarity and may also be ionic. FD is suitable to analyze molecules up to 2000–3000 u, depending on their thermal stability.

Analytes for LIFDI-MS

Analytes should preferably be soluble in standard solvents (DMF and DMSO should be avoided due to insufficient volatility). Solutions of 0.1–0.2 mg ml^{-1} are suitable for transfer through the fused silica capillary. Suspensions or emulsion are to be avoided. The analyte may have low to high polarity and may also be ionic. As LIFDI offers sample deposition under inert conditions, the sample can be highly sensitive to air and/or moisture. The mass range of FD applies analogously.

Polarity
FI exclusively generates positive ions. Apart from some rare exceptions, FD and LIFDI are exclusively operated in positive-ion mode. Anions of salts can be identified due to cluster ion formation.

Softness of Ionization
FI and FD are extremely soft ionization methods as the process of ionization does not impart energy onto the incipient molecular ions. Fragmentation, if any, generally occurs as a result of thermal energy required to effect evaporation or desorption/ionization of larger analyte species. Occasionally, field-induced dissociation or collision-induced dissociation during ion transfer into the mass analyzer may also result in fragmentation or ion losses.

Instrumentation
For decades, magnetic sector instruments have been the classic mass analyzers for FI and FD. Time-of-flight instruments have replaced many of them. Attachment of FD or LIFDI to FT-ICR or Orbitrap analyzers is still an exception but highly attractive in terms of resolving power and mass accuracy.

Accurate Mass
High-resolution and, more importantly, accurate mass data is difficult to obtain if internal mass calibration is required as is the case with magnetic sector instruments. Often, it is just impossible to effect ionization of both analyte and calibration compound simultaneously. The use of single-point corrections (lock mass) on TOF analyzers provides a notable advantage. Best results are to be expected in conjunction with FT-ICR and Orbitrap instruments, which allow to rely on external calibration.

Dissemination and Availability
FI, FD, and LIFDI are generally available as optional ionization techniques of instruments otherwise equipped with vacuum ion sources such as electron ionization (EI) or chemical ionization (CI). Adaptions to other systems can be provided upon request. The use of these techniques is not as widespread as EI, ESI, MALDI, and related ionization methods.

References

1. Müller EW (1953) Feldemission. Ergebn Exakt Naturw 27:290–360. doi:10.1007/BFb0110808
2. Gomer R, Inghram MG (1955) Applications of Field Ionization to Mass Spectrometry. J Am Chem Soc 77:500. doi:10.1021/ja01607a096

3. Inghram MG, Gomer R (1954) Mass-Spectrometric Analysis of Ions from the Field Microscope. J Chem Phys 22:1279–1280. doi:10.1063/1.1740380
4. Inghram MG, Gomer R (1955) Mass-Spectrometric Investigation of the Field Emission of Positive Ions. Z Naturforsch A 10:863–872. doi:10.1515/zna-1955-1113
5. Beckey HD (1959) Mass Spectrographic Investigations, Using a Field Emission Ion Source. Z Naturforsch A 14:712–721. doi:10.1515/zna-1959-0805
6. Beckey HD (1962) Field-Ionization Mass Spectra of Organic Molecules. Normal C_1 to C_9 Paraffins. Z Naturforsch A 17:1103–1111. doi:10.1515/zna-1962-1211
7. Beckey HD, Wagner G (1963) Analytical Use of an Ion Field Mass Spectrometer. Fresenius Z Anal Chem 197:58–80. doi:10.1007/BF00468727
8. Beckey HD (1963) Mass Spectrometric Analysis with a New Source for the Production of Ion Fields at Thin Wires or Metal Edges. Fresenius Z Anal Chem 197:80–90. doi:10.1007/BF00468728
9. Beckey HD, Wagner G (1965) Field Ionization Mass Spectra of Organic Molecules. II. Amines. Z Naturforsch A 20:169–175. doi:10.1515/zna-1965-0201
10. Beckey HD, Schulze P (1965) Field Ionization Mass Spectra of Organic Molecules. III. *N*-Paraffins Up to C_{16} and Branched Paraffins. Z Naturforsch A 20:1329–1335. doi:10.1515/zna-1965-1017
11. Beckey HD (1965) Analysis of Solid Organic Natural Products by Field Ionization Mass Spectrometry. Fresenius Z Anal Chem 207:99–104. doi:10.1007/BF00573238
12. Beckey HD (1966) Comparison of Field Ionization and Chemical Ionization Mass Spectra of Decane Isomers. J Am Chem Soc 88:5333–5335. doi:10.1021/ja00974a061
13. Beckey HD (1969) Field Desorption Mass Spectrometry: A Technique for the Study of Thermally Unstable Substances of Low Volatility. Int J Mass Spectrom Ion Phys 2:500–503. doi:10.1016/0020-7381(69)80047-1
14. Beckey HD, Heindrichs A, Winkler HU (1970) New Field Desorption Techniques. Int J Mass Spectrom Ion Phys 3:A9–A11. doi:10.1016/0020-7381(70)80009-2
15. Beckey HD (1971) Field-Ionization Mass Spectrometry. Pergamon, Elmsford
16. Sammons MC, Bursey MM, White CK (1975) Field Desorption Mass Spectrometry of Onium Salts. Anal Chem 47:1165–1166. doi:10.1021/ac60357a051
17. Beckey HD, Schulten HR (1975) Field Desorption Mass Spectrometry. Angew Chem Int Ed 14:403–415. doi:10.1002/anie.197504031
18. Lehmann WD, Schulten HR (1976) Physikalische Methoden in der Chemie: Massenspektrometrie II CI-, FI- und FD-MS. Chem Unserer Zeit 10:163–174. doi:10.1002/ciuz.19760100602
19. Beckey HD (1977) Principles of Field Desorption and Field Ionization Mass Spectrometry. Pergamon Press, Oxford
20. Larsen E, Egsgaard H, Holmen H (1978) Field Desorption Mass Spectrometry of 1-Methylpyridinium Salts. Org Mass Spectrom 13:417–424. doi:10.1002/oms.1210130710
21. Wood GW (1982) Field Desorption Mass Spectrometry: Applications. Mass Spectrom Rev 1:63–102. doi:10.1002/mas.1280010106
22. Schulten HR (1983) Analytical Applications of Field Desorption Mass Spectrometry. In: Benninghoven A (ed) Ion Formation from Organic Solids. Springer, Heidelberg
23. Lattimer RP, Schulten HR (1989) Field Ionization and Field Desorption Mass Spectrometry: Past, Present, and Future. Anal Chem 61:1201A–1215A. doi:10.1021/ac00196a721
24. Olson KL, Rinehart KL (1993) Field Desorption, Field Ionization, and Chemical Ionization Mass Spectrometry. Methods Carbohyd Chem 9:143–164
25. Del Rio JC, Philp RP (1999) Field Ionization Mass Spectrometric Study of High Molecular Weight Hydrocarbons in a Crude Oil and a Solid Bitumen. Org Geochem 30:279–286. doi:10.1016/S0146-6380(99)00014-5
26. Guo X, Fokkens RH, Peeters HJW, Nibbering NMM, de Koster CG (1999) Multiple Cationization of Polyethylene Glycols in Field Desorption Mass Spectrometry: A New Approach to Extend the Mass Scale on Sector Mass Spectrometers. Rapid Commun Mass

Spectrom 13:2223–2226. doi:10.1002/(SICI)1097-0231(19991115)13:21<2223::AID-RCM756>3.0.CO;2-C

27. Lattimer RP (2001) Field ionization (FI-MS) and field desorption (FD-MS). In: Montaudo G, Lattimer RP (eds) Mass Spectrometry of Polymers. CRC Press, Boca Raton
28. Linden HB (2002) Quick Soft Analysis of Sensitive Samples Under Inert Conditions by In-Source Liquid Injection FD. Proc 50th Ann Conf Mass Spectrom Allied Topics, MPL 373. 2002. Orlando, ASMS
29. Linden HB (2004) Liquid Injection Field Desorption Ionization: A New Tool for Soft Ionization of Samples Including Air-Sensitive Catalysts and Non-Polar Hydrocarbons. Eur J Mass Spectrom 10:459–468. doi:10.1255/ejms.655
30. Hsu CS, Green M (2001) Fragment-Free Accurate Mass Measurement of Complex Mixture Components by Gas Chromatography/Field Ionization-Orthogonal Acceleration Time-of-Flight Mass Spectrometry: An Unprecedented Capability for Mixture Analysis. Rapid Commun Mass Spectrom 15:236–239. doi:10.1002/1097-0231(20010215)15:3<236::AID-RCM197>3.0.CO;2-B
31. Qian K, Dechert GJ (2002) Recent Advances in Petroleum Characterization by GC Field Ionization Time-of-Flight High-Resolution Mass Spectrometry. Anal Chem 74:3977–3983. doi:10.1021/ac020166d
32. Schaub TM, Hendrickson CL, Qian K, Quinn JP, Marshall AG (2003) High-Resolution Field Desorption/Ionization Fourier Transform Ion Cyclotron Resonance Mass Analysis of Non-polar Molecules. Anal Chem 75:2172–2176. doi:10.1021/ac020627v
33. Schaub TM, Linden HB, Hendrickson CL, Marshall AG (2004) Continuous-Flow Sample Introduction for Field Desorption/Ionization Mass Spectrometry. Rapid Commun Mass Spectrom 18:1641–1644. doi:10.1002/rcm.1523
34. Linden HB, Gross JH (2011) A Liquid Injection Field Desorption/Ionization-Electrospray Ionization Combination Source for a Fourier Transform Ion Cyclotron Resonance Mass Spectrometer. J Am Soc Mass Spectrom 22:2137–2144. doi:10.1007/s13361-011-0259-9
35. Linden HB, Gross JH (2012) Reduced Fragmentation in Liquid Injection Field Desorption/Ionization-Fourier Transform Ion Cyclotron Resonance Mass Spectrometry by Use of Helium for the Thermalization of Molecular Ions. Rapid Commun Mass Spectrom 26:336–344. doi:10.1002/rcm.5335
36. Gomer R (1994) Field Emission, Field Ionization, and Field Desorption. Surf Sci 299 (300):129–152. doi:10.1016/0039-6028(94)90651-3
37. Prókai L (1990) Field Desorption Mass Spectrometry. Marcel Dekker, New York
38. Todd JFJ (1995) Recommendations for Nomenclature and Symbolism for Mass Spectroscopy Including an Appendix of Terms Used in Vacuum Technology. Int J Mass Spectrom Ion Proc 142:211–240. doi:10.1016/0168-1176(95)93811-F
39. Ligon WV Jr (1979) Molecular Analysis by Mass Spectrometry. Science 205:151–159. doi:10.1126/science.205.4402.151
40. Miyamoto K, Fujimaki S, Ueda Y (2009) Development of a New Electron Ionization/Field Ionization Ion Source for Gas Chromatography/Time-of-Flight Mass Spectrometry. Rapid Commun Mass Spectrom 23:3350–3354. doi:10.1002/rcm.4256
41. Schröder E (1991) Massenspektrometrie – Begriffe und Definitionen. Springer, Heidelberg
42. Derrick PJ, Robertson AJB (1973) Field Ionization Mass Spectrometry with Conditioned Razor Blades. Int J Mass Spectrom Ion Phys 10:315–321. doi:10.1016/0020-7381(73)83009-8
43. Giessmann U, Heinen HJ, Röllgen FW (1979) Field Desorption of Nonelectrolytes Using Simply Activated Wire Emitters. Org Mass Spectrom 14:177–179. doi:10.1002/oms.1210140314
44. Heinen HJ, Giessmann U, Röllgen FW (1977) Field Desorption of Electrolytic Solutions Using Untreated Wire Emitters. Org Mass Spectrom 12:710–715. doi:10.1002/oms.1210121112

45. Beckey HD, Krone H, Röllgen FW (1968) Comparison of Tips, Thin Wires, and Sharp Metal Edges as Emitters for Field Ionization Mass Spectrometry. J Sci Instrum 1:118–120. doi:10.1088/0022-3735/1/2/308
46. Beckey HD, Hilt E, Schulten HR (1973) High Temperature Activation of Emitters for Field Ionization and Field Desorption Spectrometry. J Phys E:Sci Instrum 6:1043–1044. doi:10.1088/0022-3735/6/10/028
47. Linden HB, Hilt E, Beckey HD (1978) High-Rate Growth of Dendrites on Thin Wire Anodes for Field Desorption Mass Spectrometry. J Phys E:Sci Instrum 11:1033–1036. doi:10.1088/0022-3735/11/10/019
48. Rabrenovic M, Ast T, Kramer V (1981) Alternative Organic Substances for Generation of Carbon Emitters for Field Desorption Mass Spectrometry. Int J Mass Spectrom Ion Phys 37:297–307. doi:10.1016/0020-7381(81)80051-4
49. Linden HB, Beckey HD, Okuyama F (1980) On the Mechanism of Cathodic Growth of Tungsten Needles by Decomposition of Hexacarbonyltungsten Under High-Field Conditions. Appl Phys 22:83–87. doi:10.1007/BF00897937
50. Bursey MM, Rechsteiner CE, Sammons MC, Hinton DM, Colpitts T, Tvaronas KM (1976) Electrochemically Deposited Cobalt Emitters for Field Ionization and Field Desorption Mass Spectrometry. J Phys E Sci Instrum 9:145–147. doi:10.1088/0022-3735/9/2/026
51. Matsuo T, Matsuda H, Katakuse I (1979) Silicon Emitter for Field Desorption Mass Spectrometry. Anal Chem 51:69–72. doi:10.1021/ac50037a025
52. Okuyama F, Shen GH (1981) Ion Formation Mechanisms in Field-Desorption Mass Spectrometry of Semirefractory Metal Elements. Int J Mass Spectrom Ion Phys 39:327–337. doi:10.1016/0020-7381(81)87006-4
53. Kümmler D, Schulten HR (1975) Correlation Between Emitter Heating Current and Emitter Temperature in Field Desorption Mass Spectrometry. Org Mass Spectrom 10:813–816. doi:10.1002/oms.1210100918
54. Winkler HU, Linden B (1976) On the Determination of Desorption Temperatures in Field Desorption Mass Spectrometry. Org Mass Spectrom 11:327–329. doi:10.1002/oms.1210110314
55. Schulten HR, Lehmann WD (1977) High-Resolution Field Desorption Mass Spectrometry. Part VII. Explosives and Explosive Mixtures. Anal Chim Acta 93:19–31. doi:10.1016/0003-2670(77)80003-2
56. Schulten HR, Nibbering NMM (1977) An Emission-Controlled Field Desorption and Electron Impact Spectrometry Study of Some *N*-Substituted Propane and Butane Sultams. Biomed Mass Spectrom 4:55–61. doi:10.1002/bms.1200040108
57. Schulten HR (1978) Recent Advances in Field Desorption Mass Spectrometry. Adv Mass Spectrom 7A:83–97
58. Beckey HD (1964) Molecule Dissociation by High Electric Fields. Z Naturforsch A 19:71–83. doi:10.1515/zna-1964-0114
59. Severin D (1976) Molecular Ion Mass Spectrometry for the Analysis of High- and Nonboiling Hydrocarbon Mixtures. Erdöl und Kohle Erdgas Petrochemie Vereinigt mit Brennstoff-Chemie 29:13–18
60. Mead L (1968) Field Ionization Mass Spectrometry of Heavy Petroleum Fractions. Waxes. Anal Chem 40:743–747. doi:10.1021/ac60260a040
61. Scheppele SE, Hsu CS, Marriott TD, Benson PA, Detwiler KN, Perreira NB (1978) Field-Ionization Relative Sensitivities for the Analysis of Saturated Hydrocarbons from Fossil-Energy-Related Materials. Int J Mass Spectrom Ion Phys 28:335–346. doi:10.1016/0020-7381(78)80077-1
62. Gross JH (2008) Molecular Ions of Ionic Liquids in the Gas Phase. J Am Soc Mass Spectrom 19:1347–1352. doi:10.1016/j.jasms.2008.06.002
63. Röllgen FW, Beckey HD (1970) Surface Reactions Induced by Field Ionization of Organic Molecules. Surf Sci 23:69–87. doi:10.1016/0039-6028(70)90006-3

64. Schulten HR, Beckey HD (1974) Criteria for Distinguishing Between $M^{+\cdot}$ and $[M+H]^+$ Ions in Field Desorption Mass Spectra. Org Mass Spectrom 9:1154–1155. doi:10.1002/oms.1210091111
65. Goldenfeld IV, Korostyshevsky IZ, Nazarenko VA (1973) Multiple Field Ionization. Int J Mass Spectrom Ion Phys 11:9–16. doi:10.1016/0020-7381(73)80050-6
66. Helal AI, Zahran NF (1988) Field Ionization of Indene on Tungsten. Int J Mass Spectrom Ion Proc 85:187–193. doi:10.1016/0168-1176(88)83014-3
67. Röllgen FW, Heinen HJ (1975) Formation of Multiply Charged Ions in a Field Ionization Mass Spectrometer. Int J Mass Spectrom Ion Phys 17:92–95. doi:10.1016/0020-7381(75)80010-6
68. Röllgen FW, Heinen HJ (1975) Energetics of Formation of Doubly Charged Benzene Ions by Field Ionization. Z Naturforsch A 30:918–920. doi:10.1515/zna-1975-6-735
69. Röllgen FW, Heinen HJ, Levsen K (1976) Doubly-Charged Fragment Ions in the Field Ionization Mass Spectra of Alkylbenzenes. Org Mass Spectrom 11:780–782. doi:10.1002/oms.1210110712
70. Neumann GM, Cullis PG, Derrick PJ (1980) Mass Spectrometry of Polymers: Polypropylene Glycol. Z Naturforsch A 35:1090–1097. doi:10.1515/zna-1980-1015
71. McCrae CE, Derrick PJ (1983) The Role of the Field in Field Desorption Fragmentation of Polyethylene Glycol. Org Mass Spectrom 18:321–323. doi:10.1002/oms.1210180802
72. Heine CE, Geddes MM (1994) Field-Dependent $[M\text{-}2H]^{+\cdot}$ Formation in the Field Desorption Mass Spectrometric Analysis of Hydrocarbon Samples. Org Mass Spectrom 29:277–284. doi:10.1002/oms.1210290603
73. Klesper G, Röllgen FW (1996) Field-Induced Ion Chemistry Leading to the Formation of $[M\text{-}2_nH]^{+\cdot}$ and $[2M\text{-}2_mH]^{+\cdot}$ Ions in Field Desorption Mass Spectrometry of Saturated Hydrocarbons. J Mass Spectrom 31:383–388. doi:10.1002/(SICI)1096-9888(199604)31:4<383::AID-JMS311>3.0.CO;2-1
74. Evans WJ, DeCoster DM, Greaves J (1995) Field Desorption Mass Spectrometry Studies of the Samarium-Catalyzed Polymerization of Ethylene Under Hydrogen. Macromolecules 28:7929–7936. doi:10.1021/ma00127a046
75. Evans WJ, DeCoster DM, Greaves J (1996) Evaluation of Field Desorption Mass Spectrometry for the Analysis of Polyethylene. J Am Soc Mass Spectrom 7:1070–1074. doi:10.1016/1044-0305(96)00043-8
76. Gross JH, Vékey K, Dallos A (2001) Field Desorption Mass Spectrometry of Large Multiply Branched Saturated Hydrocarbons. J Mass Spectrom 36:522–528. doi:10.1002/jms.151
77. Gross JH, Weidner SM (2000) Influence of Electric Field Strength and Emitter Temperature on Dehydrogenation and C-C Cleavage in Field Desorption Mass Spectrometry of Polyethylene Oligomers. Eur J Mass Spectrom 6:11–17. doi:10.1255/ejms.300
78. Chait EM, Shannon TW, Perry WO, Van Lear GE, McLafferty FW (1969) High-Resolution Field-Ionization Mass Spectrometry. Int J Mass Spectrom Ion Phys 2:141–155. doi:10.1016/0020-7381(69)80014-8
79. Forehand JB, Kuhn WF (1970) High Resolution Field Ionization Mass Spectrometry of the Condensable Phase of Cigaret Smoke. Anal Chem 42:1839–1841. doi:10.1021/ac50160a073
80. Schulten HR, Beckey HD, Meuzelaar HLC, Boerboom AJH (1973) High-Resolution Field Ionization Mass Spectrometry of Bacterial Pyrolysis Products. Anal Chem 45:191–195. doi:10.1021/ac60323a039
81. Schulten HR, Marzec A, Simmleit N, Dyla P, Mueller R (1989) Thermal Behavior and Degradation Products of Differently Ranked Coals Studied by Thermogravimetry and High-Resolution Field-Ionization Mass Spectrometry. Energy Fuel 3:481–487. doi:10.1021/ef00016a010
82. Games DE, Jackson AH, Millington DS (1973) Applications of Field Ionization Mass Spectrometry in the Analysis of Organic Mixtures. Tetrahedron Lett 14:3063–3066. doi:10.1016/S0040-4039(01)96320-8

83. Damico JN, Barron RP (1971) Application of Field Ionization to Gas-Liquid Chromatography-Mass Spectrometry (GLC-MS) Studies. Anal Chem 43:17–21. doi:10.1021/ac60296a032
84. Briker Y, Ring Z, Iacchelli A, McLean N, Rahimi PM, Fairbridge C, Malhotra R, Coggiola MA, Young SE (2001) Diesel Fuel Analysis by GC-FIMS: Aromatics, *n*-Paraffins, and Isoparaffins. Energy Fuel 15:23–37. doi:10.1021/ef000106f
85. Qian K, Dechert GJ, Edwards KE (2007) Deducing Molecular Compositions of Petroleum Products Using GC-Field Ionization High Resolution Time of Flight Mass Spectrometry. Int J Mass Spectrom 265:230–236. doi:10.1016/j.ijms.2007.02.012
86. Hejazi L, Ebrahimi D, Hibbert DB, Guilhaus M (2009) Compatibility of Electron Ionization and Soft Ionization Methods in Gas Chromatography/Orthogonal Time-of-Flight Mass Spectrometry. Rapid Commun Mass Spectrom 23:2181–2189. doi:10.1002/rcm.4131
87. Kane-Maguire LAP, Kanitz R, Sheil MM (1995) Comparison of Electrospray Mass Spectrometry with Other Soft Ionization Techniques for the Characterization of Cationic Π-Hydrocarbon Organometallic Complexes. J Organomet Chem 486:243–248. doi:10.1016/0022-328X(94)05041-9
88. Rogers DE, Derrick PJ (1984) Mechanisms of Ion Formation in Field Desorption of Oligosaccharides. Org Mass Spectrom 19:490–495. doi:10.1002/oms.1210191006
89. Derrick PJ, Nguyen T-T, Rogers DEC (1985) Concerning the Mechanism of Ion Formation in Field Desorption. Org Mass Spectrom 11:690. doi:10.1002/oms.1210201108
90. Veith HJ, Röllgen FW (1985) On the Ionization of Oligosaccharides. Org Mass Spectrom 11:689–690. doi:10.1002/oms.1210201108
91. Schulten HR, Beckey HD (1972) Field Desorption Mass Spectrometry with High-Temperature Activated Emitters. Org Mass Spectrom 6:885–895. doi:10.1002/oms.1210060808
92. Davis SC, Neumann GM, Derrick PJ (1987) Field Desorption Mass Spectrometry with Suppression of the High Field. Anal Chem 59:1360–1362. doi:10.1021/ac00136a021
93. Veith HJ (1977) Alkali Ion Addition in FD Mass Spectrometry. Cationization and Protonation-Ionization Methods in the Application of Nonactivated Emitters. Tetrahedron 33:2825–2828. doi:10.1016/0040-4020(77)80275-5
94. Giessmann U, Röllgen FW (1981) Electrodynamic Effects in Field Desorption Mass Spectrometry. Int J Mass Spectrom Ion Phys 38:267–279. doi:10.1016/0020-7381(81)80072-1
95. Röllgen FW (1983) Principles of field desorption mass spectrometry. In: Benninghoven A (ed) Ion Formation from Organic Solids. Springer, Heidelberg
96. Wong SS, Giessmann U, Karas M, Röllgen FW (1984) Field Desorption of Sucrose Studied by Combined Optical Microscopy and Mass Spectrometry. Int J Mass Spectrom Ion Proc 56:139–150. doi:10.1016/0168-1176(84)85038-7
97. Derrick PJ (1986) Mass Spectroscopy at High Mass. Fresenius Z Anal Chem 324:486–491. doi:10.1007/BF00474121
98. Davis SC, Natoli V, Neumann GM, Derrick PJ (1987) A Model of Ion Evaporation Tested Through Field Desorption Experiments on Glucose Mixed with Alkali Metal Salts. Int J Mass Spectrom Ion Proc 78:17–35. doi:10.1016/0168-1176(87)87039-8
99. Reichert H (1997) Monodesoxygenierte Glucosid-Synthese und Kinetikstudien der enzymatischen Spaltung. PhD Thesis. Organisch-Chemisches Institut, Heidelberg University
100. Veith HJ (1976) Field Desorption Mass Spectrometry of Quaternary Ammonium Salts: Cluster Ion Formation. Org Mass Spectrom 11:629–633. doi:10.1002/oms.1210110609
101. Veith HJ (1983) Mass Spectrometry of Ammonium and Iminium Salts. Mass Spectrom Rev 2:419–446. doi:10.1002/mas.1280020402
102. Veith HJ (1980) Collision-Induced Fragmentations of Field-Desorbed Cations. 4. Collision-Induced Fragmentations of Alkylideneammonium Ions. Angew Chem Int Ed 19:541–542. doi:10.1002/anie.198005411

103. Fischer M, Veith HJ (1981) Collision-Induced Fragmentations of Field-Desorbed Cations. 5. Reactions of 2- and 3-Phenyl Substituted Alkylalkylidene Iminium Ions in the Gas Phase. Helv Chim Acta 64:1083–1091. doi:10.1002/hlca.19810640413
104. Miermans CJH, Fokkens RH, Nibbering NMM (1997) A Study of the Applicability of Various Ionization Methods and Tandem Mass Spectrometry in the Analyses of Triphenyltin Compounds. Anal Chim Acta 340:5–20. doi:10.1016/S0003-2670(96)00541-7
105. Röllgen FW, Giessmann U, Heinen HJ (1976) Ion Formation in Field Desorption of Salts. Z Naturforsch A 31:1729–1730. doi:10.1515/zna-1976-1245
106. Röllgen FW, Ott KH (1980) On the Formation of Cluster Ions and Molecular Ions in Field Desorption of Salts. Int J Mass Spectrom Ion Phys 32:363–367. doi:10.1016/0020-7381(80)80019-2
107. Lehmann WD, Schulten HR (1977) Determination of Alkali Elements by Field Desorption Mass Spectrometry. Anal Chem 49:1744–1746. doi:10.1021/ac50020a028
108. Schulten HR, Bohl B, Bahr U, Mueller R, Palavinskas R (1981) Qualitative and Quantitative Trace-Metal Analysis in Physiological Fluids of Multiple Sclerosis Patients by Field Desorption Mass Spectrometer. Int J Mass Spectrom Ion Phys 38:281–295. doi:10.1016/0020-7381(81)80073-3
109. Keough T, DeStefano AJ (1981) Acid-Enhanced Field Desorption Mass Spectrometry of Zwitterions. Anal Chem 53:25–29. doi:10.1021/ac00224a009
110. Gross JH (2007) Liquid Injection Field Desorption/Ionization Mass Spectrometry of Ionic Liquids. J Am Soc Mass Spectrom 18:2254–2262. doi:10.1016/j.jasms.2007.09.019
111. Frauenkron M, Berkessel A, Gross JH (1997) Analysis of Ruthenium Carbonyl-Porphyrin Complexes: A Comparison of Matrix-Assisted Laser Desorption/Ionization Time-of-Flight, Fast-Atom Bombardment and Field Desorption Mass Spectrometry. Eur Mass Spectrom 3:427–438. doi:10.1255/ejms.177
112. Lattimer RP, Harmon DJ, Welch KR (1979) Characterization of Low Molecular Weight Polymers by Liquid Chromatography and Field Desorption Mass Spectroscopy. Anal Chem 51:293–296. doi:10.1021/ac50044a040
113. Craig AC, Cullis PG, Derrick PJ (1981) Field Desorption of Polymers: Polybutadiene. Int J Mass Spectrom Ion Phys 38:297–304. doi:10.1016/0020-7381(81)80074-5
114. Lattimer RP, Schulten HR (1983) Field Desorption of Hydrocarbon Polymers. Int J Mass Spectrom Ion Phys 52:105–116. doi:10.1016/0020-7381(83)85094-3
115. Matsuo T, Matsuda H, Katakuse I (1979) Use of Field Desorption Mass Spectra of Polystyrene and Polypropylene Glycol as Mass References Up to Mass 10000. Anal Chem 51:1329–1331. doi:10.1021/ac50044a050
116. Ott KH, Röllgen FW, Zwinselmann JJ, Fokkens RH, Nibbering NMM (1980) Negative Ion Field Desorption Mass Spectra of Some Inorganic and Organic Compounds. Org Mass Spectrom 15:419–422. doi:10.1002/oms.1210150805
117. Daehling P, Röllgen FW, Zwinselmann JJ, Fokkens RH, Nibbering NMM (1982) Negative Ion Field Desorption Mass Spectrometry of Anionic Surfactants. Fresenius Z Anal Chem 312:335–337. doi:10.1007/BF00470387
118. Mes GF, Van der Greef J, Nibbering NMM, Ott KH, Röllgen FW (1980) The Formation of Negative Ions by Field Ionization. Int J Mass Spectrom Ion Phys 34:295–301. doi:10.1016/0020-7381(80)85043-1
119. Dähling P, Ott KH, Röllgen FW, Zwinselmann JJ, Fokkens RH, Nibbering NMM (1983) Ionization by Proton Abstraction in Negative Ion Field Desorption Mass Spectrometry. Int J Mass Spectrom Ion Phys 46:301–304. doi:10.1016/0020-7381(83)80112-0
120. Linden HB (2001) Electric field-induced ionization of analytes in mass spectrometer by desorption from microdendrite substrates, German Patent No. DE 99-19963317
121. Gross JH, Nieth N, Linden HB, Blumbach U, Richter FJ, Tauchert ME, Tompers R, Hofmann P (2006) Liquid Injection Field Desorption/Ionization of Reactive Transition Metal Complexes. Anal Bioanal Chem 386:52–58. doi:10.1007/s00216-006-0524-0

122. Monillas WH, Yap GPH, Theopold KH (2007) A Tale of Two Isomers: A Stable Phenyl Hydride and a High-Spin ($S = 3$) Benzene Complex of Chromium. Angew Chem Int Ed 46:6692–6694. doi:10.1002/anie.200701933
123. Schaub TM, Hendrickson CL, Quinn JP, Rodgers RP, Marshall AG (2005) Instrumentation and Method for Ultrahigh Resolution Field Desorption Ionization Fourier Transform Ion Cyclotron Resonance Mass Spectrometry of Nonpolar Species. Anal Chem 77:1317–1324. doi:10.1021/ac048766v
124. Fu J, Klein GC, Smith DF, Kim S, Rodgers RP, Hendrickson CL, Marshall AG (2006) Comprehensive Compositional Analysis of Hydrotreated and Untreated Nitrogen-Concentrated Fractions from Syncrude Oil by Electron Ionization, Field Desorption Ionization, and Electrospray Ionization Ultrahigh-Resolution FT-ICR Mass Spectrometry. Energy Fuel 20:1235–1241. doi:10.1021/ef060012r
125. Stanford LA, Rodgers RP, Marshall AG, Czarnecki J, Wu XA (2007) Compositional Characterization of Bitumen/Water Emulsion Films by Negative- and Positive-Ion Electrospray Ionization and Field Desorption/Ionization Fourier Transform Ion Cyclotron Resonance Mass Spectrometry. Energy Fuel 21:963–972. doi:10.1021/ef060291i
126. Schaub TM, Rodgers RP, Marshall AG, Qian K, Green LA, Olmstead WN (2005) Speciation of Aromatic Compounds in Petroleum Refinery Streams by Continuous Flow Field Desorption Ionization FT-ICR Mass Spectrometry. Energy Fuel 19:1566–1573. doi:10.1021/ef049734d
127. Smith DF, Schaub TM, Rodgers RP, Hendrickson CL, Marshall AG (2008) Automated Liquid Injection Field Desorption/Ionization for Fourier Transform Ion Cyclotron Resonance Mass Spectrometry. Anal Chem 80:7379–7382. doi:10.1021/ac801085r
128. Heinen HJ, Hötzel C, Beckey HD (1974) Combination of a Field Desorption Ion Source with a Quadrupole Mass Analyzer. Int J Mass Spectrom Ion Phys 13:55–62. doi:10.1016/0020-7381(74)83005-6
129. Gierlich HH, Heinen HJ, Beckey HD (1975) The Application of Quadrupole Mass Filters in Field Desorption Mass Spectrometry. Biomed Mass Spectrom 2:31–35. doi:10.1002/bms.1200020107
130. Smith DF, Rahimi P, Teclemariam A, Rodgers RP, Marshall AG (2008) Characterization of Athabasca Bitumen Heavy Vacuum Gas Oil Distillation Cuts by Negative/Positive Electrospray Ionization and Automated Liquid Injection Field Desorption Ionization Fourier Transform Ion Cyclotron Resonance Mass Spectrometry. Energy Fuel 22:3118–3125. doi:10.1021/ef8000357
131. Miyabayashi K, Naito Y, Miyake M (2009) Characterization of Heavy Oil by FT-ICR MS Coupled with Various Ionization Techniques. J Jpn Pet Inst 52:159–171. doi:10.1627/jpi.52.159

Tandem Mass Spectrometry

9

Learning Objectives

- Tandem MS – concepts and terminology
- Modes of operation
- Different instrumental platforms
- Methods of ion activation to induce dissociation
- Applications to analytical problems
- Versatile tool for gas phase ion chemistry

Electron ionization mass spectra show a wealth of fragment ion peaks allowing to retrieve structural information, often though at the expense of abundance of the molecular ion. For decades, EI has served as the one and only ionization method of organic mass spectrometry. With the advent of soft ionization methods such as CI or FD we just dealt with, spectra exhibiting minor or even no fragment ion signals could be generated. While highly advantageous at first sight, in the long run, the lack of structural information presents a severe drawback for analytical applications. The development of numerous new techniques to store, manipulate, activate, fragment, and re-analyze ions in the gas phase by means of mass spectrometry have been driven both by the desire to understand the energetics, reactivity, and detailed fragmentation pathways of ions and the strong need for techniques to derive structural information from soft ionization mass spectra.

9.1 Concepts of Tandem Mass Spectrometry

The term *tandem mass spectrometry*, or briefly *tandem MS*, encompasses the numerous techniques where mass-selected ions are subjected to a second mass spectrometric analysis [1, 2]. Tandem mass spectrometry comprises the acquisition

J.H. Gross, *Mass Spectrometry*, DOI 10.1007/978-3-319-54398-7_9

and study of the spectra of ionic products or precursors of *m/z*-selected ions, or of precursor ions of a selected neutral mass loss. Tandem MS is also denoted as *mass spectrometry/mass spectrometry* from which the common acronym MS/MS is derived.

A mass spectrometer designed for MS/MS, also termed *tandem mass spectrometer*, requires to incorporate at least two stages of *m/z* analysis, often referred to as MS1 and MS2, respectively. Thus, many aspects of tandem MS are closely related to instrumentation [3]. In retrospect, we recognize that tandem MS has already been anticipated in some sections of the instrumentation chapter (Sects. 4.4.4, 4.5, 4.7.12, 4.8.4 and 4.9). Here, more principal considerations of the topic will follow.

9.1.1 Tandem-in-Space and Tandem-in-Time

There are two basic instrumental concepts for MS/MS. The first is *tandem mass spectrometry in space* (or *tandem-in-space* MS) [4]. In order to perform two consecutive mass-analyzing steps, two mass analyzers may be mounted in tandem. Thus, tandem-in-space refers to MS/MS instrumentation where product ion spectra are recorded using spatially separated *m/z* analyzers. Specific *m/z* separation is performed so that in one section of the instrument ions are selected, then dissociated in an intermediate region, and the products thereof are finally transmitted to a second analyzer for mass analysis (Fig. 9.1). All beam transmitting devices, e.g., multiple sector, ReTOF, TOF/TOF, QqQ, and QqTOF instruments follow this route to tandem MS (Fig. 9.2) [5]. The second approach, *tandem mass spectrometry in time* (or *tandem-in-time* MS), employs a single *m/z* analyzer (QIT, LIT, FT-ICR) that may be operated by executing the discrete steps of ion selection, activation, and product ion analysis in the very same place but sequentially in time [5].

In principle, both instrumental concepts can be expanded to allow for multiple-stage mass spectrometry, i.e., multiple stages of precursor ion selection followed by product ion detection for successive *n*th generation product ions [7]. While it is convenient to talk about MS/MS, acronyms like MS/MS/MS are clearly out of place. Therefore, it is common practice to use MS^2, MS^3, and generally MS^n to denote the number of stages of a tandem mass spectrometric experiment. Accordingly, in the sequential fragmentation scheme

$$m_1^+ \rightarrow m_2^+ \rightarrow m_3^+ \rightarrow m_4^+ \rightarrow m_5^+ \tag{9.1}$$

m_4^+ is the precursor ion of m_5^+, m_4^+ is a 1st generation product ion of m_3^+, a 2nd generation product ion of m_2^+, and also a 3rd generation product ion of m_1^+ [8, 9]. The corresponding spectra are analogously termed *n*th generation product ion spectra.

Clearly, the vast majority of tandem MS experiments is designed to deliver fragment ion data. Nonetheless, selected ions may also be allowed to react with neutrals in ion–molecule reactions to form products with a gain in mass (Sect. 2.13):

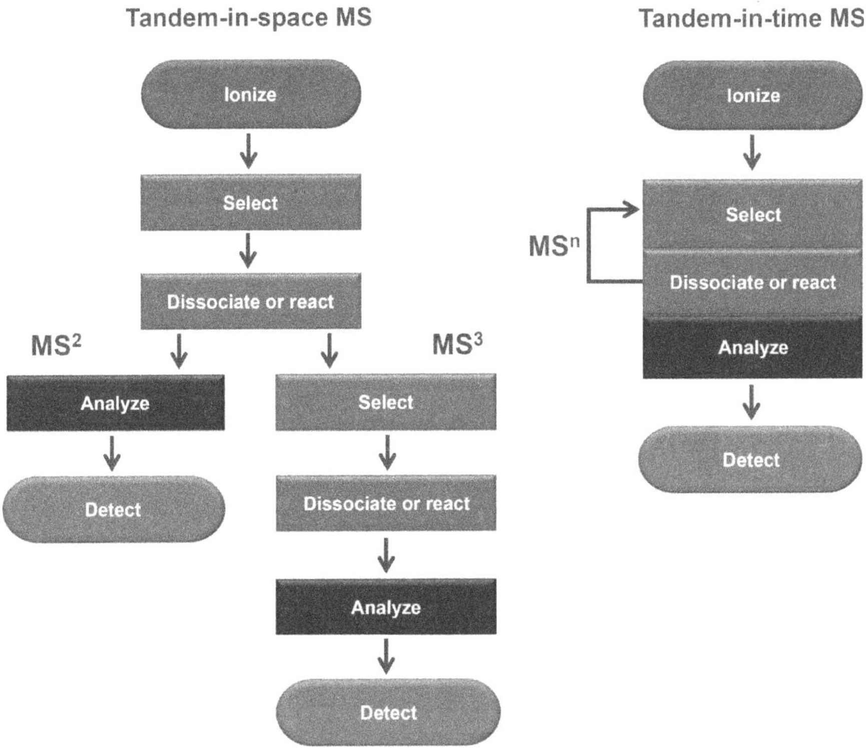

Fig. 9.1 Comparison of tandem-in-space and tandem-in-time MS. Obviously, higher order MS^n can be better realized by tandem-in-time setups, whereas tandem-in-space instrumentation is usually designed for MS^2 with MS^3 representing already the rare exception

$$m_1{}^+ + n \rightarrow m_2{}^+ \tag{9.2}$$

Ion–molecule reactions can thus be conducted under carefully controlled conditions. This sort of tandem MS is frequently employed in fundamental studies of ion reactivity.

Tandem MS is highly variable

Obviously, tandem MS experiments can be adapted according to need. They can set up as ion fragmentations, typically by energetic collisions of fast ions with an inert gas (Sect. 9.3) or as addition reactions with an according increase in precursor ion mass by addition of a reactive gaseous neutral upon very low-energy collisions (Sect. 9.18). However, ion–neutral collisions can even be soft and still nonreactive as exploited for thermalizing ions by multiple low-energy collisions with a buffer gas (Sect. 4.4.4).

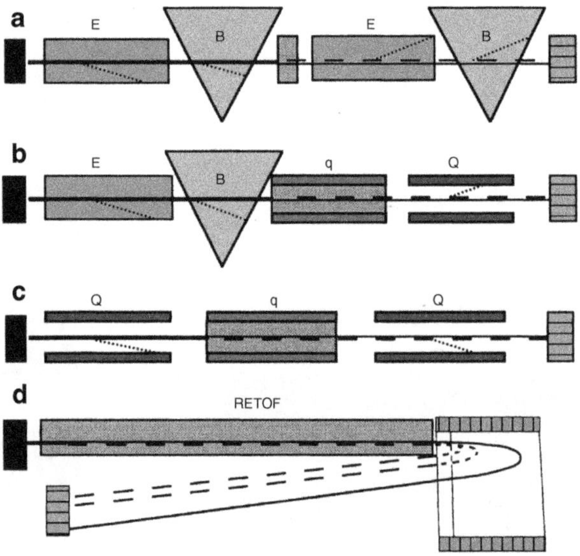

Fig. 9.2 Tandem-in-space setups for different beam instruments: (**a**) magnetic four-sector instrument of EB-EB geometry, (**b**) magnetic sector–quadrupole hybrid of EB-qQ geometry, (**c**) triple quadrupole (includes QqQ, QhQ, QoQ setups), and (**d**) ReTOF instrument. The line styles indicate —— stable precursor ions, - - - transmitted ions, and ······· non-transmitted fragment ions. *Orange* areas show the region of analytically useful ion dissociations (Adapted from Ref. [6] with permission. © Elsevier Science, 1994)

9.1.2 Pictograms for Tandem MS

To facilitate the evaluation of tandem mass spectra, the particular type of experiment can be described by pictograms. Following a simplistic notation [7, 10, 11], the chosen analyzer (or stage of experiment) may be indicated by ●, a scanning analyzer (or stage of experiment) by ○. Information such as precursor ion mass, type of ion activation, or neutral loss may be indicated as required (Table 9.1).

Dissociations in transit through the mass analyzer may either occur spontaneously (*metastable*, Sect. 9.2) or can result from intentionally supplied additional activation, typically from collisions with neutrals (Sect. 9.3). Below follows a description of methods for activating or reacting otherwise stable ions in the *field-free region* (FFR) between the first stage, *m*/*z*-selection (MS1), and product ion analysis (MS2).

Thus, to include ionization mode, type of mass analyzers, scan mode, and conditions of ion activation, a more elaborate set of pictograms has been suggested by Lehmann (Fig. 9.3) [12]. Since then, such pictorial presentations of basic experimental parameters are occasionally given along with tandem mass spectra. Unfortunately, neither an authorized "character set" nor an update to include current equipment and modes are available.

Table 9.1 Pictogram symbols for tandem MS experiments [7]

Mode	Product ion mode	Product ion mode	Precursor ion mode	Neutral loss scan
Level	MS^2	MS^3	MS^2	MS^2
Pictogram	● ↓ ○	● 228 ↓ ● 200 ↓ ○	○ ↓ CID ●	○ ↓ 32 ○
Notes		The *m/z* values of the selected ions may be noted	Conditions for activation may be added to arrow	Neutral loss can be indicated on arrow

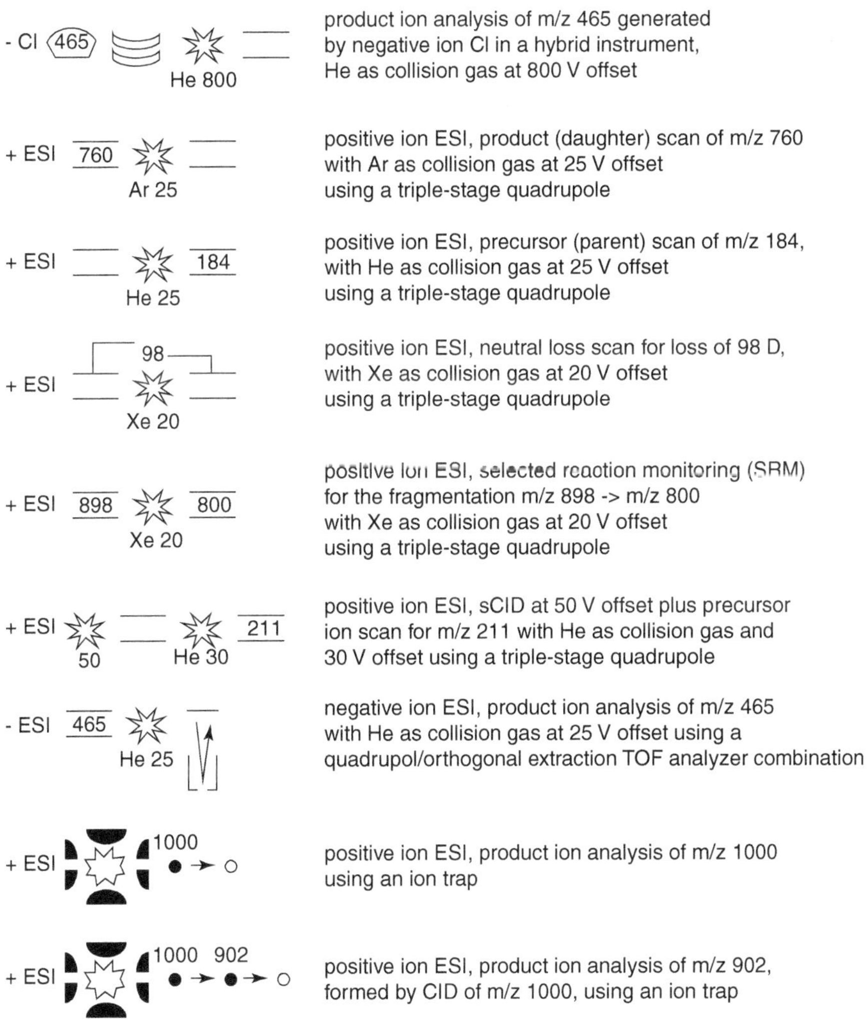

Fig. 9.3 Pictograms for tandem MS (Reproduced from Ref. [12] with permission. © Elsevier Science Inc., 1997)

Tandem MS modes are defined by mass analyzers
There is a close relationship between the type of mass analyzer and choice of method of ion activation that can be applied to the respective instrumental platform. It is therefore unfavorable to strictly separate the discussion of ion activation from that of instrumental setups and their modes of operation. Thus, the following passages of this chapter will reflect these mutual dependences by alternating discussions of activation methods and instrumental details in a way that is supposed to deliver convenient access to the subject matter.

9.1.3 Terminology for Tandem Mass Spectrometry

Here are the basic terminological conventions for tandem mass spectrometry [4]:

- The term tandem *mass spectrometry* or *mass spectrometry/mass spectrometry* collectively describes mass spectrometric experiments where mass-analyzed ions are subjected to fragmentations or ion–molecule reactions and the products thereof are collected and mass-analyzed by a second stage.
- Instruments are accordingly referred to as *tandem mass spectrometers*; their stages are denoted MS1, MS2 etc.
- Tandem MS is often abbreviated as MS/MS or MS^2. Tandem MS experiments of higher order are referred to as MS^3, MS^4, ... or generally as MS^n.
- Ions emerging from MS1 are termed *precursor ions*, those entering MS2 are called *product ions*; in higher-order experiments, one may refer to them as *n*th generation product ions. (The old terms *parent ion* and *daughter ion* are deprecated.)
- Spectra are called *tandem mass spectra* (never MS/MS spectra).

9.2 Metastable Ion Dissociation

The success of any tandem mass spectrometric experiment depends on the occurrence of some kind of reaction between the consecutive steps of precursor ion selection and product ion analysis. This demands that ions entering the zone and/or period for reaction either possess or receive sufficient internal energy for doing so; alternatively, a partner for reaction may be presented.

As dealt with in Sect. 2.6, ions reacting sufficiently fast to dissociate while transiting the analyzer are termed *metastable ions* [13]. In classical beam instruments, this is correlated to lifetimes of roughly 10^{-6}–10^{-5} s, and thus, requires rate constants of unimolecular dissociation in the order of 10^6–10^5 s^{-1}. EI, CI, and MALDI can provide a respectable fraction of ions, as to say in the afterglow of the ion source, falling into this range of internal energy and therefore into the lifetime of metastable decomposition. The fraction of metastable ion dissociations occurring in the *field-free region* (FFR) between MS1 and MS2 is accessible by means of tandem MS. Ions fragmenting during the very step of mass analysis are lost.

It is a generally accepted assumption that metastable ions possess internal energy only slightly above threshold of ion dissociation. Interestingly, there are still differences even among metastable ion populations, depending on whether they are observed in close proximity to the ion source (1.FFR) or further away (2.FFR). Metastable ion spectra represent one of the indispensable tools for studying the mechanism and thermochemistry of ion dissociations [13, 14]. Examples are given in the section on tandem MS on magnetic sector instruments.

9.3 Collision-Induced Dissociation

Even though collisions of ions with neutral gas atoms or molecules appear contradictory to the conditions of high vacuum, most mass spectrometers are equipped (or can be upgraded) to allow for their study. Consequently, fundamental and analytical studies make use of activating or reactive collisions within the mass spectrometer. The most prominent collision technique is *collision-induced dissociation* (CID) [15, 16]; the terms *collisionally activated dissociation* (CAD) or *collisional activation* (CA) are also being used. CID allows for the fragmentation of gaseous ions that were otherwise perfectly stable. Thus, CID is especially useful for elucidating the structure of ions of low internal energy as for those created by soft ionization methods.

9.3.1 Effecting Collisions in a Mass Spectrometer

CID is generally realized by passing an ion beam through a *collision cell* where the collision gas (He, N_2, Ar) is set to a pressure considerably above that of the surrounding high vacuum. This can be achieved by introducing the gas via a needle valve into a comparatively tight compartment with narrow entrance and exit slits for the ion beam (Fig. 9.4). A nearby vacuum pump removes effusing gas, thereby creating a *differentially pumped* region, due to the lack of laminar flow at some 10^{-4} Pa. Instead, expansion of the gas is diffusion-controlled. The reading of a pressure gauge can serve to reproduce the pressure adjustment, but it does not show the actual pressure inside the cell [17].

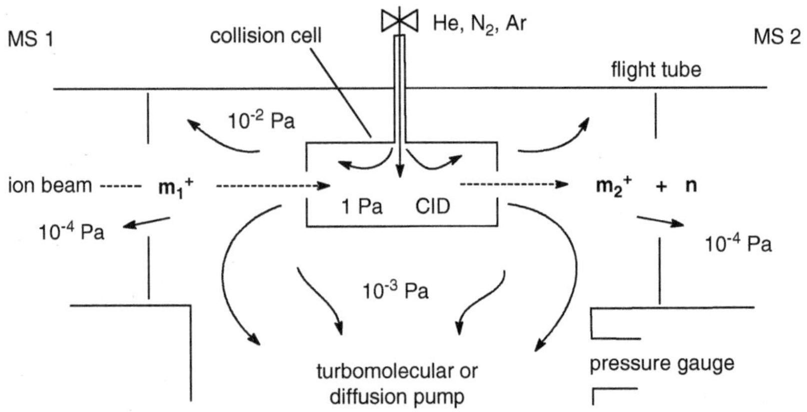

Fig. 9.4 Schematic of a collision cell for CID experiments in a beam instrument. Ions mass-selected in MS1 enter from the left

9.3.2 Energy Transfer During Collisions

The collision of an ion AB^+ carrying some kiloelectronvolts of kinetic energy with a neutral N takes about 10^{-15} s. This allows to apply the assumptions of QET analogously to electron ionization (Sect. 2.1) [14, 18–21]. The collision-induced dissociation of AB^+ can therefore be regarded as a two-step process [22]. First, the activated species AB^{+*} is formed. Second, after randomization of the internal energy has occurred, AB^{+*} will dissociate along any fragmentation pathway available at this specific level of internal energy:

$$AB^+ + N \rightarrow AB^{+*} + N \rightarrow A^+ + B + N \tag{9.3}$$

The internal energy E_{AB+*} is composed of the internal energy prior to the collision, E_{AB+}, and of the amount of energy Q transferred during the collision:

$$E_{AB+*} = E_{AB+} + Q \tag{9.4}$$

Thus, the collision marks a restart of the time scale for the activated ion. As $Q > E_{AB+}$ generally holds, the internal energy prior to the collision is of minor relevance – though not generally negligible – for the behavior of the activated ion. As may be expected, the CID spectra of stable molecular ions exhibit marked similarity to the 70-eV EI spectra of the respective compounds [15, 16].

CID causes vibrational excitation Except for the intensities relative to the precursor ion, the B/E-linked scan CID spectrum of the toluene molecular ion, *m/z* 92, closely resembles the 70-eV EI mass spectrum (Fig. 9.5; for EI cf. Sect. 6.4.3). Here, all fragments are due to CID because the molecular ion was generated by field ionization and did not show any metastable decomposition, i.e., $E_{AB+} = 0$ and $E_{AB+*} = Q$.

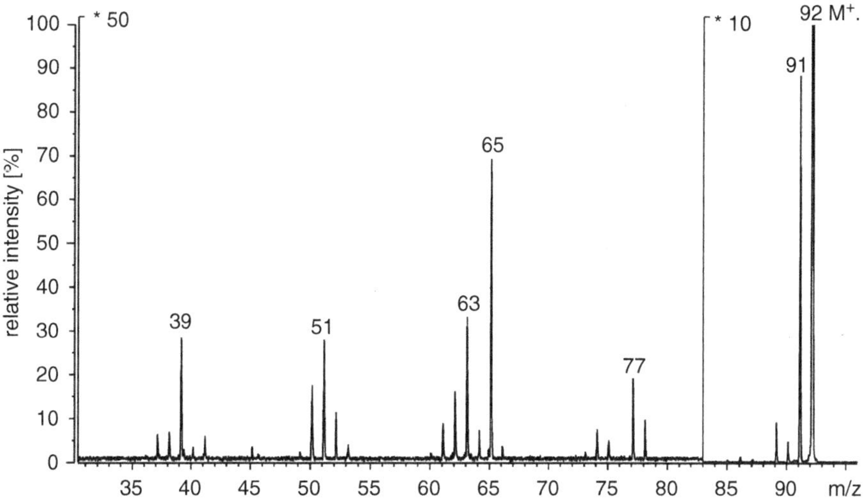

Fig. 9.5 CID spectrum of toluene molecular ion, *m/z* 92 ($E_{lab} = 10$ keV, B/E = *const.* linked scan on magnetic sector instrument (cf. Sect. 9.6.4), collision gas He at about 50% transmission)

The absolute upper limit for the value of *Q* is defined by the *center-of-mass collision energy*, E_{CM} [18, 19],

$$E_{CM} = E_{LAB}\frac{m_N}{m_N + m_{AB}} \tag{9.5}$$

where m_N is the mass of the neutral, m_{AB} the mass of the ion, and E_{LAB}, the *ion kinetic energy in the laboratory frame of reference.*

Laboratory frame of reference

E_{LAB}, the ion kinetic energy in the laboratory frame of reference, simply represents the kinetic energy of the ion as received from passing through an acceleration stage that defines its kinetic energy, e.g., a singly charged ion initially at rest will have $E_{LAB} = 10$ eV after passing through a potential of 10 V. The collision event of the ion–neutral pair, however, is also determined by both ion mass, m_{AB}, and neutral mass, m_N, as expressed by the ratio $m_N / (m_N + m_{AB})$. The neutral is commonly treated as being at rest, which is a good approximation for the collision gas at thermal energy.

For a polyatomic ion consisting of both the atom B actually, involved in the collision process, and the remainder A, the maximum of *Q* is calculated to have a lower value than E_{CM}. Assuming central collisions we obtain [19]:

$$E_{\text{int max}} = 4E_{LAB}\, m_A\, m_B \left(\frac{m_N}{m_{AB}\,(m_B + m_N)}\right)^2 \tag{9.6}$$

However, most collisions are not "head-on", but occur at some angle θ. Increasing m_{AB} makes $E_{int\,max}$ decrease, whereas larger m_N is beneficial for energy transfer. In CID-MIKES the center of the peak is shifted to the low mass side, i.e., to the low ion translational energy side, because the uptake Q originates from a loss in E_{LAB} [23–28]. The relationship between ΔE_{LAB} and Q can be expressed as [25]:

$$Q = \frac{\Delta E_{LAB}(m_{AB} + m_N)}{m_N} - \left[\left(\frac{2m_{AB}E_{LAB}}{m_N}\right)\left(1 - \sqrt{\frac{E_{LAB} - \Delta E_{LAB}}{E_{LAB}}}\cos\theta\right)\right] \quad (9.7)$$

Several conclusions can be drawn from Eq. 9.7:

- Q has a broad distribution (0–15 eV) due to variations in θ and typically is in the order of some electronvolts [29].
- Up to a certain ionic mass, the neutral penetrates the incident ion, i.e., the activated ion leaves the neutral behind (forward-scattered ion), but beyond the limit (> 10^2 atoms) the neutral is expelled in the direction of ion motion (backward-scattered ion) [25].
- At about *m/z* 1500 the translational energy loss is fully converted into vibrational excitation of the ion ($\Delta E_{LAB} = Q$).
- Q decreases beyond *m/z* 1500, thus explaining the difficulties in fragmenting heavy singly charged ions by CID (Fig. 9.6) [21, 25, 30].

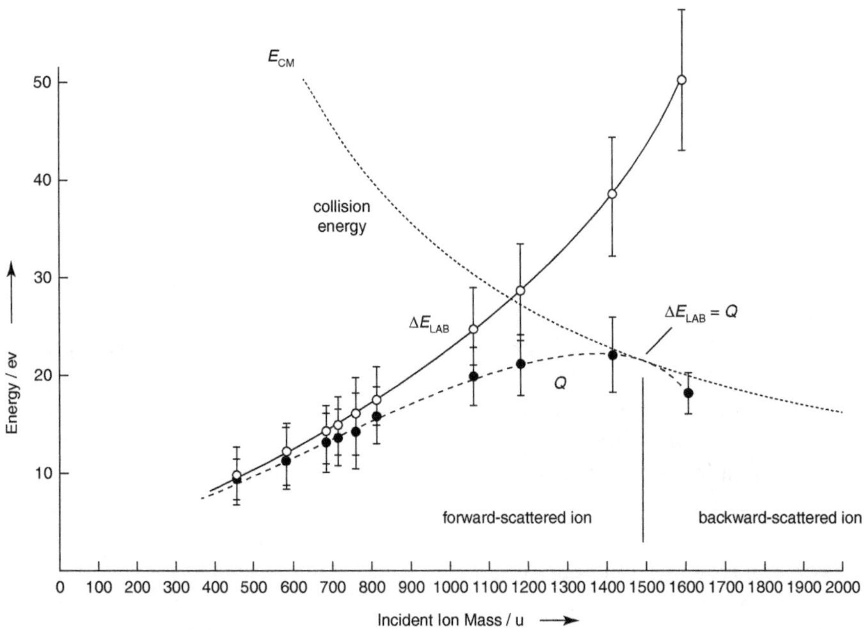

Fig. 9.6 The relationship between E_{CM}, ΔE_{LAB}, and Q (Adapted from Ref. [25] with permission. © Verlag der Zeitschrift für Naturforschung, 1984)

Selection of collision gases
In magnetic sector and TOF instruments, He is typically used as the collision gas because $E_{int\ max}$ from *high-energy collisions* (keV) is still comparatively large, and He reduces the risk of charge transfer due to its high *IE*. In the *low collision energy regime* [19] of quadrupole and ion trapping instruments (1–200 eV), heavier gases are frequently employed (N_2, Ar, Xe) to make CID more effective.

9.3.3 Single and Multiple Collisions in CID

Generally, the collision gas pressure is indirectly adjusted via the attenuation of the beam of mass-selected ions undergoing collisions. As the so-called *main beam* becomes increasingly attenuated, the probability for multiple collisions rises and so does the yield of fragments resulting from high activation energy processes. In a typical high-energy collision experiment a transmission of 90% for the main beam translates into 95% of the colliding ions to undergo single collisions while only about 5% encounter double collisions. At 50% transmission, about 68% of the colliding ions encounter a single, 23% two, and the remaining even three and four collisions (Fig. 9.7) [17]. To achieve sufficient activation of the ions in the low-energy collision regime, elongated collision cells are employed where Q is accumulated from numerous collision events.

In beam-type analyzers, the collision event leading to ion activation can be considered in terms of the Lambert-Beer law, because the precursor ion beam flux $[M_p]_0$ is exponentially reduced when passing through a collision chamber of length l containing gas at target number density n

$$[M_P] = [M_P]_0 \times e^{-n\sigma l} \tag{9.8}$$

where σ is the collision cross section of the event [31].

In tandem-in-time experiments as performed in trapping instruments a description in terms of rate constants and reaction times is more appropriate, which leads to the expression

$$[M_P]_t = [M_P]_0 \times e^{-nkt} \tag{9.9}$$

where t is the activation time span, and k sums the rate constants of all processes leading to reduction in $[M_p]_0$, i.e., it includes fragmentation and scattering losses.

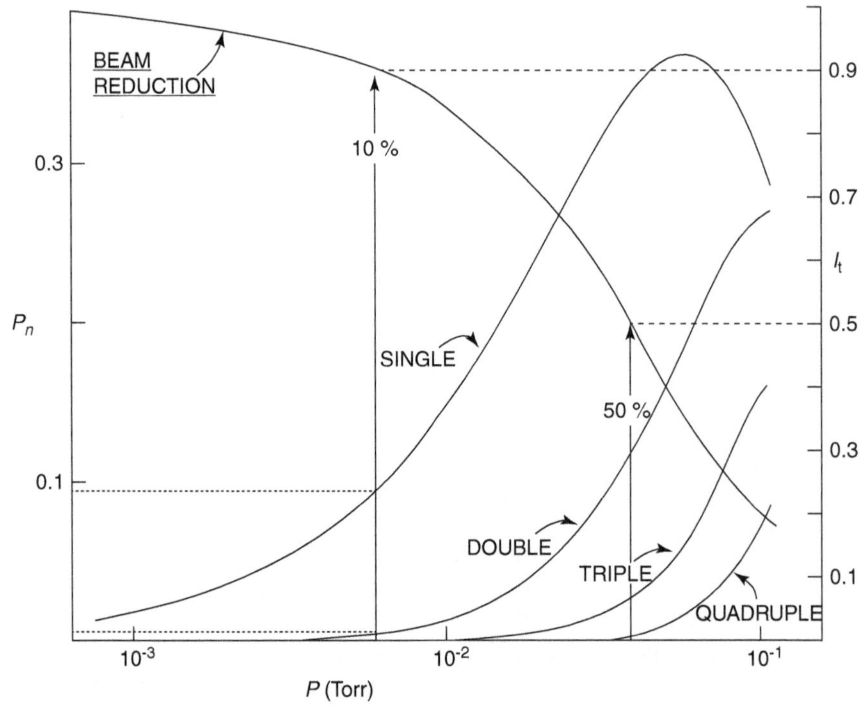

Fig. 9.7 Total collision probability P_n (*left* ordinate) and fractions of single, double, triple, and quadruple collisions vs. collision gas pressure. The transmission of the main beam I_t is given on the *right* ordinate. *Dotted lines* mark beam transmission and collision probabilities for 90% and 50% transmission, respectively. Values are calculated for an ion of collision cross section 5×10^{-16} cm^2 and 1 cm collision path; 10^{-2} Torr = 1.33 Pa (Adapted from Ref. [17] with permission. © John Wiley & Sons, 1985)

Adjusting the collision gas pressure

It has turned out that medium transmission is optimal for structure elucidation. Too strong reduction of the main beam favors ion losses due to scattering, charge exchange ($M^{+\bullet} + N \rightarrow M + N^{+\bullet}$) or charge stripping processes ($M^{+\bullet} + N \rightarrow M^{2+} + N^{+\bullet}$) instead of delivering additional structural information.

9.3.4 Time Scale of Ion Activating Processes

Collisions of energetic ions with gaseous molecules are very fast. Nonetheless, there is a considerable variation of the effective activation period, i.e., single collisions of ions of keV energy occur in the femtosecond range while those at eV energies tend to take picoseconds. If multiple collisions occur within one activation stage, the time scale is extended, because the span between collisions is then ruling the overall duration. Other activation techniques go along with even millisecond to second time spans (Fig. 9.8) [31]; most of these techniques will be addressed in this chapter [3]. While the fast ones can be treated by QET analogous to the event of electron ionization, the slower processes (SORI-CID, IRMPD, BIRD) tend to achieve an equilibrium of ion internal energy prior to dissociation.

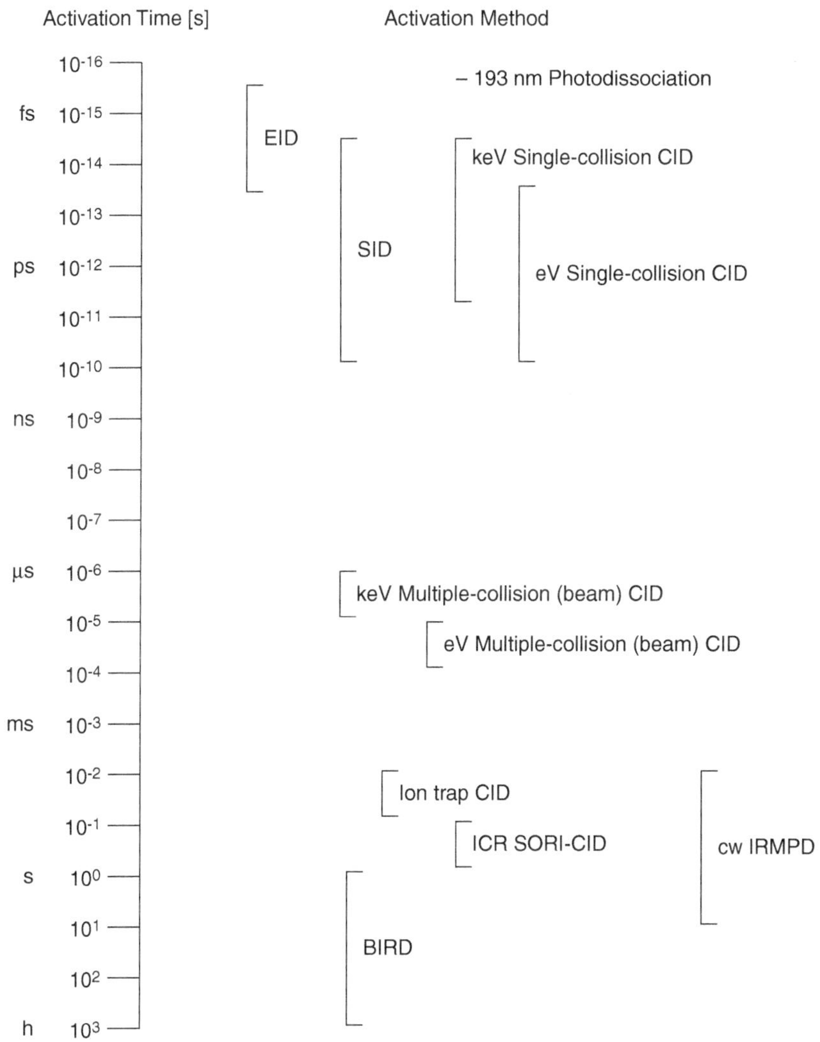

Fig. 9.8 Time scale of ion activation processes for tandem mass spectrometry (Adapted from Ref. [31] with permission. © Wiley & Sons, Ltd., 1997)

9.4 Surface-Induced Dissociation

Collisions with solid surfaces can be employed to induce dissociation of the incident ions similar to collisions with gaseous collision partners. This technique has become known as *surface-induced dissociation* (SID) [32, 33]. In SID, ions of some tens to a hundred electronvolts of kinetic energy are collided with a solid surface at an angle of about 45°. By variation of the SID target potential, the SID setup allows to control the energy of the incident ions, and therefore to adjust the degree of fragmentation. The first SID setup employed a linear quadrupole mass analyzer at right angles to the incident ion beam for fragment ion analysis (Fig. 9.9) [32, 34, 35].

SID conditions can be tuned to deliver spectra resembling either high- or low-energy CID spectra [32]. The absence of collision gas presents an advantage of SID over CID because losses of resolution due to high background pressure are avoided. However, apart from the quadrupole ion trap [36], SID requires substantial modifications of the instrumental hardware.

Fluorinated self-assembled monolayers (FSAM) are frequently employed surfaces for SID which are prepared on thin gold layers applied onto glass slides [37]. The perfluorinated alkyl groups in the top layer of the SID target serve to reduce ion losses by neutralization and improve energy transfer to the incident ions.

SID was never commercialized, and thus, SID lags behind the countless applications of CID. Nonetheless, SID is still developed further and implemented in modern instruments [37–41]. The Waters Synapt G2 may serve as an example (Fig. 9.10 and Sect. 4.10.4). In this particular instrument, the original transfer

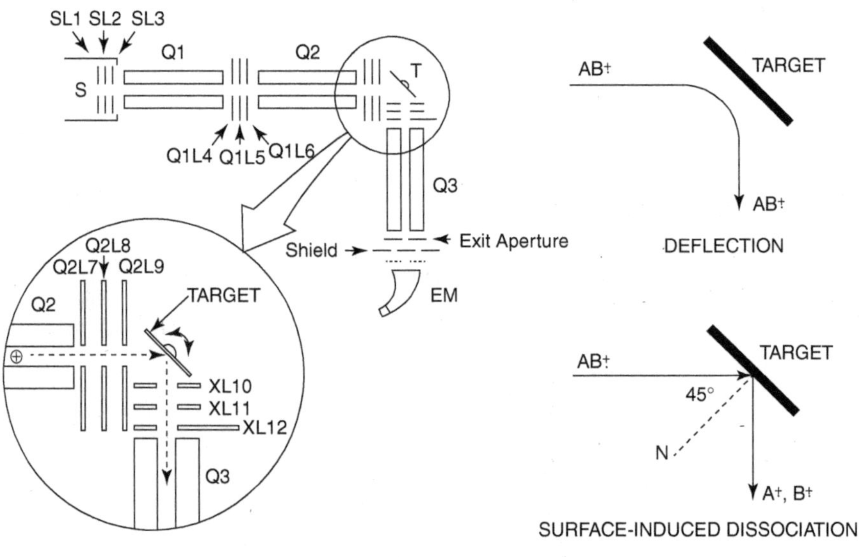

Fig. 9.9 Apparatus (*left*) and modes of operation (*right*) for SID with a modified triple quadrupole mass spectrometer (Reproduced from Ref. [34] with permission. © Elsevier Science, 1987)

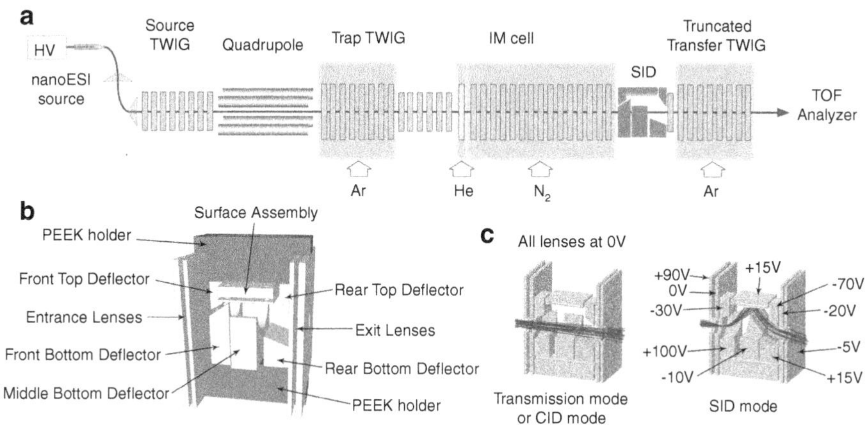

Fig. 9.10 Waters Synapt G2 modified to incorporate a SID device in front of the transfer TWIG. (**a**) Setup of the instrument (dimensions of the ion optics are not to scale). (**b**) 3D perspective view of the SID device assembly. (**c**) Cutaway views of a SIMION simulation showing the ion paths in transmission mode versus SID mode. The voltages on the SID lenses are given relative to the potential on the transfer TWIG (Reproduced from Ref. [40] with permission. © American Chemical Society, 2012)

TWIG (Sect. 4.10.3) was truncated to accommodate the SID device. The SID device itself comprises several compact electrodes to focus and deflect the entering ion beam onto the collision surface that is aligned parallel to the beam. The optimal voltages in SID experiments vary at different collision energies [40]. Switching off the deflection voltage also allows for transmitting ions through the SID device without collisions to the surface.

The reason for prefering SID over CID lays in the different processes of energy transfer to the precursor ions. Low-energy CID as used in modern hybrid instruments leads to vibrational excitation of the precursor ion via multiple collisions. SID, in contrast, causes energy to be impacted during a single fast event [37, 38]. The simplified reaction pathway for dissociation of a noncovalent protein complex via CID or SID illustrates how in CID multistep activation permits time for structural rearrangement, finally resulting in the formation of an unfolded subunit (Fig. 9.11). In SID, rapid energy deposition is proposed to induce dissociation faster than protein unfolding via different dissociation pathways [37].

Such differences in product ion formation are always observed when switching from very fast energy uptake (EI, high-energy CID, ECD) to slow heating (low-energy CID, SORI-CID, IRMPD, Sect. 9.3.4) [42]. Generally, pathways having high activation barriers are only accessibly by fast energy transfer, while slow heating fosters the selection of low-energy transition states.

Subunits of human serum amyloid P Human serum amyloid P (SAP) is a glycoprotein with an oligomerization behavior that is strongly dependent on the conditions in solution. It occurs in both a compact and a less compact SAP decamer

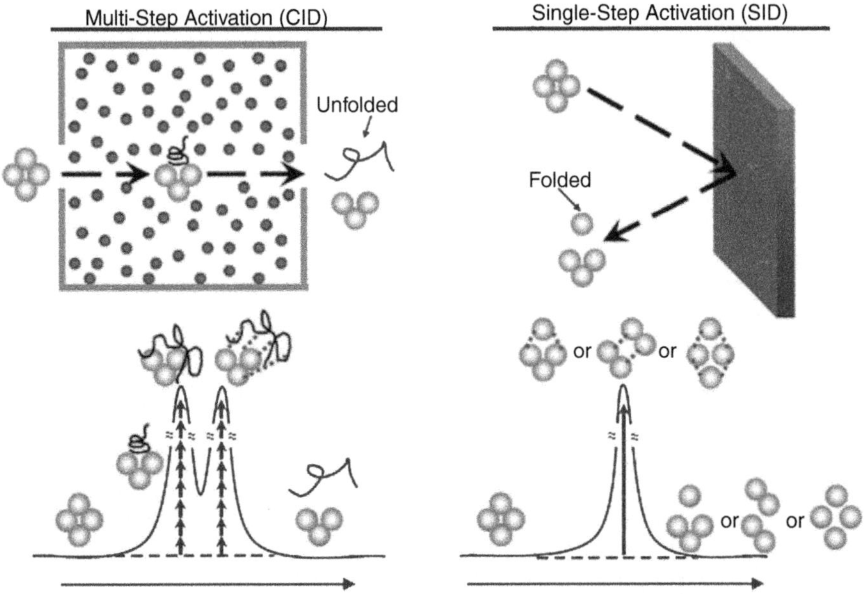

Fig. 9.11 Comparison of CID and SID experiments illustrating the differences in energy uptake (*top*) and the effect on fragmentation of a noncovalent protein complex. The reaction coordinate (*bottom*, *x* axis) is plotted versus energy (*y* axis). The actual energies needed and achieved, and numbers of rearrangements or of noncovalent bonds broken are, of course, unknown (Reproduced from Ref. [37] with permission. © American Chemical Society, 2009)

protein complex. These SAP decamers have been examined by CID at 160 V collision offset and by SID at 120 V offset. CID and SID spectra using the instrument shown in Fig. 9.10 reveal different product ion distributions (Fig. 9.12) [40]. However, the CID spectra of the two decamers are almost identical while their SID spectra show marked differences that help in distinguishing the complexes.

9.5 Tandem MS on TOF Instruments

9.5.1 Utilizing a ReTOF for Tandem MS

Consider an ion m_1^+ decomposing in transit through a field-free region. Its kinetic energy is distributed among the product ion m_2^+ and the neutral fragment n according to their relative contribution to the mass of the precursor ion:

$$E_{kin(m2+)} = E_{kin(m1+)}\frac{m_{i2}}{m_{i1}} \quad \text{and} \quad E_{kin(n)} = E_{kin(m1+)}\left(1 - \frac{m_{i2}}{m_{i1}}\right) \tag{9.10}$$

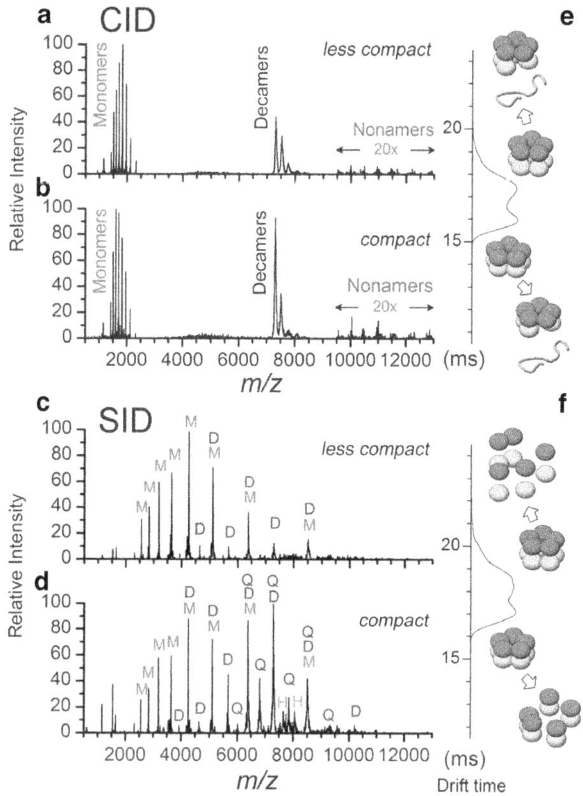

Fig. 9.12 Fragment ion spectra of SAP decamers. (**a**) CID of the less compact and (**b**) the compact decamer at 160 V. (**c**) SID of the less compact and (**d**) the compact decamer at 120 V. Major peaks are labeled in the spectra (*M* monomer; *D* dimer, *Q* tetramer, *H* hexamer). Parts (**e**) and (**f**) show the corresponding IMS drift time distributions with some separation of CID or SID products from less compact and compact SAP decamers and schematic representations for plausible dissociation pathways (Reproduced from Ref. [40] with permission. © American Chemical Society, 2012)

Fragment ions generated on the flight from the ion source to the reflector will have kinetic energies lower than intact precursor ions (Fig. 9.13). While the kinetic energy changes upon dissociation, the ion velocity remains constant, as already noted in the discussion on linear TOF (Sect. 4.2.3). A reflector is capable of handling ions bearing down to 70–90% of the energy to which it has been adjusted ($0.7\text{–}0.9 \times E_{kin(m1+)}$). Stepwise reduction of the reflector potential allows acquisition of partial fragment ion spectra each covering several percent of the precursor ion mass [6, 43, 44]. Piecing the data together yields a spectrum of the product ions formed by metastable dissociation of m_1^+. To cover the range from m_1 to $0.1 \times m_{i1}$ the reflector must be stepped down from its potential V_0 to $0.1 \times V_0$ in some 10–20 increments.

For tandem MS, the ReTOF analyzer itself only provides the field-free region and MS2 of the setup. Without further modification, the metastable dissociations of all potential precursor ion species leaving the ion source would be detected simultaneously and overlapping.

The precursor ion selection (MS1) follows a simple – although technically demanding – principle, i.e., a deflector electrode is placed adjacent to the flight

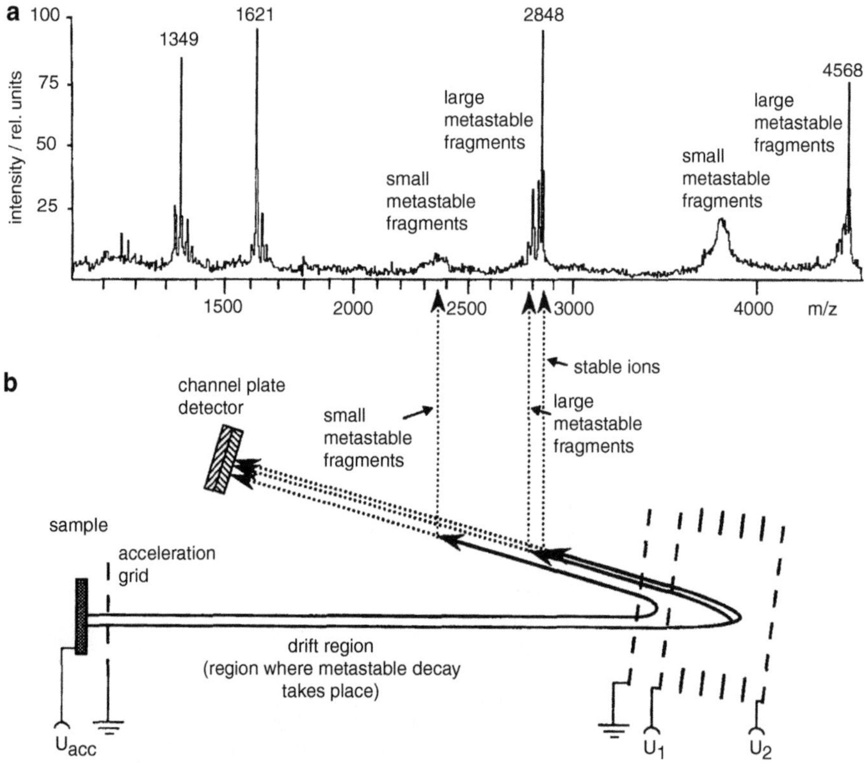

Fig. 9.13 Explanation of PSD fragments in MALDI-ReTOF spectra. (**a**) The occurrence of peaks due to ions of different origin is indicated above the schematic in the MADLI spectrum of a mixture showing $[M+H]^+$ ions of substance P, *m/z* 1348, bombesin, *m/z* 1621, melittin, *m/z* 2848, and ACTH, *m/z* 4568. (**b**) The PSD mode translates the diffuse fragment ion peaks into analytically useful signals. While the precursor ion and fragments of closely related mass penetrate deep into the reflector, those ions resulting from larger neutral losses return in the fringe field close to the reflector entry and are not properly focused onto the detector. To make these ions enter the useful reflector region, the reflector potential needs to be stepped down to successively lower values (Reproduced from Ref. [43] with permission. © John Wiley & Sons, Ltd. 1992)

path. To select precursor ions, ions below the selected precursor *m/z* value are electrostatically deflected, then the deflector is briefly turned off to transmit the precursor ions, and finally the high voltage is switched on again to deflect ions of higher *m/z*. As the deflector gate is located rather close to the ion source, it acts as a short TOF analyzer providing only moderate precursor ion resolution. An early velocity-dependent ion selector has been introduced by Bradbury and Nielsen, thus often called *Bradbury-Nielsen gate* [45]. In modern instrumentation the term *timed ion selector* (TIS) is commonly used for the precursor ion-selecting device. The entire procedure has become known as *fragment analysis and structural TOF* (FAST) [6, 43, 44].

Despite the comparatively poor precursor ion resolution and being a time- and sample-consuming FAST procedure, MS/MS of *post-source decay* (PSD) ions on the ReTOF has been one of the major tools of early MALDI biomolecule sequencing for ions in the *m/z* 500–3000 range. However, since the advent of tandem TOF instruments, the application of the FAST methodology has become rather rare.

Odd terminology
In particular the MALDI-TOF community has coined some sort of own terminology, e.g., *in-source decay* (ISD) for all fragmentations occurring within the ion source, *post-source decay* (PSD) instead of metastable ion dissociation, and *fragment analysis and structural TOF* (FAST) for the specific mode of operation of a ReTOF to detect metastable ions.

Historic remark on metastable ions in ReTOFs
Methods for the detection of metastable ion dissociations in ReTOF-MS in combination with *secondary ion mass spectrometry* (SIMS) and ^{252}Cf *plasma desorption* (^{252}Cf-PD) mass spectrometry were known before the advent of MALDI [46–49].

9.5.2 Curved-Field Reflectron

The laborious stepwise acquisition of PSD spectra can be avoided by using by the *curved-field reflectron* [50–53]. It offers advantages in speed and simplicity of operation when metastable fragmentations are to be studied, as in peptide sequencing by MALDI-TOF. Shimadzu employs curved-field reflectrons in the Axima series of MALDI-TOF instruments.

The curved-field reflectron extends over a long section of the flight tube, where it creates a nonlinear electric field that increases with its depth by steadily increasing the voltage difference between a comparatively large number of lenses. This type of ion reflector is capable of simultaneously focusing PSD fragments over the entire range of kinetic energies from 0.1–1.0 × $E_{\mathrm{kin(m1+)}}$. As it acts as a divergent ion mirror, it causes more ion losses as compared to two-stage reflectors.

The curved-field reflectron of a coaxial ReTOF instrument occupies a large portion (D) of the total flight path ($s = l_1 + D$). A prototype instrument used 86 lens elements whose voltages were set by 85 precision potentiometers located between them (Fig. 9.14) [52]. The distance l_1 between ion source and reflector entrance provided a sufficiently field-free flight path for metastable dissociations. To enhance fragmentation of precursor ions via CID, a collision cell can be placed anywhere in the short flight path in front of the precursor ion-selecting gate [53].

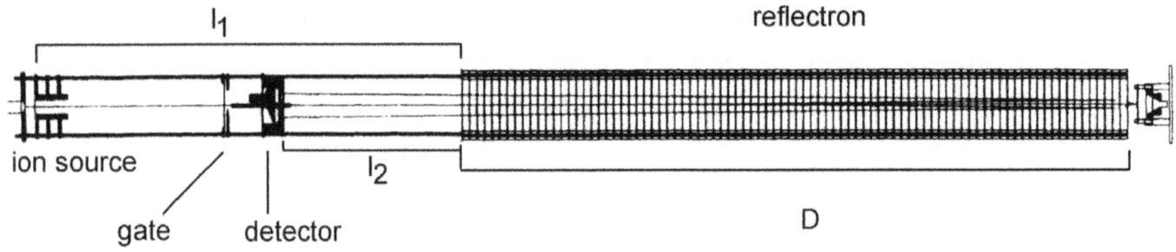

Fig. 9.14 Coaxial curved-field reflectron TOF spectrometer. The total length is about 1 m (Adapted from Ref. [52] with permission. © John Wiley & Sons, 1995)

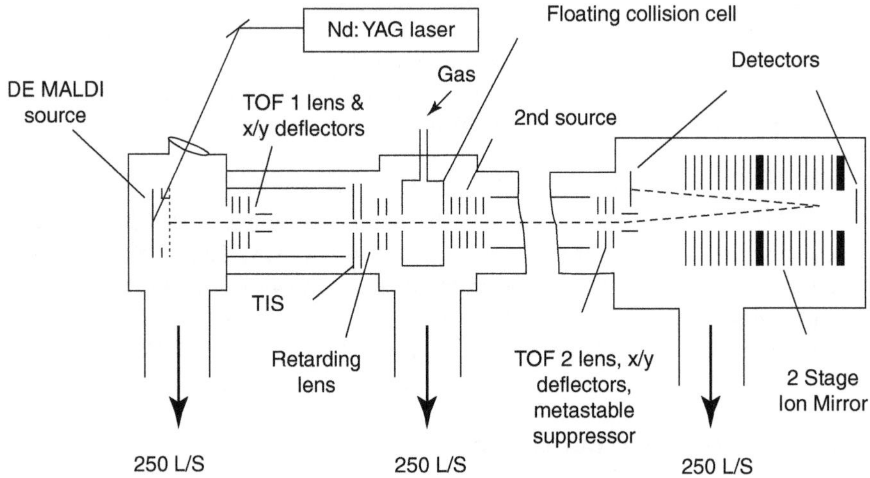

Fig. 9.15 Tandem TOF analyzer with linear TOF1 and ReTOF2. The ions from TOF1 are *m/z*-selected by a timed ion selector, decelerated, fragmented by CID, accelerated, and then passed into ReTOF2 (Reproduced from Ref. [54] with permission. © Elsevier Science, 2002)

9.5.3 Tandem MS on True Tandem TOF Instruments

Both limited precursor ion resolution and the need for stepwise acquisition of tandem mass spectra have driven the development of TOF/TOF instrumentation. Here, the MS1 functionality is achieved by a distinguished short linear TOF analyzer delivering ions *m/z*-selected by a *timed ion selector* (TIS) to a collision cell from where fragments are accelerated in a well-defined manner into the second flight tube that belongs to a ReTOF system. The first commercial TOF/TOF instruments of that class were available from Applied Biosystems [54] and Bruker Daltonik [55, 56]. Although differing in detail, the basic idea of these TOF/TOF instruments is to operate TOF1 at comparatively low acceleration voltage and to accelerate fragment ions into a high-resolving ReTOF acting as MS2 designed to analyze ions of 20–27 keV kinetic energy (Fig. 9.15).

The lower velocity of precursor ions in TOF1 does not only simplify the operation of the TIS, it also permits sufficient time for the ions to dissociate

(10–20 μs) [56] and it results in a narrow spread of the kinetic energies of the fragment ions arising thereof. After fragmentation, typically enforced by CID [57], the ions are passed into a second acceleration stage located behind the collision cell. By "lifting" all ions by a certain amount of kinetic energy, their relative spread in kinetic energy is reduced. For example, a precursor ion of 5 keV might yield fragments having 0.5–5 keV. Addition of another 15 keV to all fragment ions lifts them to 15.5–20 keV. In fact, the assembly comprising collision cell and acceleration lenses acts like a second DE ion source. Given a reflector of sufficient energy acceptance they can be analyzed without tedious stepping of the reflector voltage. The Bruker system employs 8-keV ions in TOF1 that are accelerated by another 19 kV after collision. For standard MALDI-MS operation, the ions are fully accelerated in the ion source and the TIS–collision cell–LIFT assembly is switched off (grounded). The Applied Biosystems instruments decelerate mass-analyzed ions to 1–2 keV prior to CID and then accelerate them to 20 keV for the ReTOF. Both concepts make use of delayed extraction for each stage and both require a metastable ion suppressor in the tube between collision cell and reflector. The metastable ion suppressor deflects precursor ions having survived the CID cell analogous to the TIS operation, because the 2.FFR metastable ions would otherwise interfere with the spectrum in the same way as shown in Fig. 9.13 [53, 57].

9.6 Tandem MS with Magnetic Sector Instruments

There are multiple ways of detecting metastable and collision-induced dissociations with magnetic sector instruments [13]. In fact, the whole phenomenon of so-called "diffuse peaks" in mass spectra was discovered with this particular type of mass analyzer (Sect. 4.3.2). In the mid-1940s, these broad signals were correctly interpreted as ions decomposing in transit [58, 59]. Metastable ion spectra still represent one of the indispensable tools for studying the mechanism and thermochemistry of ion dissociations [1, 2, 13, 14].

9.6.1 Dissociations in the FFR Preceding the Magnetic Sector

Peaks from metastable ion decompositions are detected at non-integral *m/z* values. Instead, the peak corresponding to a fragment m_2^+ formed from m_1^+ upon decomposition in the field-free region in front of the magnetic sector is located at a magnet setting m* which is described by the relationship $m^* = m_2^2/m_1$ [58, 59]. This is because dissociation in a *field-free region* (FFR) not only causes partitioning of ion kinetic energy (Eq. 9.10), but also goes with partitioning of momentum *p*

$$p_{(m2+)} = p_{(m1+)} \frac{m_{i2}}{m_{i1}} \tag{9.11}$$

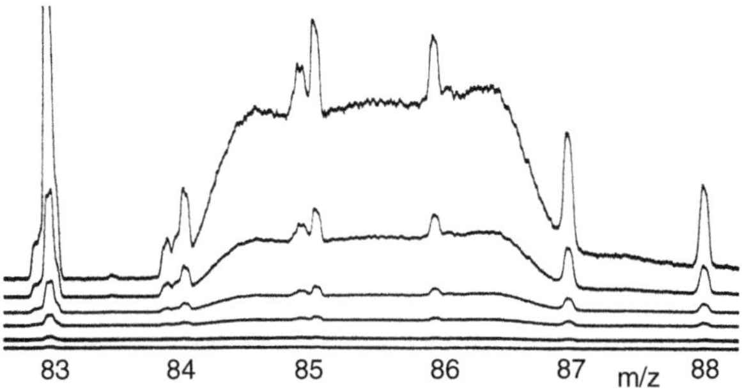

Fig. 9.16 Peak due to metastable NO loss of the *o*-nitrophenol molecular ion. The multiple traces correspond to different amplifier settings of a multi-channel recorder (Adapted from Ref. [60] with permission. © Verlag der Zeitschrift für Naturforschung, 1965)

Due to conservation of velocity, i.e., $v_1 = v_2 \equiv v$, the momentum of a fragment ion m_2^+ formed in a FFR preceding the magnetic sector is different from that of such a fragment ion arising from the ion source. The ion formed by metastable ion dissociation thus passes the magnet as if it had the virtual mass m*

$$m* = \frac{m_2^2}{m_1} \tag{9.12}$$

This explains "diffuse" peaks at fractional *m/z* values in the *B* scan spectra of B and EB instruments as a result of metastable ion dissociations [58, 59]. In turn, the mass spectra obtained from BE instruments do not show any metastable ion peaks in normal operation.

Observation of a very broad peak The metastable decay of the *o*-nitrophenol molecular ion, *m/z* 139, by loss of NO to yield the $[M–NO]^+$ ion, *m/z* 109, has been studied on a single-focusing magnetic sector instrument (Fig. 9.16) [60]. The mass spectrum shows a flat-topped peak of low intensity expanding over three mass units. Some minor and narrow "regular" peaks corresponding to fragment ions formed within the ion source are observed beside and on top of it. The peak due to the metastable dissociation is centered at *m/z* 85.5 which can be explained by the simple calculation $m* = m_2^2/m_1 = 109^2/139 = 85.5$.

9.6.2 Mass-analyzed Ion Kinetic Energy Spectra

Mass-analyzed ion kinetic energy spectra (MIKES) [61, 62] can be measured on BE geometry instruments only. The precursor ion is selected by the magnet and the fragments from dissociations of m_1^+ in the 2.FFR are analyzed by the ESA due to their kinetic energy. This is possible because the kinetic energy of the precursor is distributed among the product ion and the neutral. Derived from Eq. 9.10 we have

$$\frac{E_2}{E_1} = \frac{m_{i2}}{m_{i1}} = \frac{m_{i2}v^2}{m_{i1}v^2} \tag{9.13}$$

Thus, scanning of the electric field (*E* scan) yields an energy spectrum which allows for the determination of the *kinetic energy release* (KER) from the peak width. The MIKE technique provides good precursor ion resolution, but poor product ion resolution due to the influence of KER on peak shapes.

Abscissa of MIKE spectra
In MIKES E_1 represents the full electric field necessary to transmit the precursor ion m_1^+ through the ESA, and E_1 is often denoted as starting value E_0. Then, the abscissa of MIKE spectra is divided into units of $E/E_0 = m_2/m_1$.

9.6.3 Determination of Kinetic Energy Release

We just saw that peaks due to metastable ion dissociations are much broader than "regular" peaks (Fig. 9.16). In Sect. 2.8 we dealt with the *activation energy of the reverse reaction*, E_{or}, and *energy partitioning* as the thermochemical reasons for the occurrence of *kinetic energy release* (KER). The peak broadening is caused by the kinetic energy from KER grafted onto the kinetic energy of the ion beam as it passes through the mass analyzer. Due to the free rotation of the dissociating ion, there is no preferred orientation of this superimposed motion. Given a suitable experimental setup of the analyzer system that allows to obtain a kinetic energy spectrum, the *x*-component of KER, i.e., along the flight axis, can be calculated from the peak width of metastable ion decompositions. *Mass-analyzed ion kinetic energy spectrometry* (MIKES) is an established technique for doing so (Fig. 9.17). The peak width at half height is related to KER by [13, 14]:

$$T = \frac{m_2 U_b \; e}{16n} \left(\frac{\Delta E}{E}\right)^2 \tag{9.14}$$

where T is the average kinetic energy released, m_2 is mass of the fragment ion, n the mass of the neutral, U_b the acceleration voltage, e the electron charge, E gives the position and ΔE the width of the peak on the kinetic energy scale. Correction of the width of the metastable peak, w_{50meta}, for the width of the main beam, w_{50main}, should be applied for smaller values of T [63, 64]:

$$w_{50corr} = \sqrt{{w_{50meta}}^2 - {w_{50main}}^2} \tag{9.15}$$

KER of McLafferty rearrangements The observed KER values and also peak shapes may change dramatically as E_{0r} decreases (Fig. 9.17). In the McLafferty rearrangement of immonium ions (Sect. 6.12.1) the leaving alkene grows from

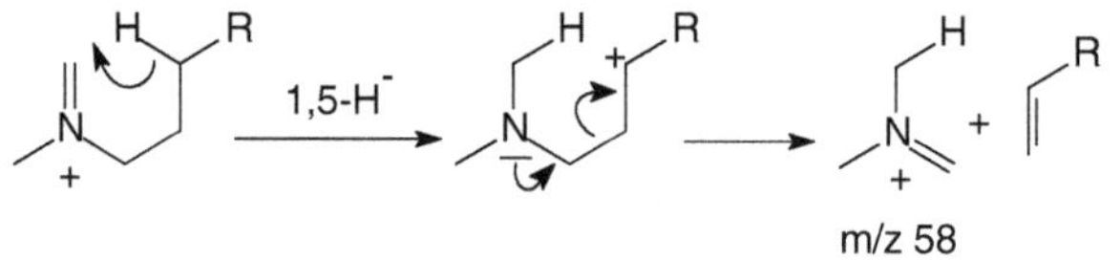

Scheme 9.1

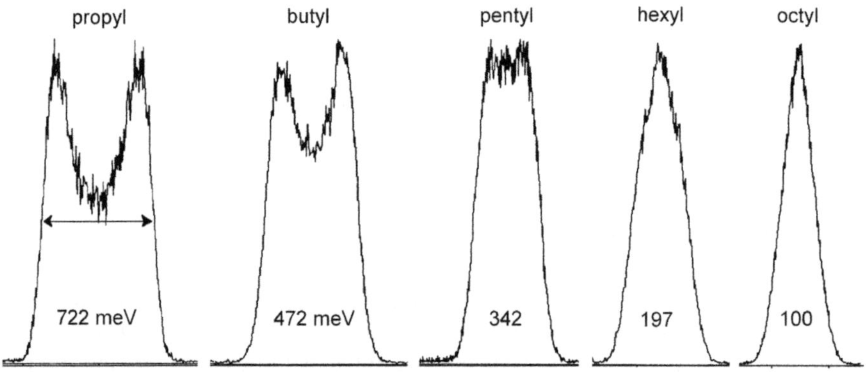

Fig. 9.17 Effect of decreasing E_{0r} on KER. The peaks from MIKE measurements result from the *m/z* 58 ion product ion of alkene loss via McL (ethene to hexene) from homologous iminium ions. The KER is determined from peak width at half height

ethene to hexene as the substituent varies from propyl to octyl. Nonetheless, the mechanism of the reaction by which the product ion at *m/z* 58 is formed remains unaffected [65] (Scheme 9.1).

Adjusting to an established standard
Before performing KER measurements, a "calibration" of the instrument (al parameters) against a well-established standard is recommended. Allylmethylether molecular ions, for example, decompose to yield three peaks of different shape and position in the spectrum [65–67].

9.6.4 B/E = *Const.* Linked Scan

Ions decomposing in the 1.FFR of BE and EB instruments can be detected using the $B/E = const.$ linked scan [68]. Due to the proportionality of B and p ($r_m = mv_i/qB$) ions are transmitted through the magnet if

$$\frac{B_2}{B_1} = \frac{m_2 v}{m_1 v} = \frac{p_2}{p_1} = \frac{m_2}{m_1} \quad (9.16)$$

where m_1 and m_2 denote the masses of the precursor and the product ion and v is their equal velocity. For their subsequent passage through the ESA, Eq. 9.13 has to be satisfied. Therefore, we have for the passage through both fields

$$\frac{B_2}{B_1} = \frac{E_2}{E_1} = \frac{m_2}{m_1} \tag{9.17}$$

which defines the conditions for a scan as $B/E = const.$ Thus, B and E have to be scanned together, i.e., in a *linked* fashion. The $B/E = const.$ linked scan provides good fragment ion resolution (R ≈ 1000) but poor precursor ion resolution (R ≈ 200). As with all linked scans, there is a risk of artefact peaks [69–72] because linked scan techniques represent no true tandem MS where MS1 and MS2 are clearly separate. The use of two complementary scan modes is therefore suggested to avoid ambiguities [70].

9.6.5 Additional Linked Scan Functions

Whereas TOF instruments solely allow for the detection of product ions of a selected precursor, sector instruments offer additional modes of operation: (*i*) to exclusively identify product ions of a particular precursor ion, so-called *precursor ion scans* [73, 74], or (*ii*) to detect only ions formed by loss of a specific neutral mass, so-called *constant neutral loss* (CNL) scan [75]. This can be achieved by some technically more demanding linked scans (Table 9.2) [76–79].

Table 9.2 Common scan laws for the detection of metastable ion dissociations on magnetic sector mass spectrometers

Selected mass	Scan law	KER from peak width?	Analyzer and FFR	Properties
m_1	$B = B_{m1}$, and $E/E_0 = m_2/m_1$	Yes	BE 2.FFR	Mass-analyzed ion kinetic energy spectrum (MIKES), E is scanned
m_1	$B/E = B_{0(1)}/E_0$ i.e., $B/E = const.$	No	BE or EB 1.FFR	Linked scan, poor precursor but good product ion resolution
m_2	$B^2/E = B_2{}^2/E_0$ i.e., $B^2/E = const.$	Yes	BE or EB 1.FFR	Linked scan, poor product but good precursor ion resolution, demands precise control of B
m_2	$B^2 \times E = B_{0(2)} \times E_0$ i.e., $B^2 \times E = const.$	No	BE 2.FFR	Linked scan, resolution controlled by that of B, needs precise control of B
m_n	$(B/E) \times [1–(E/E_0)]^{1/2}$ i.e., $E/E_0 = m_2/m_1 = 1–(m_n/m_1)$	No	BE or EB 1.FFR	Constant neutral loss (CNL), linked scan

All scans listed use constant acceleration voltage U. Scanning of U offers additional scan modes. However, scanning of U over a wide range causes detuning of the ion source

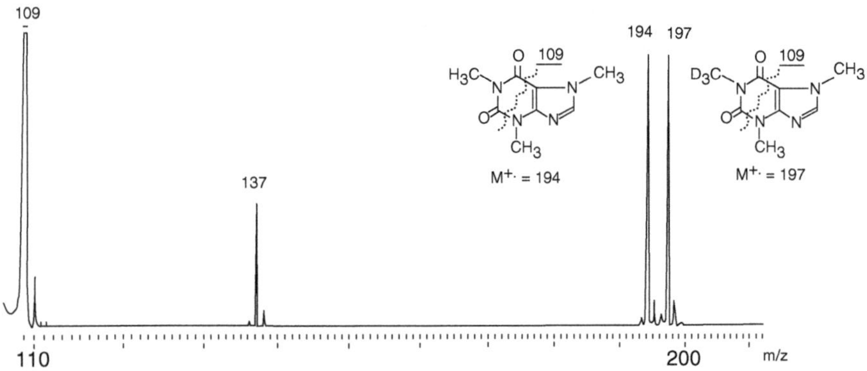

Fig. 9.18 CID B^2E spectrum of the ion m/z 109 of a caffeinated softdrink (cola) with [D_3]caffeine as internal standard. Different brands yielded 73–158 mg l^{-1} (Adapted from Ref. [80] with permission. © John Wiley & Sons, 1983)

Analytical use of the $\boldsymbol{B^2E = const.}$ **linked scan** The $B^2E = const.$ linked scan [74] has been employed to quantify the caffeine content of coffee, black tea, and caffeinated softdrinks [80]. Caffeine, $M^{+\bullet} = 194$, was determined by spiking the sample with a known concentration of [D_3]caffeine, $M^{+\bullet} = 197$, as internal standard. Both molecular ions dissociate to form a fragment ion at m/z 109 which was selected as m_2^+. Then, the precursor ion scan showed both molecular ion, m_1^+ and [D_3]m_1^+, as precursor of the ion at m/z 109. The ratio of peak intensities was taken as a measure for the relative concentration of analyte and labeled standard (Fig. 9.18). A modern approach would certainly involve a triple quadrupole instrument (Sect. 9.7).

Scan into the past?

Precursor ion scanning suggests some sort of measuring into the past. One should be aware that also in precursor ion scans the product ions are detected, but this is accomplished in a way that only fragments of a selected precursor ion mass can reach the detector, hence the term.

9.6.6 Multi-sector Instruments

Multi-sector instruments, typically four-sector machines, were developed in the 1980s to combine high precursor ion resolution with high fragment ion resolution [81, 82]. Their major field of application was sequencing of biomolecules by

FAB-CID-MS/MS. Commercial representatives are (were) the JEOL HX110/HX110A (EBEB), the JEOL MStation-T (BEBE), or the Micromass AutospecT (EBEBE). Today, all types of hybrid instruments have replaced these impressing "dinosaurs" weighing some 4–5 tons and having about 3 × 5 m footprint. A few custom-built four-sector instruments are still being used in laboratories devoted to gas-phase ion chemistry [83].

FAB and peptide sequencing The FAB-CID-MS/MS spectrum of thymosin-T1 $[M+H]^+$ ions, *m/z* 1427.7, as obtained from a magnetic four-sector instrument [84] shows numerous fragment ions due to *N*-terminal, *C*-terminal, and internal fragmentations (Fig. 9.19) [85]. It would be almost impossible to obtain sequence information from such a spectrum without generalizing rules to follow [86–91]. The most abundant ions obtained from the fragmenting peptide ion usually belong to six series named **a**, **b**, and **c** if the proton (charge) is kept in the *N*-terminus or **x**, **y**, and **z**, respectively, where the proton is located in the *C*-terminal part. Within each series the mass difference should only be one amino acid. Ideally, one can then count down the amino acids.

Tandem MS for mixtures
One of the advantages of MS/MS techniques is that they do not require the full isolation of all compounds of interest, because the precursor ion selection of MS1 excludes accompanying ions from contributing to the CID spectrum of the actually selected precursor ion as acquired by MS2 (Sect. 14.7).

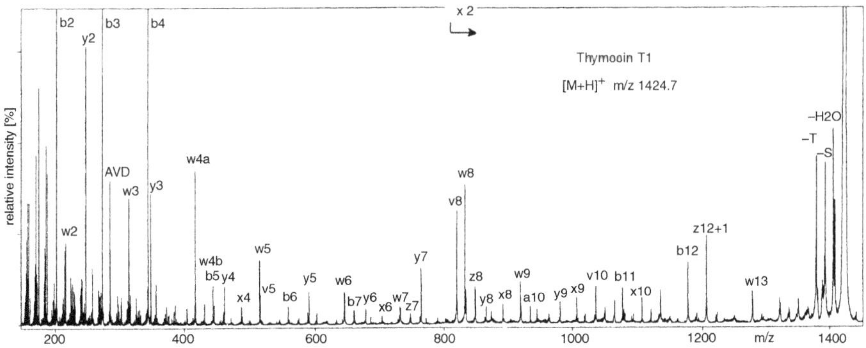

Fig. 9.19 FAB-CID tandem mass spectrum of thymosin-T1 $[M+H]^+$ ions, *m/z* 1427.7 (Reproduced from Ref. [85] by permission. © American Chemical Society, 1993)

9.7 Tandem MS with Linear Quadrupole Analyzers

9.7.1 Triple Quadrupole Mass Spectrometers

Triple quadrupole mass spectrometers, QqQ, are becoming a standard analytical tool for GC-MS/MS and LC-MS/MS applications, in particular for cases where accurate quantitation is desired (Sect. 14.3). Ever since their introduction [92–94], they have continuously been improved in terms of mass range, resolution, and sensitivity [95–97]. In early triple quadrupole mass spectrometers, Q_1 served as MS1, followed by an intermediate RF-only quadrupole, q_2, acting as "field-free region" with ion-guiding capabilities for metastable dissociations or more often as collision cell for CID experiments, and finally Q_3 to analyze the fragment ions exiting from q_2 (Fig. 9.20). The transition of ions through the QqQ instrument is normally supported by Einzel lenses in the gaps separating the quadrupoles [98, 99].

Guidance requested

Collision cells of simple short tube design like in tandem TOF or magnetic sector instruments (Sect. 9.3.1) cannot be combined with quadrupoles since the ions are rather dispersed at the exit and would be lost upon further collisional scattering.

In recent instruments, the collision region between MS1 and MS2 is not anymore an RF-only quadrupole, but a hexapole or octapole due to their steeper potential well (Sect. 4.4.4), which greatly improves their ion-guiding capabilities as compared to a true quadrupole. Today, most "triple quadrupole instruments" essentially

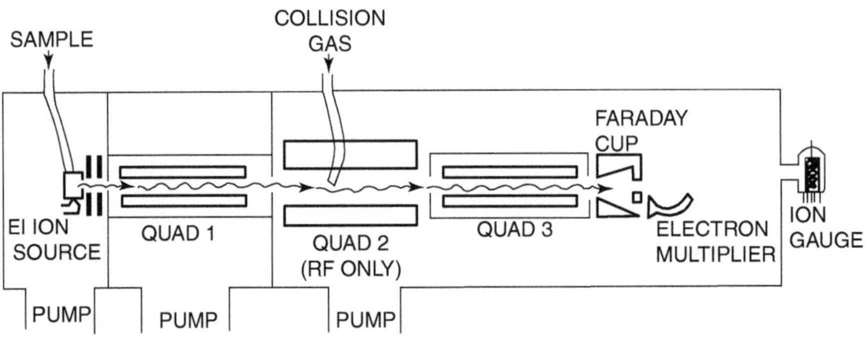

Fig. 9.20 Schematic of an early triple quadrupole mass spectrometer (QqQ) (Reproduced from Ref. [93] with permission. © Elsevier Science, 1979)

present QhQ or QoQ designs. Since the introduction of the *traveling wave ion guide* (TWIG, Sect. 4.10.2), there are also instruments featuring a Q-TWIG-Q geometry like the Waters Xevo TQ-XS or the Waters Vion IMS-Q-TOF.

In MS/MS operation, the mass-selected ions emerging from Q_1 are accelerated into the ion guide collision cell by a potential offset of typically 5–50 V where the collision gas (N_2, Ar) is provided at a pressure of 0.1–0.3 Pa. Careful optimization of all parameters allows for major improvements of CID efficiency and resolution [100]. If MS/MS is not intended, either Q_1 or Q_3 may be set to RF-only mode, thereby reducing its function to that of a simple flight tube with ion-guiding capabilities. The instrument then behaves as though it was a single quadrupole mass spectrometer.

QqQ in "normal" scanning
At first sight, there is no difference whether Q_1 or Q_3 is switched to RF-only for MS mode. However, for EI it seems better to operate Q_3 in RF-only mode. Otherwise, the ion source would effectively extend up to the entrance of Q_3 making fragment ions more abundant due to elongated time for dissociations. Soft ionization methods do not show such differences.

9.7.2 Scan Modes for Tandem MS with Triple Quadrupole Instruments

In triple quadrupole instruments Q_1 and Q_3 are operated independently as MS1 and MS2, respectively, making MS/MS straightforward. The experimental setups for product ion, precursor ion, and neutral loss scanning are summarized in Table 9.3 and depicted in Fig. 9.21. Definitely, this instrument class offers the most easily understandable tandem MS modes of operation.

Table 9.3 Scan modes of triple quadrupole instruments

Scan mode[a]	Operation of Q_1	Operation of q_2	Operation of Q_3
Product ion, define m_1	No scan, select m_1	Metastable or CID	Scan up to m_1 to collect its fragments
Precursor ion, define m_2	Scan from m_2 upwards to cover potential precursors	Metastable or CID	No scan, select m_2
Constant neutral loss, define n	Scan desired range	Metastable or CID	Scan range shifted by Δm to low mass

[a]Masses for reaction $m_1^+ \rightarrow m_2^+ + n$

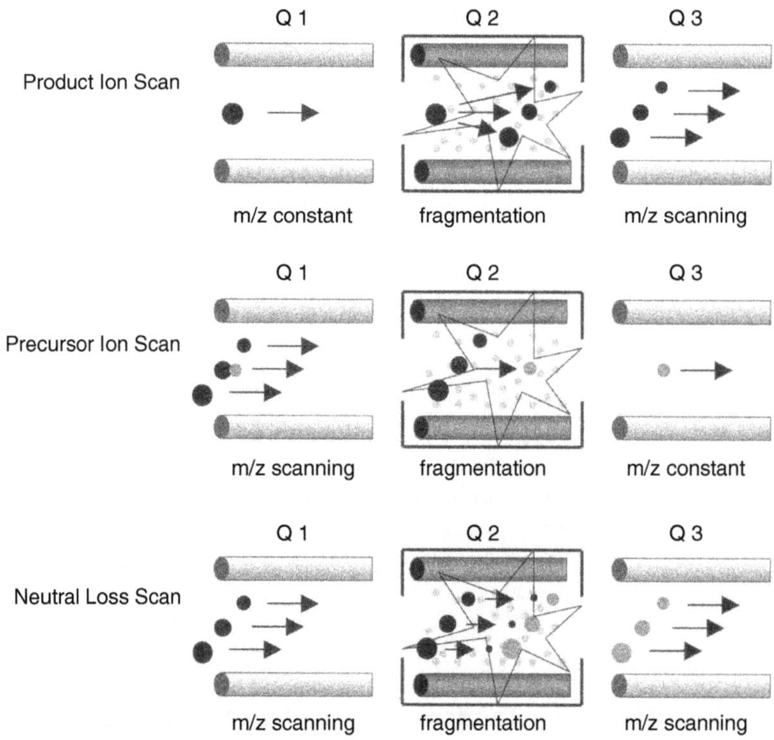

Fig. 9.21 Scan modes of triple quadrupole mass spectrometers (Adapted from Ref. [101] with permission. © Springer-Verlag, 2004)

9.7.3 Penta Quadrupole Instruments

The concept of the triple quadrupole instrument may be expanded by adding another RF-only quadrupole and a third mass-analyzing quadrupole to build a QqQqQ instrument. The penta quadrupole represents one of the rare tandem-in-space concepts to achieve MS^3. A commercial penta quadrupole instrument has once been offered by Extrel, but remained fairly exotic. Nonetheless, the penta quadrupole instrument may serve as a versatile tool for the study of gas phase ion chemistry and in particular ion–molecule reactions [102–105]. For the latter application the effective spatial separation of the zone with neutral reagent from that of preparation of the *m/z*-selected precursor ion presents a clear advantage over tandem-in-time concepts.

9.8 Tandem MS with the Quadrupole Ion Trap

Ion traps are *tandem-in-time* instruments, i.e., they perform the steps of precursor ion selection, ion activation, and acquisition of fragment ion spectra in the very same place. This advantageous property allows the multiple use of a single QIT to perform not only MS^2 but also MS^3 and higher order MS^n experiments – indeed a very economic concept. Depending on the abundance of the initial precursor ion, its fragmentation behavior – and of course, on the performance of the QIT – MS^6 experiments are possible [106].

In the QIT, MS^n is accomplished by using appropriate scan functions for the fundamental RF and the auxiliary modulation voltage (Sect. 4.6.7) [106–108]. At a sufficient level of sophistication, e.g., by combining slow and fast forward and reverse RF voltage scans with suitable settings of the auxiliary voltage, monoisotopic precursor ions can even be isolated in case of triply charged ions (Figs. 9.22 and 9.23) [109]. The resonance excitation provided by moderate

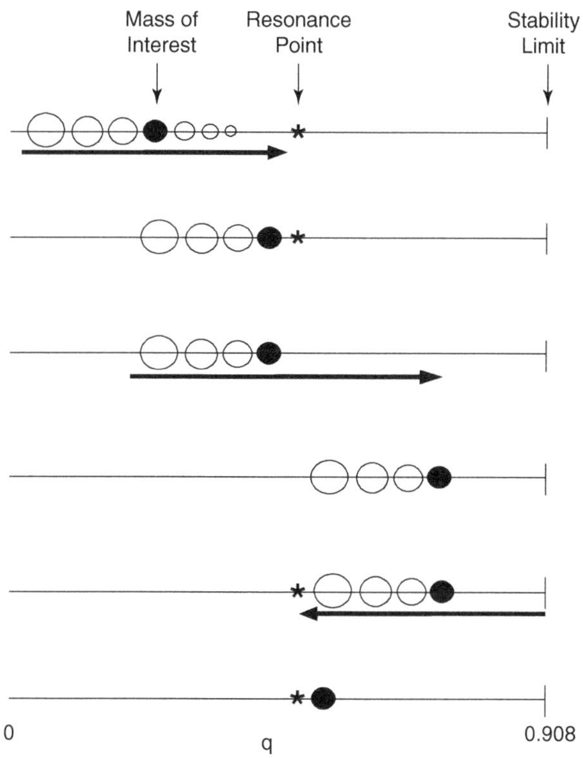

Fig. 9.22 The principle of isolation of a precursor ion by using forward and reverse scanning of a QIT. Ions smaller than the precursor are ejected by exciting them above the stability limit at $q = 0.908$, then settings are changed so that reduction of the RF amplitude causes ejection of the heavier ions (Reproduced from Ref. [109] with permission. © John Wiley & Sons, 1992)

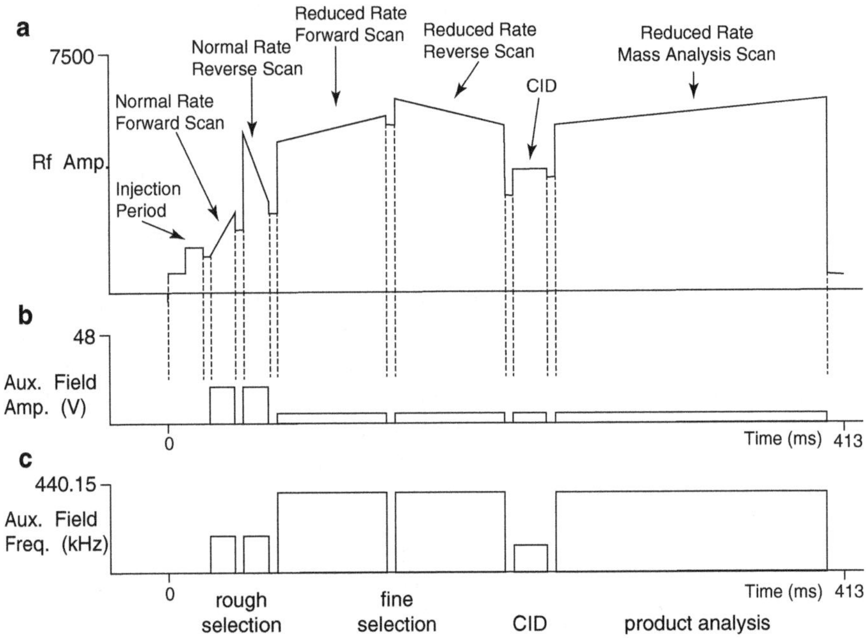

Fig. 9.23 Sequence of changes of (**a**) RF amplitude, (**b**) auxiliary voltage amplitude, and (**c**) auxiliary voltage frequency to first achieve a rough precursor ion selection, then a fine selection by repetition at slow rates, followed by CID, and product ion scan (Adapted from Ref. [109] with permission. © John Wiley & Sons, 1992)

auxiliary voltages can be employed to effect low-energy CID of the trapped ions due to activating collisions with the buffer gas [110], i.e., no additional collision gas is required in a QIT. A full description of the numerous approaches to continuously improving scans can be found in the literature [109, 111–116].

Unfortunately, there is one major disadvantage of QITs for fragment ion analysis in that they cannot simultaneously store ions over the full *m/z* range. It is a commonly accepted property of QITs to loose ions below an *m/z* value of about one third of the precursor ion. This phenomenon is known as *low-mass cutoff* (LMCO) [116].

Tandem MS on a QIT The positive-ion electrospray tandem mass spectrum of the $[M+2H]^{2+}$ ion of the β-casein tryptic phosphopeptide FQpSEEQQQTEDELQDK was obtained on a Bruker Esquire 3000 quadrupole ion trap (Fig. 9.24) [101]. Sequential amino acid residue losses from both terminal ends of the peptide are labeled according to the b- and y-ion nomenclature. Due to the phosphoserine, the C- and N-terminal peptide ions ($b_3 - b_{15}$ and $y - y_{14}$) exhibit an increase of 80 u

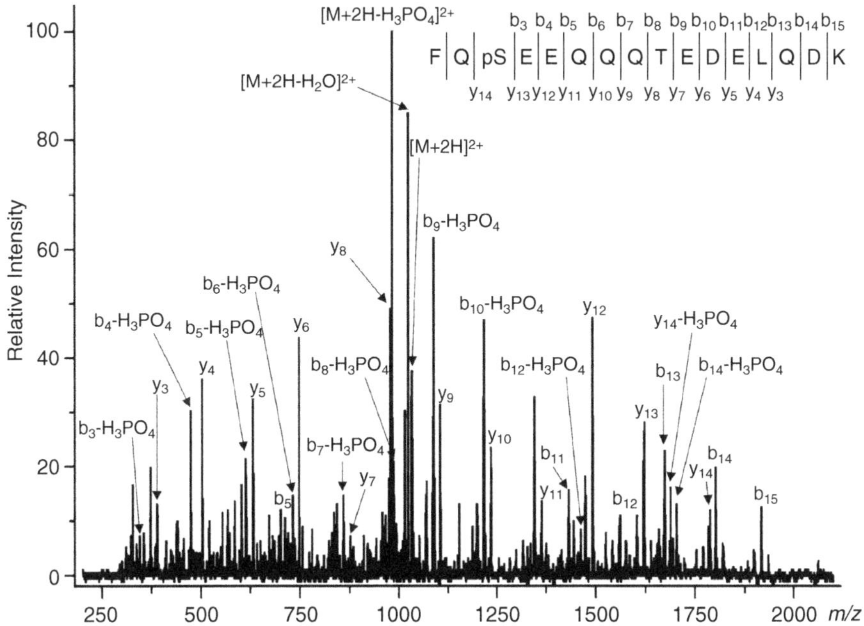

Fig. 9.24 Positive-ion electrospray tandem mass spectrum of the $[M+2H]^{2+}$ ion of the β-casein tryptic phosphopeptide FQpSEEQQQTEDELQDK as obtained upon HPLC coupling to a quadrupole ion trap (Reproduced from Ref. [101] with permission. © Springer-Verlag, 2004)

in mass as compared to the unphosphorylated form. In addition, most ions are accompanied by the corresponding fragments from H_3PO_4 loss (98 u).

QIT for MS^n MS^4 on a QIT was used for the identification of beauverolides, cyclic peptides from the fermentation broth of *Beauveria bassiana*, a pathogenic fungus of insects [117]. All MS^n (ESI-CID-QIT) experiments started from singly charged $[M+H]^+$ precursor ions (Fig. 9.25).

Limitation of tandem-in-time

In contrast to tandem-in-space instruments, tandem-in-time instruments neither support precursor ion nor constant neutral loss scanning. While product ion scans just need a precursor to be isolated prior to its fragmentation, both precursor ion and constant neutral loss scan rely on the simultaneous application of selection plus scanning or double scanning, respectively. Fulfilling two criteria at the same time requires two distinct analyzers at work.

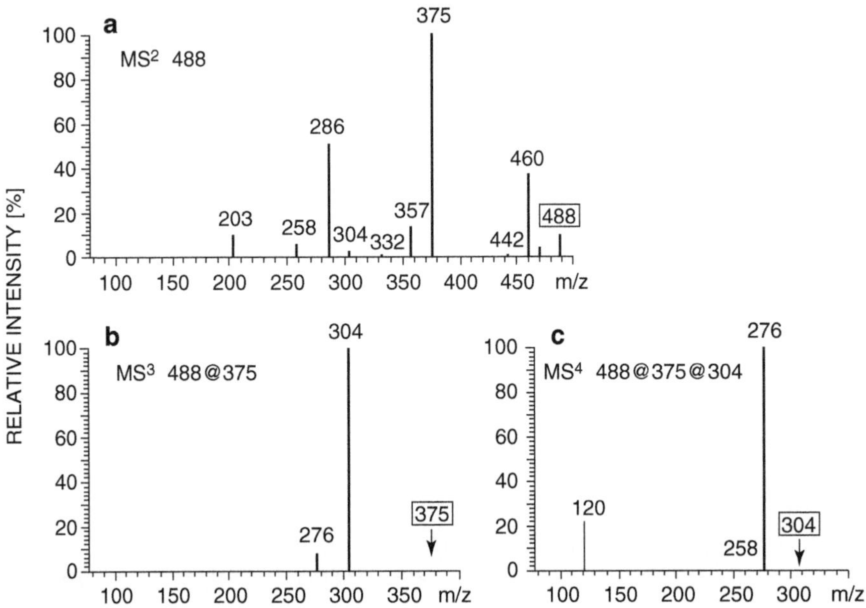

Fig. 9.25 Sequence of ESI-CID-QIT mass spectra of a beauverolide: (**a**) MS^2 of $[M+H]^+$, *m/z* 488, selected out of a full scan spectrum, (**b**) MS^3 of *m/z* 375 selected from (**a**), and (**c**) MS^4 of *m/z* 304 selected from (**b**) (Adapted from Ref. [117] by permission. © John Wiley & Sons, 2001)

9.9 Tandem MS with Linear Quadrupole Ion Traps

Mass spectrometers incorporating a linear quadrupole ion trap are highly flexible instruments. As discussed in Sect. 4.5, there are two competing concepts available on the market, one employing a LIT with axial ejection as part of a hybrid instrument [118], and another, featuring a pure LIT design with radial ejection [119, 120].

9.9.1 Tandem MS on QqLIT Instruments

The QqLIT design basically presents a triple quadrupole instrument having Q3 exchanged for a linear ion trap. As such, it offers all scan modes and properties typical for QqQ instruments (Sect. 9.7) plus those additional ones that are enabled by the LIT, i.e., higher-order tandem MS and combinations of ion accumulation and subsequent scanning for enhanced sensitivity (Fig. 9.26) [118, 121–123].

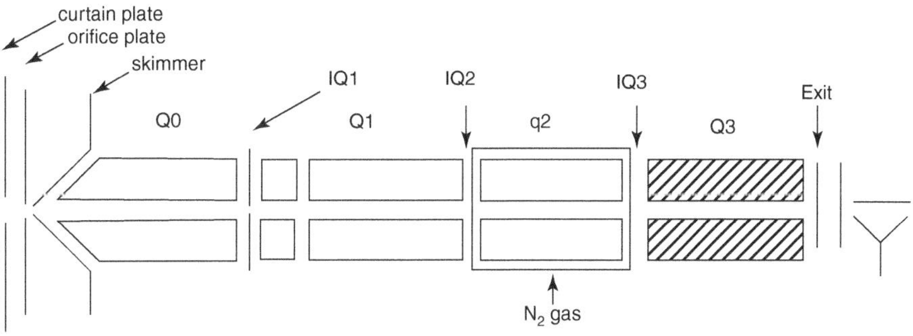

Scan Type	Q1	q2	Q3
Q1 Scan	Resolving (Scan)	RF-only	RF-only
Q3 Scan	RF-only	RF-only	Resolving (Scan)
Product Ion Scan (PIS)	Resolving (Fixed)	Fragment	Resolving (Scan)
Precursor Ion Scan (PI)	Resolving (Scan)	Fragment	Resolving (Fixed)
Neutral Loss Scan (NL)	Resolving (Scan)	Fragment	Resolving (Scan Offset)
Selected Reaction Monitoring mode (SRM)	Resolving (Fixed)	Fragment	Resolving (Fixed)
Enhanced Product Ion (EPI)	Resolving (Fixed)	Fragment	Trap/scan
MS3	Resolving (Fixed)	Fragment	Isolation/frag trap/scan
Time delayed frag capture Product Ion (TDF)	Resolving (Fixed)	Trap/No frag	Frag/trap/scan
Enhanced Q3 Single MS (EMS)	RF-only	No frag	Trap/scan
Enhanced Resolution Q3 Single MS (ERMS)	RF-only	No frag	Trap/scan
Enhanced Multiply Charge (EMC)	RF-only	No frag	Trap/empty/scan

Fig. 9.26 Correlation of the instrumental setup of a QqLIT instrument (Applied Biosystems Q-Trap series) with the description of its various scan modes. The *upper part* of the table lists scan modes that are identical to triple quadrupole instruments, whereas the *lower part* contains those unique to the specific instrument design (Reproduced from Ref. [118] with permission. © John Wiley and Sons, Ltd., 2003)

Elucidating fragmentation pathways The fragmentation pathways of ions of Trocade™, an anti-rheumatoid drug, $[\text{trocade+H}]^+$, *m/z* 437, were elucidated by sequential tandem MS up to MS^4 on a QqLIT instrument (Fig. 9.27). The protonated molecule first eliminates hydroxylamine, 33 u, to yield the acylium ion fragment at *m/z* 404, which in turn cleaves off the imidazolidinedione substituent at the α-carbon prior to loss of CO from the fragment ion at *m/z* 262 [118].

9.9.2 Tandem MS on LITs with Radial Ejection

A single LIT alone offers tandem MS along the tandem-in-time route. Improved trapping efficiency, more effective fragmentation, and trapping can be achieved when the LIT is operated with a higher buffer gas pressure, while higher scan rates

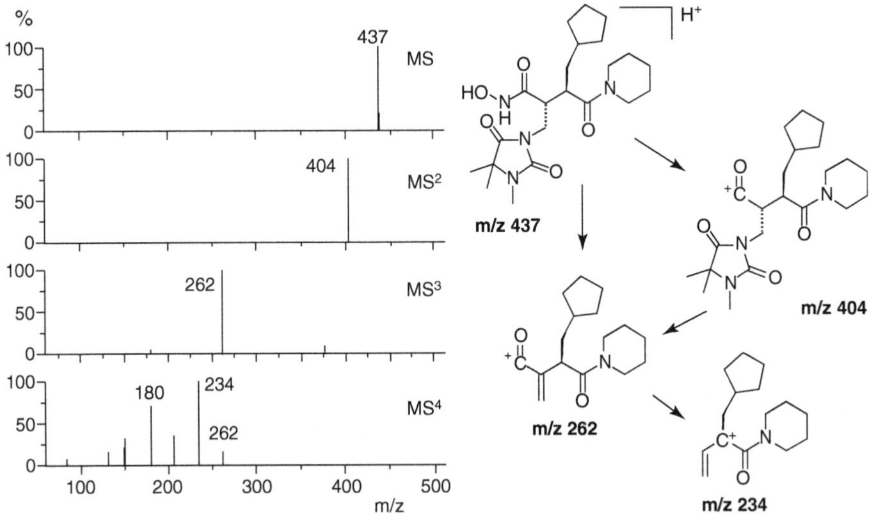

Fig. 9.27 Fragmentation pathways of [trocade+H]$^+$ ions, *m/z* 437, as elucidated by sequential tandem mass spectrometry up to MS^4 on a QqLIT instrument (Adapted from Ref. [118] with permission. © John Wiley and Sons, Ltd., 2003)

and resolving power are obtained at lower pressure. The recent *dual-LIT* design introduced by the Thermo Fisher LTQ Velos™ series unites these requirements by operating two identical LITs in tandem that are connected to the same RF and auxiliary AC power supplies, whereas the DC offset for trapping is delivered separately. Admission of the helium buffer gas into the high-pressure LIT allows to reduce its pressure in the neighboring mass-analyzing LIT (Fig. 9.28) [119]. The functional separation between the LITs not only allows to maintain unit resolution up to a scan rate of 33,000 u s^{-1}, it also more than doubles resolving power of the single-LIT version up to 25,000 when operated at very slow scan rates over a narrow *m/z* range. Such a dual-LIT design has also been incorporated in other hybrid instruments of this manufacturer that make use of LITs as MS1 (LTQ-Orbitrap Velos™ [124], LTQ-FT Velos™).

In space or in time?
With the introduction of QqLIT and dual-LIT instruments, even the concepts of tandem-in-space and tandem-in-time MS start to intermingle, because both tandem characteristics are part of each of these instruments. Once more, this demonstrates the ongoing highly dynamic development of mass spectrometry instrumentation.

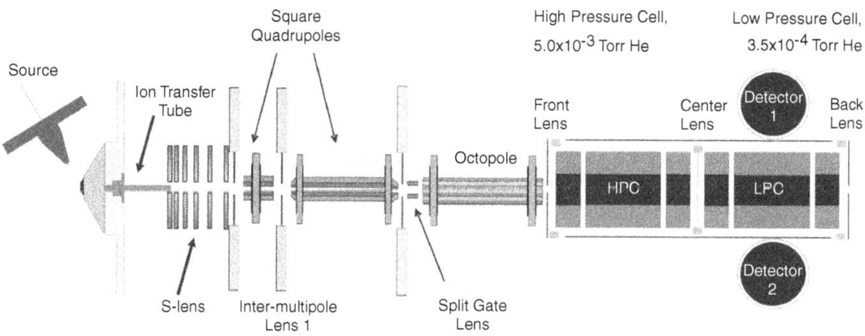

Fig. 9.28 The Thermo Fisher LTQ Velos instruments have a dual linear ion trap, the first section of which is operated at higher pressure (HPC), the second is run at lower pressure to achieve better resolving power (LPC). The dual LIT design also increases the speed of operation, because the first LIT can already prepare ions for the second while this is still mass-analyzing fragments from the previous cycle (Reprinted from Ref. [119] with permission. © American Chemical Society, 2009)

9.10 Tandem MS with Orbitrap Instruments

The Orbitrap analyzer itself does not provide for a mode of tandem MS operation. Instead, the steps of precursor ion isolation and dissociation are performed in a dedicated LIT as MS1 (Sect. 4.8.4) prior to high-resolution and accurate mass analysis of the fragments by the Orbitrap. Multiple-collision CID (Sect. 9.3) in the LIT of the LTQ-Orbitrap instrument is sometimes not hard enough to achieve fragmentation of comparatively stable precursor ions, e.g., it can be insufficient to generate immonium ion fragments from protonated peptides.

9.10.1 Higher-Energy C-Trap Dissociation

One approach towards harsher CID is to use the C-trap as a collision cell simply by raising the RF voltage from the standard setting of 1500 V peak-to-peak to 2500 V. The nitrogen present at about 1.3×10^{-3} mbar is sufficient to serve as the collision gas. After several oscillations, most of the precursor ions have undergone dissociating fragmentation, and all ions accumulate in the middle of the C-trap being confined by voltages on the gate aperture and trapping plate. This procedure has been termed *higher-energy C-trap dissociation* (HCD, Fig. 9.29a) [125]. An increase in RF voltage of the C-trap unfortunately goes along with a decrease in the *m*/*z* range that can be stored simultaneously in the C-trap.

These disadvantages are avoided by attaching an RF-only octopole collision cell with nitrogen at 5 mbar to the back end of the C-trap. To use this collision cell the C-trap passes through the ions from the LIT rather than ejecting them directly into the Orbitrap. This octopole collision cell provides fragment trapping over a

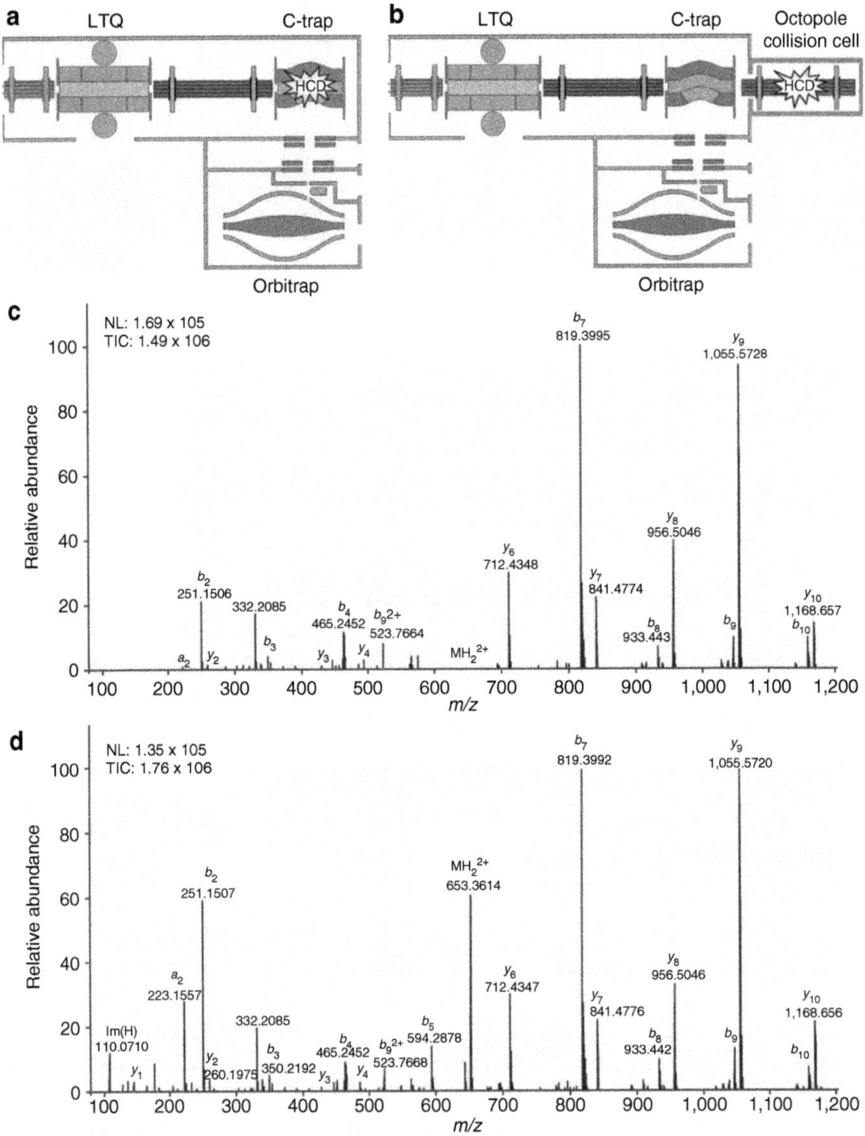

Fig. 9.29 Schematic of the hybrid LIT–Orbitrap instrument indicating the electrostatic potentials used in HCD and comparison of CID spectra. (**a**) HCD operation of the C-trap; (**b**) with an additional dedicated octopole collision cell; (**c**) CID spectrum of peptide $[HLVDEPQNLIK+2H]^{2+}$ ions from HCD as in (**a**); (**d**) spectrum as obtained by setup (**b**). NL: intensity in counts normalized to 1 s; TIC: total ion current (Reproduced from Ref. [125] with permission. © Nature Publishing Group, London, 2007)

wide *m*/*z* range. The fragments generated are then filled back into the C-trap, thermalized, and transferred into the Orbitrap for final *m*/*z* analysis (Fig. 9.29b) [125]. Such an instrument geometry is being offered as LTQ-OrbitrapXL™.

HCD for peptide ions Peptide ions, $[HLVDEPQNLIK+2H]^{2+}$, *m*/*z* 653.36, were selected as precursor ions, accumulated and isolated in the LIT until 10^5 ions were reached. With HCD setup (**a**) spectrum (**c**) was obtained. Using the dedicated octopole collision cell as depicted in (**b**) delivered the spectrum shown as (**d**) that exhibits stronger and more fragment ion signals in the lower *m*/*z* range. In particular, the immonium fragment ion of histidine can be observed at *m*/*z* 110 (Fig. 9.29) [126].

9.10.2 Extended LIT-Orbitrap Hybrid Instruments

It makes sense to extend the HCD geometry towards the dual-LIT MS1 to arrive at an advanced hybrid instrument design that combines MS^n in several modes with a powerful final *m*/*z* analysis [124]. Such an instrument has become available in the form of the Thermo Fisher LTQ Orbitrap Velos (Fig. 9.30). One of the most important advantages of this instrumentation is speed for proteomics analysis, e.g., within 1.0 s the dual-LIT can deliver five complete tandem mass spectra simultaneously with the Orbitrap running one high-resolution accurate mass scan of the whole *m*/*z* range.

Parallelized tandem MS in proteomics The coverage of the analyzed proteome and the identification of peptides have been strongly coupled to the detection limits and spectral acquisition rates of mass spectrometers. The spectral acquisition rate is primarily limited by the duration of the ion accumulation and analysis steps. Extensive parallelization of the acquisition process using a Q-Orbitrap-tandem LIT analyzer (Orbitrap Fusion tribrid, Sect. 4.9) significantly increases the spectral acquisition rate [127, 128]. The instrument's architecture permits a multitude of

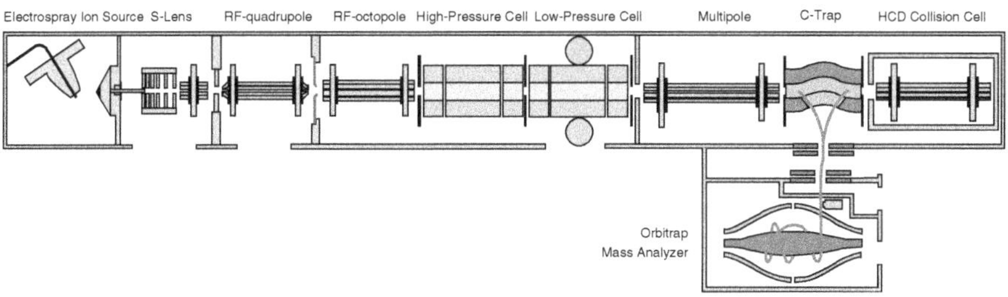

Fig. 9.30 Schematic of the Thermo Scientific LTQ Orbitrap Velos hybrid FT mass spectrometer combining dual-LIT and HCD with an Orbitrap analyzer (Courtesy of Thermo Fisher Scientific, Bremen)

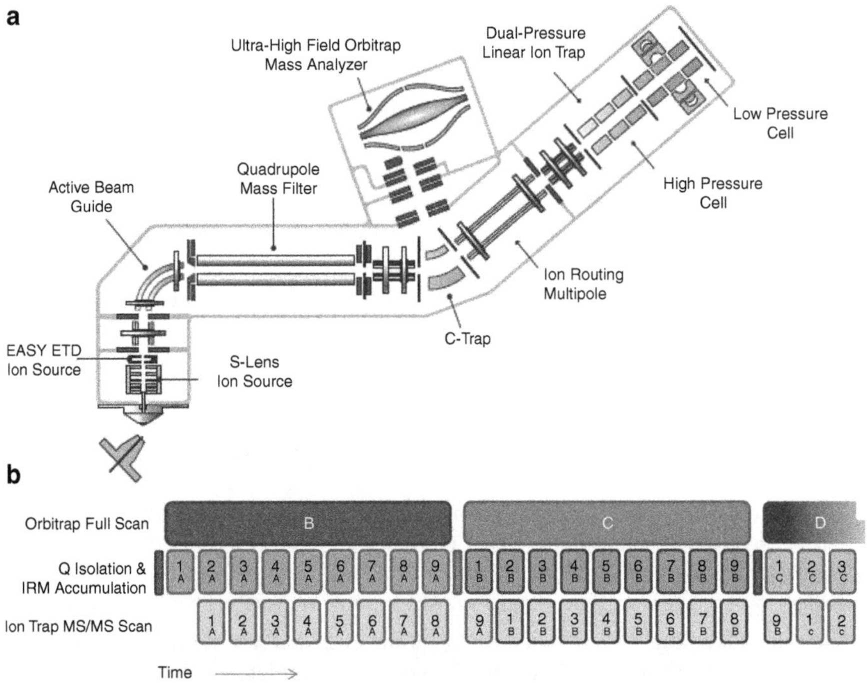

Fig. 9.31 Three processes running in parallel on the Orbitrap Fusion Lumos tribrid mass spectrometer. (**a**) Schematic of the instrument, (**b**) parallelized operation of three modes. The high-resolution accurate mass full scan of the Orbitrap takes several times longer (0.5 s) than precursor ion selection by the quadrupole and subsequent fragmentation plus fragment ion analysis in the tandem LIT (each ca. 0.06 s). The *darker-colored narrow* bars in the second row mark the ion accumulation for the Orbitrap, whereas ion accumulation for MS/MS takes longer to provide a larger precursor ion population to the tandem LIT (Reprinted with kind permission from Thermo Fisher. © Thermo Fisher Scientific, Bremen, 2015)

operational modes that allow tandem MS experiments to be run in parallel while a full range survey scan delivers accurate mass data of the next package of precursors to be interrogated (Fig. 9.31). This mode delivers survey spectra at about 2 Hz and tandem mass spectra of selected precursor ions at 15–20 Hz.

9.11 Tandem MS with FT-ICR Instruments – Part I

As ion trapping devices, FT-ICR mass spectrometers belong to the *tandem-in-time* class of instruments. Precursor ion selection (MS1) is accomplished by selectively storing the ions of interest, whereas all others are ejected by means of a suitably tailored excitation pulse. For this purpose, the SWIFT technique [129] or *correlated sweep excitation* (CHEF) [130, 131] are used (Sect. 4.7.7). Both methods generate tailored waveforms that cause excitation of all but the selected ions. Like QITs and LITs, FT-ICR analyzers are also capable of MS^n.

Although hybrid designs such as Qh-FT-ICR or LIT-FT-ICR are prevalent in modern FT-ICR instrumentation (Sects. 4.7.11 and 4.9.1), there is still the need for tandem MS experiments inside the ICR cell. Its dedicated abilities of very precise precursor ion selection, elongated ion storage in the order of tens of seconds, and possibility to admit gaseous reactants to perform even slow ion-molecule reactions make the ICR cell a unique tool [3].

9.11.1 Sustained Off-Resonance Irradiation-CID in ICR Cells

CID still is widely used as an activation technique for tandem MS in FT-ICR instruments. The collision gas is admitted into the ICR cell through a pulsed valve. To avoid detrimental effects of the collision gas on the ultra-high vacuum of the ICR cell ($\approx 10^{-10}$ mbar) the gas is admitted from a low pressure vessel ($\approx$10 mbar) in short pulses (5–50 ms). While the admitted gas causes the cell pressure to rise ($\approx 10^{-8}$ mbar), this still does not diminish the resolving power and mass accuracy of FT-ICR to an extent that would negatively affect this type of experiment. To further reduce the interference with collision gas, a pump delay (1–5 s) can be inserted between CID and *m*/*z* analysis. Generally, a set of such cycles is accumulated to obtain a spectrum.

For effective dissociation, CID requires that the ions collide sufficiently fast with the collision gas. The increase in ion kinetic energy is classically effected by short (0.1–0.5 ms) excitation at the cyclotron frequency of the precursor ion [132, 133]. This is known as *resonance excitation* (RE). The uptake of kinetic energy by resonance excitation occurs very fast, and thus, care has to be taken to avoid ion ejection from the cell. On the other hand, RE offers access to fragmentation channels requiring comparatively high activation energy.

Nowadays, *sustained off-resonance irradiation* (SORI) has established as the standard CID method in FT-ICR [134, 135], although there are others of comparable effect [136, 137]. Irradiating slightly off resonance ($\Delta\nu \approx 1\%$ or 500–1500 Hz) makes ions undergo acceleration–deceleration cycles throughout the duration of the RF pulse (Fig. 9.32). The principle behind off-resonance irradiation is the occurrence of a beat frequency f_b induced by the alternating positive and negative interference of cyclotron frequency f_c and excitation frequency f_{exc} as given by

$$f_b = f_{exc} - f_c \qquad (9.18)$$

As a consequence, the orbit does not exceed the cell dimensions but still maintains a high average translational energy for an extended activation period during which only small increments of internal energy are transferred to the ions. The ions can therefore be irradiated for a sustained period (0.1–1 s) without causing ejection, that otherwise at f_c was unavoidable. SORI-CID results in sequential

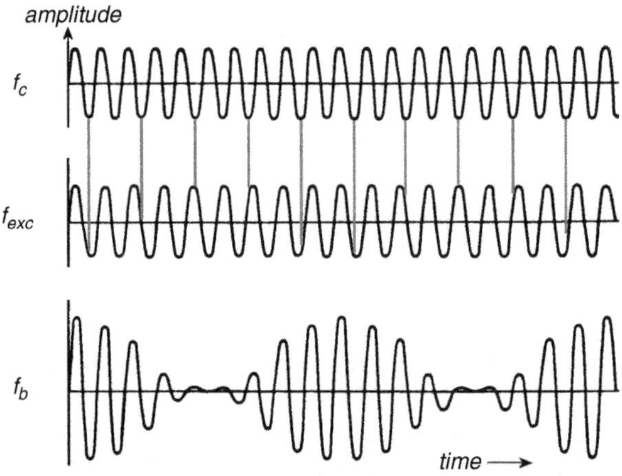

Fig. 9.32 Generation of an oscillation of ion kinetic energy as defined by a beat frequency due to off-resonance excitation; vertical connections are to locate points of positive and negative interferences, respectively. The larger the amplitude of f_b the more kinetic energy is contained in the circulating ions. One SORI-CID experiment consists of hundreds of beats

activation of ions by multiple collisions of low (<10 eV) kinetic energy ions with the collision gas, i.e., SORI-CID exploits slow internal heating of the ions [138]. Hence, SORI-CID addresses those fragmentation routes requiring rather low activation energy but benefit from sufficient reaction time.

Selective precursor ion activation
Both, RE-CID and SORI-CID are highly selective in precursor ion *m/z*, and therefore, activate only the precursor ion itself, normally even just a selected isotopolog. As a result, special pulse shapes are required to achieve activation of all isotopologs to preserve isotopic information in the fragment ion spectra. Furthermore, the high *m/z* selectivity causes only the precursor ion to dissociate while fragment ions do not receive any further energy to trigger second-generation cleavages.

SORI at work MALDI-SORI-FT-ICR spectra of the 2-aminobenzamide derivative of an unknown oligosaccharide were used for structure elucidation. First, the $[M+Na]^+$ ion, *m/z* 1240.5, was selected and fragmented (MS^2, Fig. 9.33a), then selected fragments thereof were subjected to further dissociation; to illustrate the principle, only one of these has been included here (MS^3, Fig. 9.33b). The frequency for SORI was chosen at 1.5% distant from the respective precursor ion's cyclotron frequency and supplied with an amplitude $V_{SORI} = 10$ V [138].

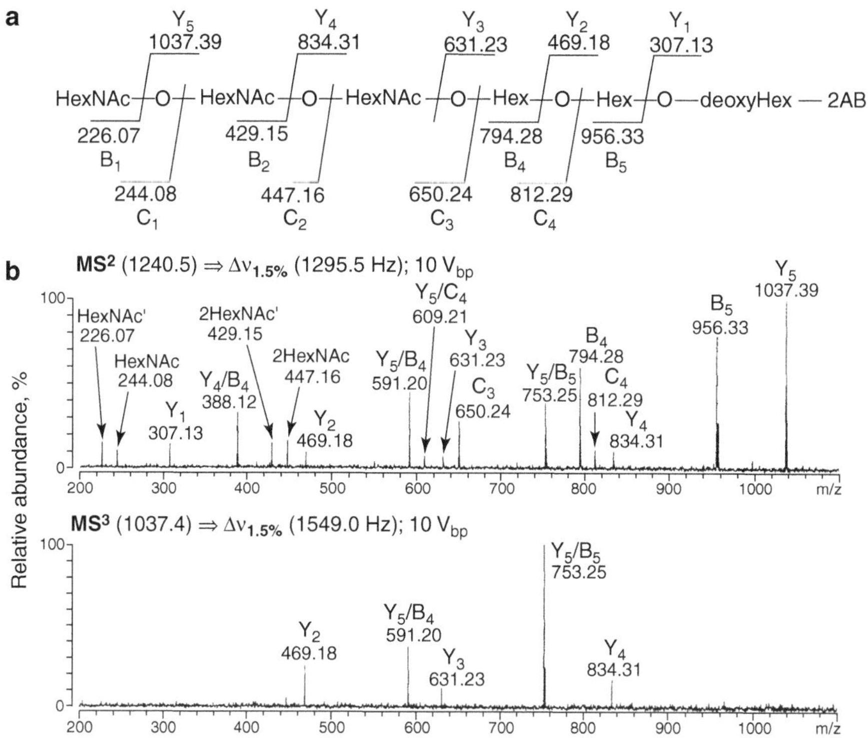

Fig. 9.33 MALDI-SORI-FT-ICR spectra of the $[M+Na]^+$ ion, *m/z* 1240.5, of the 2-aminobenzamide derivative of an unknown oligosaccharide (MS^2, **a**), and of the fragment at *m/z* 1037.4 obtained thereof (MS^3, **b**) (Adapted from Ref. [139] with permission. © Elsevier Science Publishers, 2002)

Dosing gas into ICR cells

CID can rather easily be implemented on FT-ICR instruments because it only demands for a pulse valve and a reservoir. Although the collision gas in SORI-CID can be easily handled, its use is nonetheless in contradiction to the high vacuum requirements of the ICR cell. Thus, alternative ion activation techniques without the use of gas are desirable.

9.12 Infrared Multiphoton Dissociation

The energy received from multiple photon absorption may also be used to activate and dissociate otherwise stable gaseous ions [140]:

$$m_1^+ + x \times h\nu \rightarrow m_2^+ + n \qquad (9.19)$$

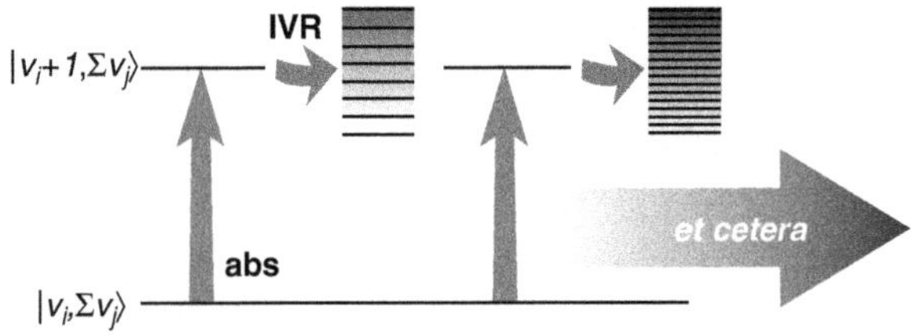

Fig. 9.34 IRMPD mechanism involving intramolecular vibrational relaxation (IVR) (Reproduced from Ref. [144] with permission. © John Wiley Periodicals, Inc., 2009)

Infrared multiphoton dissociation (IRMPD) was first described along with the dissociation of weakly bound protonated diethylether cluster ions [140]:

$$\left[(\mathrm{Et_2O})_2 + \mathrm{H}\right]^+ + x\,\mathrm{h}\nu \rightarrow [\mathrm{Et_2O} + \mathrm{H}]^+ + \mathrm{Et_2O} \tag{9.20}$$

IRMPD is a technique that can be conveniently applied to trapped ions as is the case in ICR cells. IRMPD normally employs a continuous wave carbon dioxide laser of 10.6 μm wavelength (2.83×10^{13} Hz) having a power of 25–40 W which is passed into the ICR cell through a ZnSe or BaF_2 window [141, 142]. It is advantageous to combine FT-ICR with IRMPD because the amount of energy applied to the ions can be varied via the duration of laser irradiation, typically in the range of 5–300 ms [143]. This allows for the application of IRMPD to small ions [140] as well as to medium-sized [143] or high-mass ions [142].

Absorption of photon energy by a single normal mode of the ion is usually followed by dissipation among other vibrational modes, i.e., by *intramolecular vibrational relaxation* (IVR). The initial absorbing mode thereby returns to its ground state and gets ready to absorb another IR photon and so on (Fig. 9.34) [144]. IRMPD is regarded as a *slow heating method* because a large number of IR photons must be absorbed to effect fragmentation. In case of the usual carbon dioxide laser the energy of a single photon is just 0.116 eV, i.e., per electronvolt the absorption of nine photons is required [145, 146].

Safety note

For IRMPD, care must be taken to block the IR laser from abandoning its assigned optical path. The IR laser is extremely powerful and can instantaneously ignite objects or cause injuries from burns.

9.12.1 IRMPD in QITs and LITs

IRMPD is a valuable tool for gas phase ion studies and analytical applications that often do not require the full power of a highly expensive FT-ICR instrument. Therefore, efforts have been made to implement IRMPD on three-dimensional (Fig. 9.35) [145–148] and linear quadrupole ion traps [149–152].

Collisional cooling by the buffer gas required for quadrupole ion trap operation counteracts the accumulation of the ion internal energy by slow collisional

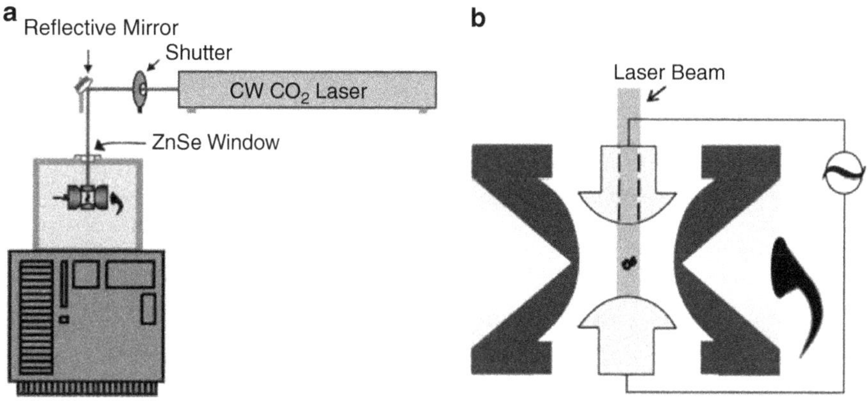

Fig. 9.35 IRMPD in a quadrupole ion trap (**a**) relative to the entire instrument and (**b**) with beam passage through a hole in the ring electrode of the QIT (Reproduced from Ref. [145] with permission. © John Wiley Periodicals, 2009)

activation. To avoid this problem, a dynamic pressure operation mode has been developed for IRMPD in QITs where initial ion storage and precursor ion selection are run at standard QIT pressure (3×10^{-2} mbar) while the buffer gas flow is interrupted several milliseconds prior to IRMPD ($<10^{-4}$ mbar) and subsequent product ion scanning [42, 146]. Alternatively, the energy drain by collisional cooling is strongly reduced by IRMPD in a tandem linear ion trap as in the Thermo LTQ Velos instruments (Fig. 9.30). The low-pressure cell is then employed for IRMPD, while the high-pressure cell only serves for CID [150].

9.13 Electron Capture Dissociation

9.13.1 Principles of Electron Capture Dissociation

For an ion, the cross section for *electron capture* (EC) roughly increases with the square of the ionic charge [153]. This makes multiply charged ions as produced by *electrospray ionization* (ESI, Chap. 12) the ideal targets for this process. When a UV laser of 193 nm wavelength (6.4 eV per photon) in the course of *ultraviolet photon dissociation* (UVPD) experiments erroneously hit a metal surface, electrons were deliberated inside the ICR cell. Electron capture by the formed multiply charged protein ions shifted their charge state from 11^+ to 10^+ without affecting mass [153]:

$$[M + 11H]^{11+} + e^- \rightarrow [M + 11H]^{10+\bullet} \qquad (9.21)$$

The product of EC is a radical ion (Fig. 9.36). The energy from neutralization of one ionic charge (5–7 eV) is transformed into ion internal energy that causes immediate fragmentation, so-called *electron capture dissociation* (ECD).

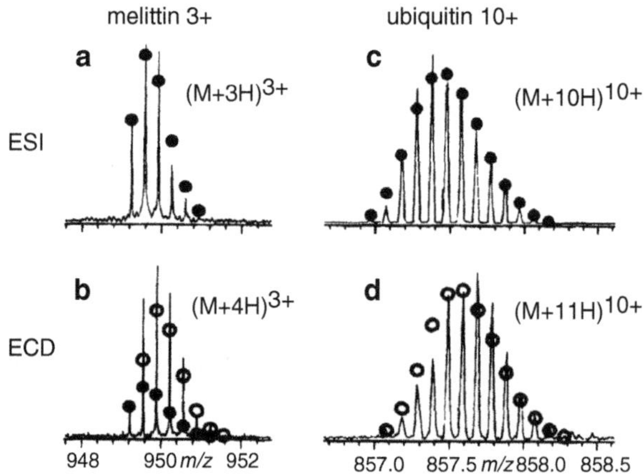

Fig. 9.36 Discovery of ECD by comparison of electrospray ionization (ESI) mass spectra of protein ions with those obtained when the UV laser was switched on to generate thermal electrons from the inner walls of the ICR cell. *Closed circles* mark the theoretically predicted isotopic abundances for the closed-shell ions of n^+ charge state, while *open circles* show those for the $(n-1)^{+\bullet}$ radical ions. The experimental patterns clearly show superimpositions of both (Reproduced from Ref. [153] with permission. © American Chemical Society, 1998)

Again, ECD is a technique for trapped ions only. To effectively achieve ECD the electrons must have energies <0.2 eV. Therefore, they are supplied analogously to EI from a carefully regulated heated filament [154] externally mounted to the ICR cell. Although a rather recent discovery [153, 155], ECD is now widely applied in biomolecule sequencing by means of ESI-FT-ICR-MS [154, 156]. The motivation for those numerous ECD applications is due to the fact that ECD yields information complementary to CID [157] and IRMPD [141].

ECD requires multiply charged precursors
As one electron charge is neutralized upon EC, the precursor ion for ECD must at least be a doubly charged positive even-electron ion to yield a singly charged radical ion for subsequent dissociation.

9.13.2 Peptide Ion Cleavages Upon ECD

In contrast to the prevalent generation of *b*- and *y*-type fragment ions from slow-heating activation methods, the fragmentation patterns in ECD contain mostly *c*- and *z*-type ions. These are generated by cleavage of an amine bond (N–C_α bond cleavage). Assuming a peptide ion $[M+zH]^{z+}$ having a lysine (Lys) residue, one can write the mechanism of ECD-induced peptide cleavage as depicted in Fig. 9.37 [158]. This scheme follows the most widely used model for the ECD mechanism,

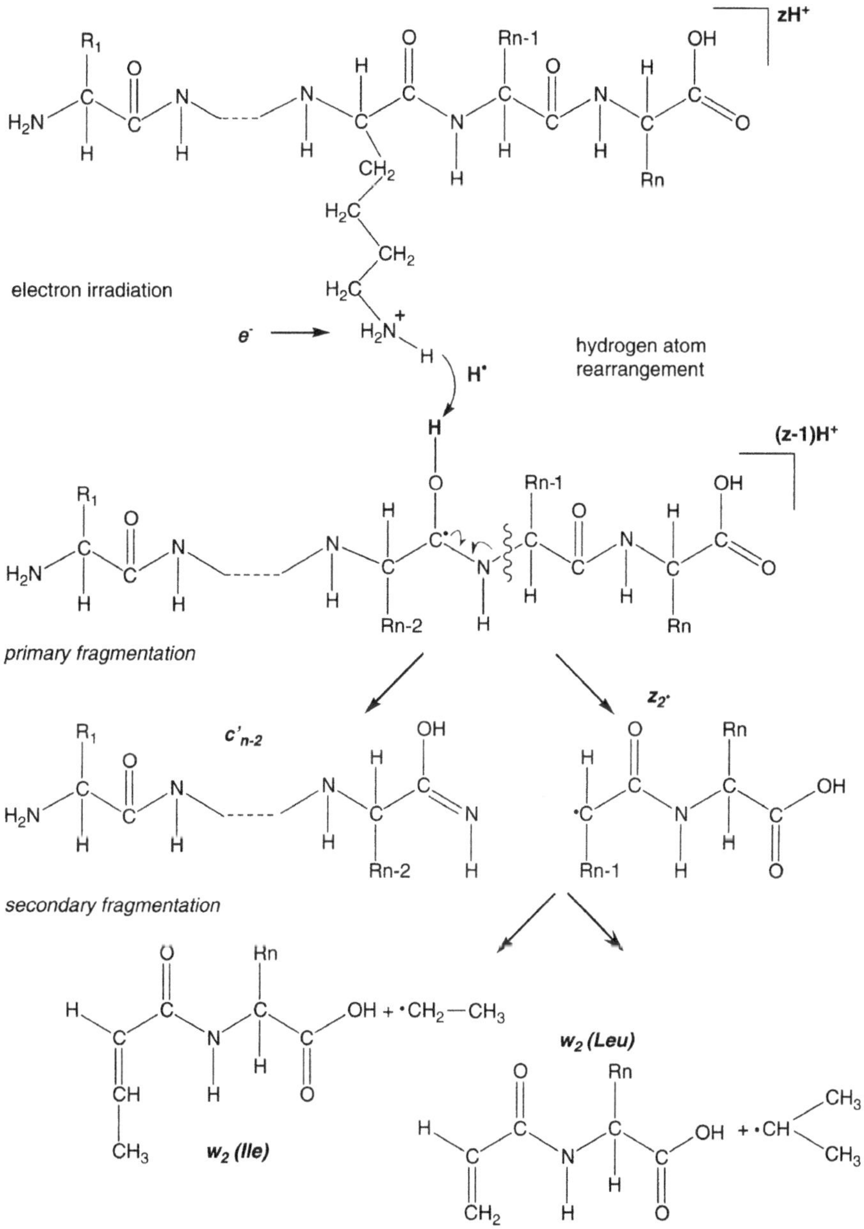

Fig. 9.37 Mechanism of fragmentation upon ECD following the hot hydrogen atom model. In this example, a protonated lysine residue captures the electron and immediately transfers a hydrogen atom to its neighboring carbonyl-O. Primary and secondary fragmentation pathways of the peptide ions are shown (Adapted from Ref. [158] with permission. © John Wiley & Sons, Ltd., 2004)

the so-called *hot hydrogen atom model*, which states that the electron is captured in a high Rydberg state by action of a charged site in the ion. Typically, the charges reside on basic amino acid residues, i.e., on arginine (Arg), lysine (Lys), or histidine (His), or on *N*-terminal amino groups. The primary odd-electron ion immediately cleaves off a hydrogen radical by N–H bond cleavage, thereby creating a hydrogen atom with an excess energy of about 6 eV. This "hot" hydrogen atom may be transferred along the peptide chain to any amide carbonyl group or to disulfide groups [159, 160]. Now, one of the electrons of the carbonyl-carbon atom is unpaired. Due to the excess energy this radical can dissociate by N–C_α bond cleavage. Thus, the amine-terminal peptide fragments are forming *c*-type fragment ions while the carboxylate-terminal fragments belong to the *z*-type fragment ion series.

The mechanism of peptide fragmentation upon ECD is still a matter of debate [160–162]. In particular, there is a discussion as to whether the ECD process is *nonergodic* (so fast that there is no internal equilibration of energy prior to dissociation) [153, 155] or ergodic (following QET) [162].

Annotating a H shift
Peptide fragments formed after transfer of a hydrogen (atom) are marked by a prime after the letter, e.g., the fragments from ECD are c' and z' ions [160].

9.14 Tandem MS with FT-ICR Instruments – Part II

As obvious from the preceding pages, both IRMPD and ECD are intimately connected with FT-ICR instrumentation. Now having considered these methods for ion activation in some detail we may focus our attention on their practical realization on the FT-ICR platform and some illustrative applications.

9.14.1 IRMPD in FT-ICR-MS

In contrast to CID conditions, the absence of a collision gas maintains the ultra-high vacuum inside the ICR cell, and thus, avoids time-consuming pump delays in the sequence of an experiment. The ultra-high vacuum environment also cancels collisional cooling as observed in QITs or LITs (Sect. 9.12.1). IRMPD was optionally available on the Bruker Apex series of FT-ICR instruments, while it has been abandoned on the more recent Solarix series, seemingly for safety of operation. Thermo LTQ-FT and LTQ-FT Ultra FT-ICR instruments still are optionally equipped with IRMPD.

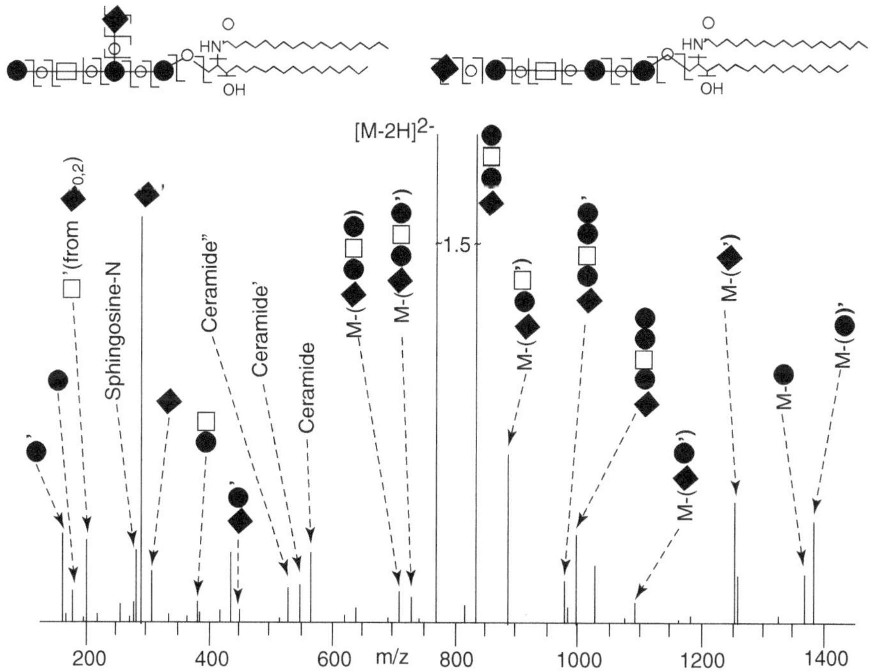

Fig. 9.38 IRMPD (200 ms, 14 W, 100 scans) spectrum of doubly deprotonated ganglioside GM1, $[M–2H]^{2–}$, occurring in two isomeric forms (Reproduced from Ref. [163] with permission. © Elsevier Science Publishers, 2005)

IRMPD application Gangliosides such as GM1 contain a hydrophobic ceramide moiety that consists of sphingosine, a long-chain amino alcohol, which is acylated with a fatty acid on the amino group. The molecule has a polar oligosaccharide head that contains sialic acid. GM1 exists as two isomeric forms, GM1a and GM1b, differing in that the sialic acid is in branched or terminal position, respectively. The negative-ion IRMPD (200 ms, 14 W, 100 scans) spectrum of doubly deprotonated ganglioside GM1, $[M–2H]^{2–}$, exhibits a cleavage within the ceramide moiety that causes loss of the fatty acid. The presence of GM1b as a minor component is evident from (*i*) the fragment ion peak at *m*/*z* 1091.722, which corresponds to a loss of the disaccharide HexNeuAc' from the precursor and (*ii*) its complementary peak at *m*/*z* 452.141 due to the disaccharide (Fig. 9.38) [163].

9.14.2 Infrared Photodissociation Spectroscopy

Provided a tunable laser light source is available, the IRMPD experiment can be performed in a wavelength-dependent manner to reveal the absorption characteristics of gaseous ions. Different from IR spectroscopy of condensed

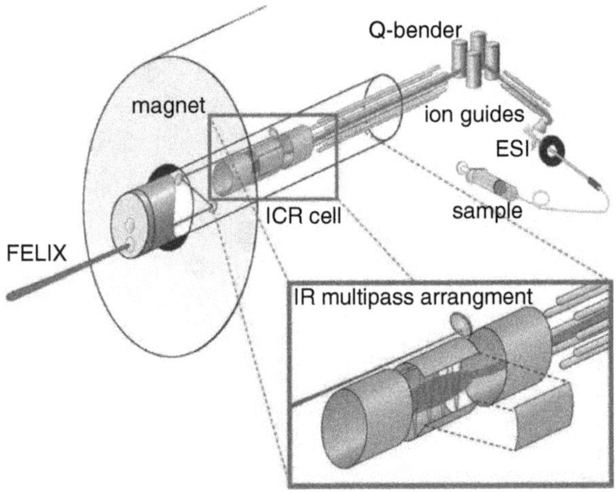

Fig. 9.39 Setup for infrared photodissociation spectroscopy. In this particular setup (FELIX at Utrecht, Netherlands) the light from a free-electron laser is guided into an open cylindrical ICR cell in a way that the IR light undergoes multiple reflections on the inner surfaces to extend its path for absorption by the ions inside the cell (Reproduced from Ref. [144] with permission. © John Wiley Periodicals, Inc., 2009)

phase samples, in mass spectrometry the occurrence of IR absorption is observed by detection of specific fragment ions and their abundances as a function of laser wavelength. This technique is known as *infrared photodissociation spectroscopy* (IRPD) [144, 164].

Unfortunately, powerful IR lasers tunable over a significant frequency range are difficult to obtain. Currently, the most effective but highly demanding approach to this end is represented by the *free-electron laser* (FEL). FEL facilities are limited and offer access for researchers to perform their experiments at dedicated ports on a tight schedule (Fig. 9.39). Alternatively, *optical parametric oscillator/amplifiers* (OPO/As) can serve as tunable IR light sources [144, 164].

9.14.3 Blackbody Infrared Radiative Dissociation

Even under essentially perfect vacuum where collisional activation is virtually absent ($<10^{-9}$ mbar) ions can undergo slow unimolecular dissociation. As the energy for these fragmentations is provided by the emission of infrared photons by blackbody radiation of the vacuum housing, this process is termed *blackbody infrared radiative dissociation* (BIRD) [165]. Blackbody infrared radiation is always present above non-zero temperatures. BIRD dissociations are characterized by reaction times in the order of several seconds to even minutes. Therefore, ICR cells provide the most suitable environment for their study. To vary the wavelength and intensity of IR radiation both the ICR cell and the surrounding vacuum manifold have to be uniformly heated. Typically, temperatures up to about 250 °C can be reached in dedicated instruments. This allows to study reaction kinetics where bonds of low to moderate strength are involved [165].

BIRD is quite exotic
Routine FT-ICR instruments are not suited for BIRD studies because of restrictions in heat resistance of electronic circuitry in proximity to the ICR cell and complications with the superconducting cryomagnet. BIRD requires wide-bore magnets (160 mm) that can accommodate the heated ICR cell housing plus a water-cooled mantle around it to prevent dissipation of heat to the magnet.

9.14.4 ECD for Tandem FT-ICR-MS

The implementation of ECD on ICR cells is nicely compatible with IRMPD. One approach is to use a hollow cathode [166] instead of a filament to deliver electrons for ECD. The hollow cathode also offers a wide electron beam that enlarges the volume where ECD can occur within the ICR cell. The IR laser then may pass through the central hole – a setup that exerts some restrictions to the ICR radii where ions can interact with the laser beam. Several cathode designs are in use (Figs. 9.40 and 9.41) [167].

ECD to locate postranslational peptide modifications The direct bond cleavages upon ECD can be used to locate postranslational peptide modifications that would be disguised in CID or IRMPD spectra. The difference between CID and IRMPD on one side and ECD on the other arises from the loss of most posttranslational modifications prior to backbone cleavage to from *b*- and *y*-type ions, while in ECD the chain is immediately cleaved to yield *c*- and *z*-type ions, independent of the peptide sequence [168]. Thus, the neutral loss reflects the mass of the modification, e.g., additional 80 u (HPO_3) in case of the phosphorylation that can be identified to occur at the tyrosine of the peptide RLpYIFSCFR (Fig. 9.42)

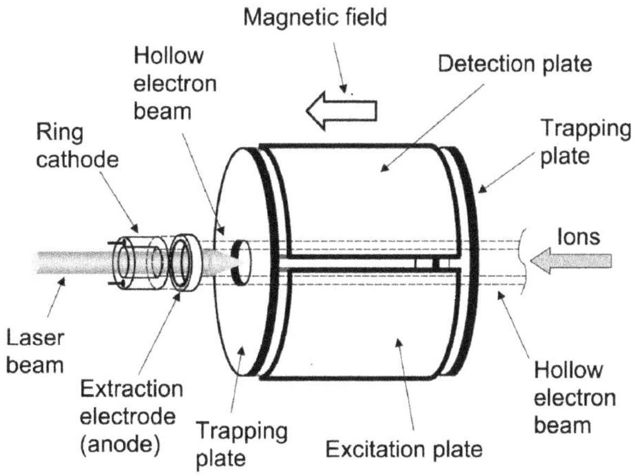

Fig. 9.40 A combined ECD and IRMPD setup for FT-ICR-MS. The IR laser is transmitted into the cell via the central hole of indirectly heated ring dispenser cathode mounted to the rear trapping plate of an ICR cell (Reproduced from Ref. [167] by permission. © John Wiley & Sons, 2003)

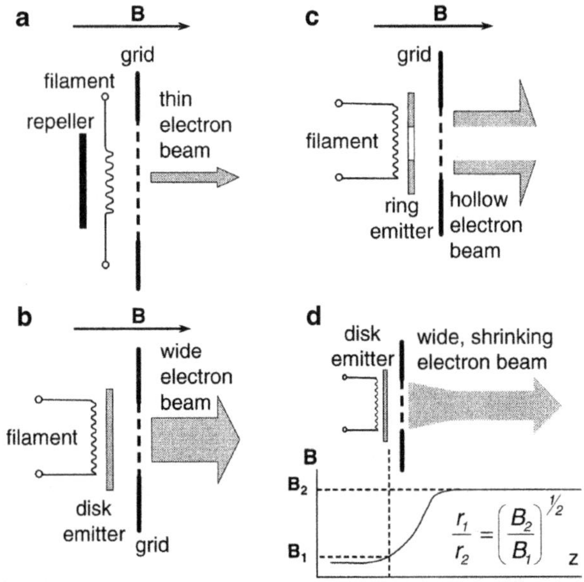

Fig. 9.41 Electron injection systems for ECD-FT-ICR instruments: (**a**) directly heated filament in homogeneous magnetic field, (**b**) disk-shaped indirectly heated cathode in homogeneous magnetic field, (**c**) ring-shaped indirectly heated cathode, and (**d**) cathode in fringing magnetic field region with beam collimation (Reproduced from Ref. [158] with permission. © John Wiley & Sons, Ltd., 2004)

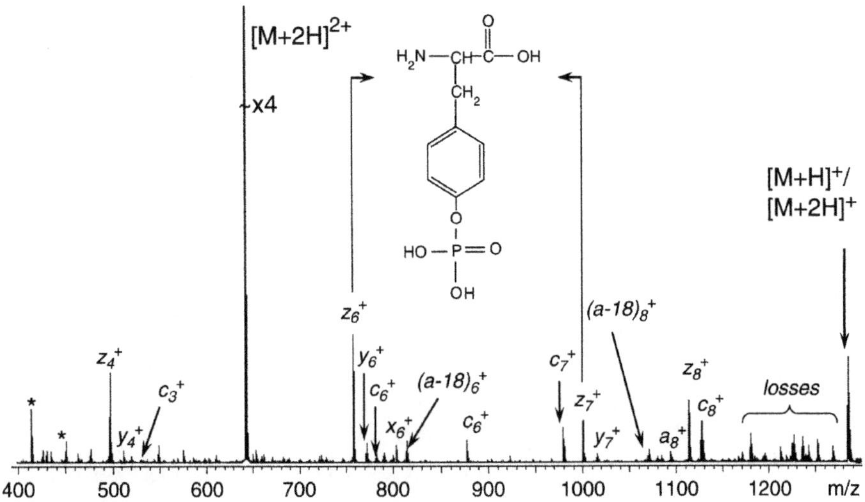

Fig. 9.42 Upon ECD, the $[M+2H]^{2+}$ ion of the peptide RLpYIFSCFR exhibits an increased mass difference of 80 u between its z_6^+ and z_7^+ fragments due to tyrosine phosphorylation (Adapted from Ref. [158] with permission. © John Wiley & Sons, Ltd., 2004)

[158]. The opportunity to obtain complementary peptide sequence information is the reason why CID or IRMPD spectra are sometimes combined with ECD spectra for structure elucidation of peptides [141, 157, 169].

9.15 Electron Transfer Dissociation

ECD can only take place in the ultra-high vacuum of FT-ICR mass spectrometers, while it is not possible to simultaneously store thermal electrons and peptide cations in quadrupole ion traps that utilize RF fields for ion manipulation and trapping. Furthermore, thermal electrons absorb energy from the RF field within milliseconds to become energetic. On the other hand, LITs can be operated as to store oppositely charged ions. Attempts for applying the advantages of ECD to LITs therefore make use of electron transfer via cation–anion reactions. In contrast to ECD, electron transfer may then occur at relatively high pressures ($\approx 10^{-3}$ mbar) [170]. This technique is termed *electron-transfer dissociation* (ETD) [168].

Anthracene radical anions as obtained by electron capture in a chemical ionization source with methane reagent gas were formerly employed as anions [168, 171]. Meanwhile, fluoranthene has become more widely used (Scheme 9.2) [172, 173].

Thus, ETD lends the capabilities of ECD to linear ion trap mass spectrometers. The individual steps involved in the operation of an LTQ instrument in ETD mode (Fig. 9.43) are: injection of multiply protonated peptides as delivered by an ESI source; application of a DC offset to store these ions in the front section of the LIT followed by injection of reagent anions from the CI source into the center of the LIT. Then all but the peptide precursor ions and the electron-donor reagent ions are ejected. Next the DC potential well is switched off and a secondary RF voltage is applied to the end lens plates of the LIT causing positive and negative ion populations to mix and react. The reaction period is ended by axial ejection of reagent anions while positive product ions are retained in the center section of the LIT. Finally, mass-selective radial ejection as usual yields the ETD spectrum

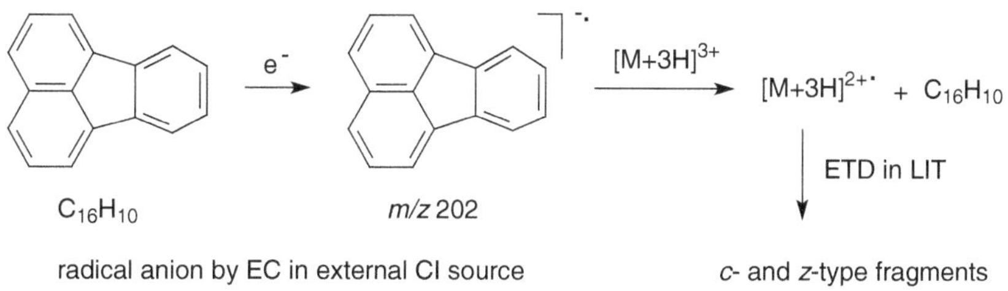

Scheme 9.2

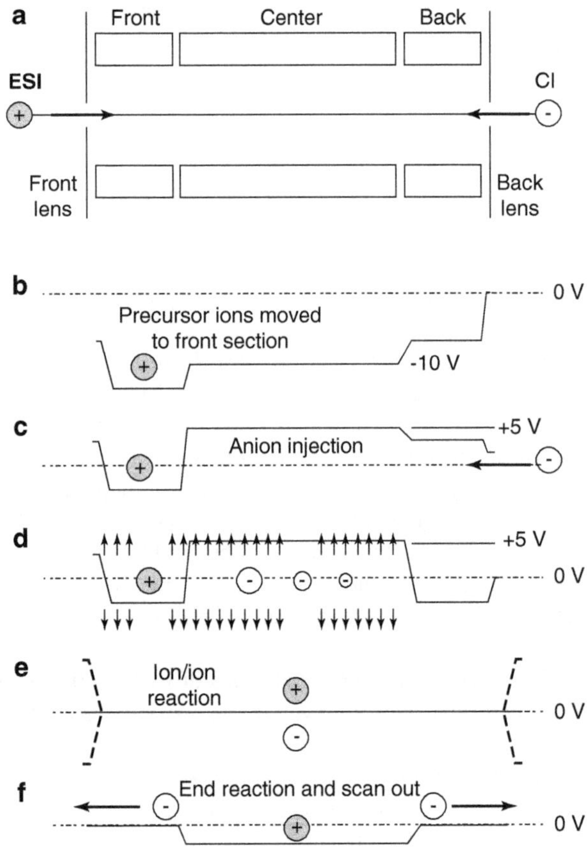

Fig. 9.43 Sequence of events to trap both positive peptide ions and reagent anions in a LIT, to react them, and to obtain an ETD spectrum showing the product ions. (**a**) Setup of the segmented LIT for ETD, (**b**) trapping of precursor ions in the front section, (**c**) admitting negative reagent ions, (**d**) anion storage in the center, (**e**) ETD reaction, and (**f**) scan for product ions (Reproduced from Ref. [168] with permission. © The National Academy of Sciences of the USA, 2004)

[168]. The attractive ETD technique has also been implemented on LITs with axial ejection [151, 174] and on LIT-Orbitrap hybrids [175–177].

Unfortunately, ETD has limited applicability to doubly protonated peptide precursor ions, $[M+2H]^{2+}$, while triply protonated ions fragment to reveal the full sequence due to the higher exothermicity of the electron capture (Fig. 9.44) [170].

9.16 Electron Detachment Dissociation

Both ECD and ETD cause direct backbone cleavages in multiply positive peptide ions to deliver *c*- and *z*-type fragments which are highly informative for mass spectral sequencing. Especially when occurring more than once on a molecule, post-translational modifications like phosphorylation or sulfonation, reduce its tendency to form multiply protonated ions. Such analytes are best studied as negative ions, which are of course not amenable to ECD [178]. If the primary

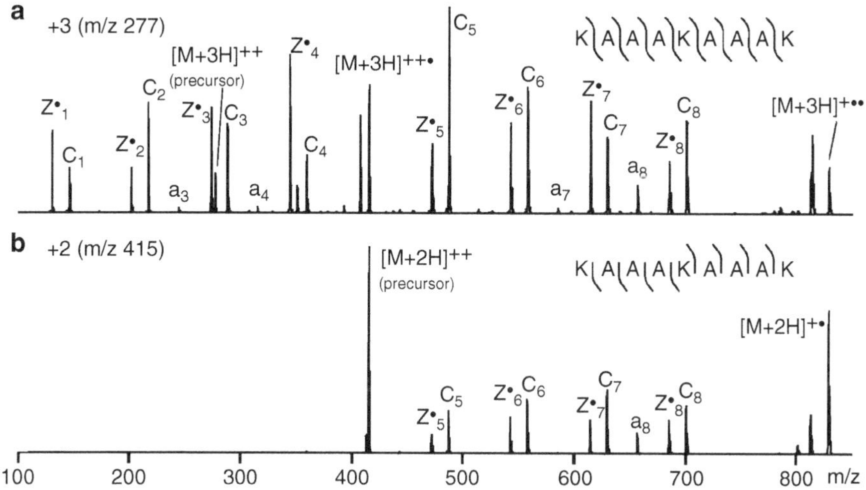

Fig. 9.44 Effect of precursor ion charge state on ETD product ion spectra of (**a**) the triply protonated peptide ion $[KAAAKAAAK+H]^{3+}$ and (**b**) the doubly protonated ion of the same peptide which only produces half of the possible *c*- and *z*-type fragments (Reproduced from Ref. [170] with permission. © American Chemical Society, 2007)

electrons are energetic (about 20 eV) rather than thermal, there is a substantial chance to promote *electron detachment* from the anion [179]. In fact, the overall process can be regarded as electron ionization of an anion, which leads+ to formation of a neutral radical site (Sect. 6.3.1).

$$[M - nH]^{n-} + e^{-} \rightarrow [M - nH]^{(n-1)-\bullet} + 2e^{-} \qquad (9.22)$$

Alternatively, electron ionization can occur anywhere along a polypeptide chain to locally form a positive radical ion that also may be regarded as an electron hole. This will attract an excess electron from one of the anionic sites of the ion and end up in mutual neutralization. The released energy effects electronic excitation, that, in turn, causes backbone cleavage [179]. This technique is termed *electron detachment dissociation* (EDD, Scheme 9.3) [178–181].

EDD is not only useful for acidic peptides but also for oligonucleotides [182] and other analytes [160]. EDD has also been adapted to QITs [180]. Nonetheless, EDD is clearly less relevant in bioanalytical work than ECD or ETD.

A variation of EDD, termed *negative electron transfer dissociation* (NETD) employs fluoranthene, $C_{16}H_{10}^{+\bullet}$, or $Xe^{+\bullet}$ ions instead of energetic electrons to induce radical cationic sites by charge transfer rather than by electron ionization [183]. NETD yields selective backbone cleavage at the C_α–C bonds, similar to EDD, but leaves the phosphorylation sites intact, thereby enabling the localization of posttranslational modifications (PTMs).

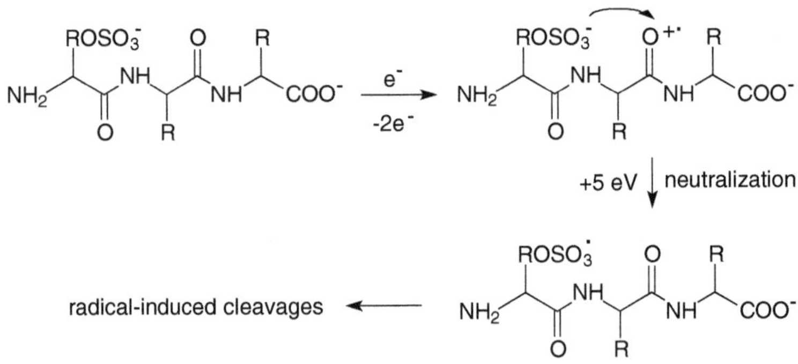

Scheme 9.3

9.17 Special Applications of Tandem MS

Bimolecular reactions may take place when gaseous ions collide with neutrals at *thermal energy* rather than at multi- or even kiloelectronvolt energy. Proton transfer is one of the prominent representatives of an *ion–molecule reaction* in the gas phase. It is employed for the determination of *GB*s and *PA*s as described below. More sophisticated studies are enabled by reactions of gaseous ions with more complex reagents in the gas phase and the immediate mass spectral analysis of the reaction products [3].

9.17.1 Ion–Molecule Reactions in Catalytic Studies

The catalytic activities of a large pool of transition-metal carbene complexes have been screened by means of ion–molecule reactions in tandem-MS experiments [184–186]. Reactions of bare or solvated metal ions with organic molecules have been studied using mass spectrometers as reaction vessels [187–190]. In contrast to the concepts and methods discussed so far, the latter experiments are not designed to study the fundamentals of mass spectrometry. Instead, sophisticated methods of modern mass spectrometry are now employed to reveal the secrets of other complex chemical systems.

Activation of methane Reaction of mass-selected $[Ni(H)(OH)]^+$ ions, *m/z* 76, with methane at 0 eV collision energy in the laboratory frame of reference yields a CH_2 insertion product, $[Ni(CH_3)(OH)]^+$, *m/z* 90. The experiments were carried out by using a QhQ mass spectrometer with an electrospray ion source. $[NiL]^+$ reactand ions were produced by ESI from solutions of NiL_2 (L = F, Cl, Br, I) in pure methanol and $[NiOH]^+$ ions from NiI_2 in H_2O. For the methane-activation study, the ions containing ^{58}Ni were mass selected in Q1 and reacted at thermal

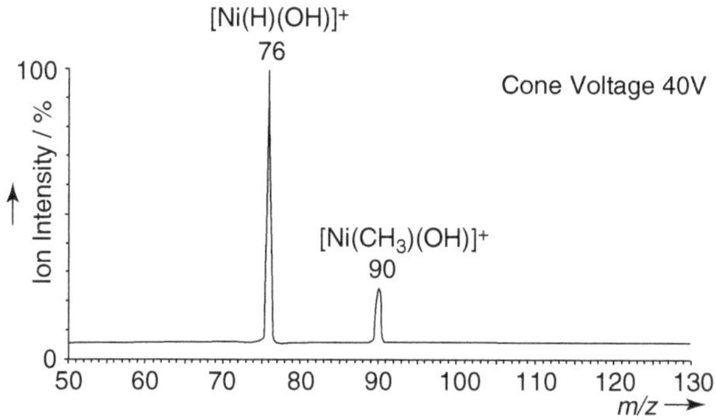

Fig. 9.45 Reaction of mass-selected $[Ni(H)(OH)]^+$ ions, *m/z* 76, with methane at 0 eV collision energy in the laboratory frame of reference yields a CH_2 insertion product, *m/z* 90. The cone voltage refers to the ESI conditions to produce optimum precursor ion abundance from Ni salt solutions (Reproduced from Ref. [190] with permission. © Wiley-VCH Verlag, Weinheim, 2007)

energy with methane in the RF-only hexapole at about 10^{-4} mbar. The ionic products were then detected by Q2 (Fig. 9.45) [190].

9.17.2 Gas Phase Hydrogen–Deuterium Exchange

Deuterium and other isotopic labeling prior to mass spectrometric analysis has been known from the early days of mass spectrometry (Sects. 2.9 and 3.3). Modern methodology even allows labeling of gaseous ions, thereby yielding insight into mechanistic details of reactions in a much more convenient way than by complicated synthetic routes. Furthermore, the gas phase exchange of hydrogen for deuterium can be applied to transient species that would otherwise remain inaccessible. So *hydrogen–deuterium exchange* (HDX) can be accomplished not only in solution (Chaps. 6 and 7 in [191]), e.g., prior to analysis by electrospray ionization, but also in the gas phase. This is best achieved on ion traps of any kind as these provide extended and easily variable reaction times – circumstances that also enable kinetic studies.

HDX in peptide fragmentation Gas phase HDX has been used to probe complete parent and fragment ion populations generated by CID of multiply charged protonated peptides [192]. The peptide ions were monoisotopically selected, dissociated by SORI-CID, and then subjected to HDX by repeated pulsed admission of CD_3OD to the ICR cell. Finally, the products were analyzed by FT-ICR-MS. HDX for variable reaction times revealed distinguished exchange kinetics for different types of ions, which allowed to deduce information on their structures. For example, *b*-type ions exhibited fast HDX while *a*-type ions showed only restricted exchange even at longer reaction times (Fig. 9.46) [192, 193]. The

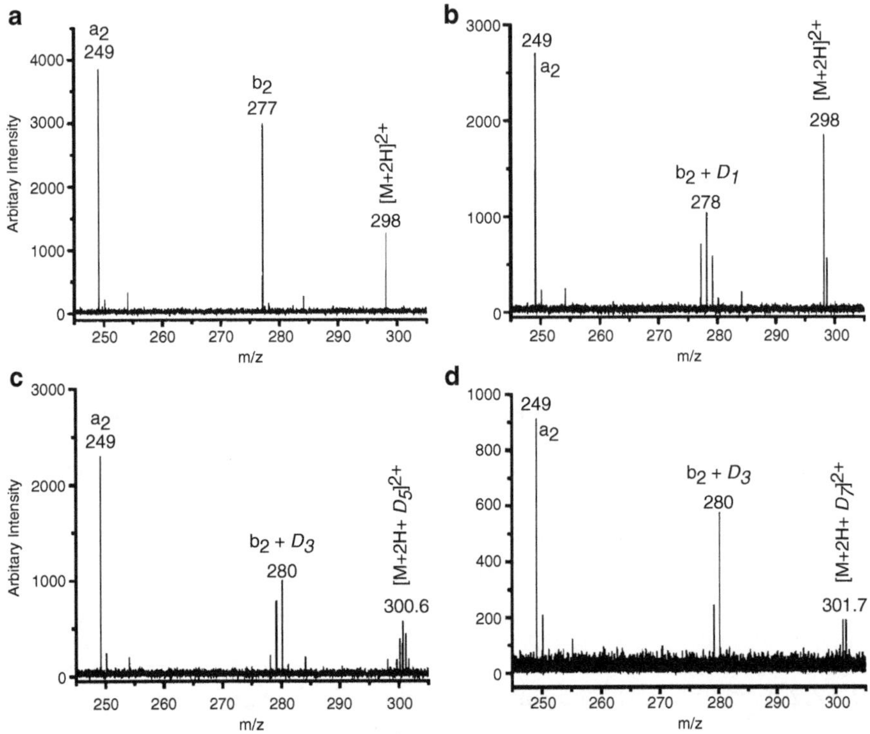

Fig. 9.46 The a_2-b_2 region of the product ion spectrum of doubly protonated YIGSR after (**a**) 0 s, (**b**) 1 s, (**c**) 10 s, and (**d**) 60 s gas phase HDX in an ICR cell. The uptake of deuterium is denoted by D_n in the formulas (Reproduced from Ref. [193] with permission. © Elsevier Science Publishers, 2009).

observed exchange behavior was used to argue in favor of a oxazolone structure of the b_2 ions.

9.17.3 Determination of Gas Phase Basicities and Proton Affinities

The methods for the determination of *GB*s and *PA*s (Sect. 2.12) make use of their relation to K_{eq} (Eq. 9.23) and the shift of K_{eq} upon change of $[AH]^+$ or B, respectively [194, 195]. Basically, the value of *GB* or *PA* is bracketed by measuring K_{eq} with a series of several reference bases ranging from lower to higher *GB* than the unknown. There are two methods we should address in brief, a detailed treatment of the topic being beyond the scope of the present book, however. The *kinetic method* makes use of the dissociation of proton-bound heterodimers, and the *thermokinetic method* determines the equilibrium constant of the acid-base reaction of gaseous ions. In general, proton transfer plays a crucial role in the formation of protonated molecules, e.g., in positive-ion chemical ionization mass spectrometry (Chap. 7).

The *kinetic method* [196–199] compares the relative rates of the competitive dissociations of a proton-bound adduct $[A–H–B]^+$ formed by admitting a mixture of A and B to a CI ion source [196, 197]. There, the proton-bound adduct $[A–H–B]^+$ is generated amongst other products such as $[AH]^+$ and $[BH]^+$. Using standard tandem MS techniques, e.g., MIKES, the cluster ion $[A–H–B_{ref}]^+$ is selected and allowed to undergo metastable decomposition:

$$[AH]^+ + B_{ref} \leftarrow [A - H - B_{ref}]^+ \rightarrow A + [B_{ref}H]^+ \tag{9.23}$$

The relative intensities of the products $[AH]^+$ and $[B_{ref}H]^+$ are then used as a measure of relative rate constants of the competing reactions. In case the *PA* of the unknown was equal to that of the reference, both peaks would be of equal intensity. As this will almost never be the case, a series of reference bases is employed instead, and *PA* is determined by interpolation. The value of $PA_{(A)}$ is obtained from a plot of $\ln[AH]^+/[B_{ref}H]^+$ versus $PA_{(B)}$ at $\ln[AH]^+/[B_{ref}H]^+ = 0$.

The *thermokinetic method* [200, 201] uses the measurement of the forward rate constant of the equilibrium

$$[AH]^+ + B_{ref} \rightleftharpoons A + [B_{ref}H]^+ \tag{9.24}$$

The thermokinetic method takes advantage of the correlation observed between k_{exp} and $\Delta G_2{}^0$ through the relationship

$$\frac{k_{exp}}{k_{coll}} = \frac{1}{1 + \exp\left[\left(\Delta G_2^0 + \Delta G_a^0\right)/RT\right]} \tag{9.25}$$

where k_{coll} is the collision rate constant and $\Delta G_a{}^0$ a term close to *RT*. The *GB* of the unknown is then obtained from $\Delta G_2{}^0 = GB - GB_{ref}$. The task to establish a proper value of the reaction efficiency, $R_{eff} = k_{exp}/k_{coll}$, is solved by plotting the experimental values of R_{eff} versus $GB_{(B)}$ and interpolating these points with a parametric function. Although this can be done with high accuracy, it is still a matter of debate as to which value of R_{eff} yields the most realistic *GB*, suggestions being $R_{eff} =$ 0.1–0.5 [194].

Determination of *GB* and *PA* *GB* and *PA* of cyclohexanecarboxamide were determined by both experimental methods. The kinetic method based on both metastable dissociation and CID yielded $GB = 862 \pm 7$ kJ mol^{-1} and $PA = 896 \pm$ 5 kJ mol^{-1}, while the thermokinetic method gave $GB = 860 \pm 5$ kJ mol^{-1} and $PA =$ 891 ± 5 kJ mol^{-1}, i.e., both methods yield comparable results (Fig. 9.47).

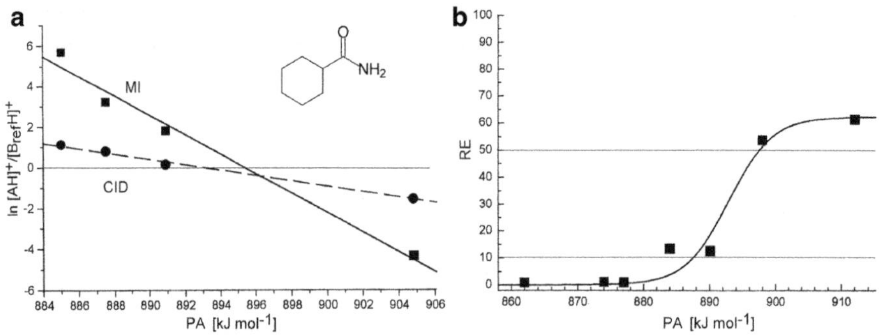

Fig. 9.47 Determination of the proton affinity of cyclohexanecarboxamide (**a**) by the kinetic method, and (**b**) by the thermokinetic method. The *horizontal lines* show the indicative values ln $[AH]^+/[B_{ref}H]^+ = 0$ in (**a**) and *RE*s according to different authors in (**b**) [194] (Adapted from Ref. [202] by permission. © IM Publications, 2003)

9.17.4 Neutralization-Reionization Mass Spectrometry

In CID, charge exchange between the ions and the collision gas is an unwanted side reaction. However, it may become useful when employed in combination with a subsequent reionization step as in *neutralization-reionization mass spectrometry* (NR-MS) [203–211]. In NR-MS, the precursor ion of some kiloelectronvolts of kinetic energy is mass-selected in MS1 and passed through a first collision cell containing a reducing collision gas. A certain fraction of these ions will be reduced by charge exchange to become neutrals. As these neutrals basically retain their initial kinetic energy and direction, they leave the first collision cell along with the precursor ion beam. Remaining ions can then be removed from the beam by electrostatic deflection. Having traveled for some microseconds along a short path through the field-free region, the neutrals are subjected to ionizing collisions in a second collision cell. Finally, the mass spectrum of the reionized species is detected by means of MS2.

For neutralization one can employ:

- noble gases of low *IE* such as Xe (12.1 eV) [205],
- metal vapors effusing from an oven, e.g., Hg (10.4 eV), Zn (9.3 eV), and Cd (9.0 eV) [203, 212],
- volatile organic molecules, e.g., benzene (9.2 eV) or triphenylamine (6.8 eV) [213].

Reionization of the neutrals in the second collision cell can be achieved using:

- O_2 (12.1 eV) or He (24.6 eV) [212, 213],
- ionization methods such as electron ionization or field ionization [207].

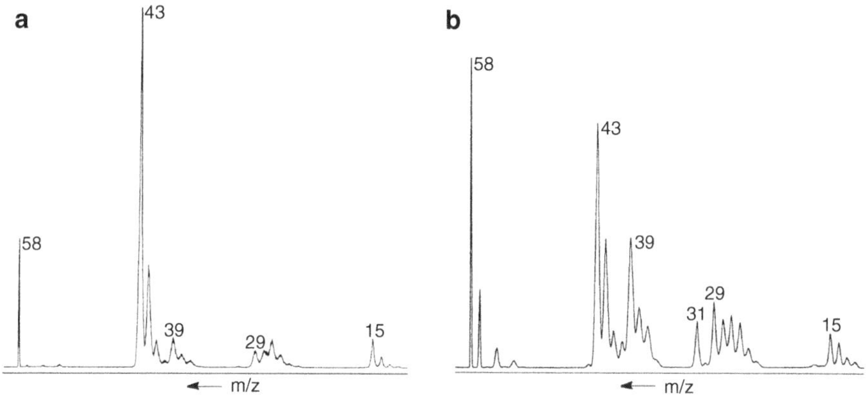

Fig. 9.48 NR-MS (Xe–He) of acetone (**a**) and its enol (**b**) from neutralization of the corresponding ions (Adapted from Ref. [205] with permission. © Elsevier Science, 1985)

NR-MS is applied in numerous ways [208, 213–215]. In particular, NR-MS is a powerful tool where the existence of short-lived and otherwise unstable species has to be proven [216–218].

NR-MS of acetone The NR mass spectrum of acetone closely resembles its 70-eV EI mass spectrum (Sect. 6.2.1), thereby demonstrating that the molecular ion basically retains the structure of the neutral (Fig. 9.48) [205]. However, the isomeric $C_3H_6O^{+\bullet}$ ions formed by McLafferty rearrangement of 2-hexanone molecular ion are expected to have enol structure (Sect. 6.8.1), and thus the corresponding NR mass spectrum is easily distinguished from that of acetone.

9.18 Tandem Mass Spectrometry Condensed

Terminology in Tandem Mass Spectrometry

The terms *tandem mass spectrometry*, also *mass spectrometry/mass spectrometry*, collectively describes mass spectrometric experiments where ions that are mass-analyzed in MS1 are subjected to fragmentations or ion–molecule reactions and the products thereof are collected and analyzed by a second stage, MS2. Tandem MS is often abbreviated as MS/MS or MS^2. Tandem MS experiments of higher order are referred to as MS^3, MS^4, ... or generally as MS^n.
Ions emerging from MS1 are termed *precursor ions*, those entering MS2 are called *product ions*; in higher-order experiments, one may refer to them as n^{th} generation product ions.

Mass Analyzers for Tandem MS

A tandem mass spectrometer can either be composed of – mostly independent – mass analyzers in serial connection or can be achieved by operating the same analyzer to sequentially perform the stages of the tandem MS experiment. The first mode of tandem MS is described as *tandem MS in space*, the second as *tandem MS in time*. Beam instruments (BE, EB, QqQ, ReTOF, QqTOF, TOF/TOF) provide tandem MS in space, ion trap analyzers (QIT, LIT, FT-ICR) yield tandem MS in time. Orbitraps cannot be operated in a tandem MS mode; they exclusively serve as MS2 to analyze fragment ions delivered by a Q- or LIT-type MS1.

Ion Activation Techniques

Ideally, a single all-purpose ion activation method would suffice to generate fragment ions for structure elucidation of any compound class. Moreover, the charge state of the precursor ion, its mass, and other characteristics would not interfere. In reality, however, no such method exists [170]. In case of peptides, for example, there is no single successful activation technique for delivering a sufficient number of sequence-informative product ions for sequence identification; instead, the amino acid composition and posttranslational modifications exhibit a strong influence on the fragmentation pattern – justifying all the previous methods. Commonly available ion activation techniques are summarized and briefly described in Table 9.4 [31, 219].

Table 9.4 Common ion activation techniques for tandem MS

Method	Instrumental platforms	Ionic charge and species accessible	Description and properties
CID	BE, ReTOF, TOF-TOF	+/– Precursor and fragments	Collisions at keV-energies with inert gas. Several eV energy transfer in single collision within a femtosecond
	QqQ, QqTOF, QqLIT, etc.	+/– Precursor and fragments	Tens of eV-collisions with inert gas About eV energy transfer per collision; several events within about a millisecond
	FT-ICR	+/– Selected precursor only	Several eV-collisions with inert gas; about eV energy transfer per collision; several events within a second.
SID	QqQ, IMS-QqTOF etc.	+/– Selected precursor only	Single collision at several tens of eV with inert surface within some picoseconds
IRMPD	FT-ICR (QIT)	+/– Precursor and fragments	Rather low-energy activation by IR laser; compatible with ECD
BIRD	FT-ICR	+/– Precursor and fragments	Slow, low-energy activation by IR blackbody radiation close to equilibrium; to study kinetics and thermodynamics
ECD	FT-ICR	Multiply + Precursor and fragments	Energy from partial neutralization by thermal electrons; extremely fast process causes radical ion cleavages
ETD	LIT and hybrids with LIT	Multiply + Precursor and fragments	Energy from partial neutralization transferred by cation–anion reaction; result similar to ECD
EDD	FT-ICR	Multiply – Precursor and fragments	Energy from partial neutralization delivered by electron detachment; results like "ECD for anions"

Applications

Tandem MS was initially developed as a tool for gas phase ion chemistry to track dissociation pathways and to determine thermodynamic properties of gaseous ions. Then, structure elucidation started to also play a role in analytical mass spectrometry. Step by step, tandem MS instruments were constructed and modes of operation were developed that allowed to use almost any type of mass analyzer.

The tremendous commercial success of all sorts of hybrid instruments is due to their effectivity in tandem MS. Today, tandem MS has a plethora of applications, mostly in biomolecule sequencing and in trace analysis to increase selectivity for the detection and eventually quantification of target compounds (Sects. 14.2 and 14.3).

References

1. McLafferty FW (ed) (1983) Tandem Mass Spectrometry. John Wiley & Sons, New York
2. Busch KL, Glish GL, McLuckey SA (1988) Mass Spectrometry/Mass Spectrometry. Wiley VCH, New York
3. Schalley CA, Springer A (2009) Mass Spectrometry and Gas-Phase Chemistry of Non-Covalent Complexes. John Wiley & Sons, Hoboken
4. Murray KK, Boyd RK, Eberlin MN, Langley GJ, Li L, Naito Y (2013) Definitions of Terms Relating to Mass Spectrometry (IUPAC Recommendations 2013). Pure Appl Chem 85:1515–1609. doi:10.1351/PAC-REC-06-04-06
5. Johnson JV, Yost RA, Kelley PE, Bradford DC (1990) Tandem-in-Space and Tandem-in-Time Mass Spectrometry: Triple Quadrupoles and Quadrupole Ion Traps. Anal Chem 62:2162–2172. doi:10.1021/ac00219a003
6. Kaufmann R, Kirsch D, Spengler B (1994) Sequencing of Peptides in a Time-of-Flight Mass Spectrometer: Evaluation of Postsource Decay Following Matrix-Assisted Laser Desorption Ionization (MALDI). Int J Mass Spectrom Ion Proc 131:355–385. doi:10.1016/0168-1176(93)03876-N
7. Glish GL (1994) Multiple Stage Mass Spectrometry: The Next Generation Tandem Mass Spectrometry Experiment. Analyst 119:533–537. doi:10.1039/AN9941900533
8. Glish G (1991) Letter to the Editor [Concerning Terms in Mass Spectrometry]. J Am Soc Mass Spectrom 2:349. doi:10.1016/1044-0305(91)80026-4
9. Thorne GC, Ballard KD, Gaskell SJ (1990) Metastable Decomposition of Peptide $[M+H]^+$ Ions via Rearrangement Involving Loss of C-Terminal Amino Acid Residue. J Am Soc Mass Spectrom 1:249–257. doi:10.1016/1044-0305(90)85042-K
10. Louris JN, Wright LG, Cooks RG, Schoen AE (1985) New Scan Modes Accessed with a Hybrid Mass Spectrometer. Anal Chem 57:2918–2924. doi:10.1021/ac00291a039
11. Glish GL, Burinsky DJ (2008) Hybrid Mass Spectrometers for Tandem Mass Spectrometry. J Am Soc Mass Spectrom 19:161–172. doi:10.1016/j.jasms.2007.11.013
12. Lehmann WD (1997) Pictograms for Experimental Parameters in Mass Spectrometry. J Am Soc Mass Spectrom 8:756–759. doi:10.1016/S1044-0305(97)00028-7
13. Cooks RG, Beynon JH, Caprioli RM (1973) Metastable Ions. Elsevier, Amsterdam
14. Levsen K (1978) Fundamental Aspects of Organic Mass Spectrometry. Weinheim, Verlag Chemie
15. McLafferty FW, Bente PFI, Kornfeld R, Tsai SC, Howe I (1973) Collisional Activation Spectra of Organic Ions. J Am Chem Soc 95:2120–2129. doi:10.1021/ja00788a007
16. Levsen K, Schwarz H (1976) Collisional Activation Mass Spectrometry – A New Probe for Structure Determination of Ions in the Gaseous Phase. Angew Chem 88:589–601. doi:10.1002/ange.19760881802

17. Holmes JL (1985) Assigning Structures to Ions in the Gas Phase. Org Mass Spectrom 20:169–183. doi:10.1002/oms.1210200302
18. Levsen K, Schwarz H (1983) Gas-Phase Chemistry of Collisionally Activated Ions. Mass Spectrom Rev 2:77–148. doi:10.1002/mas.1280020104
19. Bordas-Nagy J, Jennings KR (1990) Collision-Induced Decomposition of Ions. Int J Mass Spectrom Ion Proc 100:105–131. doi:10.1016/0168-1176(90)85071-9
20. McLuckey SA (1992) Principles of Collisional Activation in Analytical Mass Spectrometry. J Am Soc Mass Spectrom 3:599–614. doi:10.1016/1044-0305(92)85001-Z
21. Shukla AK, Futrell JH (2000) Tandem Mass Spectrometry: Dissociation of Ions by Collisional Activation. J Mass Spectrom 35:1069–1090. doi:10.1002/1096-9888(200009)35:9<1069::AID-JMS54>3.0.CO;2-C
22. Guevremont R, Boyd RK (1988) Are Derrick Shifts Real? An Investigation by Tandem Mass Spectrometry. Rapid Commun Mass Spectrom 2:1–5. doi:10.1002/rcm.1290020102
23. Bradley CD, Derrick PJ (1991) Collision-Induced Decomposition of Peptides. An Investigation into the Effect of Collision Gas Pressure on Translational Energy Losses. Org Mass Spectrom 26:395–401. doi:10.1002/oms.1210260507
24. Bradley CD, Derrick PJ (1993) Collision-Induced Decomposition of Large Organic Ions and Inorganic Cluster Ions. Effects of Pressure on Energy Losses. Org Mass Spectrom 28:390–394. doi:10.1002/oms.1210280421
25. Neumann GM, Sheil MM, Derrick PJ (1984) Collision-Induced Decomposition of Multiatomic Ions. Z Naturforsch A 39:584–592. doi:10.1515/zna-1984-0612
26. Alexander AJ, Thibault P, Boyd RK (1990) Target Gas Excitation in Collision-Induced Dissociation: A Reinvestigation of Energy Loss in Collisional Activation of Molecular Ions of Chlorophyll-a. J Am Chem Soc 112:2484–2491. doi:10.1021/ja00163a003
27. Kim BJ, Kim MS (1990) Peak Shape Analysis for Collisionally Activated Dissociation in Mass-Analyzed Ion Kinetic Energy Spectrometry. Int J Mass Spectrom Ion Proc 98:193–207. doi:10.1016/0168-1176(90)80001-J
28. Vékey K, Czira G (1993) Large Translational Energy Loss and Scattering in Collision-Induced Dissociation Processes. Org Mass Spectrom 28:546–551. doi:10.1002/oms.1210280513
29. Wysocki VH, Kenttämaa H, Cooks RG (1987) Internal Energy Distributions of Isolated Ions After Activation by Various Methods. Int J Mass Spectrom Ion Proc 75:181–208. doi:10.1016/0168-1176(87)83054-9
30. Bradley CD, Curtis JM, Derrick PJ, Wright B (1992) Tandem Mass Spectrometry of Peptides Using a Magnetic Sector/Quadrupole Hybrid-the Case for Higher Collision Energy and Higher Radio-Frequency Power. Anal Chem 64:2628–2635. doi:10.1021/ac00045a028
31. McLuckey SA, Goeringer DE (1997) Slow Heating Methods in Tandem Mass Spectrometry. J Mass Spectrom 32:461–474. doi:10.1002/(SICI)1096-9888(199705)32:5<461::AID-JMS515>3.0.CO;2-H
32. Mabud MA, Dekrey MJ, Cooks RG (1985) Surface-Induced Dissociation of Molecular Ions. Int J Mass Spectrom Ion Proc 67:285–294. doi:10.1016/0168-1176(85)83024-X
33. Cooks RG, Hoke SH II, Morand KL, Lammert SA (1992) Mass Spectrometers: Instrumentation. Int J Mass Spectrom Ion Proc 118-119:1–36. doi:10.1016/0168-1176(92)85057-7
34. Bier ME, Amy JW, Cooks RG, Syka JEP, Ceja P, Stafford G (1987) A Tandem Quadrupole Mass Spectrometer for the Study of Surface-Induced Dissociation. Int J Mass Spectrom Ion Proc 77:31–47. doi:10.1016/0168-1176(87)83022-7
35. Wysocki VH, Ding JM, Jones JL, Callahan JH, King FL (1992) Surface-Induced Dissociation in Tandem Quadrupole Mass Spectrometers: a Comparison of Three Designs. J Am Soc Mass Spectrom 3:27–32. doi:10.1016/1044-0305(92)85015-C
36. Lammert SA, Cooks RG (1991) Surface-Induced Dissociation of Molecular Ions in a Quadrupole Ion Trap Mass Spectrometer. J Am Soc Mass Spectrom 2:487–491. doi:10.1016/1044-0305(91)80036-7
37. Beardsley RL, Jones CM, Galhena AS, Wysocki VH (2009) Noncovalent Protein Tetramers and Pentamers with "n" Charges Yield Monomers with n/4 and n/5 Charges. Anal Chem 81:1347–1356. doi:10.1021/ac801883k

38. Laskin J (2004) Energetics and Dynamics of Peptide Fragmentation from Multiple-Collision Activation and Surface-Induced Dissociation Studies. Eur J Mass Spectrom 10:259–267. doi:10.1255/ejms.641
39. Wysocki VH, Joyce KE, Jones CM, Beardsley RL (2008) Surface-Induced Dissociation of Small Molecules, Peptides, and Non-Covalent Protein Complexes. J Am Soc Mass Spectrom 19:190–208. doi:10.1016/j.jasms.2007.11.005
40. Zhou M, Huang C, Wysocki VH (2012) Surface-Induced Dissociation of Ion Mobility-Separated Noncovalent Complexes in a Quadrupole/Time-of-Flight Mass Spectrometer. Anal Chem 84:6016–6023. doi:10.1021/ac300810u
41. Zhou M, Wysocki VH (2014) Surface Induced Dissociation: Dissecting Noncovalent Protein Complexes in the Gas Phase. Acc Chem Res 47:1010–1018. doi:10.1021/ar400223t
42. Brodbelt JS (2016) Ion Activation Methods for Peptides and Proteins. Anal Chem 88:30–51. doi:10.1021/acs.analchem.5b04563
43. Spengler B, Kirsch D, Kaufmann R, Jaeger E (1992) Peptide Sequencing by Matrix-Assisted Laser-Desorption Mass Spectrometry. Rapid Commun Mass Spectrom 6:105–108. doi:10.1002/rcm.1290060207
44. Boesl U, Weinkauf R, Schlag E (1992) Reflectron Time-of-Flight Mass Spectrometry and Laser Excitation for the Analysis of Neutrals, Ionized Molecules and Secondary Fragments. Int J Mass Spectrom Ion Proc 112:121–166. doi:10.1016/0168-1176(92)80001-H
45. Bradbury NE, Nielsen RA (1936) Absolute Values of the Electron Mobility in Hydrogen. Phys Rev 49:388–393. doi:10.1103/PhysRev.49.388
46. Tang X, Ens W, Standing KG, Westmore JB (1988) Daughter Ion Mass Spectra from Cationized Molecules of Small Oligopeptides in a Reflecting Time-of-Flight Mass Spectrometer. Anal Chem 60:1791–1799. doi:10.1021/ac00168a029
47. Tang X, Ens W, Mayer F, Standing KG, Westmore JB (1989) Measurement of Unimolecular Decay in Peptides of Masses Greater Than 1200 Units by a Reflecting Time-of-Flight Mass Spectrometer. Rapid Commun Mass Spectrom 3:443–448. doi:10.1002/rcm.1290031210
48. Schueler B, Beavis R, Ens W, Main DE, Tang X, Standing KG (1989) Unimolecular Decay Measurements of Secondary Ions from Organic Molecules by Time-of-Flight Mass Spectrometry. Int J Mass Spectrom Ion Proc 92:185–194. doi:10.1016/0168-1176(89)83027-7
49. Brunelle A, Della-Negra S, Depauw J, Joret H, LeBeyec Y (1991) Time-of-Flight Mass Spectrometry with a Compact Two-Stage Electrostatic Mirror: Metastable-Ion Studies with High Mass Resolution and Ion Emission from Thick Insulators. Rapid Commun Mass Spectrom 5:40–43. doi:10.1002/rcm.1290050112
50. Cornish TJ, Cotter RJ (1993) A Curved-Field Reflectron for Improved Energy Focusing of Product Ions in Time-of-Flight Mass Spectrometry. Rapid Commun Mass Spectrom 7:1037–1040. doi:10.1002/rcm.1290071114
51. Cornish TJ, Cotter RJ (1994) A Curved Field Reflection Time-of-Flight Mass Spectrometer for the Simultaneous Focusing of Metastable Product Ions. Rapid Commun Mass Spectrom 8:781–785. doi:10.1002/rcm.1290080924
52. Cordero MM, Cornish TJ, Cotter RJ, Lys IA (1995) Sequencing Peptides Without Scanning the Reflectron: Post-Source Decay with a Curved-Field Reflectron Time-of-Flight Spectrometer. Rapid Commun Mass Spectrom 9:1356–1361. doi:10.1002/rcm.1290091407
53. Cotter RJ, Gardner BD, Iltchenko S, English RD (2004) Tandem Time-of-Flight Mass Spectrometry with a Curved Field Reflectron. Anal Chem 76:1976–1981. doi:10.1021/ac0349431
54. Yergey AL, Coorssen JR, Backlund PS, Blank PS, Humphrey GA, Zimmerberg J, Campbell JM, Vestal ML (2002) De Novo Sequencing of Peptides Using MALDI/TOF-TOF. J Am Soc Mass Spectrom 13:784–791. doi:10.1016/S1044-0305(02)00393-8
55. Schnaible V, Wefing S, Resemann A, Suckau D, Bücker A, Wolf-Kümmeth S, Hoffmann D (2002) Screening for Disulfide Bonds in Proteins by MALDI In-Source Decay and LIFT-TOF/TOF-MS. Anal Chem 74:4980–4988. doi:10.1021/ac025807j

56. Suckau D, Resemann A, Schuerenberg M, Hufnagel P, Franzen J, Holle A (2003) A Novel MALDI LIFT-TOF/TOF Mass Spectrometer for Proteomics. Anal Bioanal Chem 376:952–965. doi:10.1007/s00216-003-2057-0
57. Moneti G, Francese S, Mastrobuoni G, Pieraccini G, Seraglia R, Valitutti G, Traldi P (2007) Do Collisions Inside the Collision Cell Play a Relevant Role in CID-LIFT Experiments? J Mass Spectrom 42:117–126. doi:10.1002/jms.1151
58. Hipple JA, Condon EU (1945) Detection of Metastable Ions with the Mass Spectrometer. Phys Rev 68:54–55. doi:10.1103/PhysRev.68.54
59. Hipple JA, Fox RE, Condon EU (1946) Metastable Ions Formed by Electron Impact in Hydrocarbon Gases. Phys Rev 69:347–356. doi:10.1103/PhysRev.69.347
60. Beynon JH, Saunders RA, Williams AE (1965) Formation of Metastable Ions in Mass Spectrometers with Release of Internal Energy. Z Naturforsch A 20:180–183. doi:10.1515/zna-1965-0203
61. Beynon JH, Cooks RG, Amy JW, Baitinger WE, Ridley TY (1973) Design and Performance of a Mass-Analyzed Ion Kinetic Energy (MIKE) Spectrometer. Anal Chem 45:1023A–1031A. doi:10.1021/ac60334a763
62. Amy JW, Baitinger WE, Cooks RG (1990) Building Mass Spectrometers and a Philosophy of Research. J Am Soc Mass Spectrom 1:119–128. doi:10.1016/1044-0305(90)85047-P
63. Ottinger C (1965) Fragmentation Energies of Metastable Organic Ions. Phys Lett 17:269–271. doi:10.1016/0031-9163(65)90526-3
64. Baldwin MA, Derrick PJ, Morgan RP (1976) Correction of Metastable Peak Shapes to Allow for Instrumental Broadening and the Translational Energy Spread of the Parent Ion. Org Mass Spectrom 11:440–442. doi:10.1002/oms.1210110418
65. Gross JH, Veith HJ (1993) Unimolecular Fragmentations of Long-Chain Aliphatic Iminium Ions. Org Mass Spectrom 28:867–872. doi:10.1002/oms.1210280808
66. Bowen RD, Wright AD, Derrick PJ (1992) Unimolecular Reactions of Ionized Methyl Allyl Ether. Org Mass Spectrom 27:905–915. doi:10.1002/oms.1210270812
67. Cao JR, George M, Holmes JL (1992) Fragmentation of 1- and 3-Methoxypropene Ions. Another Part of the $[C_4H_8O]^{+\cdot}$ Cation Radical Potential Energy Surface. J Am Soc Mass Spectrom 3:99–107. doi:10.1016/1044-0305(92)87042-W
68. Millington DS, Smith JA (1977) Fragmentation Patterns by Fast Linked Electric and Magnetic Field Scanning. Org Mass Spectrom 12:264–265. doi:10.1002/oms.1210120418
69. Morgan RP, Porter CJ, Beynon JH (1977) On the Formation of Artefact Peaks in Linked Scans of the Magnet and Electric Sector Fields in a Mass Spectrometer. Org Mass Spectrom 12:735–738. doi:10.1002/oms.1210121206
70. Lacey MJ, Macdonald CG (1980) The Use of Two Linked Scanning Modes in Alternation to Analyze Metastable Peaks. Org Mass Spectrom 15:134–137. doi:10.1002/oms.1210150306
71. Lacey MJ, Macdonald CG (1980) Interpreting Metastable Peaks from Double Focusing Mass Spectrometers. Org Mass Spectrom 15:484–485. doi:10.1002/oms.1210150306
72. Mouget Y, Bertrand MJ (1995) Graphical Method for Artefact Peak Interpretation, and Methods for Their Rejection, Using Double and Triple Sector Magnetic Mass Spectrometers. Rapid Commun Mass Spectrom 9:387–396. doi:10.1002/rcm.1290090506
73. Evers EAIM, Noest AJ, Akkerman OS (1977) Deconvolution of Composite Metastable Peaks: A New Method for the Determination of Metastable Transitions Occurring in the First Field Free Region. Org Mass Spectrom 12:419–420. doi:10.1002/oms.1210120702
74. Boyd RK, Porter CJ, Beynon JH (1981) A New Linked Scan for Reversed Geometry Mass Spectrometers. Org Mass Spectrom 16:490–494. doi:10.1002/oms.1210161104
75. Lacey MJ, Macdonald CG (1979) Constant Neutral Spectrum in Mass Spectrometry. Anal Chem 51:691–695. doi:10.1021/ac50042a027
76. Boyd RK, Beynon JH (1977) Scanning of Sector Mass Spectrometers to Observe the Fragmentations of Metastable Ions. Org Mass Spectrom 12:163–165. doi:10.1002/oms.1210120311
77. Jennings KR (1984) Scanning methods for double-focusing mass spectrometers. In: Almoster Ferreira MA (ed) Ion Processes in the Gas Phase. D. Reidel Publishing, Dordrecht, pp 7–21

78. Fraefel A, Seibl J (1984) Selective Analysis of Metastable Ions. Mass Spectrom Rev 4:151–221. doi:10.1002/mas.1280040202
79. Boyd RK (1994) Linked-Scan Techniques for MS/MS Using Tandem-in-Space Instruments. Mass Spectrom Rev 13:359–410. doi:10.1002/mas.1280130502
80. Walther H, Schlunegger UP, Friedli F (1983) Quantitative Determination of Compounds in Mixtures by $B^2E = const.$ Linked Scans. Org Mass Spectrom 18:572–575. doi:10.1002/oms.1210181215
81. Futrell JH (2000) Development of Tandem Mass Spectrometry. One Perspective. Int J Mass Spectrom 200:495–508. doi:10.1016/S1387-3806(00)00353-5
82. Fenselau C (1992) Tandem Mass Spectrometry: The Competitive Edge for Pharmacology. Annu Rev Pharmacol Toxicol 32:555–578. doi:10.1146/annurev.pa.32.040192.003011
83. Srinivas R, Sülzle D, Weiske T, Schwarz H (1991) Generation and Characterization of Neutral and Cationic 3-Silacyclopropenylidene in the Gas Phase. Description of a New BEBE Tandem Mass Spectrometer. Int J Mass Spectrom Ion Proc 107:369–376. doi:10.1016/0168-1176(91)80071-T
84. Bordaz-Nagy J, Despeyroux D, Jennings KR, Gaskell SJ (1992) Experimental Aspects of the Collision-Induced Decomposition of Ions in a Four-Sector Tandem Mass Spectrometer. Org Mass Spectrom 27:406–415. doi:10.1002/oms.1210270410
85. Stults JT, Lai J, McCune S, Wetzel R (1993) Simplification of High-Energy Collision Spectra of Peptides by Amino-Terminal Derivatization. Anal Chem 65:1703–1708. doi:10.1021/ac00061a012
86. Biemann K, Papyannopoulos IA (1994) Amino Acid Sequencing of Proteins. Acc Chem Res 27:370–378. doi:10.1021/ar00047a008
87. Papyannopoulos IA (1995) The Interpretation of Collision-Induced Dissociation Tandem Mass Spectra of Peptides. Mass Spectrom Rev 14:49–73. doi:10.1002/mas.1280140104
88. Lehmann WD (1996) Massenspektrometrie in der Biochemie. Spektrum Akademischer Verlag, Heidelberg
89. Chapman JR (ed) (2000) Mass Spectrometry of Proteins and Peptides. Humana Press, Totowa
90. Snyder AP (2000) Interpreting Protein Mass Spectra. Oxford University Press, New York
91. Kinter M, Sherman NE (2000) Protein Sequencing and Identification Using Tandem Mass Spectrometry. John Wiley & Sons, Chichester
92. Yost RA, Enke CG (1978) Selected Ion Fragmentation with a Tandem Quadrupole Mass Spectrometer. J Am Chem Soc 100:2274–2275. doi:10.1021/ja00475a072
93. Yost RA, Enke CG, McGilvery DC, Smith D, Morrison JD (1979) High Efficiency Collision-Induced Dissociation in an Rf-Only Quadrupole. Int J Mass Spectrom Ion Phys 30:127–136. doi:10.1016/0020-7381(79)80090-X
94. Yost RA, Enke CG (1979) Triple Quadrupole Mass Spectrometry for Direct Mixture Analysis and Structure Elucidation. Anal Chem 51:1251A–1262A. doi:10.1021/ac50048a002
95. Hunt DF, Shabanowitz J, Giordani AB (1980) Collision Activated Decompositions in Mixture Analysis with a Triple Quadrupole Mass Spectrometer. Anal Chem 52:386–390. doi:10.1021/ac50053a004
96. Dawson PH, French JB, Buckley JA, Douglas DJ, Simmons D (1982) The Use of Triple Quadrupoles for Sequential Mass Spectrometry: The Instrument Parameters. Org Mass Spectrom 17:205–211. doi:10.1002/oms.1210170503
97. Dawson PH, French JB, Buckley JA, Douglas DJ, Simmons D (1982) The Use of Triple Quadrupoles for Sequential Mass Spectrometry: A Detailed Case Study. Org Mass Spectrom 17:212–219. doi:10.1002/oms.1210170504
98. Inglebert RL, Hennequin JF (1980) Overall Transmission of Quadrupole Mass Spectrometers. Adv Mass Spectrom 8B:1764–1770
99. Cerezo A, Miller MK (1991) Einzel Lenses in Atom Probe Designs. Surf Sci 246:450–456. doi:10.1016/0039-6028(91)90450-7
100. Thomson BA, Douglas DJ, Corr JJ, Hager JW, Jolliffe CL (1995) Improved Collisionally Activated Dissociation Efficiency and Mass Resolution on a Triple Quadrupole Mass Spectrometer System. Anal Chem 67:1696–1704. doi:10.1021/ac00106a008

101. Zeller M, Koenig S (2004) The Impact of Chromatography and Mass Spectrometry on the Analysis of Protein Phosphorylation Sites. Mass Spectrometric Phosphorylation Analysis. Anal Bioanal Chem 378:889–909. doi:10.1007/s00216-003-2391-2
102. Schwartz JC, Schey KL, Cooks RG (1990) A Penta-Quadrupole Instrument for Reaction Intermediate Scans and Other MS-MS-MS Experiments. Int J Mass Spectrom Ion Proc 101:1–20. doi:10.1016/0168-1176(90)80017-W
103. Gozzo FC, Sorrilha AEPM, Eberlin MN (1996) The Generation, Stability, Dissociation and Ion/Molecule Chemistry of Sulfinyl Cations in the Gas Phase. J Chem Soc Perkin Trans 2:587–596. doi:10.1039/P29960000587
104. Juliano VF, Gozzo FC, Eberlin MN, Kascheres C, do Lago CL (1996) Fast Multidimensional (3D and 4D) MS^2 and MS^3 Scans in a High-Transmission Pentaquadrupole Mass Spectrometer. Anal Chem 68:1328–1334. doi:10.1021/ac9508659
105. Eberlin MN (1997) Triple-Stage Pentaquadrupole (QqQqQ) Mass Spectrometry and Ion/Molecule Reactions. Mass Spectrom Rev 16:113–144. doi:10.1002/(SICI)1098-2787(1997)16:3<113::AID-MAS1>3.0.CO;2-K
106. March RE (1998) Quadrupole Ion Trap Mass Spectrometry: Theory, Simulation, Recent Developments and Applications. Rapid Commun Mass Spectrom 12:1543–1554. doi:10.1002/(SICI)1097-0231(19981030)12:20<1543::AID-RCM343>3.0.CO;2-T
107. Griffiths IW (1990) Recent Advances in Ion-Trap Technology. Rapid Commun Mass Spectrom 4:69–73. doi:10.1002/rcm.1290040302
108. Siethoff C, Wagner-Redeker W, Schäfer M, Linscheid M (1999) HPLC-MS with an Ion Trap Mass Spectrometer. Chimia 53:484–491
109. Schwartz JC, Jardine I (1992) High-Resolution Parent-Ion Selection/Isolation Using a Quadrupole Ion-Trap Mass Spectrometer. Rapid Commun Mass Spectrom 6:313–317. doi:10.1002/rcm.1290060419
110. Remes PM, Glish GL (2009) On The Time Scale of Internal Energy Relaxation of AP-MALDI and Nano-ESI Ions in a Quadrupole Ion Trap. J Am Soc Mass Spectrom 20:1801–1812. doi:10.1016/j.jasms.2009.05.018
111. Louris JN, Cooks RG, Syka JEP, Kelley PE, Stafford GC Jr, Todd JFJ (1987) Instrumentation, Applications, and Energy Deposition in Quadrupole Ion-Trap Tandem Mass Spectrometry. Anal Chem 59:1677–1685. doi:10.1021/ac00140a021
112. McLuckey SA, Glish GL, Kelley PE (1987) Collision-Activated Dissociation of Negative Ions in an Ion Trap Mass Spectrometer. Anal Chem 59:1670–1674. doi:10.1021/ac00140a019
113. Cooks RG, Amy JW, Bier M, Schwartz JC, Schey K (1989) New mass spectrometers. Adv Mass Spectrom 11A:33–52
114. Murrell J, Konn DO, Underwood NJ, Despeyroux D (2003) Studies into the Selective Accumulation of Multiply Charged Protein Ions in a Quadrupole Ion Trap Mass Spectrometer. Int J Mass Spectrom 227:223–234. doi:10.1016/S1387-3806(03)00109-X
115. Hashimoto Y, Hasegawa H, Yoshinari K (2003) Collision-Activated Infrared Multiphoton Dissociation in a Quadrupole Ion Trap Mass Spectrometer. Anal Chem 75:420–425. doi:10.1021/ac025866x
116. March RE, Todd JFJ (2005) Quadrupole Ion Trap Mass Spectrometry. John Wiley & Sons, Hoboken
117. Kuzma M, Jegorov A, Kacer P, Havlícek V (2001) Sequencing of New Beauverolides by High-Performance Liquid Chromatography and Mass Spectrometry. J Mass Spectrom 36:1108–1115. doi:10.1002/jms.213
118. Hopfgartner G, Husser C, Zell M (2003) Rapid Screening and Characterization of Drug Metabolites Using a New Quadrupole-Linear Ion Trap Mass Spectrometer. J Mass Spectrom 38:138–150. doi:10.1002/jms.420
119. Pekar Second T, Blethrow JD, Schwartz JC, Merrihew GE, MacCoss MJ, Swaney DL, Russell JD, Coon JJ, Zabrouskov V (2009) Dual-Pressure Linear Ion Trap Mass Spectrometer Improving the Analysis of Complex Protein Mixtures. Anal Chem 81:7757–7765. doi:10.1021/ac901278y

120. Magparangalan DP, Garrett TJ, Drexler DM, Yost RA (2010) Analysis of Large Peptides by MALDI Using a Linear Quadrupole Ion Trap with Mass Range Extension. Anal Chem 82:930–934. doi:10.1021/ac9021488
121. Londry FA, Hager JW (2003) Mass Selective Axial Ion Ejection from a Linear Quadrupole Ion Trap. J Am Soc Mass Spectrom 14:1130–1147. doi:10.1016/S1044-0305(03)00446-X
122. Hopfgartner G, Varesio E, Tschaeppaet V, Grivet C, Bourgogne E, Leuthold LA (2004) Triple Quadrupole Linear Ion Trap Mass Spectrometer for the Analysis of Small Molecules and Macromolecules. J Mass Spectrom 39:845–855. doi:10.1002/jms.659
123. Moberg M, Markides KE, Bylund D (2005) Multi-Parameter Investigation of Tandem Mass Spectrometry in a Linear Ion Trap Using Response Surface Modelling. J Mass Spectrom 40:317–324. doi:10.1002/jms.787
124. Olsen JV, Schwartz JC, Griep-Raming J, Nielsen ML, Damoc E, Denisov E, Lange O, Remes P, Taylor D, Splendore M, Wouters ER, Senko M, Makarov A, Mann M, Horning S (2009) A Dual Pressure Linear Ion Trap Orbitrap Instrument with Very High Sequencing Speed. Mol Cell Proteomics 8:2759–2769. doi:10.1074/mcp.M900375-MCP200
125. Olsen JV, Macek B, Lange O, Makarov A, Horning S, Mann M (2007) Higher-Energy C-Trap Dissociation for Peptide Modification Analysis. Nat Methods 4:709–712. doi:10.1038/nmeth1060
126. Olsen JV, de Godoy LMF, Li G, Macek B, Mortensen P, Pesch R, Makarov A, Lange O, Horning S, Mann M (2005) Parts Per Million Mass Accuracy on an Orbitrap Mass Spectrometer via Lock Mass Injection into a C-Trap. Mol Cell Proteomics 4:2010–2021. doi:10.1074/mcp.T500030-MCP200
127. Senko MW, Remes PM, Canterbury JD, Mathur R, Song Q, Eliuk SM, Mullen C, Earley L, Hardman M, Blethrow JD, Bui H, Specht A, Lange O, Denisov E, Makarov A, Horning S, Zabrouskov V (2013) Novel Parallelized Quadrupole/Linear Ion Trap/Orbitrap Tribrid Mass Spectrometer Improving Proteome Coverage and Peptide Identification Rates. Anal Chem 85:11710–11714. doi:10.1021/ac403115c
128. Lebedev AT, Damoc E, Makarov AA, Samgina TY (2014) Discrimination of Leucine and Isoleucine in Peptides Sequencing with Orbitrap Fusion Mass Spectrometer. Anal Chem 86:7017–7022. doi:10.1021/ac501200h
129. Guan S, Marshall AG (1996) Stored Waveform Inverse Fourier Transform (SWIFT) Ion Excitation in Trapped Ion Mass Spectrometry: Theory and Applications. Int J Mass Spectrom Ion Proc 157(158):5–37. doi:10.1016/S0168-1176(96)04461-8
130. Heck AJR, Derrick PJ (1997) Ultrahigh Mass Accuracy in Isotope-Selective Collision-Induced Dissociation Using Correlated Sweep Excitation and Sustained Off-Resonance Irradiation: A Fourier Transform Ion Cyclotron Resonance Mass Spectrometry Case Study on the $[M+2H]^{2+}$ Ion of Bradykinin. Anal Chem 69:3603–3607. doi:10.1021/ac970254b
131. Heck AJR, Derrick PJ (1998) Selective Fragmentation of Single Isotopic Ions of Proteins Up to 17 KDa Using 9.4 Tesla Fourier Transform Ion Cyclotron Resonance. Eur Mass Spectrom 4:181–188. doi:10.1255/ejms.207
132. Cody RB, Freiser BS (1982) Collision-Induced Dissociation in a Fourier-Transform Mass Spectrometer. Int J Mass Spectrom Ion Phys 41:199–204. doi:10.1016/0020-7381(82)85035-3
133. Cody RB, Burnier RC, Freiser BS (1982) Collision-Induced Dissociation with Fourier Transform Mass Spectrometry. Anal Chem 54:96–101. doi:10.1021/ac00238a029
134. Gauthier JW, Trautman TR, Jacobson DB (1991) Sustained Off-Resonance Irradiation for Collision-Activated Dissociation Involving FT-ICR-MS. CID Technique that Emulates Infrared Multiphoton Dissociation. Anal Chim Acta 246:211–225. doi:10.1016/0003-2670(91)80053-V
135. Senko MW, Speir JP, McLafferty FW (1994) Collisional Activation of Large Multiply Charged Ions Using Fourier Transform Mass Spectrometry. Anal Chem 66:2801–2808. doi:10.1021/ac00090a003

136. Boering KA, Rolfe J, Brauman JI (1992) Control of Ion Kinetic Energy in Ion Cyclotron Resonance Spectrometry: Very-Low-Energy Collision-Induced Dissociation. Rapid Commun Mass Spectrom 6:303–305. doi:10.1002/rcm.1290060416
137. Lee SA, Jiao CQ, Huang Y, Freiser BS (1993) Multiple Excitation Collisional Activation in Fourier-Transform Mass Spectrometry. Rapid Commun Mass Spectrom 7:819–821. doi:10.1002/rcm.1290070908
138. Mihalca R, van der Burgt YEM, Heck AJR, Heeren RMA (2007) Disulfide Bond Cleavages Observed in SORI-CID of Three Nonapeptides Complexed with Divalent Transition-Metal Cations. J Mass Spectrom 42:450–458. doi:10.1002/jms.1175
139. Mirgorodskaya E, O'Connor PB, Costello CE (2002) A General Method for Precalculation of Parameters for Sustained Off Resonance Irradiation/Collision-Induced Dissociation. J Am Soc Mass Spectrom 13:318–324. doi:10.1016/S1044-0305(02)00340-9
140. Woodin RL, Bomse DS, Beauchamp JL (1978) Multiphoton Dissociation of Molecules with Low Power Continuous Wave Infrared Laser Radiation. J Am Chem Soc 100:3248–3250. doi:10.1021/ja00478a065
141. Håkansson K, Cooper HJ, Emmet MR, Costello CE, Marshall AG, Nilsson CL (2001) Electron Capture Dissociation and Infrared Multiphoton Dissociation MS/MS of an *N*-Glycosylated Tryptic Peptic to Yield Complementary Sequence Information. Anal Chem 73:4530–4536. doi:10.1021/ac0103470
142. Little DP, Senko MW, O'Conner PB, McLafferty FW (1994) Infrared Multiphoton Dissociation of Large Multiply-Charged Ions for Biomolecule Sequencing. Anal Chem 66:2809–2815. doi:10.1021/ac00090a004
143. Watson CH, Baykut G, Eyler JR (1987) Laser Photodissociation of Gaseous Ions Formed by Laser Desorption. Anal Chem 59:1133–1138. doi:10.1021/ac00135a015
144. Eyler JR (2009) Infrared Multiple Photon Dissociation Spectroscopy of Ions in Penning Traps. Mass Spectrom Rev 28:448–467. doi:10.1002/mas.20217
145. Brodbelt JS, Wilson JJ (2009) Infrared Multiphoton Dissociation in Quadrupole Ion Traps. Mass Spectrom Rev 28:390–424. doi:10.1002/mas.20216
146. Hashimoto Y, Hasegawa H, Waki I (2004) High Sensitivity and Broad Dynamic Range Infrared Multiphoton Dissociation for a Quadrupole Ion Trap. Rapid Commun Mass Spectrom 18:2255–2259. doi:10.1002/rcm.1619
147. Newsome GA, Glish GL (2009) Improving IRMPD in a Quadrupole Ion Trap. J Am Soc Mass Spectrom 20:1127–1131. doi:10.1016/j.jasms.2009.02.003
148. Newsome GA, Glish GL (2011) A New Approach to IRMPD Using Selective Ion Dissociation in a Quadrupole Ion Trap. J Am Soc Mass Spectrom 22:207–213. doi:10.1007/s13361-010-0039-y
149. Madsen JA, Gardner MW, Smith SI, Ledvina AR, Coon JJ, Schwartz JC, Stafford GC, Brodbelt JS (2009) Top-Down Protein Fragmentation by Infrared Multiphoton Dissociation in a Dual Pressure Linear Ion Trap. Anal Chem 81:8677–8686. doi:10.1021/ac901554z
150. Gardner MW, Smith SI, Ledvina AR, Madsen JA, Coon JJ, Schwartz JC, Stafford GC, Brodbelt JS (2009) Infrared Multiphoton Dissociation of Peptide Cations in a Dual Pressure Linear Ion Trap Mass Spectrometer. Anal Chem 81:8109–8118. doi:10.1021/ac901313m
151. Campbell JL, Hager JW, Le Blanc JCY (2009) On Performing Simultaneous Electron Transfer Dissociation and Collision-Induced Dissociation on Multiply Protonated Peptides in a Linear Ion Trap. J Am Soc Mass Spectrom 20:1672–1683. doi:10.1016/j.jasms.2009.05.009
152. Ledvina AR, Lee MV, McAlister GC, Westphall MS, Coon JJ (2012) Infrared Multiphoton Dissociation for Quantitative Shotgun Proteomics. Anal Chem 84:4513–4519. doi:10.1021/ac300367p
153. Zubarev RA, Kelleher NL, McLafferty FW (1998) Electron Capture Dissociation of Multiply Charged Protein Cations. A Nonergodic Process. J Am Chem Soc 120:3265–3266. doi:10.1021/ja973478k

154. Axelsson J, Palmblad M, Håkansson K, Håkansson P (1999) Electron Capture Dissociation of Substance P Using a Commercially Available Fourier Transform Ion Cyclotron Resonance Mass Spectrometer. Rapid Commun Mass Spectrom 13:474–477. doi:10.1002/(SICI)1097-0231(19990330)13:6<474::AID-RCM505>3.0.CO;2-1
155. Cerda BA, Horn DM, Breuker K, Carpenter BK, McLafferty FW (1999) Electron Capture Dissociation of Multiply-Charged Oxygenated Cations. A Nonergodic Process. Eur Mass Spectrom 5:335–338. doi:10.1255/ejms.293
156. Håkansson K, Emmet MR, Hendrickson CL, Marshall AG (2001) High-Sensitivity Electron Capture Dissociation Tandem FTICR Mass Spectrometry of Microelectrosprayed Peptides. Anal Chem 73:3605–3610. doi:10.1021/ac010141z
157. Leymarie N, Berg EA, McComb ME, O'Conner PB, Grogan J, Oppenheim FG, Costello CE (2002) Tandem Mass Spectrometry for Structural Characterization of Proline-Rich Proteins: Application to Salivary PRP-3. Anal Chem 74:4124–4132. doi:10.1021/ac0255835
158. Tsybin YO, Ramstroem M, Witt M, Baykut G, Hakansson P (2004) Peptide and Protein Characterization by High-Rate Electron Capture Dissociation Fourier Transform Ion Cyclotron Resonance Mass Spectrometry. J Mass Spectrom 39:719–729. doi:10.1002/jms.658
159. Zubarev RA, Horn DM, Fridriksson EK, Kelleher NL, Kruger NA, Lewis MA, Carpenter BK, McLafferty FW (2000) Electron Capture Dissociation for Structural Characterization of Multiply Charged Protein Cations. Anal Chem 72:563–573. doi:10.1021/ac990811p
160. Zubarev RA (2003) Reactions of Polypeptide Ions with Electrons in the Gas Phase. Mass Spectrom Rev 22:57–77. doi:10.1002/mas.10042
161. Leymarie N, Costello CE, O'Connor PB (2003) Electron Capture Dissociation Initiates a Free Radical Reaction Cascade. J Am Chem Soc 125:8949–8958. doi:10.1021/ja028831n
162. Turecek F (2003) N-C_{α} Bond Dissociation Energies and Kinetics in Amide and Peptide Radicals. Is the Dissociation a Non-Ergodic Process? J Am Chem Soc 125:5954–5963. doi:10.1021/ja021323t
163. McFarland MA, Marshall AG, Hendrickson CL, Nilsson CL, Fredman P, Mansson JE (2005) Structural Characterization of the GM1 Ganglioside by Infrared Multiphoton Dissociation, Electron Capture Dissociation, and Electron Detachment Dissociation Electrospray Ionization FT-ICR MS/MS. J Am Soc Mass Spectrom 16:752–762. doi:10.1016/j.jasms.2005.02.001
164. Oh HB, Lin C, Hwang HY, Zhai H, Breuker K, Zabrouskov V, Carpenter BK, McLafferty FW (2005) Infrared Photodissociation Spectroscopy of Electrosprayed Ions in a Fourier Transform Mass Spectrometer. J Am Chem Soc 127:4076–4083. doi:10.1021/ja040136n
165. Dunbar RC (2004) BIRD (Blackbody Infrared Radiative Dissociation): Evolution, Principles, and Applications. Mass Spectrom Rev 23:127–158. doi:10.1002/mas.10074
166. Tsybin YO, Hakansson P, Budnik BA, Haselmann KF, Kjeldsen F, Gorshkov M, Zubarev RA (2001) Improved Low-Energy Electron Injection Systems for High Rate Electron Capture Dissociation in Fourier Transform Ion Cyclotron Resonance Mass Spectrometry. Rapid Commun Mass Spectrom 15:1849–1854. doi:10.1002/rcm.448
167. Tsybin YO, Witt M, Baykut G, Kjeldsen F, Hakansson P (2003) Combined Infrared Multiphoton Dissociation and Electron Capture Dissociation with a Hollow Electron Beam in Fourier Transform Ion Cyclotron Resonance Mass Spectrometry. Rapid Commun Mass Spectrom 17:1759–1768. doi:10.1002/rcm.1118
168. Syka JEP, Coon JJ, Schroeder MJ, Shabanowitz J, Hunt DF (2004) Peptide and Protein Sequence Analysis by Electron Transfer Dissociation Mass Spectrometry. Proc Natl Acad Sci U S A 101:9528–9533. doi:10.1073/pnas.0402700101
169. Cooper HJ, Hakansson K, Marshall AG (2005) The Role of Electron Capture Dissociation in Biomolecular Analysis. Mass Spectrom Rev 24:201–222. doi:10.1002/mas.20014
170. Swaney DL, McAlister GC, Wirtala M, Schwartz JC, Syka JEP, Coon JJ (2007) Supplemental Activation Method for High-Efficiency Electron-Transfer Dissociation of Doubly Protonated Peptide Precursors. Anal Chem 79:477–485. doi:10.1021/ac061457f
171. Coon JJ, Syka JEP, Schwartz JC, Shabanowitz J, Hunt DF (2004) Anion Dependence in the Partitioning Between Proton and Electron Transfer in Ion/Ion Reactions. Int J Mass Spectrom 236:33–42. doi:10.1016/j.ijms.2004.05.005

172. Good DM, Wirtala M, McAlister GC, Coon JJ (2007) Performance Characteristics of Electron Transfer Dissociation Mass Spectrometry. Mol Cell Proteomics 6:1942–1951. doi:10.1074/mcp.M700073-MCP200
173. Chi A, Huttenhower C, Geer LY, Coon JJ, Syka JEP, Bai DL, Shabanowitz J, Burke DJ, Troyanskaya OG, Hunt DF (2007) Analysis of Phosphorylation Sites on Proteins from Saccharomyces Cerevisiae by Electron Transfer Dissociation (ETD) Mass Spectrometry. Proc Natl Acad Sci U S A 104:2193–2198. doi:10.1073/pnas.0607084104
174. Liang X, Hager JW, McLuckey SA (2007) Transmission Mode Ion/Ion Electron-Transfer Dissociation in a Linear Ion Trap. Anal Chem 79:3363–3370. doi:10.1021/ac062295q
175. McAlister GC, Berggren WT, Griep-Raming J, Horning S, Makarov A, Phanstiel D, Stafford G, Swaney DL, Syka JEP, Zabrouskov V, Coon JJ (2008) A Proteomics Grade Electron Transfer Dissociation-Enabled Hybrid Linear Ion Trap-Orbitrap Mass Spectrometer. J Proteome Res 7:3127–3136. doi:10.1021/pr800264t
176. Williams DK Jr, McAlister GC, Good DM, Coon JJ, Muddiman DC (2007) Dual Electrospray Ion Source for Electron-Transfer Dissociation on a Hybrid Linear Ion Trap-Orbitrap Mass Spectrometer. Anal Chem 79:7916–7919. doi:10.1021/ac071444h
177. McAlister GC, Phanstiel D, Good DM, Berggren WT, Coon JJ (2007) Implementation of Electron-Transfer Dissociation on a Hybrid Linear Ion Trap-Orbitrap Mass Spectrometer. Anal Chem 79:3525–3534. doi:10.1021/ac070020k
178. Haselmann KF, Budnik BA, Kjeldsen F, Nielsen ML, Olsen JV, Zubarev RA (2002) Electronic Excitation Gives Informative Fragmentation of Polypeptide Cations and Anions. Eur J Mass Spectrom 8:117–121. doi:10.1255/ejms.479
179. Budnik BA, Haselmann KF, Zubarev RA (2001) Electron Detachment Dissociation of Peptide Di-Anions: An Electron-Hole Recombination Phenomenon. Chem Phys Lett 342:299–302. doi:10.1016/S0009-2614(01)00501-2
180. Kjeldsen F, Silivra OA, Ivonin IA, Haselmann KF, Gorshkov M, Zubarev RA (2005) C_α-C Backbone Fragmentation Dominates in Electron Detachment Dissociation of Gas-Phase Polypeptide Polyanions. Chem Eur J 11:1803–1812. doi:10.1002/chem.200400806
181. Anusiewicz I, Jasionowski M, Skurski P, Simons J (2005) Backbone and Side-Chain Cleavages in Electron Detachment Dissociation (EDD). J Chem Phys A 109:11332–11337. doi:10.1021/jp055018g
182. Yang J, Mo J, Adamson JT, Haakansson K (2005) Characterization of Oligodeoxynucleotides by Electron Detachment Dissociation Fourier Transform Ion Cyclotron Resonance Mass Spectrometry. Anal Chem 77:1876–1882. doi:10.1021/ac048415g
183. Huzarska M, Ugalde I, Kaplan DA, Hartmer R, Easterling ML, Polfer NC (2010) Negative Electron Transfer Dissociation of Deprotonated Phosphopeptide Anions: Choice of Radical Cation Reagent and Competition Between Electron and Proton Transfer. Anal Chem 82:2873–2878. doi:10.1021/ac9028592
184. Adlhart C, Hinderling C, Baumann H, Chen P (2000) Mechanistic Studies of Olefin Metathesis by Ruthenium Carbene Complexes Using Electrospray Ionization Tandem Mass Spectrometry. J Am Chem Soc 122:8204–8214. doi:10.1021/ja9938231
185. Hinderling C, Adlhart C, Chen P (2000) Mechanism-Based High-Throughput Screening of Catalysts. Chimia 54:232–235
186. Volland MAO, Adlhart C, Kiener CA, Chen P, Hofmann P (2001) Catalyst Screening by Electrospray Ionization Tandem Mass Spectrometry: Hofmann Carbenes for Olefin Metathesis. Chem Eur J 7:4621–4632. doi:10.1002/1521-3765(20011105)7:21<4621::AID-CHEM4621>3.0.CO;2-C
187. Schwarz H (2003) Relativistic Effects in Gas-Phase Ion Chemistry: An Experimentalist's View. Angew Chem Int Ed 42:4442–4454. doi:10.1002/anie.200300572
188. Schwarz H (2004) On the Spin-Forbiddeness of Gas-Phase Ion-Molecule Reactions: A Fruitful Intersection of Experimental and Computational Studies. Int J Mass Spectrom 237:75–105. doi:10.1016/j.ijms.2004.06.006

189. Boehme DK, Schwarz H (2005) Gas-Phase Catalysis by Atomic and Cluster Metal Ions: The Ultimate Single-Site Catalysts. Angew Chem Int Ed 44:2336–2354. doi:10.1002/chin.200525226
190. Schlangen M, Schroeder D, Schwarz H (2007) Pronounced Ligand Effects and the Role of Formal Oxidation States in the Nickel-Mediated Thermal Activation of Methane. Angew Chem Int Ed 46:1641–1644. doi:10.1002/anie.200603266
191. Kaltashov IA, Eyles SJ (2005) Mass Spectrometry in Biophysics: Conformation and Dynamics of Biomolecules. John Wiley & Sons, Hoboken
192. Somogyi A (2008) Probing Peptide Fragment Ion Structures by Combining Sustained Off-Resonance Collision-Induced Dissociation and Gas-Phase H/D Exchange (SORI-HDX) in Fourier Transform Ion-Cyclotron Resonance (FT-ICR) Instruments. J Am Soc Mass Spectrom 19:1771–1775. doi:10.1016/j.jasms.2008.08.012
193. Bythell BJ, Somogyi A, Paizs B (2009) What Is the Structure of B_2 Ions Generated from Doubly Protonated Tryptic Peptides? J Am Soc Mass Spectrom 20:618–624. doi:10.1016/j.jasms.2008.11.021
194. Harrison AG (1997) The Gas-Phase Basicities and Proton Affinities of Amino Acids and Peptides. Mass Spectrom Rev 16:201–217. doi:10.1002/(SICI)1098-2787(1997)16:4<201::AID-MAS3>3.0.CO;2-L
195. McMahon TB (2000) Thermochemical Ladders: Scaling the Ramparts of Gaseous Ion Energetics. Int J Mass Spectrom 200:187–199. doi:10.1016/S1387-3806(00)00308-0
196. Cooks RG, Kruger TL (1977) Intrinsic Basicity Determination Using Metastable Ions. J Am Chem Soc 99:1279–1281. doi:10.1021/ja00446a059
197. Cooks RG, Wong PSH (1998) Kinetic Method of Making Thermochemical Determinations: Advances and Applications. Acc Chem Res 31:379–386. doi:10.1021/ar960242x
198. Cooks RG, Patrick JS, Kotiaho T, McLuckey SA (1994) Thermochemical Determinations by the Kinetic Method. Mass Spectrom Rev 13:287–339. doi:10.1002/mas.1280130402
199. Kukol A, Strehle F, Thielking G, Grützmacher HF (1993) Methyl Group Effect on the Proton Affinity of Methylated Acetophenones Studied by Two Mass Spectrometric Techniques. Org Mass Spectrom 28:1107–1110. doi:10.1002/oms.1210281021
200. Bouchoux G, Salpin JY (1996) Gas-Phase Basicity and Heat of Formation of Sulfine $CH_2{=}S{=}O$. J Am Chem Soc 118:6516–6517. doi:10.1021/ja9610601
201. Bouchoux G, Salpin JY, Leblanc D (1996) A Relationship Between the Kinetics and Thermochemistry of Proton Transfer Reactions in the Gas Phase. Int J Mass Spectrom Ion Proc 153:37–48. doi:10.1016/0168-1176(95)04353-5
202. Witt M, Kreft D, Grützmacher HF (2003) Effects of Internal Hydrogen Bonds Between Amide Groups: Protonation of Alicyclic Diamides. Eur J Mass Spectrom 9:81–95. doi:10.1255/ejms.535
203. Danis PO, Wesdemiotis C, McLafferty FW (1983) Neutralization-Reionization Mass Spectrometry (NRMS). J Am Chem Soc 105:7454–7456. doi:10.1021/ja00363a048
204. Gellene GI, Porter RF (1983) Neutralized Ion-Beam Spectroscopy. Acc Chem Res 16:200–207. doi:10.1021/ar00090a003
205. Terlouw JK, Kieskamp WM, Holmes JL, Mommers AA, Burgers PC (1985) The Neutralization and Reionization of Mass-Selected Positive Ions by Inert Gas Atoms. Int J Mass Spectrom Ion Proc 64:245–250. doi:10.1016/0168-1176(85)85013-8
206. Holmes JL, Mommers AA, Terlouw JK, Hop CECA (1986) The Mass Spectrometry of Neutral Species Produced from Mass-Selected Ions by Collision and by Charge Exchange. Experiments with Tandem Collision Gas Cells. Int J Mass Spectrom Ion Proc 68:249–264. doi:10.1016/0168-1176(86)87051-3
207. Blanchette MC, Holmes JL, Hop CECA, Mommers AA (1988) The Ionization of Fast Neutrals by Electron Impact in the Second Field-Free Region of a Mass Spectrometer of Reversed Geometry. Org Mass Spectrom 23:495–498. doi:10.1002/oms.1210230611
208. McLafferty FW (1992) Neutralization-Reionization Mass Spectrometry. Int J Mass Spectrom Ion Proc 118(119):221–235. doi:10.1016/0168-1176(92)85063-6

209. Goldberg N, Schwarz H (1994) Neutralization-Reionization Mass Spectrometry: a Powerful "Laboratory" to Generate and Probe Elusive Neutral Molecules. Acc Chem Res 27:347–352. doi:10.1021/ar00047a005
210. Schalley CA, Hornung G, Schroder D, Schwarz H (1998) Mass Spectrometry As a Tool to Probe the Gas-Phase Reactivity of Neutral Molecules. Int J Mass Spectrom Ion Proc 172:181–208. doi:10.1016/S0168-1176(97)00115-8
211. Schalley CA, Hornung G, Schroder D, Schwarz H (1998) Mass Spectrometric Approaches to the Reactivity of Transient Neutrals. Chem Soc Rev 27:91–104. doi:10.1039/A827091Z
212. Blanchette MC, Bordas-Nagy J, Holmes JL, Hop CECA, Mommers AA, Terlouw JK (1988) Neutralization-Reionization Experiments: A Simple Metal Vapor Cell for VG Analytical ZAB-2F Mass Spectrometers. Org Mass Spectrom 23:804–807. doi:10.1002/oms.1210231114
213. Zhang MY, McLafferty FW (1992) Organic Neutralization Agents for Neutralization-Reionization Mass Spectrometry. J Am Soc Mass Spectrom 3:108–112. doi:10.1016/1044-0305(92)87043-X
214. Zagorevskii DV, Holmes JL (1994) Neutralization-Reionization Mass Spectrometry Applied to Organometallic and Coordination Chemistry. Mass Spectrom Rev 13:133–154. doi:10.1002/mas.1280130203
215. Zagorevskii DV, Holmes JL (1999) Neutralization-Reionization Mass Spectrometry Applied to Organometallic and Coordination Chemistry (Update: 1994–1998). Mass Spectrom Rev 18:87–118. doi:10.1002/(SICI)1098-2787(1999)18:2<87::AID-MAS1>3.0.CO;2-J
216. Weiske T, Wong T, Krätschmer W, Terlouw JK, Schwarz H (1992) Proof of the Existence of an Endohedral Helium-Fullerene (He@C_{60}) Structure via Gas-Phase Neutralization of $[HeC_{60}]^{+}$. Angew Chem Int Ed 31:183–185. doi:10.1002/anie.199201831
217. Keck H, Kuchen W, Tommes P, Terlouw JK, Wong T (1992) The Phosphonium Ylide CH_2PH_3 Is Stable in Gas Phase. Angew Chem Int Ed 31:86–87. doi:10.1002/anie.199200861
218. Schröder D, Schwarz H, Wulf M, Sievers H, Jutzi P, Reiher M (1999) Experimental Evidence for the Existence of Neutral P_6: A New Allotrope of Phosphorus. Angew Chem Int Ed 38:313–315. doi:10.1002/(SICI)1521-3773(19991203)38:23<3513::AID-ANIE3513>3.0.CO;2-I
219. Sleno L, Volmer DA (2004) Ion Activation Methods for Tandem Mass Spectrometry. J Mass Spectrom 39:1091–1112. doi:10.1002/jms.703

Fast Atom Bombardment 10

Learning Objectives

- Ablating action of energetic particles on surfaces
- Secondary ion formation by impact of primary ions and neutrals
- Desorption of ions from condensed phase into the gas phase
- Moderating effect of a liquid matrix
- FAB and LSIMS – general properties and applications
- Air- and moisture-sensitive samples
- Related desorption/ionization techniques based on particle impact

Particles impinging on surfaces with kinetic energies in the range of kilo- or even megaelectronvolts cause the ejection of neutrals along with a small fraction of ions from the surface material exposed to their bombardment. The impacting particles are either atoms, molecules, or clusters and it is generally irrelevant whether these are neutrals or ions – what matters is their high kinetic energy. Such ions bombarding the surface are called *primary ions*, those originating from and released by the surface material are referred to as *secondary ions*.

10.1 Brief Historical Sketch

Secondary ion mass spectrometry (SIMS) employing the sputtering effect of a beam of impacting ions was first applied to bulk, inorganic materials. As outlined in the reviews of Benninghoven [1] and Honig [2, 3] the technique had only sparsely been used and mentioned until the end of the 1960s (Chap. 15). Later, attempts were made to also use SIMS for the analysis of organic solids [4, 5]. Prior to this, biomacromolecules had only been analyzed by ^{252}*Californium* (^{252}Cf) *plasma desorption* (PD) time-of-flight (TOF) mass spectrometry (Sect. 10.7). Another

J.H. Gross, *Mass Spectrometry*, DOI 10.1007/978-3-319-54398-7_10

technique called *molecular beam solid analysis* (MBSA) which employed impacting energetic neutrals had also been available at that time but was not widely used in laboratories, at least not under its original name [6, 7]. Unfortunately, SIMS conditions caused electrostatic charging of organic surfaces upon ion impact, and thus this led to a disadvantageous interfering with ion source potentials. Employing a beam of energetic neutral atoms in analogy to the MBSA technique eliminated such problems and promoted further developments of this promising method [8, 9] – the technique was later named *fast atom bombardment* (FAB) [8–10].

It turned out that ions of intact molecular species could be generated even in case of highly polar compounds that definitely were no candidates for electron ionization (EI, Chaps. 5 and 6) or chemical ionization (CI, Chap. 7). Early FAB-MS suffered from rapid radiolytic decomposition of the samples caused by irradiation and from the comparatively harsh conditions of desorption/ionization. The use of a *liquid matrix* in which the analyte was dissolved meant a major breakthrough [11, 12]. Today one would refer to this as "matrix-assisted fast atom bombardment" [13, 14]. FAB-MS soon became the major competitor of field desorption (Chap. 8). It turned out that the properties of the liquid matrix are of key importance for the resulting FAB spectra [15–17]. Due to some electric conductivity of the matrix, primary ions could now again be employed successfully [18–21].

When primary ions instead of neutrals are used to provide the energy for secondary ion ejection from the liquid matrix, the technique is termed *liquid secondary ion mass spectrometry* (LSIMS, Table 10.1). Next to FAB and LSIMS, "inorganic" SIMS has tremendously developed to become a versatile method for surface analysis and more recently for molecular imaging applications (Sect. 15.6).

Table 10.1 Desorption/ionization methods employing impact of energetic particles

Method	Acronym	Principle
Secondary ion mass spectrometry	SIMS	Sputtering and ionization by a beam of ions impacting on solids with keV-energies [1–3]
Plasma desorption	PD-MS	Desorption/ionization of biomolecules by impact of single megaelectronvolt nuclear fission fragments [22–24]
Molecular beam solid analysis	MBSA	Ion formation by impact of neutral molecules with keV-energies on organic solids [6, 7]
Fast atom bombardment	FAB	Desorption/ionization from solids and most importantly liquid matrices by a beam of neutral atoms with keV-energies [8, 9]
Liquid secondary ion mass spectrometry	LSIMS	Desorption/ionization from samples dissolved in a liquid matrix by a beam of ions with keV-energies [18, 19]
Massive cluster impact	MCI	Generation of secondary ions by bombardment with massive clusters of up to 10^8 u [25]

Any energetic particle will do
Apart from kinetic energy and momentum, the characteristics of the primary particles is of lower importance [26] because only minor differences are observed between FAB and LSIMS spectra. In the following, because of the otherwise small differences between the two methods, reference to FAB will be meant to include LSIMS.

10.2 Molecular Beam Solid Analysis

Molecular beam solid analysis (MBSA) was the first technique to use a beam of energetic neutrals to achieve sputtering – or ablation as this is called nowadays – and ionization of solid samples [6, 7]. The MBSA technique employed argon and krypton for primary beam generation. The noble gas was first ionized in a primary ion source, the ions were accelerated by a high voltage of several kV and then neutralized by transmitting the primary ion beam through a charge transfer cell with the neutral gas of the same species. While losing their charge, the primary particles did not suffer a notable change in kinetic energy (Fig. 10.1 and cf. Sect. 10.3). The neutral beam then hit the analyte material on a target in the analytical ion source where analyte got ablated and – at least some small fraction of it – becoming ionized. The ions were then extracted for mass analysis in a magnetic sector analyzer.

Analysis of inorganic salts by MBSA Let's take a look at the positive-ion secondary ion mass spectrum of a piece of filter paper after deposition and evaporation of an equimolar solution of LiF, NaCl, RbBr, and CsI (0.01 M each) as shown below (Fig. 10.2). Argon was used to generate the primary beam. By MBSA, the alkali cations are efficiently desorbed into the gas phase along with some other ions generated from the paper, e.g., $C^{+\bullet}$, *m/z* 12. Also note the characteristic isotopic patterns caused by the pairs of $^{6}Li/^{7}Li$ and $^{85}Rb/^{87}Rb$ in contrast to the monoisotopic ions of ^{23}Na and ^{133}Cs. Similarly, MBSA had also been applied successfully to metals and minerals.

MBSA application to organic compounds Organic molecules have also been successfully analyzed by MBSA. The sample needed to be of low volatility and had to have a molecular weight of less than about 500 u. MBSA spectra of diphenylamine and *N*-(2-nitrophenyl-)aniline show prominent molecular ion peaks of the respective compound (Fig. 10.3), i.e., *m/z* 169 corresponding to $[C_{12}H_{11}N]^{+\bullet}$ and *m/z* 214 due to $[C_{12}H_{10}N_2O_2]^{+\bullet}$ [7]. The peak at *m/z* 168 in b) corresponds to a loss of NO_2 from the molecular ion. Overall, the degree of fragmentation appears comparable to that observed in chemical ionization.

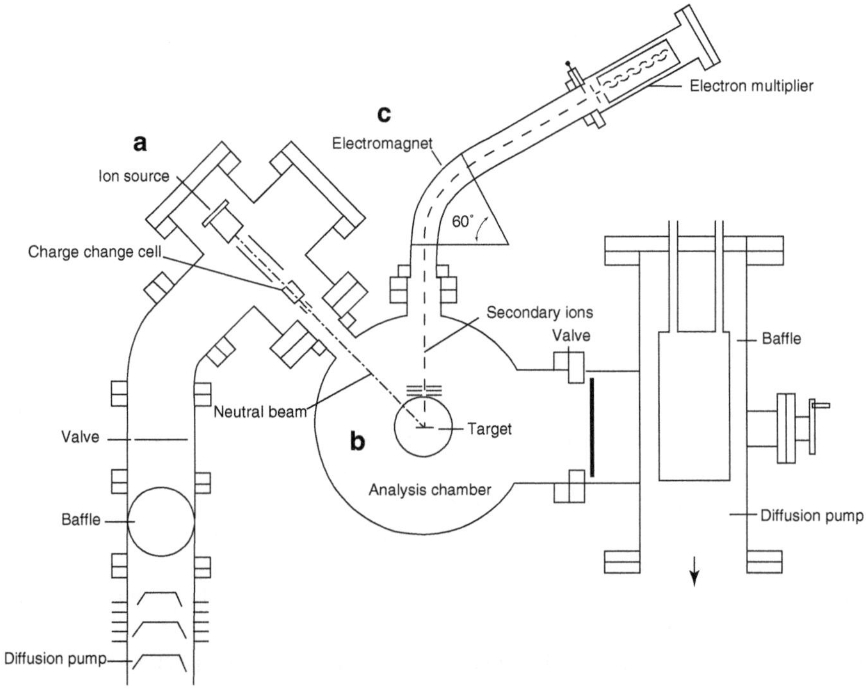

Fig. 10.1 MBSA instrument. The noble gas is ionized in the primary ion source (**a**) and ions of the gas are accelerated and guided through a charge transfer cell. The neutral beam hits a target in the analytical ion source (**b**) where sample material gets sputtered and ionized. Ions are extracted for mass analysis into a magnetic sector analyzer (**c**) (Reproduced from Ref. [7] by permission. © Wiley, 1982)

10.3 Ion Sources for FAB and LSIMS

10.3.1 FAB Ion Sources

An ion source for FAB can be constructed by suitable modification of an EI ion source (Sect. 5.1). Most importantly, the source needs to be modified to give free access to the fast atom beam. The electron-emitting filament and the ion source heaters are switched off during FAB operation (Fig. 10.4). The FAB gas is introduced via a needle valve into the lower part of the *FAB gun* mounted above the ion source. From there, it effuses into the ionization chamber of the FAB gun and into the ion source housing. The *saddle field gun* [27] is the most common type of FAB gun, delivering a primary particle flux of some $10^{10}\ s^{-1}\ mm^{-2}$ [28, 29]. The gas is ionized and the ions are accelerated by a high voltage (4–8 kV) and focused onto the sample [8, 10, 14, 30]. Neutralization of the energetic noble gas ions is effected by charge transfer with incoming neutrals (Sects. 7.4 and 9.17.4). The kinetic energy of the atoms is mostly conserved during charge transfer, and thus the

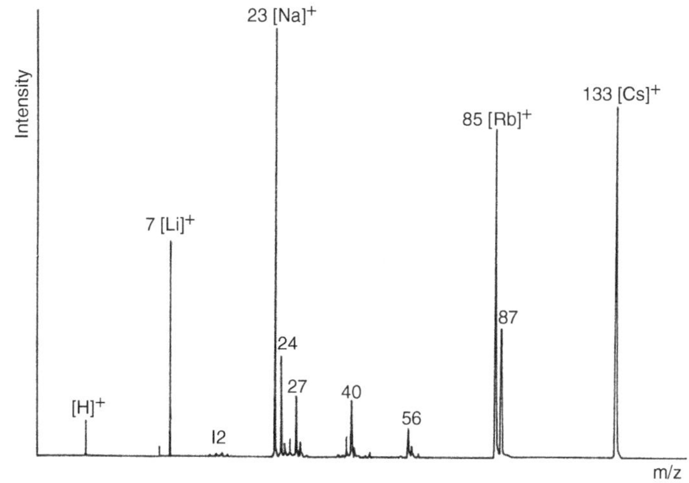

Fig. 10.2 Application of MBSA to inorganic analysis demonstrated by the positive secondary ion mass spectrum resulting after evaporation of an equimolar solution of LiF, NaCl, RbBr, and CsI (0.01 M each) on filter paper. Note the isotopic patterns by the pairs of $^{6}Li/^{7}Li$ and $^{85}Rb/^{87}Rb$ (Reproduced from Ref. [7] by permission. © Wiley, 1982)

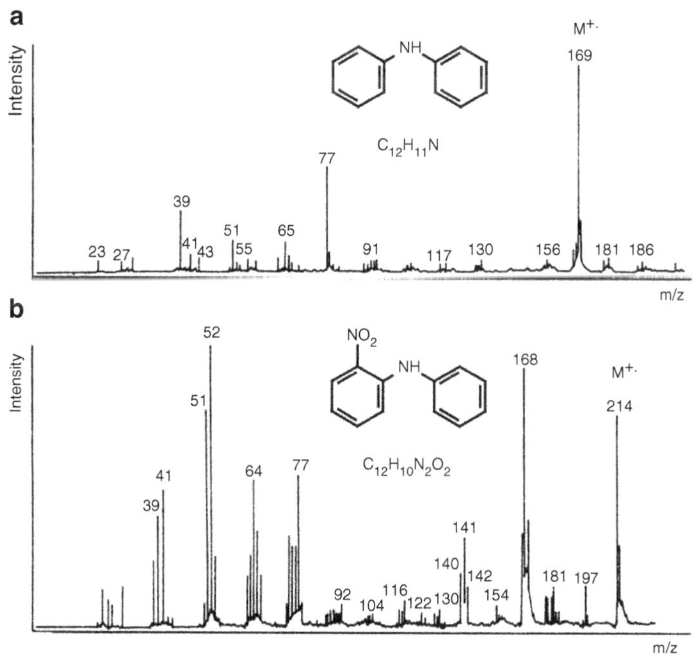

Fig. 10.3 MBSA spectra of (**a**) diphenylamine and (**b**) *N*-(2-nitrophenyl-)aniline. Both spectra show prominent molecular ion peaks of the compounds, i.e., in (**a**) *m/z* 169 corresponding to $[C_{12}H_{11}N]^{+\bullet}$ and in (**b**) *m/z* 214 due to $[C_{12}H_{10}N_2O_2]^{+\bullet}$ (Adapted from Ref. [7] by permission. © Wiley, 1982)

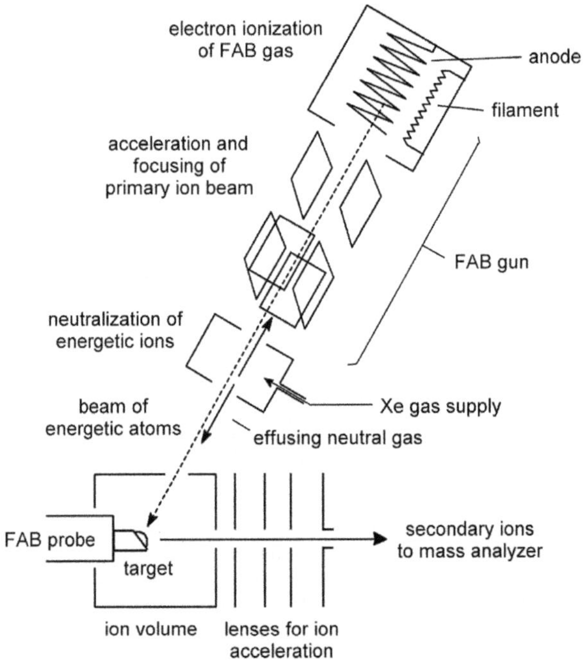

Fig. 10.4 Schematic of a FAB ion source and a FAB gun

neutrals hit the exposed surface with high kinetic energy. The fact that neutralization is not quantitative is not an issue as long electrostatic charging of the sample is avoided [26]. Ion guns for the generation of energetic noble gas ions can therefore be employed without disadvantage [31]. Xenon is preferred over argon and neon as FAB gas [32, 33], because it transfers a higher momentum when impacting onto the surface at equal kinetic energy (Fig. 10.5).

Similarity of FAB and MBSA

Having read the description on the design and operation of the FAB gun and the FAB ion source, you will have noticed the close similarities of MBSA and early FAB instrumentation. The Barber group developed the technique to full maturity and introduced the liquid matrix as the decisive detail enabling the analysis of high-mass, polar, and even ionic analytes by FAB-MS.

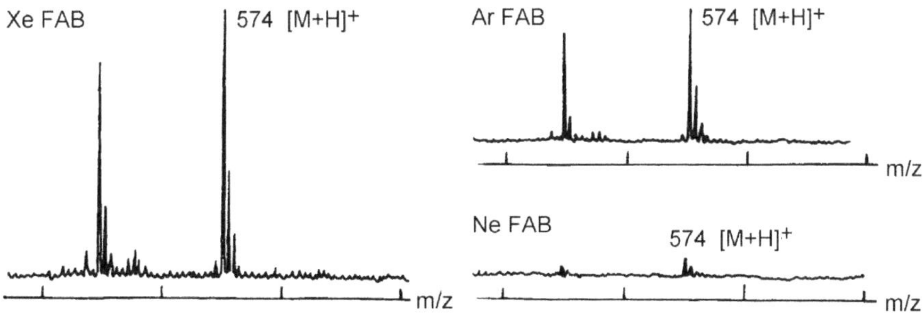

Fig. 10.5 Comparison of the efficiency of xenon, argon, and neon FAB gas for the FAB mass spectrum of the small peptide Met-enkephalin. The intensities are in scale (Reproduced from Ref. [32] by permission. © Elsevier Science, 1983)

Load to the vacuum system

Effusing FAB gas and evaporating matrix present an additional load to the high vacuum pump of the ion source housing, necessitating sufficient pumping speed (300–500 l s^{-1}) for stable operation. In contrast to EI and CI ion sources, FAB ion sources are operated without heating to reduce evaporation of the matrix and thermal stress of the analyte. Accordingly, the ion source is contaminated with matrix. Often, ion sources are constructed as EI/CI/FAB combination ion sources. After FAB measurements, it is therefore recommended to heat and pump the ion source overnight prior to EI or CI operation.

10.3.2 LSIMS Ion Sources

As mentioned before, primary ions can also be employed to provide the energy for secondary ion emission when organic compounds are admixed to a liquid matrix [18–20]. Cs^+ ions are preferentially used in organic *liquid secondary ion mass spectrometry* (LSIMS). The Cs^+ ions are produced by *thermal ionization* (Sect. 15.2) from a surface coated with cesium alumina silicate or other cesium salts [18]. Temperatures of about 1000°C are necessary to generate a sufficient flow of primary ions, and thus precautions must be taken to shield the LSIMS ion source from that heat. The Cs^+ ions are extracted, accelerated, and focused onto the target as usual by electrostatic lenses [34–36]. An advantage of Cs^+ ion guns is that the beam energy can be more widely varied, e.g., in the 5–25 keV range, in order to adjust for optimized secondary ion emission [36]. Especially with high-mass analytes, Cs^+ ion guns generally yield superior ion emission as compared to Xe FAB [26]. In order to further increase the momentum of the primary ions, gold negative atomic ions [37], as well as molecular and massive cluster ions (Sect. 10.8) have been used as primary ions.

10.3.3 FAB Probes

The analyte, either solid or admixed to some liquid matrix, is introduced into the FAB ion source by means of a probe bearing a sample holder or *FAB target*. The FAB target usually is a stainless steel or copper tip that exposes the analyte at some angle (30–60°) to the fast atom beam. The target can have a plane or more specifically cup-shaped surface to hold a 1–3 μl drop of matrix/analyte mixture (Fig. 10.6). Normally, the target is maintained at ion source temperature, i.e., only slightly above ambient temperature. Heating or – more importantly – cooling can be provided with special FAB probes only (Sect. 10.6.5).

10.3.4 Sample Preparation for FAB and LSIMS

Despite the fact that the small amount of matrix on the tip of the probe employed to introduce the sample into the ion source, sample preparation for FAB or LSIMS is quite simple.

Sample preparation usually works best when the analyte can be dissolved in a suitable solvent as to produce a solution of about 1 mg ml^{-1} which is then admixed to the matrix. This can directly be performed on the tip by placing 1–2 μl of analyte solution on top of a 1–3 μl drop of matrix.

The probe is inserted into the vacuum lock after most of the solvent has evaporated, which generally takes just half a minute. Residual solvent is quickly removed during roughing just before the lock opens towards the high vacuum of the ion source housing.

Alternatively, some tiny crystals of the analyte may directly be dissolved in the matrix. To do so, the tip of a fine pin or needle is first dipped into the analyte and

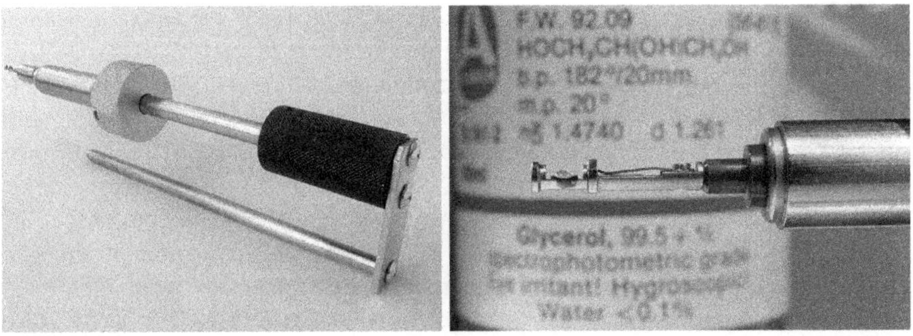

Fig. 10.6 FAB probe of a JEOL JMS-700 magnetic sector instrument (*left*). The probe tip with a drop of glycerol placed onto the exchangeable stainless steel FAB target (*right*)

then transferred and dipped into the matrix. Gentle stirring of the matrix drop helps to dissipate and dissolve the analyte. This may analogously be applied to high-boiling liquid or viscous samples.

10.4 Ion Formation in FAB and LSIMS

10.4.1 Ion Formation from Inorganic Samples

The energy provided by the impacting primary particle causes a collision cascade in the upper atomic or molecular layers of the sample. Within 30–60 ps, a cylindrical expansion is effected in the sample along the path of penetration [19]. Not all of this energy is dissipated and absorbed in deeper sample layers. A portion is directed toward the surface, where it effects ejection of material into the vacuum (Fig. 10.7) [21]. Due to the primary particle flux employed, this mode of operation corresponds to the *dynamic SIMS* mode as described in Sect. 15.6 in more detail.

In case of a bulk inorganic salt such as cesium iodide, Cs^+ and I^- ions are heading away from the surface [38]. Those ions having the suitable polarity are attracted by the extraction/acceleration voltage, those of opposite charge sign are pushed back onto the surface. Held together by strong interionic forces, ionic clusters may desorb as such or dissociate in the liquid–gas interface layer due to their internal energy content.

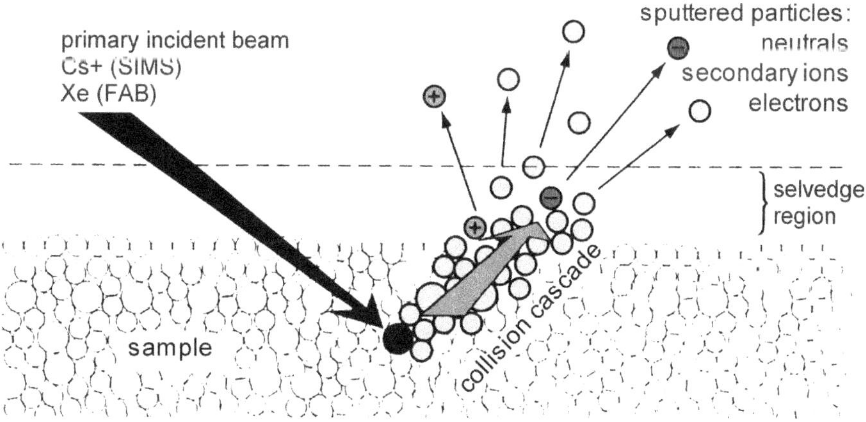

Fig. 10.7 Simple illustration of an instantaneous collision cascade generated as a result of primary particle impact in desorption/ionization mass spectrometry (Adapted from Ref. [21] by permission. © John Wiley & Sons, 1995)

FAB/SIMS of inorganic compounds Bombardment of cesium iodide or gold delivers cluster ion series which are useful for mass calibration of the instrument over a wide range. CsI works equally well in positive- and negative-ion mode to yield $[(CsI)_nCs]^+$ and $[(CsI)_nI]^-$ cluster ions, respectively (Fig. 10.8). Starting from $n = 0$, $[(CsI)_nCs]^+$ cluster ions have been observed up to *m/z* 90,000 [38]. Larger $[(CsI)_nCs]^+$ cluster ions dissociate to yield smaller ones: $[(CsI)_nCs]^+ \rightarrow [(CsI)_{n-x}Cs]^+ + (CsI)_x$ [39]. Gold produces a negative $Au_n^{-\bullet}$ cluster ion series up to about *m/z* 10,000 [40].

Monoisotopic standards
Cs, I, and Au are all monoisotopic. This presents an advantage in that it assures the peak top to exactly represent the theoretical isotopic mass of the respective cluster ion, independent of its *m/z* ratio or actual resolution (Sects. 3.2 and 3.4). CsI, KI, and other alkali salts that provide more narrow-spaced cluster ion series can alternatively be employed as saturated solutions in glycerol [41–43].

10.4.2 Ion Formation from Organic Samples

According to Todd "it is a common feature of FAB and LSIMS that they defy any generally acceptable mechanistic description" [44]. Unlike EI or CI, where ions are generated from gaseous molecules, desorption/ionization techniques involve a state transition from liquid or solid to the gas phase *and* ionization of neutral molecules. Nonetheless, reviews dealing with the processes of desorption and ion formation

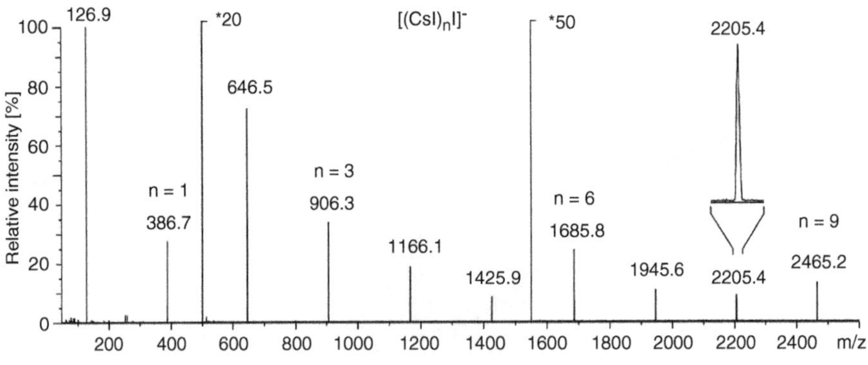

Fig. 10.8 Negative-ion FAB spectrum of solid CsI. The monoisotopic $[(CsI)_nI]^-$ cluster ion series (cf. expanded view of *m/z* 2205.4) is well suited for calibrating a wide mass range

under FAB and LSIMS conditions offer some insight [19–21]. Basically, there are two major concepts, the *chemical ionization model* on one side [44–48], and the *precursor model* on the other [48–52].

The *chemical ionization model* of FAB assumes the formation of analyte ions to occur in the liquid–gas interface layer some micrometers above the liquid matrix. In this space, a plasma state similar to the reagent gas plasma in chemical ionization can exist powered by the quasi-continuous supply of energy from a stream of impacting primary particles. The present reactive species may undergo numerous bimolecular reactions, the most interesting of them being the protonation of analyte molecules to yield $[M + H]^+$ ions. Plasma conditions could also explain the observation of $M^{+\bullet}$ and $M^{-\bullet}$ radical ions as formed in case of low-polarity analytes. Here, the primary particle beam serves to sputter material from the liquid surface and to subsequently ionize neutrals by particle impact (cf. EI, Sect 5.1) in the gas phase. Matrix molecules, preferably ionized for statistical reasons, may then act as reagent ions to effect CI of the gaseous analyte. Striking arguments for this model are the facts that ion formation largely depends on the presence of gaseous matrix [45, 46], and that FAB spectra of volatile analytes are closely similar to the corresponding CI spectra [48].

The *precursor model* of FAB applies well to ionic analytes and samples that are easily converted to ionic species within the liquid matrix, e.g., by protonation or deprotonation or due to cationization. Those *preformed ions* would simply have to be desorbed into the gas phase (Fig. 10.9). The promoting effect of decreasing pH (added acid) on $[M + H]^+$ ion yield of porphyrins and other analytes supports the precursor ion model [51, 52]. The relative intensities of $[M + H]^+$ ions in FAB spectra of aliphatic amine mixtures also do not depend to the partial pressure of the amines in the gas phase, but are sensitive on the acidity of the matrix [53]. Furthermore, incomplete desolvation of preformed ions nicely explains the observation of matrix (Ma) adducts such as $[M + Ma + H]^+$ ions. The precursor model bears some similarities to ion evaporation in field desorption (Sect. 8.6).

Many neutrals, few ions

It has been estimated that a single impact causes the eruption of about 10^3 secondary neutrals, but yields only 0.02–1.5 ions [42, 44, 53, 54]. The ions are then heading away from the surface in a *supersonic expansion* at speeds of about 1000 m s^{-1} [19, 42].

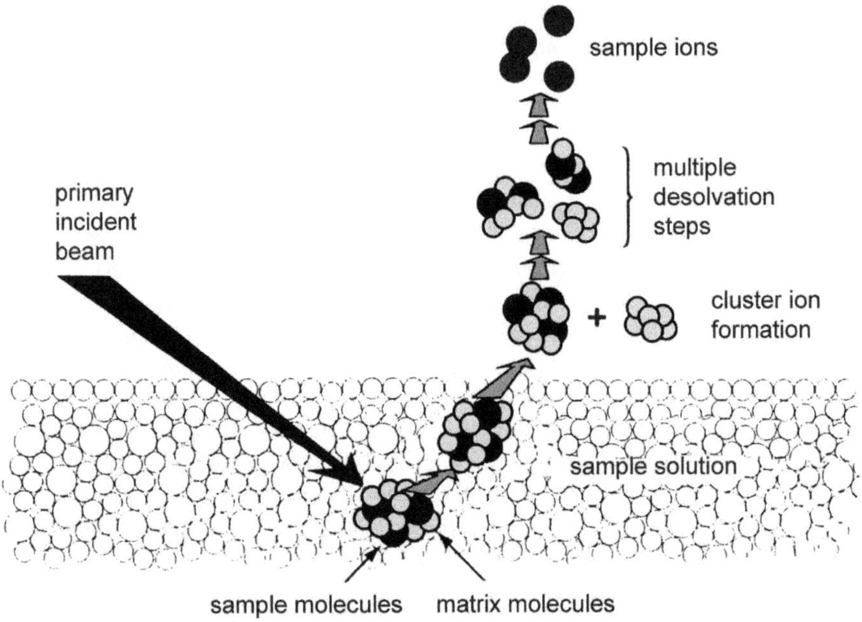

Fig. 10.9 In LSIMS and FAB, sample–matrix cluster ion formation and desolvation processes occur on a longer time scale (Adapted from Ref. [21] by permission. © John Wiley & Sons, 1995)

10.5 Liquid Matrices for FAB and LSIMS

10.5.1 The Role of the Liquid Matrix

Soon after the first use of a glycerol matrix, the importance of a liquid matrix for FAB was recognized [14]. Other organic solvents of low volatility were explored in order to obtain better spectra. The tasks of the matrix are numerous [19, 20, 33, 55, 56]:

- It has to absorb the primary energy.
- By solvation it helps to overcome intermolecular forces between analyte molecules or ions.
- The liquid matrix provides a continuously refreshing and long-lasting supply of analyte.
- It assists analyte ion formation, e.g., by yielding proton donating/accepting or electron donating/accepting species upon bombardment.

Nowadays, numerous matrices are in use (Table 10.2). Several reviews on FAB matrices in general [16, 17, 55–57] and papers on special matrices [15, 58, 59] have been published.

Table 10.2 Matrices for FAB-MS

Matrix	Uses	References
3-Nitrobenzyl alcohol (NBA)	Highly versatile, general purpose, medium polarity, first trial	[60–62]
2-Nitrophenyl octylether (NPOE)	General purpose, aprotic matrix	[15, 60]
Glycerol	Polar matrix, good for internal calibration on matrix signals	
Thioglycerol	Peptides, reductive character	[13]
"Magic bullet" (eutectic 5:1 mixture of dithiothreitol/dithioerythritol)	Peptides, small proteins, reductive character	[63]
Triethanolamine (TEA)	Basic, highly polar matrix, good for $[M - H]^-$ production	[15]
Di-, tri-, and tetraethyleneglycols	Polar, less volatile than glycerol	[13, 15]
Liquid paraffin	Aprotic, inert	[64–66]
Sulfolane	Effective solvent, rather volatile	[67, 68]
Concentrated sulfuric acid	Highly acidic, good for internal calibration on matrix signals	[69]

Scheme 10.1

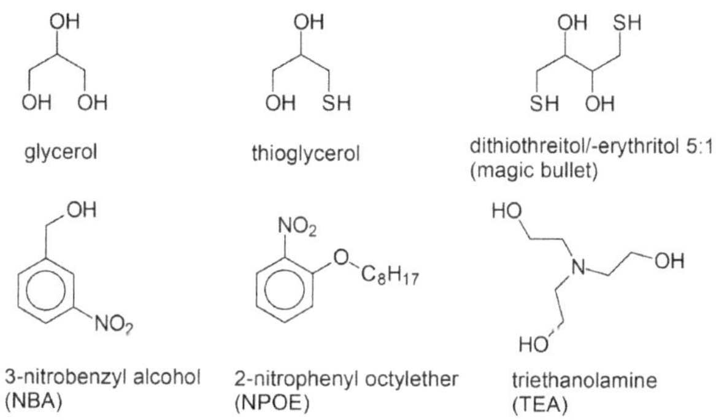

An ideal FAB matrix should fulfill the following criteria [19, 20, 33, 55, 56] (Scheme 10.1):

- The analyte should be soluble in the matrix. Otherwise, addition of co-solvents, e.g., dimethylformamide (DMF), dimethylsulfoxide (DMSO), or other additives [70, 71] can become necessary.
- Only low-vapor pressure solvents can be easily used as a matrix in FAB. In principle, volatile solvents can be employed, provided a stable surface can be obtained on the time scale of recording a mass spectrum.
- The viscosity of the solvent must be low enough to ensure the diffusion of the solutes to the surface [72].
- Ions from the matrix itself should be as unobtrusive as possible in the resulting FAB spectrum.
- The matrix itself has to be chemically inert. However, specific ion formation reactions promoting secondary ion yield are advantageous.

Note

A great advantage of FAB is that the matrix can be perfectly adapted to the analyte's requirements. On the other hand, using the wrong matrix can result in complete suppression of analytically useful signals.

10.5.2 FAB Matrix Spectra: General Characteristics

FAB matrix spectra are generally characterized by a series of matrix (Ma) cluster ions accompanied by some more abundant fragment ions in the lower *m*/*z* range. In positive-ion FAB, $[Ma_n + H]^+$ cluster ions predominate, while $[Ma_n - H]^-$ cluster ions are preferably formed in negative-ion FAB (Fig. 10.10). The principal ion series may be accompanied by $[Ma_n + alkali]^+$ ions and some fragments of minor intensity, e.g., $[Ma_n + H - H_2O]^+$. The fragment ions detected below the $[Ma + H]^+$ ion, which normally also gives rise to the base peak, are almost the same as

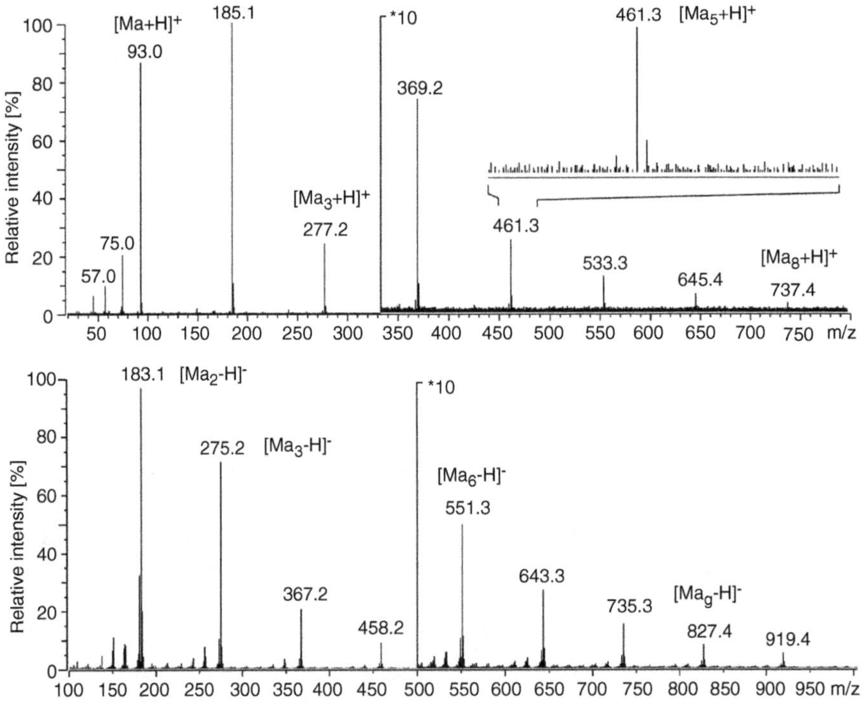

Fig. 10.10 FAB spectra of neat glycerol, $M_r = 92$ u. (**a**) Positive ions (for the positive-ion CI spectrum of glycerol, see Sect. 7.2.5); (**b**) negative ions. The expanded view in (**a**) shows the "peak at every *m*/*z*-character" of FAB spectra

observed in the positive-ion CI mass spectrum of the respective matrix compound [42].

In addition to the prominent cluster ions, radiolytic decomposition of the matrix generates an enormous number of different ions, radicals, and cluster ions resulting thereof [73, 74]. Despite being of minor intensity, they contribute to the "peak at every *m/z*-character" of FAB spectra, i.e., there is significant *chemical noise* (Sects. 1.6 and 5.2.4) [75, 76]. During elongated measurements, the changes of the matrix spectrum due to increasing radiolytic decay are clearly visible [73]. High kinetic energy of impacting primary particles combined with reduced particle flux seem to diminish destructive effects of irradiation [77].

10.5.3 Unwanted Reactions in FAB-MS

The conditions of the FAB process also promote unwanted reactions between analyte and matrix. Even though such processes are not relevant in the majority of FAB measurements, one should be aware of them. Besides addition or condensation reactions with matrix fragment ions [78, 79], reduction [80–83] and dehalogenation [84, 85] of the analyte represent the more prominent side-reactions in FAB. Electron transfer causing the reduction of otherwise doubly charged ions have also been observed [43].

10.6 Applications of FAB-MS

10.6.1 FAB-MS of Analytes of Low to Medium Polarity

The FAB plasma provides conditions that allow to ionize molecules by either loss or addition of an electron to form positive molecular ions, $M^{+\bullet}$ [48, 86], or negative molecular ions, $M^{-\bullet}$, respectively. Alternatively, protonation or deprotonation may result in $[M + H]^+$ or $[M - H]^-$ ions. Their occurrence is determined by the respective basicity or acidity of analyte and matrix. Cationization, preferably with alkali metal ions, is also frequently observed. Often, $[M + H]^+$ ions are accompanied by $[M + Na]^+$ and $[M + K]^+$ ions as already noted with FD-MS (Sect. 8.6). Furthermore, the joint occurrence of both $M^{+\bullet}$ and $[M + H]^+$ ions of one compound is not unusual [48]. In case of simple aromatic amines, for example, the peak intensity ratio $M^{+\bullet}/[M + H]^+$ increases as the ionization energy of the substrate decreases, whereas 4-substituted benzophenones show preferential formation of $[M + H]^+$ ions, regardless of the nature of the substituents [87]. It can be assumed that protonation is initiated when the benzophenone carbonyl groups form hydrogen bonds with the matrix.

Exchangeable protons can be replaced by alkali ions without affecting the charge state of a molecule. Thus, $[M - H_n + \text{alkali}_{n+1}]^+$ and $[M - H_n + \text{alkali}_{n-1}]^-$ ions can also be observed if one or more acidic hydrogens are easily exchanged [5, 18, 43, 71, 88, 89]. The addition of cation exchange resins or crown ethers may help to reduce alkali ion contaminations [90]. Double protonation to yield $[M + 2H]^{2+}$ ions or double cationization [43] are only observed with high-mass analytes [91, 92] and otherwise remain an exception in FAB. Which of the above processes will most effectively contribute to the total ion yield strongly depends on the actual analyte–matrix pair.

FAB spectrum of tetramesitylporphyrin The positive-ion FAB spectrum of tetramesitylporphyrin, $C_{56}H_{54}N_4$, in NBA matrix exhibits $M^{+\bullet}$ and $[M + H]^+$ ions (Fig. 10.11) [93]. The presence of both species can be recognized by comparison of experimental and calculated M + 1 ion intensity. This difference is due to about 20% $[M + H]^+$ ion formation. The diffuse groups of signals around *m/z* 900 reveal the formation of some adduct ions with the matrix, e.g., $[M + Ma + H - H_2O]^+$ at *m/z* 918.

FAB spectra of polyethyleneglycols Polyethyleneglycols (PEGs) of average molecular weights up to about 2,000 u are well soluble in NBA. Resulting from their flexible polyether chain, $H(OCH_2CH_2)_nOH$, PEGs are easily cationized by loose complexation with Na^+ or K^+ ions. Traces of alkali salts are sufficient to prefer $[M + alkali]^+$ over $[M + H]^+$ ions. The positive-ion FAB spectrum of PEG 600 in NBA nicely shows the molecular weight distribution of the oligomer (Fig. 10.12). The peaks belonging to the same series are displayed at 44 u distance.

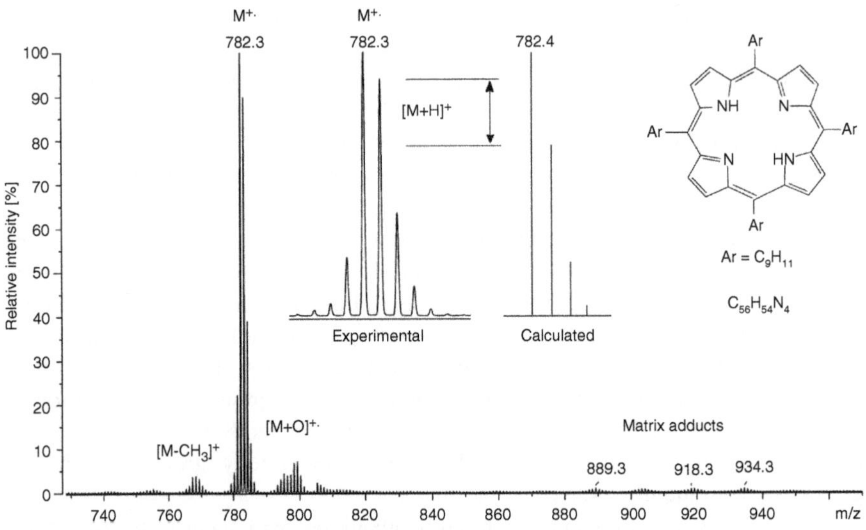

Fig. 10.11 Partial positive-ion FAB spectrum of a tetramesitylporphyrin in NBA matrix. Comparison of the experimental and calculated isotopic patterns reveals the presence of $M^{+\bullet}$ and $[M + H]^+$ ions (Adapted from Ref. [93] by permission. © IM Publications, 1997)

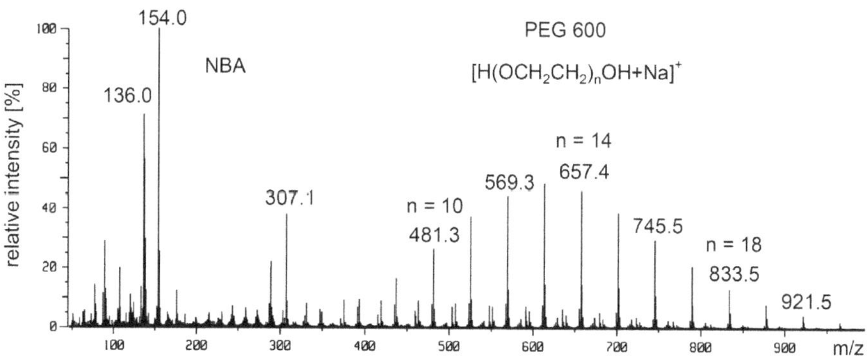

Fig. 10.12 Positive-ion FAB spectrum of polyethyleneglycol of average molecular weight 600 u (PEG 600) in NBA matrix

10.6.2 FAB-MS of Ionic Analytes

FAB is well suited for the analysis of ionic analytes. In positive-ion mode, the spectrum is usually dominated by the cationic species, C^+, which is accompanied by cluster ions of the general composition $[C_n + A_{n-1}]^+$. Thus, the distance between these signals corresponds to the complete salt [CA], i.e., yields its "molecular" weight. This behavior is perfectly analogous to FD (Sect. 8.6). In negative-ion FAB, the anion A^- will cause the base peak of the spectrum, and accordingly, cluster ions of the type $[C_{n-1} + A_n]^-$ are formed in addition. Consequently, both cation and anion are usually identified from the same FAB spectrum, irrespective of the chosen polarity. Nonetheless, it is common practice to select the polarity of the more interesting ion for the measurement.

Provided the salt is sufficiently soluble in the matrix, the signals normally exhibit high intensity as compared to those of the matrix. This result is consistent with the model of preformed ions in solution that only need to be desorbed into the gas phase.

Organic salts analysis by positive-ion FAB-MS The positive-ion FAB spectrum of an immonium perchlorate, $[C_{14}H_{16}N]^+ \; ClO_4^-$ [94], dissolved in NBA is dominated by the immonium ion (C^+) at *m/z* 198 (Fig. 10.13). The perchlorate counterion can well be identified from the cluster ions $[2C + A]^+$, *m/z* 495, and $[3C + 2A]^+$, *m/z* 792. The signal at *m/z* 495 is expanded to demonstrate that chlorine is readily recognized from its isotopic pattern (Sect. 3.2.4).

Organic salts analysis by negative-ion FAB-MS The Bunte salt $[CH_3(CH_2)_{15}S\text{-}SO_3]^- \; Na^+$ yields a very useful negative-ion FAB spectrum from NBA matrix (Fig. 10.14). NBA forms $[Ma - H]^-$ and $Ma^{-\bullet}$ ions. The salt anion contributes the base peak at *m/z* 337.3. $[C + 2A]^-$, *m/z* 697.5, and $[2C + 3A]^-$, *m/z* 1057.6, cluster

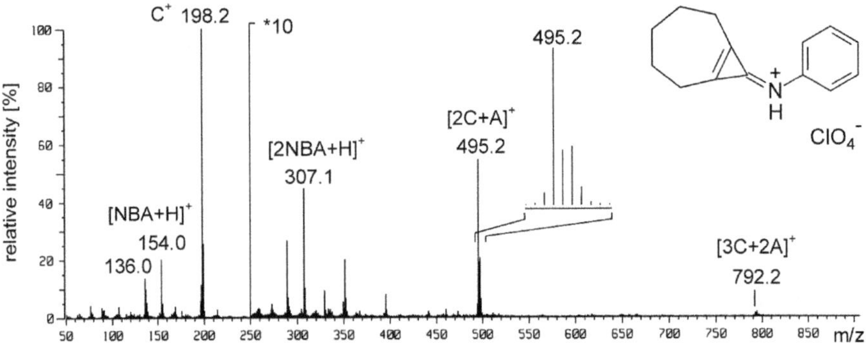

Fig. 10.13 Positive-ion FAB spectrum of an immonium salt [94]. The perchlorate counterion can well be identified from the first and second cluster ion (By courtesy of H. Irngartinger, University of Heidelberg)

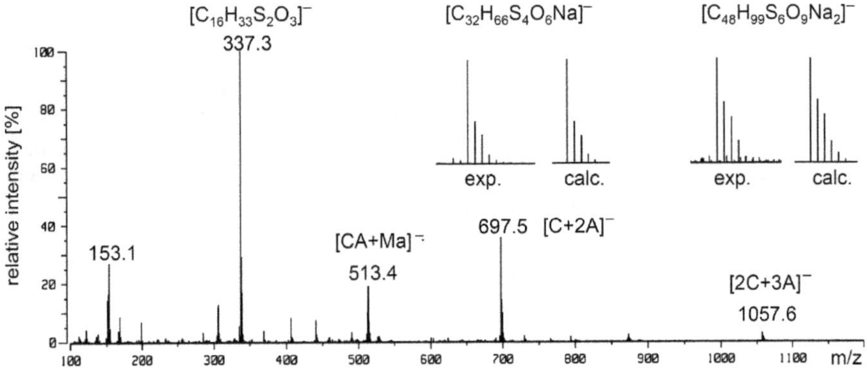

Fig. 10.14 Negative-ion FAB mass spectra of a Bunte salt. The *insets* compare experimental and calculated isotopic patterns of the $[C + 2A]^-$ and $[2C + 3A]^-$ cluster ions (By courtesy of M. Grunze, University of Heidelberg)

ions are observed in addition, their isotopic patterns being in good agreement with theoretical expectation. It is noteworthy that the matrix adduct at *m/z* 513.4 is a negative radical ion.

10.6.3 High-Mass Analytes in FAB-MS

FAB is chiefly applied to analytes up to about *m/z* 3000, but significantly heavier ions are sometimes accessible. The upper limit surely has been demonstrated by the detection of $[(CsI)_nCs]^+$ cluster ions up to *m/z* 90,000 [38]. In case of organic molecules, $[M + H]^+$, $[M + 2H]^{2+}$, and $[M + 3H]^{3+}$ of porcine trypsin, a protein of $M_r = 23{,}463$ u, have been the highest hitherto detected ions on record [92]. FAB spectra of peptides and small proteins in the *m/z* 3000–6000 range are more commonly reported [13, 91, 95], and the FAB spectrum of a dendrimer of 7,000 u has also been published [96].

Supramolecular chemistry Inclusion complexes of [60]fullerene, C_{60} [63], of its oxides $C_{60}O$, $C_{60}O_2$, and $C_{60}O_3$ [97], and of several cycloaddition products of the fullerene [98] in γ-cyclodextrin (γ-CD) can be analyzed by negative-ion FAB-MS using "magic bullet" matrix [63]. As one fullerene molecule is enclosed between two γ-CD units, the $[M - H]^-$ ions of these host-guest complexes [99] are detected starting from $[C_{156}H_{159}O_{80}]^-$ (peak of monoisotopic ion expected at *m/z* 3311.8, Fig. 10.15).

Selecting the matrix
The choice of the matrix is determined by the outer sphere of the analyte molecules, i.e., by γ-CD in case of the above inclusion complexes [60]. Fullerene and its oxides yield poor spectra in "magic bullet", but work well with less polar matrices such as NBA and NPOE.

10.6.4 Accurate Mass Measurements in FAB Mode

FAB produces long-lasting signals of sufficient intensity, thereby allowing to set magnetic sector instruments to 5,000–10,000 resolving power as needed for

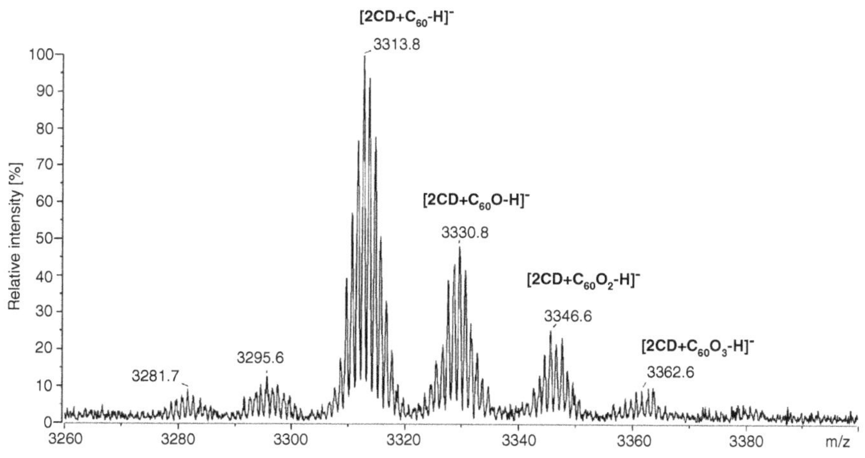

Fig. 10.15 Partial negative-ion FAB spectrum of γ–CD fullerene complexes in "magic bullet" matrix (Reproduced from Ref. [97] by permission. © IM Publications, 1998)

accurate mass measurements. In the range up to about *m*/*z* 600, internal calibration can sometimes be achieved by using the matrix peaks as mass reference, but the admixture of other mass calibrants to the matrix–analyte solution is normally preferred. PEGs are frequently employed for calibration purposes. Then, mass reference peaks are evenly spaced over the *m*/*z* range of interest (44 u distant in case of PEG, cf. Fig. 10.12) and their intensity can be adjusted to approximate those of the analyte. However, the mass calibrant can only be admixed if unwanted reactions with the analyte do not occur. In particular, in case of badly soluble analytes, complete suppression of the analyte signals by the added calibrant may pose a problem.

Accurate mass measurements The positive-ion high-resolution (HR) FAB spectrum of a cationic fluorescent marker dye shows the signal of the analyte ion enclosed by a set of mass reference peaks due to the admixture of PEG 600 (Fig. 10.16). The elemental composition of the analyte can be assigned with good accuracy: exp. *m*/*z* 663.3182, calc. *m*/*z* 663.3153 for $[C_{37}H_{42}O_4N_4F_3]^+$; exp. *m*/*z* 664.3189, calc. *m*/*z* 664.3184 for $[^{13}C^{12}C_{36}H_{42}O_4N_4F_3]^+$.

Provided a (magnetic sector) mass spectrometer offers very good scan-to-scan reproducibility of mass calibration, there is no absolute necessity to admix the mass calibrant to the analyte. Instead, alternating scans on analyte and calibrant offer almost the same level of accuracy. The simplest technical realization of such a *pseudo-internal calibration* is changing the target without interruption of the measurement [100]. The use of a *dual-target* FAB probe (DTP), having a split or double-sided target offering two separated positions, is preferable [101]. Switching between both positions is then achieved by rotating the probe axially between successive scans. The resulting *total ion chromatogram* (TIC) typically has a saw-tooth appearance (Fig. 10.17). Calibration of the analyte spectra is performed by transferring the internal calibration of the mass reference scan(s) to the successive scan(s) on the analyte. The advantages of a DTP are:

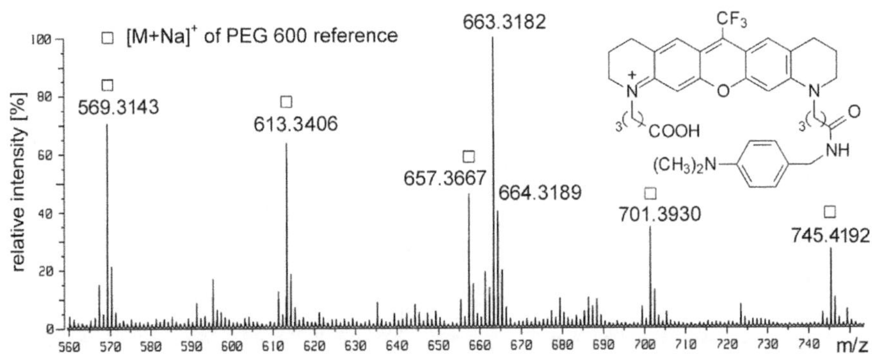

Fig. 10.16 Positive-ion FAB spectrum of a cationic fluorescent marker dye with PEG 600 admixed for internal mass calibration (By courtesy of K. H. Drexhage, University of Siegen and J. Wolfrum, Heidelberg University)

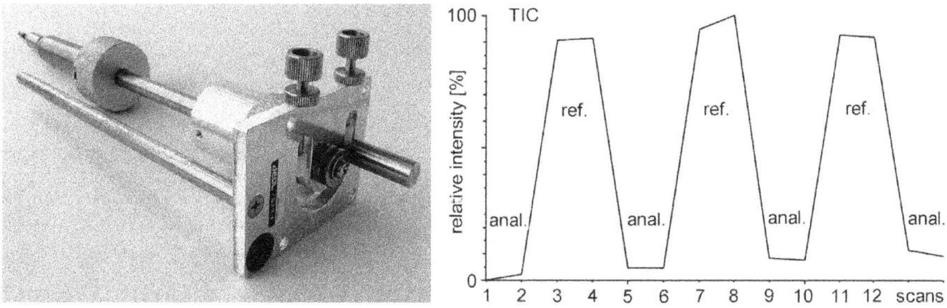

Fig. 10.17 FAB dual-target probe with handle for 180° axial turns (*left*) and TIC of a HR-FAB measurement using this probe (*right*)

- Interference of reference and analyte signals is excluded independent of the resolving power used.
- Mutual suppression of reference and analyte are avoided.
- There is no need to adjust the relative intensities of analyte and calibrant peaks very closely.
- Even otherwise reactive calibrants can be employed due to spatial separation from the analyte [102].

Magnets need time to accommodate
Scanning of a magnet is affected by hysteresis. This improves the reproducibility of mass calibration after several scan cycles. For best results with dual-target probes, it is therefore recommended to skip the first few scans.

10.6.5 Low-Temperature FAB

Originally, cooled FAB probes were designed to prolong the acquisition time for FAB measurements with more volatile matrices [103]. Research on sputtering processes from solid gases [104, 105] and studies of cluster ion formation from solid or deeply cooled liquid alcohols [106–108] have contributed to FAB at cryogenic temperatures [109, 110]. *Low-temperature fast atom bombardment* (LT-FAB) of frozen aqueous solutions of metal salts provides a source of abundant hydrated metal ions [111–113]. Organic molecules can also be detected from their frozen solutions [114]. Such LT-FAB applications are particularly interesting when enabling the detection of species that would otherwise not be accessible by mass spectrometry, because they are either extremely air- and/or water-sensitive [115, 116] as the phosphaoxetane intermediate of the Wittig reaction [117] or insoluble in standard FAB matrices [102, 118].

LT-FAB consumes somewhat higher amounts of sample than FAB at ambient temperature because standard solvents are less effective than conventional matrices. Thus, the analytes should be dissolved to yield 0.5–3.0 μg μl^{-1} solutions. About 3 μl of solution are deposited on the FAB probe tip and frozen. There are two modes for freezing the sample–matrix mixture: (i) by cooling the target with cold nitrogen gas inside a custom-made vacuum lock before application of the sample [115, 117] or (ii) by simply immersing the target with the drop of solution into liquid nitrogen for about 30 s prior to transfer into the vacuum lock (Fig. 10.18) [102, 109, 110, 116, 119]. LT-FAB mass spectra are then obtained during thawing of frozen solutions inside the FAB ion source, which allows to employ almost any solvent as matrix in LT-FAB-MS. Consequently, neither volatility nor unwanted chemical reactions with the matrix restrict the choice of a matrix. Instead, the solvent matrix may be tailored to the analyte's requirements.

LT-FAB for highly reactive species Selective activation of C–H bonds is rarely observed in saturated alkyl groups. However, iridium complex **1** simply reacts by C–H insertion of the metal into a ligand bond upon treatment with LiBr in solution. The reaction can be tracked by LT-FAB-MS (Fig. 10.19). Decreasing intensity of the molecular ion of **1**, *m*/*z* 812.4, and increasing intensity of $M^{+\bullet}$ of **2**, *m*/*z* 856.4, indicate the progress of this reaction. Furthermore, the halogen exchange is reflected by the changing isotopic pattern.

10.6.6 FAB-MS and Peptide Sequencing

The ability of FAB mass spectra to deliver peptide sequence information was soon recognized [12, 120]. Initially, the sequence was derived from fragment ions observed in the full scan spectra [12, 95]. Another approach to sequence information is to subject the protein to enzymatic hydrolysis by a mixture of several carboxy-peptidases to produce a series of truncated molecules, i.e. of peptides.

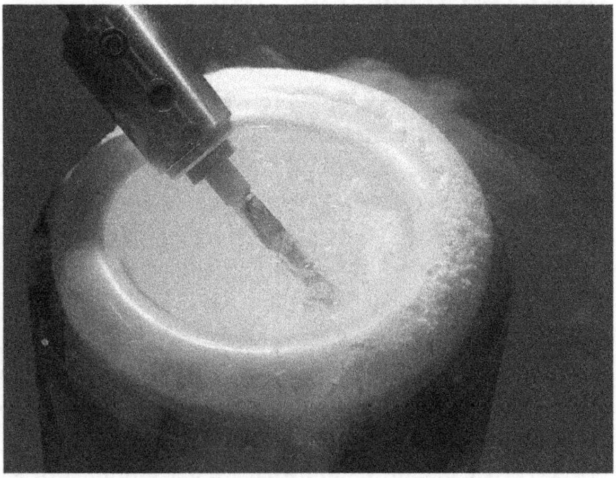

Fig. 10.18 Getting ready for LT-FAB by immersion of a FAB target with sample solution into liquid nitrogen. After about 30 s the solvent matrix is deeply frozen and the tip is cooled to allow for transfer of the probe into the vacuum lock and further into the ion source whilst avoiding untimely thawing of the solvent

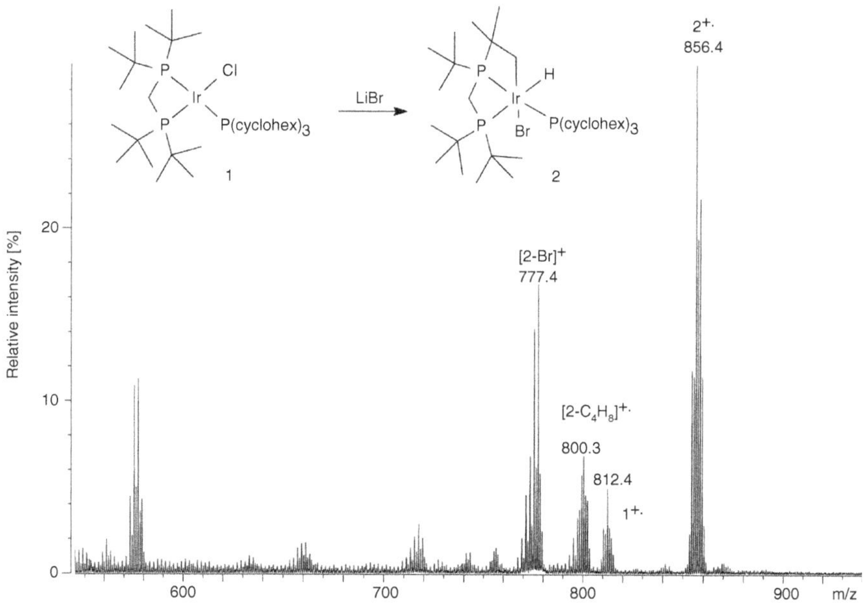

Fig. 10.19 Partial LT-FAB mass spectrum of the reaction mixture containing the iridium complexes **1** and **2** in toluene. In addition to the changes in mass, the isotopic pattern changes upon exchange of Cl by Br (By courtesy of P. Hofmann, Heidelberg University)

The FAB spectrum of the peptide mixture then reveals the *C*-terminal sequence [121, 122]. In the MALDI community, this approach became known as *peptide ladder sequencing* [123].

As protein ions are too big to effect fragmentation by collision-induced dissociation (CID, Sect. 9.3), they are enzymatically degraded to peptides prior to their mass spectrometric examination, e.g., by tryptic digestion [124]. The digest may be used directly to obtain MS/MS spectra of peptide $[M + H]^+$ or $[M + Na]^+$ ions. Alternatively, the peptides may be separated by *liquid chromatography* (LC), *capillary electrophoresis* (CE) [125], or *2D gel electrophoresis* prior to MS.

Nowadays, sequencing of peptides and other biopolymers by tandem mass spectrometry represents a major field of work for many mass spectrometrists [126–129]; FAB and LSIMS no longer play a role here (for an example of peptide sequencing by FAB-MS cf. Sect. 9.6.6).

10.7 FAB and LSIMS: General Characteristics

10.7.1 Sensitivity of FAB-MS

In FAB mode, the sensitivity (Sect. 1.6) is more difficult to specify than for other ionization methods, because the intensity of a signal strongly depends on the actual preparation on the target. Magnetic sector instruments yield ion currents of about 10^{-11}–10^{-10} A on matrix ions at $R = 1000$. Significantly lower Figs. (10^{-15}–10^{-14} A) are obtained for the $[M + H]^+$ ion of bovine insulin, *m/z* 5734.6, at $R = 6000$. Accordingly, the detection limits vary depending on the solubility of the analyte and the ease to achieve some sort of ionization if not already ionic at all.

10.7.2 Types of Ions in FAB-MS

FAB produces a variety of ions depending on the polarity and on the ionization energy of the analyte as well as on the presence or absence of impurities such as alkali metal ions [126]. However, with some knowledge of the types of ions formed, reasonable compositions can be assigned to the signals (Table 10.3).

10.7.3 Analytes for FAB-MS

For FAB/LSIMS, the analyte should be soluble to at least 0.1 mg ml^{-1} in some solvent or even better directly in the matrix; concentrations of 0.1–3 μg $μl^{-1}$ in the matrix are ideal. In case of extremely low solubility, additives such as other solvents, acids, or surfactants can help [71].

The analyte may be neutral or ionic. Solutions containing metal salts, e.g., from buffers or excess of non-complexed metals, may cause a confusingly large number of signals due to multiple proton/metal exchange and adduct ion formation [88]. The mass range up to 3,000 u is easily covered by FAB, samples reaching up to about twice that mass still may work if sufficient solubility and some ease of ionization are combined.

Table 10.3 Ions formed by FAB/LSIMS

Analytes	Positive ions	Negative ions
Nonpolar	$M^{+\bullet}$	$M^{-\bullet}$
Medium polarity	$M^{+\bullet}$ and/or $[M + H]^+$, $[M + alkali]^+$ *Clusters* $[2 M]^{+\bullet}$ and/or $[2 M + H]^+$, $[2 M + alkali]^+$ *Adducts* $[M + Ma + H]^+$, $[M + Ma + alkali]^+$	$M^{-\bullet}$ and/or $[M - H]^-$ *Clusters* $[2 M]^{-\bullet}$ and/or $[2 M - H]^-$ *Adducts* $[M + Ma]^{-\bullet}$, $[M + Ma - H]^-$
Polar	$[M + H]^+$, $[M + alkali]^+$ *Clusters* $[nM + H]^+$, $[nM + alkali]^+$ *Adducts* $[M + Ma + H]^+$, $[M + Ma + alkali]^+$ *Exchange* $[M - H_n + alkali_{n+1}]^+$ *High-mass anal.* $[M + 2H]^{2+}$, $[M + 2alkali]^{2+}$	$[M - H]^-$ *Clusters* $[nM - H]^-$ *Adducts* $[M + Ma - H]^-$ *Exchange* $[M - H_n + alkali_{n-1}]^-$
Ionic[a]	C^+, $[C_n + A_{n-1}]^+$, rarely $[CA]^{+\bullet}$	A^-, $[C_{n-1} + A_n]^-$, rarely $[CA]^{-\bullet}$

[a]comprising cation C^+ and anion A^-

10.7.4 Mass Analyzers for FAB-MS

Double-focusing magnetic sector instruments represent the standard in FAB-MS, because they combine a suitable mass range with the ability to perform high-resolution and accurate mass measurements. Until the advent of ESI and MALDI, FAB-MS/MS on magnetic four-sector instruments was the method of choice for biomolecule sequencing [130–132]. Linear quadrupole [133] and triple quadrupole instruments have also been adapted to FAB ion sources. Other types of mass analyzers are rare exceptions with FAB or LSIMS ion sources.

10.7.5 Future Perspective for FAB and LSIMS

The strong interrelationship of double-focusing magnetic sector instruments and FAB or LSIMS is most probably the main cause of the extremely diminishing use of this otherwise valuable technique. Clearly, FAB and LSIMs were of highest relevance in the 1990s when the technique had reached maturity (Fig. 10.20). Similarly, as this type of mass analyzer has mostly been replaced by either oaTOF, Orbitrap, or FT-ICR systems, FAB is phasing out from mass spectrometry. This may very well be the last mass spectrometry textbook to include a dedicated chapter on FAB-MS and closely related techniques based on particle impact.

While FAB and LSIMS are highly useful and versatile "soft" methods, they have widely been replaced by matrix-assisted laser desorption/ionization (MALDI,

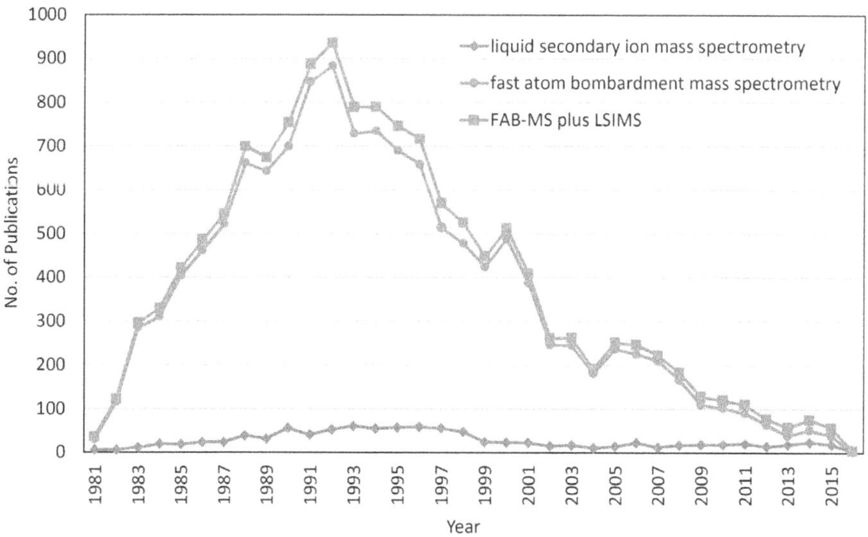

Fig. 10.20 Number of annual publications employing fast atom bombardment mass spectrometry or liquid secondary ion mass spectrometry along with total number of both techniques. Clearly, FAB dominated, while LSIMS had been playing a minor role; both had their greatest impact on MS in the 1990s (Data retrieved using CAS SciFinder software)

Chap. 11), electrospray ionization (ESI, Chap. 12), and related API techniques like atmospheric pressure chemical ionization (APCI), atmospheric pressure photoionization (APPI), direct analysis in real time (DART), and others.

10.8 Massive Cluster Impact

Massive cluster impact (MCI) mass spectrometry presents an additional means of generating secondary ions by bombardment of a surface [25]. Massive clusters of up to 10^8 u are generated by electrohydrodynamic ionization (Sect. 12.1) of an electrolyte/glycerol solution, e.g., 0.75 M ammonium acetate in glycerol. The resulting clusters consisting of about 10^6 glycerol molecules and bearing about 200 electron charges on the average are accelerated by a 10–20 kV high voltage [134]. Although those highly charged microdroplets carry megaelectronvolt kinetic energies, the translational energy per nucleon is only in the order of 1 eV, whereas it is about 50 eV per nucleon in the case of Xe FAB. A shock wave model is proposed to explain ion formation in MCI [135]. According to this model both the impacting cluster and the surface of the bulk or matrix-dissolved analyte are compressed to gigapascal pressures upon impact. Some mixing of analyte and impacting microdroplet can be demonstrated by the occurrence of analyte species cationized by the same ions used as electrolyte in the solution from which the massive clusters are generated. Nonetheless, a matrix effect due to accumulation of a thin layer of glycerol on the surface can be excluded [134]. Instead, dry sample preparations work equally well in MCI [134].

MCI has successfully been applied to analyze proteins up to about 17,000 u [136]. These form multiply charged ions, e.g., $[M + 6Na]^{6+}$, under the conditions of MCI [136]. Especially in the mass range of about 10^4 u, MCI is superior to FAB and LSIMS because it combines good signal intensity due to the enormous momentum of the impinging species with a remarkably low degree of ion fragmentation. Despite of its promising capabilities, MCI has been superseded by MALDI and ESI before it could receive widespread acceptance.

10.9 ^{252}Californium Plasma Desorption

Historically, ^{252}*Californium plasma desorption* (^{252}Cf-PD) was the next desorption /ionization method to be introduced in mass spectrometry after SIMS and MBSA. ^{252}Cf-PD dates back to 1973 [19, 22–24, 137–139] and was the first method to yield ions of bovine insulin [140]. Practically, ^{252}Cf-PD served for protein characterization, an application which is nowadays completely in the hands of MALDI or ESI (Chaps. 11 and 12) [141]. Based on how it was used, PD-MS is rather the precursor of MALDI, based on the principle of ion generation, it is closer to SIMS and FAB.

In ^{252}Cf-PD-MS, particles of megaelectronvolt translational energy are created from radioactive decay of ^{252}Cf nuclides, the nuclear process being the source of their kinetic energy. Each event yields two nuclides of varying identity, the sum of their masses being the mass of the former nucleus. The fission fragments of similar mass are travelling in opposite directions. Thus, only one of each pair can be employed to effect desorption of ions from a thin film of analyte on a support foil. The ionization process in ^{252}Cf-PD is different from FAB with some closer relations to dry SIMS. The incident particles are normally travelling from the backside through a thin sample layer on a support foil [21, 142]. The initial interaction of the fission fragment with a solid produces approximately 300 electron–hole pairs per angstrom along its track. Recombination of these pairs releases a large amount of energy to the surrounding medium. Within an organic layer, the resulting sudden heat is dissipated by lattice vibrations (phonons) that finally effect desorption of ions from that layer [24, 143, 144]. In addition to spontaneous ion desorption, ionization processes can occur on the nanosecond timescale in the gas phase [145].

Deposition of the analyte on nitrocellulose films instead of metal foils allows the removal of alkali ion contaminations by washing of the sample layer which results in better PD spectra [146]. Further improvements can be achieved by adsorption of the analyte molecules on top of an organic low-molecular-weight matrix layer [147, 148].

Obviously, ^{252}Cf-PD creates ions in a pulsed manner – one burst of ions per fission event – analogous to laser desorption, a fact that restricted the adaptation of ^{252}Cf-PD to time-of-flight (TOF) analyzers (Sect. 4.2). The second fission fragment is not wasted as it serves to trigger the time measurement of the TOF analyzer if the fission fragment source is placed between sample and fission fragment detector (Fig. 10.21) [21, 143].

^{252}Cf-PD mass spectrum of bovine insulin The ^{252}Cf-PD mass spectrum of bovine insulin exhibits the $[M + H]^+$ ion as well as the doubly charged $[M + 2H]^{2+}$ and triply charged $[M + 3H]^{3+}$ ion (Fig. 10.22) [139]. In addition, there are fragment ions corresponding to the A and B chain as well as some **a**-type peptide fragments ions.

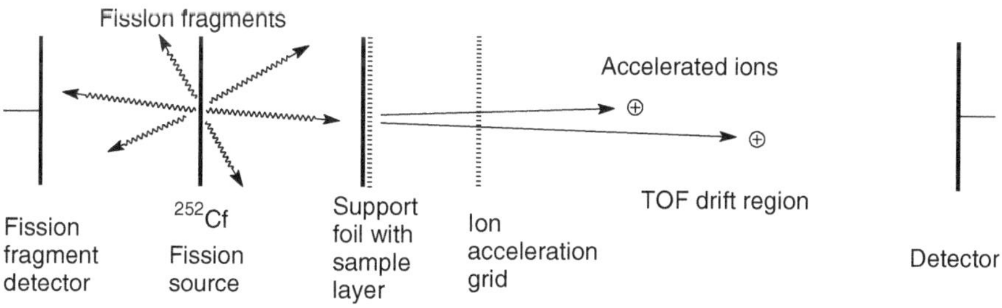

Fig. 10.21 Schematic of a ^{252}Cf-plasma desorption TOF instrument [143]

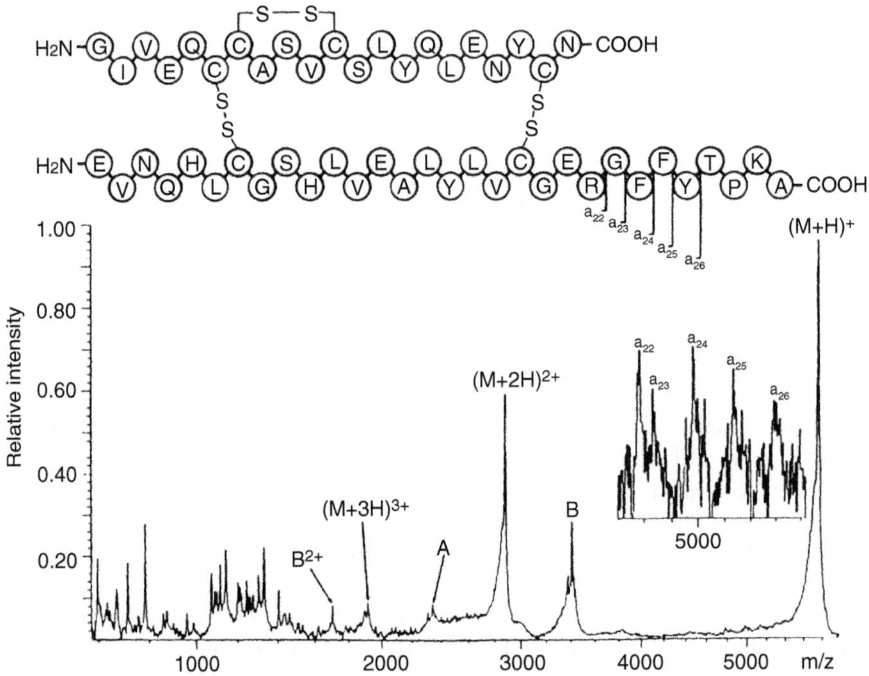

Fig. 10.22 ^{252}Cf-PD mass spectrum of oxidized insulin. Note the extremely uneven baseline and the tailing of the peaks towards the low-mass side, which is due to fragmentation (Reproduced from Ref. [139] by permission. © John Wiley and Sons, 1994)

10.10 Ionization by Particle Impact at a Glance

Basic Principle

The ionization techniques discussed in this chapter share the feature that they all rely on the impact of energetic primary particles to effect ablation and eventually ionization of neutrals. These techniques include *secondary ion mass spectrometry* (SIMS), ^{252}*Californium* (^{252}Cf) *plasma desorption* (PD), *molecular beam solid analysis* (MBSA), *fast atom bombardment* (FAB), and *liquid secondary ion mass spectrometry* (LSIMS). SIMS paved the way to all the other mentioned techniques. SIMS uses primary ions to induce the generation of secondary ions and still is profitably used in inorganic MS, most importantly, for imaging applications (Sect. 15.6). MBSA was the first method to use a primary beam of neutrals and was later established in organic MS as FAB. The versatility and softness of FAB is based on the use of a liquid matrix, which acts as a solvent for the analyte and as a moderator for the energy of the primary neutrals. Other than employing primary ions, SIMS is practically identical to FAB.

Analytes for FAB and LSIMS

Analytes need to be soluble in the organic solvent matrix. FAB and LSIMS likewise can be employed for nonpolar, polar, and ionic analytes. Exposure of a drop of the analyte–matrix mixture to the primary beam is performed on the tip of a probe.

Analytes should preferably be soluble in standard solvents including DMF and DMSO. Solutions of 0.3–3.0 mg ml^{-1} are suitable for admixture to the matrix. FAB and LSIMS are capable of analyzing molecules up to 2,000–4,000 u, depending on their solubility in the matrix. Low-mass analytes may interfere with matrix peaks.

Analytes for PD-MS
PD-MS has been used to analyze (bio)macromolecules. PD-MS is strictly linked to TOF analyzers and requires dedicated instruments. With the advent of ESI and MALDI, PD-MS has essentially disappeared from practical use.

Polarity
FAB and LSIMS both generate positive as well as negative ions. The analyte can be detected as molecular ions or adduct ions, e.g., $M^{+\bullet}$, $[M + H]^+$, $[M + \text{cation}]^+$, $M^{-\bullet}$, $[M - H]^-$, $[M + \text{anion}]^-$. The choice of ion polarity is usually based on the properties of the analyte, i.e., depends on its acidity or basicity, ionization energy or electron affinity.

Softness of Ionization
FAB and LSIMS are soft desorption/ionization methods. Often, only species reflecting the intact analyte molecule are observed. The softness of ionization allows for matrix adduct ions to occur. Nonetheless, some fragmentation can occasionally be observed as a result of energy imparted onto the ions by collisions in the selvedge region between condensed phase and gas phase.

Instrumentation
Magnetic sector instruments are normally used in combination with FAB and LSIMS. The fact that this type of mass analyzer is vanishing from organic and life science MS laboratories causes FAB and LSIMS to disappear from the repertoire of ionization methods in use.

Accurate Mass
Due to stable and long-lasting ion currents, FAB and LISMS are well suited for high-resolution and accurate mass measurements. Internal mass calibration is required when magnetic sector instruments are used. Often, it is just sufficient to admix a calibration compound to the analyte–matrix solution. If admixture cannot be achieved, dual target probes provide pseudo-internal calibration.

Dissemination and Availability
In the late 1980s and 1990s, magnetic sector instruments were sold with FAB or LSIMS as optional ionization methods. Nowadays, FAB and LSIMS have mostly been superseded by ESI, APCI, MALDI, and also by ambient ionization techniques.

References

1. Benninghoven A (2011) The Development of SIMS and International SIMS Conferences: A Personal Retrospective View. Surf Interface Anal 43:2–11. doi:10.1002/sia.3688

2. Honig RE (1985) The Development of Secondary Ion Mass Spectrometry (SIMS): a Retrospective. Int J Mass Spectrom Ion Proc 66:31–54. doi:10.1016/0168-1176(85)83018-4
3. Honig RE (1995) Stone-Age Mass Spectrometry: The Beginnings of "SIMS" at RCA Laboratories, Princeton. Int J Mass Spectrom Ion Proc 143:1–10. doi:10.1016/0168-1176(94)04130-Y
4. Barber M, Vickerman JC, Wolstenholme J (1980) Secondary Ion Mass Spectra of Some Simple Organic Molecules. J Chem Soc Faraday Trans 1(76):549–559. doi:10.1039/F19807600549
5. Benninghoven A (1983) Secondary ion mass spectrometry of organic compounds. In: Benninghoven A (ed) Ion Formation from Organic Solids. Springer, Heidelberg
6. Devienne FM (1967) Different Uses of High Energy Molecular Beams. Entropie 18:61–67
7. Devienne FM, Roustan JC (1982) "Fast Atom Bombardment" – A Rediscovered Method for Mass Spectrometry. Org Mass Spectrom 17:173–181. doi:10.1002/oms.1210170405
8. Barber M, Bordoli RS, Sedgwick RD, Tyler AN (1981) Fast Atom Bombardment of Solids as an Ion Source in Mass Spectrometry. Nature 293:270–275. doi:10.1038/293270a0
9. Barber M, Bordoli RS, Sedgwick RD, Tyler AN (1981) Fast Atom Bombardment Mass Spectrometry of Cobalamines. Biomed Mass Spectrom 8:492–495. doi:10.1002/bms.1200081005
10. Surman DJ, Vickerman JC (1981) Fast Atom Bombardment Quadrupole Mass Spectrometry. J Chem Soc Chem Commun:324–325. doi:10.1039/C39810000324
11. Barber M, Bordoli RS, Sedgwick RD, Tyler AN, Bycroft BW (1981) Fast Atom Bombardment Mass Spectrometry of Bleomycin A2 and B2 and Their Metal Complexes. Biochem Biophys Res Commun 101:632–638. doi:10.1016/0006-291X(81)91305-X
12. Morris HR, Panico M, Barber M, Bordoli RS, Sedgwick RD, Tyler AN (1981) Fast Atom Bombardment: A New Mass Spectrometric Method for Peptide Sequence Analysis. Biochem Biophys Res Commun 101:623–631. doi:10.1016/0006-291X(81)91304-8
13. Barber M, Bordoli RS, Elliott GJ, Sedgwick RD, Tyler AN, Green BN (1982) Fast Atom Bombardment Mass Spectrometry of Bovine Insulin and Other Large Peptides. J Chem Soc Chem Commun:936–938. doi:10.1039/C39820000936
14. Barber M, Bordoli RS, Elliott GJ, Sedgwick RD, Tyler AN (1982) Fast Atom Bombardment Mass Spectrometry. Anal Chem 54:645A–657A. doi:10.1021/ac00241a817
15. Meili J, Seibl J (1983) Matrix Effects in Fast Atom Bombardment (FAB) Mass Spectrometry. Int J Mass Spectrom Ion Phys 46:367–370. doi:10.1016/0020-7381(83)80128-4
16. Gower LJ (1985) Matrix Compounds for Fast Atom Bombardment Mass Spectrometry. Biomed Mass Spectrom 12:191–196. doi:10.1002/bms.1200120502
17. De Pauw E, Agnello A, Derwa F (1991) Liquid Matrices for Liquid Secondary Ion Mass Spectrometry-Fast Atom Bombardment [LSIMS-FAB]: An Update. Mass Spectrom Rev 10:283–301. doi:10.1002/mas.1280100402
18. Aberth W, Straub KM, Burlingame AL (1982) Secondary Ion Mass Spectrometry with Cesium Ion Primary Beam and Liquid Target Matrix for Analysis of Bioorganic Compounds. Anal Chem 54:2029–2034. doi:10.1021/ac00249a028
19. Sundqvist BUR (1992) Desorption Methods in Mass Spectrometry. Int J Mass Spectrom Ion Proc 118(119):265–287. doi:10.1016/0168-1176(92)85065-8
20. Sunner J (1993) Ionization in Liquid Secondary Ion Mass Spectrometry (LSIMS). Org Mass Spectrom 28:805–823. doi:10.1002/oms.1210280802
21. Busch KL (1995) Desorption Ionization Mass Spectrometry. J Mass Spectrom 30:233–240. doi:10.1002/jms.1190300202
22. Macfarlane RD, Torgerson DF (1976) Californium-252-Plasma Desorption Time-of-Flight Mass Spectrometry. Int J Mass Spectrom Ion Phys 21:81–92. doi:10.1016/0020-7381(76)80068-X
23. Macfarlane RD, Torgerson DF (1976) Californium-252 Plasma Desorption Mass Spectroscopy. Science 191:920–925. doi:10.1126/science.1251202

24. Macfarlane RD (1983) High energy heavy-ion induced desorption. In: Benninghoven A (ed) Ion Formation from Organic Solids. Springer, Heidelberg
25. Mahoney JF, Perel J, Ruatta SA, Martino PA, Husain S, Lee TD (1991) Massive Cluster Impact Mass Spectrometry: A New Desorption Method for the Analysis of Large Biomolecules. Rapid Commun Mass Spectrom 5:441–445. doi:10.1002/rcm.1290051004
26. Miller JM (1989) Fast Atom Bombardment Mass Spectrometry of Organometallic, Coordination, and Related Compounds. Mass Spectrom Rev 9:319–347. doi:10.1002/mas.1280090304
27. Franks J, Ghander AM (1974) Saddle Field Ion Source of Spherical Configuration for Etching and Thinning Applications. Vacuum 24:489–491. doi:10.1016/0042-207X(74)90015-3
28. Alexander AJ, Hogg AM (1986) Characterization of a Saddle-Field Discharge Gun for FABMS Using Different Discharge Vapors. Int J Mass Spectrom Ion Proc 69:297–311. doi:10.1016/0168-1176(86)87021-5
29. Boggess B, Cook KD (1994) Determination of Flux from a Saddle Field Fast-Atom Bombardment Gun. J Am Soc Mass Spectrom 5:100–105. doi:10.1016/1044-0305(94)85041-0
30. Barber M, Bordoli RS, Sedgwick RD, Tyler AN (1981) Fast Atom Bombardment of Solids (F.A.B.): A New Ion Source for Mass Spectrometry. J Chem Soc Chem Commun 7:325–327. doi:10.1039/C39810000325
31. McDowell RA, Morris HR (1983) Fast Atom Bombardment Mass Spectrometry: Biological Analysis Using an Ion Gun. Int J Mass Spectrom Ion Phys 46:443–446. doi:10.1016/0020-7381(83)80147-8
32. Morris HR, Panico M, Haskins NJ (1983) Comparison of Ionization Gases in FAB Mass Spectra. Int J Mass Spectrom Ion Phys 46:363–366. doi:10.1016/0020-7381(83)80127-2
33. Fenselau C (1983) Fast Atom Bombardment. In: Benninghoven A (ed) Ion Formation from Organic Solids. Springer, Heidelberg
34. Burlingame AL, Aberth W (1983) Use of a cesium primary beam for liquid SIMS analysis of bio-organic compounds. In: Benninghoven A (ed) Ion Formation from Organic Solids. Springer, Heidelberg
35. Aberth W, Burlingame AL (1984) Comparison of Three Geometries for a Cesium Primary Beam Liquid Secondary Ion Mass Spectrometry Source. Anal Chem 56:2915–2918. doi:10.1021/ac00278a066
36. Aberth WH, Burlingame AL (1988) Effect of Primary Beam Energy on the Secondary-Ion Sputtering Efficiency of Liquid Secondary-Ionization Mass Spectrometry in the 5–30-keV Range. Anal Chem 60:1426–1428. doi:10.1021/ac00165a016
37. McEwen CN, Hass JR (1985) Negative Gold Ion Gun for Liquid Secondary Ion Mass Spectrometry. Anal Chem 57:890–892. doi:10.1021/ac00281a025
38. Katakuse I, Nakabushi H, Ichihara T, Sakurai T, Matsuo T, Matsuda H (1984) Generation and Detection of Cluster Ions $[(CsI)_NCs]^+$ Ranging up to $m/z = 90{,}000$. Int J Mass Spectrom Ion Proc 57:239–243. doi:10.1016/0168-1176(84)85180-0
39. Katakuse I, Nakabushi H, Ichihara T, Sakurai T, Matsuo T, Matsuda H (1984) Metastable Decay of Cesium Iodide Cluster Ions. Int J Mass Spectrom Ion Proc 62:17–23. doi:10.1016/0168-1176(84)80066-X
40. Sim PG, Boyd RK (1991) Calibration and Mass Measurement in Negative-Ion Fast-Atom Bombardment Mass Spectrometry. Rapid Commun Mass Spectrom 5:538–542. doi:10.1002/rcm.1290051111
41. Rapp U, Kaufmann H, Höhn M, Pesch R (1983) Exact Mass Determinations Under FAB Conditions. Int J Mass Spectrom Ion Phys 46:371–374. doi:10.1016/0020-7381(83)80129-6
42. Sunner J (1993) Role of Ion-Ion Recombination for Alkali Chloride Cluster Formation in Liquid Secondary Ion Mass Spectrometry. J Am Soc Mass Spectrom 4:410–418. doi:10.1016/1044-0305(93)85006-J
43. Cao Y, Haseltine JN, Busch KL (1996) Double Cationization with Alkali Ions in Liquid Secondary Ion Mass Spectrometry. Spectroscopy Lett 29:583–589. doi:10.1080/00387019608007053

44. Todd PJ (1988) Secondary Ion Emission from Glycerol Under Continuous and Pulsed Primary Ion Current. Org Mass Spectrom 23:419–424. doi:10.1002/oms.1210230521
45. Schröder E, Münster H, Budzikiewicz H (1986) Ionization by Fast Atom Bombardment - a Chemical Ionization (Matrix) Process Ion the Gas Phase? Org Mass Spectrom 21:707–715. doi:10.1002/oms.1210211016
46. Münster H, Theobald F, Budzikiewicz H (1987) The Formation of a Matrix Plasma in the Gas Phase Under Fast Atom Bombardment Conditions. Int J Mass Spectrom Ion Proc 79:73–79. doi:10.1016/0168-1176(87)80024-1
47. Rosen RT, Hartmann TG, Rosen JD, Ho CT (1988) Fast-Atom-Bombardment Mass Spectra of Low-Molecular-Weight Alcohols and Other Compounds. Evidence for a Chemical-Ionization Process in the Gas Phase. Rapid Commun Mass Spectrom 2:21–23. doi:10.1002/rcm.1290020108
48. Miller JM, Balasanmugam K (1989) Fast Atom Bombardment Mass Spectrometry of Some Nonpolar Compounds. Anal Chem 61:1293–1295. doi:10.1021/ac00186a022
49. Benninghoven A (1983) Organic Secondary Ion Mass Spectrometry (SIMS) and Its Relation to Fast Atom Bombardment (FAB). Int J Mass Spectrom Ion Phys 46:459–462. doi:10.1016/0020-7381(83)80151-X
50. van Breemen RB, Snow M, Cotter RJ (1983) Time-Resolved Laser Desorption Mass Spectrometry. I. Desorption of Preformed Ions. Int J Mass Spectrom Ion Phys 49:35–50. doi:10.1016/0020-7381(83)85074-8
51. Musselman B, Watson JT, Chang CK (1986) Direct Evidence for Preformed Ions of Porphyrins in the Solvent Matrix for Fast Atom Bombardment Mass Spectrometry. Org Mass Spectrom 21:215–219. doi:10.1002/oms.1210210408
52. Shiea J, Sunner J (1991) The Acid Effect in Fast Atom Bombardment. Org Mass Spectrom 26:38–44. doi:10.1002/oms.1210260107
53. Todd PJ (1991) Solution Chemistry and Secondary Ion Emission from Amine-Glycerol Solutions. J Am Soc Mass Spectrom 2:33–44. doi:10.1016/1044-0305(91)80059-G
54. Wong SS, Röllgen FW (1986) Sputtering of Large Molecular Ions by Low Energy Particle Impact. Nulc Instrum Methods Phys Res B B14:436–447. doi:10.1016/0168-583X(86)90139-4
55. Baczynskyi L (1985) New Matrices for Fast Atom Bombardment Mass Spectrometry. Adv Mass Spectrom 10:1611–1612
56. De Pauw E, Agnello A, Derwa F (1986) Liquid Matrices for Liquid Secondary Ion Mass Spectrometry. Mass Spectrom Rev 5:191–212. doi:10.1002/mas.1280050204
57. Gower LJ (1985) Matrix Compounds for Fast Atom Bombardment: A Further Review. Adv Mass Spectrom 10:1537–1538
58. Staempfli AA, Schlunegger UP (1991) A New Matrix for Fast-Atom Bombardment Analysis of Corrins. Rapid Commun Mass Spectrom 5:30–31. doi:10.1002/rcm.1290050108
59. Visentini J, Nguyen PM, Bertrand MJ (1991) The Use of 4-Hydroxybenzenesulfonic Acid as a Reduction-Inhibiting Matrix in Liquid Secondary-Ion Mass Spectrometry. Rapid Commun Mass Spectrom 5:586–590. doi:10.1002/rcm.1290051204
60. Meili J, Seibl J (1984) A New Versatile Matrix for Fast Atom Bombardment Analysis. Org Mass Spectrom 19:581–582. doi:10.1002/oms.1210191111
61. Barber M, Bell D, Eckersley M, Morris M, Tetler L (1988) The Use of *meta*-Nitrobenzyl Alcohol as a Matrix in Fast Atom Bombardment Mass Spectrometry. Rapid Commun Mass Spectrom 2:18–21. doi:10.1002/rcm.1290020107
62. Aubagnac J-L (1990) Use of *M*-Nitrobenzyl Alcohol As a Matrix in Fast-Atom-Bombardment Negative-Ion Mass Spectrometry of Polar Compounds. Rapid Commun Mass Spectrom 4:114–116. doi:10.1002/rcm.1290040405
63. Andersson T, Westman G, Stenhagen G, Sundahl M, Wennerström O (1995) A Gas Phase Container for C_{60}: a γ-Cyclodextrin Dimer. Tetrahedron Lett 36:597–600. doi:10.1016/0040-4039(94)02282-G

64. Dube G (1984) The Behavior of Aromatic Hydrocarbons Under Fast Atom Bombardment. Org Mass Spectrom 19:242–243. doi:10.1002/oms.1210190510
65. Abdul-Sada AK, Greenway AM, Seddon KR (1989) The Extent of Aggregation of Air-Sensitive Alkyllithium Compounds as Determined by Fast-Atom-Bombardment Mass Spectrometry. J Organomet Chem 375:C17–C19. doi:10.1016/0022-328X(89)85099-5
66. Abdul-Sada AK, Greenway AM, Seddon KR (1996) The Application of Liquid Paraffin and 3,4-Dimethoxybenzyl Alcohol as Matrix Compounds to Fast Atom Bombardment Mass Spectrometry. Eur Mass Spectrom 2:77–78. doi:10.1255/ejms.82
67. Bandini AL, Banditelli G, Minghetti G, Pelli B, Traldi P (1989) Fast Atom Bombardment Induced Decomposition Pattern of the Gold(III) Bis(Carbene) Complex [[(*p*-MeC_6H_4NH)(EtO)C]$_2$AuI_2]ClO_4, a Retrosynthetic Process? Organometallics 8:590–593. doi:10.1021/om00105a003
68. Dobson JC, Taube H (1989) Coordination Chemistry and Redox Properties of Polypyridyl Complexes of Vanadium(II). Inorg Chem 28:1310–1315. doi:10.1021/ic00306a021
69. Leibman CP, Todd PJ, Mamantov G (1988) Enhanced Positive Secondary Ion Emission from Substituted Polynuclear Aromatic Hydrocarbon/Sulfuric Acid Solutions. Org Mass Spectrom 23:634–642. doi:10.1002/oms.1210230903
70. Rozenski J, Herdewijn P (1995) The Effect of Addition of Carbon Powder to Samples in Liquid Secondary Ion Mass Spectrometry: Improved Ionization of Apolar Compounds. Rapid Commun Mass Spectrom 9:1499–1501. doi:10.1002/rcm.1290091507
71. Huang ZH, Shyong BJ, Gage DA, Noon KR, Allison J (1994) *N*-Alkylnicotinium Halides: A Class of Cationic Matrix Additives for Enhancing the Sensitivity in Negative Ion Fast-Atom Bombardment Mass Spectrometry of Polyanionic Analytes. J Am Soc Mass Spectrom 5:935–948. doi:10.1016/1044-0305(94)87019-5
72. Shiea JT, Sunner J (1990) Effects of Matrix Viscosity on FAB Spectra. Int J Mass Spectrom Ion Proc 96:243–265. doi:10.1016/0168-1176(90)85126-M
73. Field FH (1982) Fast Atom Bombardment Study of Glycerol: Mass Spectra and Radiation Chemistry. J Phys Chem 86:5115–5123. doi:10.1021/j100223a013
74. Caldwell KA, Gross ML (1994) Origins and Structures of Background Ions Produced by Fast-Atom Bombardment of Glycerol. J Am Soc Mass Spectrom 5:72–91. doi:10.1016/1044-0305(94)85039-9
75. Busch KL (2002) Chemical Noise in Mass Spectrometry. Part I. Spectroscopy 17:32–37
76. Busch KL (2003) Chemical Noise in Mass Spectrometry. Part II – Effects of Choices in Ionization Methods on Chemical Noise. Spectroscopy 18:56–62
77. Reynolds JD, Cook KD (1990) Improving Fast Atom Bombardment Mass Spectra: the Influence of Some Controllable Parameters on Spectral Quality. J Am Soc Mass Spectrom 1:149–157. doi:10.1016/1044-0305(90)85051-M
78. Barber M, Bell DJ, Morris M, Tetler LW, Woods MD, Monaghan JJ, Morden WE (1988) The Interaction of *meta*-Nitrobenzyl Alcohol with Compounds Under Fast-Atom-Bombardment Conditions. Rapid Commun Mass Spectrom 2:181–183. doi:10.1002/rcm.1290020905
79. Tuinman AA, Cook KD (1992) Fast Atom Bombardment-Induced Condensation of Glycerol with Ammonium Surfactants. I. Regioselectivity of the Adduct Formation. J Am Soc Mass Spectrom 3:318–325. doi:10.1016/1044-0305(92)87059-8
80. Aubagnac JL, Claramunt RM, Sanz D (1990) Reduction Phenomenon on the FAB Mass Spectra of *N*-Aminoazoles with a Glycerol Matrix. Org Mass Spectrom 25:293–295. doi:10.1002/oms.1210250511
81. Murthy VS, Miller JM (1993) Suppression Effects on a Reduction Process in Fast-Atom Bombardment Mass Spectrometry. Rapid Commun Mass Spectrom 7:874–881. doi:10.1002/rcm.1290071004
82. Aubagnac J-L, Gilles I, Lazaro R, Claramunt R-M, Gosselin G, Martinez J (1995) Reduction Phenomenon in Frit Fast-Atom Bombardment Mass Spectrometry. Rapid Commun Mass Spectrom 9:509–511. doi:10.1002/rcm.1290090607

83. Aubagnac J-L, Gilles I, Claramunt RM, Escolastico C, Sanz D, Elguero J (1995) Reduction of Aromatic Fluorine Compounds in Fast-Atom Bombardment Mass Spectrometry. Rapid Commun Mass Spectrom 9:156–159. doi:10.1002/rcm.1290090210
84. Théberge R, Bertrand MJ (1995) Beam-Induced Dehalogenation in LSIMS: Effect of Halogen Type and Matrix Chemistry. J Mass Spectrom 30:163–171. doi:10.1002/jms.1190300125
85. Théberge R, Bertrand MJ (1998) An Investigation of the Relationship Between Analyte Surface Concentration and the Extent of Beam-Induced Dehalogenation in Liquid Secondary Ion Mass Spectrometry. Rapid Commun Mass Spectrom 12:2004–2010. doi:10.1002/(SICI)1097-0231(19981230)12:24<2004::AID-RCM427>3.0.CO;2-P
86. Vetter W, Meister W (1985) Fast Atom Bombardment Mass Spectrum of β-Carotene. Org Mass Spectrom 20:266–267. doi:10.1002/oms.1210200321
87. Nakata H, Tanaka K (1994) Structural and Substituent Effects on $M^{+\cdot}$ vs. $[M + H]^+$ Formation in Fast Atom Bombardment Mass Spectra of Simple Organic Compounds. Org Mass Spectrom 29:283–288. doi:10.1002/oms.1210290604
88. Moon DC, Kelly JA (1988) A Simple Desalting Procedure for Fast Atom Bombardment Mass Spectrometry. Biomed Mass Spectrom 17:229–237. doi:10.1002/bms.1200170312
89. Prókai L, Hsu BH, Farag H, Bodor N (1989) Desorption Chemical Ionization, Thermospray, and Fast Atom Bombardment Mass Spectrometry of Dihydropyridine – Pyridinium Salt-Type Redox Systems. Anal Chem 61:1723–1728. doi:10.1021/ac00190a026
90. Kolli VSK, York WS, Orlando R (1998) Fast Atom Bombardment Mass Spectrometry of Carbohydrates Contaminated with Inorganic Salts Using a Crown Ether. J Mass Spectrom 33:680–682. doi:10.1002/(SICI)1096-9888(199807)33:7<680::AID-JMS673>3.0.CO;2-Y
91. Desiderio DM, Katakuse I (1984) Fast Atom Bombardment Mass Spectrometry of Insulin, Insulin A-Chain, Insulin B-Chain, and Glucagon. Biomed Mass Spectrom 11:55–59. doi:10.1002/bms.1200110202
92. Barber M, Green BN (1987) The Analysis of Small Proteins in the Molecular Weight Range 10–24 kDa by Magnetic Sector Mass Spectrometry. Rapid Commun Mass Spectrom 1:80–83. doi:10.1002/rcm.1290010505
93. Frauenkron M, Berkessel A, Gross JH (1997) Analysis of Ruthenium Carbonyl-Porphyrin Complexes: A Comparison of Matrix-Assisted Laser Desorption/Ionization Time-of-Flight, Fast-Atom Bombardment and Field Desorption Mass Spectrometry. Eur Mass Spectrom 3:427–438. doi:10.1255/ejms.177
94. Irngartinger H, Altreuther A, Sommerfeld T, Stojanik T (2000) Pyramidalization in Derivatives of Bicyclo[5.1.0]oct-1(7)-enes and 2,2,5,5-Tetramethylbicyclo[4.1.0]hept-1(6)-enes. Eur J Org Chem 2000:4059–4070. doi:10.1002/1099-0690(200012)2000:24<4059::AID-EJOC4059>3.0.CO;2-V
95. Barber M, Bordoli RS, Elliott GJ, Tyler AN, Bill JC, Green BN (1984) Fast Atom Bombardment (FAB) Mass Spectrometry: A Mass Spectral Investigation of Some of the Insulins. Biomed Mass Spectrom 11:182–186. doi:10.1002/bms.1200110409
96. Rajca A, Wongsriratanakul J, Rajca S, Cerny R (1998) A Dendritic Macrocyclic Organic Polyradical with a Very High Spin of $S = 10$. Angew Chem Int Ed 37:1229–1232. doi:10.1002/(SICI)1521-3773(19980518)37:9<1229::AID-ANIE1229>3.0.CO;2-%23
97. Giesa S, Gross JH, Krätschmer W, Gleiter R (1998) Experiments Towards an Analytical Application of Host-Guest Complexes of [60] Fullerene and Its Derivatives. Eur Mass Spectrom 4:189–196. doi:10.1255/ejms.208
98. Juo CG, Shiu LL, Shen CKF, Luh TJ, Her GR (1995) Analysis of C_{60} Derivatives by Fast-Atom Bombardment Mass Spectrometry As Γ-Cyclodextrin Inclusion Complexes. Rapid Commun Mass Spectrom 9:604–608. doi:10.1002/rcm.1290090714
99. Vincenti M (1995) Host-Guest Chemistry in the Mass Spectrometer. J Mass Spectrom 30:925–939. doi:10.1002/jms.1190300702
100. Morgan RP, Reed ML (1982) Fast Atom Bombardment (FAB)-Accurate Mass Measurement. Org Mass Spectrom 17:537. doi:10.1002/oms.1210171015

101. Münster H, Budzikiewicz H, Schröder E (1987) A Modified Target for FAB Measurements. Org Mass Spectrom 22:384–385. doi:10.1002/oms.1210220616
102. Gross JH, Giesa S, Krätschmer W (1999) Negative-Ion Low-Temperature Fast-Atom Bombardment Mass Spectrometry of Monomeric and Dimeric [60]Fullerene Compounds. Rapid Commun Mass Spectrom 13:815–820. doi:10.1002/(SICI)1097-0231(19990515)13:9<815::AID-RCM572>3.0.CO;2-L
103. Falick AM, Walls FC, Laine RA (1986) Cooled Sample Introduction Probe for Liquid Secondary Ionization Mass Spectrometry. Anal Biochem 159:132–137. doi:10.1016/0003-2697(86)90317-9
104. Jonkman HT, Michl J (1981) Secondary Ion Mass Spectrometry of Small-Molecule Solids at Cryogenic Temperatures. 1. Nitrogen and Carbon Monoxide. J Am Chem Soc 103:733–737. doi:10.1021/ja00394a001
105. Orth RG, Jonkman HT, Michl J (1981) Secondary Ion Mass Spectrometry of Small-Molecule Solids at Cryogenic Temperatures. 2. Rare Gas Solids. J Am Chem Soc 103:6026–6030. doi:10.1021/ja00410a006
106. Katz RN, Chaudhary T, Field FH (1986) Particle Bombardment (FAB) Mass Spectra of Methanol at Sub-Ambient Temperatures. J Am Chem Soc 108:3897–3903. doi:10.1021/ja00274a007
107. Katz RN, Chaudhary T, Field FH (1987) Particle Bombardment (KeV) Mass Spectra of Ethylene Glycol, Glycerol, and Water at Sub-Ambient Temperatures. Int J Mass Spectrom Ion Proc 78:85–97. doi:10.1016/0168-1176(87)87043-X
108. Johnstone RAW, Wilby AH (1989) Fast Atom Bombardment at Low Temperatures. Part 2. Polymerization in the Matrix. Int J Mass Spectrom Ion Proc 89:249–264. doi:10.1016/0168-1176(89)83063-0
109. Kosevich MV, Czira G, Boryak OA, Shelkovsky VS, Vékey K (1997) Comparison of Positive and Negative Ion Clusters of Methanol and Ethanol Observed by Low Temperature Secondary Ion Mass Spectrometry. Rapid Commun Mass Spectrom 11:1411–1416. doi:10.1002/(SICI)1097-0231(19970830)11:13<1411::AID-RCM967>3.0.CO;2-8
110. Kosevich MV, Czira G, Boryak OA, Shelkovsky VS, Vékey K (1998) Temperature Dependences of Ion Currents of Alcohol Clusters Under Low-Temperature Secondary Ion Mass Spectrometric Conditions. J Mass Spectrom 33:843–849. doi:10.1002/(SICI)1096-9888(199809)33:9<843::AID-JMS695>3.0.CO;2-7
111. Magnera TF, David DE, Stulik D, Orth RG, Jonkman HT, Michl J (1989) Production of Hydrated Metal Ions by Fast Ion or Atom Beam Sputtering. Collision-Induced Dissociation and Successive Hydration Energies of Gaseous Cu^+ with 1-4 Water Molecules. J Am Chem Soc 111:5036–5043. doi:10.1021/ja00196a003
112. Boryak OA, Stepanov IO, Kosevich MV, Shelkovsky VS, Orlov VV, Blagoy YP (1996) Origin of Clusters. I. Correlation of Low Temperature Fast Atom Bombardment Mass Spectra with the Phase Diagram of NaCl-Water Solutions. Eur Mass Spectrom 2:329–339. doi:10.1255/ejms.43
113. Kosevich MV, Boryak OA, Stepanov IO, Shelkovsky VS (1997) Origin of Clusters. II. Distinction of Two Different Processes of Formation of Mixed Metal/Water Clusters Under Low-Temperature Fast Atom Bombardment. Eur Mass Spectrom 3:11–17. doi:10.1255/ejms.28
114. Boryak OA, Kosevich MV, Shelkovsky VS, Blagoy YP (1996) Study of Frozen Solutions of Nucleic Acid Nitrogen Bases by Means of Low Temperature Fast-Atom-Bombardment Mass Spectrometry. Rapid Commun Mass Spectrom 10:197–199. doi:10.1002/(SICI)1097-0231(19960131)10:2<197::AID-RCM457>3.0.CO;2-G
115. Huang M-W, Chei HL, Huang JP, Shiea J (1999) Application of Organic Solvents As Matrixes to Detect Air-Sensitive and Less Polar Compounds Using Low-Temperature Secondary Ion Mass Spectrometry. Anal Chem 71:2901–2907. doi:10.1021/ac980516p
116. Hofmann P, Volland MAO, Hansen SM, Eisenträger F, Gross JH, Stengel K (2000) Isolation and Characterization of a Monomeric, Solvent Coordinated Ruthenium(II) Carbene Cation

Relevant to Olefin Metathesis. J Organomet Chem 606:88–92. doi:10.1016/S0022-328X(00)00288-6

117. Wang CH, Huang MW, Lee CY, Chei HL, Huang JP, Shiea J (1998) Detection of a Thermally Unstable Intermediate in the Wittig Reaction Using Low-Temperature Liquid Secondary Ion and Atmospheric Pressure Ionization Mass Spectrometry. J Am Soc Mass Spectrom 9:1168–1174. doi:10.1016/S1044-0305(98)00089-0
118. Giesa S, Gross JH, Hull WE, Lebedkin S, Gromov A, Krätschmer W, Gleiter R (1999) $C_{120}OS$: The First Sulfur-Containing Dimeric [60]Fullerene Derivative. Chem Commun:465–466. doi:10.1039/a809831j
119. Gross JH (1998) Use of Protic and Aprotic Solvents of High Volatility As Matrixes in Analytical Low-Temperature Fast-Atom Bombardment Mass Spectrometry. Rapid Commun Mass Spectrom 12:1833–1838. doi:10.1002/(SICI)1097-0231(19981215)12:23<1833::AID-RCM401>3.0.CO;2-O
120. König WA, Aydin M, Schulze U, Rapp U, Höhn M, Pesch R, Kalikhevitch VN (1983) Fast-Atom-Bombardment for Peptide Sequencing – A Comparison with Conventional Ionization Techniques. Int J Mass Spectrom Ion Phys 46:403–406. doi:10.1016/0020-7381(83)80137-5
121. Caprioli RM (1987) Enzymes and Mass Spectrometry: A Dynamic Combination. Mass Spectrom Rev 6:237–287. doi:10.1002/mas.1280060202
122. Caprioli RM (1988) Analysis of Biochemical Reactions with Molecular Specificity Using Fast Atom Bombardment Mass Spectrometry. Biochemistry 27:513–521. doi:10.1021/bi00402a001
123. Chait BT, Wang R, Beavis RC, Kent SB (1993) Protein Ladder Sequencing. Science 262:89–92. doi:10.1126/science.8211132
124. Naylor S, Findeis AF, Gibson BW, Williams DH (1985) An Approach Towards the Complete FAB Analysis of Enzymic Digests of Peptides and Proteins. J Am Chem Soc 108:6359–6363. doi:10.1021/ja00280a037
125. Deterding LJ, Tomer KB, Wellemans JMY, Cerny RL, Gross ML (1999) Capillary Electrophoresis/Tandem Mass Spectrometry with Array Detection. Eur Mass Spectrom 5:33–40. doi:10.1255/ejms.247
126. Lehmann WD (1996) Massenspektrometrie in der Biochemie. Spektrum Akademischer Verlag, Heidelberg
127. Chapman JR (ed) (2000) Mass Spectrometry of Proteins and Peptides. Humana Press, Totowa
128. Snyder AP (2000) Interpreting Protein Mass Spectra. Oxford University Press, New York
129. Kinter M, Sherman NE (2000) Protein Sequencing and Identification Using Tandem Mass Spectrometry. Wiley, Chichester
130. Stults JT, Lai J, McCune S, Wetzel R (1993) Simplification of High-Energy Collision Spectra of Peptides by Amino-Terminal Derivatization. Anal Chem 65:1703–1708. doi:10.1021/ac00061a012
131. Bordaz-Nagy J, Despeyroux D, Jennings KR, Gaskell SJ (1992) Experimental Aspects of the Collision-Induced Decomposition of Ions in a Four-Sector Tandem Mass Spectrometer. Org Mass Spectrom 27:406–415. doi:10.1002/oms.1210270410
132. Karlsson NG, Karlsson H, Hansson GC (1996) Sulfated Mucin Oligosaccharides from Porcine Small Intestine Analyzed by Four-Sector Tandem Mass Spectrometry. J Mass Spectrom 31:560–572. doi:10.1002/(SICI)1096-9888(199605)31:5<560::AID-JMS331>3.0.CO;2-0
133. Caprioli RM, Beckner CF, Smith LA (1983) Performance of a Fast-Atom Bombardment Source on a Quadrupole Mass Spectrometer. Biomed Mass Spectrom 10:94–97. doi:10.1002/bms.1200100209
134. Cornett DS, Lee TD, Mahoney JF (1994) Matrix-Free Desorption of Biomolecules Using Massive Cluster Impact. Rapid Commun Mass Spectrom 8:996–1000. doi:10.1002/rcm.1290081218

135. Mahoney JF, Perel J, Lee TD, Martino PA, Williams P (1992) Shock Wave Model for Sputtering Biomolecules Using Massive Cluster Impact. J Am Soc Mass Spectrom 3:311–317. doi:10.1016/1044-0305(92)87058-7
136. Mahoney JF, Cornett DS, Lee TD (1994) Formation of Multiply Charged Ions from Large Molecules Using Massive-Cluster Impact. Rapid Commun Mass Spectrom 8:403–406. doi:10.1002/rcm.1290080513
137. Sundqvist B, Macfarlane RD (1985) Californium-252-Plasma Desorption Mass Spectrometry. Mass Spectrom Rev 4:421–460. doi:10.1002/mas.1280040403
138. Macfarlane RD (1993) Californium-252-Plasma Desorption Mass Spectrometry I – A Historical Perspective. Biol Mass Spectrom 22:677–680. doi:10.1002/bms.1200221202
139. Macfarlane RD, Hu ZH, Song S, Pittenauer E, Schmid ER, Allmaier G, Metzger JO, Tuszynski W (1994) ^{252}Cf-Plasma Desorption Mass Spectrometry II – A Perspective of New Directions. Biol Mass Spectrom 23:117–130. doi:10.1002/bms.1200230302
140. Håkansson P, Kamensky I, Sundqvist B, Fohlman J, Peterson P, McNeal CJ, Macfarlane RD (1982) Iodine-127-Plasma Desorption Mass Spectrometry of Insulin. J Am Chem Soc 104:2948–2949. doi:10.1021/ja00374a053
141. Macfarlane RD (1999) Mass Spectrometry of Biomolecules: from PDMS to MALDI. Brazilian J Phys 29:415–421. doi:10.1590/S0103-97331999000300003
142. Sundqvist B, Håkansson P, Kamensky I, Kjellberg J (1983) Fast heavy ion induced desorption of molecular ions from small proteins. In: Benninghoven A (ed) Ion Formation from Organic Solids. Springer, Heidelberg
143. Macfarlane RD (1981) ^{252}Californium Plasma Desorption Mass Spectrometry. Biomed Mass Spectrom 8:449–453. doi:10.1002/bms.1200080918
144. Wien K, Becker O (1983) Secondary ion emission from metals under fission fragment bombardment. In: Benninghoven A (ed) Ion Formation from Organic Solids. Springer, Heidelberg
145. Zubarev RA, Abeywarna UK, Demirev P, Eriksson J, Papaléo R, Håkansson P, Sundqvist BUR (1997) Delayed, Gas-Phase Ion Formation in Plasma Desorption Mass Spectrometry. Rapid Commun Mass Spectrom 11:963–972. doi:10.1002/(SICI)1097-0231(19970615) 11:9<963::AID-RCM878>3.0.CO;2-%23
146. Jonsson GP, Hedin AB, Håkansson P, Sundqvist BUR, Säve BGS, Nielsen P, Roepstorff P, Johansson KE, Kamensky I, Lindberg MSL (1986) Plasma Desorption Mass Spectrometry of Peptides and Proteins Adsorbed on Nitrocellulose. Anal Chem 58:1084–1087. doi:10.1021/ac00297a023
147. Wolf B, Macfarlane RD (1991) Small Molecules as Substrates for Adsorption/Desorption in Californium-252 Plasma Desorption Mass Spectrometry. J Am Soc Mass Spectrom 2:29–32. doi:10.1016/1044-0305(91)80058-F
148. Song S, Macfarlane RD (2002) PDMS-Chemistry of Angiotensin II and Insulin in Glucose Glass Thin Films. Anal Bioanal Chem 373:647–655. doi:10.1007/s00216-002-1361-4

11 Matrix-Assisted Laser Desorption/ Ionization

Learning Objectives

- Pulsed laser light as a source of energy for desorption and ionization
- Ion formation from thin solid layers
- Matrix assistance as a key to soft desorption/ionization
- Ionization in an inherently pulsed mode
- Applications for small molecules, synthetic polymers, and biomolecules
- Vacuum and atmospheric pressure sources for MALDI
- MALDI imaging techniques

Laser desorption/ionization (LDI) was introduced in the late 1960s [1–3], long before the advent of field desorption (FD, Chap. 8), *californium plasma desorption* (^{252}Cf-PD, Sect. 10.8) or *fast atom bombardment* (FAB, Chap. 10). While low-mass organic salts and light-absorbing organic molecules are easily accessible by LDI [2, 3], it takes a serious effort to obtain useful mass spectra of biomolecules [4], in particular when the mass of the analyte exceeds 2000 u [5, 6]. FAB and ^{252}Cf-PD therefore represented the standard in all life science-related fields of mass spectrometry until the late 1980s, while LDI was regarded rather exotic [7].

The admixture of strongly light-absorbing compounds to the sample prior to preparation for laser desorption effected a tremendous change of what was possible in mass spectrometry. Two approaches were independently developed: (*i*) the admixture of ultrafine cobalt powder (particle size about 30 nm) to analyte solutions in glycerol [8, 9], and (*ii*) the cocrystallization of the analyte with an organic matrix [10–13]. When combined with a *time-of-flight* (TOF, Sect. 4.2) mass analyzer, both methods are capable of producing mass spectra of proteins of about 100,000 u molecular weight. Nonetheless, the application of the "*ultrafine-metal-plus-liquid-matrix*" method remained an exception because the versatility of an organic matrix

J.H. Gross, *Mass Spectrometry*, DOI 10.1007/978-3-319-54398-7_11

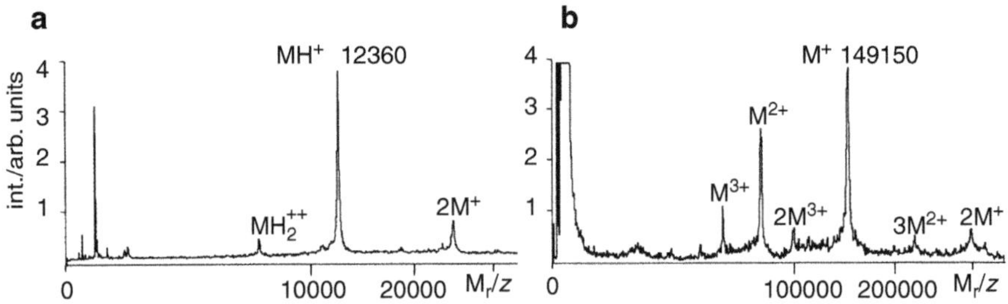

Fig. 11.1 MALDI-TOF mass spectra of (**a**) porcine cytochrome C from 2,5-dihydroxybenzoic acid matrix at a laser wavelength of 337 nm and (**b**) a monoclonal antibody from nicotinic acid matrix at 266 nm. These spectra from one of the landmark papers during the early phase of MALDI development impressively demonstrate the enormous potential of the method (Reproduced from Ref. [16] by permission. © John Wiley & Sons, 1991)

and the sensitivity of *matrix-assisted laser desorption/ionization* (MALDI) [10, 11, 14, 15] made it by far superior to the admixture of cobalt powder (Fig. 11.1) [16–19]. In its present state, MALDI represents a major analytical tool in the modern life sciences [20–25] and in polymer science [24–27].

11.1 Ion Sources for LDI and MALDI

The basic setup of LDI/MALDI ion sources is comparatively simple (Fig. 11.2) [28]. Both LDI and MALDI make use of the absorption of laser light by a solid sample layer. The energy uptake upon laser irradiation then causes evaporation and eventually ionization of the sample. The pulse of laser light is focused onto a small spot which is typically 0.05–0.2 mm in diameter [29]. As laser irradiance is a critical parameter in MALDI, a variable beam attenuator in the laser optical path is employed to adjust the irradiance. Then, the laser attenuation is individually optimized for each measurement. LDI/MALDI ion sources are generally operated at ambient temperature.

Although lasers of both ultraviolet (UV) and infrared (IR) wavelengths are in use, UV lasers are by far the most important light sources in analytical LDI-MS and MALDI-MS. Among these, nitrogen lasers and frequency-tripled or quadrupled Nd:Yag lasers serve for the majority of applications [30]. IR-MALDI is dominated by Er:Yag lasers [30, 31] while TEA-CO_2 lasers (cf. IRMPD in Sect. 9.12) are rarely used (Table 11.1) [17, 32].

Photon energy We can calculate the energy per photon of the widely employed frequency-tripled Nd:Yag laser by using the relationship $E = h\nu$ and substituting $\nu = c/\lambda$ (Sect. 2.10.6). For a wavelength $\lambda = 355$ nm and with $h = 4.14 \times 10^{-15}$ eVs ($= 6.63 \times 10^{-34}$ Js) we obtain $E = 4.14 \times 10^{-15}$ eVs $\times$ (2.99×10^{8} m s^{-1}/ 3.55×10^{-7} m) = 3.49 eV (Table 11.1). This tells us, on the one hand, that the photon energy is substantial, but on the other, that a single photon

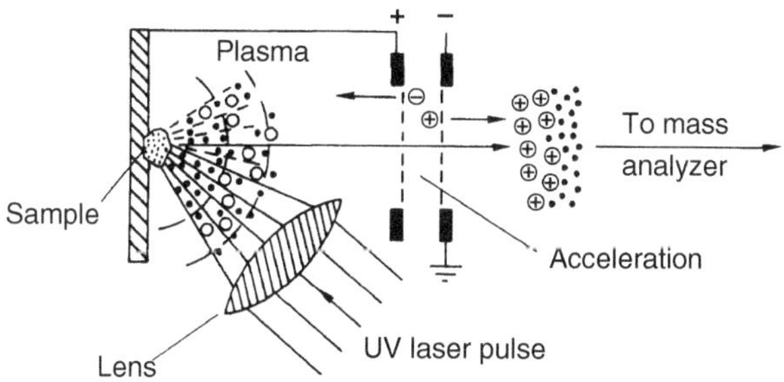

Fig. 11.2 Simplistic laser desorption ion source for nonresonant light absorption by a solid; in practice, the solid is supplied as a thin microcrystalline layer. Here, positive ions are continuously being extracted as long as the supply is sustained by the laser desorption plasma (Reproduced from Ref. [28] by permission. © Elsevier Science, 1994)

Table 11.1 Lasers for laser desorption/ionization

Spectral range	Wavelength	Photon energy	Laser type
UV	193 nm	6.4 eV	ArF Excimer laser
UV	248 nm	5.0 eV	KrF Excimer laser
UV	266 nm	4.7 eV	Frequency-quadrupled Nd:YAG laser
UV	308 nm	3.8 eV	XeCl Excimer laser
UV	337 nm	3.7 eV	Nitrogen laser[a]
UV	355 nm	3.5 eV	Frequency-tripled Nd:YAG laser[a]
IR	1.06 μm	1.2 eV	Nd:YAG laser[b]
IR	2.94 μm	0.4 eV	Er:YAG laser[b]
IR	1.7–2.5 μm	0.7–0.5 eV	Optical parametric oscillator (OPO) laser
IR	10.6 μm	0.1 eV	CO_2 laser

[a]most frequently used UV lasers
[b]most frequently used IR lasers

will not be able to cause ionization. Unlike photoionization, MALDI relies on the coincidence of a large number of photon absorptions across a macroscopic area.

UV lasers are emitting pulses of 3–10 ns duration, while those of IR lasers are in the range of 6–200 ns. Short pulses are needed to effect sudden ablation of the sample layer. In addition, an extremely short time interval of ion generation basically avoids thermal degradation of the analyte, e.g., a 10 ns laser pulse would require the high rate constant of 10^8 s^{-1} to complete decomposition. On the other hand, substantially longer irradiation would simply cause heating of the bulk material. In case of IR-MALDI, a slight decrease in threshold fluence has been observed with shorter laser pulses [33]. Furthermore, a short time interval of ion generation means a better definition of the starting pulse, which is relevant when a TOF analyzer is being used. Fortunately, the introduction of delayed extraction techniques (Sect. 4.2.6) has greatly reduced the influence of the laser pulse duration on resolving power and mass accuracy [33].

Mostly UV MALDI
The majority of MALDI applications are run with UV lasers. IR-MALDI has been restricted to applications where the deeper penetration of IR radiation offers advantages, e.g., for the direct desorption of analytes from *sodium dodecyl sulfate* (SDS) gels or *thin layer chromatography* (TLC) plates.

11.2 Ion Formation

The mechanisms of ion formation in MALDI are a subject of continuing research [34–39]. The major concerns are the relationship between ion yield and laser fluence [29, 40], the temporal evolution of the desorption process and its implications upon ion formation [41], the initial velocity of the desorbing ions [33, 42, 43], and the question whether preformed ions or ions generated in the gas phase provide the major source of the ionic species detected in MALDI [44–46].

11.2.1 Ion Yield and Laser Fluence

Ion formation does not occur below a *threshold laser irradiance* of about 10^6 W cm^{-2}. At threshold, a sharp onset of desorption/ionization occurs and ion abundances rise to a high power (5th to 9th) of laser irradiance [17, 40, 47]. The threshold *laser fluence* for the detection of matrix and analyte ions not only depends on the actual matrix, but also on the molar matrix-to-analyte ratio, e.g., the minimum threshold laser fluence for cytochrome C was found at a molar matrix-to-sample ratio of 4000 : 1. Significantly higher or lower ratios require almost twice that laser fluence (Fig. 11.3) [48]. The increase at low analyte concentrations can be attributed to a decreasing detection efficiency because a larger volume of material has to be ablated in order to generate a sufficient number of analyte ions. At high analyte concentrations, the energy absorption per volume is reduced as the matrix becomes diluted with analyte molecules causing a higher threshold fluence. The total particle yield from laser desorption as a function of *laser fluence* has been determined by collecting the desorbed neutrals on a quartz crystal microbalance [49]. The study by Quist *et al.* [29] indicates that the desorption of neutrals occurs by thermal evaporation starting at laser fluences of about 11 mJ cm^{-2}. However, the ion-to-neutral ratio of the MALDI process was determined to be less than 10^{-5} [49].

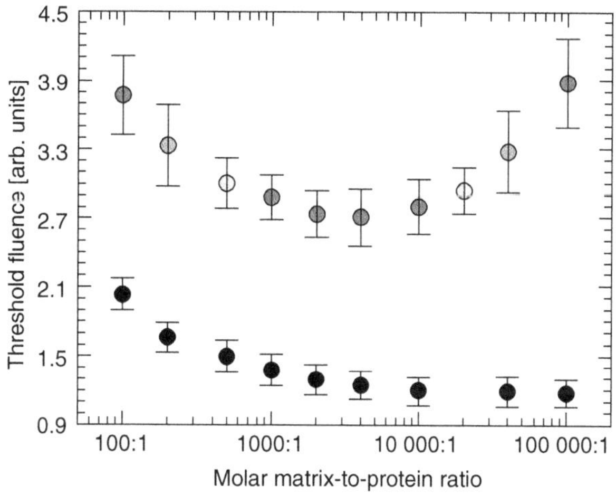

Fig. 11.3 Threshold fluence for positive ions of (*colored* ○) cytochrome c and (●) sinapinic acid as a function of the molar matrix-to-protein ratio. The range indicated by *green circles* provides optimum performance in terms of resolution and signal-to-noise ratio (Adapted from Ref. [48] by permission. © John Wiley & Sons, 1994)

Fluence and irradiance

The *fluence* is defined as energy per unit area; in MALDI typical fluences are in the range of 10–100 mJ cm^{-2}. The *irradiance* is fluence divided by the laser pulse duration; in MALDI the irradiances are in the range of 10^6–10^7 W cm^{-2} [37].

11.2.2 Effect of Laser Irradiation on the Surface

Best MALDI spectra in terms of resolution and low to absent ion fragmentation are obtained slightly above threshold for analyte ion formation [17, 47]. An evenly distributed shallow ablation of material from the upper layers of the sample is achieved if a comparatively homogeneous laser fluence is irradiated onto the target [29, 40, 50]. Ideal laser spot sizes are 100–200 µm as realized by 100–200 mm focal length of the commonly employed lenses [51]. Numerous single-shot spectra are then obtained from one spot. Such a laser spot size is also advantageous because a number of micrometer-sized crystrals are illuminated simultaneously thereby averaging out the effects of mutual orientation of crystal surfaces and laser beam axis [50, 52, 53]. On the other hand, an extremely sharp laser spot causes the eruption of material from a small area upon formation of a deep crater (Fig. 11.4). The MALDI spectra of cytochrome C (M_r = 12,360 u) demonstrate the superior quality of spectra obtained using an optimized spot size [54].

Although established over the years, nitrogen lasers inherently possess disadvantages in that *i*) their maximum repetition rate is limited to about 50 Hz, and *ii*) their average lifespan is only several 10^7 shots. Diode-pumped solid-state lasers such as the frequency-tripled Nd:YAG laser can deliver rates of > 1 kHz and have a hundred times longer lifespan. Especially in MALDI imaging and automated

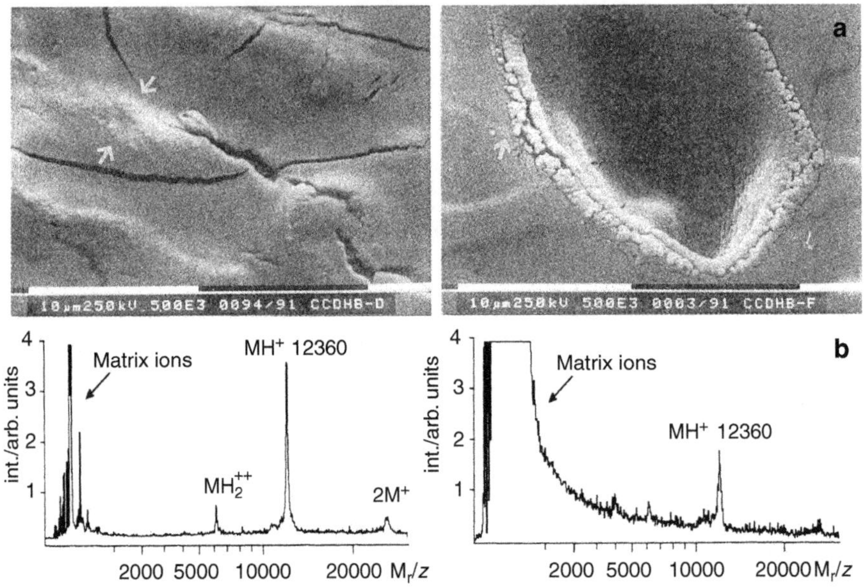

Fig. 11.4 Effect of focused and defocused laser beam. (**a**) SEM micrographs of DHB single crystals after exposure to 10 laser shots (337 nm) under focused (*right column*) and defocused (*left column*) irradiation with corresponding sum spectra of horse heart cytochrome C (M_r = 12,360 u); *black and white bars* correspond to 10 μm. (**b**) Resulting MALDI spectra (Reproduced from Ref. [54] by permission. © Elsevier Science, 1991)

high-throughput proteomics this number of shots is easily reached. Frequency-tripled Nd:YAG lasers unfortunately suffer from poor MALDI performance, e.g., they are of limited use with certain matrices and with highly relevant thin layer preparations. Their inferiority is not caused by the slight change from 337 nm to 355 nm wavelength but simply by their too small spot size. While nitrogen lasers deliver a moderately focused beam profile that also varies from shot to shot (Fig. 11.5), frequency-tripled Nd:YAG lasers yield sharp and too small irradiated spots. The insertion of a beam modulator to create beam profiles delivering a diffuse multispot pattern of similar overall diameter as a nitrogen laser solves this problem. This way, Bruker's Smartbeam™ Nd:YAG lasers even surpass the MALDI performance of nitrogen lasers (Fig. 11.6) [39, 55].

Use low laser fluence and acquire thousands of shots

MALDI spectra are acquired just above the threshold laser fluence for ion formation. Single-shot spectra therefore tend to exhibit a low signal-to-noise ratio (Sect. 1.6.3) due to poor ion statistics. With the 10–50 Hz repetition rates of nitrogen lasers, it was common to accumulate 50–200 single-shot spectra to create the final spectrum [53]. Nowadays, kHz shot rates of Nd:YAG lasers allow thousands of laser shots to be accumulated per final MALDI spectrum.

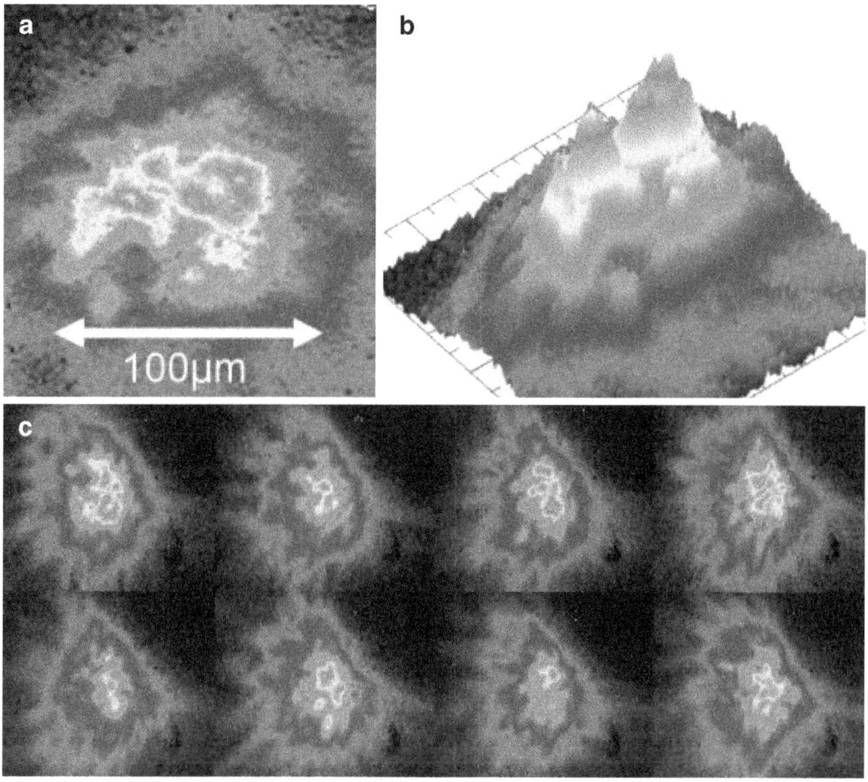

Fig. 11.5 Typical profile of a nitrogen laser. (**a**) View from top, (**b**) 3D view from the side, (**c**) beam profile of eight consecutive laser shots, demonstrating the shot-to-shot variation in the profile of the nitrogen laser. Different colors represent different intensities (Reproduced from Ref. [55] with permission. © Wiley, 2006)

11.2.3 Temporal Evolution of a Laser Desorption Plume

The desorption of ions and neutrals into the vacuum upon irradiation of a laser pulse proceeds as a jet-like *supersonic expansion* [43]: a small, but initially hot and very rapidly expanding plume is generated [15, 56]. The description of MALDI as an *energy-sudden* method [46] nicely expresses the explosive character of the plume formed by the nanosecond laser pulse. As the expansion is adiabatic, the process is accompanied by fast cooling of the plume [43].

Although the initial velocity of the desorbed ions is difficult to measure, reported values generally are in the range of 400–1200 m s^{-1}. The initial velocity is almost independent of the mass of the analyte ions but dependent on the matrix [37, 41–43, 52, 57, 58]. On the other hand, the initial analyte ion velocity is not independent of

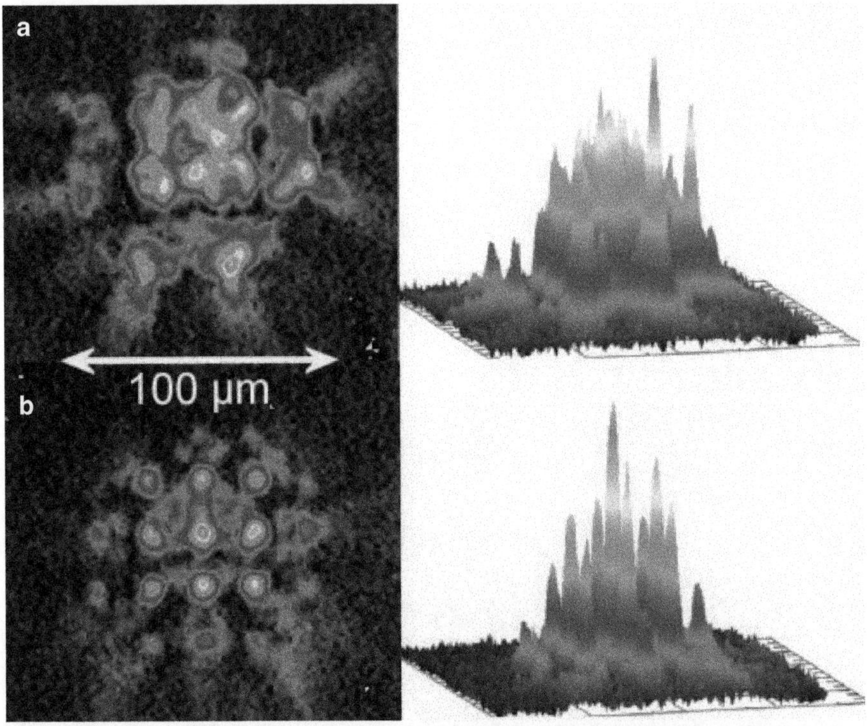

Fig. 11.6 Beam profiles of two differently structured beams of an Nd:YAG laser as employed in Bruker's Smartbeam lasers, (**a**) structured with FWHM of a Gaussian fit of the envelope of 60 µm and (**b**) with fit of 45 µm. The overlapping local maxima and the pattern are clearly visible (Reproduced from Ref. [55] with permission. © Wiley, 2006)

the compound class, i.e., peptides show a behavior different from oligosaccharides [15, 58]. The essential independence of mean ion velocities on the molecular weight of the analyte leads to an approximate linear increase of the mean initial kinetic energies of the analyte ions with mass. High-mass ions therefore carry tens of electronvolts of translational energy *before* ion acceleration [37, 47, 57]. The initial velocity of the ions is superimposed onto that obtained from ion acceleration, thereby causing considerable losses in resolution with continuous extraction TOF analyzers, in particular when operated in the linear mode.

Photographs of the plume Laser flash light photographs of the temporal evolution of a laser desorption plume are highly illustrative [59, 60]. The plume shown in Fig. 11.7 was generated from neat glycerol by an Er:Yag (2.94 µm) laser of 100 ns pulse width. Such laser pulse durations are typical for IR-MALDI. Glycerol was employed as a liquid matrix to provide a homogeneous sample and reproducible plume formation. Pulses of a frequency-doubled Nd:YAG laser (532 nm, 8 ns

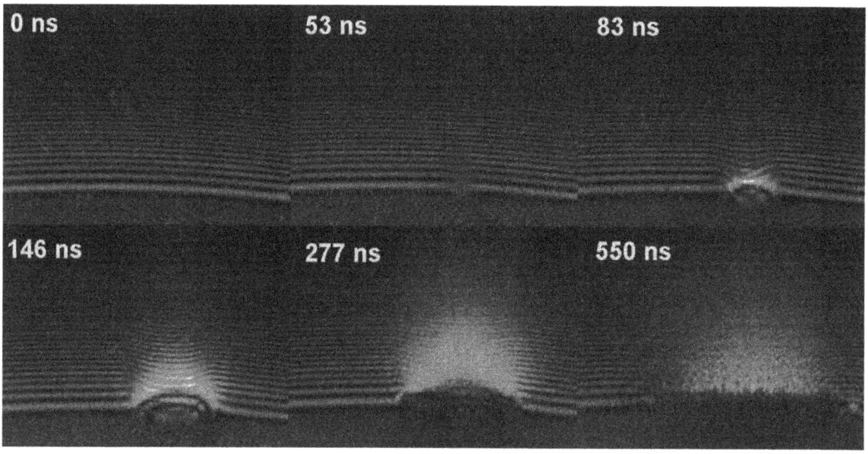

Fig. 11.7 Temporal evolution of a laser desorption plume generated by a 100-ns Er:Yag (2.94 μm) laser pulse from neat glycerol [60] (By courtesy of F. Hillenkamp and A. Leisner, University of Münster)

duration) served as the flashing light source for obtaining the photographs. Dark-field illumination was used to show the particulate components of the plume. In the beginning, the plume appears to consist of a continuous cloud of material of varying density, whereas individual micrometer-sized particles dominate later images. Interestingly, even after the exposure there was still some ejection of material observed [61].

Always vacuum MALDI?

Based on the understanding that mass analyzers require ions to be generated in vacuum, MALDI was initially developed as a vacuum ionization technique. In fact, most MALDI sources are operated in high vacuum and in combination with TOF analyzers. The MALDI-TOF-MS combination still defines the gold standard of MALDI-MS. Accordingly, most of this chapter implicitly is about vacuum MALDI. Nonetheless, it turned out that the MALDI process tolerates mbar-pressures and can also be performed at atmospheric pressure; the latter is referred to as atmospheric pressure MALDI (AP-MALDI, Sect. 11.8). The presence of gas can provide some collisional cooling of the freshly formed ions (cf. vacuum CI versus APCI in Sect. 7.8). This effect may even be increased at super-atmospheric pressure as demonstrated by running MALDI at 4–5 bar [62]. While from the user's perspective both vacuum MALDI and AP-MALDI may appear to work the same way, there are differences in the microscopic processes.

11.2.4 Processes of Ion Formation in MALDI

The pathways of ion formation in MALDI are numerous, i.e., no single process applies [15, 45, 46]. The promoting effect of decreasing pH of matrix-analyte solutions upon peptide ion yield indicates desorption of preformed $[M + H]^+$ ions. Similar observations are made for cationization products such as $[M + \text{alkali}]^+$ ions from oxygen-rich analytes. Nonetheless, gas phase processes – essentially some sort of CI in the dense desorption plume – cannot be excluded, because ions may be formed in the plasma plume even some hundred micrometers above the sample surface [63, 64]. Another study reveals a gradual increase of the initial ion velocities as the mass of oligosaccharides and synthetic polymers increases; they may even reach the high level characteristic for peptides and proteins. Introduction of a charged functional group via derivatization has the same effect on small oligosaccharides. This indicates that typical MALDI analytes require their incorporation as preformed ions into the matrix crystal to effectively become released into the gas phase, while gas phase cationization is viable for low-molecular-weight neutrals [43]. When non-carboxylic acid matrices are being used to protonate slightly basic analyte molecules, excited states of the matrix molecules may account for proton transfer [64, 65].

In case of UV light-absorbing analytes, direct photoionization can also occur. The frequently observed positive and negative radical ions $M^{+\bullet}$ [66, 67] and $M^{-\bullet}$ [68–70] can only be generated by removal or capture of an electron. Thus, $M^{+\bullet}$ and $M^{-\bullet}$ ions point towards the occurrence of photoionization [66], charge transfer, and electron capture in the gas phase [46, 66]. Which of the above processes contributes most to ion formation depends on the actual combination of matrix, analyte, and possibly present additives or contaminants.

11.2.5 "Lucky Survivor" Model of Ion Formation

The plasma emerging from a surface upon laser irradiation contains both positive and negative ions – it is neutral in total. Depending only on the polarity of the acceleration voltage one may either extract positive or negative ions, a situation similar to CI where an isobutane reagent gas plasma works equally well to deliver protonated species in PICI or deprotonated ions in NICI (Sect. 7.5). The starting conditions in MALDI, however, are quite different in that the analyte can be *multiply* protonated, deprotonated or otherwise charged by ion attachment in solution before its incorporation into the matrix crystals [15, 46]. Proof of multiple charging of macromolecules in solution phase is directly obtained from electrospray ionization mass spectra (Chap. 12).

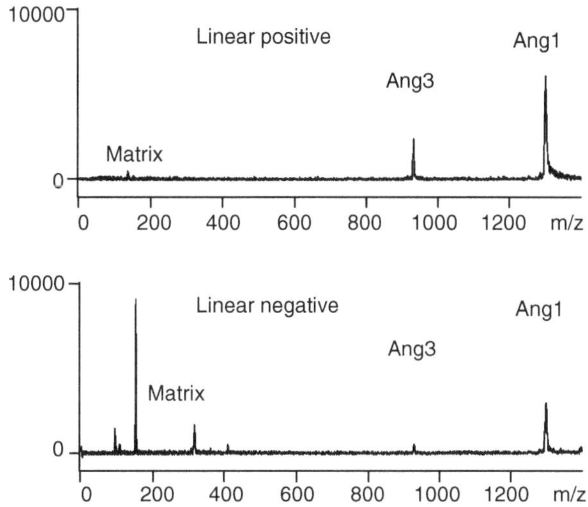

Fig. 11.8 MALDI mass spectra of a mixture of the small peptides angiotensin 1 (Ang1) and angiotensin 3 (Ang3) from DHB matrix as obtained on a linear TOF instrument in (**a**) positive-ion and (**b**) negative-ion mode under otherwise identical conditions (Reproduced from Ref. [46] with permission. © John Wiley & Sons, Ltd., 2000)

Peptide ion formation Although peptides and proteins are generally prepared for MALDI from acidified solutions, both singly protonated or deprotonated ions can normally be observed solely depending on the polarity of the extraction voltage. However, negative ion spectra tend to be less intensive for the same laser fluence, i.e., positive- and negative-ion mass spectra are not analogous (Fig. 11.8). Interestingly, the relative ion yields of both polarities are basically independent of the solvent composition, its pH, and of the solution phase acidity/basicity of the analyte.

In order to explain the above observations, we have to answer the following questions concerning the ionization process:

- Why are singly charged ions the (almost) only species observed in MALDI?
- How can charge separation be accomplished when mutual neutralization is considered to be the preferred process inside the plume?
- What are the fundamental processes limiting the ionic charge state to just one – either positive or negative?

The so-called *lucky survivor model* [46] explains this behavior in terms of mutual neutralization by recombination of cationic and anionic components of the plasma. Re-neutralization rates are higher, the higher the initial charge state of an ion. Thus, re-neutralization is slower for singly charged ions representing a late stage of the sequence, and therefore less probable to occur. Hence, singly charged ions generally are the "lucky survivors of the re-neutralization conflict" inside the laser plume (Fig. 11.9). As the fast moving electrons are most rapidly lost from the laser plume, an excess positive charge is established over time, which explains the lower abundance of negative ions in MALDI.

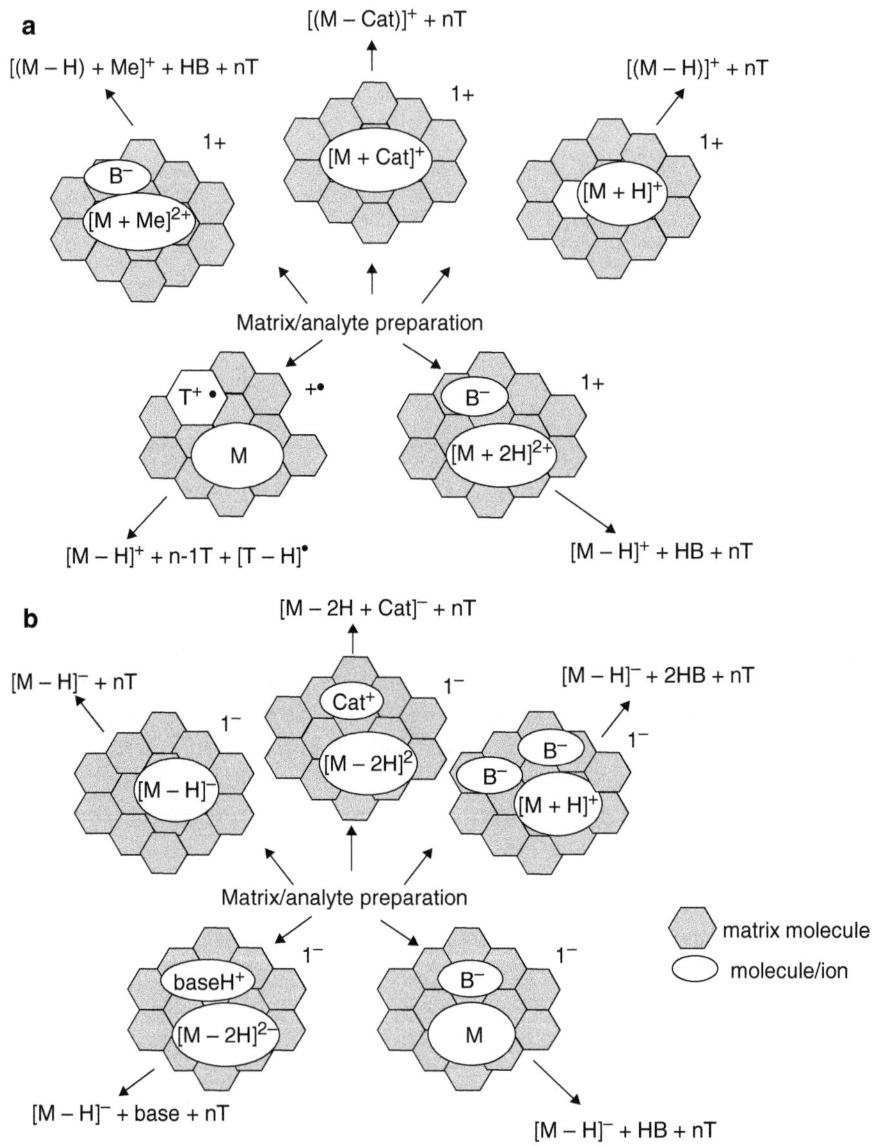

Fig. 11.9 Pathways of formation of singly charged ions from sample–matrix preparations according to the lucky survivor model. (**a**) Positive ion formation, (**b**) negative ion formation; M: analyte molecule, T: matrix molecule, Cat: small cation, Me: metal^{2+}, B: base (Adapted from Ref. [46] with permission. © John Wiley & Sons., Ltd., 2000)

11.3 MALDI Matrices

11.3.1 Role of the Solid Matrix

The role of the matrix in MALDI is analogous to that in FAB (Sect. 10.3). In contrast to FAB, MALDI matrices are generally crystalline solids of low vapor pressure in order not to be volatized in the ion source vacuum. While in principle any liquid can serve as a FAB matrix to moderate the energy of the impacting primary particles, the matrix in MALDI has to effectively absorb the laser light of the wavelength intended for use [71]. In UV-MALDI, the molecules need to possess a suitable chromophore, because energy uptake is based on the strong absorption, and thus the resulting electronic excitation of the matrices. Therefore, the structure of UV-MALDI matrices is based on some aromatic core suitably functionalized to achieve the desired properties.

In case of IR-MALDI, fewer restrictions apply because wavelengths around 3 µm are effectively absorbed by O–H and N–H stretch vibrations, while wavelengths around 10 µm cause excitation of C–O stretch and O–H bending vibrations [33, 36]. Therefore, malonic acid, succinic acid, malic acid, urea, and glycerol serve well as matrices in IR-MALDI [31, 32]. A matrix can serve as protonating or deprotonating agent or as electron-donating or -accepting agent.

Job of the matrix

It is evident that the first function of the matrix essentially is to dilute and isolate analyte molecules from each other. This occurs during solvent evaporation and concomitant formation of a solid solution. Then, upon laser irradiation, it functions as a mediator for energy absorption [46].

11.3.2 Matrices in UV-MALDI

Nicotinic acid (NA) was the first organic compound to be successfully employed as a matrix in UV-MALDI of peptides and proteins [12–14]. Ever since, better matrices have been sought, some of which now being widespread in use (Table 11.2 and Fig. 11.10). The currently most relevant matrices for UV-MALDI are HCCA, DHB, SA, DHAP, 3-HPA, DCTB, and dithranol. Nonetheless, even [60]fullerene [72] and porphyrins [73] have been used. Ionic liquids (ILs) have been employed as liquid MALDI matrices to achieve long-lasting signals on the same spot [74, 75].

Table 11.2 UV-MALDI matrices

Compound	Acronym	Application to	References
Nicotinic acid	NA	Peptides, proteins	[12–14]
Picolinic acid	PA	Oligonucleotides, DNA	[76]
3-Hydroxypicolinic acid	HPA, 3-HPA	Oligonucleotides, DNA	[77]
3-Aminopicolinic acid	3-APA	Oligonucleotides, DNA	[78]
6-Aza-2-thiothymine	ATT	Oligonucleotides, DNA	[79–81]
2,5-Dihydroxybenzoic acid	DHB	Proteins, oligosaccharides	[17, 54]
DHB-based mixtures	DHB/XY and super-DHB	Proteins, oligosaccharides	[82–86]
3-Aminoquinoline	3-AQ	Oligosaccharides	[87–89]
α-Cyano-4-hydroxycinnamic acid	α-CHC, α-CHCA, 4-HCCA, CHCA	Peptides, smaller proteins, triacylglycerols, numerous other compounds	[90–93]
4-Chloro-α-cyano-cinnamic acid	ClCCA	Peptides	[94, 95]
3,5-Dimethoxy-4-hydroxycinnamic acid	SA	Proteins	[96]
2-(4-Hydroxyphenylazo) benzoic acid	HABA	Peptides, proteins, glycoproteins, polystyrene	[71, 97]
2-Mercaptobenzothiazole	MBT	Peptides, proteins, synthetic polymers	[98]
5-Chloro-2-mercaptobenzothiazole	CMBT	Glycopeptides, phosphopeptides, and proteins	[98]
2,6-Dihydroxyacetophenone	DHAP	Glycopeptides, phosphopeptides, proteins	[99, 100]
2,4,6-Trihydroxyacetophenone	THAP	Solid-supported oligonucleotides	[101]
Dithranol (1,8,9-anthracenetriol)	None	Synthetic polymers	[102, 103]
9-Nitroanthracene	9-NA	Fullerenes and derivatives	[70, 104, 105]
Benzo[a]pyrene	None	Fullerenes and derivatives	[69]
2-[(2*E*)-3-(4-*tert*-Butylphenyl)-2-methylprop-2-enylidene]malonitrile	DCTB	Oligomers, polymers, dendrimers, small molecules	[106, 107]

Acronyms for matrices

It is common to use acronyms rather than compound names for most UV-MALDI matrices. However, these are not always consistently used, e.g., α-CHC, 4-HCCA, CHCA, and CCA all refer to α-cyano-4-hydroxycinnamic acid. Others may be easily confused, e.g., nicotinic acid (NA) and

(continued)

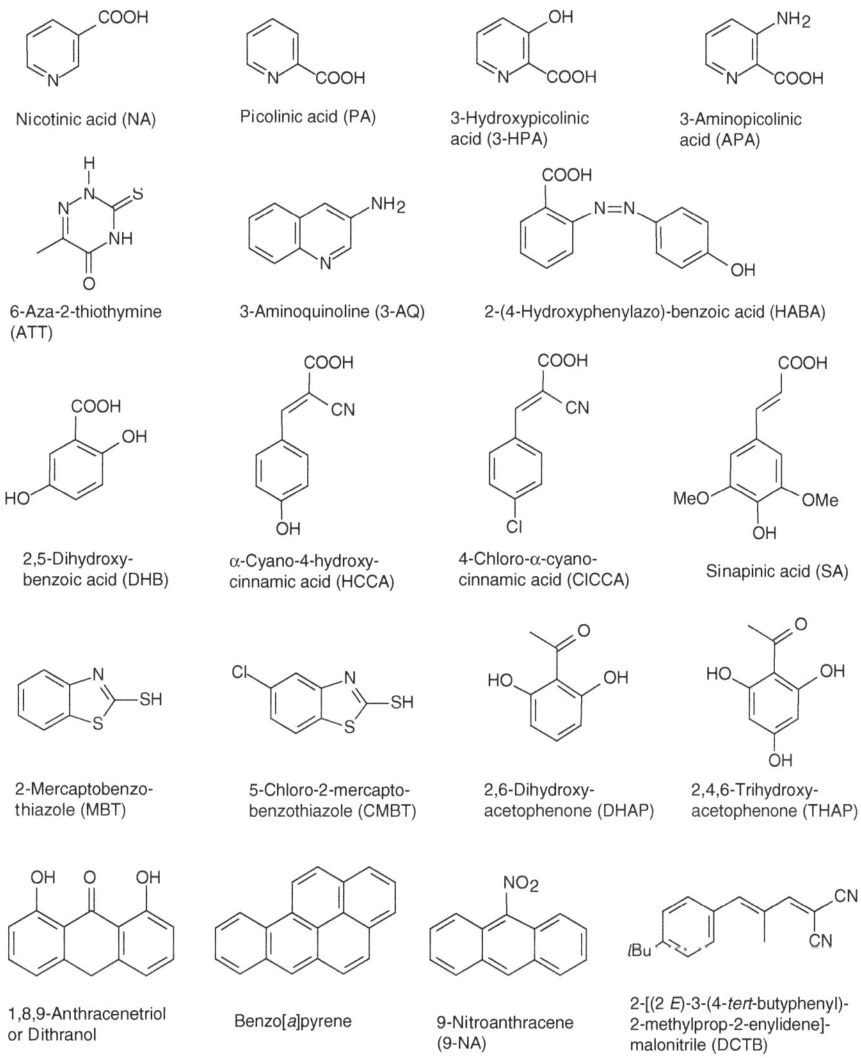

Fig. 11.10 Structures, names, and acronyms of common UV-MALDI matrices

9-nitroanthracene (9-NA), while some like dithranol or benzopyrene do not have an acronym, and others in fact can appear mysterious (DCTB).

Matrix is key to success

The choice of the right matrix is key to success in MALDI – and at the same time appears to be some kind of magic. For a first approach to a new analytical problem, it is recommended to try a matrix from the above

(continued)

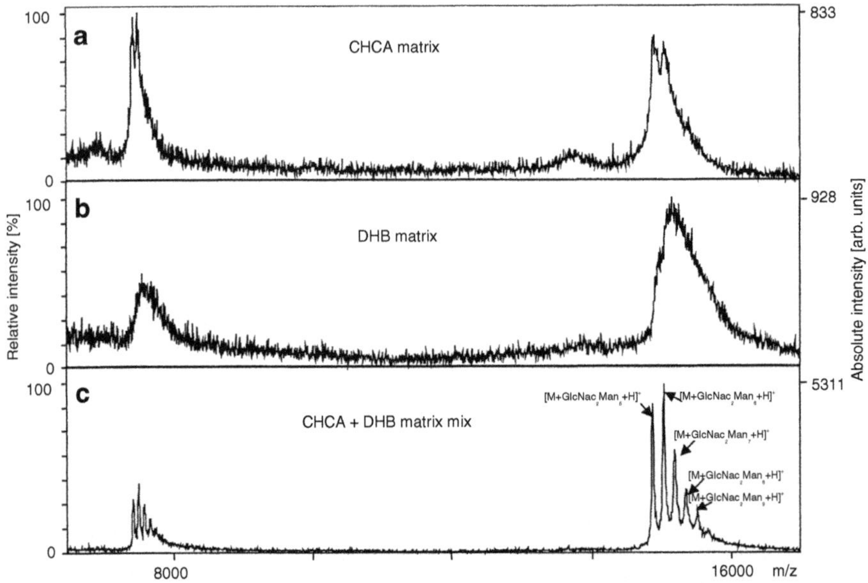

Fig. 11.11 Linear mode positive-ion MALDI-TOF spectra of ribonuclease B in 80 mM urea. (**a**) 300 fmol in CHCA, (**b**) 600 fmol in DHB, and (**c**) 300 fmol in CHCA/DHB matrix mix (Reproduced from Ref. [85] by permission. © Elsevier Science, 2003)

compilation. In general, highly polar analytes work better with highly polar matrices, and nonpolar analytes are preferably combined with nonpolar matrices. Matrix acidity data may help to judge its protonating effect [94, 108, 109]. While many compound classes may be analyzed using a variety of matrices, in less fortunate cases, only one specific analyte–matrix combination might yield useful MALDI spectra.

Only with the right matrix The choice of a matrix and optimized conditions of sample preparation have substantial influence on the analytical value of MALDI spectra. Even when employing standard matrices such as CHCA or DHB, significant improvements can be achieved, e.g., by appropriate mixing of the two matrices to analyze ribonuclease B (Fig. 11.11) [85].

11.3.3 Characteristics of MALDI Matrix Spectra

MALDI matrix (Ma) spectra are characterized by strong molecular and/or ions from protonation, cationization etc. The signals are accompanied by series of matrix cluster ions and some more abundant fragment ions [36]. In positive-ion MALDI, $[Ma_n + H]^+$ cluster ions predominate, while $[Ma_n - H]^-$ cluster ions are preferably formed in negative-ion MALDI. The principal ion series may be accompanied by $[Ma_n + alkali]^+$ ions and some fragments of minor intensity, e.g., $[Ma_n + H - H_2O]^+$. In particular with aprotic matrices, radical ions tend to dominate. In addition, a "continuous" background is formed by clustering of radiolytic decomposition products of the matrix. In general, the spectrum of the neat matrix, i.e., its LDI spectrum, strongly depends on the actual laser fluence and on the presence of impurities. Thus, the "correct" LDI spectrum of the matrix compound largely differs from what is obtained under conditions applied to form analyte ions from that matrix, because then, a 10–100-fold increased matrix ion density causes numerous secondary processes to occur. This dramatic change in mass spectral appearance bears some similarity to the transition observed from EI to CI spectra of reagent gases (Sect. 7.2.2).

11.4 Sample Preparation

The standard method of sample preparation in LDI and MALDI involves deposition and subsequent evaporation of 0.5–2 μl of dilute sample(–matrix) solution on the surface of a *sample holder* or *MALDI target*, as it is often referred to. Both composition of the solution and surface characteristics of the target strongly effect the outcome of the MALDI-MS experiment.

11.4.1 MALDI Target

Sample introduction has undergone a dramatic change in MALDI. In first experiments, single samples were supplied on MALDI probes designed similar to FAB probes (Sect. 10.3). Soon, multi-sample probes were developed. Early commercial products provided approximately twenty spots on one target which could be rotated, shifted, or freely moved in *x*- and *y*-directions to bring any spot on its surface into the laser's focus. Driven by the needs of combinatorial chemistry, 96-spot targets were developed to allow for the transfer of samples from a complete standard well plate. Soon after, the current standard of 384-spot, occasionally even 1536-spot, targets was established (Fig. 11.12). To take full advantage of such targets it is recommended to combine robotic sample preparation with automated measurement of the MALDI spectra.

The spot size of MALDI preparations and thus the amount of sample necessary to yield a useful layer can be substantially reduced by so-called *AnchorChip*™ targets (Bruker Daltonik). Such targets bear small hydrophilic spots on a hydrophobic surface. As a result, the evaporating drop of matrix–analyte solution is "anchored" to such a point where it shrinks until the onset of crystallization exactly within this hydrophilic area (Fig. 11.13c) [110]. The resulting preparation covers a much smaller surface than that from a freely spreading drop. In addition to improved detection limits, this technique simplifies automated spot finding due to their precisely defined location on the target.

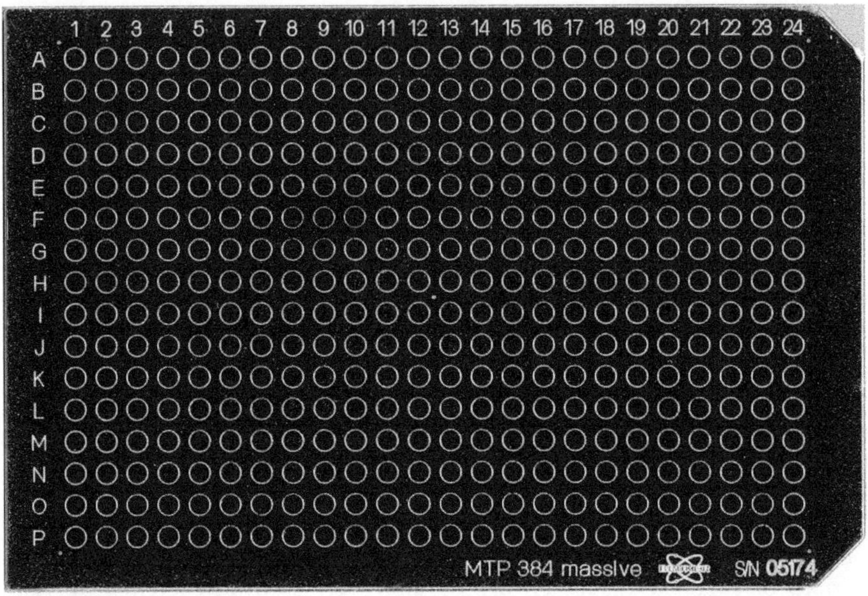

Fig. 11.12 Typical MALDI target: Bruker Scout384™ target offers a 16 × 24 spot array with up to 384 positions for sample preparation. Here, a standard nickel-coated massive aluminum version is shown; its dimensions are 84 × 128 mm with engraved marks of 3 mm in diameter

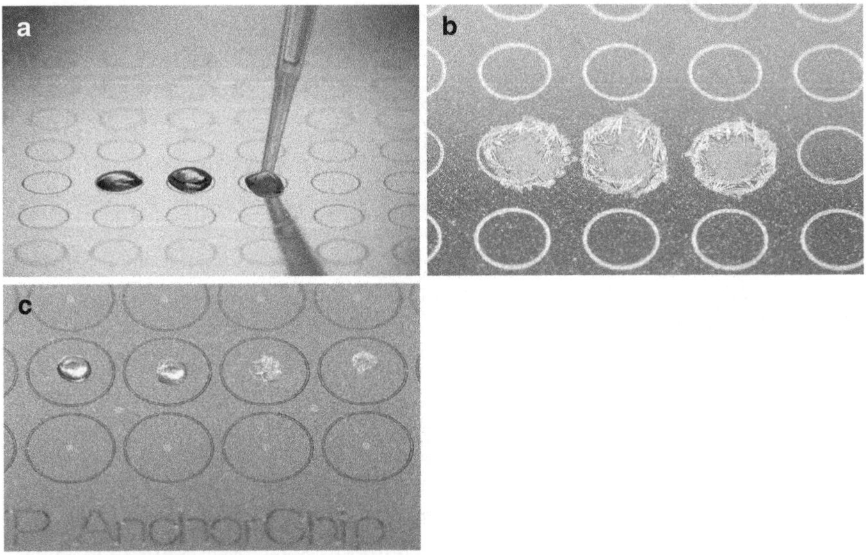

Fig. 11.13 Sample preparation for MALDI. (**a**) Pipetting of 1 μl of sample–matrix solution onto a standard MALDI target; (**b**) same spots after DHB has crystallized show large crystals on the rim and evenly distributed small crystals in the center; (**c**) cummulative effect of hydrophilic spots (*bright areas in circles*) present on a hydrophobic surface of an AnchorChip™ target on crystallizing DHB matrix

11.4.2 Standard Sample Preparation

The analyte should be soluble to at least about 0.1 mg ml^{-1} in some solvent. If a matrix is used, the matrix is dissolved to yield either a saturated solution or a concentration of about 10 mg ml^{-1}. The solution of the analyte is then admixed to that of the matrix. For optimized MALDI spectra, the molar matrix-to-analyte ratio is normally adjusted as to fall into the range from 1000 : 1 to 100,000 : 1 [16, 17, 54]. In this range, a good signal-to-noise ratio and a low degree of ion fragmentation are preserved. At very high sample concentrations the "matrix effect" is diminished and the spectra start resembling LDI spectra. Too low sample concentrations require additional laser irradiance for sufficient analyte ion production [48]. However, given a proper preparation, even a molar matrix-to-analyte ratio of 10^8 : 1 can produce useful results. A sufficient miscibility of analyte and matrix is also required [102].

Sample consumption Assuming a typical MALDI matrix with an M_r of about 200 g mol^{-1}, dissolution at 10 mg ml^{-1} in a suitable solvent yields a matrix solution that is 0.05 M in concentration, which is equal to 5×10^{-8} mol μl^{-1}. An average peptide of M_r around 2000 g mol^{-1} dissolved at 0.01 mg ml^{-1} results in 5×10^{-12} mol μl^{-1} (5 pmol μl^{-1}). Mixing the matrix with the analyte solution 1:1 (v/v) results in a molar matrix-to-analyte ratio of 10,000 : 1 for preparation on a target. Pipetting 1 μl of this mixture per spot onto a MALDI target corresponds to 2.5 pmol of sample per spot (Fig. 11.13). In fact, MALDI-TOF-MS of peptides can be extended to 1/1000th of this amount, and thus, may routinely deliver useful spectra down to a few fmol of peptide per spot, which is equal to a molar matrix-to-analyte ratio of 10,000,000 : 1.

The crystallization process is a critical parameter in LDI and MALDI sample preparation [54, 111, 112]. The conventional co-crystallization is usually termed *dried droplet preparation*. Dried droplet preparation yields comparatively large crystals, especially when slow evaporation, e.g., from aqueous solutions, is involved. Unfortunately, large crystals are detrimental for good shot-to-shot reproducibility and mass accuracy.

Evenly distributed thin layers of microcrystallites are therefore preferred [111, 113]. The original so-called *thin layer technique* involves preparation of a thin HCHA layer from solution in acetone on top of which the analyte is placed in a second step without re-dissolving the matrix [114, 115]. The formation of thin layers can also be assisted by (*i*) using volatile solvent(s) such as acetone, (*ii*) by eventually enforcing evaporation by gentle heating of the target or by a softly blowing hair dryer, and finally (*iii*) by using polished targets. Thus, the thin layer technique had a significant impact on MALDI sample preparation [114, 116].

Finally, (nano)electrospray deposition can be used to deposit the analytes onto different kinds of predeposited matrix layers. MALDI sample preparations where the analyte solution is deposited on top of a previously prepared matrix layer are generally termed *sandwich methods*. The base layer of matrix may be prepared either by the standard dried droplet technique or by thin layer preparation. For (nano)electrospray deposition of peptides, for example, a 10^{-5} M solution is sprayed from a (nano)electrospray capillary onto the solid matrix layer. The advantage of nanoelectrospray over conventional electrospray is that very small droplets are formed, which arrive at the target as dry particles, and thus, do not wet and re-dissolve the matrix surface [45].

11.4.3 Cationization

Metal ions, in particular singly charged ions such as Na^+, K^+, Cs^+, and Ag^+ are sometimes added to the matrix–analyte solution to effect cationization of the neutral analyte [117]. This is advantageous when the analyte has a high affinity to a certain metal ion, e.g., towards alkali ions in case of oligosaccharides [6]. Addition of individual cations can also lead to a concentration of ions of a particular kind, e.g., promoting $[M + K]^+$ ions over all other alkali ion adducts upon addition of a potassium salt (Fig. 11.14).

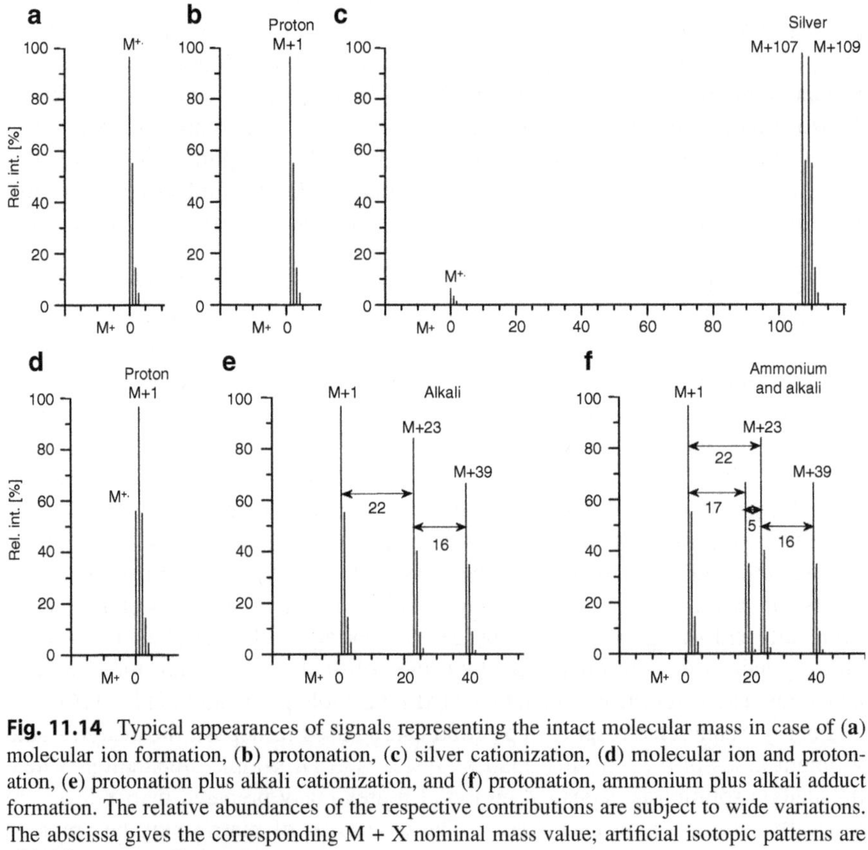

Fig. 11.14 Typical appearances of signals representing the intact molecular mass in case of (**a**) molecular ion formation, (**b**) protonation, (**c**) silver cationization, (**d**) molecular ion and protonation, (**e**) protonation plus alkali cationization, and (**f**) protonation, ammonium plus alkali adduct formation. The relative abundances of the respective contributions are subject to wide variations. The abscissa gives the corresponding M + X nominal mass value; artificial isotopic patterns are added for more realistic appearance

Silver ions (from silver trifluoroacetate or trifluoromethanesulfonate), Cu^+, and other transition metal ions in their 1+ oxidation state [118, 119] are frequently employed to obtain $[M + metal]^+$ ions from nonfunctionalized or at least nonpolar hydrocarbons [120], polyethylene [121, 122], or polystyrene (for an example see Sect. 11.6.1) [118, 119, 123–125].

Na^+ and K^+ are everywhere
Sodium and potassium are ubiquitous and the corresponding adducts are almost omnipresent given the analyte has some alkali ion affinity [126]. It is therefore advisable to know these typical mass differences by heart. Searching a spectrum for those frequent peak distances, e.g., +22 u and +16 u in case of $[M + Na]^+$ and $[M + K]^+$ ions accompanying $[M + H]^+$, reveals the true molecular mass. Other cations, e.g., Li^+ or Ag^+, are easily identifiable by their isotopic pattern.

Accurate mass data provided, the $\Delta(m/z)$ values between suspect pairs of peaks can be used to unequivocally identify $[M + Na]^+$, $[M + K]^+$, and other frequent cationization product ions the same way as we used the corresponding differences to verify the presence of certain elements by their characteristic $\Delta(m/z)$ between isotopes (Table 3.2) [127]. The most frequent pairs to be distinguished are collected below (Table 11.3).

11.4.4 Cation Exchange and the Need for Cation Removal

If an analyte molecule contains several acidic hydrogens, these can be exchanged by alkali ions without generating a charged species, e.g., [M – H + K] or [M – 2H + 2Na]. As a result, a single analyte species will form numerous ionic species thereby significantly decreasing the abundance of each species involved, e.g., $[M - 2H + Na]^-$, $[M - 2H + K]^-$, $[M - 3H + Na + K]^-$ etc. Fortunately, in MALDI, we only need to consider singly charged ions.

Challenging multiple cation exchange Oligonucleotides are important representatives of this type of compounds. Their extreme polarity and poly-anionic character alone make them very hard to analyze. Additionally, each added

Table 11.3 Characteristic mass differences to identify frequent cationization products

Pair of ions	Δm [u]
$M^{+\bullet}$ vs. ^{13}C-$M^{+\bullet}$	1.0033
$M^{+\bullet}$ vs. $[M + H]^+$	1.0078
$[M + H]^+$ vs. $[M + NH_4]^+$	17.0265
$[M + H]^+$ vs. $[M + Na]^+$	21.9819
$[M + H]^+$ vs. $[M + K]^+$	37.9559
$[M + Na]^+$ vs. $[M + K]^+$	15.9739
$[M + H]^+$ vs. $[M + O + H]^+$	15.9949

nucleoside imports another exchangeable hydrogen via the phosphate residue. An oligonucleotide 11mer, for example, can theoretically appear as any ion from $[M-H]^-$, $[M-2H+Na]^-$ up to $[M-10H+9Na]^-$, and, provided these are present, can repeat this exchange scheme with K^+ and NH_4^+ ions. Further, products of mixed exchange like $[M-6H+3Na+2K]^-$ have to be considered. Thus, hydrogen-to-metal exchange may finally result in complete suppression of a useful signal as numerous, eventually unresolved, peaks each of very low intensity can appear just as a slight and broad bump in the baseline of the spectrum [128]. Mass spectral analysis of oligonucleotides is alternatively performed by electrospray ionization (ESI) and their sequencing is also dealt with in that context (Sect. 12.6.4).

On-target washing presents a simple but very effective approach to reduce the alkali ion content of MALDI sample preparations [129, 130]. For this purpose, 2–5 µl of alkali ion-free water containing 0.1–1% formic or trifluoroacetic acid is placed on top of the crystalline layer and removed after a few seconds by a microliter pipette or by blowing it off with a stream of pressurized air. The acidification avoids dissolution of the crystals in case of carboxylic acid matrix preparations.

Cation exchange resins can be added prior to preparation to substitute alkali ions for ammonium (Fig. 11.15) [30]. To take full effect, it is important to keep the cation exchange beads even on the target in order to capture the alkali ion contamination of the metal surface, too. No useful signals are obtained when the laser hits the cation exchange beads. Furthermore, there is a risk of ion source contamination as beads may occasionally fall off the surface, even as a result of laser shots.

Another approach is to use tips of microliter pipettes as miniature columns by filling them with *size exclusion chromatography* (SEC) stationary phase material or standard C_{18} reversed phase material [131, 132]. Such tips are also commercially available as ZipTips™ [128]. There is a risk of sample absorption on the column

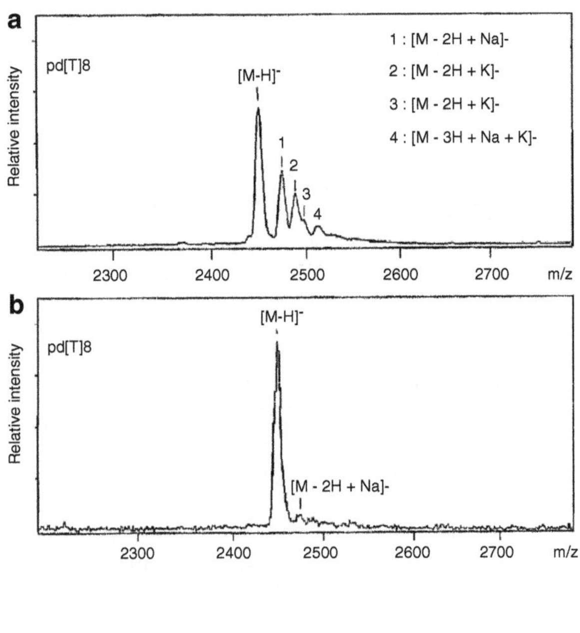

Fig. 11.15 Negative-ion MALDI spectra of the oligonucleotide pd[T]$_8$; (**a**) 5 pmol, (**b**) same as (**a**) after addition of 5–10 cation exchange beads to the sample preparation (Adapted from Ref. [30] by permission. © John Wiley & Sons, 1992)

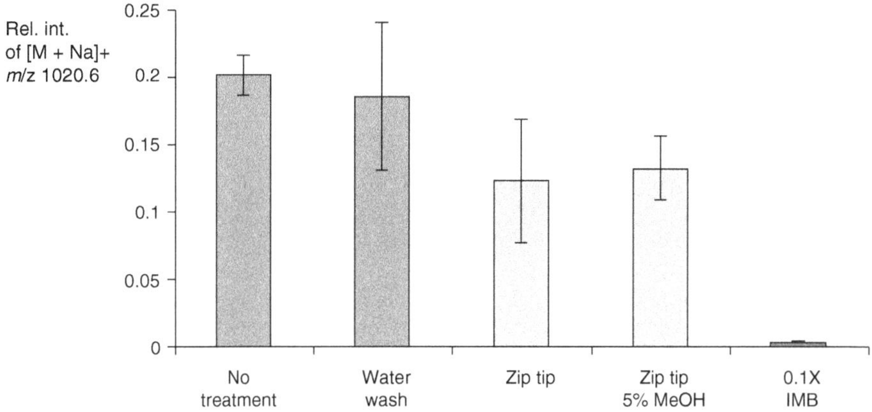

Fig. 11.16 Comparison of common alkali adduct suppression techniques. The ratio of the intensity of a peptide $[M + Na]^+$ peak, *m/z* 1020.6, to the sum of $[M + H]^+$ and $[M + Na]^+$ signal intensities is shown. *Error bars* represent standard deviation of three measurements (Adapted from Ref. [133] with permission. © John Wiley & Sons, Ltd, 2004)

material, which is particularly critical for minor components of complex mixtures – and the cost factor of these consumables should also be kept in mind.

Finally, it is advantageous to add a surfactant blend (Invitrosol-MALDI protein solubilizer B, IMB) prior to preparation (Fig. 11.16) [133].

Equally, sodium dodecyl sulfate contaminations should be removed from 2D gel electrophoresis before subjecting samples to MALDI-MS [134].

11.4.5 Anion Adducts

In negative-ion MALDI, analyte molecules do not exclusively form $[M - H]^-$ ions but also anion adducts with $[M + Cl]^-$, $[M + COOH]^-$, and $[M + CF_3COO]^-$ being most likely. Formiate and triflate adducts can be formed when matrix solutions are acidified by use of formic acid or trifluoroacetic acid (HTFA), respectively. Additionally, open-electron ions can be formed by electron capture (Sect. 7.6). It is therefore helpful to have accurate mass differences for their identification at hand (Table 11.4).

11.4.6 Solvent-Free Sample Preparation

If an analyte is absolutely insoluble or only soluble in solvents that are not acceptable for the standard MALDI sample preparation technique, it can alternatively be ground together with the solid matrix, preferably in a vibrating ball mill. The resulting fine powder is then spread onto the target. To avoid contamination, non-adherent material should be gently blown away from the target before insertion into the ion source [122, 135, 136] (Fig. 11.17).

Table 11.4 Characteristic mass differences to identify frequent negative adduct ions

Pair of ions	Δm [u]
$M^{-\bullet}$ vs. $^{13}C\text{-}M^{-\bullet}$	1.0033
$[M-H]^-$ vs. $M^{-\bullet}$	1.0078
$[M-H]^-$ vs. $[M+OH]^-$	18.0106
$[M-H]^-$ vs. $[M+{}^{35}Cl]^-$	35.9767
$[M-H]^-$ vs. $[M+COOH]^-$	46.0055
$[M-H]^-$ vs. $[M+{}^{79}Br]^-$	79.9261
$[M-H]^-$ vs. $[M+CF_3COO]^-$	113.9928

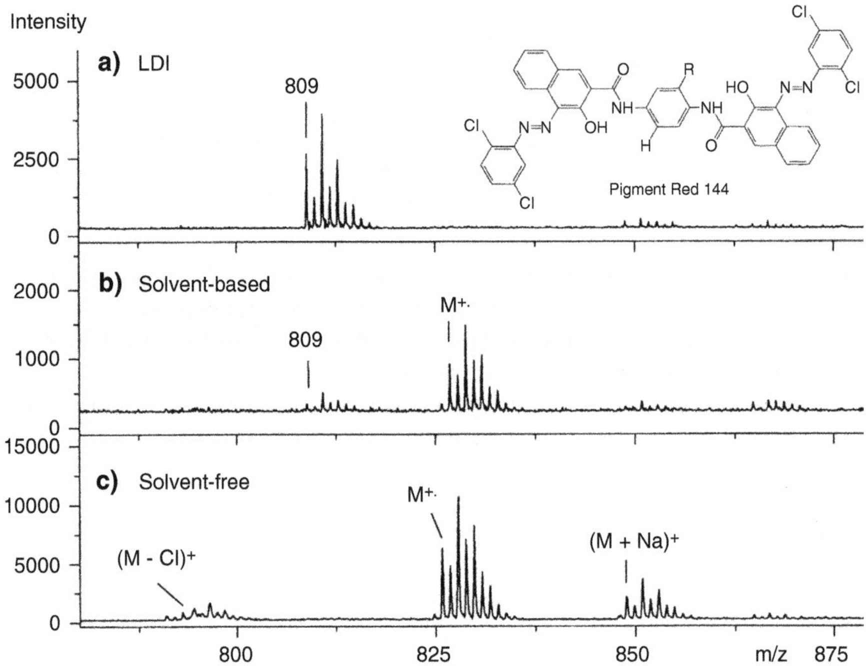

Fig. 11.17 Comparison of spectra of the organic dye Pigment Red 144 as obtained by (**a**) LDI, (**b**) solvent-based, and (**c**) solvent-free MALDI sample preparation (Adapted from Ref. [136] by permission. © John Wiley & Sons, 2001)

MALDI of an insoluble pigment The organic dye Pigment Red 144, has been subjected to mass analysis by LDI, solvent-based MALDI, and solvent-free MALDI [136]. Its monoisotopic molecular ion, $[C_{40}H_{23}Cl_5O_4N_6]^{+\bullet}$, is expected at *m/z* 826.0. Due to the strong light absorption of the pigment, the uptake of energy in LDI causes quantitative fragmentation to yield solely $[M-OH]^+$ ions. Here, solvent-based MALDI results in a poor sample preparation because of the unfavorable solvents needed, whereas solvent-free sample preparation yields a better spectrum exhibiting mainly $M^{+\bullet}$ and $[M+Na]^+$ ions of the pigment (Fig. 11.15).

11.4.7 Additional Methods of Sample Supply

Surface-adsorbed analytes can be examined by laser desorption techniques if they are supplied on a metal foil, a TLC plate [137], or at least on semiconducting material. Even the foil itself can be subject to LDI. This requires the foil to be fixed on top of a sample target, e.g., by means of (conducting) double-sided adhesive tape or some general-purpose adhesive. Care has to be taken not to produce sharp edges protruding from the surface because these might cause discharges in the ion source when the accelerating voltage is switched on. Furthermore, the mass calibration can be affected by such an unusually thick "sample layer". The latter two limitations are only relevant in case of on-axis MALDI-TOF analysis, while oaTOF analyzers and other setups with external MALDI ion sources are by far more robust in this respect.

Safety notice
Unconventional sample supply techniques on commercial MALDI instruments afford great care. Possible pitfalls include (*i*) blocking of the vacuum lock due to unacceptable thickness of the target, (*ii*) loss of the sample inside the ion source or inside the vacuum lock, (*iii*) damage to the instrument from electric discharges. It is therefore highly recommended to use dedicated sample holders when such are supplied by the instrument manufacturer.

11.5 Applications of LDI

Although LDI is also possible for peptides [5] and oligosaccharides [4, 6], it is suited much better for analyzing organic and inorganic salts [138–140], molecules with large conjugated π-electron systems [141–143], organic dyes as contained in ballpoint pen inks [144], porphyrins [145], or UV light-absorbing synthetic polymers [5, 56]. As interferences with matrix ions are excluded, LDI presents a useful and quick alternative to MALDI in the low-mass range. In addition, solvent-free sample preparation can be employed with insoluble analytes by simply grinding the solid onto the sample holder. However, LDI is a "harder" ionization method than MALDI and fragmentation has to be taken into account.

LDI of a polycyclic aromatic hydrocarbon Polycyclic aromatic hydrocarbons (PAHs) are easily detected by LDI due to their strong UV absorbance. The positive-ion LDI-TOF mass spectrum of 1,2,3,4,5,6-hexahydrophenanthro[1,10,9,8-*opqra*] perylene exclusively presents the molecular ion at *m/z* 356 (Fig. 11.18; for the EI spectrum cf. Sect. 2.1) [143].

Fullerene soot analyzed by LDI Fullerene soot as obtained by the Huffman-Krätschmer synthesis [146] can be characterized by positive- as well as negative-

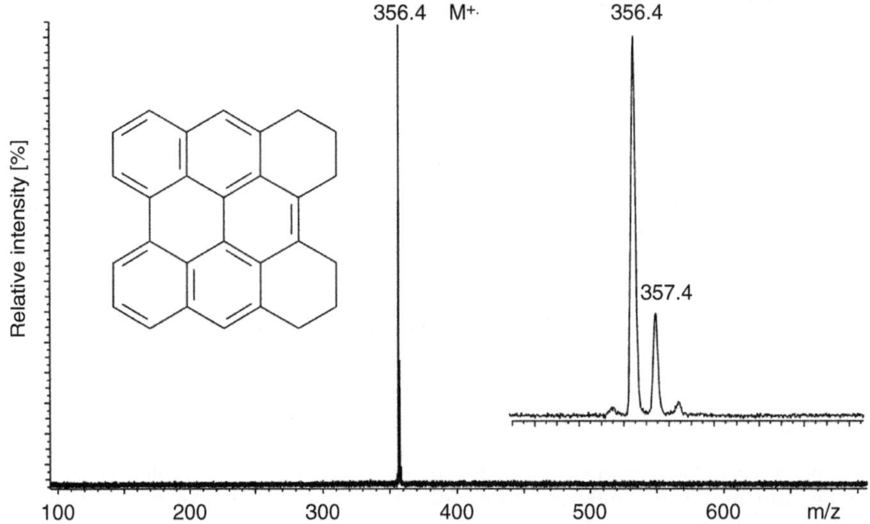

Fig. 11.18 Positive-ion LDI-TOF mass spectrum of 1,2,3,4,5,6-hexahydrophenanthro[1,10,9,8-*opqra*]perylene. The *inset* shows an expanded view of the molecular ion signal (Adapted from Ref. [143] with permission. © Elsevier Science, 2002)

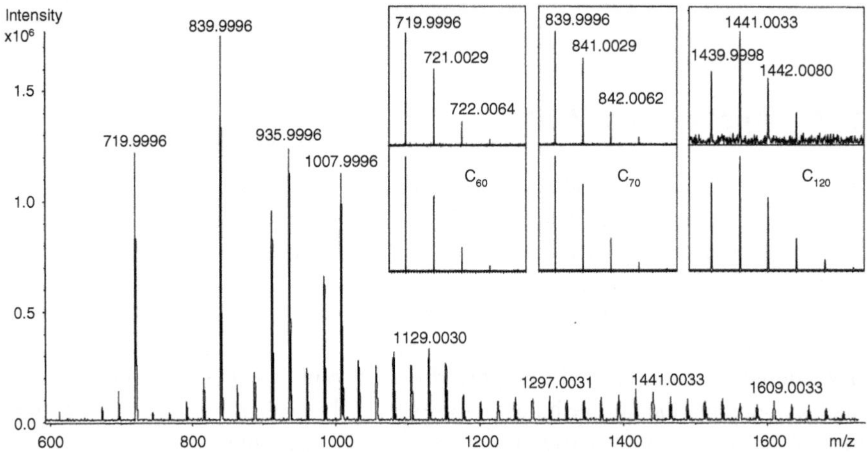

Fig. 11.19 Positive-ion LDI-FT-ICR mass spectrum of a fullerene soot. The *insets* show expanded views of the experimental (*upper parts*) and calculated (*lower parts*) isotopic patterns of $C_{60}^{+\bullet}$, $C_{70}^{+\bullet}$, and $C_{120}^{+\bullet}$. Sample courtesy of W. Krätschmer, Max Planck Institute for Nuclear Physics, Heidelberg (Reproduced from Ref. [148] by permission. © Wiley-VCH, Weinheim, 2009)

ion LDI-MS [141]. Such LDI spectra can exhibit fullerene molecular ion signals well beyond *m*/*z* 3000; among these, $C_{60}^{+\bullet}$ and $C_{70}^{+\bullet}$ are clearly accentuated (Fig. 11.19). Furthermore, such samples provide experimental carbon-only isotopic patterns over a wide mass range (Sect. 3.2.1). The spectrum below was obtained on a FT-ICR mass spectrometer; hence the resolution is 175,000 at *m/z* 840, i.e., almost by a factor of 1000 higher than on early TOF instruments as used for the discovery of C_{60} and larger fullerenes [147]. The insets show expanded views of the $M^{+\bullet}$ ions for C_{60}, C_{70}, and C_{120} together with the corresponding calculated isotopic patterns. Note, that the accurate masses are lower than the nominal values by the mass of an electron, while the difference in mass of 1.0033 u between ^{12}C and ^{13}C can be recognized from the mass increment of the 1st and 2nd isotopic peaks, respectively.

11.6 Applications of MALDI

MALDI applications are growing at a rapid pace with thousands of publications annually. A single book chapter thus can impossibly cover all aspects of these developments. However, there are several excellent monographs on different aspects of MALDI that are highly recommended to anyone intending to pursue further studies of MALDI-MS [23–26, 149–152]. The following section will merely outline selected flagship applications of MALDI-MS.

11.6.1 General Protein Analysis by MALDI-MS

The success story of MALDI started with the demonstration of intact protein analysis by MALDI-TOF-MS. In their seminal work, F. Hillenkamp and M. Karas showed that MALDI is unique in that it can combine the ability for:

- desorbing ions of biomacromolecules into the gas phase,
- preserving their structural integrity, and
- being perfectly compatible with mass analyzers with almost unlimited *m/z* range and extraordinary sensitivity (Figs. 11.1 and 11.4) [11, 13, 14].

The analysis of intact proteins is often the first step in a series of analytical procedures revealing characteristics of cells, physiological pathways, diseases, or other aspects of interest in a biological or biomedical context. Often, the proteins are separated prior to MALDI-MS, e.g., by 2D gel electrophoresis. MALDI experiments must be carried out with highly purified proteins or mixtures containing only a limited number of proteins. In cases where the full mass range of proteins is needed, MALDI-TOF-MS would be the preferred choice.

The most commonly used matrices for MALDI of proteins are 3,5-dimethoxy-4-hydroxycinnamic acid (generally known as sinapinic acid (SA) [96]) and 2,5-dihydroxybenzoic acid (DHB) [17, 54]. Alternatively, for peptides, proteins, and glycoproteins one can use 2-(4-hydroxyphenylazo)benzoic acid (HABA) [71], 2-mercaptobenzothiazole (MBT), and 5-chloro-2-mercaptobenzothiazole (CMBT). For smaller proteins of up to about 6000 u good results can also be obtained using α-cyano-4-hydroxycinnamic acid (α-CHCA) [90].

11.6.2 Protein Fingerprints and MALDI Biotyping

Any organism bears a characteristic *protein fingerprint*. Protein fingerprints (and also those of carbohydrates) can be readily obtained by means of MALDI-MS. The necessary purification steps prior to MALDI analysis depend on the individual sample. For instance, the protein composition of a Mozzarella cheese will be able to reveal whether it was made from cow's milk or of that of a water buffalo [153], or whether feta cheese is "contaminated" with cow's milk [154]. MALDI spectra of protein extracts from different *Bacillus* species can be used to distinguish pathogenic from nonpathogenic bacteria, e.g., the protein fingerprints of chemically lysed *B. anthracis* (Sterne), *B. thuringiensis* (4A1), and *B. cereus* (6E1) are clearly different [155]; even different strains are distinguishable on the basis of particular biomarker proteins.

This field of MALDI-based mass spectrometry for the identification of biological species is known as *MALDI biotyping*. Instruments optimized for use in the clinical laboratory are available, e.g., the Bruker MALDI biotyper, a compact linear-mode MALDI instrument. MALDI biotyping is now well established for the identification of bacteria as it offers much faster and also cheaper means than immunoassays [156–158].

Microorganisms on fish In food analysis of fish and seafood products, differentiating between individual species of pathogenic and food-spoilage microorganisms and their rapid identification are particularly important. MALDI-TOF-MS protein fingerprinting was used to characterize the main 26 species responsible for seafood spoilage and associated pathogenic bacteria such as *Acinetobacter baumanii* and *Pseudomonas* species (Fig. 11.20) [159]. For this purpose, low-mass proteins were extracted from intact bacterial cells and subjected to MALDI analysis using α-CHCA matrix on a linear TOF instrument. Then, a library of specific MS fingerprints was compiled by comparing 10–35 characteristic peaks per organism in a range of *m/z* 2,000–10,000 from the protein fingerprint MALDI spectra.

MALDI-TOF spectra of intact parasites The selection of the proper matrix and the technique of sample preparation also matters in MALDI biotyping as is impressively demonstrated by the comparison of matrices for the identification of *Trypanosoma cruzi*, a protozoan flagellate parasite that causes Chagas disease (American trypanosomiasis). In this study, positive-ion MALDI spectra were obtained after using dried droplets or thin layer preparation in combination with DHB, SA, and CHCA [157]. Microscopic images of the preparations with SA and CHCA already showed differences in uniformity (Fig. 11.21). The superiority of SA by thin layer technique was directly reflected in the quality of the MALDI spectrum (Fig. 11.22). DHB neither formed a crystalline layer nor was it able to yield a useful spectrum.

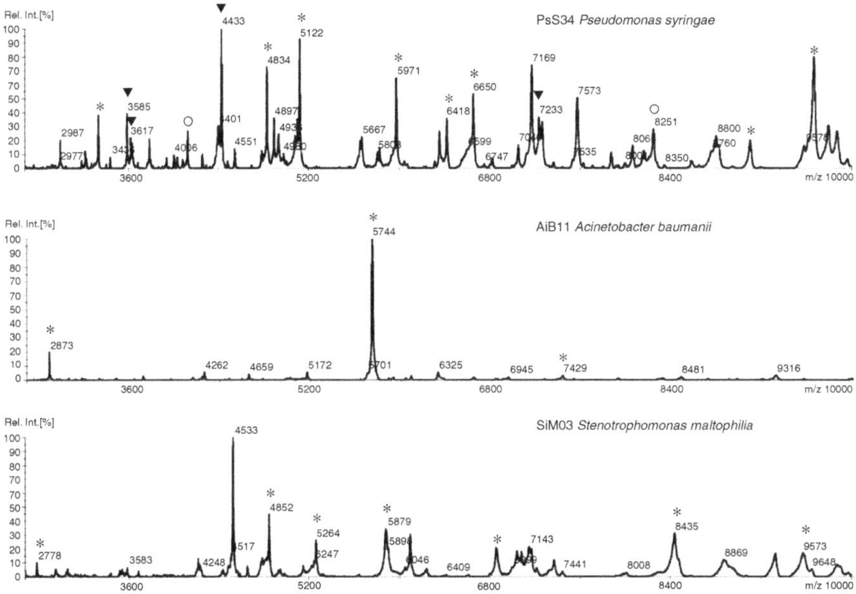

Fig. 11.20 Protein fingerprint MALDI-TOF spectra of *Pseudomonas syringae* (*top*), *Acetinobacter baumannii* (*center*) and *Stenotrophomonas maltophilia* (*bottom*) have clearly different appearances; species-specific peaks are indicated by *, genus-specific peaks by O, and other characteristic peaks by ▼ (Adapted from Ref. [159] with permission. © American Chemical Society, 2010)

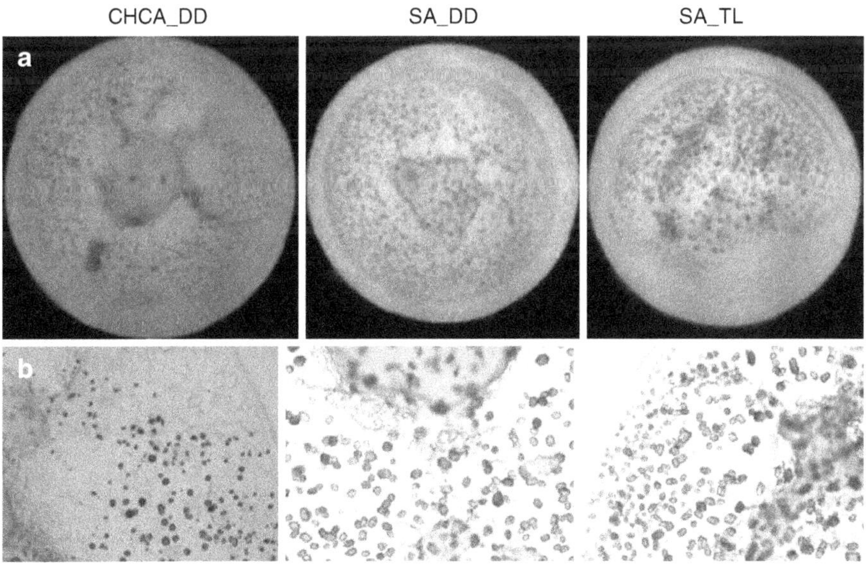

Fig. 11.21 Microscopic images of intact parasite cells embedded in different matrices imaged at two levels of resolution (**a**) ×10 and (**b**) ×100; DD: dried droplet preparation, TL: thin layer method. Matrices were dissolved in acetonitrile : water = 7 : 3 with 0.1% of trifluoroacetic acid. The superior uniformity of the thin layer sample deposition is visible and notably affects the quality of the MALDI spectrum (Fig. 11.22) (Adapted from Ref. [157] with permission. © Wiley, 2016)

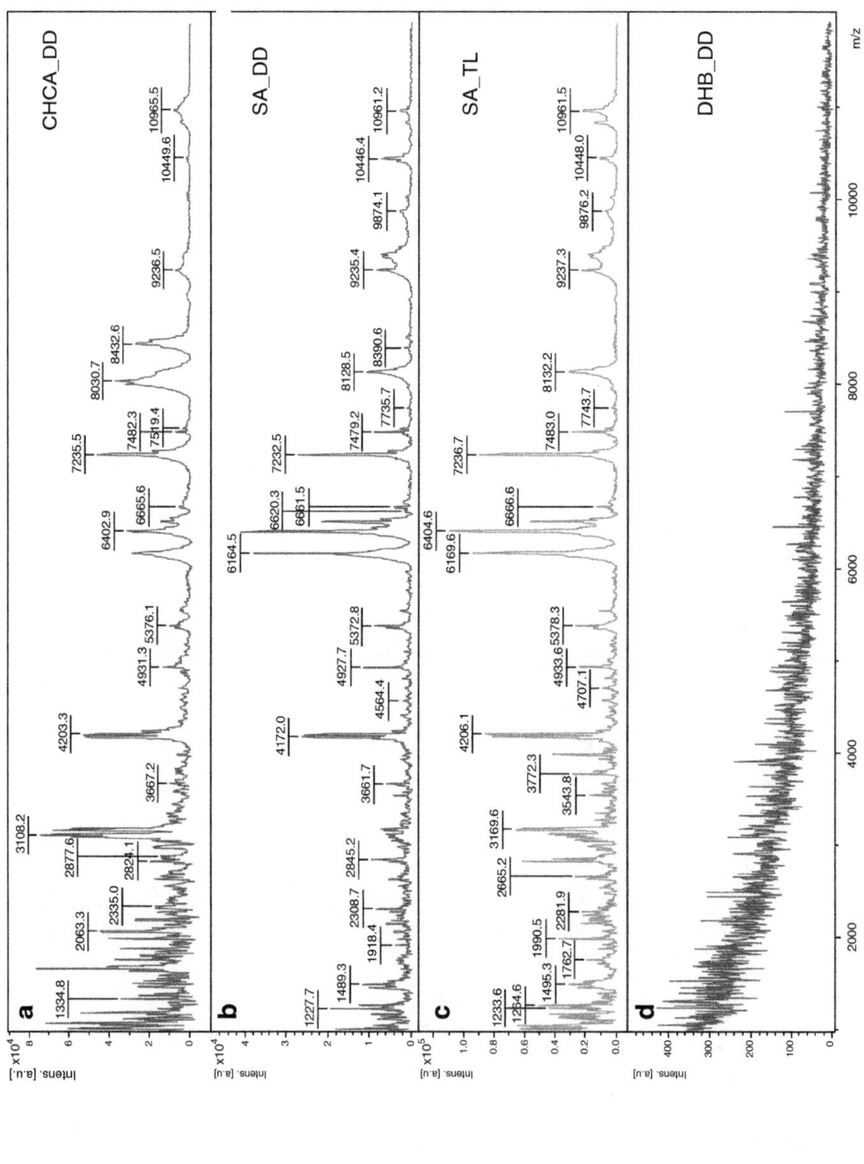

Fig. 11.22 MALDI biotyping of *Trypanosoma cruzi* using **(a)** CHCA DD, **(b)** SA DD, **(c)** SA TL, and **(d)** DHB DD (DD: dried droplet preparation, TL: thin layer method). SA TL delivers best results in terms of number of signals and intensity while DHB totally fails here (Adapted from Ref. [157] with permission. © Wiley, 2016)

11.6.3 Peptide Sequencing and Proteomics

Analysis of the total of all proteins expressed by a living organism, a type of tissue, or certain cells is a tremendous task, as we are dealing with thousands of proteins with relative abundances in range of $> 1000 : 1$. This field of research called *proteomics* aims at quantitative analysis of entire proteomes of individual organisms, ,and requires complex analytical approaches involving different separation techniques along with MS and MS/MS [160–169]. Of course, in proteomics there are no restrictions as to ionization methods, while MALDI (together with ESI; see Chap. 12) accomplish 99.9% of all MS analyses in proteomics.

A standardized workflow for the complete analysis of a protein by using a pure MALDI strategy comprises several steps (Fig. 11.23). It commences with the measurement of the intact protein's mass, preferably by MALDI-TOF-MS as this combination offers inexpensive and reliable access to the full *m*/*z* range where proteins may occur. Next, a proteolytic digestion is performed to cut the macromolecule into smaller peptide subunits, typically in the range of 800–2500 u. Generally, the enzyme trypsin is employed to deliver these peptides, a so-called *tryptic digest*, which are then analyzed in a survey measurement by MALDI-TOF-MS. The resulting MALDI spectrum presents a so-called *peptide mass map*. Such peptide mass maps usually suffice to identify the protein [170].

The next stage is to subject as many as possible peptides of the peptide mass map to tandem MS to reveal their individual amino acid sequences. Interpreting the amino acid sequences requires substantial knowledge of the fragmentation behavior of peptide ions [164, 168, 171]. Provided some basic information on the fragmentation pathways of peptide ions is available, computer algorithms can be developed that allow to derive substantial, however not necessarily complete, sequence information. Automated MALDI-TOF/TOF peptide sequencing is thus widely used. The procedure includes automated precursor ion selection for tandem MS, e.g., by selecting several abundant $[M + H]^+$ ions of a survey spectrum and generating peak lists from those tandem mass spectra. The experimental results are finally compared with large peptide databases. The number of potential proteins and its tryptic peptides can further be narrowed down using accurate mass data of the protein and the peptides. While MALDI-MS and MALDI-MS/MS could serve this pupose almost alone, electrospray ionization and liquid chromatography coupling to MS today contribute to a larger extent to the instrumental and methodological mix in proteomics, because the LC-MS technique is more efficient in detecting trace proteins than approaches starting from 2D gels [22–25, 152, 172, 173].

Only the peptide subunits of a protein can be efficiently fragmented by CID for tandem MS analysis. Identifying a protein from such a peptide "jumble" is called *bottom-up* protein analysis. The corresponding tandem MS of the entire protein ions is called *top-down* protein analysis. As the *top-down* approach requires larger amounts of purified protein, it is more widely applied in protein biochemistry. ECD-FT-ICR-MS, assisted by IRMPD heating of the protein ions, is currently the exclusive tool for this purpose (Sect. 9.14.4).

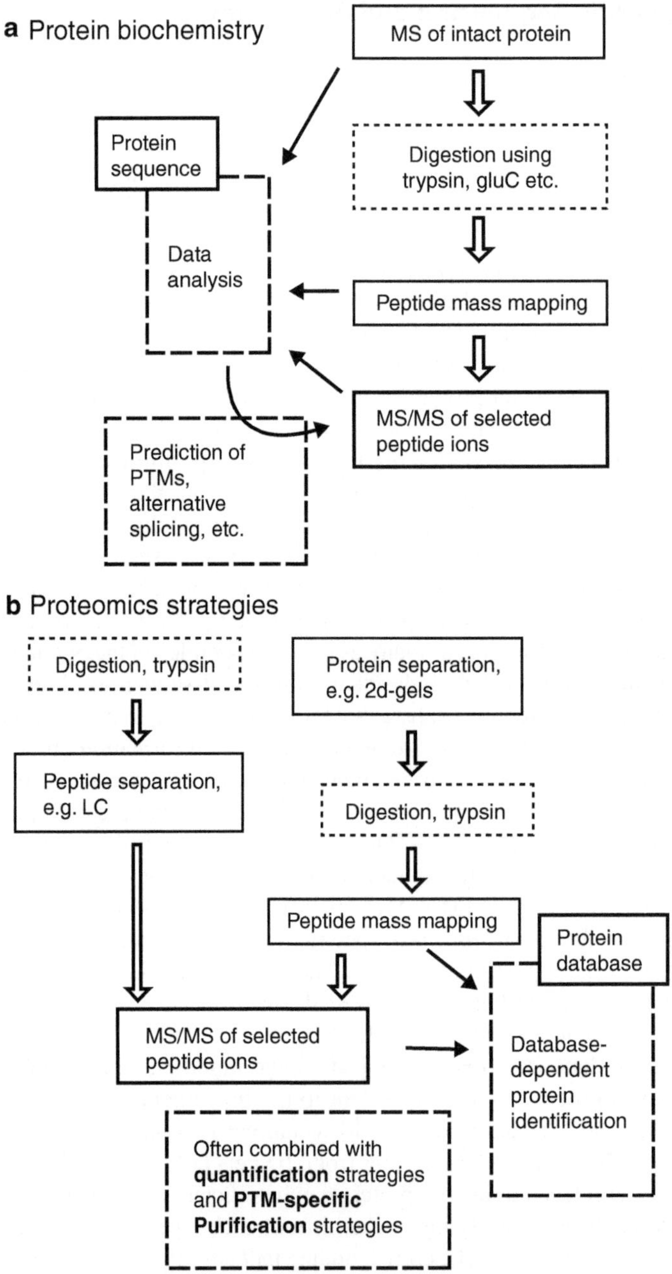

Fig. 11.23 Analytical strategies in (**a**) protein biochemistry requiring highly purified proteins and (**b**) proteomics addressing the entire proteome of a living cell. (Adapted from Chap. 3 by Hjernø and Jensen in Ref. [15] by permission. © Wiley-VCH, Weinheim, 2007)

Peptide fragmentations
Examples and mechanistic aspects of peptide fragmentation are also covered in the context of tandem MS (see Sects. 9.6.6, 9.8, and 9.10.1). The mechanism of peptide cleavage upon ECD is discussed in Sect. 9.13.2 with an example in Sect. 9.14.4; peptide ETD spectra are given in Sect. 9.15. Some further examples will follow in Chap. 12.

Peptide ions are comparatively large, and thus assume various fragmentation pathways. The most obvious and analytically useful fragmentation routes involve the cleavage of the peptide backbone. Following the nomenclature for peptide backbone cleavages originally suggested by Roepstoff and Fohlman [174] and modified by Biemann [175] fragments bearing the charge (due to protonation) at the N-terminus are denoted as a-, b-, and c-ions depending on the actual bond cleaved. If C-terminal fragment ions are formed, the ions are termed x-, y-, and z-ions, respectively (Scheme 11.1). Further, a number index counting from 1 to n–1 for a peptide composed of n amino acids is used to indicate which bond is cleaved. Within each ion series, peaks are seperated by $\Delta m/z$ values directly reflecting the amino acid residue (Table A.11 in Appendix) between them.

The base fragment ion series due to amide bond cleavages are formed by b-ions on the N-terminus and y-ions on the C-terminus. The signals of the a-ions are set off to lower mass by 28 u (CO loss) from the b-ions, while c-ions are 17 u (NH_3) heavier than b-ions as the adjacent N–C_α bond is cleaved. The x-ions of the C-terminal series are by 26 u lighter than y-ions (minus CO, plus H_2) and z-ions are again by 17 u (NH_3) heavier than y-ions.

CID of peptide ions Scheme 11.1 depicts the most likely structures for the main peptide fragment ions. For example, the nominal acylium form of the b_3 ions is not stable, rather it is stabilized by formation of a 5-membered oxazolone ring [176–179] at its C-terminus. Note that this ion contains the amino acid residues up to the third (R^3) including the carbonyl group of R^3 and that the charge is carried by the nitrogen of the ring. The corresponding a_3 ion is formed by elimination of the carbonyl group (CO) from the oxazolone ring.

Fragmentation of [QAMNKFTF–NH_2+H]$^+$ The purified octapeptide QAMNKFTF–NH_2 was subjected to positive-ion MALDI-TOF/TOF analysis. The spectrum shown (Fig. 11.24) was obtained from the [M + H]$^+$ precursor ion, m/z 985.53. The fragment at m/z 968.33 corresponds to ammonia loss from [M + H]$^+$. All seven ions belonging to the b-ion series are detected at m/z 821.25, 720.23, 573.19, 445.12, 331.08, 200.04, and 129.02. In addition b–NH_3 ions, referred to as b* ions, accompany the first four ions at m/z 804.24, 703.22, 556.17, and 428,10 because the N-terminal glutamine (Q) has a tendency to lose NH_3.Thus, we have ions consistent with the expected b_7 to b_1 and b_7* to b_4* fragments, although the ion at m/z 129 can also be formed from lysine (K). The four additional fragment ions at

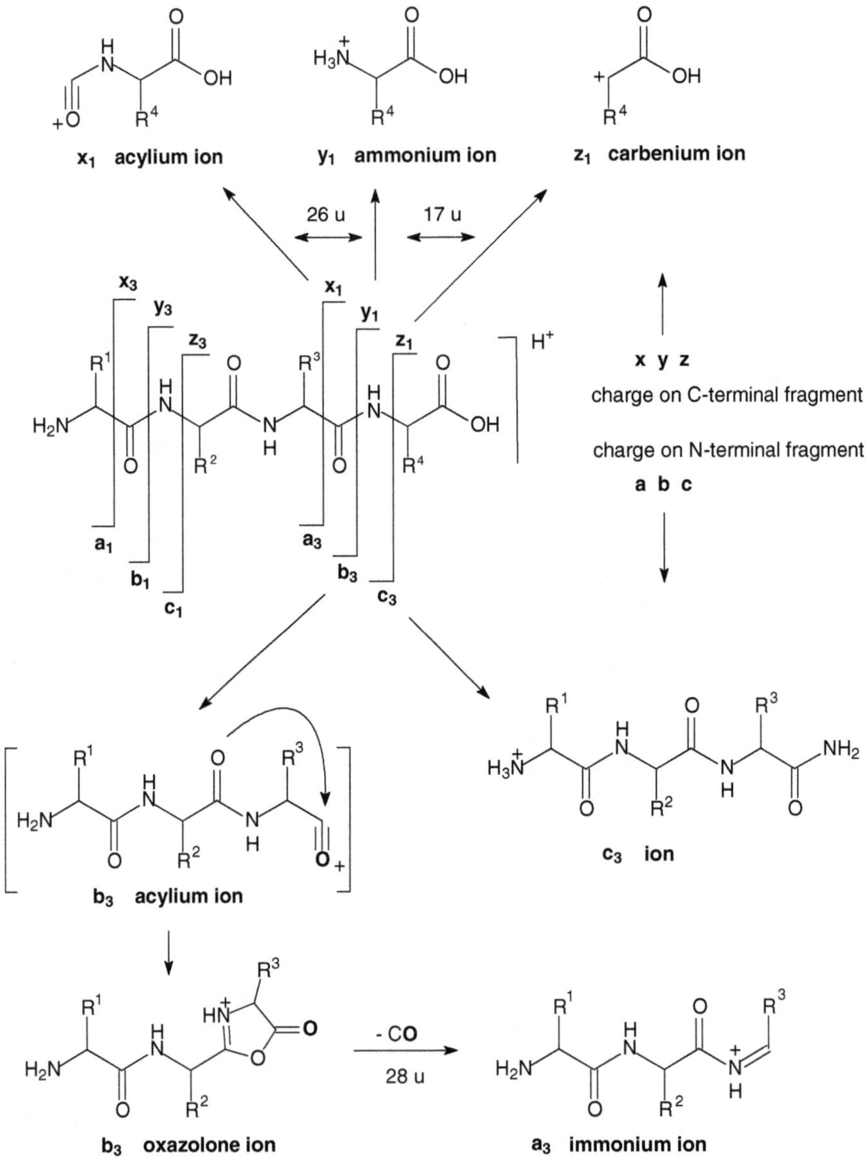

Scheme 11.1 (One carbonyl-*O* is set in bold for better tracking)

m/*z* 857.29, 786.25, 655.25, and 541.23 belong to the y-series and represent the y_7 to y_4 ions, whereas smaller y ions are absent (only their hypothetical positions are indicated as y_1^a to y_3^a) [180].

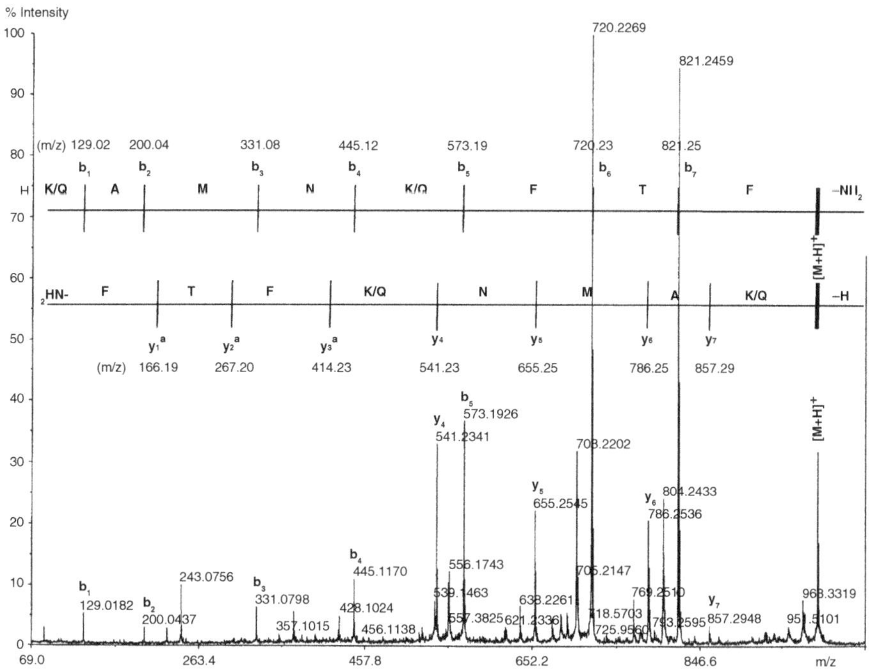

Fig. 11.24 MALDI-TOF/TOF mass spectrum of the purified octapeptide H-QAMNKFTF-NH_2 showing the experimental b_j and y_j peptide fragment ion series; y^a ions are only hypothetical in this case (Adapted from Ref. [180] with permission. © John Wiley & Sons, 2010)

It needs to be emphasized that the actual appearance of a tandem mass spectrum acquired of one and the same compound may be subject to substantial variation for several reasons:

- The spectrum depends to some extent on the ionization method employed to generate a $[M + H]^+$ precursor ion. Ions from MALDI are entering the activation stage with already somewhat higher internal energy than those from ESI.
- The charge state of the selected precursor ion is of utmost importance. With increasing number of charges the Coulombic repulsion also contributes to drive the incipient fragments apart, and thus, less energy needs to be provided by the activation method used.
- The particular activation technique, i.e., low-energy multiple-collision CID versus high-energy single-collision CID versus IRMPD, for example, influences the internal energy and lifetime of decomposing ions, and thus, the selection of fragmentation pathways and/or the relative abundance of fragment ions.
- Instrumental factors such as ion lifetime or internal energy distribution also effect the appearance of the spectrum. In tandem MS, quadrupole ion trap analyzers tend to suppress the lower third of the m/z range, whereas TOF and magnetic sector analyzers do not.

In combination with the intrinsic properties of the ion under study these specific differences introduced into the sequencing experiment cause certain fragments to occur in the final spectrum while others may be missed. This is commonly referred to as *sequence coverage* of a given instrumental configuration.

Peptides aren't all the same
Peptides show marked differences, though having a great deal in common. Biochemists always emphasize the enormous variability of peptides and proteins assembled from as just twenty amino acids and the plethora of resulting functional characteristics. Accordingly, one should stay aware of the fact, that every (peptide) molecule has intrinsic properties also determining their fragmentation into ions.

11.6.4 Carbohydrate Analysis by MALDI-MS

Starting from simple mono- and disaccharides to oligo- and polysaccharides, carbohydrates play an important role in organisms and nutrition. MALDI-MS (typically using DHB or some DHB-containing matrix [17, 82–84, 86]), is a powerful tool for their characterization [181]. Applications include the characterization of maltose chains in "gummy bears" [82], fructans in onions [182], high-molecular-weight oligosaccharides in human milk [83, 84], and others [117, 183]. MALDI-MS of carbohydrates from fungal spores [184] allows for the characterization of the corresponding fungus.

Carbohydrates form alkali adduct ions
Carbohydrates possess a high affinity towards alkali metal ions, and thus in MALDI spectra $[M + Na]^+$ and/or $[M + K]^+$ are normally observed instead of or sometimes in addition to $[M + H]^+$ ions of very low abundance. It generally depends on the relative amount of alkali ion impurities which ionic species will dominate within the spectrum. As NH_4^+ and K^+ ions share the same ionic radius, $[M + NH_4]^+$ adducts may also occur. Radical ions are not observed.

Gummy bear spectrum The maltose chains in the confectionery "gummy bears" consist of up to about 30 maltose units that can easily be extracted into water and analyzed by MALDI-MS [82]. To do so, it is sufficient to allow a gummy bear to take a short bath in water and to admix 1 μl of this extract to about 60 μl of 10 mg ml^{-1} DHB in water : acetonitrile = 1 : 1 (v/v) with 0.1 % of trifluoroacetic acid (Fig. 11.25). Next, 1 μl of this maltose–matrix solution is spotted onto a target and allowed to crystallize (Fig. 11.13). The positive-ion linear mode MALDI-TOF spectrum then exhibits signals due to $[M + Na]^+$ ions of the maltose chains. Linear mode is recommended, as oligosaccharides of > 2000 u tend to fragment even in

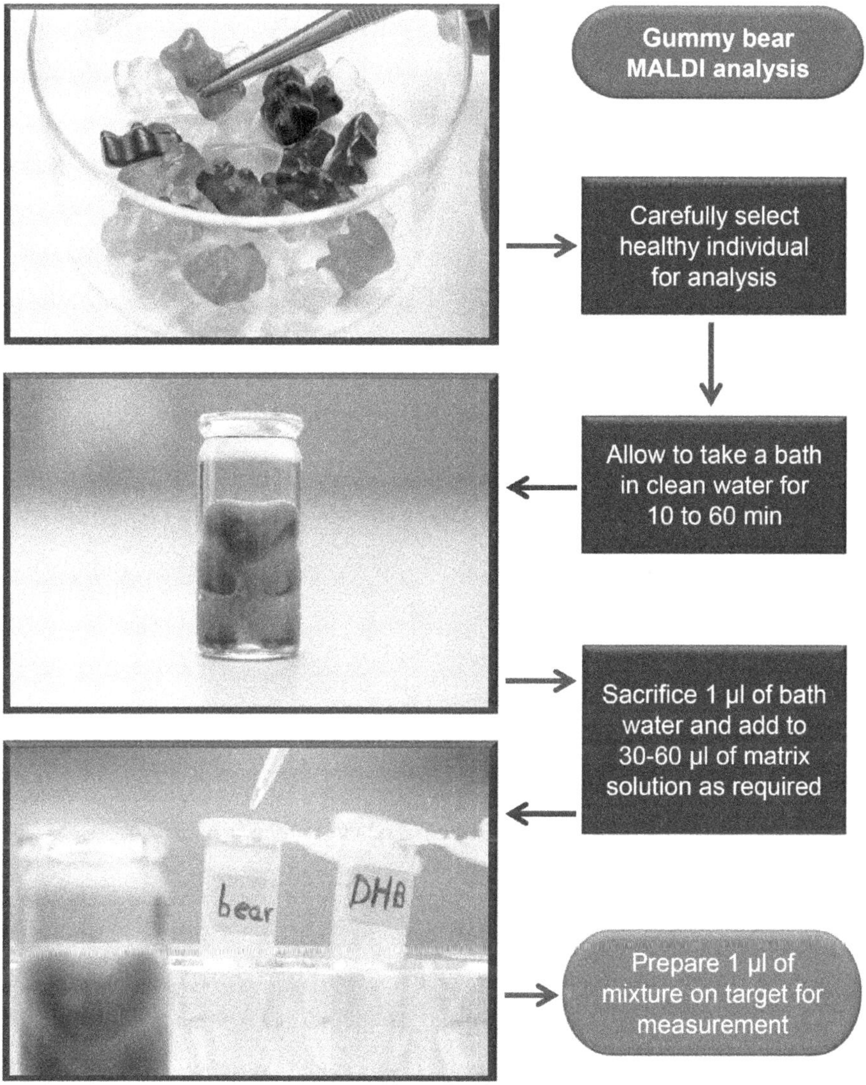

Fig. 11.25 Procedure to measure oligosaccharides of a gummy bear by MALDI-MS. The resulting spectrum is shown in Fig. 11.26

MALDI precluding their detection in reflector mode. Oligosaccharide ions have the formula $[C_6H_{12}O_6 + (C_6H_{10}O_5)_n + Na]^+$, and thus, occur in the spectrum at $\Delta(m/z) = 162$, i.e., by $C_6H_{10}O_5$ monomer units apart (Fig. 11.26). The MALDI-TOF spectrum covering the range *m/z* 400–5000 shows peaks belonging to the 3mer at *m/z* 527 up to the 30mer at *m/z* 4905.

The structure of linear as well as complex branched oligosaccharides can be sequenced by tandem MS analogous to peptide sequencing [181, 185]. If the

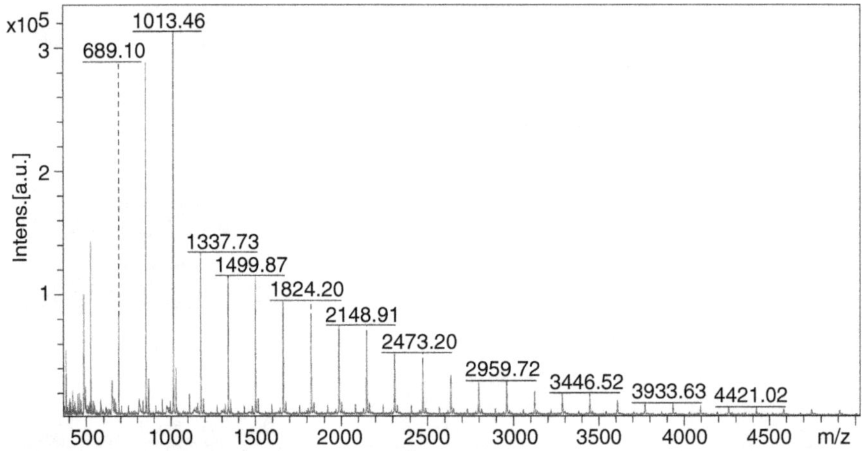

Fig. 11.26 Positive-ion linear mode MALDI-TOF spectrum of the maltose chains extracted from the red gummy bears shown in Fig. 11.25 in the range *m/z* 400–5000. The $[M + Na]^+$ ion peaks of the oligosaccharides occur at $\Delta(m/z) = 162$

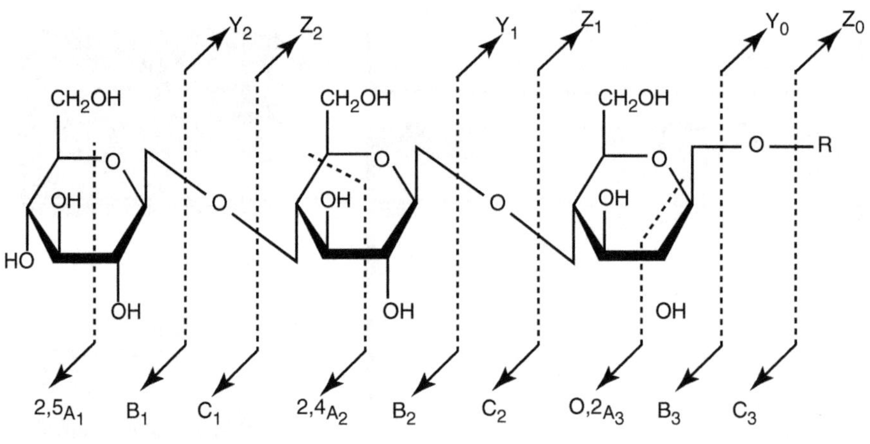

Scheme 11.2 Carbohydrate fragmentation and naming of fragment ions

carbohydrate ions are generated by MALDI, sufficient energy for their fragmentation can be provided in two ways: (*i*) Higher laser irradiance can effect *in-source decay* (ISD) or *metastable dissociation* [124]; the latter being termed *post-source decay* (PSD) in the MALDI-TOF community. (*ii*) *Collision-induced dissociation* (CID) of selected precursor ions can be employed alternatively. (Of course, other compound classes such as peptides, oligonucleotides, or synthetic polymers can be treated analogously.) The general scheme of carbohydrate fragmentation is as follows (from Ref. [181] by permission, © Elsevier Science, 2003) Scheme 11.2.

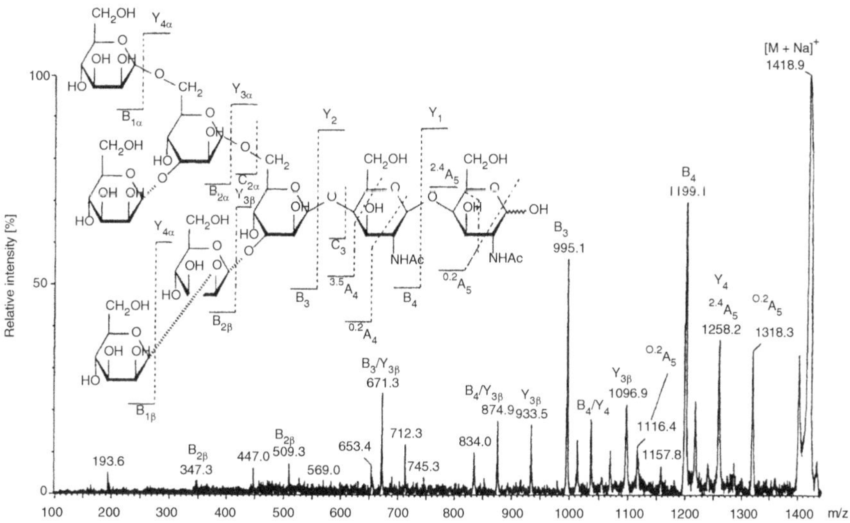

Fig. 11.27 PSD-MALDI-TOF spectrum of *N*-linked glycan $(Man)_6(GlcNAc)_2$ from chicken ovalbumin (Reproduced from Ref. [181] by permission. © Elsevier Science, 2003)

Fragmentation of a glycan The PSD-MALDI-TOF spectrum of the $[M + Na]^+$ ion, *m/z* 1418.9, of high-mannose *N*-linked glycan $(Man)_6(GlcNAc)_2$ from chicken ovalbumin shows distinct cleavages of the branched carbohydrate skeleton (Fig. 11.27) [181]. The spectrum was obtained using DHB matrix.

11.6.5 Oligonucleotide Analysis by MALDI-MS

Oligonucleotides and DNA represent the highest polarity class of biopolymers. Therefore, it is of special importance that isolation in an organic matrix allows to overcome their strong intermolecular interaction. MALDI analysis of oligonucleotides is further complicated by the numerous acidic hydrogens present in a single molecule. In particular the phosphate groups easily exchange protons with the ubiqitous alkali ions [30]. Thus, MALDI of this compound class requires to follow proven experimental protocols to obtain clean spectra of ions representing the intact macromolecules. The acidity of the phosphates makes oligonucleotides and DNA accessible as $[M - H]^-$ ions if measured in the negative ion mode [30].

Due to their numerous acidic hydrogens, oligonucleotides require desalting prior to MALDI, e.g., by using cation exchange resins [30]. Similar procedures are necessary when other ionization methods are applied to this compound class [81, 101, 186, 187].

Deoxynucleotide 5mer The negative- and positive-ion mode MALDI-TOF spectra of the solid-supported 5-meric oligodeoxynucleotide *po*-CNE 5′-GACTT-3′

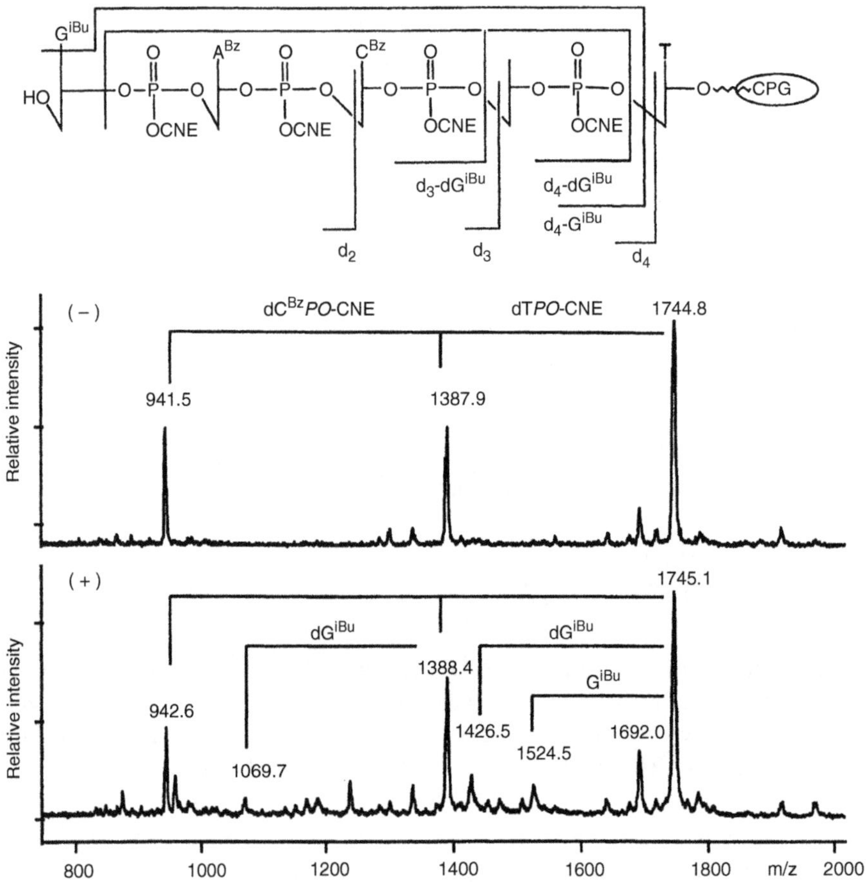

Fig. 11.28 Comparison of the negative- and positive-ion mode MALDI-TOF spectra of the 5-meric *po*-CNE 5′-GACTT-3′ oligodeoxynucleotide. Both show fragment ions by ISD (Adapted from Ref. [101] by permission. © John Wiley & Sons, 2000)

[101]: comparison shows that both exhibit fragment ions due to cleavages of the phosphotriester backbone (Fig. 11.28). As oligonucleotides normally do not exhibit such a distinct level of ISD in MALDI spectra, it has been argued that the linking to the solid support plays a role for the generation of this mass ladder of peaks which differ by one nucleotide residue.

11.6.6 MALDI-MS of Synthetic Polymers

MALDI is the method of choice for the analysis of synthetic polymers. MALDI is soft enough to provide intact molecular ions or intimately related ions by cationization and gives access to an essentially unlimited mass range [26, 27,

151]. As ions from MALDI are almost always singly charged [46] the spectrum may represent a very good approximation to the molecular weight distribution of the examined polymer. While polar polymers such as poly(methylmethacrylate) (PMMA) [102, 188], polyethylene glycol (PEG) [188, 189], and others [98, 190, 191] readily form $[M + H]^+$ or $[M + alkali]^+$ ions, nonpolar polymers like polystyrene (PS) [118, 119, 124, 125] or nonfunctionalized polymers like polyethylene (PE) [121, 122] can only be cationized by transition metal ions in their 1+ oxidation state [118, 119]. The formation of evenly spaced oligomer ion series can also be employed to establish an internal mass calibration of a spectrum [190].

The most important parameters that can be determined by MALDI are *number-average molecular weight* (M_n), *weight-average molecular weight* (M_w), and the molecular weight distribution expressed as *polydispersity* (*PD*) [125, 192]:

$$M_n = \frac{\sum M_i I_i}{\sum I_i} \tag{11.1}$$

$$M_w = \frac{\sum M_i^2 I_i}{\sum M_i I_i} \tag{11.2}$$

$$PD = \frac{M_w}{M_n} \tag{11.3}$$

where M_i and I_i represent the molecular weights of the oligomeric components and their signal intensities (assuming a linear relationship between number of ions and signal intensity) of the detected species. The formula for M_n is identical to that used for the calculation of the molecular weight from isotopic masses and their abundances as represented by an isotopic pattern (Eq. 3.2 in Sect. 3.1.5).

Silver adduct formation Polystyrenes ranging from PS 2200 to PS 12500 form $[M + metal]^+$ ions with Ag^+ and Cu^+ ions when silver or copper(I) salts are admixed to the sample preparation. In case of PS 12500, both metal ions were found to effect cationization equally well, i.e., without causing differences in average molecular weight or ionic abundances (Fig. 11.29) [125].

How to determine endgroups If the mass of the monomer is not already known prior to MALDI-MS, it is obtained from $\Delta(m/z)$ of adjacent peaks within the series of signals. Averaging of multiple measurements improves the accuracy of the value. Next, integer multiples of $\Delta(m/z)$ are subtracted from the m/z value of a peak at the low-mass side of the distribution until the remainder roughly attains the mass of the monomer. The mass of the sum of both endgroups, possibly including the charge bearing adduct ion, is thus obtained. However, the value is not unambiguous, because large endgroups may be misinterpreted as mass of a monomer plus a smaller endgroup. Polyethylene glycol 600 serves as a simple example: Peaks representing $[M + Na]^+$ ions at m/z 305.16, 349.19, 393.21, 437.24, ... deliver an average of $\Delta(m/z) = 44.03$. Subtracting 22.99 u for sodium and multiples (6) of

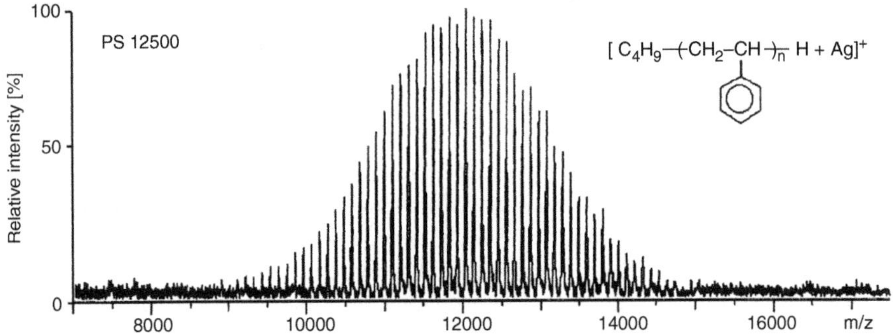

Fig. 11.29 Linear-mode positive-ion MALDI-TOF spectrum of polystyrene 12500 doped with Ag^+ ions. Subtraction of the Ag^+ ion mass (average of 108 u for the nonresolved pair of ^{107}Ag and ^{109}Ag) is therefore required to derive the correct molecular mass of the individual species. The isotopic pattern of silver does not affect the spectrum as isotopic resolution here is not achieved anyway (Adapted from Ref. [125] by permission. © John Wiley & Sons, 2001)

44.03 u from *m/z* 305.16 yields 17.99 u for the endgroups, i.e., 18 u point towards H and OH in this case.

In addition, the determination of a polymer's endgroup(s) [193, 194] and the analysis of random and block-copolymers [195, 196] can be achieved by MALDI. However, care has to be taken when judging the MALDI spectra because of the mass-dependent desorption and detection characteristics of the experiment. In case of higher polydispersity ($PD > 1.1$) high-mass ions are underestimated from MALDI spectra [112, 192]. The current practice to deal with such samples is to fractionate them by *gel permeation chromatography* (GPC) [191] or *size-exclusion chromatography* (SEC) prior to MALDI analysis [192, 197].

Polymer mixture Extracted and synthesized oligo(ethylene terephthalate)s were compared by MALDI-MS [194]. Using the symbols G for ethylene glycol units, GG for diethylene glycol units, and T for terephthalic acid units, the detected oligomers were (*i*) cyclic oligomers $[GT]_n$, (*ii*) linear chains H-$[GT]_n$-G, and (*iii*) some other distributions such as linear H-$[GH]_n$-OH and H-$[GGT]_1$-$[GT]_{n-1}$-G oligomers and cyclic H-$[GGT]_1$-$[GT]_{n-1}$ oligomers. Type (*i*) was mainly contained in technical yarns and tiles, whereas types (*ii*) and (*iii*) were constituents of the model oligomers (Fig. 11.30).

MALDI-MS of a block copolymer An ethylene oxide (EO)–propylene oxide (PO) block copolymer has been analyzed by MALDI-MS. Interferences are likely to occur, as ion series caused by different EO/PO ratios are going to superimpose in the spectrum. Using a JEOL SpiralTOF instrument, a design offering very high resolving power (Sect. 4.2.11) [198], allowed to separate overlapping isotopic patterns of the monoisotopic $[M+Na]^+$ ion of (EO_4–PO_{14}) and of the $^{13}C_2$ isotopic ion of (EO_0–PO_{17}) as present in the range *m/z* 1027.2–1033.2, for example. Due to $R = 80{,}000$, the instrument was still able to separate the doublet at *m/z* 1029.7 with peaks at $\Delta(m/z) = 0.03$ (Fig. 11.31).

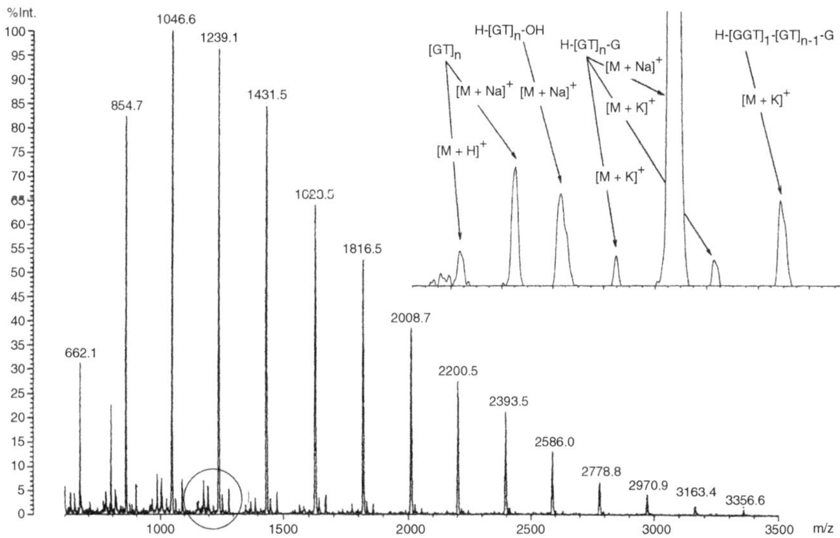

Fig. 11.30 Oligo(ethylene terephthalate diol)s: MALDI-TOF spectrum of the model compound. The *inset* shows an expanded view of the low-intensity peaks *m/z* 940–1120 (*circled*) (Adapted from Ref. [194] by permission. © John Wiley & Sons, 1995)

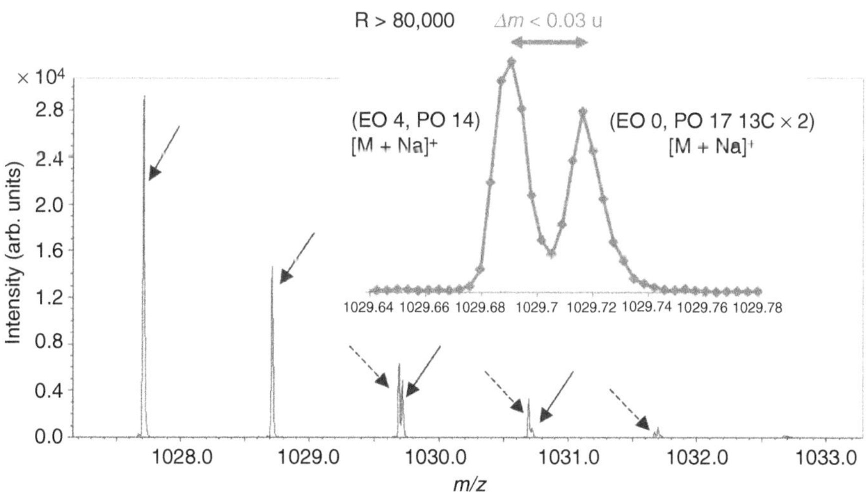

Fig. 11.31 Partial MALDI mass spectrum of an EO–PO block copolymer at *m/z* 1027.2–1033.2 as obtained on a JEOL SpiralTOF instrument. *Solid arrows* indicate the isotopic pattern of (EO0–PO17), and the *dotted arrows* indicate that of (EO4–PO14). The *inset* shows an expanded view of the doublet at *m/z* 1029.7; the *diamonds* on the line correspond to data points (Sect. 4.10) (Adapted with permission from Ref. [198] © Mass Spectrometry Society of Japan, 2014)

MALDI of dendrimers In terms of their behavior in MALDI-MS, dendrimers exhibit some resemblance to polymers. The molecular weight of dendrimers quickly increases as the molecules grow with each generation of branching. As dendrimer syntheses tend to yield "imperfect" by-products, the restriction of MALDI to form singly charged ions is beneficial in that it results in spectra that reveal all components at a glance. A MALDI-TOF spectrum of a dendrimer mixture has already been discussed in the context of mass calibration (Sect. 3.7.4) [199–201].

11.7 Special Surfaces to Mimic the Matrix Effect

MALDI is so unique in offering a wide range of applications from small molecule analysis over peptides and synthetic polymers to large biomacromolecules that efforts have been made to mimic the matrix effect in other ways without having the specific disadvantages of matrixes, such as background peaks (which are particularly disturbing in the low-mass range). Here, alternative techniques are briefly discussed.

11.7.1 Desorption/Ionization on Silicon

In *desorption/ionization on silicon* (DIOS), the analyte is absorbed by a micrometers-thick porous surface layer on a silicon chip, i.e., the porous silicon is used as substitute of an organic matrix [202, 203]. Porous silicon surfaces with high UV absorptivity can be generated with varying properties from flat crystalline silicon by using a galvanostatic etching procedure [204]. Stabilization of the freshly prepared surfaces is achieved by hydrosilylation. Porous silicon surfaces can be reused several times after washing. Arrays of 100–1000 sample positions can be realized on a 3 × 3 cm silicon chip [204]. The DIOS technique offers picomole detection limits for peptides, comparatively simple sample preparation, and – most importantly for small molecule analysis – the absence of matrix peaks in the spectra [205, 206].

DIOS of a tryptic digest DIOS-TOF/TOF experiments on the tryptic digest of 100 fmol of the protein bovine serum albumine (BSA) demonstrate this technique. Using conductive tape the DIOS chip was directly attached to the MALDI target plate of an Applied Biosystems 4700 tandem TOF instrument equipped with a frequency-tripled Nd:YAG laser (355 nm). The resulting DIOS-TOF spectrum of the digest and the DIOS-TOF/TOF spectrum of one selected peptide, $[YLYEIAR + H]^+$, m/z 927.5 are shown in Fig. 11.32. The tandem mass spectrum provides complete detection of the y and b ion series [206].

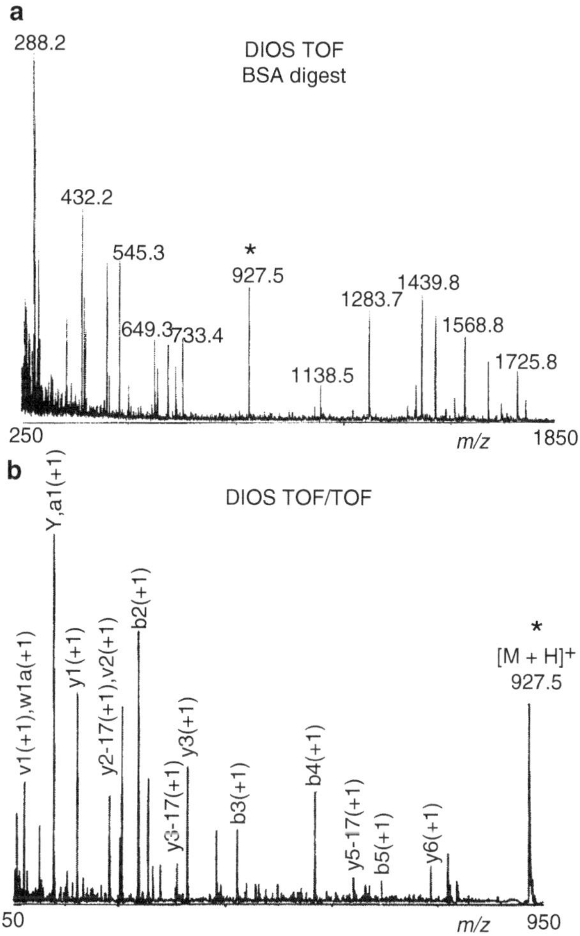

Fig. 11.32 DIOS applied to a tryptic BSA digest. (**a**) DIOS spectrum of the tryptic peptides from BSA; (**b**) DIOS tandem mass spectrum of the $[YLEIAR + H]^+$ peptide ion, *m*/*z* 927.5, to demonstrate sensitivity and sequence coverage of DIOS (Adapted from Ref. [206] with permission. © American Chemical Society, 2003)

11.7.2 Nano-assisted Laser Desorption/Ionization

A more recent approach, also from the Suizdak group, is to modify silicon surfaces with *single-crystal silicon nanowires* (SiNWs), which also happen to provide a good platform for surface-based mass spectrometry. Those silicon nanowires are directly synthesized on the surface of a silicon wafer. The formation of SiNW can be well controlled to define physical dimensions, composition, density, and position of the nanowires on the surface [207, 208].

The synthesis of SiNWs starts from gold nanoparticles with diameters of 10, 20, or 40 nm that are distributed on a silicon substrate. The nanoclusters are required to catalyze SiNW growth. The method employs an elaborate series of steps of growth, etching, oxidation, and finally silylation to generate a perfluorophenyl-derivatized SiNW surface. Like DIOS targets, the SiNW-coated plates are attached to a

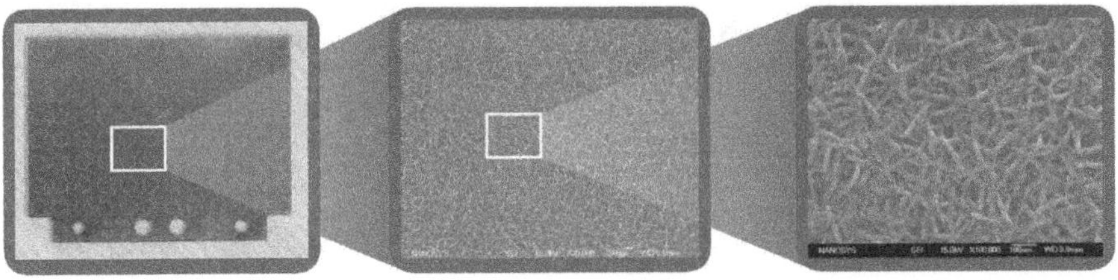

Fig. 11.33 NALDI target plate. The figure shows the NALDI target plate (*left*) and increasing magnification SEM images (*center* and *right*) of the nanostructured coating that provides the active surface for desorption/ionization of deposited analytes (Courtesy of Bruker Daltonik GmbH, Bremen)

modified sample plate. The procedure of measuring a spectrum is then analogous to LDI or DIOS, i.e., the special surface replaces the organic matrix.

The term *nano-assisted laser desorption/ionization* (NALDI) [209, 210] has been coined for techniques using nanostructured surfaces to mimic MALDI. The NALDI™ sample plates have become commerically available from a major manufacturer of MALDI-TOF instrumentation (Fig. 11.33). Like DIOS, NALDI is particularly useful for small molecule analysis in high-throughput analytics [209, 210]. In contrast to DIOS, NALDI is still in use.

11.7.3 Further Variations of the MALDI Theme

The properties of a surface may to a certain extent be tailored to optimize its performance for a particular field of application. Basically, the matrix–analyte pair is replaced by a customized surface–analyte pair that is subjected to laser irradiation. While this approach, on the one hand, simplifies sample preparation, on the other it necessitates preparation of a set of delicate surfaces to be used for different needs.

Silica gel can be derivatized in multiple ways, e.g., by covalently binding ligands via Si–O bonds to its surface. Both *surface-enhanced laser desorption/ionization* (SELDI) and *material-enhanced laser desorption/ionization* (MELDI) make use of the presence of metal complexes on a silica gel surface to selectively adsorb target compounds via complex formation from solution to a target surface [211]. Besides silica gel, also cellulose or glycidyl methacrylate particles, and even diamond powder have been employed as carriers for the metal complex-functionalized groups [212, 213].

Delicate surfaces
Surfaces for DIOS, NALDI, or MELDI are active and rather sensitive. They require proper storage, handling, and processing, e.g., washing, before use. As the sample holder is of one type of customized surface only, this sort of

(continued)

targets is merely useful when performing a large number of very similar analyses. Increased cost at reduced robustness as compared to simple stainless steel plates have to be taken into account.

11.8 MALDI Mass Spectral Imaging

11.8.1 Methodology of MALDI Imaging

MALDI-MS can be used to generate ion images of samples thus providing the capability of mapping specific molecules to two-dimensional coordinates of the original sample [214]. This approach to surface analysis has long been known in *secondary ion mass spectrometry* (SIMS, Sect. 15.6) and was introduced in MALDI-MS as *MALDI imaging* by the Caprioli group in 1997 [214]. Since then, MALDI imaging has undergone a tremendous development [215–218] (see Chap. 4 in [15] and Chap. 12 in [219]). The high sensitivity of the technique ranging down to the low femtomole to even attomole levels for proteins and peptides gives access to the study of intricate biochemical processes. In fact, MALDI imaging is most frequently used to map local concentrations of target analytes in tissue samples, but it can also be applied to analyze paint or ink on paper or valuable artwork.

IMS or IMS or MSI?

The term *imaging mass spectrometry* (IMS) is correlated to the same acronym as *ion mobility spectrometry* (IMS, Sect. 4.10), thus one must be aware of the context in which IMS is being used. The more recent term *mass spectral imaging* (MSI) resolves this ambiguity.

The preparation procedure is critical for the outcome of MALDI imaging. It consists of coating of the tissue section or a blotted imprint of the section with an evenly distributed thin matrix layer before the sample can be placed into the mass spectrometer (Fig. 11.34) [220]. The matrix solution is preferably sprayed onto the sample, e.g., by a pneumatic or electrostatic nebulizer delivering very fine droplets to assure homogeneous coating [221]. Alternatively, a picoliter volume spotter can be used to deposit matrix spots in a fixed pattern onto the sample slice [215]. Variations in matrix crystallization or layer thickness result in erroneous images, because the intensity of the signals would rather be determined by the quality of the matrix layer on the actual pixel than by the concentration of the analyte underneath. Microcrystalline layers and laser spot focus diameter also determine the spatial resolution of the imaging process, which can resolve structures to about 10 μm [216, 221, 222].

MALDI imaging creates an array of mass spectra, i.e., each "pixel" of the image, often of an 256 × 256 spot array, is represented by a MALDI spectrum of its own.

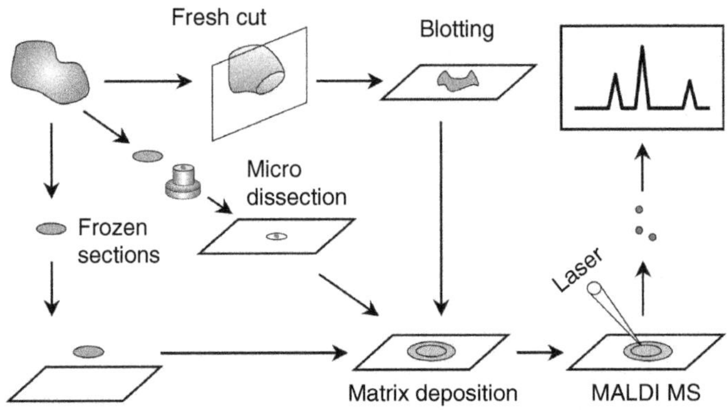

Fig. 11.34 Sample preparation strategies for MALDI imaging of tissues (Reprduced from Ref. [220] with permission. © John Wiley & Sons, Ltd., 2001)

Images are then obtained by extracting ionic abundances of certain *m*/*z* or eventually *m*/*z* ranges for display. In other words, reconstructed ion chromatograms (Sect. 1.5) are plotted two-dimensionally rather than just along a time axis. Often, color coding is used to simplify the recognition of patterns, e.g., a certain color may represent a certain compound or *m*/*z* range, its brightness may reveal the abundance of the compound. It is obvious from this approach that only a few components or compound groups can be displayed in one image at a time. This is why MALDI imaging results are often represented by a set of images each of them composed to highlight a topic of its own (Fig. 11.35). It is furthermore required to correlate the MALDI mass spectral image with the optical image of the sample as obtained by light microscopy immediately before matrix coating.

11.8.2 Instrumentation for MALDI-MSI

MSI instrumentation can be classified according to how ions are generated from the sample, i.e., either by irradiation with a pulsed laser as in MALDI or by bombardment with energetic particles as in SIMS [215]. SIMS uses a continuous particle beam that can be precisely focused, and thus, SIMS can deliver images offering a spatial resolution in the order of 100 nm, however, at the cost of fragmentation upon impact of the energetic particles. The lateral resolution of MALDI imaging is generally limited by both the laser focus and even more so by the homogeneity of the matrix coating. MALDI-MSI yields a lateral resolution of about 20 μm, but may resolve down to 5 μm in fortunate cases. As an advantage over SIMS, MALDI-TOF can access an essentially unlimited *m*/*z* range [215]. Most recently, a record of 1.4 μm lateral resolution has been achieved with an atmospheric pressure MALDI source [223].

While a few years back it took 4–12 h to acquire a MALDI image, an optimized imaging system like the Bruker rapifleX MALDI tissuetyper can collect the same amount of spectral data in about 1 h. To achieve this, the instrument has a dedicated laser optical system to allow for quick scanning of the sample surface and it

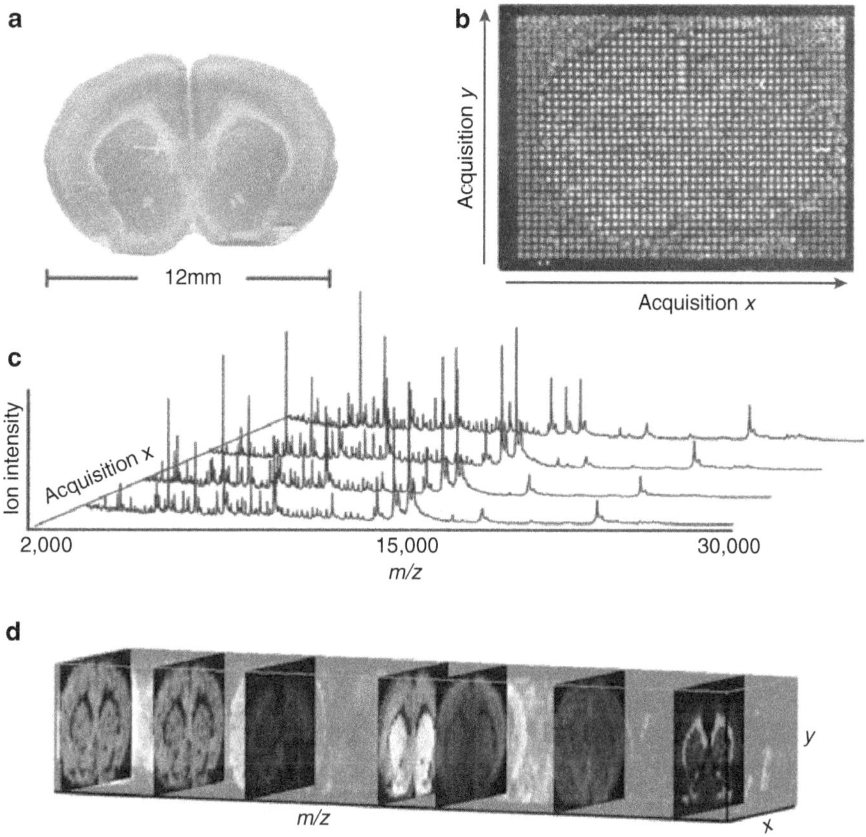

Fig. 11.35 Conceptual overview of MALDI imaging. (**a**) Freshly cut tissue section (here: mouse brain); (**b**) mounted section after application of matrix, here by a robotic picoliter volume spotter; (**c**) partial series of mass spectra along the *x*-axis of the sample; (**d**) three-dimensional volumetric plot of the complete dataset with selected *m/z* ranges per image (Reproduced from Ref. [215] with permission. © Nature Publishing Group, 2007)

operates a frequency tripled Nd:Yag laser at 10 kHz. Different from older approaches, the laser is set to deliver a 5 μm spot size and the lateral resolution of the intended image is then determined by setting the array size of the surface that is to be collected to yield data for one pixel of the MALDI image (Fig. 11.36) [224].

Even nowadays, with terabyte-capacities for data storage, MALDI-MSI presents a challenge in terms of data handling, because an array of 256 by 256 dots yields 65536 spectra. Assuming 2 MB of data per MALDI spectrum, such an image requires about 128 GB of hard disk storage. As an advantage, the data can retrospectively be interrogated for any *m/z* that turns out to be of interest.

It should also be noted that collecting such a large number of spectra goes along with a need for frequent ion source cleaning (up to daily) and with occasional replacement of the solid state laser.

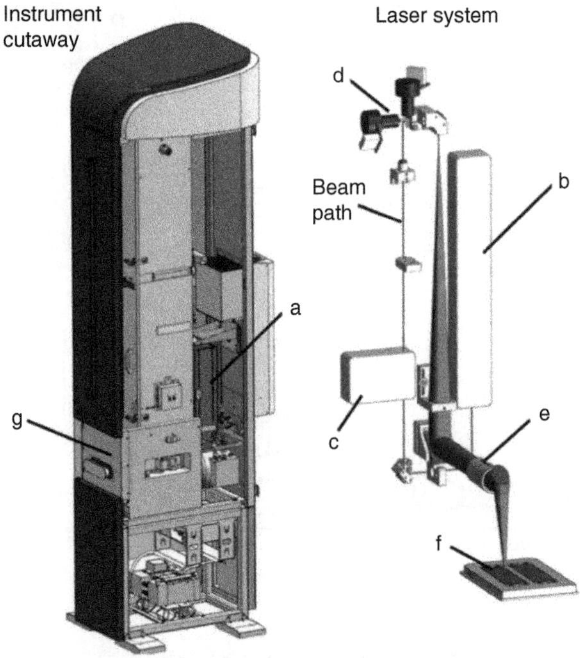

Fig. 11.36 Schematic of the RapifleX MALDI Tissuetyper instrument and its laser system employing two rotating mirrors. The laser system is mounted onto the flight tube as an enclosed box (**a**) containing the major optical elements. The beam is routed from the beam source (**b**) through the attenuator (**c**) onto the rotating mirrors (**d**) which allow fast and precise positioning of the laser spot. The laser is then focused (**e**) onto the target plate (**f**) inside the instruments source (**g**) (Adapted from Ref. [224] with permission. © Wiley, 2015)

11.8.3 Applications of MALDI-MSI

MALDI-MSI has a wide range of applications with an emphasis on intact tissue analysis. In analogy to MALDI biotyping, the field of MALDI-MSI tissuetyping has evolved. While the spectral information may be exactly the same, the imaging approach additionally delivers detailed information on the lateral distribution of the compounds of interest. An example of a MALDI image of tissue has already been shown (Fig. 11.35), another one is provided below (Fig. 11.37). The majority of MALDI-MSI applications certainly is in the life sciences and pharmaceutical development as it permits to track drugs and metabolites across organs and tissue regions [225–227].

MALDI imaging of fingerprints has evolved as an important tool in forensic science [228, 229]. In addition to an optical image of a fingerprint, the MALDI imaging approach enables to selectively interrogate fingerprint for compound classes. While the lipids image basically reflects the conventional fingerprint, MALDI offers enhanced levels of detection [228–230]. Further, MALDI-MSI enables the analysis of proteins from blood stains [231], traces of medication or illicit drugs [232], and other target compounds that may be of interest in a specific case [25].

Fingerprint MALDI images Ungroomed fingerprints obtained from different surfaces including glass, metal, wood, plastic, and leather were recovered and subjected to MALDI imaging. Rather than using conventional TiO_2 powder, the contrast-enhancing dusting was performed using CHCA matrix [228]. Then MALDI images were collected and reconstructed ion currents were plotted for selected compounds such as *m/z* 118 as marker of an endogenous amino acid (valine), *m/z* 283 for an endogenous fatty acid (oleic acid), and *m/z* 304 for

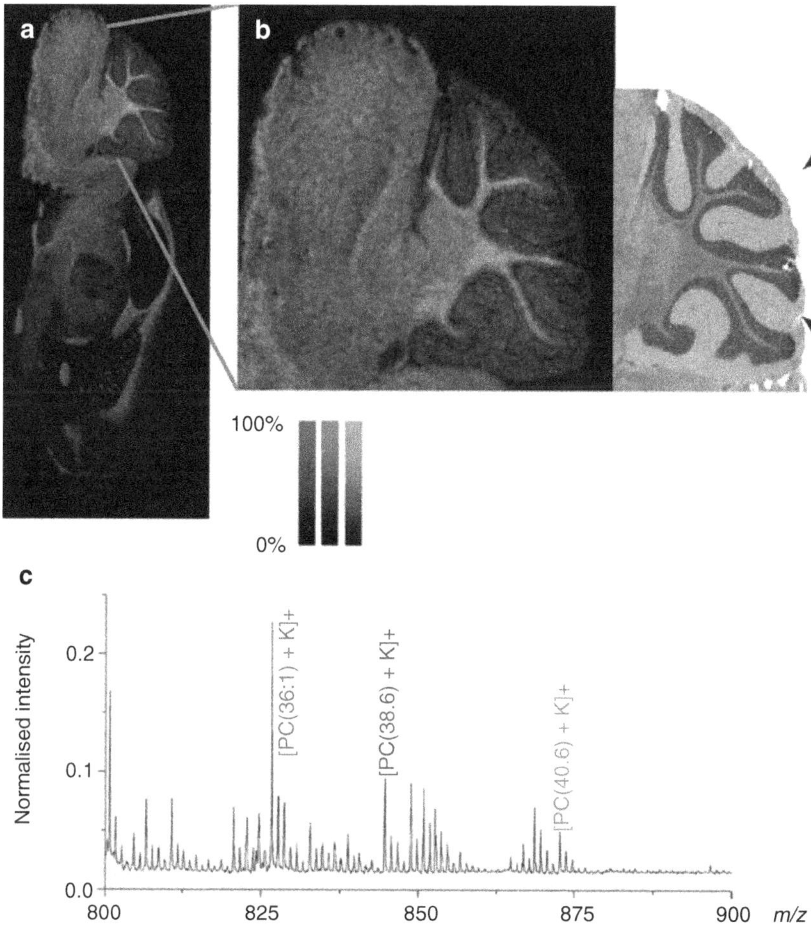

Fig. 11.37 (**a**) Positive-ion images of phosphatidylcholines (PC) in cerebellum tissue. Compounds $[PC(40{:}6) + K]^+$, $[PC(38{:}6) + K]^+$, and $[PC(36{:}1) + K]^+$ were observed at *m/z* 972, 844, and 826 and shown in *red*, *blue*, and *green*, respectively, acquired with a 20 × 20 μm raster. This image contained 181,723 pixels. (**b**) Enlarged region showing the complementary distributions of these ions in the cerebellum. The corresponding microscopic image of the stained section is shown on the right. (**c**) Overall average on tissue spectrum (Reproduced from Ref. [224] with permission. © Wiley, 2015)

dimethylbenzylammonium ion (DBA) as an exogenous compound (Fig. 11.38). It should be noted that, for ease of comparison with the dusted optical images, MALDI images were flipped left to right.

More than just nice pictures

Clearly, MALDI imaging provides pictures that often have esthetic appeal and may even have artistic quality. No wonder that such material is often showcased during conferences and company presentations. The preceding

(continued)

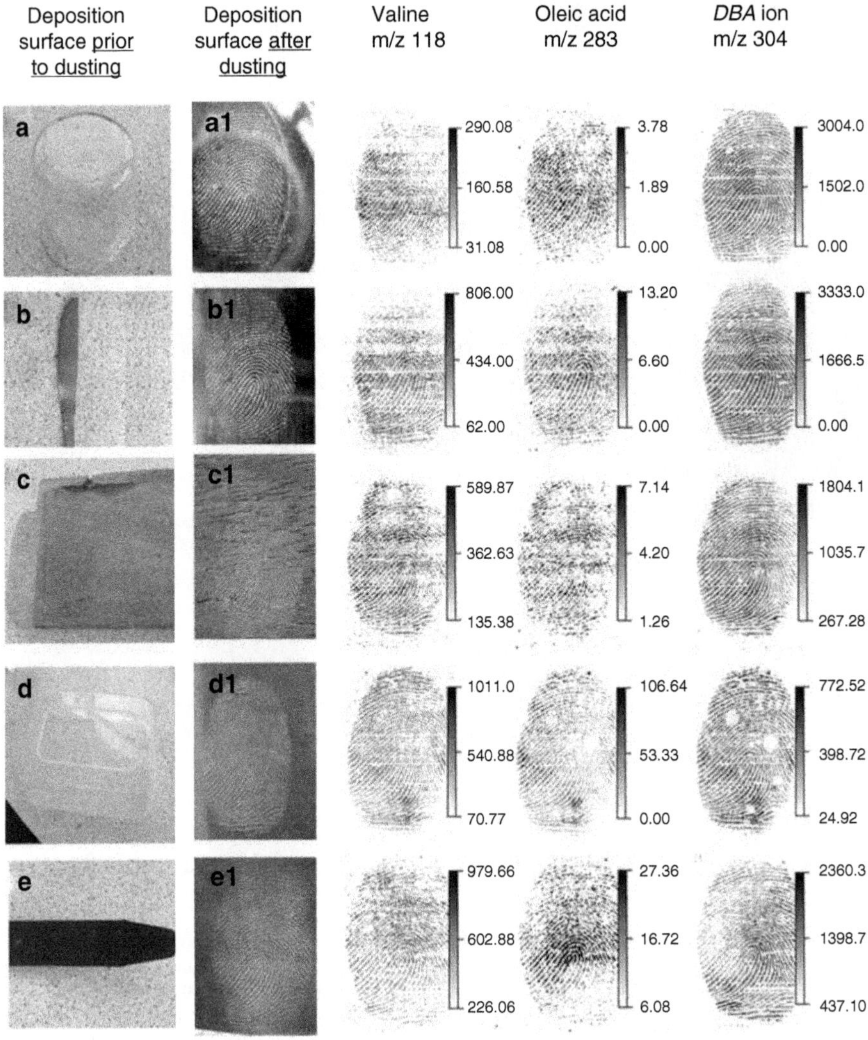

Fig. 11.38 Recovery and MALDI MSI analysis of ungroomed fingerprints obtained from (**a**) glass, (**b**) metal, (**c**) wood, (**d**) plastic, and (**e**) leather. MALDI images of three selected compounds are shown on the right of each fingerprint (Reproduced from Ref. [228] with permission. © American Chemical Society, 2011)

section should also have pointed out that these pictures are connected to a wealth of analytical information as each pixel is backed up by a complete mass spectrum. It is just not possible to depict all this information in a single picture. Typically, they display spatial distributions of a few selected compounds in a color-coded fashion; one would have to generate large numbers of them to address every possible facet of such a data set.

11.9 Atmospheric Pressure MALDI

In *atmospheric pressure MALDI* (AP-MALDI) the MALDI process takes place in dry nitrogen gas under atmospheric pressure. The desorbed ions are then transferred into the vacuum of the mass analyzer by means of an *atmospheric pressure ionization* (API) interface which is provided by any electrospray ionization (ESI, Chap. 12) interface. AP-MALDI was first presented in combination with an orthogonal acceleration TOF (oaTOF, Sect. 4.2.8) analyzer where the original ESI ion interface was modified to accommodate a MALDI target plus a laser light source instead of the ESI spray capillary [233]. While the coherence of the laser light is preserved in vacuum MALDI, the use of an optical fiber to guide the light from the laser to the sample layer results in a loss of coherence.

AP-MALDI has been adapted to a quadrupole ion trap (QIT, Sect. 4.6) [234] where an improved design was realized by extending the heated transfer capillary of a Finnigan LCQ ion trap instrument toward the MALDI target. Thus, a multi-sample target on an *xy*-movable target holder and observation optics could be incorporated on the atmospheric pressure side (Fig. 11.39) [235]. The entrance of the capillary extender is held at 1.5–3 kV to attract the ions from the target surface located about 2 mm away. Based on this development, AP-MALDI can now also be attached to QIT, LIT, Q-TOF, and Orbitrap analyzers.

Compared to vacuum MALDI, AP-MALDI has a larger tolerance to laser fluence variations and exhibits reduced fragmentation due to the collisional cooling of the expanding plume. As a result of this cooling process, clustering between

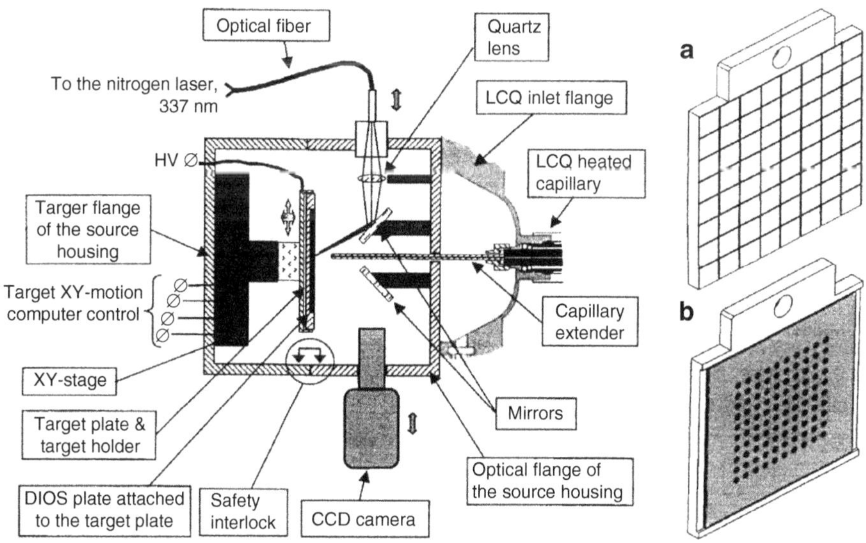

Fig. 11.39 AP-MALDI ion source with extended transfer capillary. *Insets*: (**a**) the target holder can be equipped with a 64-spot MALDI target or (**b**) a 10 × 10-spot DIOS chip (Adapted from Ref. [205] by permission. © John Wiley & Sons, 2002)

matrix and analyte ions is more pronounced. Declustering can be achieved by employing higher laser fluences or adapting the parameters of the atmospheric pressure interface [236].

AP-MALDI presents an add-on to any instrument with atmospheric pressure interface, i.e., mass spectrometers with ESI, APCI, or APPI source can also accommodate an AP-MALDI source. The limit of detection (LOD) of vacuum MALDI is 5–10 fold lower than in AP-MALDI and the laser threshold fluence is about 1.5 fold lower in vacuum MALDI compared to AP-MALDI (Fig. 11.40) [237]. Thus, AP-MALDI can increase the versatility of mass spectrometers without sacrificing too much performance.

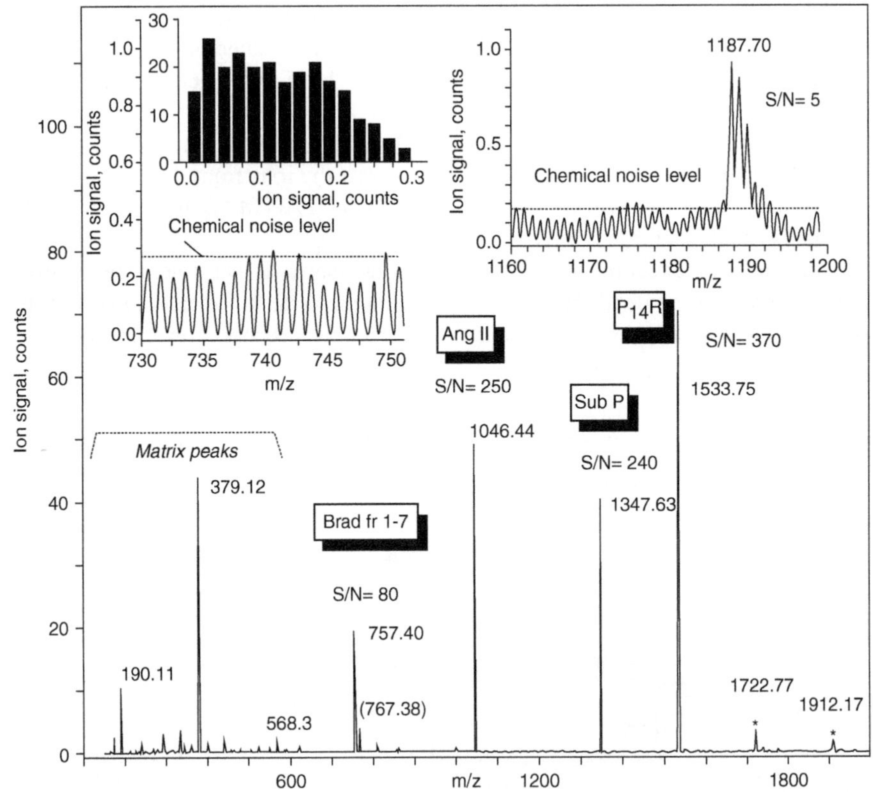

Fig. 11.40 AP-MALDI spectrum of four synthetic peptides in CHCA as obtained in a 1-min scan of a spot containing 300 fmol of bradykinin fr. 1–7 (*m/z* 757), 100 fmol of angiotensin II (*m/z* 1046), 100 fmol of $P_{14}R$ (*m/z* 1534), and 50 fmol of substance P (*m/z* 1348). Single and double matrix adducts of $P_{14}R$ are indicated by *asterisks* (*m/z* 1723, 1912). Note the doubly charged ion of $P_{14}R$ at *m/z* 767. *Inserts* show representative patterns of chemical noise in the vicinity of bradykinin and angiotensin II. The *left insert* also shows the histogram for the chemical noise signal. The *insert on the right* shows a peptide contaminant with the intensity slightly above the limit of detection (Reproduced from Ref. [237] with permission. © Elsevier, 2016)

11.10 Essentials of MALDI

Basic Principle

Laser desorption/ionization (LDI) and matrix-assisted laser desorption/ionization (MALDI) rely on the absorption of energy from light by a thin crystalline layer of sample or sample–matrix mixture, respectively. The laser may be of infrared (IR) or ultraviolet (UV) wavelength; UV lasers are by far most common. The uptake of energy from a large number of photons irradiated within several nanoseconds locally leads to the formation of a plasma. Depending on the actual analyte–matrix combination, ionization occurs via different channels such as multiphotonionization, charge transfer, protonation or deprotonation, addition of cations or anions, or electron capture. MALDI generally yields singly charged ions.

Sample Preparation and Measurement

For LDI, the analyte is preferably provided as dilute solution, about 1 µl of which is applied onto a (stainless steel) sample plate and allowed to dry.

For MALDI, a dilute sample solution (0.01–1.0 mg ml^{-1}) is admixed to an excess of matrix solution (ca. 10 mg ml^{-1}) as to achieve an analyte-to-matrix ratio preferably in the range of 1:1000 to 1:10,000. About 1 µl of the combined solutions is then pipetted onto a sample plate, allowed to dry, and crystallize.

Thin layers of homogenously distributed microcrystals are preferred for good shot-to-shot reproducibility, and thus, high mass resolution and accuracy. The laser fluence is adjusted slightly above threshold for ion formation. Individual spectra by thousands of laser shots are accumulated to yield the final MALDI spectrum.

Sample Consumption and Detection Limit

In MALDI MS, the combination of the actual analyte, the selection of the matrix, and the procedure of sample preparation essentially represent the limiting factors for sample consumption and detection limit.

The minimum sample load or the detection limit is usually specified instead of sensitivity. Sample loads of 1 fmol of a protein can normally be achieved. As thousands of single-shot spectra can be obtained from one preparation spread over some square millimeters, the sample consumption has been estimated to approximate 10^{-17} mol per laser shot, i.e., normally more than 99% of the sample can theoretically be recovered from the target. Improved ion extraction and detection as well as miniaturized sample preparation, e.g., by means of the anchor target technology, can provide attomole detection limits for peptides.

Analytes for MALDI

For standard MALDI sample preparation, the analyte should be soluble to about 0.1 mg ml^{-1} in some solvent. If an analyte is completely insoluble, solvent-free sample preparation may alternatively be applied (Sect. 11.4.3). The analyte may be medium polar to highly polar, neutral or ionic. Nonpolar compounds are hardest to analyze. Solutions containing metal salts, e.g., from buffers or excess of

Table 11.5 Ions formed by LDI and MALDI

Analytes	Positive ions	Negative ions
Nonpolar	$M^{+\bullet}$, $[M + Ag]^+$, $[M + Cs]^+$ [a]	$M^{-\bullet}$
Medium polarity	$M^{+\bullet}$ and/or $[M + H]^+$, $[M + alkali]^+$, {*clusters* $[2M]^{+\bullet}$ and/or $[2M + H]^+$, $[2M + alkali]^+$, *adducts* $[M + Ma + H]^+$, $[M + Ma + alkali]^+$}[c]	$M^{-\bullet}$ and/or $[M - H]^-$, {*clusters* $[2M]^{-\bullet}$ and/or $[2M - H]^-$*adducts* $[M + Ma]^{-\bullet}$, $[M + Ma - H]^-$}
Polar	$[M + H]^+$, $[M + alkali]^+$, *exchange* $[M - H_n + alkali_{n+1}]^+$ *high-mass anal.* $[M + 2H]^{2+}$, $[M + 2alkali]^{2+}${*clusters* $[nM + H]^+$, $[nM + alkali]^+$, *adducts* $[M + Ma + H]^+$, $[M + Ma + alkali]^+$}	$[M - H]^-$, *exchange* $[M - H_n + alkali_{n-1}]^-$ {*clusters* $[nM - H]^-$ *adducts* $[M + Ma - H]^-$}
Ionic [b]	C^+, $[C_n + A_{n-1}]^+$, {$[CA]^{+\bullet}$}	A^-, $[C_{n-1} + A_n]^-$, {$[CA]^{-\bullet}$}

[a]Silver and cesium ions can serve as a workaround for nonpolar analytes
[b]Comprising of cation C^+ and anion A^-
[c]Braces denote rarely observed species

noncomplexed metals, may cause a confusingly large number of signals due to multiple proton/metal exchange and adduct ion formation; even complete suppression of the analyte can occur.

The mass range of MALDI is theoretically almost unlimited; in practice, limits strongly depend on the compound class to be analyzed.

Types of Ions in LDI and MALDI

LDI and MALDI produce a variety of ions depending on the polarity of the analyte, its ionization energy, the characteristics of the matrix (if any) and on the presence or absence of impurities such as alkali metal ions [20, 36, 37]. The tendency to form radical ions is somewhat lower than in case of FAB/LSIMS (Table 11.5).

Mass Analyzers for MALDI-MS

Laser desorption intrinsically is a pulsed ionization process, which is therefore ideally combined with time-of-flight (TOF) analyzers (Sect. 4.2) [17, 56]. Ever since the first MALDI experiments, MALDI and TOF have been forming a unit, and the majority of MALDI applications are MALDI-TOF measurements. Vice versa, it was the success of MALDI that pushed forth the tremendous delevopment of TOF mass analyzers. More recently, MALDI has also been adapted to orthogonal acceleration TOF analyzers [238].

Fourier transform ion cyclotron resonance (FT-ICR, Sect. 4.7) can be used in combination with an external ion source [239], and thus, MALDI-FT-ICR has become a mature combination [240, 241]. Modern MALDI-FT-ICR instruments make use of collisional cooling of the plasma plume before transferring the ions into the ICR cell [242, 243].

AP-MALDI may be attached to any instrument with an atmospheric pressure ionization interface.

References

1. Fenner NC, Daly NR (1966) Laser Used for Mass Analysis. Rev Sci Instrum 37:1068–1070. doi:10.1063/1.1720410
2. Vastola FJ, Pirone AJ (1968) Ionization of Organic Solids by Laser Irradiation. Adv Mass Spectrom 4:107–111
3. Vastola FJ, Mumma RO, Pirone AJ (1970) Analysis of Organic Salts by Laser Ionization. Org Mass Spectrom 3:101–104. doi:10.1002/oms.1210030112
4. Posthumus MA, Kistemaker PG, Meuzelaar HLC, Ten Noever de Brauw MC (1978) Laser Desorption-Mass Spectrometry of Polar Nonvolatile Bio-Organic Molecules. Anal Chem 50:985–991. doi:10.1021/ac50029a040
5. Wilkins CL, Weil DA, Yang CLC, Ijames CF (1985) High Mass Analysis by Laser Desorption Fourier Transform Mass Spectrometry. Anal Chem 57:520–524. doi:10.1021/ac50001a046
6. Coates ML, Wilkins CL (1985) Laser Desorption Fourier Transform Mass Spectra of Malto-Oligosaccharides. Biomed Mass Spectrom 12:424–428. doi:10.1002/bms.1200120812
7. Macfarlane RD (1999) Mass Spectrometry of Biomolecules: From PDMS to MALDI. Brazilian J Phys 29:415–421. doi:10.1590/S0103-97331999000300003
8. Tanaka K, Waki H, Ido Y, Akita S, Yoshida Y, Yhoshida T (1988) Protein and Polymer Analyses Up to *M/z* 100,000 by Laser Ionization Time-of-Flight Mass Spectrometry. Rapid Commun Mass Spectrom 2:151–153. doi:10.1002/rcm.1290020802
9. Tanaka K (2003) The Origin of Macromolecule Ionization by Laser Irradiation (Nobel Lecture). Angew Chem Int Ed 42:3861–3870. doi:10.1002/anie.200300585
10. Karas M, Bachmann D, Hillenkamp F (1985) Influence of the Wavelength in High-Irradiance Ultraviolet Laser Desorption Mass Spectrometry of Organic Molecules. Anal Chem 57:2935–2939. doi:10.1021/ac00291a042
11. Karas M, Bachmann D, Bahr U, Hillenkamp F (1987) Matrix-Assisted Ultraviolet Laser Desorption of Non-Volatile Compounds. Int J Mass Spectrom Ion Proc 78:53–68. doi:10.1016/0168-1176(87)87041-6
12. Karas M, Hillenkamp F (1988) Laser Desorption Ionization of Proteins with Molecular Masses Exceeding 10,000 Daltons. Anal Chem 60:2299–2301. doi:10.1021/ac00171a028
13. Karas M, Bahr U, Ingendoh A, Hillenkamp F (1989) Laser-Desorption Mass Spectrometry of 100,000–250,000-Dalton Proteins. Angew Chem Int Ed 28:760–761. doi:10.1002/anie.198907601
14. Karas M, Ingendoh A, Bahr U, Hillenkamp F (1989) Ultraviolet-Laser Desorption/Ionization Mass Spectrometry of Femtomolar Amounts of Large Proteins. Biomed Environ Mass Spectrom 18:841–843. doi:10.1002/bms.1200180931
15. Hillenkamp F, Peter-Katalinic J (eds) (2007) MALDI-MS. A Practical Guide to Instrumentation, Methods and Applications. Wiley-VCH, Weinheim
16. Karas M, Bahr U, Gießmann U (1991) Matrix-Assisted Laser Desorption Ionization Mass Spectrometry. Mass Spectrom Rev 10:335–357. doi:10.1002/mas.1280100503
17. Hillenkamp F, Karas M, Beavis RC, Chait BT (1991) Matrix-Assisted Laser Desorption/Ionization Mass Spectrometry of Biopolymers. Anal Chem 63:1193A–1203A. doi:10.1021/ac00024a716
18. Beavis RC (1992) Matrix-Assisted Ultraviolet Laser Desorption: Evolution and Principles. Org Mass Spectrom 27:653–659. doi:10.1002/oms.1210270602
19. Hillenkamp F, Karas M (2000) Matrix-Assisted Laser Desorption/Ionisation, an Experience. Int J Mass Spectrom 200:71–77. doi:10.1016/S1387-3806(00)00300-6
20. Lehmann WD (1996) Massenspektrometrie in der Biochemie. Spektrum Akademischer Verlag, Heidelberg
21. Cotter RJ (1997) Time-of-Flight Mass Spectrometry: Instrumentation and Applications in Biological Research. American Chemical Society, Washington, DC

22. Siuzdak G (2006) The Expanding Role of Mass Spectrometry in Biotechnology. MCC Press, San Diego
23. Cole RB (ed) (2010) Electrospray and MALDI Mass Spectrometry: Fundamentals, Instrumentation, Practicalities, and Biological Applications. Wiley, Hoboken
24. Hillenkamp F, Peter-Katalinic J (eds) (2013) MALDI MS: A Practical Guide to Instrumentation, Methods and Applications. Wiley-VCH, Weinheim
25. Cramer R (ed) (2016) Advances in MALDI and Laser-Induced Soft Ionization Mass Spectrometry. Springer, Cham. doi:10.1007/978-3-319-04819-2
26. Montaudo G, Lattimer RP (eds) (2001) Mass Spectrometry of Polymers. CRC Press, Boca Raton
27. Murgasova R, Hercules DM (2003) MALDI of Synthetic Polymers – An Update. Int J Mass Spectrom 226:151–162. doi:10.1016/S1387-3806(02)00971-5
28. Mamyrin BA (1994) Laser Assisted Reflectron Time-of-Flight Mass Spectrometry. Int J Mass Spectrom Ion Proc 131:1–19. doi:10.1016/0168-1176(93)03891-O
29. Dreisewerd K, Schürenberg M, Karas M, Hillenkamp F (1995) Influence of the Laser Intensity and Spot Size on the Desorption of Molecules and Ions in Matrix-Assisted Laser Desorption/Ionization with a Uniform Beam Profile. Int J Mass Spectrom Ion Proc 141:127–148. doi:10.1016/0168-1176(94)04108-J
30. Nordhoff E, Ingendoh A, Cramer R, Overberg A, Stahl B, Karas M, Hillenkamp F, Crain PF (1992) Matrix-Assisted Laser Desorption/Ionization Mass Spectrometry of Nucleic Acids with Wavelengths in the Ultraviolet and Infrared. Rapid Commun Mass Spectrom 6:771–776. doi:10.1002/rcm.1290061212
31. Overberg A, Karas M, Bahr U, Kaufmann R, Hillenkamp F (1990) Matrix-Assisted Infrared-Laser (2.94 μm) Desorption/Ionization Mass Spectrometry of Large Biomolecules. Rapid Commun Mass Spectrom 4:293–296. doi:10.1002/rcm.1290040808
32. Overberg A, Karas M, Hillenkamp F (1991) Matrix-Assisted Laser Desorption of Large Biomolecules with a TEA-CO_2-Laser. Rapid Commun Mass Spectrom 5:128–131. doi:10.1002/rcm.1290050308
33. Berkenkamp S, Menzel C, Hillenkamp F, Dreisewerd K (2002) Measurements of Mean Initial Velocities of Analyte and Matrix Ions in Infrared Matrix-Assisted Laser Desorption Ionization Mass Spectrometry. J Am Soc Mass Spectrom 13:209–220. doi:10.1016/S1044-0305(01)00355-5
34. Zenobi R, Knochenmuss R (1999) Ion Formation in MALDI Mass Spectrometry. Mass Spectrom Rev 17:337–366. doi:10.1002/(SICI)1098-2787(1998)17:5<337::AID-MAS2>3.0.CO;2-S
35. Menzel C, Dreisewerd K, Berkenkamp S, Hillenkamp F (2001) Mechanisms of Energy Deposition in Infrared Matrix-Assisted Laser Desorption/Ionization Mass Spectrometry. Int J Mass Spectrom 207:73–96. doi:10.1016/S1387-3806(01)00363-3
36. Dreisewerd K, Berkenkamp S, Leisner A, Rohlfing A, Menzel C (2003) Fundamentals of Matrix-Assisted Laser Desorption/Ionization Mass Spectrometry with Pulsed Infrared Lasers. Int J Mass Spectrom 226:189–209. doi:10.1016/S1387-3806(02)00977-6
37. Dreisewerd K (2003) The Desorption Process in MALDI. Chem Rev 103:395–425. doi:10.1021/cr010375i
38. Karas M, Krüger R (2003) Ion Formation in MALDI: The Cluster Ionization Mechanism. Chem Rev 103:427–439. doi:10.1021/cr010376a
39. Dreisewerd K (2014) Recent Methodological Advances in MALDI Mass Spectrometry. Anal Bioanal Chem 406:2261–2278. doi:10.1007/s00216-014-7646-6
40. Westmacott G, Ens W, Hillenkamp F, Dreisewerd K, Schürenberg M (2002) The Influence of Laser Fluence on Ion Yield in Matrix-Assisted Laser Desorption Ionization Mass Spectrometry. Int J Mass Spectrom 221:67–81. doi:10.1016/S1387-3806(02)00898-9
41. Menzel C, Dreisewerd K, Berkenkamp S, Hillenkamp F (2002) The Role of the Laser Pulse Duration in Infrared Matrix-Assisted Laser Desorption/Ionization Mass Spectrometry. J Am Soc Mass Spectrom 13:975–984. doi:10.1016/S1044-0305(02)00397-5

42. Juhasz P, Vestal ML, Martin SA (1997) On the Initial Velocity of Ions Generated by Matrix-Assisted Laser Desorption Ionization and Its Effect on the Calibration of Delayed Extraction Time-of-Flight Mass Spectra. J Am Soc Mass Spectrom 8:209–217. doi:10.1016/S1044-0305(96)00256-5
43. Karas M, Bahr U, Fournier I, Glückmann M, Pfenninger A (2003) The Initial Ion Velocity as a Marker for Different Desorption-Ionization Mechanisms in MALDI. Int J Mass Spectrom 226:239–248. doi:10.1016/S1387-3806(02)01062-X
44. Horneffer V, Dreisewerd K, Ludemann H-C, Hillenkamp F, Lage M, Strupat K (1999) Is the Incorporation of Analytes into Matrix Crystals a Prerequisite for Matrix-Assisted Laser Desorption/Ionization Mass Spectrometry? A Study of Five Positional Isomers of Dihydroxybenzoic Acid. Int J Mass Spectrom 185(186/187):859–870. doi:10.1016/S1387-3806(98)14218-5
45. Glückmann M, Pfenninger A, Krüger R, Thierolf M, Karas M, Horneffer V, Hillenkamp F, Strupat K (2001) Mechanisms in MALDI Analysis: Surface Interaction or Incorporation of Analytes? Int J Mass Spectrom 210(211):121–132. doi:10.1016/S1387-3806(01)00450-X
46. Karas M, Gluckmann M, Schäfer J (2000) Ionization in Matrix-Assisted Laser Desorption/Ionization: Singly Charged Molecular Ions Are the Lucky Survivors. J Mass Spectrom 35:1–12. doi:10.1002/(SICI)1096-9888(200001)35:1<1::AID-JMS904>3.0.CO;2-0
47. Ens W, Mao Y, Mayer F, Standing KG (1991) Properties of Matrix-Assisted Laser Desorption. Measurements with a Time-to-Digital Converter. Rapid Commun Mass Spectrom 5:117–123. doi:10.1002/rcm.1290050306
48. Medina N, Huth-Fehre T, Westman A, Sundqvist BUR (1994) Matrix-Assisted Laser Desorption: Dependence of the Threshold Fluence on Analyte Concentration. Org Mass Spectrom 29:207–209. doi:10.1002/oms.1210290410
49. Quist AP, Huth-Fehre T, Sundqvist BUR (1994) Total Yield Measurements in Matrix-Assisted Laser Desorption Using a Quartz Crystal Microbalance. Rapid Commun Mass Spectrom 8:149–154. doi:10.1002/rcm.1290080204
50. Beavis RC, Chait BT (1989) Factors Affecting the Ultraviolet Laser Desorption of Proteins. Rapid Commun Mass Spectrom 3:233–237. doi:10.1002/rcm.1290030708
51. Ingendoh A, Karas M, Hillenkamp F, Giessmann U (1994) Factors Affecting the Resolution in Matrix-Assisted Laser Desorption-Ionization Mass Spectrometry. Int J Mass Spectrom Ion Proc 131:345–354. doi:10.1016/0168-1176(93)03873-K
52. Aksouh F, Chaurand P, Deprun C, Della-Negra S, Hoyes J, Le Beyec Y, Pinho RR (1995) Influence of the Laser Beam Direction on the Molecular Ion Ejection Angle in Matrix-Assisted Laser Desorption/Ionization. Rapid Commun Mass Spectrom 9:515–518. doi:10.1002/rcm.1290090609
53. Liao P-C, Allison J (1995) Dissecting Matrix-Assisted Laser Desorption/Ionization Mass Spectra. J Mass Spectrom 30:763–766. doi:10.1002/jms.1190300517
54. Strupat K, Karas M, Hillenkamp F (1991) 2,5-Dihydroxybenzoic Acid: A New Matrix for Laser Desorption-Ionization Mass Spectrometry. Int J Mass Spectrom Ion Proc 111:89–102. doi:10.1016/0168-1176(91)85050-V
55. Holle A, Haase A, Kayser M, Hoehndorf J (2006) Optimizing UV Laser Focus Profiles for Improved MALDI Performance. J Mass Spectrom 41:705–716. doi:10.1002/jms.1041
56. Cotter RJ (1987) Laser Mass Spectrometry: An Overview of Techniques, Instruments and Applications. Anal Chim Acta 195:45–59. doi:10.1016/S0003-2670(00)85648-2
57. Pan Y, Cotter RJ (1992) Measurement of Initial Translational Energies of Peptide Ions in Laser Desorption/Ionization Mass Spectrometry. Org Mass Spectrom 27:3–8. doi:10.1002/oms.1210270103
58. Glückmann M, Karas M (1999) The Initial Ion Velocity and Its Dependence on Matrix, Analyte and Preparation Method in Ultraviolet Matrix-Assisted Laser Desorption/Ionization. J Mass Spectrom 34:467–477. doi:10.1002/(SICI)1096-9888(199905)34:5<467::AID-JMS809>3.0.CO;2-8

59. Puretzky AA, Geohegan DB, Hurst GB, Buchanan MV, Luk'yanchuk BS (1999) Imaging of Vapor Plumes Produced by Matrix Assisted Laser Desorption: A Plume Sharpening Effect. Phys Rev Lett 83:444–447. doi:10.1103/PhysRevLett.83.444
60. Leisner A, Rohlfing A, Berkenkamp S, Röhling U, Dreisewerd K, Hillenkamp F (2003) IR-MALDI with the Matrix Glycerol: Examination of the Plume Expansion Dynamics for Lasers of Different Pulse Duration. 36. DGMS Jahrestagung: Poster
61. Leisner A, Rohlfing A, Roehling U, Dreisewerd K, Hillenkamp F (2005) Time-Resolved Imaging of the Plume Dynamics in Infrared Matrix-Assisted Laser Desorption/Ionization with a Glycerol Matrix. J Phys Chem B 109:11661–11666. doi:10.1021/jp050994l
62. Chen LC, Rahman MM, Hiraoka K (2014) Super-Atmospheric Pressure Ion Sources: Application and Coupling to API Mass Spectrometer. Mass Spectrom 3:S0024. doi:10.5702/massspectrometry.S0024
63. Wang BH, Dreisewerd K, Bahr U, Karas M, Hillenkamp F (1993) Gas-Phase Cationization and Protonation of Neutrals Generated by Matrix-Assisted Laser Desorption. J Am Soc Mass Spectrom 4:393–398. doi:10.1016/1044-0305(93)85004-H
64. Liao P-C, Allison J (1995) Ionization Processes in Matrix-Assisted Laser Desorption/Ionization Mass Spectrometry: Matrix-Dependent Formation of $[M+H]^+$ Vs. $[M+Na]^+$ Ions of Small Peptides and Some Mechanistic Comments. J Mass Spectrom 30:408–423. doi:10.1002/jms.1190300304
65. Gimon ME, Preston LM, Solouki T, White MA, Russel DH (1992) Are Proton Transfer Reactions of Excited States Involved in UV Laser Desorption Ionization? Org Mass Spectrom 27:827–830. doi:10.1002/oms.1210270711
66. Juhasz P, Costello CE (1993) Generation of Large Radical Ions from Oligometallocenes by Matrix-Assisted Laser Desorption Ionization. Rapid Commun Mass Spectrom 7:343–351. doi:10.1002/rcm.1290070508
67. Lidgard RO, McConnell BD, Black DSC, Kumar N, Duncan MW (1996) Fragmentation Observed in Continuous Extraction Linear MALDI: A Cautionary Note. J Mass Spectrom 31:1443–1445. doi:10.1002/(SICI)1096-9888(199612)31:12<1443::AID-JMS448>3.0.CO;2-J
68. Irngartinger H, Weber A (1996) Twofold Cycloaddition of [60]Fullerene to a Bifunctional Nitrile Oxide. Tertrahedron Lett 37:4137–4140. doi:10.1016/0040-4039(96)00779-4
69. Gromov A, Ballenweg S, Giesa S, Lebedkin S, Hull WE, Krätschmer W (1997) Preparation and Characterization of C_{119}. Chem Phys Lett 267:460–466. doi:10.1016/S0009-2614(97)00129-2
70. Giesa S, Gross JH, Hull WE, Lebedkin S, Gromov A, Krätschmer W, Gleiter R (1999) $C_{120}OS$: The First Sulfur-Containing Dimeric [60]Fullerene Derivative. Chem Commun:465–466. doi:10.1039/a809831j
71. Juhasz P, Costello CE, Biemann K (1993) Matrix-Assisted Laser Desorption Ionization Mass Spectrometry with 2-(4-Hydroxyphenylazo)benzoic acid Matrix. J Am Soc Mass Spectrom 4:399–409. doi:10.1016/1044-0305(93)85005-I
72. Hopwood FG, Michalak L, Alderdice DS, Fisher KJ, Willett GD (1994) C_{60}-Assisted Laser Desorption/Ionization Mass Spectrometry in the Analysis of Phosphotungstic Acid. Rapid Commun Mass Spectrom 8:881–885. doi:10.1002/rcm.1290081105
73. Jones RM, Lamb JH, Lim CK (1995) 5,10,15,20-*Meso*-Tetra(hydroxyphenyl)-chlorin as a Matrix for the Analysis of Low Molecular Weight Compounds by Matrix-Assisted Laser Desorption/Ionization Time-of-Flight Mass Spectrometry. Rapid Commun Mass Spectrom 9:968–969. doi:10.1002/rcm.1290091020
74. Armstrong DW, Zhang LK, He L, Gross ML (2001) Ionic Liquids As Matrixes for Matrix-Assisted Laser Desorption/Ionization Mass Spectrometry. Anal Chem 73:3679–3686. doi:10.1021/ac010259f
75. Li YL, Gross ML (2004) Ionic-Liquid Matrices for Quantitative Analysis by MALDI-TOF Mass Spectrometry. J Am Soc Mass Spectrom 15:1833–1837. doi:10.1016/j.jasms.2004.08.011

76. Tang K, Taranenko NI, Allman SL, Chen CH, Chang LY, Jacobson KB (1994) Picolinic Acid as a Matrix for Laser Mass Spectrometry of Nucleic Acids and Proteins. Rapid Commun Mass Spectrom 8:673–677. doi:10.1002/rcm.1290080902
77. Wu KJ, Steding A, Becker CH (1993) Matrix-Assisted Laser Desorption Time-of-Flight Mass Spectrometry of Oligonucleotides Using 3-Hydroxypicolinic Acid as an Ultraviolet-Sensitive Matrix. Rapid Commun Mass Spectrom 7:142–146. doi:10.1002/rcm.1290070206
78. Taranenko NI, Tang K, Allman SL, Ch'ang LY, Chen CH (1994) 3-Aminopicolinic Acid As a Matrix for Laser Desorption Mass Spectrometry of Biopolymers. Rapid Commun Mass Spectrom 8:1001–1006. doi:10.1002/rcm.1290081219
79. Terrier P, Tortajada J, Zin G, Buchmann W (2007) Noncovalent Complexes Between DNA and Basic Polypeptides or Polyamines by MALDI-TOF. J Am Soc Mass Spectrom 18:1977–1989. doi:10.1016/j.jasms.2007.07.028
80. Lecchi P, Le HM, Pannell LK (1995) 6-Aza-2-thiothymine: a Matrix for MALDI Spectra of Oligonucleotides. Nucl Acids Res 23:1276–1277. doi:10.1093/nar/23.7.1276
81. Taranenko NI, Potter NT, Allman SL, Golovlev VV, Chen CH (1999) Gender Identification by Matrix-Assisted Laser Desorption/Ionization Time-of-Flight Mass Spectrometry. Anal Chem 71:3974–3976. doi:10.1021/ac990150w
82. Mohr MD, Börnsen KO, Widmer HM (1995) Matrix-Assisted Laser Desorption/Ionization Mass Spectrometry: Improved Matrix for Oligosaccharides. Rapid Commun Mass Spectrom 9:809–814. doi:10.1002/rcm.1290090919
83. Finke B, Stahl B, Pfenninger A, Karas M, Daniel H, Sawatzki G (1999) Analysis of High-Molecular-Weight Oligosaccharides from Human Milk by Liquid Chromatography and MALDI-MS. Anal Chem 71:3755–3762. doi:10.1021/ac990094z
84. Pfenninger A, Karas M, Finke B, Stahl B, Sawatzki G (1999) Matrix Optimization for Matrix-Assisted Laser Desorption/Ionization Mass Spectrometry of Oligosaccharides from Human Milk. J Mass Spectrom 34:98–104. doi:10.1002/(SICI)1096-9888(199902)34:2<98::AID-JMS767>3.0.CO;2-N
85. Laugesen S, Roepstorff P (2003) Combination of Two Matrices Results in Improved Performance of MALDI MS for Peptide Mass Mapping and Protein Analysis. J Am Soc Mass Spectrom 14:992–1002. doi:10.1016/S1044-0305(03)00262-9
86. Karas M, Ehring H, Nordhoff E, Stahl B, Strupat K, Hillenkamp F, Grehl M, Krebs B (1993) Matrix-Assisted Laser Desorption/Ionization Mass Spectrometry with Additives to 2,5-Dihydroxybenzoic Acid. Org Mass Spectrom 28:1476–1481. doi:10.1002/oms.1210281219
87. Rohmer M, Meyer B, Mank M, Stahl B, Bahr U, Karas M (2010) 3-Aminoquinoline Acting As Matrix and Derivatizing Agent for MALDI MS Analysis of Oligosaccharides. Anal Chem 82:3719–3726. doi:10.1021/ac1001096
88. Stahl B, Thurl S, Zeng J, Karas M, Hillenkamp F, Steup M, Sawatzki G (1994) Oligosaccharides from Human Milk As Revealed by Matrix-Assisted Laser Desorption/Ionization Mass Spectrometry. Anal Biochem 223:218–226. doi:10.1006/abio.1994.1577
89. Metzger JO, Woisch R, Tuszynski W, Angermann R (1994) New Type of Matrix for Matrix-Assisted Laser Desorption Mass Spectrometry of Polysaccharides and Proteins. Fresenius J Anal Chem 349:473–474. doi:10.1007/BF00322937
90. Beavis RC, Chaudhary T, Chait BT (1992) α-Cyano-4-hydroxycinnamic acid As a Matrix for Matrix-Assisted Laser Desorption Mass Spectrometry. Org Mass Spectrom 27:156–158. doi:10.1002/oms.1210270217
91. Ayorinde FO, Elhilo E, Hlongwane C (1999) Matrix-Assisted Laser Desorption/Ionization Time-of-Flight Mass Spectrometry of Canola, Castor and Olive Oils. Rapid Commun Mass Spectrom 13:737–739. doi:10.1002/(SICI)1097-0231(19990430)13:8<737::AID-RCM552>3.0.CO;2-L
92. George M, Wellemans JMY, Cerny RL, Gross ML, Li K, Cavalieri EL (1994) Matrix Design for Matrix-Assisted Laser Desorption Ionization: Sensitive Determination of PAH-DNA Adducts. J Am Soc Mass Spectrom 5:1021–1025. doi:10.1016/1044-0305(94)80021-9

93. Lidgard RO, Duncan MW (1995) Utility of Matrix-Assisted Laser Desorption/Ionization Time-of-Flight Mass Spectrometry for the Analysis of Low Molecular Weight Compounds. Rapid Commun Mass Spectrom 9:128–132. doi:10.1002/rcm.1290090205
94. Soltwisch J, Jaskolla TW, Hillenkamp F, Karas M, Dreisewerd K (2012) Ion Yields in UV-MALDI Mass Spectrometry As a Function of Excitation Laser Wavelength and Optical and Physico-Chemical Properties of Classical and Halogen-Substituted MALDI Matrixes. Anal Chem 84:6567–6576. doi:10.1021/ac3008434
95. Wiegelmann M, Soltwisch J, Jaskolla TW, Dreisewerd K (2013) Matching the Laser Wavelength to the Absorption Properties of Matrices Increases the Ion Yield in UV-MALDI Mass Spectrometry. Anal Bioanal Chem 405:6925–6932. doi:10.1007/s00216-012-6478-5
96. Beavis RC, Chait BT (1989) Cinnamic Acid Derivatives as Matrices for Ultraviolet Laser Desorption Mass Spectrometry of Proteins. Rapid Commun Mass Spectrom 3:432–435. doi:10.1002/rcm.1290031207
97. Montaudo G, Montaudo MS, Puglisi C, Samperi F (1994) 2-(4-Hydroxyphenylazo)benzoic acid: A Solid Matrix for Matrix-Assisted Laser Desorption/Ionization of Polystyrene. Rapid Commun Mass Spectrom 8:1011–1015. doi:10.1002/rcm.1290081221
98. Xu N, Huang ZH, Watson JT, Gage DA (1997) Mercaptobenzothiazoles: A New Class of Matrixes for Laser Desorption Ionization Mass Spectrometry. J Am Soc Mass Spectrom 8:116–124. doi:10.1016/S1044-0305(96)00233-4
99. Pitt JJ, Gorman JJ (1996) Matrix-Assisted Laser Desorption/Ionization Time-of-Flight Mass Spectrometry of Sialylated Glycopeptides and Proteins Using 2,6-Dihydroxyacetophenone as a Matrix. Rapid Commun Mass Spectrom 10:1786–1788. doi:10.1002/(SICI)1097-0231(199611)10:14<1786::AID-RCM751>3.0.CO;2-I
100. Gorman JJ, Ferguson BL, Nguyen TB (1996) Use of 2,6-Dihydroxyacetophenone for Analysis of Fragile Peptides, Disulfide Bonding and Small Proteins by Matrix-Assisted Laser Desorption/Ionization. Rapid Commun Mass Spectrom 10:529–536. doi:10.1002/(SICI)1097-0231(19960331)10:5<529::AID-RCM522>3.0.CO;2-9
101. Meyer A, Spinelli N, Imbach JL, Vasseur J-J (2000) Analysis of Solid-Supported Oligonucleotides by Matrix-Assisted Laser Desorption/Ionization Time-of-Flight Mass Spectrometry. Rapid Commun Mass Spectrom 14:234–242. doi:10.1002/(SICI)1097-0231(20000229)14:4<234::AID-RCM874>3.0.CO;2-1
102. Kassis CM, DeSimone JM, Linton RW, Lange GW, Friedman RM (1997) An Investigation into the Importance of Polymer-Matrix Miscibility Using Surfactant Modified Matrix-Assisted Laser Desorption/Ionization Mass Spectrometry. Rapid Commun Mass Spectrom 11:1462–1466. doi:10.1002/(SICI)1097-0231(19970830)11:13<1462::AID-RCM44>3.0.CO;2-2
103. Carr RH, Jackson AT (1998) Preliminary Matrix-Assisted Laser Desorption Ionization Time-of-Flight and Field Desorption Mass Spectrometric Analyses of Polymeric Methylene Diphenylene Diisocyanate, Its Amine Precursor and a Model Polyether Prepolymer. Rapid Commun Mass Spectrom 12:2047–2050. doi:10.1002/(SICI)1097-0231(19981230)12:24<2047::AID-RCM428>3.0.CO;2-9
104. Lebedkin S, Ballenweg S, Gross JH, Taylor R, Krätschmer W (1995) Synthesis of $C_{120}O$: A New Dimeric [60]Fullerene Derivative. Tetrahedron Lett 36:4971–4974. doi:10.1016/0040-4039(95)00784-A
105. Ballenweg S, Gleiter R, Krätschmer W (1996) Chemistry at Cyclopentene Addends on [60]Fullerene. Matrix-Assisted Laser Desorption-Ionization Time-of-Flight Mass Spectrometry (MALDI-TOF MS) As a Quick and Facile Method for the Characterization of Fullerene Derivatives. Synth Met 77:209–212. doi:10.1016/0379-6779(96)80089-0
106. Ulmer L, Mattay J, Torres-Garcia HG, Luftmann H (2000) The Use of 2-[(2*E*)-3-(4-*tert*-Butylphenyl)-2-methylprop-2-enylidene]malononitrile as a Matrix for Matrix-Assisted Laser Desorption/Ionization Mass Spectrometry. Eur J Mass Spectrom 6:49–52. doi:10.1255/ejms.329
107. Brown T, Clipston NL, Simjee N, Luftmann H, Hungebühler H, Drewello T (2001) Matrix-Assisted Laser Desorption/Ionization of Amphiphilic Fullerene Derivatives. Int J Mass Spectrom 210(211):249–263. doi:10.1016/S1387-3806(01)00429-8

108. Mirza SP, Raju NP, Vairamani M (2004) Estimation of the Proton Affinity Values of Fifteen Matrix-Assisted Laser Desorption/Ionization Matrices Under Electrospray Ionization Conditions Using the Kinetic Method. J Am Soc Mass Spectrom 15:431–435. doi:10.1016/j.jasms.2003.12.001
109. Burton RD, Watson CH, Eyler JR, Lang GL, Powell DH, Avery MY (1997) Proton Affinities of Eight Matrixes Used for Matrix-Assisted Laser Desorption/Ionization. Rapid Commun Mass Spectrom 11:443–446. doi:10.1002/(SICI)1097-0231(199703)11:5<443::AID-RCM897>3.0.CO;2-3
110. Nordhoff E, Schürenberg M, Thiele G, Lübbert C, Kloeppel K-D, Theiss D, Lehrach H, Gobom J (2003) Sample Preparation Protocols for MALDI-MS of Peptides and Oligonucleotides Using Prestructured Sample Supports. Int J Mass Spectrom 226:163–180. doi:10.1016/S1387-3806(02)00978-8
111. Westman A, Huth-Fehre T, Demirev PA, Sundqvist BUR (1995) Sample Morphology Effects in Matrix-Assisted Laser Desorption/Ionization Mass Spectrometry of Proteins. J Mass Spectrom 30:206–211. doi:10.1002/jms.1190300131
112. Arakawa R, Watanabe S, Fukuo T (1999) Effects of Sample Preparation on Matrix-Assisted Laser Desorption/Ionization Time-of-Flight Mass Spectra for Sodium Polystyrene Sulfonate. Rapid Commun Mass Spectrom 13:1059–1062. doi:10.1002/(SICI)1097-0231(19990615)13:11<1059::AID-RCM608>3.0.CO;2-1
113. Chan PK, Chan T-WD (2000) Effect of Sample Preparation Methods on the Analysis of Dispersed Polysaccharides by Matrix-Assisted Laser Desorption/Ionization Time-of-Flight Mass Spectrometry. Rapid Commun Mass Spectrom 14:1841–1847. doi:10.1002/1097-0231(20001015)14:19<1841::AID-RCM104>3.0.CO;2-Q
114. Vorm O, Mann M (1994) Improved Mass Accuracy in Matrix-Assisted Laser Desorption/Ionization Time-of-Flight Mass Spectrometry of Peptides. J Am Soc Mass Spectrom 5:955–958. doi:10.1016/1044-0305(94)80013-8
115. Ayorinde FO, Keith QL Jr, Wan LW (1999) Matrix-Assisted Laser Desorption/Ionization Time-of-Flight Mass Spectrometry of Cod Liver Oil and the Effect of Analyte/Matrix Concentration on Signal Intensities. Rapid Commun Mass Spectrom 13:1762–1769. doi:10.1002/(SICI)1097-0231(19990915)13:17<1762::AID-RCM711>3.0.CO;2-8
116. Vorm O, Roepstorff P, Mann M (1994) Improved Resolution and Very High Sensitivity in MALDI-TOF of Matrix Surfaces Made by Fast Evaporation. Anal Chem 66:3281–3287. doi:10.1021/ac00091a044
117. Bashir S, Derrick PJ, Critchley P, Gates PJ, Staunton J (2003) Matrix-Assisted Laser Desorption/Ionization Time-of-Flight Mass Spectrometry of Dextran and Dextrin Derivatives. Eur J Mass Spectrom 9:61–70. doi:10.1255/ejms.510
118. Rashidezadeh H, Baochuan G (1998) Investigation of Metal Attachment to Polystyrenes in Matrix-Assisted Laser Desorption Ionization. J Am Soc Mass Spectrom 9:724–730. doi:10.1016/S1044-0305(98)00038-5
119. Rashidezadeh H, Hung K, Baochuan G (1998) Probing Polystyrene Cationization in Matrix-Assisted Laser/Desorption Ionization. Eur Mass Spectrom 4:429–433. doi:10.1255/ejms.267
120. Kühn G, Weidner S, Decker R, Holländer A (1997) Derivatization of Double Bonds Investigated by Matrix-Assisted Laser Desorption/Ionization Mass Spectrometry. Rapid Commun Mass Spectrom 11:914–918. doi:10.1002/(SICI)1097-0231(199705)11:8<914::AID-RCM920>3.0.CO;2-2
121. Kühn G, Weidner S, Just U, Hohner S (1996) Characterization of Technical Waxes. Comparison of Chromatographic Techniques and Matrix-Assisted Laser-Desorption/Ionization Mass Spectrometry. J Chromatogr A 732:111–117. doi:10.1016/0021-9673(95)01255-9
122. Pruns JK, Vietzke J-P, Strassner M, Rapp C, Hintze U, König WA (2002) Characterization of Low Molecular Weight Hydrocarbon Oligomers by Laser Desorption/Ionization Time-of-Flight Mass Spectrometry Using a Solvent-Free Sample Preparation Method. Rapid Commun Mass Spectrom 16:208–211. doi:10.1002/rcm.568

123. Mowat IA, Donovan RJ (1995) Metal-Ion Attachment to Non-Polar Polymers During Laser Desorption/Ionization at 337 Nm. Rapid Commun Mass Spectrom 9:82–90. doi:10.1002/rcm.1290090118
124. Goldschmitt RJ, Wetzel SJ, Blair WR, Guttman CM (2000) Post-Source Decay in the Analysis of Polystyrene by Matrix-Assisted Laser Desorption/Ionization Time-of-Flight Mass Spectrometry. J Am Soc Mass Spectrom 11:1095–1106. doi:10.1016/S1044-0305(00)00177-X
125. Kéki S, Deák G, Zsuga M (2001) Copper(I) Chloride: A Simple Salt for Enhancement of Polystyrene Cationization in Matrix-Assisted Laser Desorption/Ionization Mass Spectrometry. Rapid Commun Mass Spectrom 15:675–678. doi:10.1002/rcm.284
126. Zhang J, Zenobi R (2004) Matrix-Dependent Cationization in MALDI Mass Spectrometry. J Mass Spectrom 39:808–816. doi:10.1002/jms.657
127. Thurman EM, Ferrer I (2010) The Isotopic Mass Defect: a Tool for Limiting Molecular Formulas by Accurate Mass. Anal Bioanal Chem 397:2807–2816. doi:10.1007/s00216-010-3562-6
128. Salplachta J, Rehulka P, Chmelik J (2004) Identification of Proteins by Combination of Size-Exclusion Chromatography with Matrix-Assisted Laser Desorption/Ionization Time-of-Flight Mass Spectrometry and Comparison of Some Desalting Procedures for Both Intact Proteins and Their Tryptic Digests. J Mass Spectrom 39:1395–1401. doi:10.1002/jms.700
129. Jensen ON, Wilm M, Shevchenko A, Mann M (1999) Sample Preparation Methods for Mass Spectrometric Peptide Mapping Directly from 2-DE Gels. Methods Mol Biol 112:513–530
130. Rehulka P, Salplachta J, Chmelik J (2003) Improvement of Quality of Peptide Mass Spectra in Matrix-Assisted Laser Desorption/Ionization Time-of-Flight Mass Spectrometry and Post-Source Decay Analysis of Salty Protein Digests by Using on-Target Washing. J Mass Spectrom 38:1267–1269. doi:10.1002/jms.548
131. Zhang L, Orlando R (1999) Solid-Phase Extraction/MALDI-MS: Extended Ion-Pairing Surfaces for the On-Target Cleanup of Protein Samples. Anal Chem 71:4753–4757. doi:10.1021/ac990328e
132. Gobom J, Nordhoff E, Mirgorodskaya E, Ekman R, Roepstorff P (1999) Sample Purification and Preparation Technique Based on Nano-Scale Reversed-Phase Columns for the Sensitive Analysis of Complex Peptide Mixtures by Matrix-Assisted Laser Desorption/Ionization Mass Spectrometry. J Mass Spectrom 34:105–116. doi:10.1002/(SICI)1096-9888(199902)34:2<105::AID-JMS768>3.0.CO;2-4
133. Leite JF, Hajivandi MR, Diller T, Pope RM (2004) Removal of Sodium and Potassium Adducts Using a Matrix Additive During Matrix-Associated Laser Desorption/Ionization Time-of-Flight Mass Spectrometric Analysis of Peptides. Rapid Commun Mass Spectrom 18:2953–2959. doi:10.1002/rcm.1711
134. Puchades M, Westman A, Blennow K, Davidsson P (1999) Removal of Sodium Dodecyl Sulfate from Protein Samples Prior to Matrix-Assisted Laser Desorption/Ionization Mass Spectrometry. Rapid Commun Mass Spectrom 13:344–349. doi:10.1002/(SICI)1097-0231(19990315)13:5<344::AID-RCM489>3.0.CO;2-V
135. Trimpin S, Grimsdale AC, Räder HJ, Müllen K (2002) Characterization of an Insoluble Poly(9,9-diphenyl-2,7-fluorene) by Solvent-Free Sample Preparation for MALDI-TOF Mass Spectrometry. Anal Chem 74:3777–3782. doi:10.1021/ac0111863
136. Trimpin S, Rouhanipour A, Az R, Räder HJ, Müllen K (2001) New Aspects in Matrix-Assisted Laser Desorption/Ionization Time-of-Flight Mass Spectrometry: a Universal Solvent-Free Sample Preparation. Rapid Commun Mass Spectrom 15:1364–1373. doi:10.1002/rcm.372
137. Guittard J, Hronowski XL, Costello CE (1999) Direct Matrix-Assisted Laser Desorption/Ionization Mass Spectrometric Analysis of Glycosphingolipids on Thin Layer Chromatographic Plates and Transfer Membranes. Rapid Commun Mass Spectrom 13:1838–1849. doi:10.1002/(SICI)1097-0231(19990930)13:18<1838::AID-RCM726>3.0.CO;2-9

138. McCrery DA, Ledford EB Jr, Gross ML (1982) Laser Desorption Fourier Transform Mass Spectrometry. Anal Chem 54:1435–1437. doi:10.1021/ac00245a040
139. Claereboudt J, Claeys M, Geise H, Gijbels R, Vertes A (1993) Laser Microprobe Mass Spectrometry of Quaternary Phosphonium Salts: Direct Versus Matrix-Assisted Laser Desorption. J Am Soc Mass Spectrom 4:798–812. doi:10.1016/1044-0305(93)80038-Z
140. Gromer S, Gross JH (2002) Methylseleninate Is a Substrate Rather Than an Inhibitor of Mammalian Thioredoxin Reductase: Implications for the Antitumor Effects of Selenium. J Biol Chem 277:9701–9706. doi:10.1074/jbc.M109234200
141. Wood TD, Van Cleef GW, Mearini MA, Coe JV, Marshall AG (1993) Formation of Giant Fullerene Gas-Phase Ions (C_{2n}^{+}, $n = 60$–500): Laser Desorption/Electron Ionization Fourier-Transform Ion Cyclotron Resonance Mass Spectrometric Evidence. Rapid Commun Mass Spectrom 7:304–311. doi:10.1002/rcm.1290070408
142. Beck RD, Weis P, Hirsch A, Lamparth I (1994) Laser Desorption Mass Spectrometry of Fullerene Derivatives: Laser-Induced Fragmentation and Coalescence Reactions. J Phys Chem 98:9683–9687. doi:10.1021/j100090a001
143. Wolkenstein K, Gross JH, Oeser T, Schöler HF (2002) Spectroscopic Characterization and Crystal Structure of the 1,2,3,4,5,6-Hexahydrophenanthro[1,10,9,8-*opqra*]Perylene. Tetrahedron Lett 43:1653–1655. doi:10.1016/S0040-4039(02)00085-0
144. Grim DM, Siegel J, Allison J (2002) Does Ink Age Inside of a Pen Cartridge? J Forensic Sci 47:1294–1297. doi:10.1520/JFS15563J
145. Jones RM, Lamb JH, Lim CK (1995) Urinary Porphyrin Profiles by Laser Desorption/Ionization Time-of-Flight Mass Spectrometry Without the Use of Classical Matrixes. Rapid Commun Mass Spectrom 9:921–923. doi:10.1002/rcm.1290091011
146. Krätschmer W, Lamb LD, Fostiropoulos K, Huffman DR (1990) Solid C_{60}: A New Form of Carbon. Nature 347:354–358. doi:10.1038/347354a0
147. Kroto H (1997) Symmetry, Space, Stars and C_{60}. Rev Mod Phys 69:703–722. doi:10.1103/RevModPhys.69.703
148. Gross JH (2009) Mass Spectrometry. In: Andrews DL (ed) Encyclopedia of Applied Spectroscopy. Wiley-VCH, Weinheim
149. Chapman JR (ed) (2000) Mass Spectrometry of Proteins and Peptides. Humana Press, Totowa
150. Snyder AP (2000) Interpreting Protein Mass Spectra. Oxford University Press, New York
151. Pasch H, Schrepp W (2003) MALDI-TOF Mass Spectrometry of Synthetic Polymers. Springer, Heidelberg
152. Barner-Kowollik C, Gruendling T, Falkenhagen J, Weidner S (eds) (2012) Mass Spectrometry in Polymer Chemistry. Wiley-VCH, Weinheim
153. Angeletti R, Gioacchini AM, Seraglia R, Piro R, Traldi P (1998) The Potential of Matrix-Assisted Laser Desorption/Ionization Mass Spectrometry in the Quality Control of Water Buffalo Mozzarella Cheese. J Mass Spectrom 33:525–531. doi:10.1002/(SICI)1096-9888(199806)33:6<525::AID-JMS655>3.0.CO;2-S
154. Fanton C, Delogu G, Maccioni E, Podda G, Seraglia R, Traldi P (1998) Matrix-Assisted Laser Desorption/Ionization Mass Spectrometry in the Dairy Industry 2. The Protein Fingerprint of Ewe Cheese and Its Application to Detection of Adulteration by Bovine Milk. Rapid Commun Mass Spectrom 12:1569–1573. doi:10.1002/(SICI)1097-0231(19981030)12:20<1569::AID-RCM341>3.0.CO;2-F
155. Krishnamurthy T, Ross PL, Rajamani U (1996) Detection of Pathogenic and Non-Pathogenic Bacteria by Matrix-Assisted Laser Desorption/Ionization Time-of-Flight Mass Spectrometry. Rapid Commun Mass Spectrom 10:883–888. doi:10.1002/(SICI)1097-0231(19960610)10:8<883::AID-RCM594>3.0.CO;2-V
156. Egert M, Spaeth K, Weik K, Kunzelmann H, Horn C, Kohl M, Blessing F (2015) Bacteria on Smartphone Touchscreens in a German University Setting and Evaluation of Two Popular Cleaning Methods Using Commercially Available Cleaning Products. Folia Microbiol 60:159–164. doi:10.1007/s12223-014-0350-2

157. Avila CC, Almeida FG, Palmisano G (2016) Direct Identification of Trypanosomatids by Matrix-Assisted Laser Desorption Ionization–Time-of-Flight Mass Spectrometry (DIT MALDI-TOF MS). J Mass Spectrom 51:549–557. doi:10.1002/jms.3763
158. Mestas J, Quias T, Dien Bard J (2016) Direct Identification of Aerobic Bacteria by Matrix-Assisted Laser Desorption Ionization Time-of-Flight Mass Spectrometry Is Accurate and Robust. J Clin Lab Anal 30:543–551. doi:10.1002/jcla.21900
159. Bohme K, Fernandez-No IC, Barros-Velazquez J, Gallardo JM, Calo-Mata P, Canas B (2010) Species Differentiation of Seafood Spoilage and Pathogenic Gram-Negative Bacteria by MALDI-TOF Mass Fingerprinting. J Proteome Res 9:3169–3183. doi:10.1021/pr100047q
160. Gevaert K, Vandekerckhove J (2000) Protein Identification Methods in Proteomics. Electrophoresis 21:1145–1154. doi:10.1002/(SICI)1522-2683(20000401)21:6<1145::AID-ELPS1145>3.0.CO;2-Z
161. Peng J, Gygi SP (2001) Proteomics: The Move to Mixtures. J Mass Spectrom 36:1083–1096. doi:10.1002/jms.229
162. Aebersold R, Mann M (2003) Mass Spectrometry-Based Proteomics. Nature 422:198–207. doi:10.1038/nature01511
163. Reinders J, Lewandrowski U, Moebius J, Wagner Y, Sickmann A (2004) Challenges in Mass Spectrometry-Based Proteomics. Proteomics 4:3686–3703. doi:10.1002/pmic.200400869
164. Paizs B, Suhai S (2005) Fragmentation Pathways of Protonated Peptides. Mass Spectrom Rev 24:508–548. doi:10.1002/mas.20024
165. Khidekel N, Ficarro SB, Clark PM, Bryan MC, Swaney DL, Rexach JE, Sun YE, Coon JJ, Peters EC, Hsieh-Wilson LC (2007) Probing the Dynamics of *O*-GlcNAc Glycosylation in the Brain Using Quantitative Proteomics. Nature Chem Biol 3:339–348. doi:10.1038/nchembio881
166. Vestal M, Hayden K (2007) High Performance MALDI-TOF Mass Spectrometry for Proteomics. Int J Mass Spectrom 268:83–92. doi:10.1016/j.ijms.2007.06.21
167. Nesvizhskii AI, Vitek O, Aebersold R (2007) Analysis and Validation of Proteomic Data Generated by Tandem Mass Spectrometry. Nature Methods 4:787–797. doi:10.1038/nmeth1088
168. Paizs B, Van SM (2008) Editorial: Focus Issue on Peptide Fragmentation. J Am Soc Mass Spectrom 19:1717–1718. doi:10.1016/j.jasms.2008.10.009
169. Seidler J, Zinn N, Boehm ME, Lehmann WD (2010) De Novo Sequencing of Peptides by MS/MS. Proteomics 10:634–649. doi:10.1002/pmic.200900459
170. Henzel WJ, Watanabe C, Stults JT (2003) Protein Identification: The Origins of Peptide Mass Fingerprinting. J Am Soc Mass Spectrom 14:931–942. doi:10.1016/S1044-0305(03)00214-9
171. Bleiholder C, Osburn S, Williams TD, Suhai S, Van SM, Harrison AG, Paizs B (2008) Sequence-Scrambling Fragmentation Pathways of Protonated Peptides. J Am Chem Soc 130:17774–17789. doi:10.1021/ja805074d
172. Kinter M, Sherman NE (2000) Protein Sequencing and Identification Using Tandem Mass Spectrometry. Wiley, Chichester
173. Kaltashov IA, Eyles SJ (2005) Mass Spectrometry in Biophysics: Conformation and Dynamics of Biomolecules. John Wiley & Sons Inc., Hoboken
174. Roepstorff P (1984) Proposal for a Common Nomenclature for Sequence Ions in Mass Spectra of Peptides. Biomed Mass Spectrom 11:601. doi:10.1002/bms.1200111109
175. Biemann K (1988) Contributions of Mass Spectrometry to Peptide and Protein Structure. Biomed Environ Mass Spectrom 16:99–111. doi:10.1002/bms.1200160119
176. Yalcin T, Khouw C, Csizmadia IG, Peterson MR, Harrison AG (1995) Why Are b Ions Stable Species in Peptide Spectra? J Am Soc Mass Spectrom 6:1165–1174. doi:10.1016/1044-0305(95)00569-2
177. Yalcin T, Csizmadia IG, Peterson MR, Harrison AG (1996) The Structure and Fragmentation of B_n ($n >= 3$) Ions in Peptide Spectra. J Am Soc Mass Spectrom 7:233–242. doi:10.1016/1044-0305(95)00677-X

178. Harrison AG (2008) Peptide Sequence Scrambling Through Cyclization of B5 Ions. J Am Soc Mass Spectrom 19:1776–1780. doi:10.1016/j.jasms.2008.06.025
179. Harrison AG (2009) To b or Not to B: the Ongoing Saga of Peptide b Ions. Mass Spectrom Rev 28:640–654. doi:10.1002/mas.20228
180. Amadei GA, Cho CF, Lewis JD, Luyt LG (2010) A Fast, Reproducible and Low-Cost Method for Sequence Deconvolution of "on-Bead" Peptides via "on-Target" Maldi-TOF/TOF Mass Spectrometry. J Mass Spectrom 45:241–251. doi:10.1002/jms.1708
181. Harvey DJ (2003) Matrix-Assisted Laser Desorption/Ionization Mass Spectrometry of Carbohydrates and Glycoconjugates. Int J Mass Spectrom 226:1–35. doi:10.1016/S1387-3806(02)00968-5
182. Stahl B, Linos A, Karas M, Hillenkamp F, Steup M (1997) Analysis of Fructans from Higher Plants by Matrix-Assisted Laser Desorption/Ionization Mass Spectrometry. Anal Biochem 246:195–204. doi:10.1006/abio.1997.2011
183. Garrozzo D, Impallomeni G, Spina E, Sturiale L, Zanetti F (1995) Matrix-Assisted Laser Desorption/Ionization Mass Spectrometry of Polysaccharides. Rapid Commun Mass Spectrom 9:937–941. doi:10.1002/rcm.1290091014
184. Welham KJ, Domin MA, Johnson K, Jones L, Ashton DS (2000) Characterization of Fungal Spores by Laser Desorption/Ionization Time-of-Flight Mass Spectrometry. Rapid Commun Mass Spectrom 14:307–310. doi:10.1002/(SICI)1097-0231(20000315)14:5<307::AID-RCM823>3.0.CO;2-3
185. Harvey DJ, Naven TJP, Küster B, Bateman R, Green MR, Critchley G (1995) Comparison of Fragmentation Modes for the Structural Determination of Complex Oligosaccharides Ionized by Matrix-Assisted Laser Desorption/Ionization Mass Spectrometry. Rapid Commun Mass Spectrom 9:1556–1561. doi:10.1002/rcm.1290091517
186. Lin H, Hunter JM, Becker CL (1999) Laser Desorption of DNA Oligomers Larger than One Kilobase from Cooled 4-Nitrophenol. Rapid Commun Mass Spectrom 13:2335–2340. doi:10.1002/(SICI)1097-0231(19991215)13:23<2335::AID-RCM794>3.0.CO;2-1
187. Bartolini WP, Johnston MV (2000) Characterizing DNA Photo-Oxidation Reactions by High-Resolution Mass Measurements with Matrix-Assisted Laser Desorption/Ionization Time-of-Flight Mass Spectrometry. J Mass Spectrom 35:408–416. doi:10.1002/(SICI)1096-9888(200003)35:3<408::AID-JMS951>3.0.CO;2-0
188. Jackson AT, Yates HT, Scrivens JH, Critchley G, Brown J, Green MR, Bateman RH (1996) The Application of Matrix-Assisted Laser Desorption/Ionization Combined with Collision-Induced Dissociation to the Analysis of Synthetic Polymers. Rapid Commun Mass Spectrom 10:1668–1674. doi:10.1002/(SICI)1097-0231(199609)10:12<1459::AID-RCM630>3.0.CO;2-Q
189. Tang X, Dreifuss PA, Vertes A (1995) New Matrixes and Accelerating Voltage Effects in Matrix-Assisted Laser Desorption/Ionization of Synthetic Polymers. Rapid Commun Mass Spectrom 9:1141–1147. doi:10.1002/rcm.1290091212
190. Montaudo G, Montaudo MS, Puglisi C, Samperi F (1994) Self-Calibrating Property of Matrix-Assisted Laser Desorption/Ionization Time-of-Flight Spectra of Polymeric Materials. Rapid Commun Mass Spectrom 8:981–984. doi:10.1002/rcm.1290081215
191. Williams JB, Chapman TM, Hercules DM (2003) Matrix-Assisted Laser Desorption/Ionization Mass Spectrometry of Discrete Mass Poly(butylene glutarate) Oligomers. Anal Chem 75:3092–3100. doi:10.1021/ac030061q
192. Nielen MFW, Malucha S (1997) Characterization of Polydisperse Synthetic Polymers by Size-Exclusion Chromatography/Matrix-Assisted Laser Desorption/Ionization Time-of-Flight Mass Spectrometry. Rapid Commun Mass Spectrom 11:1194–1204. doi:10.1002/(SICI)1097-0231(199707)11:11<1194::AID-RCM935>3.0.CO;2-L
193. de Koster CG, Duursma MC, van Rooij GJ, Heeren RMA, Boon JJ (1995) Endgroup Analysis of Polyethylene Glycol Polymers by Matrix-Assisted Laser Desorption/Ionization Fourier-Transform Ion Cyclotron Resonance Mass Spectrometry. Rapid Commun Mass Spectrom 9:957–962. doi:10.1002/rcm.1290091018

194. Weidner S, Kühn G, Just U (1995) Characterization of Oligomers in Poly(Ethylene Terephthalate) by Matrix-Assisted Laser Desorption/Ionization Mass Spectrometry. Rapid Commun Mass Spectrom 9:697–702. doi:10.1002/rcm.1290090813
195. Montaudo MS (1999) Sequence Constraints in a Glycine-Lactic Acid Copolymer Determined by Matrix-Assisted Laser Desorption/Ionization Mass Spectrometry. Rapid Commun Mass Spectrom 13:639–644. doi:10.1002/(SICI)1097-0231(19990430)13:8<639::AID-RCM513>3.0.CO;2-J
196. Montaudo MS (2002) Mass Spectra of Copolymers. Mass Spectrom Rev 21:108–144. doi:10.1002/mas.10021
197. Murgasova R, Hercules DM (2003) Quantitative Characterization of a Polystyrene/Poly (α-methylstyrene) Blend by MALDI Mass Spectrometry and Size-Exclusion Chromatography. Anal Chem 75:3744–3750. doi:10.1021/ac020593r
198. Satoh T, Kubo A, Hazama H, Awazu K, Toyoda M (2014) Separation of Isobaric Compounds Using a Spiral Orbit Type Time-of-Flight Mass Spectrometer, MALDI-SpiralTOF. Mass Spectrom 3:S0027-1-S0027/5. doi:10.5702/massspectrometry.S0027
199. Grayson SM, Myers BK, Bengtsson J, Malkoch M (2014) Advantages of Monodisperse and Chemically Robust "SpheriCal" Polyester Dendrimers as a "Universal" MS Calibrant. J Am Soc Mass Spectrom 25:303–309. doi:10.1007/s13361-013-0777-8
200. Casey BK, Grayson SM (2015) Letter: The Potential of Amine-Containing Dendrimer Mass Standards for Internal Calibration of Peptides. Eur J Mass Spectrom 21:747–752. doi:10.1255/ejms.1394
201. Gross JH (2016) Improved Procedure for Dendrimer-Based Mass Calibration in Matrix-Assisted Laser Desorption/Ionization-Time-of-Flight-Mass Spectrometry. Anal Bioanal Chem 408:5945–5951. doi:10.1007/s00216-016-9714-6
202. Wei J, Buriak JM, Siuzdak G (1999) Desorption-Ionization Mass Spectrometry on Porous Silicon. Nature 399:243–246. doi:10.1038/20400
203. Go EP, Shen Z, Harris K, Siuzdak G (2003) Quantitative Analysis with Desorption/Ionization on Silicon Mass Spectrometry Using Electrospray Deposition. Anal Chem 75:5475–5479. doi:10.1021/ac034376h
204. Shen Z, Thomas JJ, Averbuj C, Broo KM, Engelhard M, Crowell JE, Finn MG, Siuzdak G (2001) Porous Silicon as a Versatile Platform for Laser Desorption/Ionization Mass Spectrometry. Anal Chem 73:612–619. doi:10.1021/ac000746f
205. Laiko VV, Taranenko NI, Berkout VD, Musselman BD, Doroshenko VM (2002) Atmospheric Pressure Laser Desorption/Ionization on Porous Silicon. Rapid Commun Mass Spectrom 16:1737–1742. doi:10.1002/rcm.781
206. Go EP, Prenni JE, Wei J, Jones A, Hall SC, Witkowska HE, Shen Z, Siuzdak G (2003) Desorption/Ionization on Silicon Time-of-Flight/Time-of-Flight Mass Spectrometry. Anal Chem 75:2504–2506. doi:10.1021/ac026253n
207. Kang MJ, Pyun JC, Lee JC, Choi YJ, Park JH, Park JG, Lee JG, Choi HJ (2005) Nanowire-Assisted Laser Desorption and Ionization Mass Spectrometry for Quantitative Analysis of Small Molecules. Rapid Commun Mass Spectrom 19:3166–3170. doi:10.1002/rcm.2187
208. Go EP, Apon JV, Luo G, Saghatelian A, Daniels RH, Sahi V, Dubrow R, Cravatt BF, Vertes A, Siuzdak G (2005) Desorption/Ionization on Silicon Nanowires. Anal Chem 77:1641–1646. doi:10.1021/ac048460o
209. Vidova V, Novak P, Strohalm M, Pol J, Havlicek V, Volny M (2010) Laser Desorption-Ionization of Lipid Transfers: Tissue Mass Spectrometry Imaging Without MALDI Matrix. Anal Chem 82:4994–4997. doi:10.1021/ac100661h
210. Shenar N, Cantel S, Martinez J, Enjalbal C (2009) Comparison of Inert Supports in Laser Desorption/Ionization Mass Spectrometry of Peptides: Pencil Lead, Porous Silica Gel, DIOS-Chip and NALDI Target. Rapid Commun Mass Spectrom 23:2371–2379. doi:10.1002/rcm.4158
211. Hashir MA, Stecher G, Bakry R, Kasemsook S, Blassnig B, Feuerstein I, Abel G, Popp M, Bobleter O, Bonn GK (2007) Identification of Carbohydrates by Matrix-Free Material-

Enhanced Laser Desorption/Ionisation Mass Spectrometry. Rapid Commun Mass Spectrom 21:2759–2769. doi:10.1002/rcm.3147

212. Rainer M, Muhammad NNH, Huck CW, Feuerstein I, Bakry R, Huber LA, Gjerde DT, Zou X, Qian H, Du X, Fang WG, Ke Y, Bonn GK (2006) Ultra-Fast Mass Fingerprinting by High-Affinity Capture of Peptides and Proteins on Derivatized Poly(Glycidyl Methacrylate/Divinylbenzene) for the Analysis of Serum and Cell Lysates. Rapid Commun Mass Spectrom 20:2954–2960. doi:10.1002/rcm.2673
213. Feuerstein I, Najam-ul-Haq M, Rainer M, Trojer L, Bakry R, Aprilita NH, Stecher G, Huck CW, Bonn GK, Klocker H, Bartsch G, Guttman A (2006) Material-Enhanced Laser Desorption/Ionization (MELDI)-A New Protein Profiling Tool Utilizing Specific Carrier Materials for Time-of-Flight Mass Spectrometric Analysis. J Am Soc Mass Spectrom 17:1203–1208. doi:10.1016/j.jasms.2006.04.032
214. Caprioli RM, Farmer TB, Gile J (1997) Molecular Imaging of Biological Samples: Localization of Peptides and Proteins Using MALDI-TOF MS. Anal Chem 69:4751–4760. doi:10.1021/ac970888i
215. Cornett DS, Reyzer ML, Chaurand P, Caprioli RM (2007) MALDI Imaging Mass Spectrometry: Molecular Snapshots of Biochemical Systems. Nat Methods 4:828–833. doi:10.1038/nmeth1094
216. Chaurand P, Schriver KE, Caprioli RM (2007) Instrument Design and Characterization for High Resolution MALDI-MS Imaging of Tissue Sections. J Mass Spectrom 42:476–489. doi:10.1002/jms.1180
217. Franck J, Arafah K, Elayed M, Bonnel D, Vergara D, Jacquet A, Vinatier D, Wisztorski M, Day R, Fournier I, Salzet M (2009) MALDI Imaging Mass Spectrometry: State of the Art Technology in Clinical Proteomics. Mol Cell Proteom 8:2023–2033. doi:10.1074/mcp.R800016-MCP200
218. Francese S, Dani FR, Traldi P, Mastrobuoni G, Pieraccini G, Moneti G (2009) MALDI Mass Spectrometry Imaging, from Its Origins Up to Today: The State of the Art. Comb Chem High Throughput Screening 12:156–174. doi:10.2174/138620709787315454
219. Ramanathan R (ed) (2009) Mass Spectrometry in Drug Metabolism and Pharmacokinetics. John Wiley & Sons, Inc., Hoboken
220. Todd PJ, Schaaff TG, Chaurand P, Caprioli RM (2001) Organic Ion Imaging of Biological Tissue with Secondary Ion Mass Spectrometry and Matrix-Assisted Laser Desorption/Ionization. J Mass Spectrom 36:355–369. doi:10.1002/jms.153
221. Sugiura Y, Shimma S, Setou M (2006) Two-Step Matrix Application Technique to Improve Ionization Efficiency for Matrix-Assisted Laser Desorption/Ionization in Imaging Mass Spectrometry. Anal Chem 78:8227–8235. doi:10.1021/ac060974v
222. Guenther S, Koestler M, Schulz O, Spengler B (2010) Laser Spot Size and Laser Power Dependence of Ion Formation in High Resolution MALDI Imaging. Int J Mass Spectrom 294:7–15. doi:10.1016/j.ijms.2010.03.014
223. Kompauer M, Heiles S, Spengler B (2017) Atmospheric Pressure MALDI Mass Spectrometry Imaging of Tissues and Cells at 1.4-μm Lateral Resolution. Nat Methods 14:90–96. doi:10.1038/nmeth.4071
224. Ogrinc Potocnik N, Porta T, Becker M, Heeren RMA, Ellis SR (2015) Use of Advantageous, Volatile Matrices Enabled by Next-Generation High-Speed Matrix-Assisted Laser Desorption/Ionization Time-of-Flight Imaging Employing a Scanning Laser Beam. Rapid Commun Mass Spectrom 29:2195–2203. doi:10.1002/rcm.7379
225. Spengler B (2015) Mass Spectrometry Imaging of Biomolecular Information. Anal Chem 87:64–82. doi:10.1021/ac504543v
226. Grey AC (2016) MALDI Imaging of the Eye: Mapping Lipid, Protein and Metabolite Distributions in Aging and Ocular Disease. Int J Mass Spectrom 401:31–38. doi:10.1016/j.ijms.2016.02.017
227. Heyman HM, Dubery IA (2016) The Potential of Mass Spectrometry Imaging in Plant Metabolomics: A Review. Phytochemistry Reviews 15:297–316. doi:10.1007/s11101-015-9416-2

228. Ferguson L, Bradshaw R, Wolstenholme R, Clench M, Francese S (2011) Two-Step Matrix Application for the Enhancement and Imaging of Latent Fingermarks. Anal Chem 83:5585–5591. doi:10.1021/ac200619f
229. Bradshaw R, Denison N, Francese S (2016) Development of Operational Protocols for the Analysis of Primary and Secondary Fingermark Lifts by MALDI-MS Imaging. Anal Methods 8:6795–6804. doi:10.1039/c6ay01406b
230. Emerson B, Gidden J, Lay JO Jr, Durham B (2011) Laser Desorption/Ionization Time-of-Flight Mass Spectrometry of Triacylglycerols and Other Components in Fingermark Samples. J Forensic Sci 56:381–389. doi:10.1111/j.1556-4029.2010.01655.x
231. Deininger L, Patel E, Clench MR, Sears V, Sammon C, Francese S (2016) Proteomics Goes Forensic: Detection and Mapping of Blood Signatures in Fingermarks. Proteomics 16:1707–1717. doi:10.1002/pmic.201500544
232. Groeneveld G, de Puit M, Bleay S, Bradshaw R, Francese S (2015) Detection and Mapping of Illicit Drugs and Their Metabolites in Fingermarks by MALDI MS and Compatibility with Forensic Techniques. Scientific Reports 5:11716. doi:10.1038/srep11716
233. Laiko VV, Baldwin MA, Burlingame AL (2000) Atmospheric Pressure Matrix-Assisted Laser Desorption/Ionization Mass Spectrometry. Anal Chem 72:652–657. doi:10.1021/ac990998k
234. Laiko VV, Moyer SC, Cotter RJ (2000) Atmospheric Pressure MALDI/Ion Trap Mass Spectrometry. Anal Chem 72:5239–5243. doi:10.1021/ac000530d
235. Moyer SC, Marzilli LA, Woods AS, Laiko VV, Doroshenko VM, Cotter RJ (2003) Atmospheric Pressure Matrix-Assisted Laser Desorption/Ionization (AP MALDI) on a Quadrupole Ion Trap Mass Spectrometer. Int J Mass Spectrom 226:133–150. doi:10.1016/S1387-3806(02)00972-7
236. Doroshenko VM, Laiko VV, Taranenko NI, Berkout VD, Lee HS (2002) Recent Developments in Atmospheric Pressure MALDI Mass Spectrometry. Int J Mass Spectrom 221:39–58. doi:10.1016/S1387-3806(02)00893-X
237. Moskovets E, Misharin A, Laiko V, Doroshenko V (2016) A Comparative Study on the Analytical Utility of Atmospheric and Low-Pressure MALDI Sources for the Mass Spectrometric Characterization of Peptides. Methods 104:21–32. doi:10.1016/j.ymeth.2016.02.009
238. Krutchinsky AN, Loboda AV, Spicer VL, Dworschak R, Ens W, Standing KG (1998) Orthogonal Injection of Matrix-Assisted Laser Desorption/Ionization Ions into a Time-of-Flight Spectrometer Through a Collisional Damping Interface. Rapid Commun Mass Spectrom 12:508–518. doi:10.1002/(SICI)1097-0231(19980515)12:9<508::AID-RCM197>3.0.CO;2-L
239. McIver RT Jr, Li Y, Hunter RL (1994) Matrix-Assisted Laser Desorption/Ionization with an External Ion Source Fourier-Transform Mass Spectrometer. Rapid Commun Mass Spectrom 8:237–241. doi:10.1002/rcm.1290080303
240. Li Y, McIver RT Jr, Hunter RL (1994) High-Accuracy Molecular Mass Determination for Peptides and Proteins by Fourier Transform Mass Spectrometry. Anal Chem 66:2077–2083. doi:10.1021/ac00085a024
241. Li Y, Tang K, Little DP, Koester H, McIver RT Jr (1996) High-Resolution MALDI Fourier Transform Mass Spectrometry of Oligonucleotides. Anal Chem 68:2090–2096. doi:10.1021/ac9601268
242. Baykut G, Jertz R, Witt M (2000) Matrix-Assisted Laser Desorption/Ionization Fourier Transform Ion Cyclotron Resonance Mass Spectrometry with Pulsed In-Source Collision Gas and In-Source Ion Accumulation. Rapid Commun Mass Spectrom 14:1238–1247. doi:10.1002/1097-0231(20000730)14:14<1238::AID-RCM17>3.0.CO;2-H
243. O'Connor PB, Costello CE (2001) A High Pressure Matrix-Assisted Laser Desorption/Ionization Fourier Transform Mass Spectrometry Ion Source for Thermal Stabilization of Labile Biomolecules. Rapid Commun Mass Spectrom 15:1862–1868. doi:10.1002/rcm.447

Electrospray Ionization 12

Learning Objectives

- Electrospray – a method of ion formation at atmospheric pressure
- Interfacing atmospheric pressure ionization to analyzer high vacuum
- Spraying of electrolytic solutions by action of an electrostatic field
- Processes of ion liberation from electrolytic solutions
- Formation of multiply charged ions and charge deconvolution
- Small molecules analysis by electrospray ionization
- High-mass and high-polarity capabilities of electrospray ionization

Electrospray ionization (ESI) is the most prominent technique among the group of *atmospheric pressure ionization* (API) methods, some of which have already been discussed in the context of chemical ionization at atmospheric pressure (APCI, Sects. 7.8 and 7.9). ESI is the method of choice for *liquid chromatography-mass spectrometry coupling* (LC-MS, Chap. 14) [1–4]. In fact, ESI and *matrix-assisted laser desorption/ionization* (MALDI, Chap. 11) have provided the means for expanding the application of MS into the fields of biology and the biomedical sciences, and currently, they are the most frequently employed ionization methods in MS [1, 2, 4–11].

ESI "is a soft ionization technique that accomplishes the transfer of ions from solution to the gas phase. The technique is extremely useful for the analysis of large, non-volatile, chargeable molecules such as proteins and nucleic acid polymers" [10–15]. In contrast to *fast atom bombardment* (FAB, Chap. 10), in ESI the solution is composed of a volatile solvent containing the ionic analyte at very low concentration, typically 10^{-6}–10^{-4} M. In addition, the transfer of ions from the condensed phase into the state of isolated gas-phase ions starts at atmospheric pressure and

J.H. Gross, *Mass Spectrometry*, DOI 10.1007/978-3-319-54398-7_12

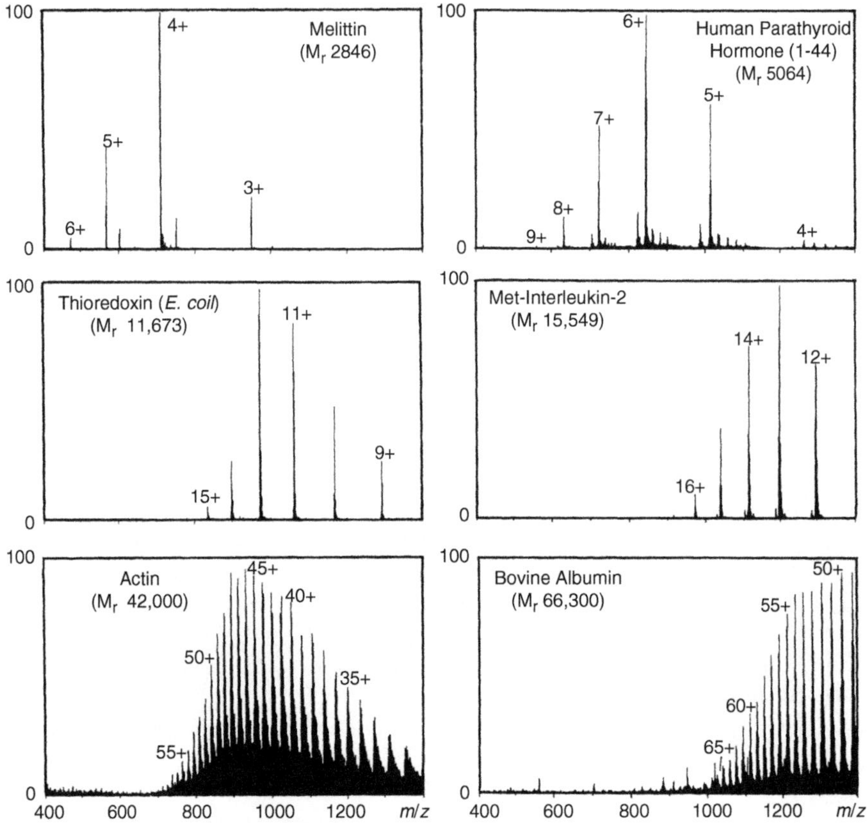

Fig. 12.1 Relationship between the mass of peptides and proteins and the number of ionic charges under ESI conditions (Adapted from Ref. [18] by permission. © American Chemical Society, 1990)

incrementally proceeds into the high vacuum of the mass analyzer [6, 16–18]. This results in a marked softness of ionization and makes ESI the "wings for molecular elephants" [19]. Another reason for the extraordinary high-mass capability of ESI [15, 20, 21] is founded in the characteristic formation of multiply charged ions in case of high-mass analytes [15, 18, 22]. Multiple charging also folds up the *m*/*z* scale by the number of charges, and thus, shifts the ions into an *m*/*z* range accessible by most mass analyzers (Fig. 12.1 and Sect. 3.8)

ESI serves equally well for small polar molecules, ionic metal complexes [23–25], and other soluble inorganic analytes [26]. So let's start exploring the ESI route with this promising outlook in mind.

Beyond the usual *m/z*: Most high-mass analytes examined by ESI readily form multiply charged ions. Normally, it is therefore sufficient in ESI-MS to cover the range up to *m/z* 3000 for the detection of ions. This does not preclude, however, that ESI can produce ions of much higher *m/z* [27, 28]; even ions at *m/z* 85,000 have been observed [29].

12.1 Route Leading to Electrospray Ionization

ESI in its current state-of-the-art has not resulted from a straightforward development. It has many predecessors, some of which having been successful at their time, while others were rather short-lived methods replaced as soon as more sensitive or more robust techniques appeared [30]. Nonetheless, the development of all those techniques aimed at both the direct coupling of liquid chromatography to mass spectrometry and the access to highly polar or even ionic analytes.

Following this historical sketch of milestones along the way to ESI, the below sections will emphasize the construction of ESI interfaces, the process of electrospray as such, and the pathways of ion liberation from the liquid phase into the state of isolated gas phase ions.

12.1.1 Atmospheric Pressure Ionization and Related Methods

The first technique, *atmospheric pressure ionization* (API), was presented as early as 1973 by the Horning group [31]. Just 1 year later, the same group introduced a largely improved variant as *atmospheric pressure chemical ionization* (APCI) [32]. In 2000, *atmospheric pressure photoionization* (APPI) was developed to expand the range of applications to analytes of lower polarity [33]. As API, APCI, and APPI essentially rely on chemical ionization processes, these were already discussed in Sects. 7.8 and 7.9. Both techniques, APCI and APPI, are frequently employed. Nowadays, *atmospheric pressure ionization* has been transformed into a collective term for all techniques where ion generation occurs at atmospheric pressure.

12.1.2 Thermospray

In *Thermospray* (TSP) [34–36] a solution of the analyte and a volatile buffer, usually 0.1 M ammonium acetate, is evaporated from a heated capillary at a liquid flow of 1–2 ml min^{-1} into a heated chamber (>600 °C), hence the term. As the solvent evaporates, the analyte starts to form adducts with ions from the buffer salt. While most of the neutrals are removed by a vacuum pump, the ions are extracted orthogonally from their main axis of motion by use of an electrostatic potential. The

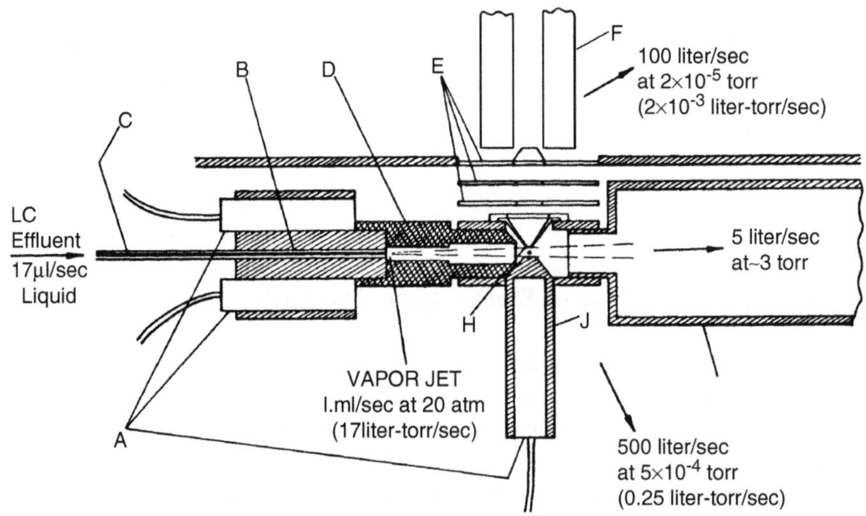

Fig. 12.2 Thermospray interface. *A* cartridge heater; *B* copper block brazed to stainless steel capillary; *C* capillary; *D* copper tube; *E* ion lenses; *F* quadrupole mass analyzer; *G* line to rotary vane pump; *H* ion exit aperture; *J* source heater (Reproduced from Ref. [35] by permission. © American Chemical Society, 1983)

ions are transferred into a quadrupole mass analyzer through a pinhole of about 25 μm in diameter (Fig. 12.2). A quadrupole is employed due to its tolerance to poor vacuum conditions.

As the pure TSP mode only works with high-polarity solvents in the presence of a buffer salt, modified modes of operation were developed to expand the use of TSP ion sources to lower-polarity systems. One approach used an electrical discharge in the vapor phase [37], while another operated an electron-emitting filament in the expanding gas cloud. Either addition essentially emulated APCI on the TSP interface. With this added versatility, TSP meant a breakthrough for LC-MS [38]. Nonetheless, with the advent of ESI, TSP interfaces vanished rather quickly from the laboratories.

Only halfway API: Strictly speaking, thermospray is not really an API method because the analyte solution is sprayed into a rough vacuum of several hundred Pa instead of spraying at full atmospheric pressure.

12.1.3 Electrohydrodynamic Ionization

An electrolytic solution of sufficiently low volatility can be transferred into the vacuum without sudden evaporation and then be sprayed from a fine capillary by the action of a strong electrostatic field. This is known as *electrohydrodynamic ionization* (EHI) [39, 40]. EHI results from the interaction of the field with the liquid meniscus at the end of the capillary tube [41, 42]. A mist of micrometer-sized electrically charged droplets expands into the vacuum at supersonic speed. The droplets shrink upon evaporation of solvent. Shrinking causes the charge density on their surface to exceed the *Rayleigh limit* of stability [43], i.e., the surface tension is overcome by electrostatic repulsion. The electric forces then tear the droplets apart. The sequence of droplet shrinking and subsequent disintegration into smaller subunits occurs repeatedly and eventually leads to the formation of isolated gas-phase ions.

Even though EHI ion sources are at hand by simply replacing the field emitter of a field desorption (FD) source with a capillary tube (Sect. 8.3) [44, 45], EHI never managed to become established in organic mass spectrometry. This is most probably due to its limitation to low-volatile solvents. Nonetheless, EHI has been applied to analyze polymers [46] and is still used to generate primary ions in massive cluster impact (MCI) mass spectrometry (Sect. 10.8).

EHI has important features in common with ESI:

- An electrolytic solution is sprayed by the mere action of an electrostatic field.
- Spraying forms a mist of electrically highly charged droplets.
- Analyte ions are liberated from solution phase into the gas phase.
- Analyte ions thus have already to exist before spraying of the solution.

12.1.4 Electrospray Ionization

The conceptual development of electrospray ionization by the Dole group [47] actually preceded API, TSP, and EHI by several years [48]. The underlying principle of ESI, which it shares with EHI, even dates back to work by Zeleny in 1917 [41] and Taylor in 1964 [42].

In ESI, similar to EHI, a mist of micrometer-sized electrically charged droplets is generated. The repetitive shrinking and droplet disintegration are also observed under ESI conditions. In contrast to EHI, the process of electrostatic spraying is sustained at atmospheric pressure. The electrostatically charged aerosol is then continuously passed into the mass analyzer by means of a differentially pumped interface. The limitation of Dole's experiments was that the ions of the electrosprayed high-molecular-weight polystyrene used by his group could not be detected with his mass spectrometers [47–49]. It took years of work for the Fenn group and lasted until the late 1980s to fully realize that analytes of 100–2000 u molecular weight can be readily analyzed with a quadrupole attached to a properly constructed ESI interface [16, 19, 50]. To avoid freezing of the aerosol droplets under the conditions of adiabatic expansion on their transition from the atmosphere into the vacuum, sufficient energy supply turned out to be crucial. The heat may either be delivered by a heated countercurrent gas stream or by a heated capillary being part of the interface. Until today, all ESI sources make use of the one or the other way of heating the aerosol. The fact that ESI can be run with almost any standard solvent is another key to its tremendous success [19].

Open to the atmosphere: Any atmospheric pressure ionization method, i.e., ESI as well as APCI and APPI, requires an uninterrupted transport of ions from ambient pressure into the high vacuum of a mass analyzer. An API interface has thus to accomplish the efficient transfer of ions while at the same time it has to remove the concomitant gas flow to preserve the analyzer vacuum. This is accomplished by means of differential pumping.

12.2 Interfaces for Electrospray Ionization

12.2.1 Basic Design Considerations

The first electrospray-mass spectrometry interface was designed by the Fenn group in the mid 1980s [16, 50–52]. In this interface, the dilute sample solution is supplied by a syringe pump through a hypodermic needle – the *spray capillary* – at a flow of 5–20 μl min^{-1}. The spray capillary is kept at a potential of 3–4 kV relative to a surrounding cylindrical electrode (Fig. 12.3). Then, the electrosprayed aerosol expands into a countercurrent stream of hot nitrogen gas serving as a heat supply for vaporization of the solvent. A small portion of the sprayed material enters the aperture of a short capillary (0.2 mm inner diameter, 60 mm length) interfacing the atmospheric pressure spray zone to the first pumping stage ($\approx 10^2$ Pa) that is entered by the gas in a free jet expansion. Most of the gas expanding from the desolvating aerosol is pumped off by a rotary vane pump as it exits from the capillary. A minor portion passes through the orifice of a skimmer (a cone-shaped electrode with a small aperture at its apex) into the high vacuum behind ($\approx 10^{-3}$–10^{-4} Pa). At this stage, desolvation of the ions is completed, while the ions are focused into a mass analyzer. Suitable potentials applied to capillary, skimmer, and lenses behind

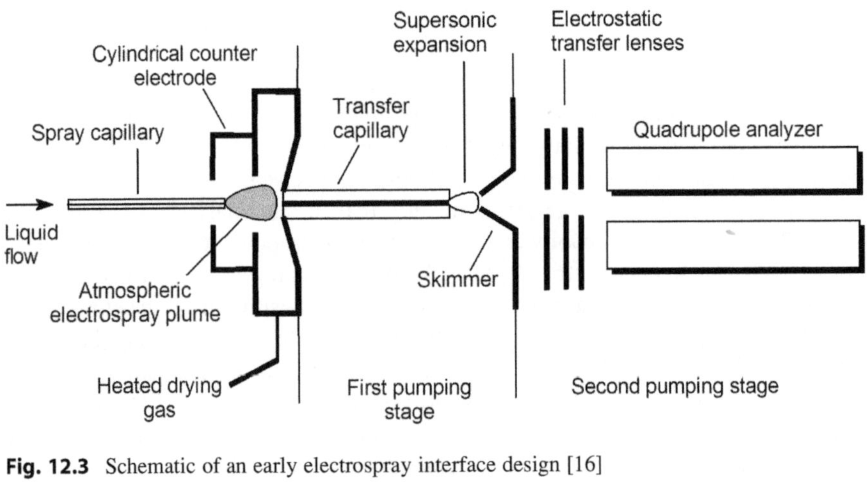

Fig. 12.3 Schematic of an early electrospray interface design [16]

provide an effective transfer of ions through the interface, while the neutral gas is not affected and exits via the vacuum system.

Modern *ESI interfaces* are designed in many variations of this basic scheme [53, 54]. They may either use a *heated transfer capillary* or a *countercurrent stream of hot nitrogen* (sometimes called *curtain gas*) to enforce solvent evaporation [55]. These differences can affect a system's robustness and the degree of cluster ion formation with a particular ESI interface [56, 57]. Whatever the details, they are all derived from a *nozzle-skimmer system* initially proposed by Kantrowitz and Grey [58] that delivers an intense cool molecular jet into the high vacuum environment [47, 50, 59].

The adiabatic expansion of the gas upon entering the first pumping stage reduces random motion of the particles due to extensive cooling. Furthermore, a portion of the thermal motion is converted into directed flow by the nozzle-skimmer arrangement. In summary, this causes the heavier analyte ion-containing solvent clusters to travel close to the center of the flight path through the interface, while light solvent molecules escape from the jet [48]. Thus, the skimmer orifice is not just statistically passed by all sorts of particles but rather selectively by ionic constituents of the adiabatically expanding plume.

A comparison of API interface concepts – all of them in use today – is provided in Fig. 12.4 [60]. A closer discussion of the particular approaches will follow later in this chapter.

Ions already have to be there: ESI requires analyte ions to be present in the sample solution because ESI does not actively create ions. In fact, ESI is rather a method of ion transfer than a true ionization method. Thus, ESI is in stark contrast to all other ionization methods currently in use (EI, CI, APCI, APPI, FAB, FD, MALDI, DART). Therefore, *electrospray ionization* (ESI) is also simply referred to as *electrospray* (ES) and *ESI ion sources* may better be termed *ESI interfaces*.

12.2.2 Adaptation of ESI to Different Flow

The actual process of "electrospraying" disperses a liquid into an aerosol, which works best at flows of 1–20 μl min^{-1}. This sets certain limits to its use as an LC-MS interface in respect to solvent properties such as volatility and polarity. Consequently, a number of sprayer design modifications have led to an expansion of the range of ESI applications (Fig. 12.5).

The design of a *pneumatically assisted* ESI interface differs from the simple electrospray interface in that it provides a pneumatic assistance for the spray process. This is achieved by supplying a concentric flow of an inert gas such as nitrogen around the electrospray plume [61–63]. Assistance by a *nebulizer gas* stream of about 1–5 l min^{-1} allows for higher liquid flow and for a reduced influence of the surface tension of the solvent [64]. Pneumatically assisted ESI can

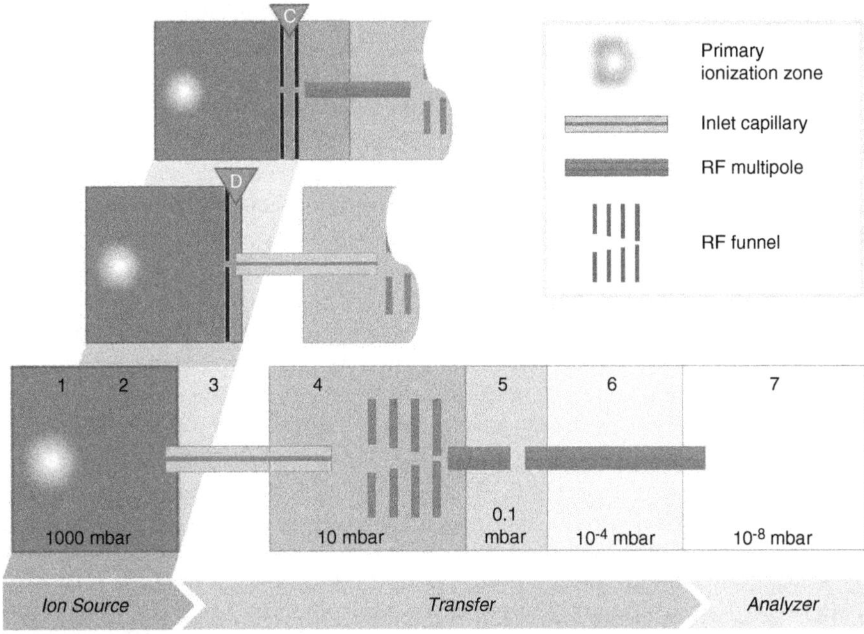

Fig. 12.4 Comparison of basic API interface designs and their functional regions: (*1*) Ion formation, (*2*) thermalization, (*3*) turbulent entry flow, (*4*) expansion into vacuum, (*5–6*) ion guides and eventually activation by CID, (*7*) mass analyzer. Indicated pressures may vary considerably. RF funnels and RF multipoles are not to scale and various voltages are normally applied to these ion optical elements. *Bottom:* ion source coupled via a capillary to the vacuum system of the analyzer, e.g., Thermo-Fisher. *Center*: same as previous but additional directed "dry" (*D*) gas flow through a biased sampling electrode, termed *spray shield* in instruments by Bruker Daltonics or Agilent Technologies. *Top*: ion source coupled via orifices to the vacuum system of the analyzer; additionally a curtain (*C*) gas flow is directed into the source, and a differential pumping stage (AB SCIEX) (Reproduced from Ref. [60] with permission. © Springer, 2014)

accommodate flows of 10–200 µl min^{-1}. In fact, all modern ESI interfaces are equipped with a nebulizer gas or *sheath gas* line enclosing the spray capillary. Thus, most routine ESI measurements are actually performed using pneumatically assisted ESI. In pneumatically assisted ESI the purpose of the high voltage is almost reduced to the mere supply of electric charging of the droplets. For highly polar solutions at very low liquid flow, nanoESI provides the better technique (next section).

For *capillary zone electrophoresis* (CZE) mass spectrometry coupling, another modification of an ESI sprayer has been developed. It uses a *sheath flow* or *make-up flow* of solvent for establishing the electrical contact at the CZE terminus, thus defining both the CZE and electrospray field gradients. The make-up flow also serves to adjust the low CZE flow to an ESI-compatible level.

This way, the composition of the electrosprayed liquid can be controlled independently of the CZE buffer, thereby enabling operation with buffers that could not

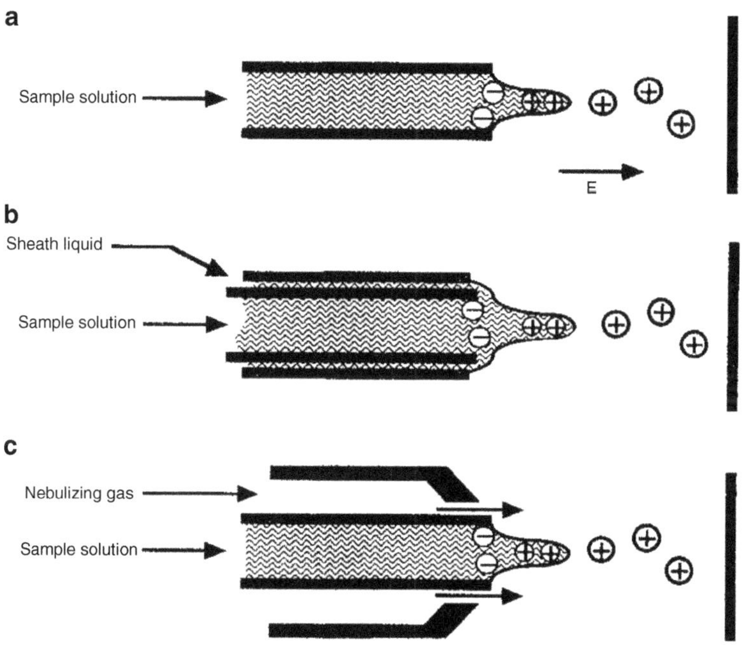

Fig. 12.5 Different sprayers for ESI. (**a**) Pure electrospray, (**b**) ESI with sheath liquid, (**c**) pneumatically-assisted ESI (Adapted from Ref. [6] (p. 109) by permission. © John Wiley & Sons, Inc., 1997)

be used previously, e.g., aqueous and high ionic strength buffers. In addition, the interface operation becomes independent of the CZE flow rate [65].

Ion spray? *Pneumatically assisted electrospray* is also termed *ion spray* (ISP). However, the term ISP is not recommended in place of pneumatically-assisted ESI because ISP represents a mere modification of the ESI setup and is a company-specific term [66].

12.2.3 Improved Electrospray Configurations

Since the publication of the original design in the 1980s by the Fenn group, the ESI interface underwent various substantial improvements in

- robustness of operation during elongated periods of unattended operation,
- ion transmission from the sprayer into the mass analyzer,
- softness for effective ion desolvation without inducing fragmentation, and
- effectiveness of differential pumping.

Nonetheless, whatever the actual design, all of those interfaces still have some basic characteristics in common:

- electrostatic spraying of an electrolytic solution at atmospheric pressure,
- heat supply for solvent evaporation and ion desolvation,
- supersonic expansion into the first pumping stage, and
- differential pumping across three or sometimes four stages.

While early interfaces were intuitively aligned along the central axis from the spray capillary to the analyzer entrance, more recent designs employ spraying at an angle to the vacuum entrance. These arrangements have the advantage of largely reducing possible contamination, especially by preventing the clogging of capillaries and skimmers, which formerly was one of the most severe problems with the otherwise easy-to-use ESI interfaces. When analytes are accompanied by nonvolatile impurities, e.g., by buffer salts used to improve liquid chromatography or organic material as present in blood or urine samples, the deposition of this material can cause the rapid breakdown of the ESI interface.

These improved designs achieve a spatial separation of the deposition site of nonvolatized material and the location of the ion entrance into the mass spectrometer. Such designs include (*i*) spraying *off-axis*, (*ii*) guiding the desolvating microdroplets through *inflected paths*, and (*iii*) spraying at an angle up to *orthogonal* (Fig. 12.6) [66]. It is a great advantage of orthogonal spraying that the entrance of the interface may selectively collect small and highly charged droplets that present the best source of analyte ions. Larger and less-charged droplets are not sufficiently attracted by the extraction field at 90° angle and therefore miss the orifice.

The first commercial ESI interface using about 90° deflection is the Waters *z-spray*™ interface (Fig. 12.7). All modern electrospray interfaces employ a closely related configuration. The entrance region of Bruker and Agilent API interfaces, for example, comprises a grounded spray capillary, a counter electrode at high voltage, and a countercurrent flow of hot nitrogen around the orifice of the ion transfer capillary that is aligned close to right angle with respect to the sprayer (Fig. 12.8). Modern interfaces are also designed with easy cleaning in mind.

12.2.4 Advanced Atmospheric Pressure Interface Designs

We have already briefly encountered some of the modern atmospheric pressure interfaces as front-ends of mass analyzers in the context of instrumentation (Chap. 4) and tandem MS (Chap. 9). The actual configuration of such interfaces largely depends on the high vacuum requirements of the mass analyzer attached, e.g., simple two-stage differential pumping is sufficient for linear quadrupoles and quadrupole ion traps, while others demand for virtual absence of residual gas. Furthermore, company-specific technologies will govern certain parts of the ion transfer optics such as RF-only ion guides (Figs. 12.4 and 12.9).

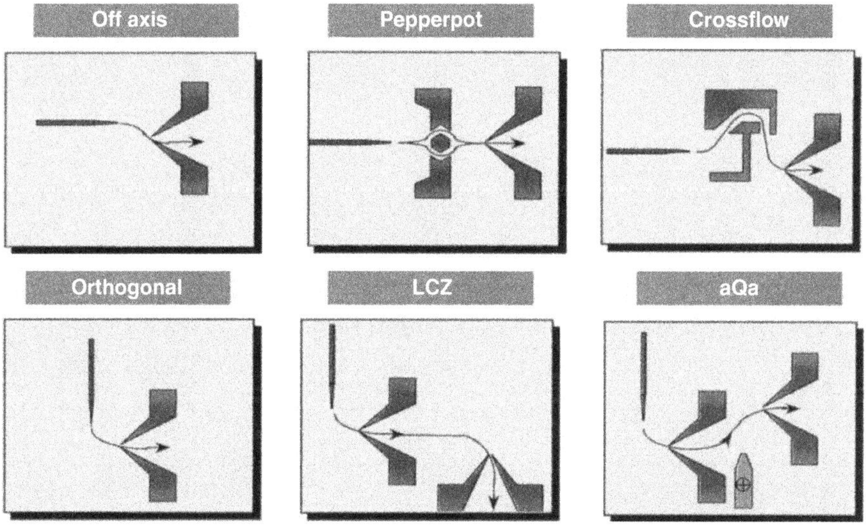

Fig. 12.6 Some strategies used in commercial API ion sources to increase solvent compatibility and system robustness. Some of these designs are (were) commercial brands: Pepperpot, Crossflow, and LCZ ("z-spray", Micromass); AQA (Thermo Finnigan) (Reproduced from Ref. [66] by permission. © John Wiley & Sons, 1999)

In recent years, so-called *ion funnels* are being used in place of the conventional skimmer cone electrode [67–69]. Ion funnels are radio frequency devices (≤1 MHz) composed of a stack of dozens of ring electrodes, typically spaced about 3 mm apart along the ion funnel axis, with a central aperture of increasingly smaller diameter, e.g., from 20 mm at the opening to 1 mm at the exit. An RF voltage of equal amplitude but opposite phase (200–400 V) is supplied between adjacent electrodes. Similar to stacked ring ion guides (Sect. 4.10) this alignment of electrodes creates a field that pushes ions down a low electric field gradient far more effectively than the field gradient alone could do. As the apertures decrease along the device the ion packages are not only transported but – more importantly – are also radially confined. This is employed to focus ion beams through narrow apertures into the next differential pumping stage or into a mass analyzer [70, 71]. As ion funnels are best operated under the conditions of collisionally damped ion motion, i.e., at rough vacuum of 1–10 mbar (Sect. 4.4.4), they are perfectly compatible with the first pumping stage of ESI interfaces. Ion funnels increase the transmission of ESI interfaces, and accordingly, result in at least tenfold-improved overall sensitivity of the mass spectrometer as compared to sources with a skimmer electrode.

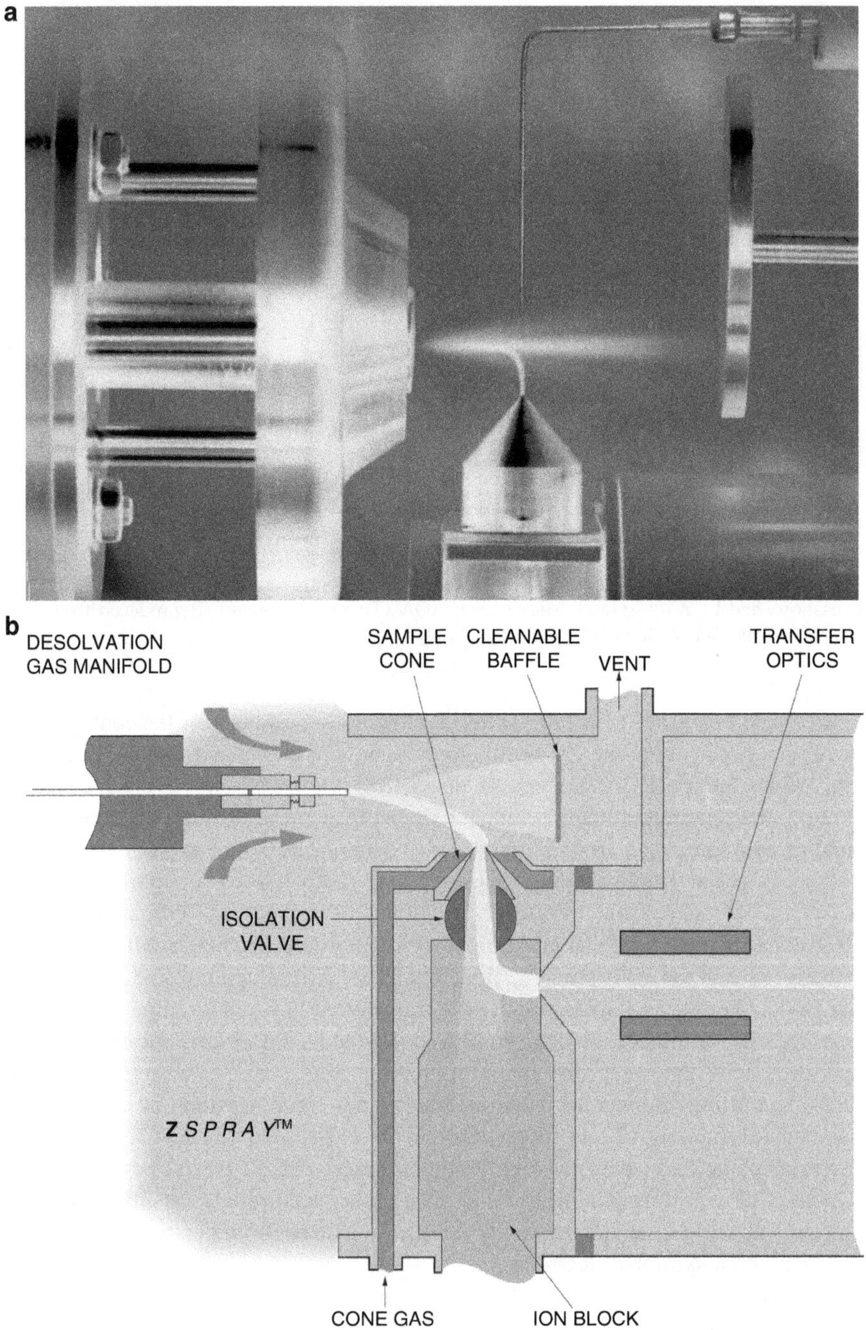

Fig. 12.7 Micromass *z*-spray interface. (**a**) Photograph of the actual spray from which charged constituents are extracted downwards into the entrance orifice. While large droplets and neutrals are traveling on a straight path toward the counter electrode, small highly charged droplets are attracted by the entrance at the cone-shaped electrode. (**b**) Schematic including the inner parts of the interface (By courtesy of Waters Corporation, MS Technologies, Manchester, UK)

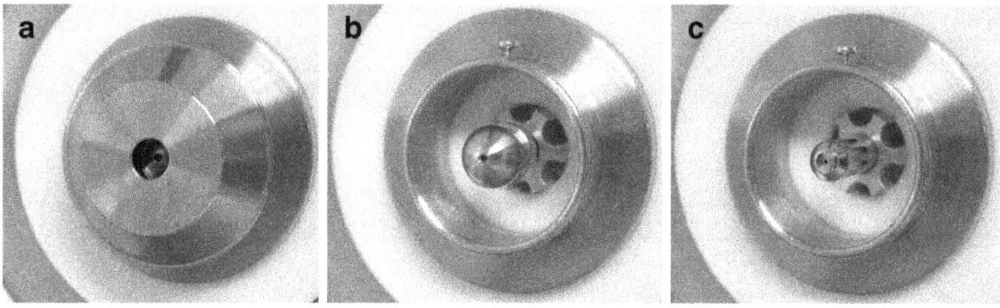

Fig. 12.8 Atmospheric pressure side of the Bruker Apollo II API interface. (**a**) Spray shield in place, (**b**) removal of the spray shield shows an aerodynamically shaped cap on top of the transfer capillary, and (**c**) metal-coated section of the glass transfer capillary. The hot desolvation gas is supplied via six concentrically aligned ports around the transfer capillary. In operation, the sprayer would be aligned close to the spray shield as to direct the aerosol from top to bottom in an orientation close to right angle with respect to the transfer capillary. For the interior layout of this interface cf. Fig. 12.12

Multi-purpose API interfaces: There are no dedicated ESI interfaces anymore. All interfaces are constructed to be compatible with any variant of atmospheric pressure ionization by simply swapping the front part, e.g., an ESI sprayer for an APCI unit. The interface from the orifice at atmospheric pressure to the entry of the mass analyzer at high vacuum remains untouched. This enables quick method switching, avoids down time by interrupted vacuum, and ensures constant levels of mass resolving power and mass accuracy.

Two-stage off-axis ion funnels The next level of achieving efficient ion collection, transfer across pumping stages, and focusing is achieved by two-stage ion funnels in an off-axis alignment. Again, this exploits the fact that ions may easily be guided along potential gradients while neutrals are not affected. Thus, ions can be pushed out of the stream to follow a different track while neutrals are directed into an exhaust pipe, e.g., as in the Waters StepWave interface (Fig. 12.10).

12.2.5 Nozzle-Skimmer Dissociation

The rough vacuum of the first pumping stage, formerly the short zone between nozzle and skimmer, of an atmospheric pressure interface does not only provide

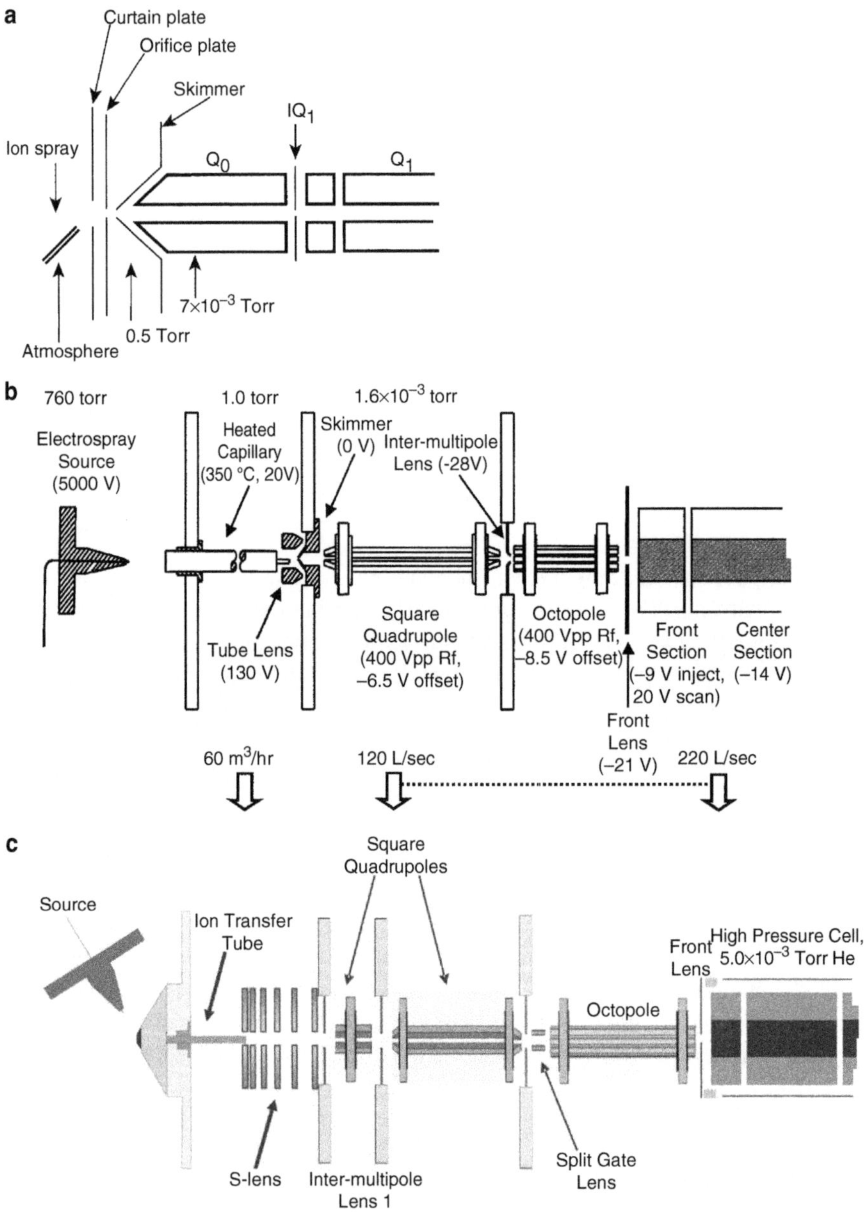

Fig. 12.9 Electrospray interfaces: (**a**) Setup for linear quadrupole and triple quadrupole instruments with 45° spray, heated countercurrent desolvation gas ("curtain gas"), orifice–skimmer setup for the first pumping stage, and RF-only quadrupole as ion guide in the second pumping stage. (**b**) On-axis spray on entrance of heated capillary serving as counter electrode, nozzle-skimmer arrangement, and RF-only multipole ion guides in front of an LIT. (**c**) Similar to (**b**) but the skimmer has been replaced by an ion-focusing lens system to improve transmission. This figure uses the front parts from Figs. 4.46, 4.50, and 9.28, respectively; reference to the according sources is given there

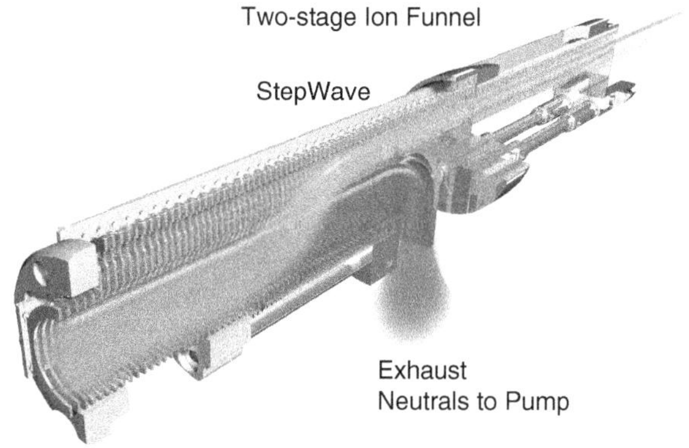

Fig. 12.10 Two-stage ion funnel with off-axis alignment for optimized transfer of ions (*orange cloud*) while neutral gas (*blue cloud*) is directed into an exhaust pipe. This particular setup is realized in the Waters StepWave interface (Adapted with permission of Waters MS Technologies, Manchester, 2016)

space for effective desolvation [72, 73], but can also be used to achieve fragmentation of the ions by *collision-induced dissociation* (CID, Sect. 9.3). While a comparatively high pressure in this region can effect collisional cooling (Sect. 4.4.4) rather than dissociative collisions [74], an increased voltage difference in this region enhances ion fragmentation by CID [72, 74, 75].

Nozzle-skimmer dissociation (NSD) or simply *skimmer CID* can

- strip off residual solvent molecules,
- achieve fragmentation of ions resulting in spectra similar to CI mode [76], and
- generate first-generation fragment ions for further tandem MS experiments.

The latter method provides a *pseudo MS*^{3} operation on triple quadrupole or Q-TOF mass spectrometers [77–79]. Real MS^3 would require mass-selection prior to the first CID stage, too (for an example of pseudo MS^3 using NSD cf. Sect. 12.5.1). A programmable CID routine delivers ESI mass spectra with a variable degree of fragmentation from a single run [75, 77, 78, 80].

Unwanted CID Even a moderate voltage drop between nozzle and skimmer can cause the elimination of weakly bonded substituents such as CO_2 in case of carbon dioxide-protected deprotonated *N*-heterocycles. In particular, $SnMe_3$-substituted anions such as 2-(trismethylstannyl)pyrrole-*N*-carbamate exhibit strong variations in the $[A–CO_2]^-/A^-$ ratio of up to a factor of 30 preventing the detection of A^- at slightly elevated voltages (Fig. 12.11) [81].

For NSD it is not required to have a true nozzle–skimmer arrangement. Instead, a potential drop of 20–100 V across a suitable pressure region of any ESI interface design suffices to induce this sort of CID. The Bruker Apollo II interface, for example, features a dual ion funnel setup with the first ion funnel in the rough vacuum of the supersonic expansion plume ($\approx$ 3–4 mbar) and the second ion funnel prior to an RF-only hexapole used to alternatively guide or accumulate ions. Here

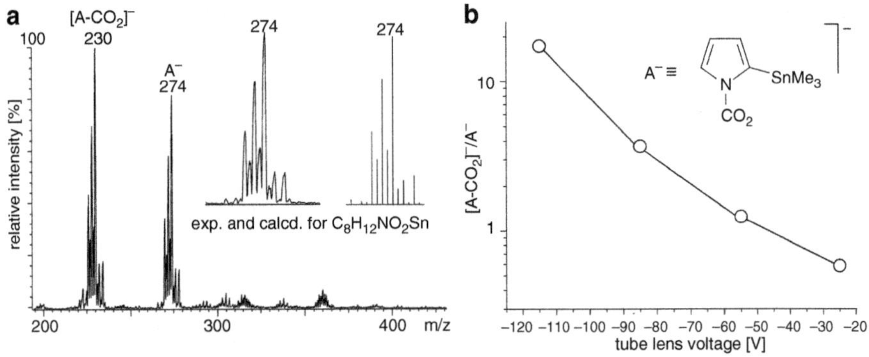

Fig. 12.11 (**a**) Partial negative-ion ESI spectrum of 2-(trismethylstannyl)pyrrole-*N*-carbamate (A^-) from tetrahydrofurane at low nozzle-skimmer voltage drop and (**b**) dependence of the $[A–CO_2]^-/A^-$ ratio variation on this voltage

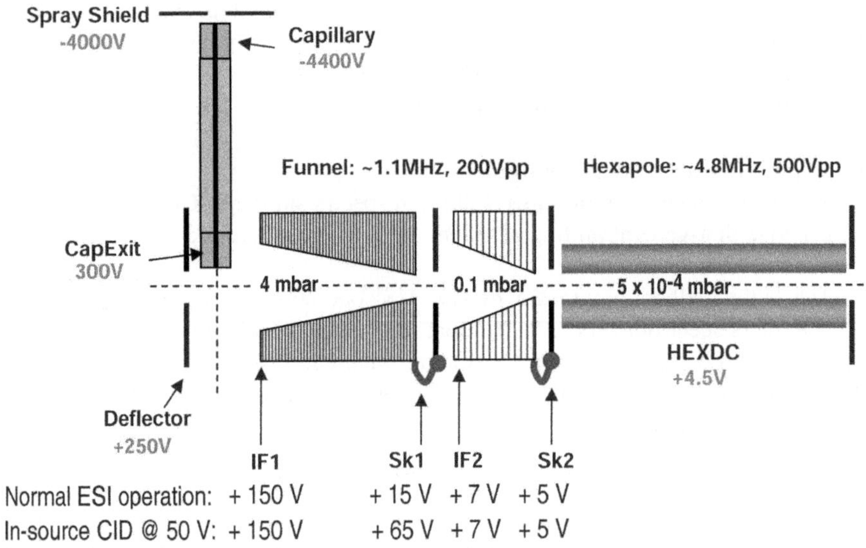

Fig. 12.12 ESI interface with differential pumping in a dual ion funnel arrangement (Bruker Apollo II™). In normal ESI operation the main DC gradient is located in the first ion funnel while ions drop only by about 8 V into the second. Lifting the exit potential of the first funnel causes the ions to enter the second ion funnel at much higher velocity, which is sufficient for NSD (Courtesy of Bruker Daltonik GmbH, Bremen)

NSD or *in-source CID* as it is termed by the manufacturer, is achieved by shifting the DC potentials as to have the largest voltage drop at the entrance into the second ion funnel where a pressure of ≈ 0.1 mbar is suitable for low-energy CID (Fig. 12.12).

12.3 Nanoelectrospray

Miniaturization of electrospray is even more attractive than access to high liquid flows. A more narrow spray capillary results in smaller droplets and, moreover, in much reduced flow, as theoretically described and experimentally demonstrated by Wilm and Mann [82]. Such a downscaling can be achieved by replacing the spray needle by a borosilicate glass capillary of some microliters volume to which a fine tip is pulled with a micropipette puller. The tip has a narrow bore exit of 1–4 μm diameter making flow rates of 20–50 nl min^{-1} sufficient to provide a stable electrospray [83]. Derived from the nanoliter-flow, the term *nanoelectrospray* (nanoESI) has become established for that technique. While conventional ESI produces initial droplets of 1–2 μm in diameter, the droplet size from nanoESI is less than 200 nm, i.e., their volume is about 100–1000 times smaller. NanoESI allows for high-polarity solvents such as pure water in both positive- and negative-ion mode, has extremely low sample consumption [84], and tolerates even higher loads with buffer salts than conventional ESI [55, 85].

Just 800 fmol of BSA consumed In the pioneering nanoESI work, the minuscule sample consumption was demonstrated along an attempt to sequence tryptic peptides (Sect. 11.6.3) of the protein bovine serum albumin (BSA, $M_r \approx 66{,}400$ u). Each of the BSA-derived peptide ions shown in the full scan spectrum (Fig. 12.13) was subjected to fragment ion analysis by means of CID-MS/MS on a triple quadrupole instrument. Merely 800 fmol of BSA was consumed for the tryptic digest used in this analysis [84], a type of nanoESI application that is still highly attractive [86].

12.3.1 Practical Considerations for NanoESI

For the measurement, the nanoESI capillary is adjusted to locate at about 1 mm distance from the entrance of the counter electrode by means of a micromanipulator. Thus, precise optical control is needed during positioning to prevent crashing of the tip or electric discharges during operation. Commercial nanoESI sources are therefore equipped with a built-in microscope or camera (Fig. 12.14). The spray voltage of 0.7–1.2 kV is normally applied via an electrically conducting coating on the outer surface of the spray capillaries, usually a sputtered gold film. Occasionally, wider capillaries with a fine metal filament inside are used. With the high voltage switched on, the liquid sample flow is solely driven by capillary forces refilling the aperture as droplets are leaving the tip. Sometimes, liquid flow is slightly supported by a gentle backing pressure on the capillary. Meanwhile, numerous specialized *nanoelectrospray emitters* – as these capillaries are often termed – have been developed to deliver optimum performance under various conditions of operation including nanoLC-MS coupling [87].

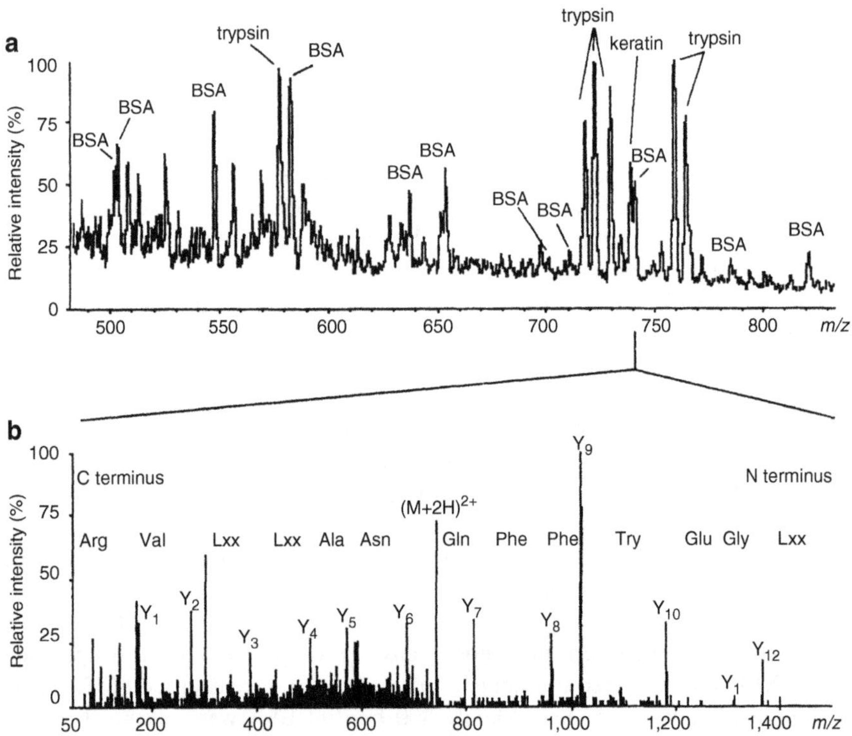

Fig. 12.13 Peptide sequencing by nanoESI-CID-MS/MS from a tryptic digest of BSA; 800 fmol of BSA were used: (**a**) full scan spectrum, (**b**) fragmentation of the selected doubly charged peptide ion at *m/z* 740.5 (Adapted from Ref. [84] by permission. © Nature Publishing Group, 1996)

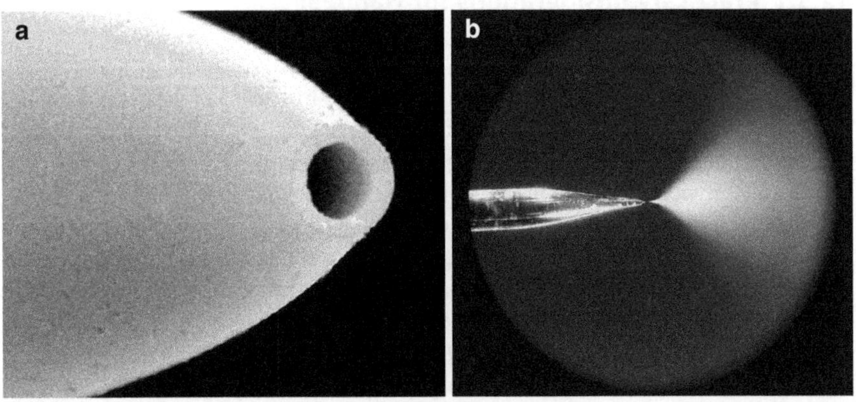

Fig. 12.14 Nanoelectrospray; (**a**) SEM micrograph of the open end of a glass nanoESI capillary having a 2-µm aperture, (**b**) microscopic view of the spray from a nanoESI capillary as provided by observations optics (By courtesy of New Objective, Woburn, MA)

Advantages of nanoESI: Besides its low sample consumption, nanoESI is free of *memory effects* because each sample is supplied in a fresh capillary by means of disposable micropipettes. Furthermore, the narrow exits of nanoESI capillaries prevent air-sensitive samples from rapid decomposition.

12.3.2 Spray Modes of NanoESI

The onset of electrospray as well as the spatial and temporal characteristics of the spray plume largely depends on the experimental parameters. Strong effects are exerted by surface tension and polarity of the solvent, sample concentration, and electric field strength at the tip of the spray capillary. The latter parameter can easily be adjusted, and as demonstrated in Fig. 12.15, demands for careful control as to avoid disadvantageous spray conditions. At low electric field strength some spray will occur, but mostly by multiple discontinuous jets (dripping mode, D) not accompanied by useful aerosol formation [88]. Increasing the spray voltage initiates the formation of the charged mist, which is still accompanied by a spindle-like jet (S) taking away most of the liquid flow. Further increase of the spray voltage forms a wide cone-jet (C) purely consisting of charged microdroplets. As the voltage exceeds a certain limit, the electrostatically driven dissipation of liquid surmounts the solvent flow attainable through the narrow capillary orifice, and thus, the cone-jet starts pulsing (P). Finally, at very high voltages any rough edge around the capillary orifice may initiate a cone-jet of its own. This multi-jet mode

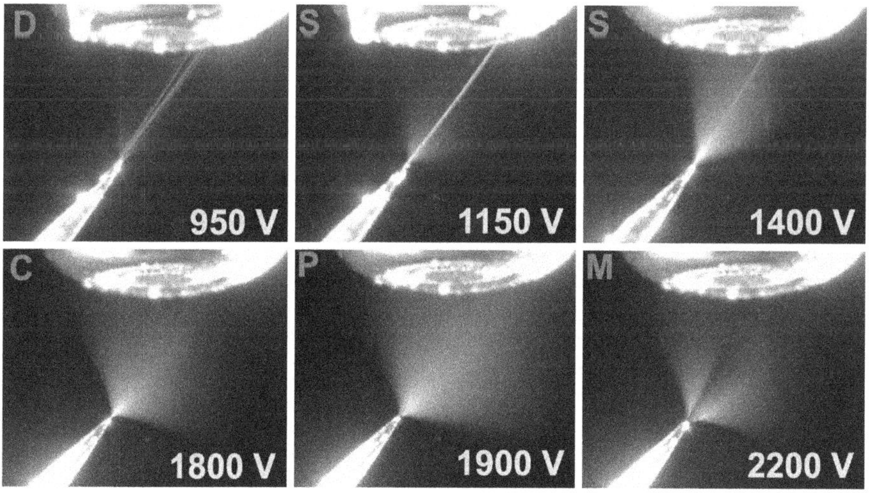

Fig. 12.15 Photographs of nanoelectrospray plumes as effected by different spray voltages. The modes observed starting from the *upper left* are dripping (***D***), spindle (***S***), cone-jet (***C***), pulsed cone-jet (***P***), and multi-jet (***M***). Only pure cone-jet mode will deliver stable electrospray for analytical work (Reproduced from Ref. [88] with permission. © Elsevier, 2004)

(M) causes losses due to overly wide dissipation of the sample flow. Any further increase of the spray voltage results in electric discharges not only detrimental for the capillary tip but eventually also causing failures of the instrument's electronics.

Applicable to ESI in general: These observations are equally relevant to (pneumatically-assisted) ESI at standard flows [89]. Then, the corresponding voltages are just higher by a factor of ≥2, which is mostly due to the increased gap between spray capillary and counter electrode to accommodate the larger plume. The optimization of the electrospray for temporal stability by adjustment of liquid flow, nebulizer gas pressure, and spray voltage is therefore necessary for any analytical ESI work.

12.3.3 Nanoelectrospray from a Chip

The sample throughput of nanoESI is limited by the comparatively time-consuming procedure of manual capillary loading. A chip-based nanoESI sprayer on an etched silicon wafer allows for the automated loading of the sprayer array by a pipetting robot (Fig. 12.16). The chip provides a 10 × 10 array of nanoESI spray nozzles of 10 μm inner diameter. Volumes up to 10 μl are supplied directly from a pipette contacting the chip from the backside. An electrically conducting coating of the pipette tip is used to connect the sprayer to high voltage. Pipetting robot and automated chip handling are united in a common housing that replaces the conventional (nano)ESI spray unit.

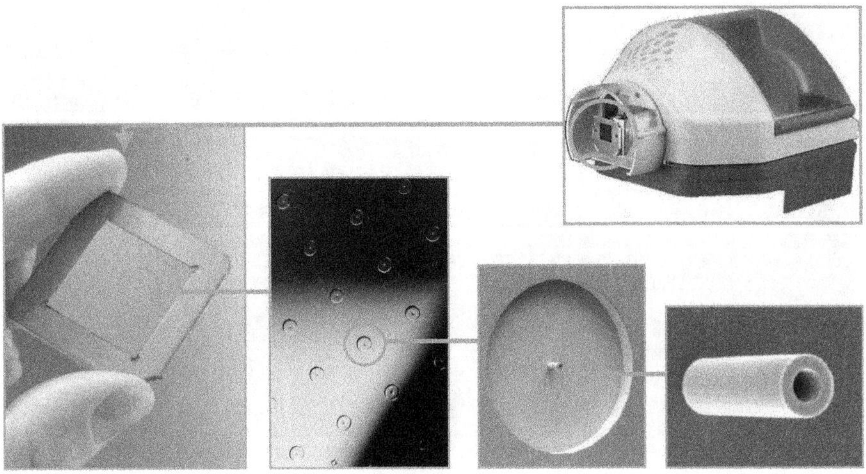

Fig. 12.16 Chip-based Advion nanoESI system. The pictures stepwise zoom in from the pipetting unit to the spray capillary on the silicon chip (By courtesy of G. Schultz, Advion BioSciences, Ithaca, NY)

12.4 Ion Formation in ESI

Until now, our discussion of electrospray was rather technical with an emphasis on interface design and occasional reference to applications. Next we shall consider the physicochemical aspects of the ESI process. This section presents answers to basic questions such as to why an electrospray does occur at all, how isolated gas phase ions are formed from droplets, and what rules are governing the charge state (distribution) of those incipient gas phase ions [89–91]. Ion formation in ESI can be considered to be composed of these steps:

- spraying of a electrostatically charged aerosol of micrometer-sized droplets,
- dramatic reduction of the droplets' size by rapid solvent evaporation,
- repeated disintegration of the microdroplets into even smaller units, and finally
- liberation of fully desolvated ions into the gas phase.

12.4.1 Formation of the Electrospray Plume

To understand the formation of a continuous spray, consider the surface of an electrolytic solution when exiting an electrically conducting capillary held at high electric potential with reference to a nearby counter electrode. In practice, the spray capillary has about 75 μm inner diameter and is kept at 3–4 kV with reference to the sampling orifice at approximately 1 cm distance. At the open end of the capillary the emerging liquid is thus exposed to an electric field of about 10^6 V m^{-1}. The electric field causes charge separation in the electrolytic solution and finally deformation of the meniscus into a cone. The phenomenon of cone formation has been discovered by Zeleny [41] and first theoretically described by Taylor [42], hence it was termed *Taylor cone*.

The process of Taylor cone formation starts when the spherical surface forms an oval under the influence of increasing field strength. In turn, a sharper curvature of the oval increases the field strength. The Taylor cone forms as soon as the critical electric field strength is reached and starts ejecting a fine jet of liquid from its apex towards the counter electrode when surface tension is overcome by the electrostatic forces [82]. The jet carries a large excess of ions of one particular charge sign, because it emerges from the point of highest charge density, i.e., from the cone's apex [92]. Such a jet, however, cannot remain stable for an elongated period of time but breaks up into small droplets (Fig. 12.17) [93]. Due to their charge, these droplets are driven apart by Coulombic repulsion. Overall, this process causes the generation of a fine spray, and thus gave rise to the term *electrospray* (Figs. 12.18). This mode of operation is termed *cone-jet mode* [6].

The ESI process overall represents an electrolytic flow cell where the connection from the spray capillary to the counter electrode is created by charge transportation via the electrically charged aerosol (Fig. 12.19) [94–96]. In positive-ion mode,

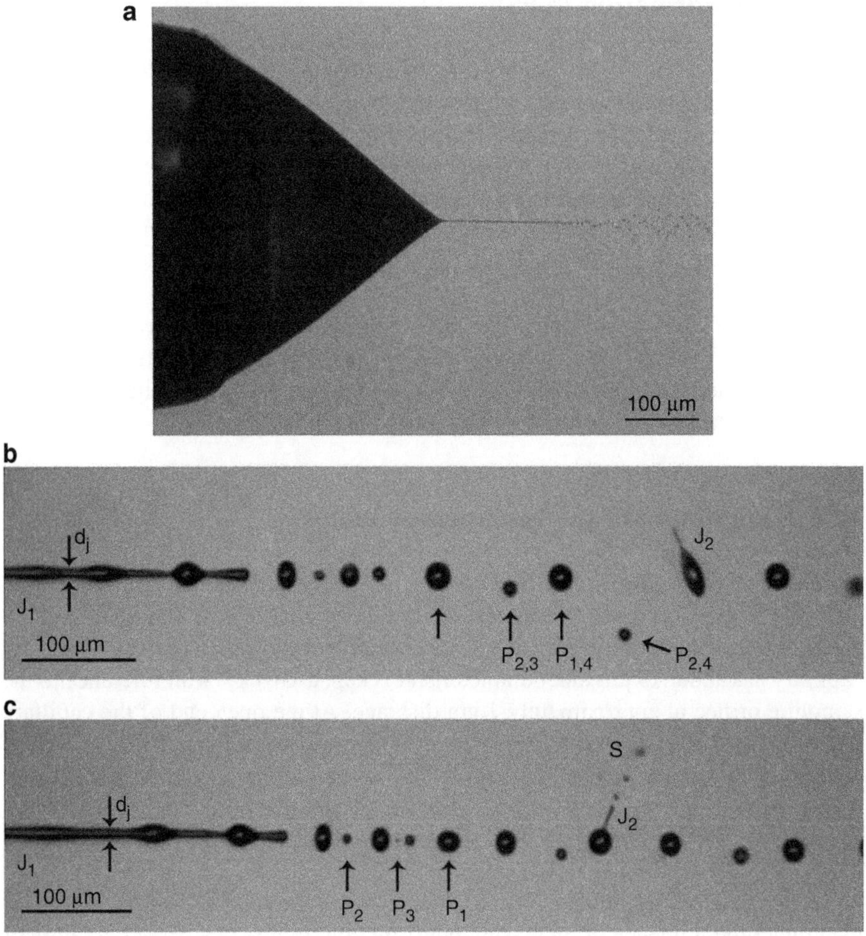

Fig. 12.17 Taylor cone and jet disintegration in ESI. (**a**) Microphotograph of the meniscus shape during electrospray in stable cone-jet mode for optimum analytical operation. The shape and the emerging jet remain stationary and continuously delivering numerous small droplets upon breaking up of the jet. Snapshots (**b**, **c**) show details of the transition from jet to droplets and their shrinking by ejection of a series of much smaller off-spring droplets (Adapted from Ref. [93] with permission. © American Chemical Society, 2007)

neutralization at the sampling orifice is effected by electrons from the high voltage power supply, which in turn originate from oxidation of anions on the inner wall of the spray capillary. In negative-ion mode, reduction of cations will occur in place of oxidation [64].

$M^{+\bullet}$ ions in ESI mode? Under rare circumstances, in ESI, molecular ions, $M^{+\bullet}$, can be formed. This requires that the electrolytic processes during electrospray cause molecular ion formation by electrolytic oxidation [96]. An electrolytic

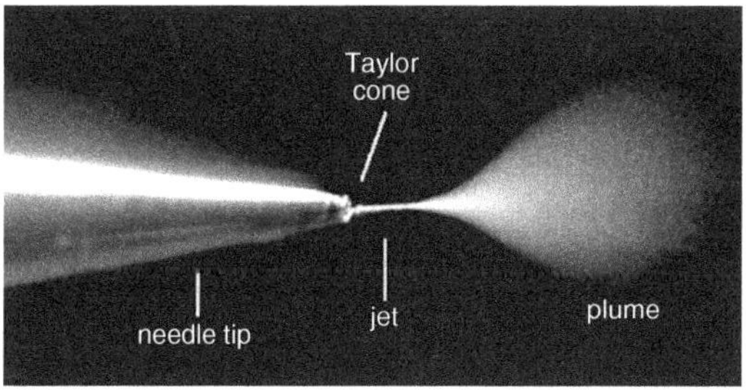

Fig. 12.18 Electrospray from a nanoESI capillary. The jet emitted from the Taylor cone is clearly visible and separate from the region of rapid expansion into a plume of microdroplets (By courtesy of New Objective, Woburn, MA)

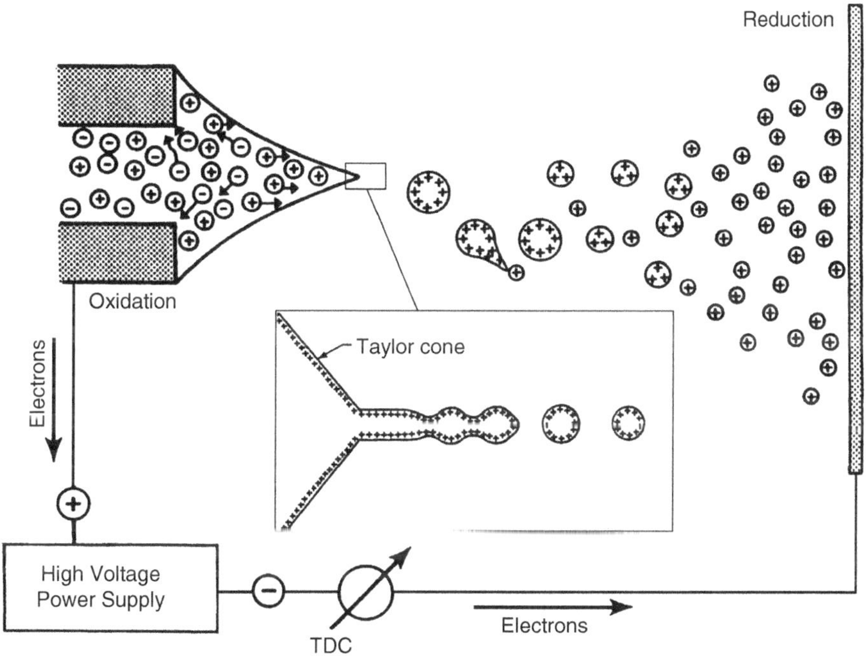

Fig. 12.19 Schematic of Taylor cone formation, ejection of a jet, and its disintegration into a fine spray. The electrochemical processes of ESI [94, 95] are also assigned (Adapted from Ref. [54] by permission of the authors)

molecular ion formation becomes more probable if nonpolar molecules of very low ionization energy are precluded from other ionization pathways such as protonation or cationization. Electrolytic $M^{+\bullet}$ ion formation normally requires perfectly dry aprotic solvents, low liquid flow for increased reaction time, and preferably metal spray capillaries rather than fused silica capillaries. ESI may also result in changes of the oxidation state of metal ions, e.g., $Ag^+ \rightarrow Ag^0$, $Cu^{2+} \rightarrow Cu^+$.

12.4.2 Disintegration of Charged Droplets

When a micrometer-sized droplet carrying a large excess of ions of one particular charge sign – some 10^4 charges can be considered to be a realistic value – evaporates some solvent, the charge density on its surface is continuously increased. As soon as electrostatic repulsion exceeds the conservative force of surface tension, disintegration of the droplet into smaller subunits will occur. The point at which this occurs is known as the *Rayleigh limit* [43]. Originally, it has been assumed that the droplets would then be degraded by *Coulomb fission* (or *Coulomb explosion*). This process then occurs repeatedly to generate increasingly smaller microdoplets. While the model of a cascading reduction in size holds valid, more recent work has demonstrated that the microdroplets do not explode, but eject a series of much smaller microdroplets from an elongated end (Figs. 12.17, 12.19, and 12.20) [54, 90, 93, 97]. The ejection from an elongated end can be explained by deformation of the flying microdroplets, i.e., they have no perfect spherical shape. Thus, the charge density on their surface is not homogeneous, but significantly increased in the region of sharper curvature. The smaller offspring droplets carry off only about 1–2% of the mass, but 10–18% of the charge of the parent droplet [90]. This process resembles the initial ejection of a jet from the Taylor cone. The concept of this so-called *droplet jet fission* is not only based on theoretical considerations but has been proven by flash microphotographs of droplet

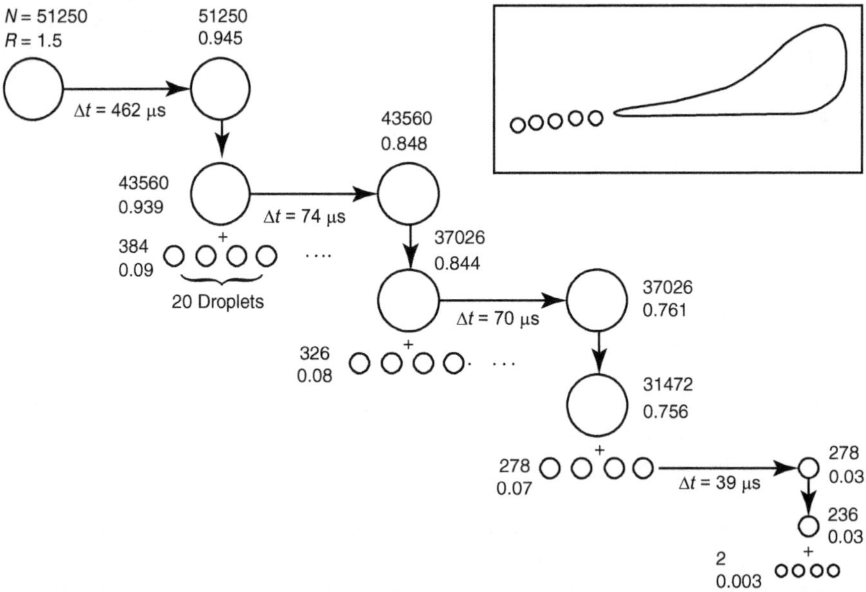

Fig. 12.20 Droplet jet fission. The average number of charges on a droplet, the radii of the droplets [μm], and the timescale of events are assigned. The *inset* shows a drawing of droplet jet fission based on an actual flash microphotograph published by Gomez and Tang [97] (Reproduced from Ref. [54] by permission of the authors)

shadows [97, 98]. The total series of events from the initially sprayed droplet to the isolated ion takes less than one millisecond. Micro-shadowgraphs also show that neutral droplets exhibit an analogous distortion of their shapes followed by ejection of off-spring droplets when field ionized by an electric field of about 2.5×10^6 V m^{-1} [99].

12.4.3 Formation of Gas-Phase Ions from Charged Droplets

The process of droplet jet fission starts on a macroscopic scale and eventually leads to states that might be regarded as large clusters or multiply solvated ions. This model does not address the final step of the creation of isolated gas phase ions from these multi-molecular entities, however.

The elder model of ion formation, the *charged-residue model* (CRM), assumes complete desolvation of ions to occur by successive loss of all solvent molecules from droplets that are sufficiently small to contain just one analyte molecule at the end of a droplet fission cascade [22, 47, 100]. The charges, e.g., protons, being part of this ultimate droplet are then transferred onto the (macro)molecule, especially if this exposes some basic sites. According to CRM, even large proteins should at least be able to form singly charged ions, although the formation of multiply charged species should be of higher probability. In fact, all charge states down to 1+ have been observed [27].

A later theory, the *ion evaporation model* (IEM) [101, 102], describes the formation of desolvated ions as direct evaporation from the surface of highly charged microdroplets [103] (for ion evaporation in FD-MS cf. Sect. 8.6). Ionic solvation energies are in the range of 3–6 eV, but at 300 K thermal energy can only contribute about 0.03 eV to their escape from solution. Thus, the electric force has to provide the energy needed. It has been calculated that a field of 10^9 V m^{-1} is required for ion evaporation, which corresponds to a final droplet diameter of 10 nm [102]. The IEM nicely corresponds to the observation that the number of charges is related to the fraction of the microdroplet's surface that a (macro)molecule can cover. Upon shrinking of the droplet, the size of such a molecule and number of droplet charges remain constant. Now, the increasing charge density brings more charges within the reach of an analyte molecule as the spacing of the surface charges decreases [104, 105]. Flat and planar molecules therefore exhibit higher average charge states than compact ones, e.g., the unfolding of (globular) proteins is accompanied by higher charge states under otherwise identical ESI conditions [106, 107].

Further support of IEM comes from the effect of the droplet evaporation rate on the charge state distribution of proteins. Fast evaporation (more drying gas, higher temperature) favors higher average charge states, while slower evaporation results in fewer charges. This is in accordance with the reduced time available for ion evaporation from the shrinking droplet. It leads to a relative enrichment of charge on the droplet, and thus, on the leaving ions [104].

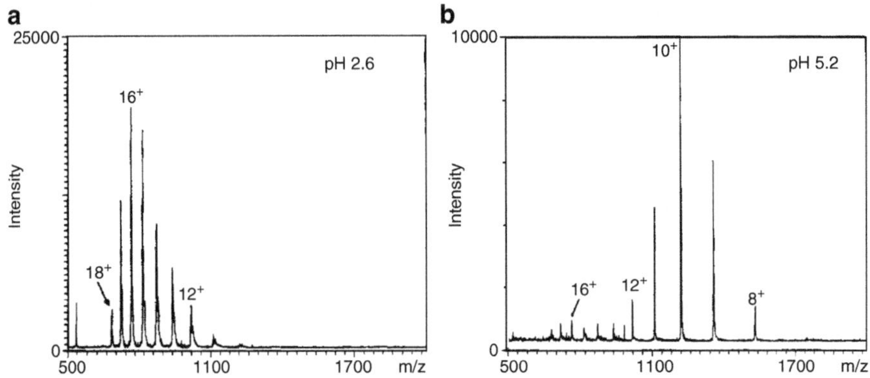

Fig. 12.21 Positive-ion ESI mass spectra of cytochrome c at different pH of the sprayed solution: (**a**) at pH 2.6, (**b**) at pH 5.2 (Adapted from Ref. [107] by permission. © American Chemical Society, 1990)

Influencing the charge state by pH The average charge state of a protein depends on whether it is denatured or not and on the actual solvent; lower pH causes more protons to be attached to the protein than neutral conditions [107, 108]. The degree of denaturization in turn depends on the pH of the electrosprayed solution. Resulting conformational changes of the protein, e.g., unfolding upon protonation, make additional basic sites accessible, thereby effecting an increase of the average charge state (Fig. 12.21) [107]. The maximum number of charges that can be placed upon peptide and protein molecules is directly related to the number of basic amino acid residues (arginine, lysine, histidine) present.

Influencing the charge state by reduction The cleavage of disulfide bonds by reduction with 1,4-dithiothreitol causes the unfolding of the protein. This exposes additional basic sites to protonation, and therefore results in higher average charge states in the corresponding positive-ion ESI spectrum (Figs. 12.22 and 12.23) [106].

In contradiction to IEM, the electric field strength locally necessary to evaporate ions from a droplet cannot be attained, because the droplet would be crossing the Rayleigh limit before [27, 109].

Other work revealed the importance of gas-phase proton transfer reactions [110–113]. This implies that multiply charged peptide ions do not exist as preformed ions in solution, but are generated by gas-phase ion–ion reactions. The proton exchange is driven by the difference in proton affinities (*PA*, Sects. 2.12 and 9.17) of the species encountered, e.g., a protonated solvent molecule of low *PA* will protonate a peptide ion with some basic sites left. Under equilibrium conditions, the process would continue until the peptide ion is "saturated" with protons, a state that also marks its maximum number of charges.

Even though the pathways of ion formation in ESI may be debatable [90, 91, 105], we can briefly summarize this as follows: CRM can be assumed to hold valid for large molecules [22], while the formation of smaller ions is better described by IEM [90, 91].

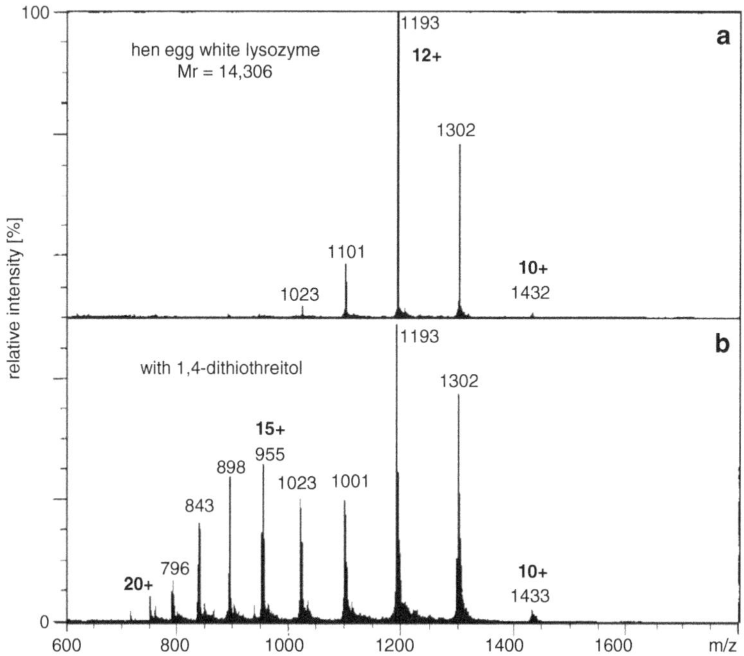

Fig. 12.22 Positive-ion ESI spectra of (**a**) hen egg white lysozyme and (**b**) the protein after addition of 1,4-dithiothreitol (Reproduced from Ref. [106] by permission. © American Chemical Society, 1990)

Independent of the "true" mechanism of ion liberation, the close correlation between the numbers of charge states and the surface a macromolecule exposes to its surrounding solvent can be used to observe these changes by ESI-MS [106–108, 114, 115].

12.5 Multiply Charged Ions and Charge Deconvolution

12.5.1 Dealing with Multiply Charged Ions

The above discussion of ion formation in ESI has revealed that – apart from compound class – the actual experimental conditions exert significant influence on the appearance of an ESI spectrum. The most influential factors are:

- pH of the sprayed solution,
- flow of sample solution,
- flow (or pressure) of nebulizing gas, and
- flow and temperature of the desolvation gas or the temperature of the heated desolvation capillary, respectively.

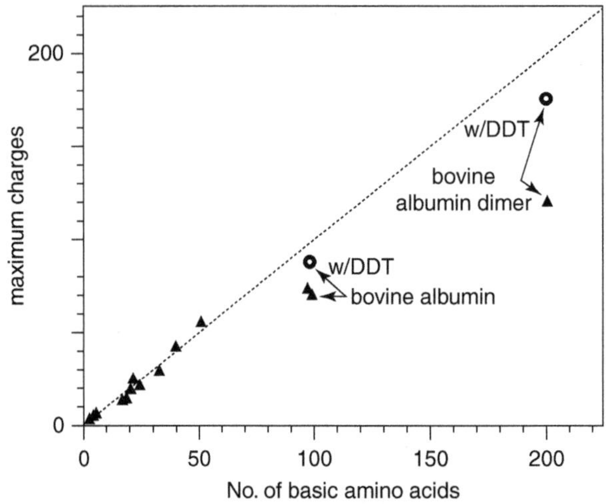

Fig. 12.23 Correlation between the number of basic amino acid residues and the maximum number of charges observed for a set of peptides and proteins under ESI conditions. Labels w/DDT indicate reduction with dithiothreitol in solution (Reproduced from Ref. [106] by permission. © American Chemical Society, 1990)

In ESI, the number of charges on a molecule basically depends on its molecular weight [22, 116] and on the number of potential charge sites available, e.g., sites for protonation [12, 22, 106, 107], deprotonation [117, 118], or cationization [119]. On the one hand, this behavior advantageously folds up the *m/z* scale to make even extremely large molecules accessible to standard mass analyzers, e.g., up to *m/z* 3000 (Fig. 12.24). On the other hand, it creates a confusingly large number of peaks and requires tools to deal with in order to enable reliable mass assignments of unknown samples.

While low-mass polymers exhibit only singly charged ions in ESI, polymers of higher mass form doubly, triply, and multiply charged ions [16]. Basically, the number of charges on those molecules increases in parallel to their average molecular weight. For example, polyethylene glycol of an average molecular mass of 400 u (PEG 400) exclusively exhibits singly charged ions in positive-ion ESI. PEG 1000 about equally forms 1+ and 2+ charge states, and with PEG 1500 the 3+ charge state starts to dominate [16, 105].

Furthermore, charge distributions depend on the sample concentration, e.g., PEG 1450 yields triply and few doubly charged ions at 0.005 mg ml^{-1} in MeOH : H_2O = 1 : 1, triply and doubly charged ions of equal abundance plus few singly charged ions at 0.05 mg ml^{-1}, but mainly doubly charged ions accompanied by few singly and triply charged ions at 0.5 mg ml^{-1} [105]. This demonstrates that a comparatively fixed number of charges in a droplet is distributed among few or many analyte molecules contained, and thus, supports IEM.

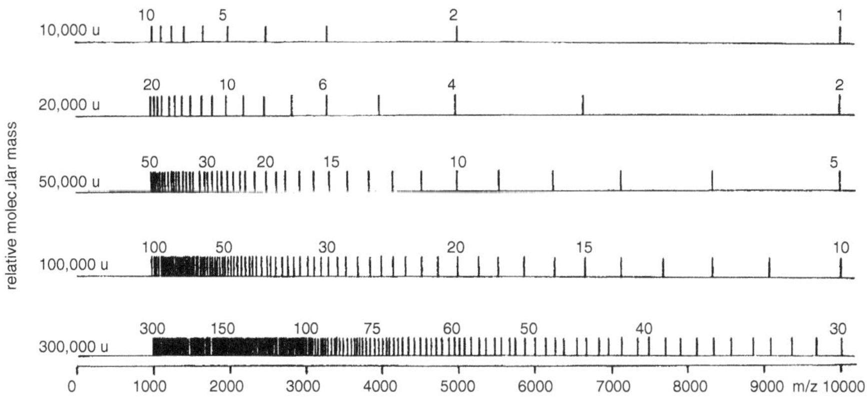

Fig. 12.24 Calculated *m/z* values for the different charge states of molecules of different molecular weight. Representative peaks are labeled with their corresponding charge state (Adapted from Ref. [116] by permission. © John Wiley & Sons, 1992)

Multiple cationization of PEG PEGs and related oxygen-rich compounds readily form $[M+alkali_n]^{n+}$ ions [16, 119, 120] or $[M+nNH_4]^{n+}$ ions. Triton X-405, a commercial detergent used in acrylic paints for stabilization of the suspension, has been analyzed by positive-ion nanoESI-MS. The molecular weight distribution appeared trifold; in this case, due to the presence of ammonium acetate as $[M+NH_4]^+$, $[M+2NH_4]^{2+}$, and $[M+3NH_4]^{3+}$ ion series (Fig. 12.25a). For endgroup analysis *nozzle-skimmer dissociation* (NSD) was applied at 60 V offset upon which only the $[M+3NH_4]^{3+}$ ions (least stable due to highest internal Coulombic repulsion) underwent significant dissociation to yield some low-mass fragment ions (Fig. 12.25b). The occurrence of $[C_8H_{17}\text{-}C_6H_4\text{-}(OC_2H_4)_n]^+$ ions at *m/z* 233 and 277 pointed towards octylphenyl endgroups. Their presence was then verified in a pseudo MS^3 experiment by CID-MS/MS of the fragment ion at *m/z* 233 at 20 V collision offset (Fig. 12.25c) [79].

Annoying superimposition: In ESI spectra of (synthetic) polymers, multiple charging causes the simultaneous occurrence of superimposing ion series each of them representing the molecular weight distribution of the polymer. Therefore, MALDI (Chap. 11) is generally preferred for polymer analysis as it delivers only singly charged ions, and thus provides mass spectra that are much easier to interpret.

12.5.2 Mathematical Charge Deconvolution

How would we be able to retrieve the correct molecular weight from ESI spectra as just presented in Figs. 12.21 and 12.22, or even worse, at the beginning of this chapter, in Fig. 12.1, if the charge states corresponding to individual peaks were not yet assigned? A systematic treatment of these ion series reveals that adjacent signal groups (to include isotopic patterns) in an ESI mass spectrum of a pure compound

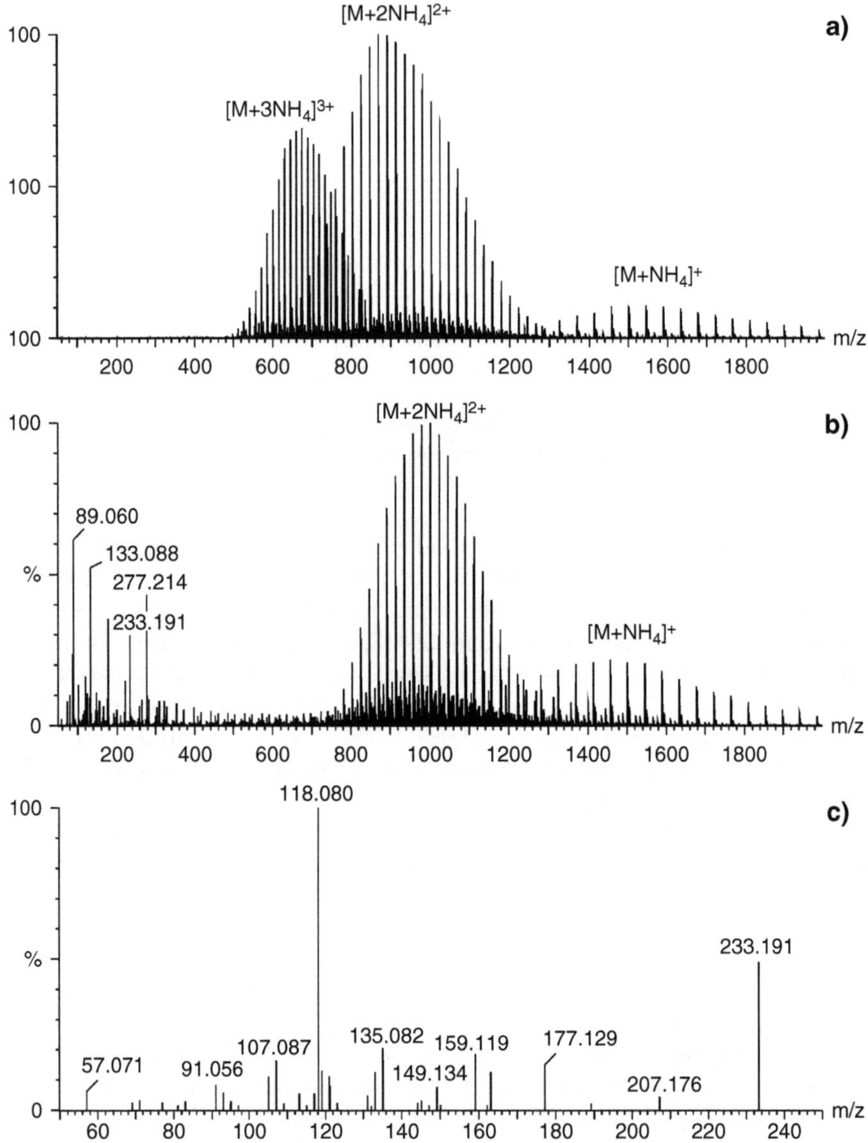

Fig. 12.25 Triton X-405 analyzed by positive-ion nanoESI-MS. (**a**) Molecular weight distribution appears trifold as $[M+NH_4]^+$, $[M+2NH_4]^{2+}$, and $[M+3NH_4]^{3+}$ ions series; (**b**) only the triply charged ions undergo significant dissociation upon NSD to yield low-mass fragment ions; (**c**) CID spectrum of fragment ion at *m/z* 233 for endgroup analysis (Reproduced from Ref. [79] with permission. © Elsevier, 2009)

belong to charge states differing exactly by one, i.e., distributions have no gaps or jumps. This renders the calculation of the number of charges corresponding to individual peaks straightforward, and thus, permits to deduce an unknown molecular weight M_r [63, 116, 121].

For the charge states of neighboring peaks belonging to a pair at m/z_1 (higher value) and m/z_2 (lower value) we have :

$$n_2 = n_1 + 1 \tag{12.1}$$

Assuming all charges from protonation and using m_H for the mass of a proton, m/z_1 is determined by

$$m/z_1 = \frac{M_r + n_1 m_H}{n_1} \tag{12.2}$$

and m/z_2 of the peak at lower mass is given by

$$m/z_2 = \frac{M_r + n_2 m_H}{n_2} = \frac{M_r + (n_1 + 1)\, m_H}{n_1 + 1} \tag{12.3}$$

where n_2 can be expressed by inserting Eq. 12.1. The charge state n_1 can then be obtained from

$$n_1 = \frac{m/z_2 - m_H}{m/z_1 - m/z_2} \tag{12.4}$$

Having calculated n_1, M_r is given by

$$M_r = n_1\,(m/z_1 - m_H) \tag{12.5}$$

In case of cationization instead of protonation, m_H has to be replaced by the corresponding mass of the cationizing agent, in most cases simply by that of NH_4^+, Na^+, or K^+. (The recognition of cationized species is addressed in Sects. 8.6 and 11.4).

Manual charge deconvolution For the ease of calculation we use nominal mass (Sect. 3.1.5) and assume the charges from protonation. Consider the first peak at m/z 1001, the second at m/z 501. Now n_1 is obtained according to Eq. 12.4 from $n_1 = (501 - 1)/(1001 - 501) = 500/500 = 1$. Therefore, M_r is calculated from Eq. 12.5 to be $M_r = 1 \times (1001 - 1) = 1000$. (The doubly protonated ion is detected at m/z 501 because $(1000 + 2)/2 = 501$.)

Averaging increases accuracy: As each pair of signals delivers an independent mass value for the hypothetical singly charged ion, mass accuracy can greatly be enhanced in ESI by multiple determination of this value and subsequent calculation of the average.

12.5.3 Computerized Charge Deconvolution

The above procedure may be time-consuming but at least it works for pure compounds. When mixtures are to be addressed, proper manual assignment of all peaks becomes increasingly difficult. Additional problems arise from the simultaneous presence of peaks due to protonation and cation attachment. Therefore, numerous refined algorithms have been developed to cope with these requirements [122–125]. Modern ESI instruments normally come with elaborate *charge deconvolution* software or offer such software as an option. The efficiency of these programs [126–128] can largely be improved by specifying some limitations, e.g., the expected range of charge numbers, the type of ions or presumed adducts, and the resolving power employed for the measurement. The resolving power is relevant to assist the algorithm in distinguishing neighboring peaks of other charge states from isotopic contributions.

ESI-MS of transferrin Transferrin, a human protein of close to 80 kDa, occurs in several glycoforms, i.e., its structure contains different antenna-shaped oligosaccharide receptors. Here, these are indicated by labels for one biantenna (Bi), two biantennas (BiBi), one biantenna plus one triantenna (BiTri), and one biantenna plus one fucosylated biantenna (BiBiF), respectively. Transferrin may also lack an *N*-glycan, even in healthy individuals, while truncated transferrin, indicated by X and Y, may occur due to inappropriate storage or handling. The positive-ion ESI mass spectrum of transferrin from a healthy individual was measured using a medium-resolution TOF mass spectrometer (QSTAR, AB Sciex). The spectrum was obtained of a solution in acetonitrile : water = 60 : 40 (v/v) with 0.1% of formic acid. Under these conditions, multiple protonation leads to a wide distribution of charge states, mainly covering the range *m/z* 1700–3000 (Fig. 12.26) [129]. However, it is hardly possible to detect all components contributing to the spectrum without charge deconvolution. After using ProMass deconvolution software (Thermo Fisher Scientific) to transform the raw data into a spectrum reflecting only singly charged ions, the individual components are easily recognized. The contributing proteins detected are X (69022 u), Y (73430 u), Bi (77363 u), BiBi (79553 u), BiBiF (79769 u), and BiTri (80205 u).

ESI-MS at different levels of resolution A mixture of the proteins bovine ubiquitin, horse cytochrome c, and horse myoglobin, each at a concentration of 10 μM, was analyzed by positive-ion ESI-FT-ICR-MS. While the first analysis was carried out with only 16 k data (LR), the second was obtained from a 512 k transient (HR), resulting in $R = 2000$ and $R = 60{,}000$, respectively (Sect. 4.7.5). Charge deconvolution by the *Zscore* algorithm delivered "zero-charge spectra" clearly separating the proteins (Fig. 12.27) [123]. The program used here handles LR spectra to yield unresolved isotopic distribution envelopes as well as HR spectra to show the full isotopic information in the resulting zero-charge spectrum.

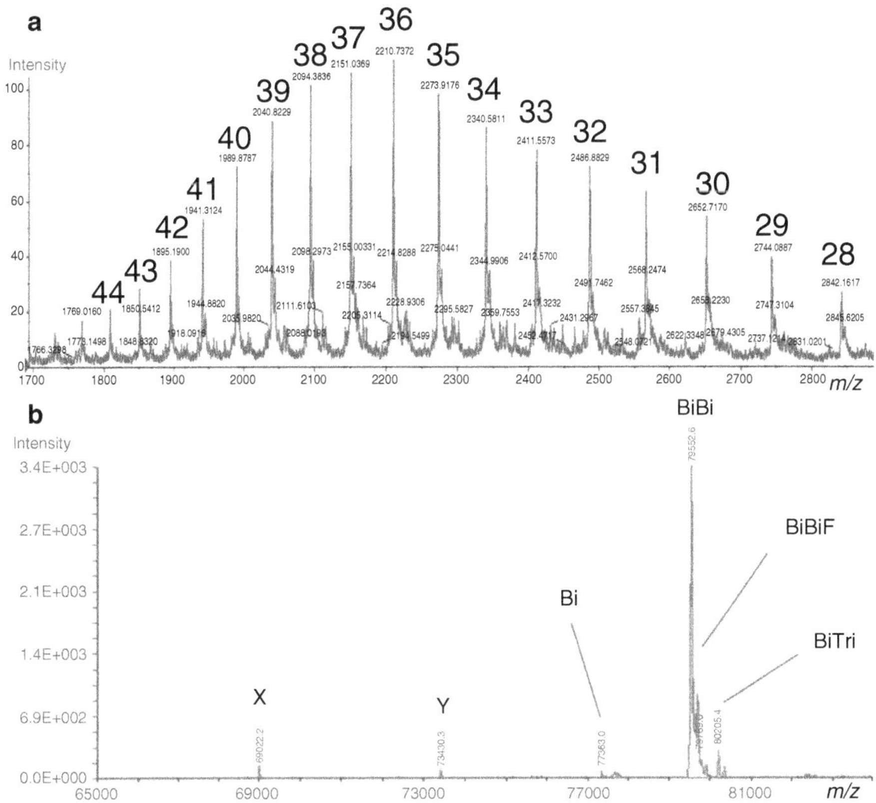

Fig. 12.26 Positive-ion ESI mass spectrum of a solution of transferrin in acetonitrile : water = 60 : 40 (v/v) with 0.1% of formic acid. (**a**) Spectrum as measured with the number of charges assigned, (**b**) after charge deconvolution to deliver a hypothetical spectrum of singly charged ions. Labels indicate one biantenna (*Bi*), two biantennas (*BiBi*), one biantenna plus one triantenna (*BiTri*), and one biantenna plus one fucosylated biantenna (*BiBiF*), respectively. Truncated transferrin is indicated by X and Y (Adapted from Ref. [129] with permission. © Springer, 2016)

Charge deconvoluted spectra: The output of computerized charge deconvolution can often be customized to either display the hypothetical mass spectrum as it would appear with singly charged ions (Fig. 12.26) or to deliver "zero-charge" spectra showing the molecular weights of the corresponding neutrals (Fig. 12.27). It is important to note that the output of neutral M_r represents the only case where the abscissa *has to be* labeled "*mass* [u]", while mass spectra strictly require "*m*/*z*" on the *x* axis!

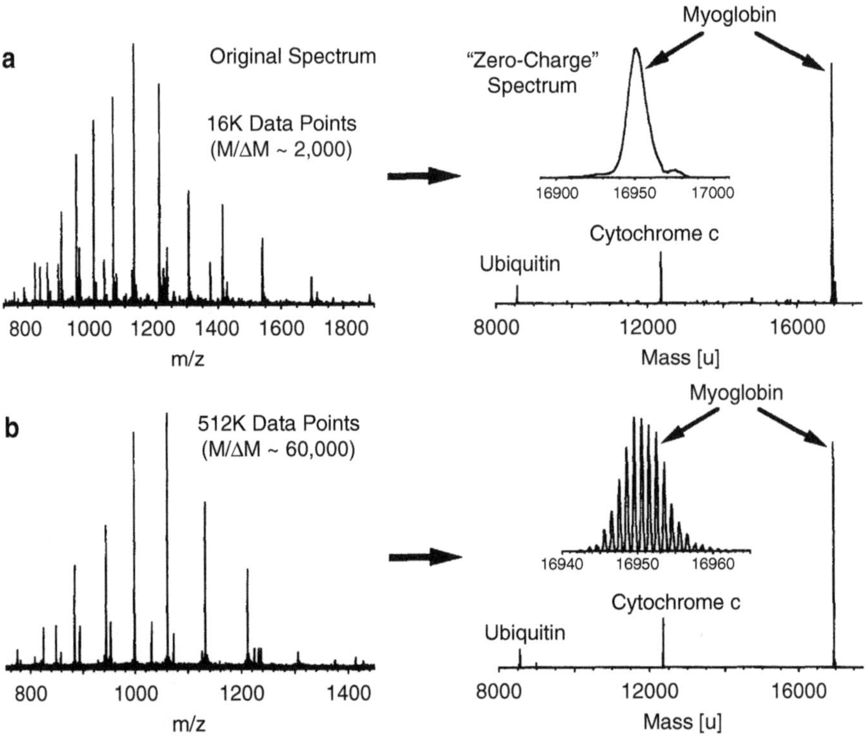

Fig. 12.27 Charge deconvolution of (**a**) LR and (**b**) HR positive-ion ESI spectra of an artificial protein mixture. The "zero-charge" peak of myoglobin is also shown in expanded view to reveal the delineation of the isotopic pattern (Adapted from Ref. [123] by permission. © Elsevier, 1998)

12.5.4 Hardware Charge Deconvolution

The most effective technique to achieve charge deconvolution of complex spectra due to multiply charged ions is to achieve the full separation between signals corresponding to different charge states and to resolve their isotopic patterns. Beyond a molecular weight of about a few thousand u this requires high-resolving mass analyzers, because the isotopic distribution of organic ions then becomes several mass units wide (Fig. 12.28). The minimum resolving power needed for full isotopic separation is always equal to the ion's mass number (Sects. 3.4, 3.7, and 3.8), independent of the charge state of the ion. Lower resolution only envelops the isotopic distribution. At insufficient resolution, the resulting peak may even be wider than the envelope [116].

Magnetic sector instruments (Sect. 4.3) were used first to demonstrate the beneficial effects of high resolution on ESI spectra of biomolecules [120, 130, 131]. Today, FT-ICR instruments (Sect. 4.7) [132, 133] and more recently orthogonal acceleration time-of-flight (oaTOF, Sects. 4.2.8 and 4.9) or Orbitrap (Sect. 4.8) analyzers offer by far more effective means to resolve such signals.

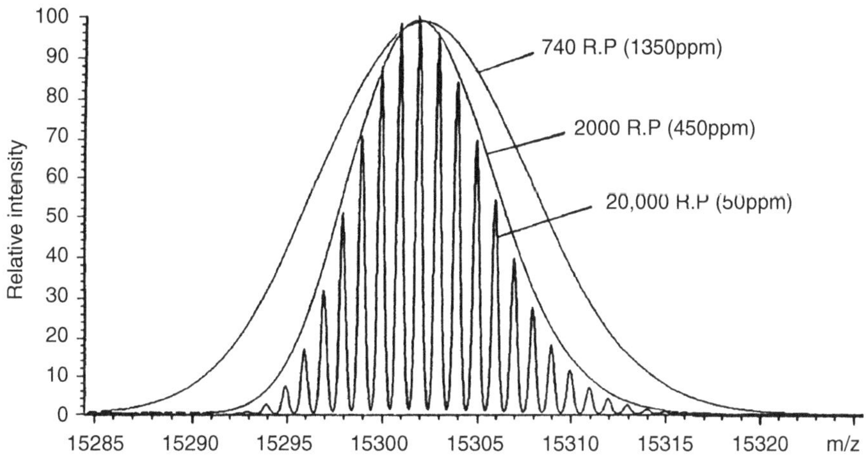

Fig. 12.28 Theoretical peak shape for a hypothetical singly charged protein ion of $M_r = 15{,}300$ u at different settings of resolution (Reproduced from Ref. [116] by permission. © John Wiley & Sons, 1992)

Rule for minimum resolving power: The mass resolving power to achieve full separation of isotopic peaks only depends on the molecular weight, M_r, of the analyte, but it is independent of the number of charges, z, of the ions. For example, the isotope peaks of the $[M+H]^+$ ion of thioredoxin (Fig. 12.1) would appear at m/z 11674 and be spaced at $\Delta(m/z) = 1$. Using $R = m/\Delta m$ (Sect. 3.4) we calculate the minimum value $R_{min} = 11674 / 1 = 11674$. For the $[M+8H]^{8+}$ ion of this protein ($z = 8$), the signals are centered at m/z 1459 and spaced at $\Delta(m/z) = 0.125$. Thus, we calculate $R_{min} = m/\Delta m = 1459 / 0.125 = 11674$. In brief, the numerical value of M_r directly reflects R_{min}.

ESI-Orbitrap mass spectra of intact proteins The positive-ion ESI-Orbitrap mass spectra of intact proteins show fully resolved isotopic patterns when 100 transients at a resolving power setting of $R = 100{,}000$ are acquired and charge deconvoluted. Figure 12.29 shows the results for the $[M+10H]^{10+}$ ion of horse heart apomyoglobin, $m = 16{,}940.965$ u (neutral mass of monoisotopic molecule) and of the $[M+21H]^{21+}$ ion of carbonic anhydrase, $m = 29{,}006.683$ u, both in very good agreement with the calculated isotopic patterns and masses [134]. A comparison with the previous example also demonstrates the great advances made in MS instrumentation that now allows to routinely resolve such signals. (Further examples are given by the ESI-ECD-FT-ICR spectra of proteins in Sect. 9.13 or by example II in the preceding Sect. 12.5.3.)

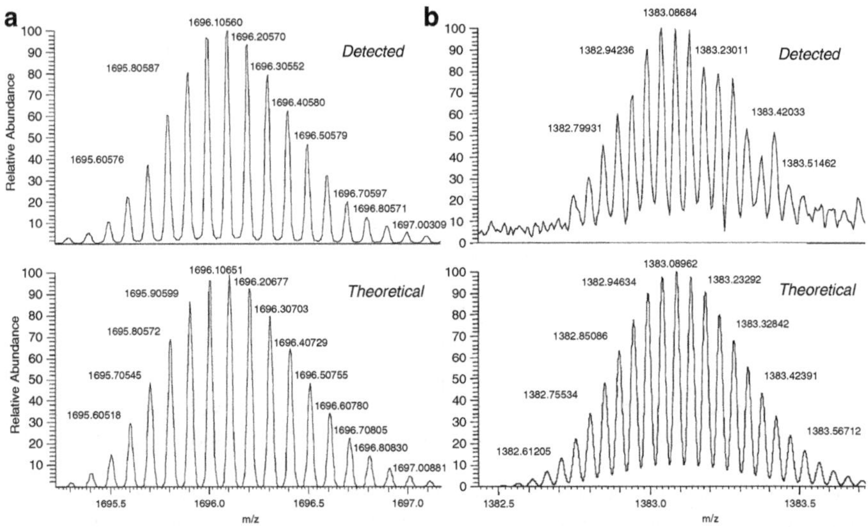

Fig. 12.29 ESI-orbitrap-MS of proteins. Fully resolved isotopic patterns as obtained upon charge deconvolution of (**a**) the $[M+10H]^{10+}$ ion of horse heart apomyoglobin, $m = 16{,}940.965$ u (neutral mass of monoisotopic molecule) and (**b**) the $[M+21H]^{21+}$ ion of carbonic anhydrase, $m = 29{,}006.683$ u (Reproduced from Ref. [134] by permission. © American Chemical Society, 2006)

12.5.5 Controlled Charge Reduction in ESI

The complexity of ESI spectra of mixtures with all components forming series of multiply charged ions is apparent. An alternative approach to high resolution and data reduction by charge deconvolution is presented by the controlled reduction of the charge states themselves. *Charge reduction electrospray* results in a significantly reduced number of peaks per component at the cost of their detection being required at substantially higher *m/z* [135, 136]. In particular oaTOF analyzers provide a sufficient mass range for such an experimental approach at reasonable cost.

Charge reduction can be accomplished by neutralizing ion–molecule reactions during the desolvation step of ESI. The reducing ions needed for such neutralizations can either be generated by irradiating the gas with a ^{210}Po α-particle source [135, 137] or much more conveniently by a corona discharge [138, 139]. Besides being nonradiative, the corona discharge offers the advantage of being tunable to achieve varying degrees of neutralization (Fig. 12.30) [138, 139].

Ion–ion chemistry of oppositely charged ions provides another access to charge reduction and charge state determination [110]. Such studies were done either by employing the region preceding the skimmer of an ESI interface as a flow reactor or inside a quadrupole ion trap. In the first case, both the substrate ion and the oppositely charged reactant ion are created by means of two separate ESI sprayers attached to a common interface [140]. The approach in a quadrupole ion trap makes

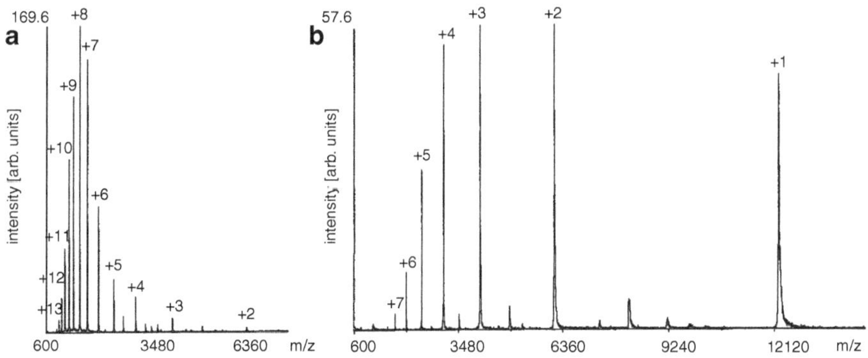

Fig. 12.30 Positive-ion ESI mass spectra of cytochrome c (**a**) under standard ESI conditions from acidic solution, (**b**) same but with medium setting of charge-reducing corona discharge (Adapted from Ref. [138] by permission. © American Chemical Society, 2000)

use of the in-trap generation of proton-transferring reactant ions, while substrate ions are admitted via the ESI interface [141]. Finally, a noninstrumental approach is to derivatize the analytes as to reduce their ability of binding protons at basic functional groups [136].

12.6 Applications of ESI-MS

ESI-MS is not only a versatile tool for any aspects of peptide and protein characterization including their complete sequencing, it also offers a tremendous variety of other applications some of which are highlighted below [4, 9–11, 25, 142–145].

12.6.1 ESI-MS of Small Molecules

Polar analytes in the *m/z* 100–1500 range are often involved in pharmaceutical analytics including metabolism studies. The types of ions formed are various and depend on the ion polarity, the pH of the solution, the presence of salts, and the concentration of the sprayed solution. Multiply charged ions are rarely observed.

Drug development The compound below represents the functional part of an effective drug (BM 50.0341) inhibiting HIV-1 infection by suppression of the unfolding of the gp120 glycoprotein (Fig. 12.31). Its positive-ion nanoESI spectrum from ethanol in the presence of ammonium chloride exhibits signals due to the formation of $[M+H]^+$, $[M+NH_4]^+$, and $[M+Na]^+$ ions. In addition, cluster ions of the type $[2M+H]^+$, $[2M+NH_4]^+$, and $[2M+Na]^+$ are observed as typical for samples at comparatively high concentration. In negative-ion mode [146–149], the $[M–H]^-$ ion is accompanied by $[M+Cl]^-$ and $[M+EtO]^-$ adduct ions; the corresponding cluster ion series is also observed.

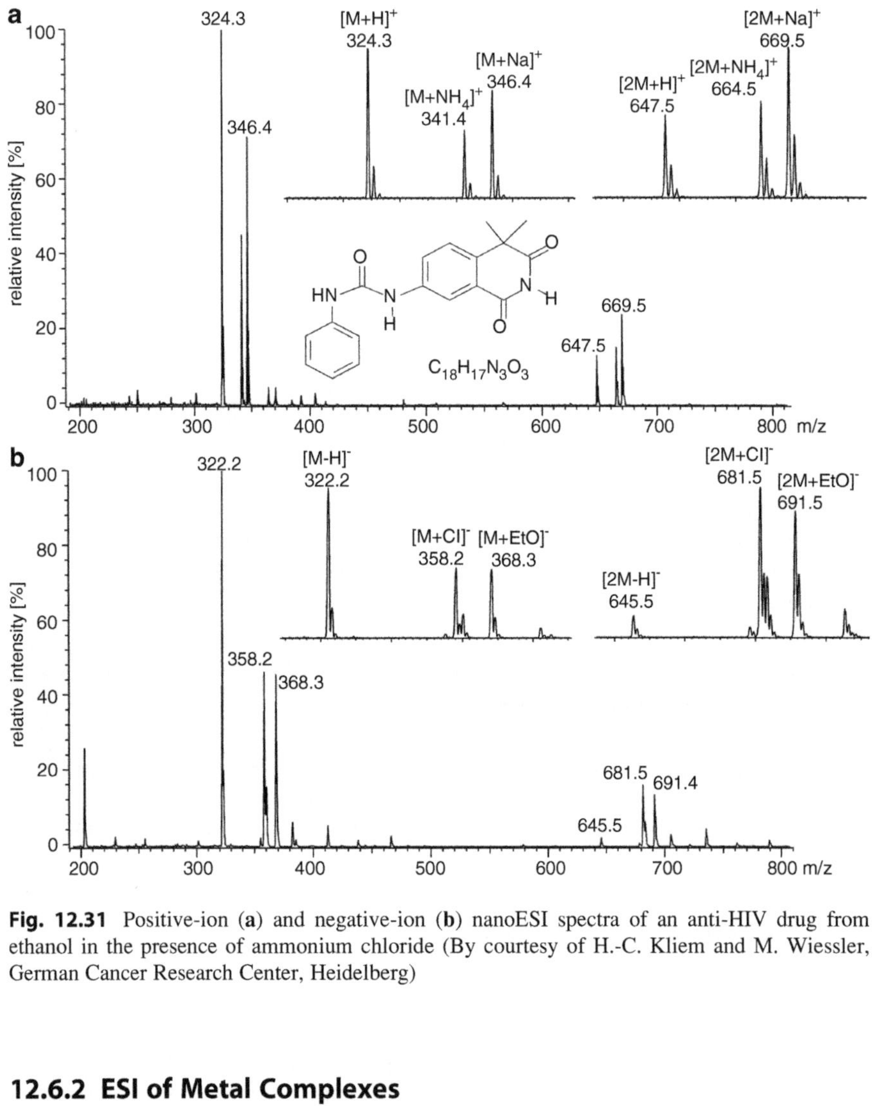

Fig. 12.31 Positive-ion (a) and negative-ion (b) nanoESI spectra of an anti-HIV drug from ethanol in the presence of ammonium chloride (By courtesy of H.-C. Kliem and M. Wiessler, German Cancer Research Center, Heidelberg)

12.6.2 ESI of Metal Complexes

In general, ESI can be well applied to ionic metal complexes and related compounds if these are soluble to at least 10^{-6} M in solvents suitable for the method [23–25]. Whether conventional or nanoESI should be employed basically depends on the tendency of the respective compounds towards decomposition. Labile complexes or compounds that are strongly adhesive to surfaces are preferably analyzed by nanoESI to avoid long-lasting contamination of the sample supply line. Illustrative examples in this field are presented by the application of ESI to isopoly metal oxyanions [150], polyphosphates [151], transition metal complexes (Fig. 12.32) [26, 152, 153], and cadmium sulfide clusters [154]. Furthermore, the

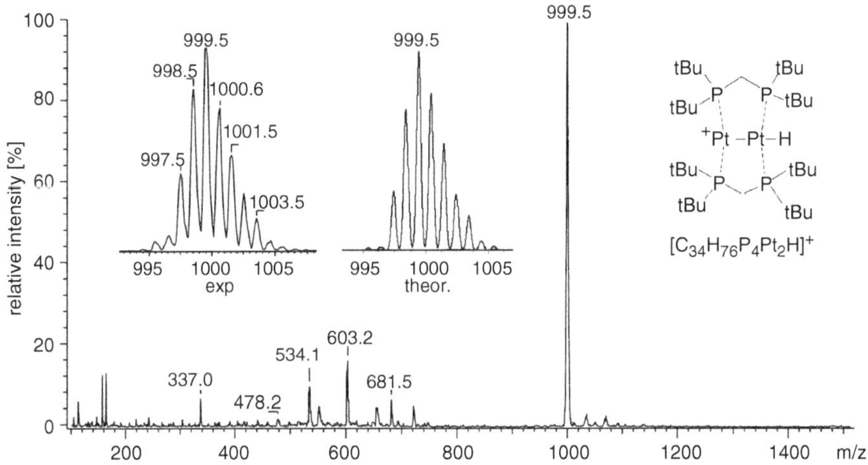

Fig. 12.32 Positive-ion ESI spectrum of a cationic dinuclear platinum hydride complex from dichloromethane solution. The *insets* compare experimental and theoretical isotopic patterns (By courtesy of P. Hofmann, Heidelberg University)

gas-phase reactions of electrosprayed metal complexes can be directly examined by tandem MS techniques (Sect. 9.17.1) [155–157].

12.6.3 ESI of Surfactants

Surfactants belong to a group of products where a low price is crucial, and therefore they are usually synthesized from coarsely defined mineral oil fractions or vegetable oils both of which represent (sometimes complex) mixtures (Fig. 12.33). Cationic and anionic surfactants are readily detected by ESI, but it also serves well for the detection of nonionic surfactants which tend to form $[M+alkali]^+$ or $[M-H]^-$ ions, respectively [158–162].

12.6.4 Oligonucleotides, DNA, and RNA

For the analysis of *oligonucleotides*, *DNA*, and *RNA* negative-ion ESI is best suited [145]. While MALDI becomes difficult beyond oligonucleotide 20-mers, ESI can handle much larger molecules [163–166]. The problems associated with mass spectrometry of oligonucleotides are due to the often multiple exchange of protons versus alkali ions (Sect. 11.5). Instead of ion exchange beads, nitrogen bases have proven very helpful in removing alkali ions from solutions [167]. In particular, the addition of 25 mM imidazole and piperidine yields very clean spectra (Fig. 12.34) [168]. Even after cation removal, these polyanionic species are demanding targets for MS.

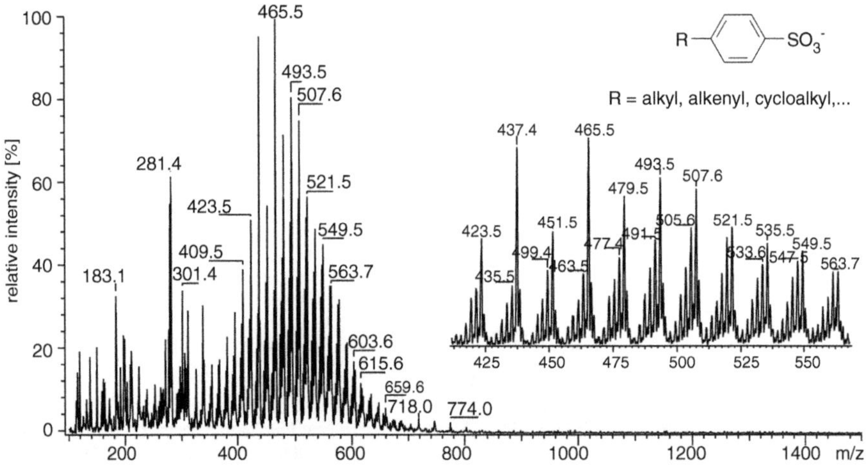

Fig. 12.33 Negative-ion ESI spectrum of an industrial cooling lubricant dissolved in 1-propanol at 1:1000. The dominant ions belong to alkylbenzene sulfonates. The *inset* expands the *m/z* 420–555 range, the most intensive peaks belonging to saturated alkyl chains (By courtesy of OMTEC GmbH, Eberbach)

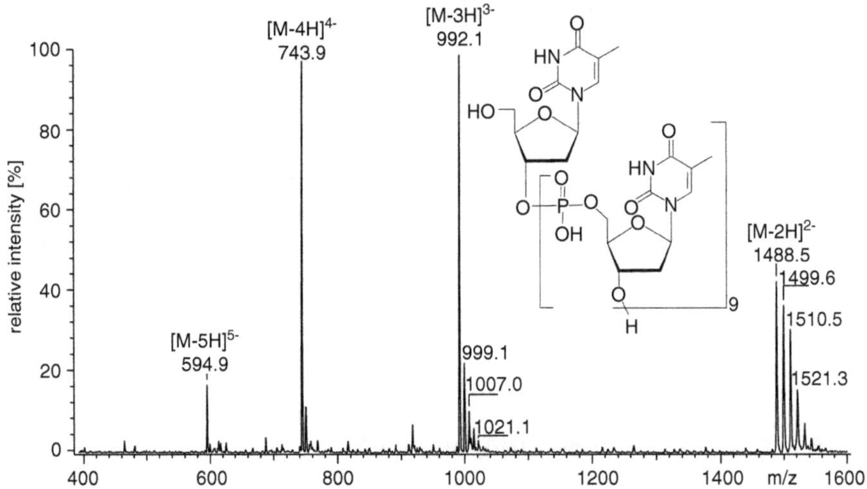

Fig. 12.34 Negative-ion ESI spectrum of the oligonucleotide dT_{10} in the presence of imidazole and piperidine. Here, H^+/Na^+ exchange is not completely suppressed (By courtesy of T. Krüger, University of Heidelberg)

Conventionally, oligonucleotides are presented by starting from the 5-hydroxyl terminus and writing along the phosphodiester chain towards the 3-hydroxyl terminus, i.e., from the 5′ to the 3′ end or from the phosphate to the ribose, respectively (Fig. 12.35). Oligonucleotides built from *nucleotides* based on the furanose ribose

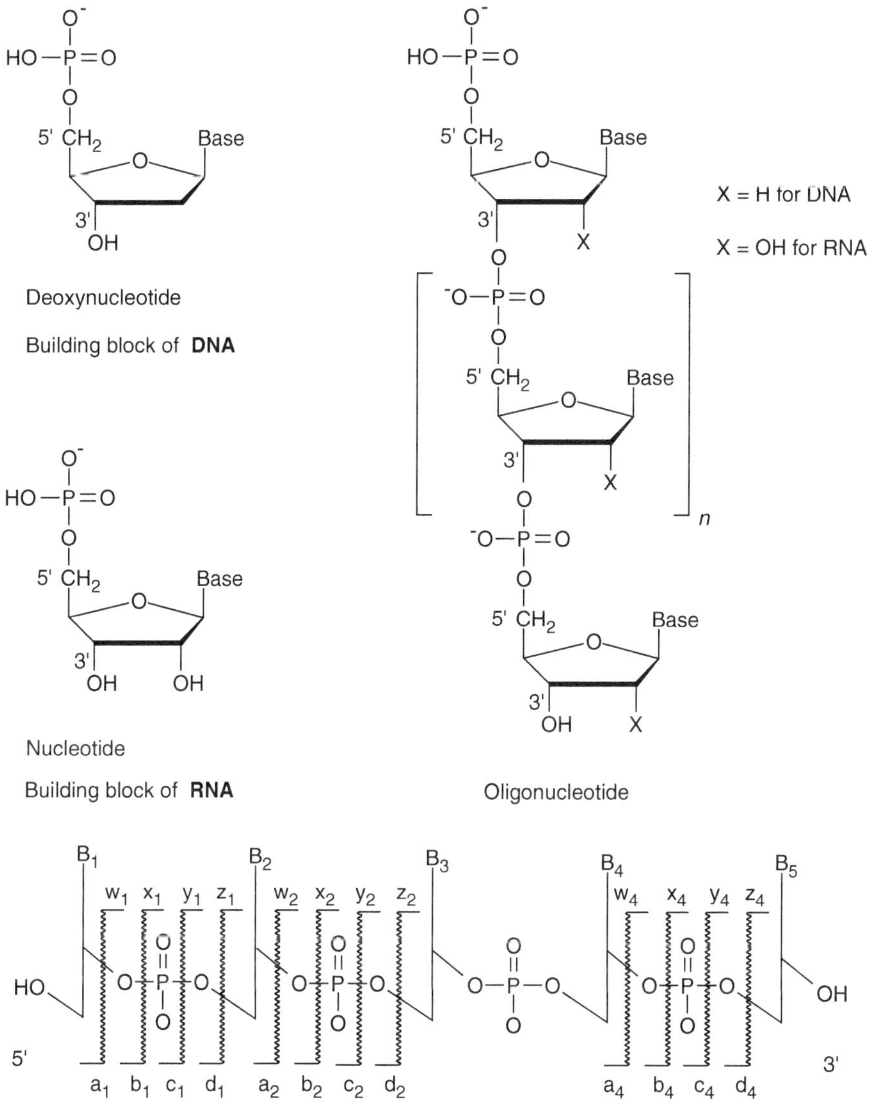

Fig. 12.35 Structures of nucleotides of DNA and RNA (*upper left*), general structure of oligonucleotides (*upper right*), and basic fragmentation scheme of oligonucleotides using the symbolized writing convention for the oligonucleotide backbone comprising furanose and *base* (*bottom*)

are termed *ribonucleic acids* (RNAs), those based on deoxyribose are termed *deoxyribonucleic acids* (DNAs). The bases attached to the pentose moieties are nitrogen-rich heterocyclic compounds.

Sequencing of oligonucleotides by ESI-MS/MS techniques is also feasible [163, 165, 169, 170]. Charged fragments of the 5′ end are denoted with letters and numerical subscripts from the beginning of the alphabet (*a*- to *d*-type ions) while fragments of the 3′ end are labeled as *w*- to *z*-type ions (Fig. 12.35) [171]. The bases on the ribose moieties are denoted either without qualification as base B_n with the subscripts starting on the 5′ end or by using the one-letter code of the entire nucleotides.

Sequence of an oligonucleotide The ESI-FT-ICR spectrum of $[M–4H]^{4-}$ ions of the phosphorothioate deoxyoligonucleotide 5′-GCCCAAGCTGGCATCCGTCA-3′ upon IRMPD exhibits numerous peaks corresponding to fragment ions of charge states from 1– to 4– (Fig. 12.36). This mass spectrum is greatly simplified upon charge deconvolution. Thanks to the resolving power of FT-ICR-MS, the assignment of charge states is absolutely reliable. In the resulting zero-charge spectrum, a_n-*B* and w_n fragment ions can be retrieved and the sequence thus derived [169].

12.6.5 ESI-MS of Oligosaccharides

Oligosaccharides [55, 74, 172, 173] as well as closely related compounds such as glycoproteins [73, 174], gangliosides [175], liposaccharides etc. are similar to oligonucleotides in that they require polar solvents and very soft ionization, in particular when the molecules are branched. As demonstrated by a large number of applications, ESI permits molecular weight determination and structure elucidation in these cases (Fig. 12.37; for a general fragmentation scheme cf. Sect. 11.5) [5].

12.6.6 Observing Supramolecular Chemistry at Work

The outstanding softness of ion formation of ESI allows to preserve noncovalent bonds during the sequence of ion liberation from solution into the gas phase. This can be observed by the formation of solvent adducts, cluster ions, and in particular, by its ability to deliver supramolecular systems into the gas phase [144, 176–180].

Formation of pseudorotaxanes The alkyl groups of secondary ammonium ions are able to barely pass through the cavity of benzo-21-crown-7 (**C7**) while phenyl groups require the wider cavity of dibenzo-24-crown-8 (**C8**) to form pseudorotaxanes. On the other side, phenyl groups suffice as stoppers to trap **C7** on the axle. The larger **C8** forms pseudorotaxanes even with secondary di*benzyl* ammonium ions. This can be directly observed by positive-ion ESI-MS of a mixture of suitably substituted ammonium ions as in case of a four-component self-sorting system consisting of **1**-H·PF6, **2**-H·PF6, **C7**, and **C8** (inset of Fig. 12.38) [178]. As anthracenyl and phenyl groups are present in **1**-H· PF6, it cannot overcome the barrier to insert into **C7**. Thus, only two peaks of high intensity are observed, i.e., for [**2**-H@**C7**]+, *m*/*z* 550, and for [**1**-H@**C8**]+, *m*/*z* 746. A weak peak indicating

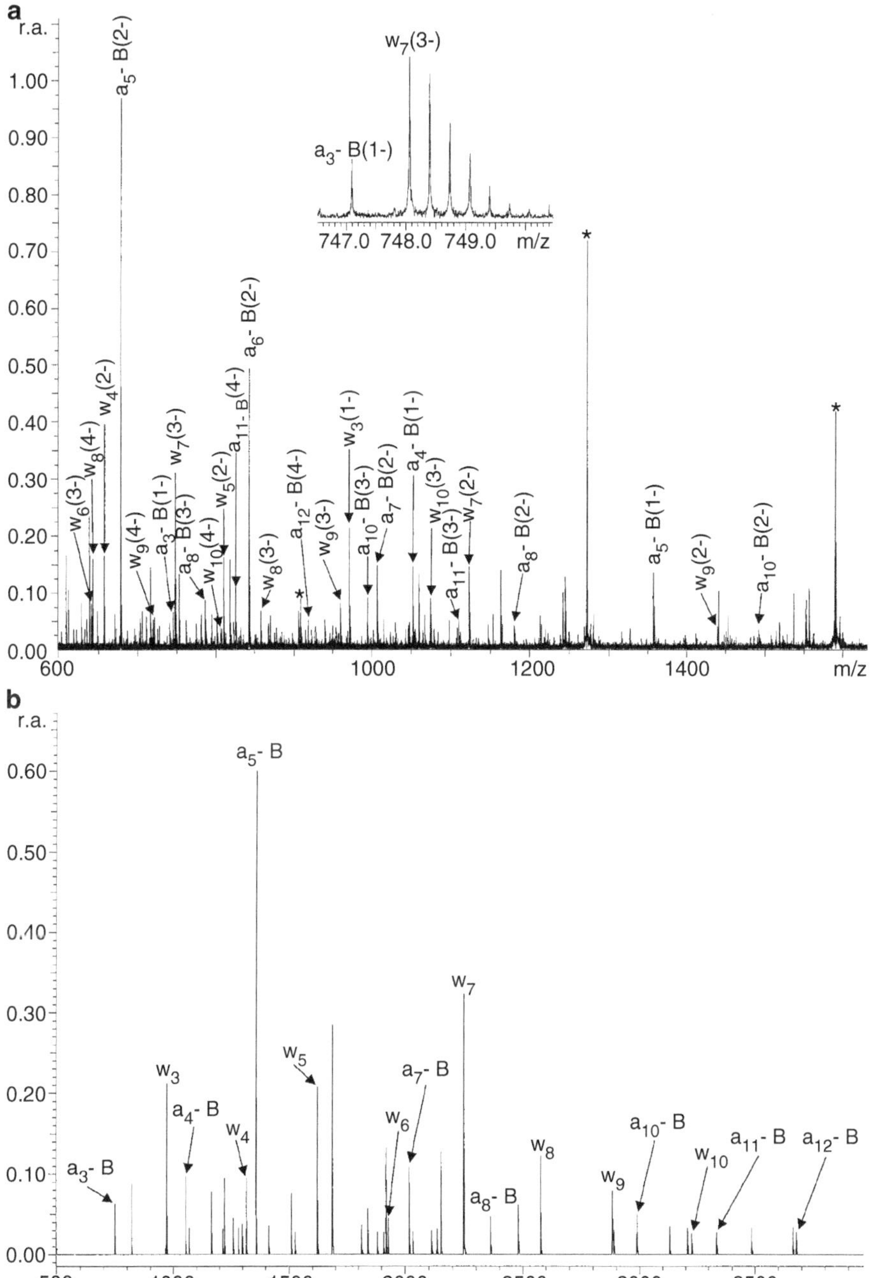

Fig. 12.36 ESI-FT-ICR IRMPD spectrum of negative ions of the phosphorothioate deoxyoligonucleotide 5′-GCCCAAGCTGGCATCCGTCA-3′. (**a**) The mass spectrum as obtained and (**b**) after charge deconvolution. Only the a_n-B and w_n fragment ions are labeled. In (**a**) peaks corresponding to residual precursor ions are labeled with an asterisk. The *inset* shows that closely spaced fragment ions can be resolved by FT-ICR-MS (Adapted from Ref. [169] with permission. © Elsevier, 2003)

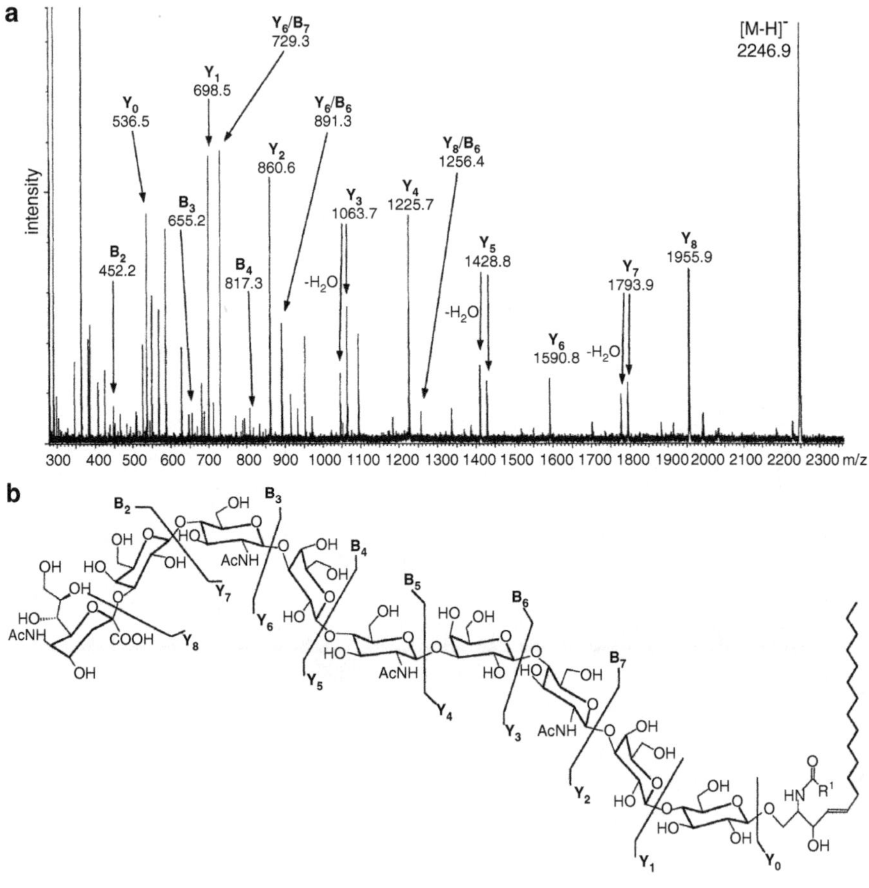

Fig. 12.37 (**a**) NanoESI-CID-MS/MS spectrum of the [M–H]$^-$ ion, *m/z* 2246.9, of a modified nonasaccharide obtained in a Q-TOF hybrid instrument and (**b**) proposed structure with fragments indicated (Reproduced from Ref. [175] by permission. © Elservier Science, 2001)

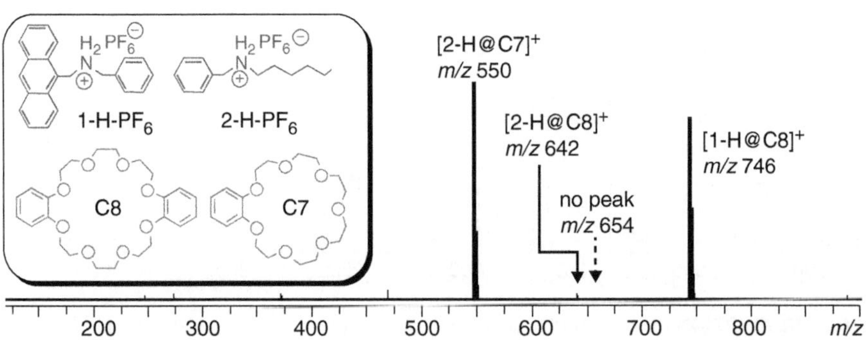

Fig. 12.38 Electrospray-ionization Fourier-transform ion-cyclotron-resonance (ESI-FT-ICR) mass spectrum of an equimolar mixture of **1**-H·PF6, **2**-H·PF6, **C7**, and **C8** in dichloromethane and their chemical structures (*inset*) (Reproduced from Ref. [178] with permission. © American Chemical Society, 2008)

[**2**-H@**C8**]+ is just visible at *m*/*z* 642. **1**-H+ and **C7,** in contrast, do not join into a complex as indicated by the missing peak at *m*/*z* 654.

12.6.7 High-Mass Proteins and Protein Complexes

The extraordinary high-mass capabilities of ESI allow for the analysis of proteins and protein complexes far beyond 10^6 u (>1 MDa) [14, 15, 21, 176, 177]. Even though the resulting ions are formed in very high charge states special mass analyzers with an expanded *m*/*z* range are required for this type of research.

Ions of 1 Mu The gram-negative spiral bacterium *Helicobacter pylori* is infecting almost half of the world's population. *H. pylori* possesses a very large multi-protein complex urease, which is essential for its survival in the acidic environment of the stomach. NanoESI has been used to establish the molecular weight of the 12-mer urease complex of 1,063,900 ± 600 u (Fig. 12.39) [15]. Spraying urease at higher

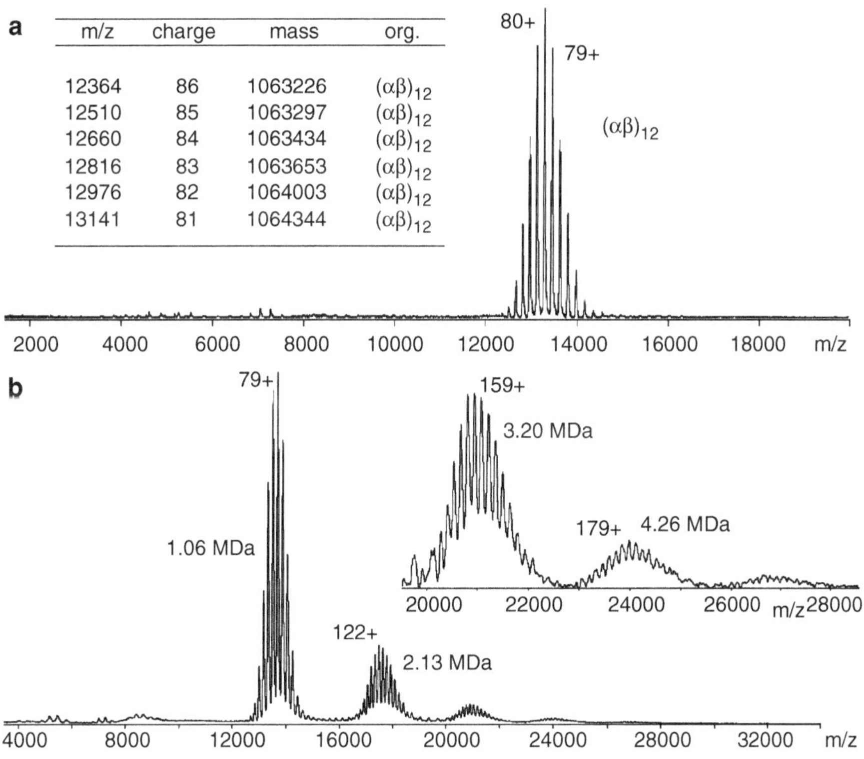

Fig. 12.39 NanoESI spectra of urease in 200 μM ammonium acetate at pH 8.0. (**a**) Using 20 μM urease mainly delivers $(\alpha\beta)_{12}$ subunits while (**b**) 40 μM concentration of the urease monomer also yield 24-, 36-, and even 48-mers (Adapted from Ref. [15] with permission. © Wiley Periodicals, Inc., 2004)

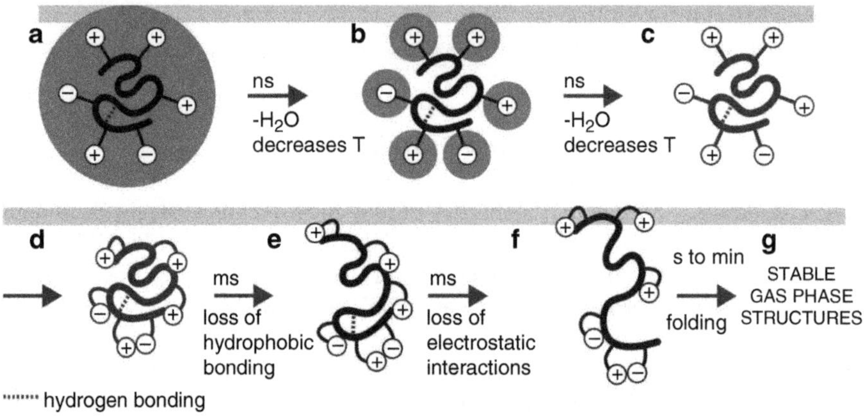

Fig. 12.40 Stepwise protein desolvation ($A \rightarrow C$), denaturization to an exterior-collapsed structure (D) and refolding to a stable gas-phase structure ($D \rightarrow G$) in transit from native solution phase to gas phase (Reproduced from Ref. [177] with permission. © The National Academy of Sciences of the USA, 2008)

concentration results in the formation of even larger protein complexes up to 48-mers of >4 Mu that are detected at up to about *m/z* 27,000 corresponding to charge states of >180+.

The question of whether or not proteins preserve their solution structure during ESI-MS has been addressed by Breuker and McLafferty [177]. According to their discussion, a protein ion loses the last hundred or so water molecules that are forming a monolayer around it during the very last steps of ion desolvation on the nanosecond timescale. The loss of water is accompanied by strong cooling of the protein ion, which finally collapses within several picoseconds as its exterior ionic interactions have been lost. Then, much slower during several milliseconds, the protein undergoes loss of hydrophobic bonding and of electrostatic interactions before it stabilizes over seconds to a final gas-phase conformation that is different from its native structure in solution. Due to the limited life time of the ions in normal ESI operation only the steps down to the cold exterior-collapsed structure can take place (Fig. 12.40).

12.7 Electrospray Roundup

Mode of Operation

In electrospray ionization an electrolytic solution is dissipated at atmospheric pressure by means of an electrostatic field to form an electrically charged aerosol. Aerosol formation is normally supported by a nebulizer gas (pneumatically-assisted ESI). Ions present in the charged droplets are liberated into the gas phase along a sequence of repeated droplet shrinking and droplet disintegration. During these steps, the mixture comprising gas, ions, and residual microdroplets is continuously transferred from the open atmosphere into the vacuum of the mass analyzer by

Table 12.1 Ions formed by ESI

Analytes	Positive ions	Negative ions
Low polarity	$[M+H]^+$, $[M+cat]^+$ if any at all[a]	$[M-H]^-$, $[M+an]^-$ if any at all[a]
Medium polarity	$[M+H]^+$, $[M+cat]^+$, $[M+alkali]^{+a}$	$[M-H]^-$, $[M+an]^{-a}$
Medium to high polarity	$[M+H]^+$, $[M+cat]^+$, $[M+alkali]^{+a}$ *exchange* $[M-H_n+alkali_{n+1}]^+$ {*clusters* $[2M+H]^+$, $[2M+alkali]^+$, *adducts* $[M+solv+H]^+$, $[M+solv+alkali]^+$}[c]	$[M-H]^-$, $[M+an]^{-a}$ *exchange* $[M-H_n+alkali_{n-1}]^-$ {*clusters* $[2M-H]^-$ *adducts* $[M+solv-H]^-$}[c]
Ionic[b]	C^+, $[C_n+A_{n-1}]^+$	A^-, $[C_{n-1}+A_n]^-$

[a]Some cation cat^+ or anion an^- incidentally present
[b]Comprising analyte cation C^+ and analyte anion A^-
[c]Braces denote less abundant species

means of an interface employing differential pumping stages. ESI is extremely soft as there is no ionization process involved that could impart energy on analyte molecules.

Analytes Suitable for Electrospray

As a general rule, ESI-MS can successfully be applied when the analyte is intrinsically ionic or can easily be transformed in solution phase to become ionic by protonation, deprotonation, cation attachment, or anion attachment. Thus, ESI can handle medium polar to ionic analytes from as low as 10 u to as high as 10^6 u in mass. ESI can deal equally well with ions of both polarities, whereas neutral nonpolar analytes are not suitable (Table 12.1).

The solvent may vary from volatile, nonpolar, and aprotic to moderately volatile, highly polar, and protic, e.g., diethylether, tetrahydrofuran, dichloromethane, trichloromethane, isopropanol, methanol, acetonitrile, water, and mixtures of these. Up to about 10% of dimethylsulfoxide or dimethylformamide can be tolerated in aqueous or methanolic solution. The addition of volatile acids or bases to promote ion formation is frequently employed. Volatile buffers and low concentrations of alkali ions ($<10^{-3}$ M) to promote cationization can be tolerated.

As a rule of thumb, less volatile solvents call for more sheath (nebulizer) gas (typical range is 1–3 l min^{-1}) and higher temperature of the desolvation gas or heated capillary (typical range is 150–250 °C), respectively. Both, insufficient desolvation and too strong desolvation will cause the ion formation to cease.

Types of Ions in ESI

Very similar to the previously introduced desorption methods ESI produces a variety of ions depending on the polarity of the analyte, the characteristics of the solvent, and on the presence or absence of impurities such as alkali metal or ammonium ions, for example. Radical ions are normally not observed (Table 12.1).

Sample Consumption

Sample consumption is chiefly determined by the concentration of the analyte solution and the liquid flow. For example, during a 1-min measurement conventional ESI consumes 4 pmol of sample when a 10^{-6} M solution is delivered at a flow of 4 μl min^{-1}. For nanoESI this reduces to 40 fmol for the same solution at 40 nl min^{-1}. Modern instruments have notably lower sample consumption, because recent interfaces transmit a much larger fraction of ions into the mass analyzer. Thus, while being operated at the same flow, very short acquisition times result in low volumes of sample solution.

Mass Analyzers for ESI

ESI and all other API sources are available in combination with all types of mass analyzers, i.e., basically one can choose any mass analyzer according to the analytical requirements. As fragment ions in ESI are often absent or at least exhibit very low abundance, analyzers capable of tandem MS and/or accurate mass measurement are preferred to provide an additional source of mass spectral information.

Comparison of ESI to APCI and APPI

The importance of ESI for LC-MS can be inferred from its wide range of analyte acceptance in terms of both polarity and mass. A graphical representation of the molecular weight and analyte polarity ranges covered by ESI, APCI, and APPI is best suited to give and impression of the preferred fields of application for these methods (Fig. 12.41). APCI and APPI, on the other hand, are very similar in coverage as both are accessing the lower left segment of the polarity-mass plane

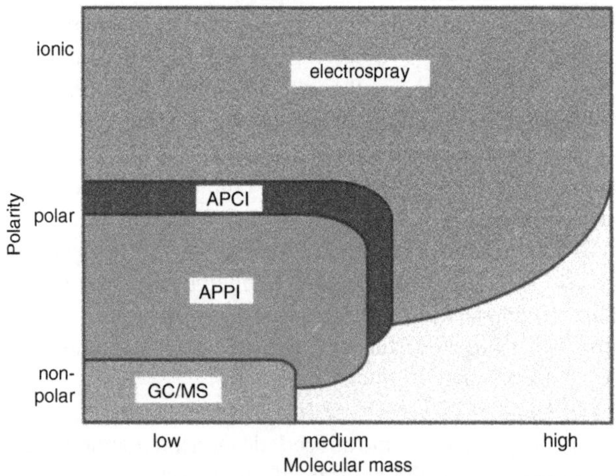

Fig. 12.41 ESI features a wide range of analyte acceptance in terms of both polarity and mass to handle medium polar to ionic analytes while APCI and APPI give access to the lower left segment of the polarity-mass plane (Adapted with permission of U. Karst from cover illustration of *Anal Bioanal Chem* 378(4), 2004. © Springer, Heidelberg, 2004)

in this illustration. APCI and APPI were discussed in the context of chemical ionization in Sects. 7.8 and 7.9.

References

1. Rossi DT, Sinz MW (eds) (2002) Mass Spectrometry in Drug Discovery. Marcel Dekker, New York
2. Schalley CA (ed) (2003) Modern Mass Spectrometry. Springer, New York
3. Ardrey RE (2003) Liquid Chromatography-Mass Spectrometry – An Introduction. Wiley, Chichester
4. Siuzdak G (2006) The Expanding Role of Mass Spectrometry in Biotechnology. MCC Press, San Diego
5. Lehmann WD (1996) Massenspektrometrie in der Biochemie. Spektrum Akademischer Verlag, Heidelberg
6. Dole RB (ed) (1997) Electrospray Ionization Mass Spectrometry – Fundamentals, Instrumentation and Applications. Wiley, Chichester. doi:10.17226/5702
7. Roboz J (1999) Mass Spectrometry in Cancer Research. CRC Press, Boca Raton. doi:10.1089/apc.1999.13.57
8. Chapman JR (ed) (2000) Mass Spectrometry of Proteins and Peptides. Humana Press, Totowa
9. Pramanik BN, Ganguly AK, Gross ML (eds) (2002) Applied Electrospray Mass Spectrometry. Marcel Dekker, New York
10. Cole RB (ed) (2010) Electrospray and MALDI Mass Spectrometry: Fundamentals, Instrumentation, Practicalities, and Biological Applications. Wiley, Hoboken
11. Lehmann WD (2010) Protein Phosphorylation Analysis by Electrospray Mass Spectrometry: A Guide to Concepts and Practice. Royal Society of Chemistry, Cambridge. doi:10.1007/s00265-010-1026-9
12. Amad MH, Cech NB, Jackson GS, Enke CG (2000) Importance of Gas-Phase Proton Affinities in Determining the Electrospray Ionization Response for Analytes and Solvents. J Mass Spectrom 35:784–789. doi:10.1002/1096-9888(200007)35:7<784::AID-JMS17>3.0.CO;2-Q
13. Schalley CA (2000) Supramolecular Chemistry Goes Gas Phase: The Mass Spectrometric Examination of Noncovalent Interactions in Host-Guest Chemistry and Molecular Recognition. Int J Mass Spectrom 194:11–39. doi:10.1016/S1387-3806(99)00243-2
14. Cristoni S, Bernardi LR (2003) Development of New Methodologies for the Mass Spectrometry Study of Bioorganic Macromolecules. Mass Spectrom Rev 22:369–406. doi:10.1002/mas.10062
15. Heck AJR, van den Heuvel RHH (2004) Investigation of Intact Protein Complexes by Mass Spectrometry. Mass Spectrom Rev 23:368–389. doi:10.1002/mas.10081
16. Fenn JB, Mann M, Meng CK, Wong SF, Whithouse CM (1989) Electrospray Ionization for Mass Spectrometry of Large Biomolecules. Science 246:64–71. doi:10.1126/science.2675315
17. Fenn JB, Mann M, Meng CK, Wong SF (1990) Electrospray Ionization – Principles and Practice. Mass Spectrom Rev 9:37–70. doi:10.1002/mas.1280090103
18. Smith RD, Loo JA, Edmonds CG, Barinaga CJ, Udseth HR (1990) New Developments in Biochemical Mass Spectrometry: Electrospray Ionization. Anal Chem 62:882–899. doi:10.1021/ac00208a002
19. Fenn JB (2003) Electrospray: Wings for Molecular Elephants (Nobel Lecture). Angew Chem, Int Ed 42:3871–3894. doi:10.1002/anie.200300605
20. Fuerstenau SD, Benner WH (1995) Molecular Weight Determination of Megadalton DNA Electrospray Ions Using Charge Detection Time-of-Flight Mass Spectrometry. Rapid Commun Mass Spectrom 9:1528–1538. doi:10.1002/rcm.1290091513

21. Fuerstenau SD, Benner WH, Thomas JJ, Brugidou C, Bothner B, Suizdak G (2001) Mass Spectrometry of an Intact Virus. Angew Chem Int Ed 40:541–544. doi:10.1002/1521-3773(20010202)40:3<541::AID-ANIE541>3.0.CO;2-K
22. Felitsyn N, Peschke M, Kebarle P (2002) Origin and Number of Charges Observed on Multiply-Protonated Native Proteins Produced by ESI. Int J Mass Spectrom 219:39–62. doi:10.1016/S1387-3806(02)00588-2
23. Colton R, D'Agostino A, Traeger JC (1995) Electrospray Mass Spectrometry Applied to Inorganic and Organometallic Chemistry. Mass Spectrom Rev 14:79–106. doi:10.1002/mas.1280140203
24. Traeger JC (2000) Electrospray Mass Spectrometry of Organometallic Compounds. Int J Mass Spectrom 200:387–401. doi:10.1016/S1387-3806(00)00346-8
25. Henderson W, McIndoe SJ (2005) Mass Spectrometry of Inorganic and Organometallic Compounds. Wiley, Chichester. doi:10.1002/cfg.467
26. Poon GK, Bisset GMF, Mistry P (1993) Electrospray Ionization Mass Spectrometry for Analysis of Low-Molecular-Weight Anticancer Drugs and Their Analogs. J Am Soc Mass Spectrom 4:588–595. doi:10.1016/1044-0305(93)85020-X
27. Winger BE, Light-Wahl KJ, Ogorzalek Loo RR, Udseth HR, Smith RD (1993) Observation and Implications of High Mass-to-Charge Ratio Ions from Electrospray Ionization Mass Spectrometry. J Am Soc Mass Spectrom 4:536–545. doi:10.1016/1044-0305(93)85015-P
28. Wang Y, Schubert M, Ingendoh A, Franzen J (2000) Analysis of Non-Covalent Protein Complexes Up to 290 kDa Using Electrospray Ionization and Ion Trap Mass Spectrometry. Rapid Commun Mass Spectrom 14:12–17. doi:10.1002/(SICI)1097-0231(20000115)14:1<12::AID-RCM825>3.0.CO;2-7
29. Sobott F, Hernández H, McCammon MG, Tito MA, Robinson CV (2002) A Tandem Mass Spectrometer for Improved Transmission and Analysis of Large Macromolecular Assemblies. Anal Chem 74:1402–1407. doi:10.1021/ac0110552
30. Covey TR, Thomson BA, Schneider BB (2009) Atmospheric Pressure Ion Sources. Mass Spectrom Rev 28:870–897. doi:10.1002/mas.20246
31. Horning EC, Horning MG, Carroll DI, Dzidic I, Stillwell RN (1973) New Picogram Detection System Based on a Mass Spectrometer with an External Ionization Source at Atmospheric Pressure. Anal Chem 45:936–943. doi:10.1021/ac60328a035
32. Horning EC, Carroll DI, Dzidic I, Haegele KD, Horning MG, Stillwell RN (1974) Atmospheric Pressure Ionization (API) Mass Spectrometry. Solvent-Mediated Ionization of Samples Introduced in Solution and in a Liquid Chromatograph Effluent Stream. J Chromatogr Sci 12:725–729. doi:10.1093/chromsci/12.11.725
33. Robb DB, Covey TR, Bruins AP (2000) Atmospheric Pressure Photoionization: an Ionization Method for Liquid Chromatography-Mass Spectrometry. Anal Chem 72:3653–3659. doi:10.1021/ac0001636
34. Blakley CR, Carmody JJ, Vestal ML (1980) A New Soft Ionization Technique for Mass Spectrometry of Complex Molecules. J Am Chem Soc 102:5931–5933. doi:10.1021/ja00538a050
35. Blakley CR, Vestal ML (1983) Thermospray Interface for Liquid Chromatography/Mass Spectrometry. Anal Chem 55:750–754. doi:10.1021/ac00255a036
36. Vestal ML (1983) Studies of Ionization Mechanisms Involved in Thermospray LC-MS. Int J Mass Spectrom Ion Phys 46:193–196. doi:10.1016/0020-7381(83)80086-2
37. Wilkes JG, Freeman JP, Heinze TM, Lay JO Jr, Vestal ML (1995) AC Corona-Discharge Aerosol-Neutralization Device Adapted to Liquid Chromatography/Particle Beam/Mass Spectrometry. Rapid Commun Mass Spectrom 9:138–142. doi:10.1002/rcm.1290090207
38. Vestal ML (1984) High-Performance Liquid Chromatography-Mass Spectrometry. Science 226:275–281. doi:10.1126/science.6385251
39. Evans CA Jr, Hendricks CD (1972) Electrohydrodynamic Ion Source for the Mass Spectrometry of Liquids. Rev Sci Inst 43:1527–1530. doi:10.1063/1.1685481

40. Simons DS, Colby BN, Evans CA Jr (1974) Electrohydrodynamic Ionization Mass Spectrometry. Ionization of Liquid Glycerol and Nonvolatile Organic Solutes. Int J Mass Spectrom Ion Phys 15:291–302. doi:10.1016/0020-7381(74)85006-0
41. Zeleny J (1917) Instability of Electrified Liquid Surfaces. Phys Rev 10:1–7. doi:10.1103/PhysRev.10.1
42. Taylor GI (1964) Disintegration of Water Drops in an Electric Field. Proc Royal Soc London A 280:383–397. doi:10.1098/rspa.1964.0151
43. Rayleigh L (1882) On the Equilibrium of Liquid Conducting Masses Charged with Electricity. Dublin Phil Mag J Sci (London/Edinburgh) 14:184–186. doi:10.1080/14786448208628425
44. Dülcks T, Röllgen FW (1995) Ionization Conditions and Ion Formation in Electrohydrodynamic Mass Spectrometry. Int J Mass Spectrom Ion Proc 148:123–144. doi:10.1016/0168-1176(95)04250-O
45. Dülcks T, Röllgen FW (1995) Ion Source for Electrohydrodynamic Mass Spectrometry. J Mass Spectrom 30:324–332. doi:10.1002/jms.1190300215
46. Cook KD (1986) Electrohydrodynamic Mass Spectrometry. Mass Spectrom Rev 5:467–519. doi:10.1002/mas.1280050404
47. Dole M, Mack LL, Hines RL, Mobley RC, Ferguson LD, Alice MB (1968) Molecular Beams of Macroions. J Chem Phys 49:2240–2249. doi:10.1063/1.1670391
48. Dole M, Hines RL, Mack LL, Mobley RC, Ferguson LD, Alice MB (1968) Gas Phase Macroions. Macromolecules 1:96–97. doi:10.1021/ma60001a017
49. Gieniec J, Mack LL, Nakamae K, Gupta C, Kumar V, Dole M (1984) Electrospray Mass Spectroscopy of Macromolecules: Application of an Ion-Drift Spectrometer. Biomed Mass Spectrom 11:259–268. doi:10.1002/bms.1200110602
50. Yamashita M, Fenn JB (1984) Electrospray Ion Source. Another Variation on the Free-Jet Theme. J Phys Chem 88:4451–4459. doi:10.1021/j150664a002
51. Yamashita M, Fenn JB (1984) Negative Ion Production with the Electrospray Ion Source. J Phys Chem 88:4671–4675. doi:10.1021/j150664a046
52. Whitehouse CM, Robert RN, Yamashita M, Fenn JB (1985) Electrospray Interface for Liquid Chromatographs and Mass Spectrometers. Anal Chem 57:675–679. doi:10.1021/ac00280a023
53. Bruins AP (1991) Mass Spectrometry with Ion Sources Operating at Atmospheric Pressure. Mass Spectrom Rev 10:53–77. doi:10.1002/mas.1280100104
54. Kebarle P, Tang L (1993) From Ions in Solution to Ions in the Gas Phase – The Mechanism of Electrospray Mass Spectrometry. Anal Chem 65:972A–986A. doi:10.1021/ac00070a001
55. Karas M, Bahr U, Dülcks T (2001) Nano-Electrospray Ionization Mass Spectrometry: Addressing Analytical Problems Beyond Routine. Fresenius J Anal Chem 366:669–676. doi:10.1007/s002160051561
56. Anacleto JF, Pleasance S, Boyd RK (1992) Calibration of Ion Spray Mass Spectra Using Cluster Ions. Org Mass Spectrom 27:660–666. doi:10.1002/oms.1210270603
57. Hop CECA (1996) Generation of High Molecular Weight Cluster Ions by Electrospray Ionization; Implications for Mass Calibration. J Mass Spectrom 31:1314–1316. doi:10.1002/(SICI)1096-9888(199611)31:11<1314::AID-JMS429>3.0.CO;2-N
58. Kantrowitz A, Grey J (1951) High Intensity Source for the Molecular Beam. I. Theoretical. Rev Sci Inst 22:328–332. doi:10.1063/1.1745921
59. Fenn JB (2000) Mass Spectrometric Implications of High-Pressure Ion Sources. Int J Mass Spectrom 200:459–478. doi:10.1016/S1387-3806(00)00328-6
60. Klee S, Derpmann V, Wissdorf W, Klopotowski S, Kersten H, Brockmann KJ, Benter T, Albrecht S, Bruins AP, Dousty F, Kauppila TJ, Kostiainen R, O'Brien R, Robb DB, Syage JA (2014) Are Clusters Important in Understanding the Mechanisms in Atmospheric Pressure Ionization? Part 1: Reagent Ion Generation and Chemical Control of Ion Populations. J Am Soc Mass Spectrom 25:1310–1321. doi:10.1007/s13361-014-0891-2

61. Bruins AP, Covey TR, Henion JD (1987) Ion Spray Interface for Combined Liquid Chromatography/Atmospheric Pressure Ionization Mass Spectrometry. Anal Chem 59:2642–2646. doi:10.1021/ac00149a003
62. Covey TR, Bruins AP, Henion JD (1988) Comparison of Thermospray and Ion Spray Mass Spectrometry in an Atmospheric Pressure Ion Source. Org Mass Spectrom 23:178–186. doi:10.1002/oms.1210230305
63. Covey TR, Bonner RF, Shushan BI, Henion JD (1988) The Determination of Protein, Oligonucleotide, and Peptide Molecular Weights by Ion-Spray Mass Spectrometry. Rapid Commun Mass Spectrom 2:249–256. doi:10.1002/rcm.1290021111
64. Ikonomou MG, Blades AT, Kebarle P (1991) Electrospray – Ion Spray: A Comparison of Mechanisms and Performance. Anal Chem 63:1989–1998. doi:10.1021/ac00018a017
65. Smith RD, Barinaga CJ, Udseth HR (1988) Improved Electrospray Ionization Interface for Capillary Zone Electrophoresis-Mass Spectrometry. Anal Chem 60:1948–1952. doi:10.1021/ac00169a022
66. Abian J (1999) The Coupling of Gas and Liquid Chromatography with Mass Spectrometry. J Mass Spectrom 34:157–168. doi:10.1002/(SICI)1096-9888(199903)34:3<157::AID-JMS804>3.0.CO;2-4
67. Shaffer SA, Tang K, Anderson GA, Prior DC, Udseth HR, Smith RD (1997) A Novel Ion Funnel for Focusing Ions at Elevated Pressure Using Electrospray Ionization Mass Spectrometry. Rapid Commun Mass Spectrom 11:1813–1817. doi:10.1002/(SICI)1097-0231(19971030)11:16<1813::AID-RCM87>3.0.CO;2-D
68. Shaffer SA, Prior DC, Anderson GA, Udseth HR, Smith RD (1998) An Ion Funnel Interface for Improved Ion Focusing and Sensitivity Using Electrospray Ionization Mass Spectrometry. Anal Chem 70:4111–4119. doi:10.1021/ac9802170
69. Kim T, Tolmachev AV, Harkewicz R, Prior DC, Anderson G, Udseth HR, Smith RD, Bailey TH, Rakov S, Futrell JH (2000) Design and Implementation of a New Electrodynamic Ion Funnel. Anal Chem 72:2247–2255. doi:10.1021/ac991412x
70. Ibrahim Y, Belov ME, Tolmachev AV, Prior DC, Smith RD (2007) Ion Funnel Trap Interface for Orthogonal Time-of-Flight Mass Spectrometry. Anal Chem 79:7845–7852. doi:10.1021/ac071091m
71. Ibrahim YM, Belov ME, Liyu AV, Smith RD (2008) Automated Gain Control Ion Funnel Trap for Orthogonal Time-of-Flight Mass Spectrometry. Anal Chem 80:5367–5376. doi:10.1021/ac8003488
72. Smith RD, Loo JA, Barinaga CJ, Edmonds CG, Udseth HR (1990) Collisional Activation and Collision-Activated Dissociation of Large Multiply Charged Polypeptides and Proteins Produced by Electrospray Ionization. J Am Soc Mass Spectrom 1:53–65. doi:10.1016/1044-0305(90)80006-9
73. Harvey DJ (2000) Collision-Induced Fragmentation of Underivatized *N*-Linked Carbohydrates Ionized by Electrospray. J Mass Spectrom 35:1178–1190. doi:10.1002/1096-9888(200010)35:10<1178::AID-JMS46>3.0.CO;2-F
74. Schmidt A, Bahr U, Karas M (2001) Influence of Pressure in the First Pumping Stage on Analyte Desolvation and Fragmentation in Nano-ESI MS. Anal Chem 71:6040–6046. doi:10.1021/ac010451h
75. Jedrzejewski PT, Lehmann WD (1997) Detection of Modified Peptides in Enzymatic Digests by Capillary Liquid Chromatography/Electrospray Mass Spectrometry and a Programmable Skimmer CID Acquisition Routine. Anal Chem 69:294–301. doi:10.1021/ac9606618
76. Weinmann W, Stoertzel M, Vogt S, Svoboda M, Schreiber A (2001) Tuning Compounds for Electrospray Ionization/in-Source Collision-Induced Dissociation and Mass Spectra Library Searching. J Mass Spectrom 36:1013–1023. doi:10.1002/jms.201
77. Huddleston MJ, Bean MF, Carr SA (1993) Collisional Fragmentation of Glycopeptides by Electrospray Ionization LC/MS and LC/MS/MS: Methods for Selective Detection of Glycopeptides in Protein Digests. Anal Chem 65:877–884. doi:10.1021/ac00055a009

78. Chen H, Tabei K, Siegel MM (2001) Biopolymer Sequencing Using a Triple Quadrupole Mass Spectrometer in the ESI Nozzle-Skimmer/Precursor Ion MS/MS Mode. J Am Soc Mass Spectrom 12:846–852. doi:10.1016/S1044-0305(01)00258-6
79. Hoogland FG, Boon JJ (2009) Development of MALDI-MS and Nano-ESI-MS Methodology for the Full Identification of Poly(ethylene glycol) Additives in Artists' Acrylic Paints. Int J Mass Spectrom 284:66–71. doi:10.1016/j.ijms.2009.03.002
80. Miao X-S, Metcalfe CD (2003) Determination of Carbamazepine and Its Metabolites in Aqueous Samples Using Liquid Chromatography-Electrospray Tandem Mass Spectrometry. Anal Chem 75:3731–3738. doi:10.1021/ac030082k
81. Gross JH, Eckert A, Siebert W (2002) Negative-Ion Electrospray Mass Spectra of Carbon Dioxide-Protected *N*-Heterocyclic Anions. J Mass Spectrom 37:541–543. doi:10.1002/jms.302
82. Wilm MS, Mann M (1994) Electrospray and Taylor-Cone Theory, Dole's Beam of Macromolecules at Last? Int J Mass Spectrom Ion Proc 136:167–180. doi:10.1016/0168-1176(94)04024-9
83. Wilm M, Mann M (1996) Analytical Properties of the Nanoelectrospray Ion Source. Anal Chem 68:1–8. doi:10.1021/ac9509519
84. Wilm M, Shevshenko A, Houthaeve T, Breit S, Schweigerer L, Fotsis T, Mann M (1996) Femtomole Sequencing of Proteins from Polyacrylamide Gels by Nano-Electrospray Mass Spectrometry. Nature 379:466–469. doi:10.1038/379466a0
85. Juraschek R, Dülcks T, Karas M (1999) Nanoelectrospray – More Than Just a Minimized-Flow Electrospray Ionization Source. J Am Soc Mass Spectrom 10:300–308. doi:10.1016/S1044-0305(98)00157-3
86. Guo M, Huang BX, Kim HY (2009) Conformational Changes in Akt1 Activation Probed by Amide Hydrogen/Deuterium Exchange and Nano-Electrospray Ionization Mass Spectrometry. Rapid Commun Mass Spectrom 23:1885–1891. doi:10.1002/rcm.4085
87. Gibson GTT, Mugo SM, Oleschuk RD (2009) Nanoelectrospray Emitters: Trends and Perspective. Mass Spectrom Rev 28:918–936. doi:10.1002/mas.20248
88. Valaskovic GA, Murphy JP, Lee MS (2004) Automated Orthogonal Control System for Electrospray Ionization. J Am Soc Mass Spectrom 15:1201–1215. doi:10.1016/j.jasms.2004.04.033
89. Kebarle P, Verkerk UH (2009) Electrospray: From Ions in Solution to Ions in the Gas Phase, What We Know Now. Mass Spectrom Rev 28:898–917. doi:10.1002/mas.20247
90. Cole RB (2000) Some Tenets Pertaining to Electrospray Ionization Mass Spectrometry. J Mass Spectrom 35:763–772. doi:10.1002/1096-9888(200007)35:7<763::AID-JMS16>3.0.CO;2-%23
91. Kebarle P (2000) A Brief Overview of the Present Status of the Mechanisms Involved in Electrospray Mass Spectrometry. J Mass Spectrom 35:804–817. doi:10.1002/1096-9888(200007)35:7<804::AID-JMS22>3.0.CO;2-Q
92. Marginean I, Nemes P, Parvin L, Vertes A (2006) How Much Charge Is There on a Pulsating Taylor Cone? Appl Phys Lett 89:064104-1-064104/3. doi:10.1063/1.2266889
93. Nemes P, Marginean I, Vertes A (2007) Spraying Mode Effect on Droplet Formation and Ion Chemistry in Electrosprays. Anal Chem 79:3105–3116. doi:10.1021/ac062382i
94. de la Mora JF, Van Berkel GJ, Enke CG, Cole RB, Martinez-Sanchez M, Fenn JB (2000) Electrochemical Processes in Electrospray Ionization Mass Spectrometry. J Mass Spectrom 35:939–952. doi:10.1002/1096-9888(200008)35:8<939::AID-JMS36>3.0.CO;2-V
95. Van Berkel GJ (2000) Electrolytic Deposition of Metals on to the High-Voltage Contact in an Electrospray Emitter: Implications for Gas-Phase Ion Formation. J Mass Spectrom 35:773–783. doi:10.1002/1096-9888(200007)35:7<773::AID-JMS4>3.0.CO;2-6
96. Schäfer M, Drayue M, Springer A, Zacharias P, Meerholz K (2007) Radical Cations in Electrospray Mass Spectrometry: Formation of Open-Shell Species, Examination of the Fragmentation Behavior in ESI-MS^n and Reaction Mechanism Studies by Detection of Transient Radical Cations. Eur J Org Chem 2007:5162–5174. doi:10.1002/ejoc.200700199

97. Gomez A, Tang K (1994) Charge and Fission of Droplets in Electrostatic Sprays. Phys Fluids 6:404–414. doi:10.1063/1.868037
98. Duft D, Achtzehn T, Müller R, Huber BA, Leisner T (2003) Coulomb Fission. Rayleigh Jets from Levitated Microdroplets. Nature 421:128. doi:10.1038/421128a
99. Grimm RL, Beauchamp JL (2005) Dynamics of Field-Induced Droplet Ionization: Time-Resolved Studies of Distortion, Jetting, and Progeny Formation from Charged and Neutral Methanol Droplets Exposed to Strong Electric Fields. J Phys Chem B 109:8244–8250. doi:10.1021/jp0450540
100. Mack LL, Kralik P, Rheude A, Dole M (1970) Molecular Beams of Macroions, II. J Chem Phys 52:4977–4986. doi:10.1063/1.1672733
101. Iribarne JV, Thomson BA (1976) On the Evaporation of Small Ions from Charged Droplets. J Chem Phys 64:2287–2294. doi:10.1063/1.432536
102. Thomson BA, Iribarne JV (1979) Field-Induced Ion Evaporation from Liquid Surfaces at Atmospheric Pressure. J Chem Phys 71:4451–4463. doi:10.1063/1.438198
103. Labowsky M, Fenn JB, de la Mora JF (2000) A Continuum Model for Ion Evaporation from a Drop: Effect of Curvature and Charge on Ion Solvation Energy. Anal Chim Acta 406:105–118. doi:10.1016/S0003-2670(99)00595-4
104. Fenn JB (1993) Ion Formation from Charged Droplets: Roles of Geometry, Energy, and Time. J Am Soc Mass Spectrom 4:524–535. doi:10.1016/1044-0305(93)85014-O
105. Fenn JB, Rosell J, Meng CK (1997) In Electrospray Ionization, How Much Pull Does an Ion Need to Escape Its Droplet Prison? J Am Soc Mass Spectrom 8:1147–1157. doi:10.1016/S1044-0305(97)00161-X
106. Loo JA, Edmonds CG, Udseth HR, Smith RD (1990) Effect of Reducing Disulfide-Containing Proteins on Electrospray Ionization Mass Spectra. Anal Chem 62:693–698. doi:10.1021/ac00206a009
107. Chowdhury SK, Katta V, Chait BT (1990) Probing Conformational Changes in Proteins by Mass Spectrometry. J Am Chem Soc 112:9012–9013. doi:10.1021/ja00180a074
108. Nemes P, Goyal S, Vertes A (2008) Conformational and Noncovalent Complexation Changes in Proteins During Electrospray Ionization. Anal Chem 80:387–395. doi:10.1021/ac0714359
109. Schmelzeisen-Redeker G, Bütfering L, Röllgen FW (1989) Desolvation of Ions and Molecules in Thermospray Mass Spectrometry. Int J Mass Spectrom Ion Proc 90:139–150. doi:10.1016/0168-1176(89)85004-9
110. Williams ER (1996) Proton Transfer Reactivity of Large Multiply Charged Ions. J Mass Spectrom 31:831–842. doi:10.1002/(SICI)1096-9888(199608)31:8<831::AID-JMS392>3.0.CO;2-7
111. Iavarone AT, Jurchen JC, Williams ER (2001) Supercharged Protein and Peptide Ions Formed by Electrospray Ionization. Anal Chem 73:1455–1460. doi:10.1021/ac001251t
112. Iavarone AT, Williams ER (2002) Supercharging in Electrospray Ionization: Effects on Signal and Charge. Int J Mass Spectrom 219:63–72. doi:10.1016/S1387-3806(02)00587-0
113. Iavarone AT, Williams ER (2003) Mechanism of Charging and Supercharging Molecules in Electrospray Ionization. J Am Chem Soc 125:2319–2327. doi:10.1021/ja021202t
114. Youhnovski N, Matecko I, Samalikova M, Grandori R (2005) Characterization of Cytochrome c Unfolding by Nano-Electrospray Ionization Time-of-Flight and Fourier Transform Ion Cyclotron Resonance Mass Spectrometry. Eur J Mass Spectrom 11:519–524. doi:10.1255/ejms.730
115. Dobo A, Kaltashov IA (2001) Detection of Multiple Protein Conformational Ensembles in Solution Via Deconvolution of Charge-State Distributions in ESI-MS. Anal Chem 73:4763–4773. doi:10.1021/ac010713f
116. Chapman JR, Gallagher RT, Barton EC, Curtis JM, Derrick PJ (1992) Advantages of High-Resolution and High-Mass Range Magnetic-Sector Mass Spectrometry for Electrospray Ionization. Org Mass Spectrom 27:195–203. doi:10.1002/oms.1210270308
117. Cole RB, Harrata AK (1993) Solvent Effect on Analyte Charge State, Signal Intensity, and Stability in Negative Ion Electrospray Mass Spectrometry – Implications for the Mechanism of Negative Ion Formation. J Am Soc Mass Spectrom 4:546–556. doi:10.1016/1044-0305(93)85016-Q

118. Straub RF, Voyksner RD (1993) Negative Ion Formation in Electrospray Mass Spectrometry. J Am Soc Mass Spectrom 4:578–587. doi:10.1016/1044-0305(93)85019-T
119. Saf R, Mirtl C, Hummel K (1994) Electrospray Mass Spectrometry Using Potassium Iodide in Aprotic Organic Solvents for the Ion Formation by Cation Attachment. Tetrahedron Lett 35:6653–6656. doi:10.1016/S0040-4039(00)73459-9
120. Cody RB, Tamura J, Musselman BD (1992) Electrospray Ionization/Magnetic Sector Mass Spectrometry: Calibration, Resolution, and Accurate Mass Measurements. Anal Chem 64:1561–1570. doi:10.1021/ac00038a012
121. Mann M, Meng CK, Fenn JB (1989) Interpreting Mass Spectra of Multiply Charged Ions. Anal Chem 61:1702–1708. doi:10.1021/ac00190a023
122. Labowsky M, Whitehouse CM, Fenn JB (1993) Three-Dimensional Deconvolution of Multiply Charged Spectra. Rapid Commun Mass Spectrom 7:71–84. doi:10.1002/rcm.1290070117
123. Zhang Z, Marshall AG (1998) A Universal Algorithm for Fast and Automated Charge State Deconvolution of Electrospray Mass-to-Charge Ratio Spectra. J Am Soc Mass Spectrom 9:225–233. doi:10.1016/S1044-0305(97)00284-5
124. Maleknia SD, Downard KM (2005) Charge Ratio Analysis Method to Interpret High Resolution Electrospray Fourier Transform-Ion Cyclotron Resonance Mass Spectra. Int J Mass Spectrom 246:1–9. doi:10.1016/j.ijms.2005.08.002
125. Maleknia SD, Downard KM (2005) Charge Ratio Analysis Method: Approach for the Deconvolution of Electrospray Mass Spectra. Anal Chem 77:111–119. doi:10.1021/ac048961+
126. Lu W, Callahan JH, Fry FS, Andrzejewski D, Musser SM, Harrington PD (2011) A Discriminant Based Charge Deconvolution Analysis Pipeline for Protein Profiling of Whole Cell Extracts Using Liquid Chromatography-Electrospray Ionization-Quadrupole Time-of-Flight Mass Spectrometry. Talanta 84:1180–1187. doi:10.1016/j.talanta.2011.03.024
127. Maleknia SD, Green DC (2010) ECRAM Computer Algorithm for Implementation of the Charge Ratio Analysis Method to Deconvolute Electrospray Ionization Mass Spectra. Int J Mass Spectrom 290:1–8. doi:10.1016/j.ijms.2009.10.005
128. Winkler R (2010) ESIprot: a Universal Tool for Charge State Determination and Molecular Weight Calculation of Proteins from Electrospray Ionization Mass Spectrometry Data. Rapid Commun Mass Spectrom 24:285–294. doi:10.1002/rcm.4384
129. Wada Y (2016) Mass Spectrometry of Transferrin and Apolipoprotein C-III for Diagnosis and Screening of Congenital Disorder of Glycosylation. Glycoconjug J 33:297–307. doi:10.1007/s10719-015-9636-0
130. Dobberstein P, Schroeder E (1993) Accurate Mass Determination of a High Molecular Weight Protein Using Electrospray Ionization with a Magnetic Sector Instrument. Rapid Commun Mass Spectrom 7:861–864. doi:10.1002/rcm.1290070916
131. Haas MJ (1999) Fully Automated Exact Mass Measurements by High-Resolution Electrospray Ionization on a Sector Instrument. Rapid Commun Mass Spectrom 13:381–383. doi:10.1002/(SICI)1097-0231(19990315)13:5<381::AID-RCM495>3.0.CO;2-A
132. Hofstadler SA, Griffey RH, Pasa-Tolic R, Smith RD (1998) The Use of a Stable Internal Mass Standard for Accurate Mass Measurements of Oligonucleotide Fragment Ions Using Electrospray Ionization Fourier Transform Ion Cyclotron Resonance Mass Spectrometry with Infrared Multiphoton Dissociation. Rapid Commun Mass Spectrom 12:1400–1404. doi:10.1002/(SICI)1097-0231(19981015)12:19<1400::AID-RCM337>3.0.CO;2-T
133. Stenson AC, Landing WM, Marshall AG, Cooper WT (2002) Ionization and Fragmentation of Humic Substances in Electrospray Ionization Fourier Transform-Ion Cyclotron Resonance Mass Spectrometry. Anal Chem 74:4397–4409. doi:10.1021/ac020019f
134. Makarov A, Denisov E, Kholomeev A, Balschun W, Lange O, Strupat K, Horning S (2006) Performance Evaluation of a Hybrid Linear Ion Trap/Orbitrap Mass Spectrometer. Anal Chem 78:2113–2120. doi:10.1021/ac0518811
135. Scalf M, Westphall MS, Krause J, Kaufmann SL, Smith LM (1999) Controlling Charge States of Large Ions. Science 283:194–197. doi:10.1126/science.283.5399.194

136. Krusemark CJ, Frey BL, Belshaw PJ, Smith LM (2009) Modifying the Charge State Distribution of Proteins in Electrospray Ionization Mass Spectrometry by Chemical Derivatization. J Am Soc Mass Spectrom 20:1617–1625. doi:10.1016/j.jasms.2009.04.017
137. Scalf M, Westphall MS, Smith LM (2000) Charge Reduction Electrospray Mass Spectrometry. Anal Chem 72:52–60. doi:10.1021/ac990878c
138. Ebeling DD, Westphall MS, Scalf M, Smith LM (2000) Corona Discharge in Charge Reduction Electrospray Mass Spectrometry. Anal Chem 72:5158–5161. doi:10.1021/ac000559h
139. Ebeling DD, Scalf M, Westphall MS, Smith LM (2001) A Cylindrical Capacitor Ionization Source: Droplet Generation and Controlled Charge Reduction for Mass Spectrometry. Rapid Commun Mass Spectrom 15:401–405. doi:10.1002/rcm.245
140. McLuckey SA, Stephenson JL Jr (1998) Ion/Ion Chemistry of High-Mass Multiply Charged Ions. Mass Spectrom Rev 17:369–407. doi:10.1002/(SICI)1098-2787(1998)17:6<369::AID-MAS1>3.0.CO;2-J
141. Herron WJ, Goeringer DE, McLuckey SA (1996) Product Ion Charge State Determination Via Ion/Ion Proton Transfer Reactions. Anal Chem 68:257–262. doi:10.1021/ac950895b
142. Schalley CA (ed) (2007) Analytical Methods in Supramolecular Chemistry. Wiley-VCH, New York. doi:10.5301/EJO.2008.2975
143. Ramanathan R (ed) (2009) Mass Spectrometry in Drug Metabolism and Pharmacokinetics. Wiley, Hoboken. doi:10.1109/TNS.2009.2019110
144. Schalley CA, Springer A (2009) Mass Spectrometry and Gas-Phase Chemistry of Non-Covalent Complexes. Wiley, Hoboken. doi:10.3762/bjoc.5.76
145. Banoub JH, Limbach PA (eds) (2009) Mass Spectrometry of Nucleosides and Nucleic Acids. CRC Press, Boca Raton. doi:10.1109/TNS.2009.2019110
146. Williams TTJ, Perreault H (2000) Selective Detection of Nitrated Polycyclic Aromatic Hydrocarbons by Electrospray Ionization Mass Spectrometry and Constant Neutral Loss Scanning. Rapid Commun Mass Spectrom 14:1474–1481. doi:10.1002/1097-0231(20000830)14:16<1474::AID-RCM46>3.0.CO;2-Z
147. Zhu J, Cole RB (2000) Formation and Decompositions of Chloride Adduct Ions, $[M+Cl]^-$, in Negative Ion Electrospray Ionization Mass Spectrometry. J Am Soc Mass Spectrom 11:932–941. doi:10.1016/S1044-0305(00)00164-1
148. Yang C, Cole RB (2002) Stabilization of Anionic Adducts in Negative Ion Electrospray Mass Spectrometry. Anal Chem 74:985–991. doi:10.1021/ac0108818
149. Schalley CA, Ghosh P, Engeser M (2004) Mass Spectrometric Evidence for Catenanes and Rotaxanes from Negative-ESI FT-ICR Tandem-MS Experiments. Int J Mass Spectrom 232:249–258. doi:10.1016/j.ijms.2004.02.003
150. Truebenbach CS, Houalla M, Hercules DM (2000) Characterization of Isopoly Metal Oxyanions Using Electrospray Time-of-Flight Mass Spectrometry. J Mass Spectrom 35:1121–1127. doi:10.1002/1096-9888(200009)35:9<1121::AID-JMS40>3.0.CO;2-7
151. Choi BK, Hercules DM, Houalla M (2000) Characterization of Polyphosphates by Electrospray Mass Spectrometry. Anal Chem 72:5087–5091. doi:10.1021/ac000044q
152. Favaro S, Pandolfo L, Traldi P (1997) The Behavior of $[Pt(H^3\text{-Allyl})XP(C_6H_5)_3]$ Complexes in Electrospray Ionization Conditions Compared with Those Achieved by Other Ionization Methods. Rapid Commun Mass Spectrom 11:1859–1866. doi:10.1002/(SICI)1097-0231(199711)11:17<1859::AID-RCM973>3.0.CO;2-P
153. Feichtinger D, Plattner DA (1997) Direct Proof for Mn^V-Oxo-Salen Complexes. Angew Chem Int Ed 36:1718–1719. doi:10.1002/anie.199717181
154. Løver T, Bowmaker GA, Henderson W, Cooney RP (1996) Electrospray Mass Spectrometry of Some Cadmium Thiophenolate Complexes and of a Thiophenolate Capped CdS Cluster. Chem Commun:683–685. doi:10.1039/CC9960000683
155. Hinderling C, Feichtinger D, Plattner DA, Chen P (1997) A Combined Gas-Phase, Solution-Phase, and Computational Study of C-H Activation by Cationic Iridium(III) Complexes. J Am Chem Soc 119:10793–10804. doi:10.1021/ja970995u

156. Reid GE, O'Hair RAJ, Styles ML, McFadyen WD, Simpson RJ (1998) Gas Phase Ion-Molecule Reactions in a Modified Ion Trap: H/D Exchange of Non-Covalent Complexes and Coordinatively Unsaturated Platinum Complexes. Rapid Commun Mass Spectrom 12:1701–1708. doi:10.1002/(SICI)1097-0231(19981130)12:22<1701::AID-RCM392>3.0.CO;2-S
157. Volland MAO, Adlhart C, Kiener CA, Chen P, Hofmann P (2001) Catalyst Screening by Electrospray Ionization Tandem Mass Spectrometry: Hofmann Carbenes for Olefin Metathesis. Chem Eur J 7:4621–4632. doi:10.1002/1521-3765(20011105)7:21<4621::AID-CHEM4621>3.0.CO;2-C
158. Jewett BN, Ramaley L, Kwak JCT (1999) Atmospheric Pressure Ionization Mass Spectrometry Techniques for the Analysis of Alkyl Ethoxysulfate Mixtures. J Am Soc Mass Spectrom 10:529–536. doi:10.1016/S1044-0305(99)00017-3
159. Benomar SH, Clench MR, Allen DW (2001) The Analysis of Alkylphenol Ethoxysulphonate Surfactants by High-Performance Liquid Chromatography, Liquid Chromatography-Electrospray Ionisation-Mass Spectrometry and Matrix-Assisted Laser Desorption Ionisation-Mass Spectrometry. Anal Chim Acta 445:255–267. doi:10.1016/S0003-2670(01)01280-6
160. Eichhorn P, Knepper TP (2001) Electrospray Ionization Mass Spectrometric Studies on the Amphoteric Surfactant Cocamidopropylbetaine. J Mass Spectrom 36:677–684. doi:10.1002/jms.170
161. Levine LH, Garland JL, Johnson JV (2002) HPLC/ESI-Quadrupole Ion Trap Mass Spectrometry for Characterization and Direct Quantification of Amphoteric and Nonionic Surfactants in Aqueous Samples. Anal Chem 74:2064–2071. doi:10.1021/ac011154f
162. Barco M, Planas C, Palacios O, Ventura F, Rivera J, Caixach J (2003) Simultaneous Quantitative Analysis of Anionic, Cationic, and Nonionic Surfactants in Water by Electrospray Ionization Mass Spectrometry with Flow Injection Analysis. Anal Chem 75:5179–5136. doi:10.1021/ac020708r
163. Little DP, Chorush RA, Speir JP, Senko MW, Kelleher NL, McLafferty FW (1994) Rapid Sequencing of Oligonucleotides by High-Resolution Mass Spectrometry. J Am Chem Soc 116:4893–4897. doi:10.1021/ja00090a039
164. Limbach PA, Crain PF, McCloskey JA (1995) Molecular Mass Measurement of Intact Ribonucleic Acids via Electrospray Ionization Quadrupole Mass Spectrometry. J Am Soc Mass Spectrom 6:27–39. doi:10.1016/1044-0305(94)00086-F
165. Little DP, Thannhauser TW, McLafferty FW (1995) Verification of 50- to 100-Mer DNA and RNA Sequences with High-Resolution Mass Spectrometry. Proc Natl Acad Sci U S A 92:2318–2322. doi:10.1073/pnas.92.6.2318
166. Hanson L, Fucini P, Ilag LL, Nierhaus KH, Robinson CV (2003) Dissociation of Intact *Escherichia Coli* Ribosomes in a Mass Spectrometer. Evidence for Conformational Change in Ribosome Elongation Factor G Complex. J Biol Chem 278:1259–1267. doi:10.1074/jbc.M208966200
167. De Bellis G, Salani G, Battaglia C, Pietta P, Rosti E, Mauri P (2000) Electrospray Ionization Mass Spectrometry of Synthetic Oligonucleotides Using 2-Propanol and Spermidine. Rapid Commun Mass Spectrom 14:243–249. doi:10.1002/(SICI)1097-0231(20000229)14:4<243::AID-RCM870>3.0.CO;2-F
168. Greig M, Griffey RH (1995) Utility of Organic Bases for Improved Electrospray Mass Spectrometry of Oligonucleotides. Rapid Commun Mass Spectrom 9:97–102. doi:10.1002/rcm.1290090121
169. Sannes-Lowery KA, Hofstadler SA (2003) Sequence Confirmation of Modified Oligonucleotides Using IRMPD in the External Ion Reservoir of an Electrospray Ionization Fourier Transform Ion Cyclotron Mass Spectrometer. J Am Soc Mass Spectrom 14:825–833. doi:10.1016/S1044-0305(03)00335-0

170. Andersen TE, Kirpekar F, Haselmann KF (2006) RNA Fragmentation in MALDI Mass Spectrometry Studied by H/D-Exchange: Mechanisms of General Applicability to Nucleic Acids. J Am Soc Mass Spectrom 17:1353–1368. doi:10.1016/j.jasms.2006.05.018
171. McLuckey SA, Van Berkel GJ, Glish GL (1992) Tandem Mass Spectrometry of Small, Multiply Charged Oligonucleotides. J Am Soc Mass Spectrom 3:60–70. doi:10.1016/1044-0305(92)85019-G
172. Pfenninger A, Karas M, Finke B, Stahl B (2002) Structural Analysis of Underivatized Neutral Human Milk Oligosaccharides in the Negative Ion Mode by Nano-Electrospray MS^n (Part 1: Methodology). J Am Soc Mass Spectrom 13:1331–1340. doi:10.1016/S1044-0305(02)00645-1
173. Pfenninger A, Karas M, Finke B, Stahl B (2002) Structural Analysis of Underivatized Neutral Human Milk Oligosaccharides in the Negative Ion Mode by Nano-Electrospray MS^n (Part 2: Application to Isomeric Mixtures). J Am Soc Mass Spectrom 13:1341–1348. doi:10.1016/S1044-0305(02)00646-3
174. Weiskopf AS, Vouros P, Harvey DJ (1998) Electrospray Ionization-Ion Trap Mass Spectrometry for Structural Analysis of Complex *N*-Linked Glycoprotein Oligosaccharides. Anal Chem 70:4441–4447. doi:10.1021/ac980289r
175. Metelmann W, Peter-Katalinic J, Müthing J (2001) Gangliosides from Human Granulocytes: A Nano-ESI QTOF Mass Spectrometry Fucosylation Study of Low Abundance Species in Complex Mixtures. J Am Soc Mass Spectrom 12:964–973. doi:10.1016/S1044-0305(01)00276-8
176. van Duijn E, Bakkes PJ, Heeren RMA, van den Heuvel RHH, van Heerikhuizen H, van der Vies SM, Heck AJR (2005) Monitoring Macromolecular Complexes Involved in the Chaperonin-Assisted Protein Folding Cycle by Mass Spectrometry. Nat Methods 2:371–376. doi:10.1038/nmeth753
177. Breuker K, McLafferty FW (2008) Stepwise Evolution of Protein Native Structure with Electrospray into the Gas Phase, 10^{-12} to 10^{2} s. Proc Natl Acad Sci U S A 105:18145–18152. doi:10.1073/pnas.0807005105
178. Jiang W, Winkler HDF, Schalley CA (2008) Integrative Self-Sorting: Construction of a Cascade-Stoppered Hetero[3]Rotaxane. J Am Chem Soc 130:13852–13853. doi:10.1021/ja806009d
179. Jiang W, Schaefer A, Mohr PC, Schalley CA (2010) Monitoring Self-Sorting by Electrospray Ionization Mass Spectrometry: Formation Intermediates and Error-Correction During the Self-Assembly of Multiply Threaded Pseudorotaxanes. J Am Chem Soc 132:2309–2320. doi:10.1021/ja9101369
180. Jiang W, Schalley CA (2010) Tandem Mass Spectrometry for the Analysis of Self-Sorted Pseudorotaxanes: The Effects of Coulomb Interactions. J Mass Spectrom 45:788–798. doi:10.1002/jms.1769

Ambient Desorption/Ionization 13

Learning Objectives

- Ion formation under ambient conditions
- Interfaces for ambient desorption/ionization-mass spectrometry
- Screening techniques for rapid quality control and safety applications
- Real time examination of samples during physical manipulation

13.1 Concept of Ambient Desorption/Ionization

All methods for the generation of ions for mass spectrometry described up to this point require the analyte for ionization to be presented either directly under high vacuum (EI, CI, FI, FD) or contained in a sort of solution from which ions are to be extracted into or generated in the gas phase (FAB, LDI, MALDI). Even the atmospheric pressure ionization techniques employ processes that create ions from dilute (solid) solutions of the sample (ESI, APCI, APPI, AP-MALDI). This chapter deals with the manifold methods and interfaces which are allowing to overcome these limitations, and which have been developing at a breathtaking pace during the last decade.

Desorption electrospray ionization (DESI) [1] was introduced at the end of 2004. The novel feature of DESI is that it allows instantaneous mass spectral analysis without sample preparation or sample pretreatment. Furthermore, the object to be analyzed is handled at atmospheric pressure, i.e., in a freely accessible open space in front of the atmospheric pressure interface [2]. Soon after in 2005, *direct analysis in real time* (DART) followed [3].

The obvious potential of both DESI and DART in high-throughput applications quickly led to the development of some "derivatives" with the intention to broaden the field of applications or to adapt the underlying methodology to specific

J.H. Gross, *Mass Spectrometry*, DOI 10.1007/978-3-319-54398-7_13

analytical needs. DESI and DART are thus the pioneers of numerous *ambient desorption/ionization* (ADI) techniques – more than thirty of which have been published since then [4]. The unifying feature of all these, of course, is the presentation of the sample under ambient conditions and without sample pretreatment. The term *ambient mass spectrometry* has thus become widely used for this group of methods [4–7]. Both terms, *ambient MS* and *ambient desorption/ionization* (ADI) are currently being used. In all these methods analyte molecules are being "wiped off" from the samples by exposing their surfaces to some ionizing gas or aerosol [8].

The nice thing about ambient MS is that it allows for the examination of untreated samples or entire objects in the open environment while maintaining sample integrity [9]. Classical atmospheric pressure ionization (API) techniques, in contrast, require a sample to be dissolved or extracted from an object or an aliquot thereof. While in ambient MS, an object is simply positioned at the entrance of a mass spectrometer and molecules released from the sample (not necessarily the entire sample) are being ionized and transferred into the mass analyzer [7]. This means that sampling is now part of the process [8]. The beauty of ambient MS is that a sample only needs to be exposed to an ionizing fluid medium under ambient conditions (Fig. 13.1).

Plenty of methods

In this chapter, we are not looking at a single ionization method but at a group of techniques that share the feature of ambient desorption/ionization. The goal of subjecting an object, essentially its surface, to immediate mass spectral analysis by simply exposing it to some sort of ion source can be achieved in numerous ways. Approaches to do so are based on ESI, APCI, APPI, combinations thereof with laser desorption, and various electrical discharges to create ionizing plasmas as employed in DART, for example.

Now, the repertoire of ADI methods includes variations of the DESI theme such as *desorption sonic spray ionization* (DeSSI) [10], later renamed *easy sonic spray ionization* (EASI) [11] or *extractive electrospray ionization* (EESI) [12, 13]. Then, there are the DESI analogs of APCI and APPI, i.e., *desorption atmospheric pressure chemical ionization* (DAPCI) [14, 15] and *desorption atmospheric pressure photoionization* (DAPPI) [16].

Analyte ions withdrawn from the sample are transported through air into the mass analyzer via a standard API interface. DESI, DART, and those numerous related methods enable the detection of surface materials like waxes, alkaloids, flavorants, or pesticides from plants as well as explosives, pharmaceuticals, or drugs of abuse from luggage or banknotes. These and many more analytical applications are readily accessible – even without harm to living organisms [17]. This simplified sample pretreatment is key to the success of ambient MS. In ambient MS, samples are accessible to observation and may even be subjected to

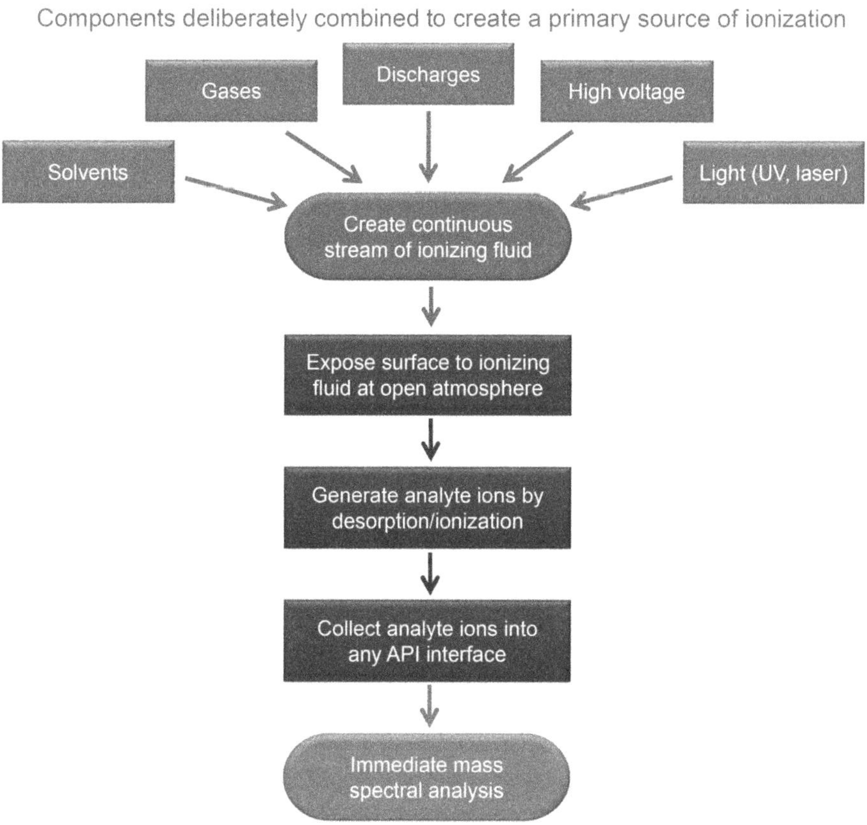

Fig. 13.1 Concept of ambient desorption/ionization mass spectrometry

some kind of processing, either mechanical manipulations or chemical treatments, while mass spectra are continuously being measured. Even a portable ion trap mass spectrometer for use with commercial DESI and DART ion sources has been designed [18].

Grounded euphoria

Although the features of DESI, DART, and many other ADI methods are in many ways superior and "revolutionary", one should be aware of intrinsic limitations. The detection of a compound largely depends on the matrix, e.g., whether it is *on* or eventually *in* skin, fruit, bark, stone etc. This also results in a limited quantification potential. However, also no other single ionization method, especially when used under just one set of conditions, can deliver ions of all constituents of a complex sample. Nonetheless, DESI, DART, and related methods can deliver a wealth of chemical information with unprecedented ease.

13.2 Desorption Electrospray Ionization

Desorption electrospray ionization (DESI) [1, 19] is applicable to solids, liquid samples, frozen solutions, and to loosely surface-bound species like adsorbed gases. It can detect low-molecular-weight organic compounds as well as comparatively large biomolecules [1, 19–21]. The material presented to DESI may be a single compound suitably prepared on a sample target analogous to LDI or it can be a complex biological material like tissue, blood, whole leaves, or fruit [22].

13.2.1 Experimental Setup for DESI

DESI is derived from electrospray ionization (ESI, Chap. 12) [23, 24] in that it employs an electrically charged aerosol that is created by pneumatically-assisted electrospray of a solvent containing some electrolyte at low concentration [1, 19]. In a standard ESI experiment the spray capillary is set to high voltage in respect to a counter electrode that is essentially represented by the atmospheric pressure entrance of the interface. Sample ions are already contained in the solution that is supplied to the sprayer. In DESI, the spray capillary is shifted away from the orifice of the API interface and only a solvent or solvent mixture is sprayed under strong pneumatic assistance onto a surface at an impact angle α, typically close to 45°. The distance between spray capillary and object is adjusted to a few millimeters and the entrance of the API interface is aligned at a similar angle and distance. Thus, sprayer, object, and orifice form a compact V-alignment. Driven by the high-velocity gas stream, the highly charged aerosol droplets receive sufficient kinetic energy to be forced onto the sample surface even while an electrostatic charge is building up there. The resulting interaction may cause surface coverage with a thin liquid film, and thus, dissolve and take up analyte ions. A surface analyzed by DESI gets "wet". This way, the solvent can also extract analytes from the object. The final release of isolated gas phase ions follows the same pathways as in ESI. Like ESI, DESI is capable of analyzing compounds from very low to high mass range while preserving the intact molecules [4].

Local electrostatic charging and the reflected gas stream now act in concert and transport analyte ions away from the surface at an angle β (Fig. 13.2). A nearby sampling orifice may then inhale a portion of the mist in the same way as it normally would do when the sample is already admixed to the solvent system. To bridge the gap between the sampling area and the entrance into the interface, a transfer line or extension tube is mounted in front of the orifice. This tube, e.g., 3 mm o.d. stainless steel, simplifies handling and particularly accessibility of the sample and also improves desolvation of the ions, probably due to different droplet sizes as compared to standard ESI conditions [1, 2]. DESI practice has shown that interfaces with a heated transfer capillary are superior to those employing a counter-current desolvation gas and corresponding modifications have been suggested [25].

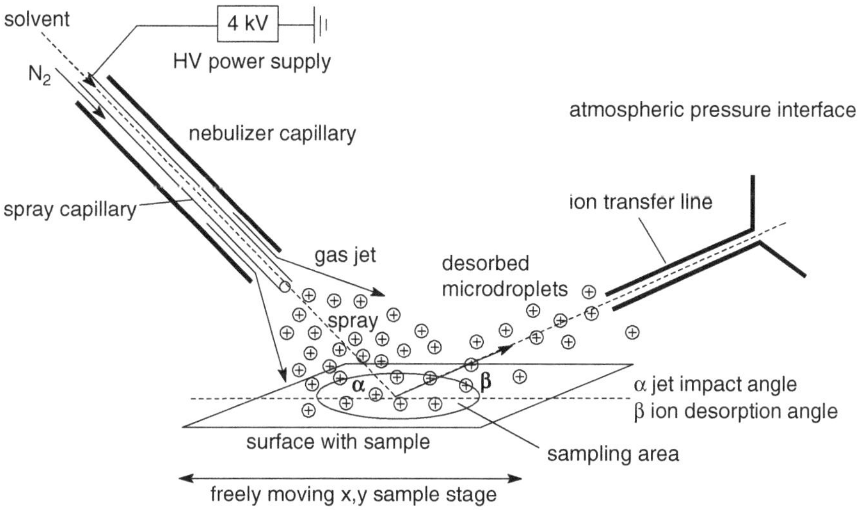

Fig. 13.2 Schematic of a DESI interface. A jet of gas and charged microdroplets is created by means of a standard pneumatic ESI sprayer and directed onto a sample surface at angle α. As a result, charged microdroplets containing ions of the surface material are created and transported away due to the action of the reflected gas stream and electric repulsion at angle β. A portion of the "secondary ESI spray" may be taken up by the atmospheric pressure interface of the mass spectrometer. Although at the expense of optimum sensitivity, an extended ion transfer line is normally employed to bridge the gap from surface to interface sampling orifice [1, 2]

Early on, commercial DESI sources have become available and have meanwhile reached a level of maturity. They feature ESI sprayers adjustable in both angle and distance towards sample plates that can be operated under data system control (Fig. 13.3).

Custom-built DESI source?
In principle, any mass spectrometer equipped with an ESI source can be modified for DESI operation by mounting the sprayer on an adjustable frame and placing a *x*,*y*-movable sample stage between sprayer and entrance of the interface [26]. For safety, a GΩ-resistor should be welded in the high-voltage supply cord. However, for successful analytical application, only sensitive modern instruments are suitable.

13.2.2 Parameters for DESI Operation

Obviously, DESI introduces new parameters to the ESI experiment. In particular, the velocity of the spray gas (represented by the supply pressure), the sprayer-to-surface and sampling orifice-to-surface distances, and the angles of impact and

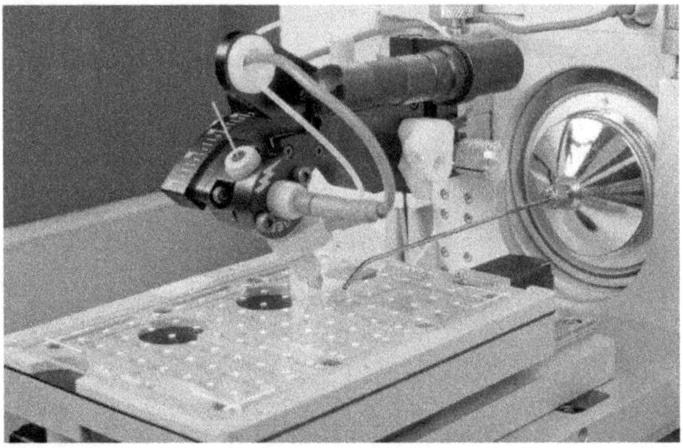

Fig. 13.3 A commercial DESI ion source. This one here is the Prosolia Omni Spray 2D source coupled to a Thermo Fisher LTQ mass spectrometer. The surface shown is a 96-spot Omni Slide HC having the standard microtiter plate dimensions. Note the extended desolvation capillary and the adjustable sprayer (Courtesy Prosolia, Inc., Indianapolis, In USA)

desorption are contributing to the affectivity of ion generation and subsequent uptake into the mass spectrometer. Accordingly, these parameters need to be carefully optimized for any DESI application as they exhibit rather wide variations (Table 13.1) [2, 22]. It has also been found that optimum settings differ between API interfaces with counter-current drying gas and those employing the heated desolvation capillary design [27]. The transit of charged particles from the sample surface into the ion transfer line of the interface is determined, among others, by the dragging action of the mass analyzer's vacuum.

Additional parameters associated with DESI are the electrical conductivity, the chemical composition, and the texture of the sample surface. Neutralization of the droplets landing at the surface must be avoided to maintain continuous release of charged particles from the surface. Conductive sample supports need to be either isolated or floated at a potential equal to or slightly lower than the spray voltage. The electrostatic properties of the surface are also relevant for an insulator, because the signal stability depends on its preferred polarity. A highly electronegative polymer like PTFE, for example, yields better signal stability in negative-ion mode, whereas PMMA performs better in positive-ion mode. The chemical composition of the surface can affect crystallization of the analyte, and thus, as observed in MALDI preparations, lead to the occurrence of "sweet spots". Therefore, high affinity of analyte molecules to the surface needs to be avoided as it is detrimental for the release of analyte. Finally, the surface texture plays a role. The use of HF etched glass slides as DESI substrates instead of untreated ones delivered a dramatic increase in signal stability and eliminated "sweet spot" effects. Generally, rough surfaces like paper or textiles give superior sensitivity [2].

Optimization of DESI conditions Examinations have been carried out on the dependence of the signal intensity of the $[M+3H]^{3+}$ ion of melittin on basic

Table 13.1 Typical parameters for DESI

Parameter	Range of useful settings
Solvent flow rate	3–5 μl min^{-1}
Nebulizer gas pressure	8–12 bar
Spray voltage	2–6 kV
Sprayer-to-surface distance	1–5 mm
Sprayer-to-surface angle	30–70°
Surface-to-desolvation capillary distance	1–5 mm
Surface-to-desolvation capillary angle	10–30°
Temperature of desolvation capillary	200–300 °C

experimental DESI parameters such as spray impact angle, spray high voltage, nebulizing gas inlet pressure, and solvent flow rate. Methanol : water = 1:1 was sprayed onto a sample of 10 ng melittin deposited on a PMMA surface at fixed spray tip-to-surface distance of 1 mm. While one parameter was varied, the others were kept constant at about their average value. The results reveal optimum conditions for each parameter that are rather typical for DESI and, as far a flow rate and spray high voltage are concerned, also for ESI (Fig. 13.4) [2].

DESI parameters can be grouped in a compound class-specific manner. It was found that proteins, for example, yield stronger signals when the spray is pointed onto the sample from close to vertical at about 1 mm distance while small molecules such as caffeine work best at an angle around 45° and several millimeters distance from the spray needle (Fig. 13.5) [2].

13.2.3 Mechanisms of Ion Formation in DESI

In DESI an electrospray plume of electrolytic solvent is usually generated by applying a potential of several kilovolts to an electrolytic solution under (strong) pneumatic assistance [2]. The mist comprising charged microdroplets, ionic clusters, and gas phase solvent ions is directed onto the sample surface. Therefore, the physical state of the sample distinguishes DESI from ESI. In this respect, DESI shows some phenomenological relationships to desorption ionization, because methods such as plasma desorption (PD), (matrix-assisted) laser desorption ionization ((MA)LDI), as well as fast atom bombardment (FAB) and its inorganic variant secondary ion mass spectrometry (SIMS, Sect. 15.6) all involve the impact of projectiles on condensed phase samples. Depending on the method, these projectiles are either photons, energetic atoms, or ions. In contrast to those desorption methods, DESI is performed in the ambient atmosphere, and therefore, the projectiles in DESI can only possess low kinetic energies.

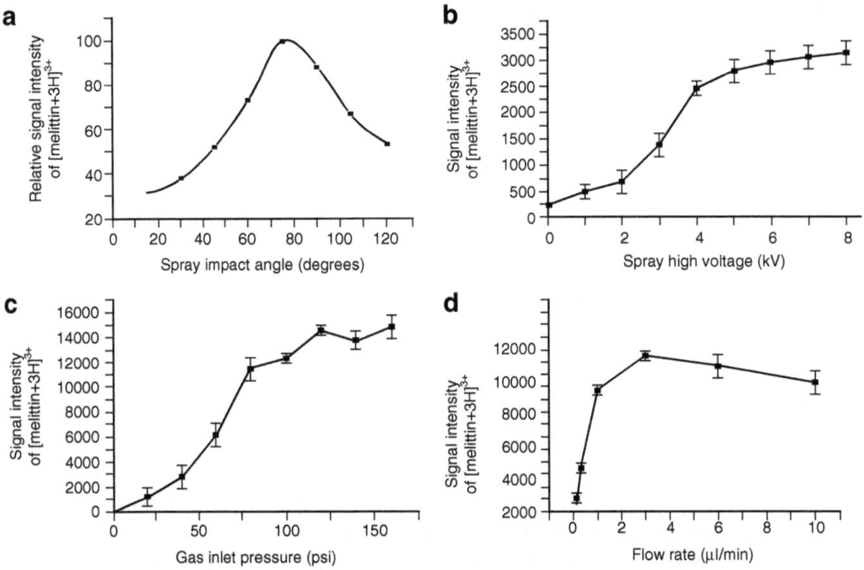

Fig. 13.4 Influence of experimental parameters on the intensity of the $[M+3H]^{3+}$ ion of melittin: (**a**) spray impact angle, (**b**) spray high voltage, (**c**) nebulizing gas pressure (14.5 psi ≈ 1 bar), (**d**) solvent flow rate (Reprinted from Ref. [2] with permission. © John Wiley & Sons, Ltd. 2005)

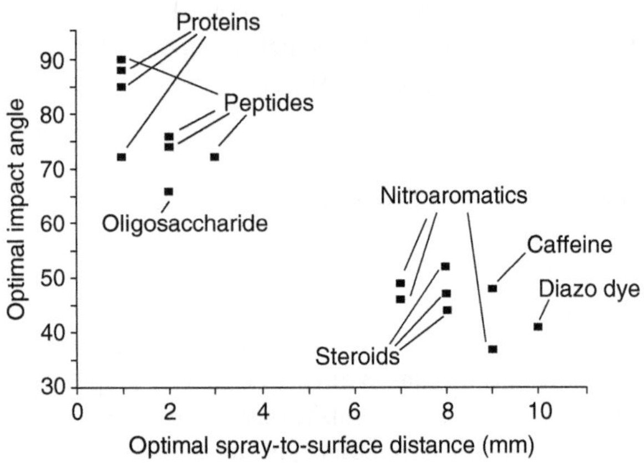

Fig. 13.5 Compound class-specific optima of spray impact angle and spray needle distance to surface. The *upper left* group of analytes would preferably be analyzed by ESI whereas the *lower right* group would rather demand for APCI (cf. Sect. 7.8) (Reprinted from Ref. [2] with permission. © John Wiley & Sons, Ltd. 2005)

Three processes of ion formation have been proposed for DESI [21]. Depending on the conditions and applied solvent-analyte pair, one of the following will predominate:

Droplet pickup *Droplet pickup* involves impact of electro sprayed droplets on the surface followed by dissolution of the analyte from the surface into the droplets. The droplets are again released from the surface and subsequent evaporation of the solvent and Coulomb fission generates ions by processes analogous to conventional ESI. The droplet pickup mechanism accounts for the similarity of DESI spectra with those of standard ESI in case of proteins. Interestingly, peptide ions can be observed even when the target and the sprayer are held at equal electrical potential. This has been attributed to the effect that offspring droplets will emerge mainly from the edges of a spreading primary droplet. In this case, charged droplet formation would essentially occur by electrospray driven by the potential between the edges and the extended desolvation capillary.

Condensed phase charge transfer When gaseous ions delivered by the electrospray interact with the analyte surface this can result in *condensed phase charge transfer*. The desorption of the analyte ions from the surface is then thought to occur by a type of *chemical sputtering*. (Chemical sputtering is a process in which ion bombardment induces chemical reactions that finally lead to the formation of volatile erosion products [28].) This way, ions can be formed by transfer of electrons, protons, or other small ions from the impacting microdroplet to the surface bearing the analyte. A surface charge builds up and the momentum delivered from the impact event may then suffice to effect direct release of analyte ions from the surface. This proceeds at very low impact energy if the reactions are exothermic, while somewhat higher energies (adjusted via gas pressure) are required to achieve lift-off in case of endothermic reactions.

Gas phase charge transfer Ion formation after volatilization or desorption of neutral species from the surface into the gas phase can lead to *gas phase charge transfer*. Ionization then proceeds via proton/electron transfer or other ion–molecule reactions at atmospheric pressure. Indeed, the assumption of ion–molecule reactions, eventually purely in the gas phase above the sample, has led to the development of an DAPCI source (Sect. 13.3), in the first place to prove this mechanism of ion formation [14]. The solvent pH can be used to positively affect the vapor pressure of the analyte, e.g., the vapor pressure of volatile plant alkaloids is increased by addition of a base.

13.2.4 Analytical Features of DESI

DESI can serve for the identification of natural products in plant material [1, 2, 22], of lipids in animal tissue [27, 29], for high-throughput analyses of pharmaceutical preparations [20], and for drug metabolite identification or even quantitation in blood and other biological fluids [2, 25], as well as for the direct monitoring of biological tissue for biomarkers and in vivo analysis [17, 27, 29]. DESI is applicable to the analysis of proteins, carbohydrates, and oligonucleotides [2], as well as small organic molecules. Potential DESI applications are also in forensics and public safety such as the detection of explosives, toxic compounds, and chemical warfare agents on a variety of common surfaces, e.g., paper, plastics, cloth or luggage [21, 30]. Plastic explosives, i.e., formulated explosive mixtures, can also be analyzed [17, 21, 30]. Even the transfer of ion-loaded gas from the sample to the API source through an up to three-meter-long stainless-steel tubing, termed non-proximate sampling, has been demonstrated [31].

The limit of detection for small peptides is in the order of 1 pg absolute or <0.1 pg mm^{-2}, for proteins in the order of <1 ng absolute or <0.1 ng mm^{-2}; small molecules such as pharmaceuticals and explosives are detectable in the range of 10–100 pg absolute or 1–10 pg mm^{-2} [2, 17]. These numbers indicate a footprint of about 10 mm^2 roughly corresponding to a circular spot of 3 mm in diameter. Smaller footprints can be realized – sample and sensitivity of the instrument permitting. The number of DESI papers is steadily growing. A few representative examples of DESI applications are compiled below.

Pharmaceuticals The negative-ion DESI mass spectrum of the over-the-counter drug acetylsalicylic acid (aspirin) was measured with a home-built DESI source attached to a seasoned triple quadrupole instrument (Fig. 13.6). The sample was presented on paper to a methanol spray. Whereas this sample even allowed tandem mass spectra of the [M–H]$^-$ ion, *m/z* 179, to be readily obtained, other samples were beyond the instrument's sensitivity limits [26].

Poisonous plants Plant alkaloids can be identified from DESI mass spectra of seeds, leaves, flowers, or roots. Here seeds of deadly nightshade (*Atropa bella-donna*) were subjected to DESI for the identification of their principal alkaloids

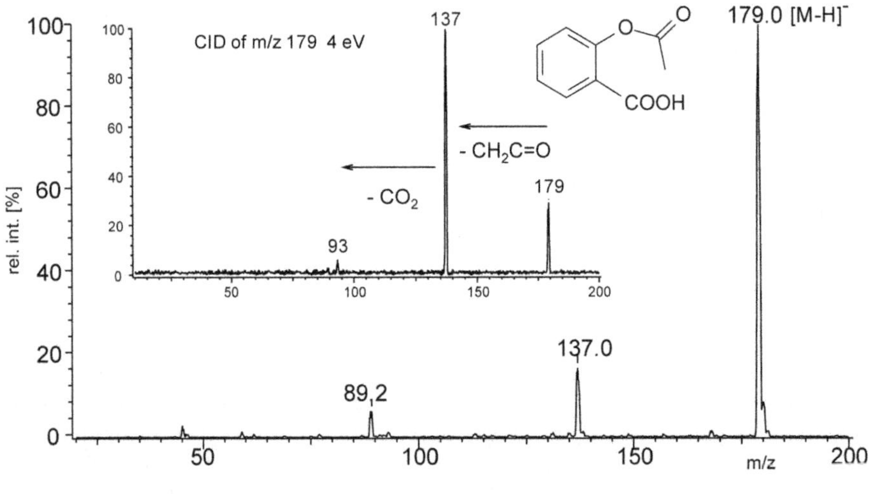

Fig. 13.6 Testing of a home-built DESI source. DESI mass spectrum of acetylsalicylic acid from paper analyzed by negative-ion DESI using methanol spray. The *inset* shows the tandem mass spectrum of the deprotonated molecule

atropine and scopolamine (Fig. 13.7) [22]. (Atropine is the name of the racemic mixture of (*R*)- and (*S*)-hyoscyamine. It is a tropane alkaloid also extracted from jimsonweed (*Datura stramonium*), mandrake (*Mandragora officinarum*) among other plants of the Solanaceae family.) The inset in Fig. 13.7 shows tandem mass spectra of the ions at *m/z* 290 and 304, thereby confirming them as corresponding to protonated hyoscyamine and scopolamine, respectively. The confirmation of the ion at *m/z* 304 as $[M+H]^+$ ion of scopolamine was obtained by comparing the tandem mass spectrum with that of the standard alkaloid.

Animal tissue Mouse liver sections were analyzed by DESI-FT-ICR-MS. The spectra of the tissue samples exhibited strong signals for phospholipids and lysophospholipids that were detected either as $[M+H]^+$, $[M+Na]^+$, or $[M+K]^+$ ions. The mass accuracy of generally 1 ppm of the FT-ICR instrument allowed for assigning unique molecular formulas to most signals (Fig. 13.8) [27].

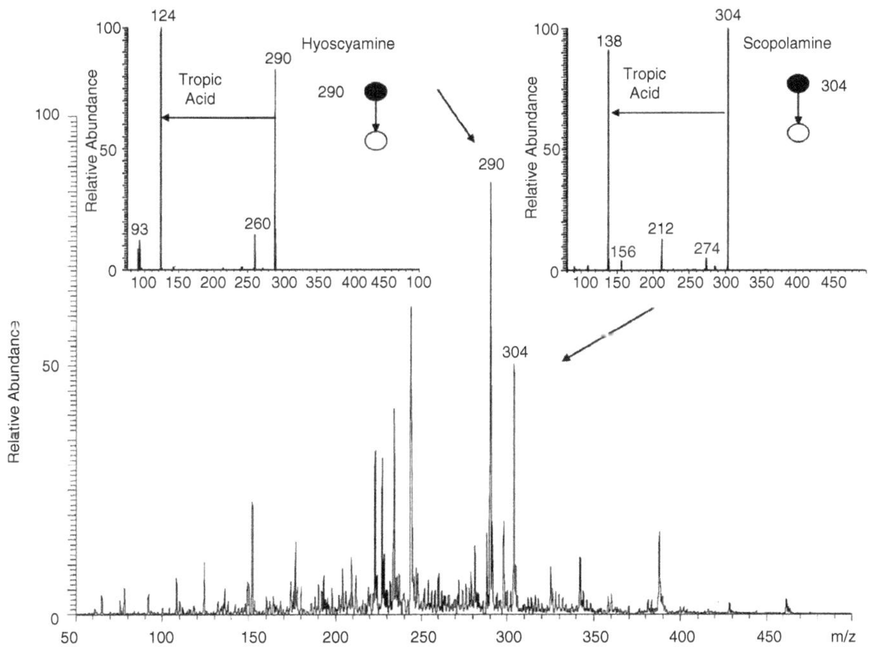

Fig. 13.7 DESI mass spectrum of *Atropa belladonna* seeds using methanol : water = 1:1 as spray solvent. The *insets* show tandem mass spectra of the protonated alkaloids hyoscamine, *m/z* 290 and scopolamine, *m/z* 304. Both protonated alkaloids have the characteristic loss of tropic acid, 166 u, in common (Reprinted from Ref. [22] with permission. © The Royal Society of Chemistry, 2005)

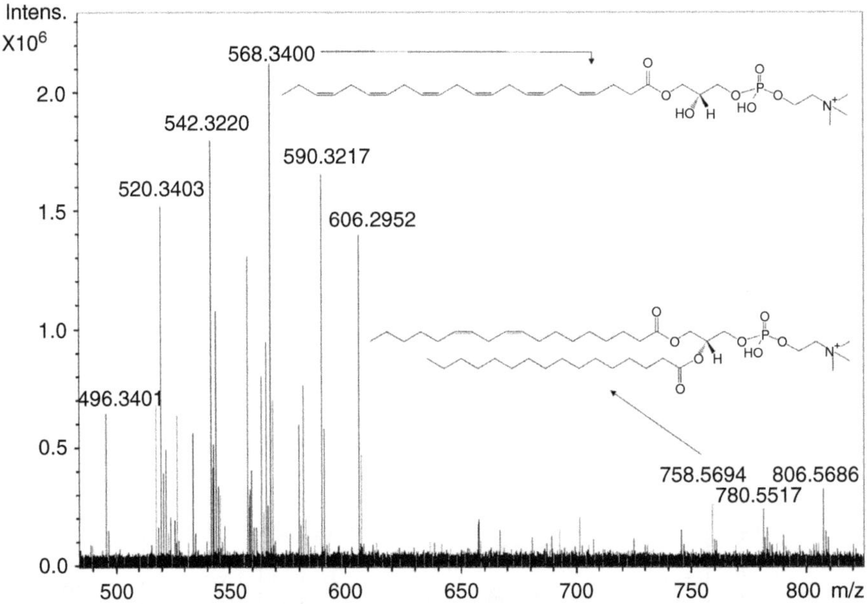

Fig. 13.8 Lipid profile of murine liver tissue sections as acquired by DESI-FT-ICR-MS using methanol : water = 1:1 (v/v) with 1% acetic acid as spray solvent (Reproduced from Ref. [27] with permission. © John Wiley & Sons, Ltd., 2008)

DESI of TLC plates Thin layer chromatography (TLC) plates were first analyzed by DESI in the van Berkel group [32]. The sprayer was positioned about 4 mm from the curtain plate of the mass spectrometer at a 50° angle relative to the TLC plate surface. The TLC plates were cut to align the sample bands with the DESI plume. Methanol was sprayed at about 5 µl min^{-1} while a *x-y-z* robotic platform and control software were used to move the TLC plate relative to the stationary DESI emitter at about 50 µm min^{-1}. The position of the TLC plate relative to the sprayer was monitored with a camera, the image of which was output to a PC so as to correlate staining, position, and DESI spectral data (Fig. 13.9).

Scrutinize the spectra

Although it appears that the results of DESI analyses (or of any other ADI technique) are almost instantaneously available, DESI spectra tend to require more thorough examination than standard ESI spectra in order to draw the right analytical conclusions.

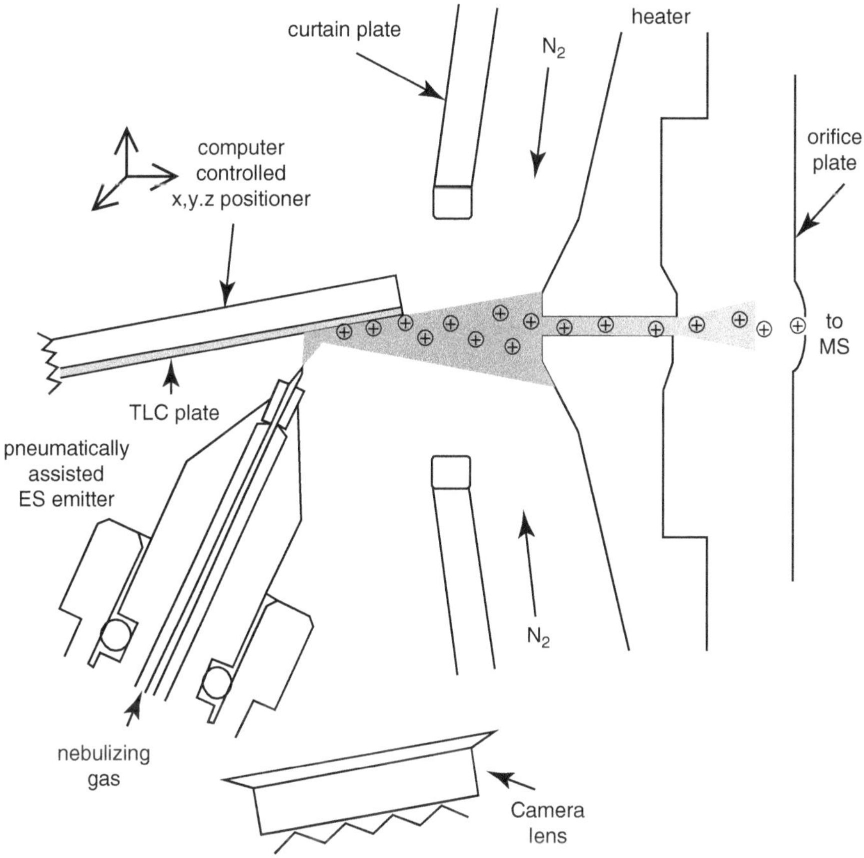

Fig. 13.9 Fully computer-controlled TLC-DESI unit attached to an ESI interface using the curtain gas design (Reprinted with permission from Ref. [32]. © The American Chemical Society, 2005)

13.3 Desorption Atmospheric Pressure Chemical Ionization

The first report on *desorption atmospheric pressure chemical ionization* (DAPCI) appeared in a paper on the analysis of nitroaromatic explosives by negative-ion DESI [14]. These molecules all possess high electron affinities and thus they are prone to electron capture and deprotonation. From the positive effect of the DAPCI mode of operation for their detection, it was inferred that a chemical ionization mechanism should be effective if analytes are volatilized in the course of DESI analysis. So the main difference between DESI and DAPCI is the substitution of the charged solvent mist by a (hot) solvent vapor and the application of a corona discharge as the initial source of electric charge in DAPCI [21]. As usual in APCI, the corona discharge is created by applying a high DC voltage (3–6 kV) to

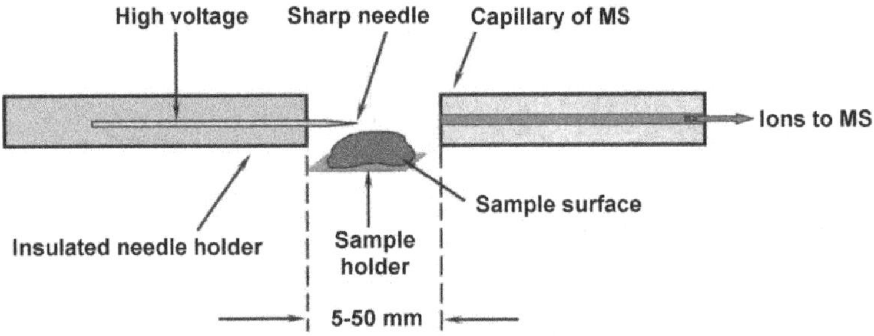

Fig. 13.10 Schematic of a DAPCI source for operation with moist ambient air as reagent gas. The sharp needle discharge electrode is coaxially centered in a capillary of 3 mm i.d. delivering humidified nitrogen gas if the ambient air is below 20% relative humidity (Adapted from Ref. [33] with permission. © John Wiley & Sons, Ltd., 2007)

a tapered tip stainless steel needle. Reactant ions are created in the solvent vapor upon passing the discharge. Then, the ionized gas streams onto the surface to be analyzed. Obviously, the droplet-pickup mechanism (Sect. 13.2.3) is precluded in DAPCI, while charge transfer to the surface and gas phase ionization of the analyte present the two possible mechanisms of ion formation [31].

It has been shown that addition of solvents can be avoided if the moisture of the ambient air is sufficient to generate H_3O^+ reagent ions [15, 33]. The setup for DAPCI (using ambient air only) is shown in Fig. 13.10. A comparison of spectra of Proctosedyl, an ointment containing cinchocaine ($M_r = 343$ u) and hydrocortisone ($M_r = 362$ u), as obtained by DESI, DAPCI with ambient air, and DAPCI with solvent is presented in Fig. 13.11.

Applications of DAPCI include the comparative analysis of different teas such as green tea, oolong, and jasmine tea by their chemical fingerprints [33, 34] and the direct rapid analysis of melamine and cyanuric acid in milk products delivering detection limits of 1–20 pg melamine mm^{-2} [35]. Furthermore, DAPCI has been successfully employed for the detection of peroxide explosives [30] or of illicit ingredients in food such as sudan red dyes in tomato sauce [33]. Analogous to DESI, DAPCI analyses can be performed with remote sampling [31].

13.4 Desorption Atmospheric Pressure Photoionization

DESI works best with polar analytes that are easy to protonate or deprotonate, although analytes of low polarity are accessible to a certain extent. This was the rationale for developing DAPCI. In order to improve the efficiency of ambient MS in the regime of low-polarity compounds even further, *desorption atmospheric pressure photoionization* (DAPPI) has been developed. DAPPI represents the adaptation of APPI for the ambient analysis of surfaces analogous to the conversion of APCI to DAPCI.

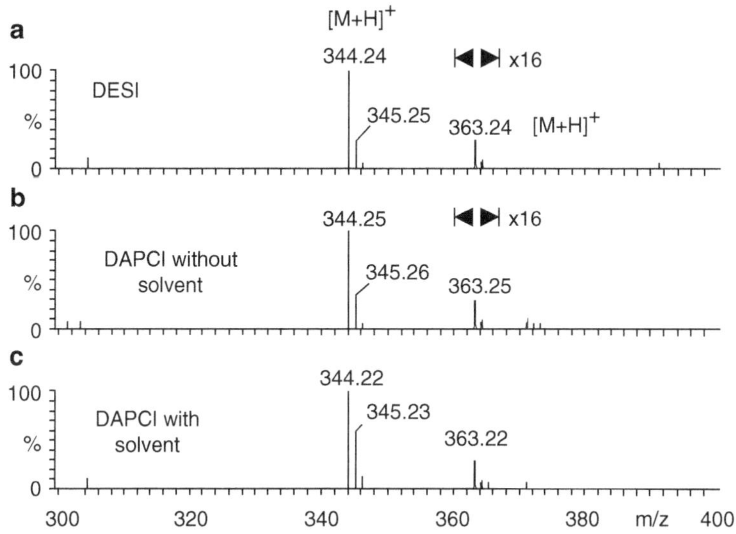

Fig. 13.11 Comparison of DESI, solvent-free DAPCI and DAPCI of Proctosedyl ointment. (**a**) Positive-ion DESI spectrum with the intensity of *m/z* 363, protonated hydrocortisone, 16-fold expanded to show the low-abundant ion. (**b**) Positive-ion DAPCI spectrum of the ointment obtained without solvent and same expansion as above. (**c**) Positive-ion DAPCI spectrum obtained with solvent (Reproduced from Ref. [15] with permission. © John Wiley & Sons, Ltd., 2006)

In DAPPI, a heated jet of solvent vapor and nebulizer gas desorbs solid analytes from the surface. Using a microchip nebulizer turned out to be advantageous for handling and for highly responsive temperature control of the gas. The microchip nebulizer is a small glass device for mixing gas and solvent flow (dopant) and for heating the fluid medium during its passage along a platinum wire (Fig. 13.12) [16]. A krypton discharge lamp is directed toward the sample so as to irradiate the vapor phase immediately above the surface with UV photons of 10 eV where ionization of the analyte occurs. Like DESI and DAPCI, DAPPI uses a standard API interface to collect the ions [16, 36].

The mechanism of ion generation in DAPPI has been proposed to be a combination of thermal and chemical processes. After thermal desorption of the analytes from the surface they can be photoionized in the gas phase. However, analytes with no UV chromophore may only be ionized by ion–molecule reactions with dopant ions. Dopant molecular ions, $D^{+\bullet}$, as formed from toluene for example, may promote charge exchange, while protonated dopant molecules, $[D+H]^+$, will yield $[M+H]^+$ ions. Acidic analytes can undergo deprotonation, while electronegative molecules are prone to anion addition or electron capture [36]. (The rules governing these processes have already been dealt with in Chap. 7). The factors influencing the desorption and ionization in DAPPI such as the microfluidic jet impinging geometry, the thermal characteristics of the surfaces subjected to DAPPI, as well as chemical aspects like spray solvent have been examined for both positive- and negative-ion mode [36].

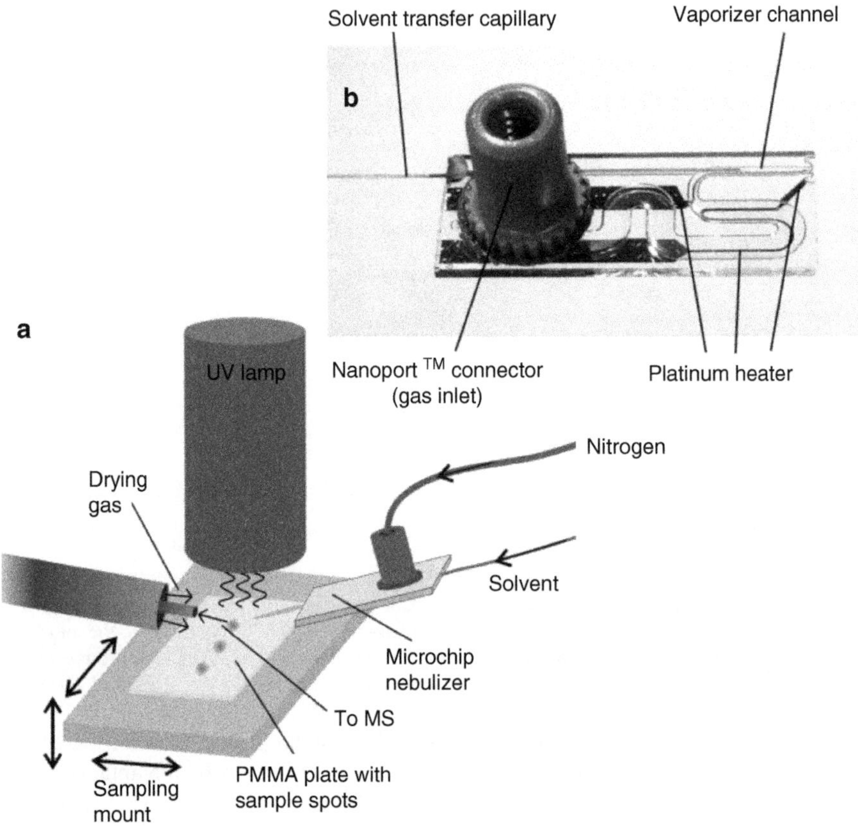

Fig. 13.12 Schematic of (**a**) the DAPPI setup and (**b**) photograph of the microchip nebulizer. The small solvent flow is mixed with nitrogen gas and vaporized in the microchip nebulizer by resistive heating of the platinum wire. The krypton UV lamp irradiates the sample surface that is in contact with the hot reagent gas (Reproduced from Ref. [16] with permission. © The American Chemical Society, 2007)

DAPPI is capable of analyzing dried sample spots of compounds of different polarities from various surfaces, may serve for the direct analysis of pharmaceuticals and illicit drugs from tablets and other preparations (Fig. 13.13), and of many other applications [16, 36–38].

13.5 Other Methods Related to DESI

Variation of the DESI theme by changing the mode of sample supply opens up a large variety of partially awe-inspiring, partially slightly odd, but always interesting analytical applications. In some cases, even the term was not finally coined at the time of their first publication.

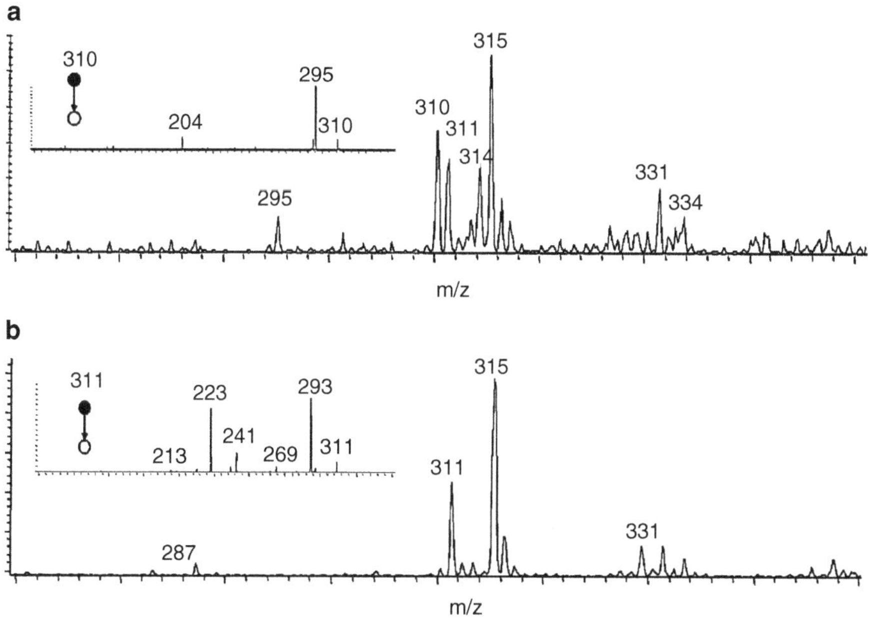

Fig. 13.13 Analysis of a hashish slab with DAPPI using toluene (**a**) and acetone (**b**) at flow rates of 2 ml min^{-1} as spray solvents. The insets show the tandem mass spectra of (**a**) the $M^{+\bullet}$ ion of cannabinol and (**b**) the $[M+H]^+$ ion of cannabinol; the ions at *m/z* 314 and 315 are attributed to the respective ionic species of tetrahydrocannabinol (THC) (Reproduced from Ref. [38] with permission. © John Wiley Sons, Ltd., 2008)

13.5.1 Desorption Sonic Spray Ionization

In ESI an electrolytic solution is sprayed mainly by the action of an electric field inducing charge separation and subsequent disintegration of a bulk liquid into an electrostatically charged mist. A nebulizing gas flow at sonic speed coaxially to the liquid flow can also create a statistical imbalance of charges, i.e., a charge separation sufficient for the purpose of forming charged droplets. This is known as *sonic spray ionization* (SSI) [39–41]. The advantage of SSI is that it operates free of a high voltage and thus appears ideal for handling under ambient conditions [10]. An adaptation of SSI for ambient mass spectrometry was thus made and initially termed *desorption sonic spray ionization* (DeSSI) [10].

Naming
Soon after its introduction, DeSSI was renamed *easy ambient sonic-spray ionization* (EASI) [42], the superfluous inclusion of the adjective "easy" and the generation of a rather blatant acronym (EASI) seem to have driven this change.

DeSSI (or EASI) requires unusually high backpressure of ca. 30 bar to achieve the sonic velocity of the nebulizer gas stream resulting in a flow of about 3 l min^{-1} to dissipate the liquid flow of 20 μl min^{-1} methanol/water solution. The curtain gas pressure of the API interface is also set to a rather high value of 5 bar.

The method has shown to deliver good results for the fingerprinting of biodiesel fuel [43] and perfumes [42], for the analysis of fabric softeners and surfactants [44], coupling to membrane inlet systems (MIMS-DeSSI) [11], and to analyze components separated on TLC plates [45]. However, the method appears to exhibit low inter-system compatibility; in some laboratories high voltages were needed to obtain a signal.

13.5.2 Extractive Electrospray Ionization

Analyte ions can also be efficiently generated when sample vapor or finely dispersed sample droplets transported by a carrier gas stream are admixed to the expanding electrospray plume. This technique, simple yet effective, has been introduced as *extractive electrospray ionization* (EESI) [46]. It utilizes two separate sprayers, one conventional ESI sprayer to provide the electrostatically charged mist and another to supply the sample vapor or mist (Fig. 13.14). While this approach is suggested for API interfaces with the heated transfer capillary design, the sample carrier stream may alternatively be passed into the desolvation gas of interfaces employing the heated curtain gas design (Fig. 13.15) [13, 47].

Instead of a separate sample sprayer, an ultrasonic nebulizer may also deliver a sample-containing aerosol, which is transported and admixed to the electrospray mist by action of a mild stream of nitrogen. As the droplets of both origins are "fused" inside a small housing enclosing the spray, this approach has been termed *fused-droplet electrospray ionization*, and thus, led to the somewhat confusing acronym FD-ESI [48, 49].

EESI has its strengths in headspace analytical applications; it has been employed to classify authentic perfumes and to detect counterfeit products from chemical

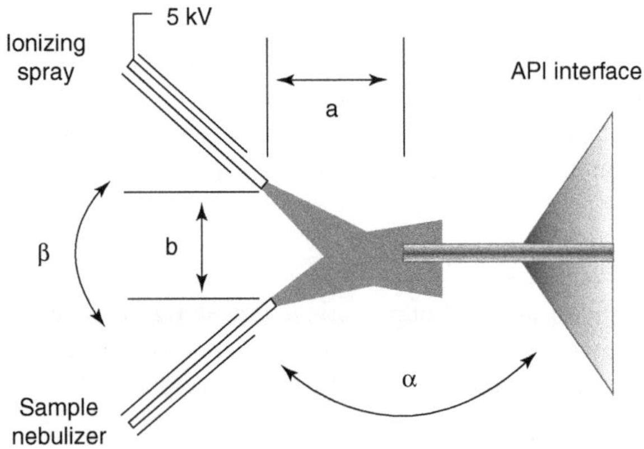

Fig. 13.14 Extractive electrospray ionization interface with two mixing sprays in front of a heated transfer capillary. The distances *a* and *b* and the angles *α* and *β* are adjusted as required for optimum signal intensity (Adapted from Ref. [46] with permission. © The Royal Society of Chemistry, 2006)

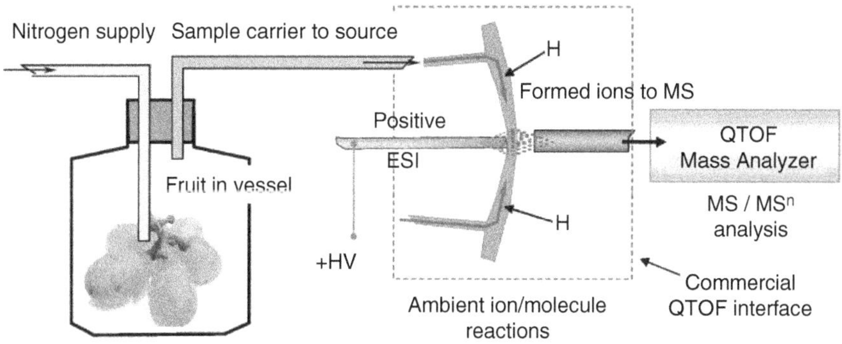

Fig. 13.15 Schematic of an EESI source where the sample carrier gas is fed into the curtain gas of the API interface. Here, the experiment is designed to determine the ripening of fruit from its headspace, i.e., odor (Adapted from Ref. [50] with permission. © The American Chemical Society, 2007)

fingerprints of the fragrances after their application on paper strips as usually performed for customer's testing [51]. It may serve for the rapid determination of the ripening of fruit via headspace analysis as pointed out in Fig. 13.15 [50], or to identify spoiled food, either vegetables or meat samples, even in the frozen state, by detection of typical degradation products or metabolites from bacterial growth [12, 47]. It is also possible to detect melamine in milk [52] (a sort of analysis one never would have assumed to be necessary until after the Olympic games in China in 2008). Finally, as the location of the extraction can be several meters away from the mass spectrometer, traces of toxic chemicals, explosives, or drugs on skin can be detected by EESI without any hazard to a person [13, 53].

13.5.3 Electrospray-Assisted Laser Desorption/Ionization

The technique of *electrospray-assisted laser desorption/ionization* (ELDI) combines two well-matured techniques of ionization for the benefit of improved analysis of samples under ambient conditions. The development of ELDI emanates from the fact that in (MA)LDI by far more neutrals than ions are released from the sample layer (Chap. 11) [54]. Consequently, post-ionization of laser-desorbed neutrals is promising and such methods have indeed been developed (cf. Refs. in [55]). The unique feature of ELDI is to laser-irradiate the sample in the ambient close to the ESI plume, wherein the neutrals are then ionized by ion–molecule reactions [55].

Standard conditions of ESI for ELDI involve a methanol : water =1:1 mixture with 0.1% acetic acid sprayed at 3–5 μl min^{-1} from a grounded needle as to pass closely over an also grounded sample support. The orifice of the API interfaces acting as the counter electrode is held at 4–5 kV negative voltage. The UV nitrogen

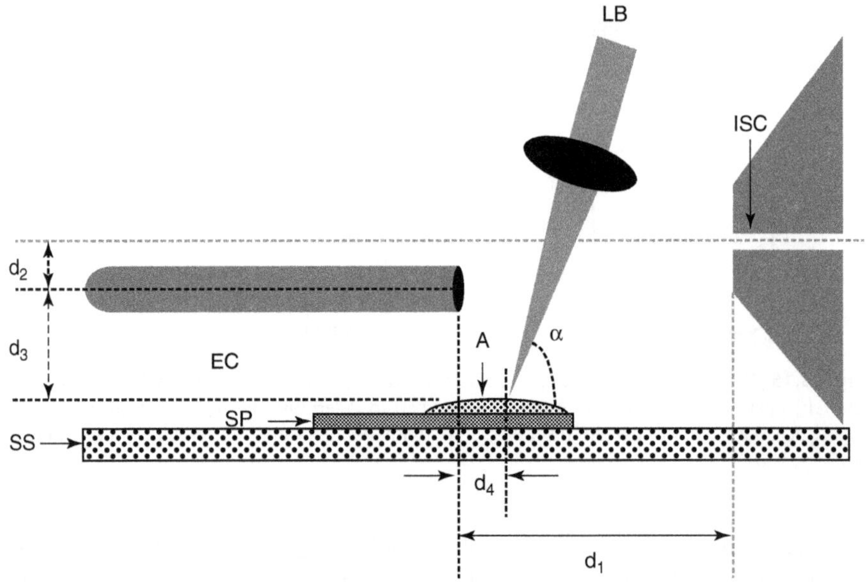

Fig. 13.16 ELDI setup. *A* analyte, SP: stainless steel sample support plate, *SS* mobile sample stage, *EC* electrospray capillary, *LB* UV laser beam, *ISC* ion sampling capillary of the API interface. The distances d_1 through d_4 are all in the order of millimeters (Reproduced from Ref. [55] with permission. © John Wiley & Sons, Ltd., 2005)

laser is adjusted to irradiate the sample sideward at an angle of about 45° while spraying (Fig. 13.16).

Effect of the laser in ELDI The combined use of ESI and LDI in ELDI is demonstrated for a sample of neat bovine cytochrome c on a stainless steel target (Fig. 13.17). The first spectrum (**A**), basically a blank spectrum, was obtained under pure LDI conditions. Spectrum **B** was measured with ESI on, but no laser irradiation. Finally, spectrum **C** was generated with both ESI and LDI active. It clearly shows the charge state distribution of the protein as typical for ESI spectra. The advantage of ELDI is that samples can be presented to the inlet nozzle directly from the outside as compared to ESI or MALDI that require additional sample preparation [55].

ELDI has also been applied to the analysis of peptides and proteins [56] even from biological media [57], to detect chemicals on different surfaces [58], and of course, for compound identification on TLC plates [59]. It has been found that addition of a matrix is beneficial for the laser desorption part of the method. This gave rise to *matrix-assisted laser desorption electrospray ionization* (MALDESI) [60].

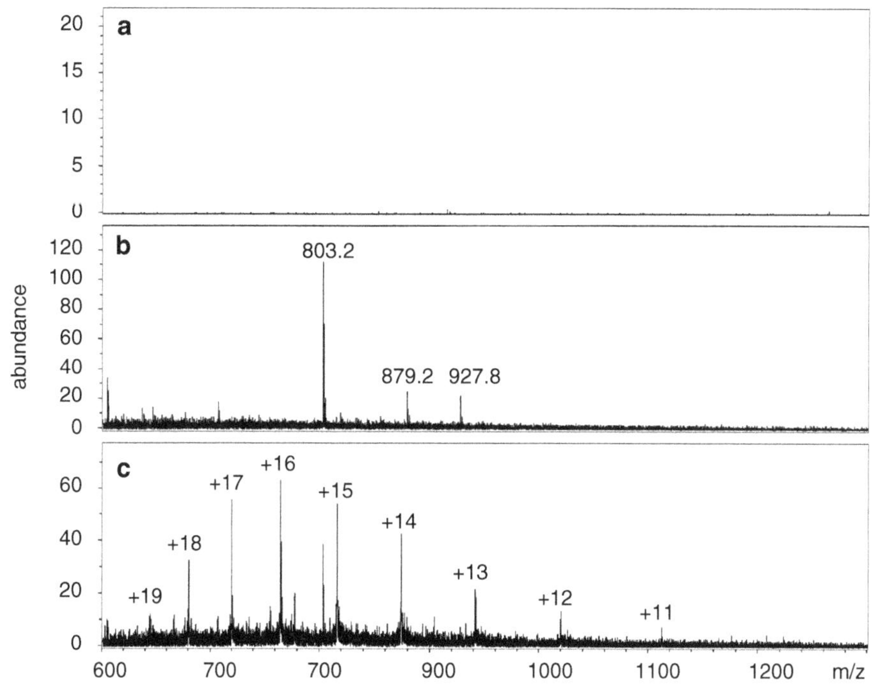

Fig. 13.17 Effect of the combined use of ESI and LDI in ELDI for a sample of neat bovine cytochrome *c*. *Spectrum* (**a**) was obtained under laser desorption only; (**b**) under ESI only; and (**c**) with both ESI and LDI active (Reproduced from Ref. [55] with permission. © John Wiley & Sons, Ltd., 2005)

13.5.4 Laser Ablation Electrospray Ionization

As just described, ELDI and MALDESI require pretreated samples, making them unfavorable for the (*in vivo*) analysis of water-rich biological samples that would preferentially be examined under ambient conditions. By replacing the UV laser with an IR laser (Er:YAG laser of 2.94 μm wavelength), the energy may directly be coupled into the OH vibrational modes of water-rich samples such as tissues. This experimental approach has been termed *laser ablation electrospray ionization* (LAESI) [61–63]. In contrast to AP-IR-MALDI, in LAESI the infrared laser only ablates neutrals from the sample, a noteworthy amount of them even in particulate state, which could be ascertained by flash shadowgraphy [61]. The laser impinging on the sample surface at 90° creates a plume that intercepts an electrospray operating in the cone-jet mode parallel to and at about 25 mm distance from the sample surface. The electrospray post-ionizes the neutrals and the particulate matter in that plume and transports the incipient analyte ions along the spray axis into the sampling orifice of an orthogonal acceleration time-of-flight (oa-TOF) mass spectrometer [61]. Apart from the IR laser, the experimental setup is sufficiently similar to ELDI to omit a schematic here.

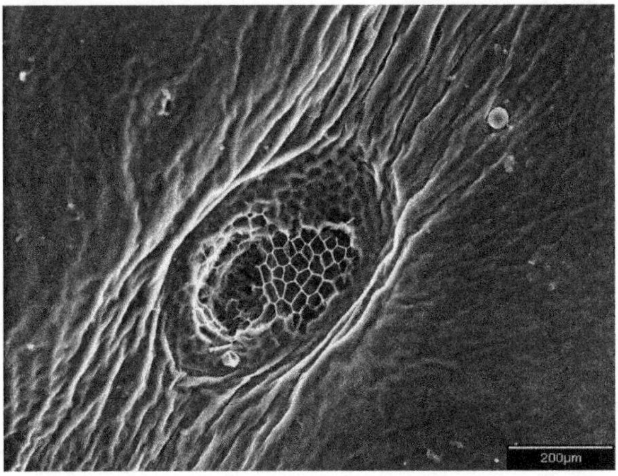

Fig. 13.18 Scanning electron microscope image of the ablation crater produced by a single laser pulse on the adaxial leaf surface of a Zebra plant (*Aphelandra squarrosa*). Scale bar corresponds to 200 μm. Multiple laser pulses penetrated deeper. The wrinkles on the cuticle were caused by the collapse of the underlying cells due to rapid water loss in the vacuum environment during SEM imaging (Adapted from Ref. [62] with permission. © The American Chemical Society, 2008)

In order to minimize the interference of external electromagnetic fields and air currents the LAESI system is shielded by a Faraday cage and a plastic enclosure, respectively. The enclosure also provides protection from potential health hazards of the fine particulates generated in the laser ablation process.

Tissue analysis by LAESI For LAESI, tissue samples are mounted on microscope slides, positioned 10–30 mm below the spray axis and 3–5 mm ahead of the emitter tip, and ablated using an Er:YAG laser with a pulse length of <100 ns and 5 Hz repetition rate. The scanning electron microscope image of the ablation crater produced by a single laser pulse on the adaxial leaf surface of a Zebra plant (*Aphelandra squarrosa*) is shown below (Fig. 13.18). The waxy cuticle and some of the upper epidermal and palisade cells were removed from a slightly elliptical area with axes of 300 and 280 μm indicating effective ablation of tissue [62]. This way, LAESI offers lateral mapping of metabolite distributions and their variations with depth on plant leaves. However, at present, LAESI cannot compete with vacuum imaging methods such as SIMS or MALDI [61].

13.6 Rapid Evaporative Ionization Mass Spectrometry

We have already discussed the impressive capabilities of biotyping and tissuetyping in the context of MALDI-MS (Sects. 11.5 and 11.7). However, MALDI bio- and tissuetyping are restricted to *in vitro* samples. What, if such valuable mass spectral information was also available in real time by use of some ambient MS technique? In fact, *rapid evaporative ionization mass spectrometry* (REIMS) permits the immediate identification of bacteria, fungi, and other microorganisms [64], and moreover, REIMS opens the road to *in situ* and *in vivo* tissue analyses [65].

13.6.1 Setup of Rapid Evaporative Ionization Mass Spectrometry

REIMS was developed for mass spectral tissue analysis in real time during surgical interventions employing electrosurgical dissection of the tissues. Electrosurgery employs high-frequency electric current for tissue ablation, cutting, and coagulation [65]. The current is directly applied onto the tissues, where it cuts due to thermal damage. Cutting is accompanied by the formation of surgical smoke containing both positively and negatively charged droplets. These charged droplets provide the basis for ion formation analogous to ESI (Sect. 12.4). The charged aerosol can be supplied to the mass spectrometer by modifying the cutting electrode to incorporate a 0.125-inch inner diameter stainless steel tubing that is connected to the API interface via an up to 2-m-long PTFE tubing. The transport of the aerosol from the electrosurgical blade to the interface is driven by a Venturi gas jet pump that aspirates the aerosol from the surgical site. The exhaust of the PTFE line is then positioned near the inlet orifice. An orthogonal orientation of the exhaust line relative to the ion transfer capillary minimizes contamination of the atmospheric pressure interface. An analogous setup with electric current applied to a bipolar forceps can be employed for bacteria and tissue samples alike (Fig. 13.19) [65, 66].

13.6.2 REIMS Spectra

Depending on the chosen polarity, REIMS of biological tissues or microbial samples either generates protonated or deprotonated molecules, mostly of lipids and their thermal degradation products, e.g., fatty acids (Fig. 13.20). When REIMS is applied to the analysis of aqueous solutions of amino acids, pharmaceuticals, or peptides it also yields protonated or deprotonated analyte molecules accompanied by alkali metal and/or ammonium ion adducts. Analogous to ESI, radical ions are not observed in REIMS spectra [65, 66].

13.6.3 REIMS in the Operating Room

As mentioned above, REIMS is intended for online monitoring of tissue being cut during surgery. The quick and unequivocal identification of carcinomatous tissue among healthy parts of an organ is of utmost importance for the surgeon. Traditional histopathological analysis means time-consuming microscopic examination of tissue sections. REIMS is sensitive enough to even allow for combination with

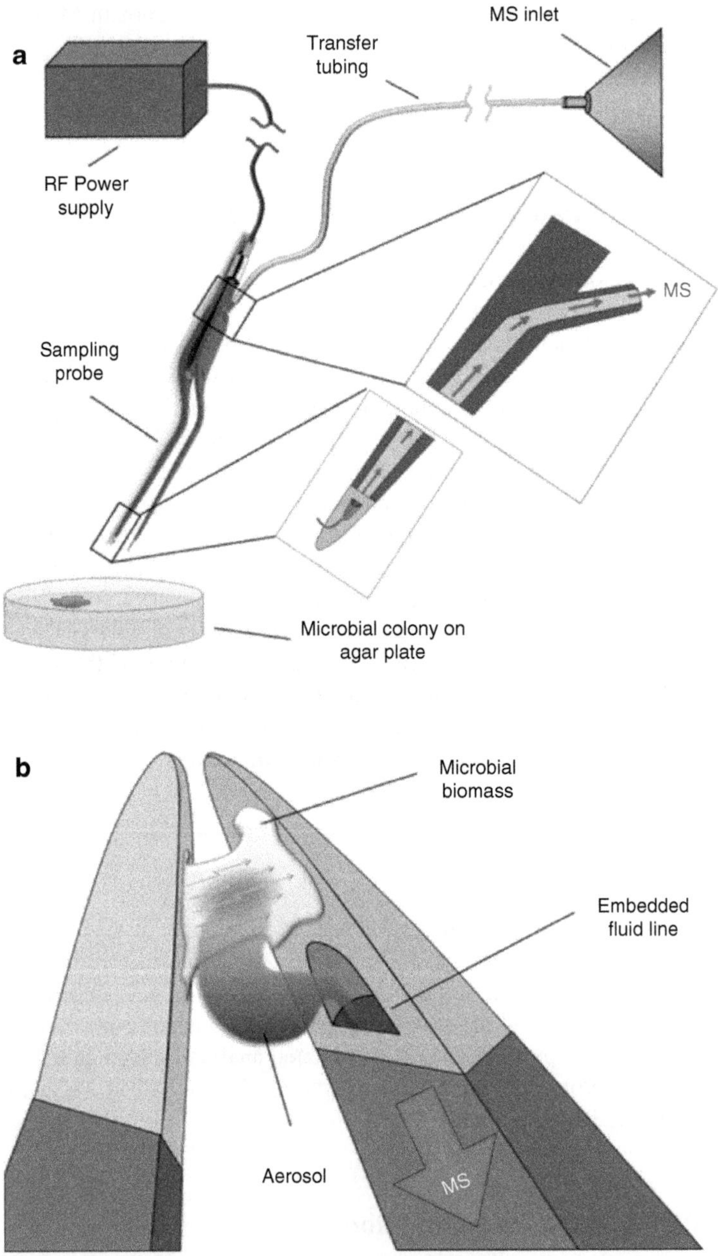

Fig. 13.19 (**a**) Setup used for analysis of bacteria by REIMS. (**b**) Scheme of analysis. Microbial biomass is held between the two electrodes of the irrigated bipolar forceps, electrical current is applied, sample is evaporated thermally, and the produced aerosol is aspirated into the opening of the embedded fluid line (Reproduced from Ref. [67] with permission. © American Chemical Society, 2014)

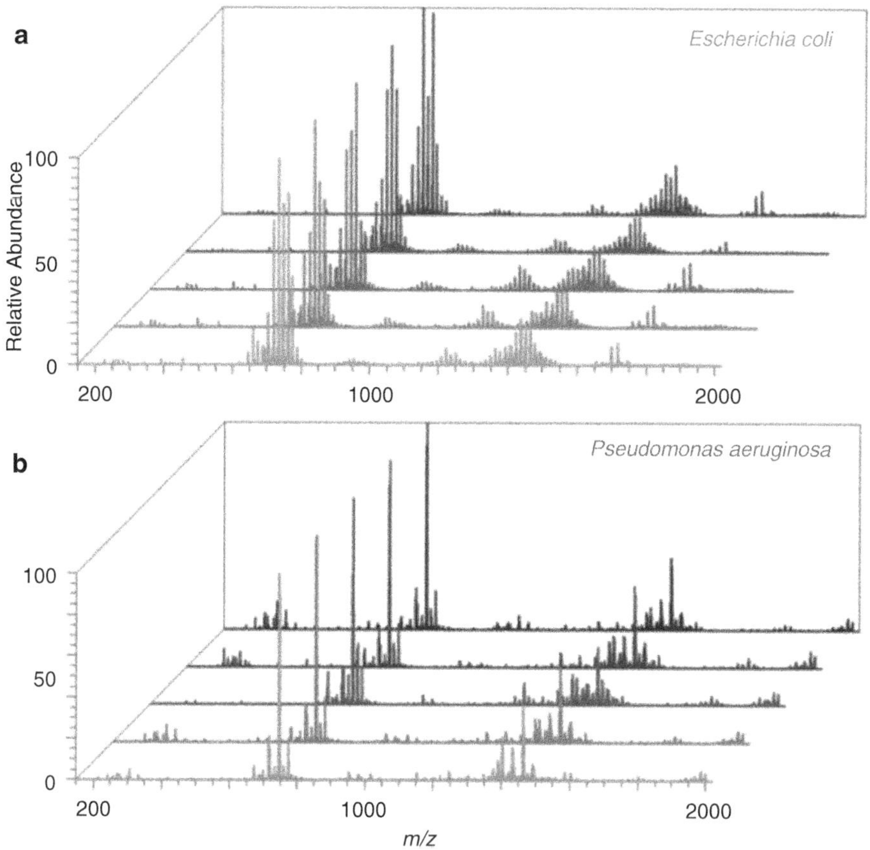

Fig. 13.20 REIMS spectra of different bacteria. (**a**) *Escherichia coli* and (**b**) *Pseudomonas aeruginosa*, each grown on five different solid growth media (Adapted from Ref. [67] with permission. © American Chemical Society, 2014)

endoscopic electrosurgery tools and it permits for mass spectra to be obtained in real time (Fig. 13.21) [66].

In the context of clinical applications, REIMS can also serve for high-throughput identification of clinically important bacteria and fungi [64] as well as for the analysis of bulk tissue and bacterial colonies on growth media [68]. Further, REIMS can be used in the detection of food fraud, e.g., to distinguish meat products from cattle, horse, or venison [69].

Whatever the origin of samples may be, their differentiation normally relies on using statistical tools such as principal component analysis (PCA), because the differences between spectra of healthy and infected tissue, for example, are often not immediately visible from the spectra.

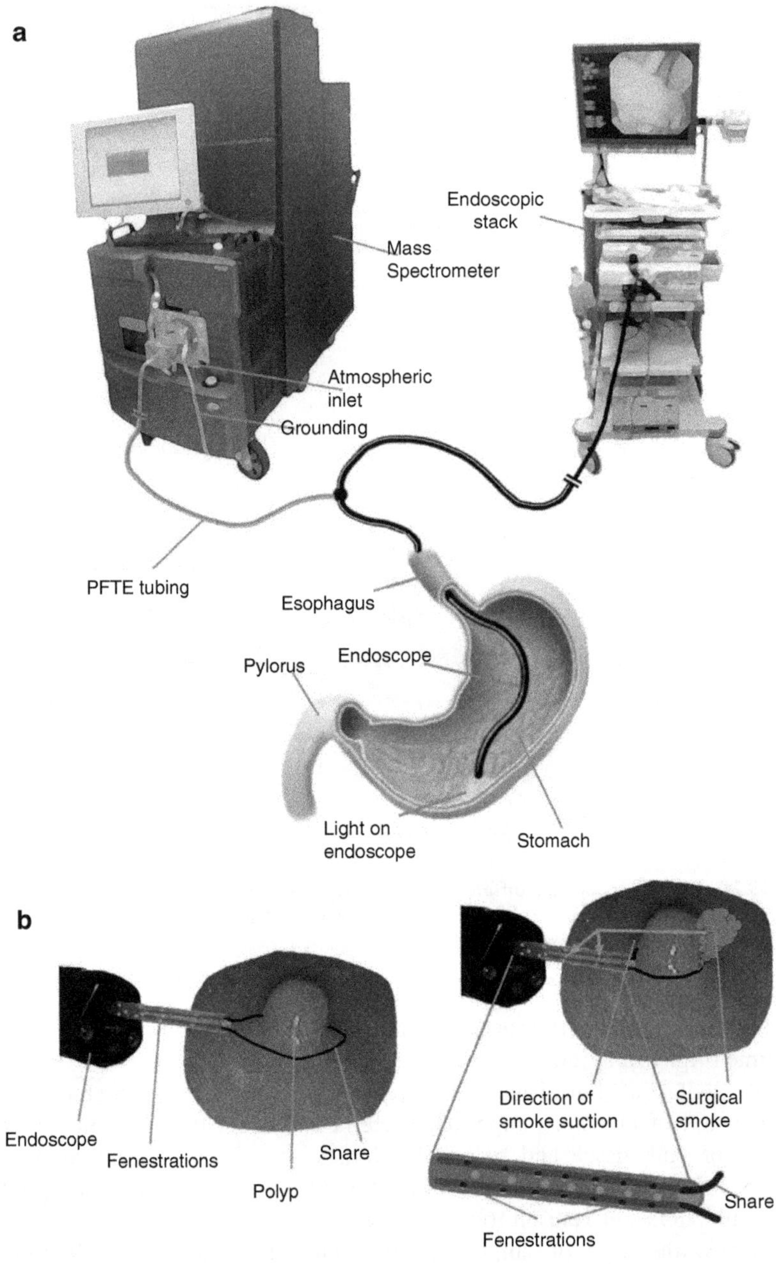

Fig. 13.21 Endoscopy experimental setup. (**a**) The polypectomy snare was equipped with an additional T-piece in order to establish direct connection between the electrode tip and the mass spectrometer for the transfer of electrosurgical aerosol. (**b**) Resection of GI polyps by using a commercial snare. The polyp is captured with the snare loop, which is tightly fastened around its base. Electrosurgical dissection is performed and the generated aerosol is aspirated through the fenestrations created on the plastic sheath of the snare (Reproduced from Ref. [66] with permission. © Wiley, 2015)

Recognizing gastric carcinoma Gastric mucosa, gastric submucosa, and adenocarcinoma tissue were analyzed by REIMS using a modified Waters Xevo G2-S Q-Tof mass spectrometer. Both, cancerous and healthy mucosal tissues were found to feature mainly phospholipids in the *m*/*z* 600–900 region, whereas submucosa mainly showed triglyceride and phosphatidylinositol species in the *m*/*z* 850–1000 region. In this case, even a visual comparison of the abundances of selected peaks shows significant differences between cancerous and healthy tissues in the range *m*/*z* 600–1000 (Fig. 13.22). Nonetheless, the recognition is notably simplified by translation of the spectral data in statistically evaluated plots (Kruskal-Wallis ANOVA test).

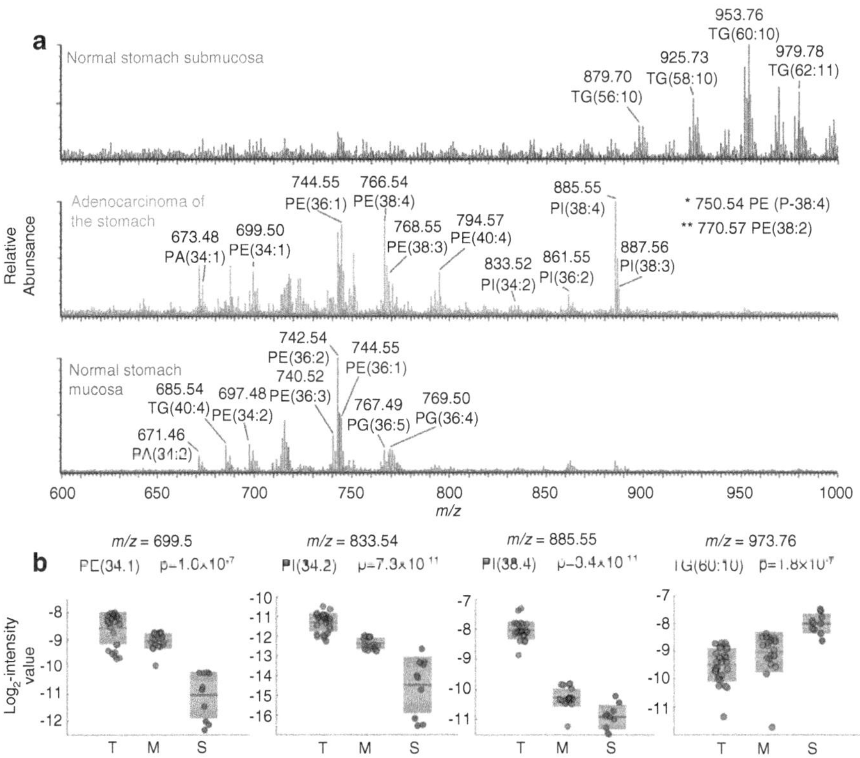

Fig. 13.22 (**a**) Mass spectra from gastric mucosa, gastric submucosa, and adenocarcinoma tissue recorded *ex vivo*. (**b**) Comparison of the abundance of selected peaks showing significant differences between cancerous and healthy tissues in the range *m*/*z* 600–1000 using Kruskal–Wallis ANOVA, $p < 0.005$. *T* tumor, *M* mucosa, *S* submucosa (Reproduced from Ref. [66] with permission. © Wiley, 2015)

13.7 Atmospheric Pressure Solids Analysis Probe

The *atmospheric pressure solids analysis probe* (ASAP) [70, 71] addresses a more classical field of organic mass spectrometry: the analysis of small organic molecules. With the successive replacement of classical EI and CI instrumentation – mostly magnetic sector instruments equipped with direct insertion probes – by APCI (Sect. 7.8), ESI (Chap. 12) or MALDI (Chap. 11) instruments, the tools to deal with samples that would previously have been run by EI-MS or CI-MS have been phased out in many MS laboratories. Based on a modification to an APCI source, ASAP offers an alternative to EI (Chap. 5) or CI (Chap. 7) Thus, ASAP can fill this gap in the MS toolbox at least to some extent [70].

13.7.1 Setup of the Atmospheric Pressure Solids Analysis Probe

In ASAP, by simply inserting a melting point tube into a stream of hot nitrogen gas, the solid is evaporated from the tube's surface and then ionized at atmospheric pressure by the corona discharge of an APCI source. The hot gas stream (350–500 °C) may either be provided by the APCI sprayer or by an ESI sprayer, provided the latter features a heated desolvation gas supply. In contrast to DESI or DAPCI, no solvent flow is employed in ASAP. Thus, the only modification of a commercial APCI source is to machine a small port into the housing around the spray region for insertion of the glass tube or to seal the hole by a plug when switching back to standard APCI or ESI operation (Fig. 13.23). ASAP devices are commercially available [72] but can also be custom-built with comparative ease [70, 73].

Not exactly ambient MS

ASAP does not strictly meet the criteria of ambient MS, in particular, if we define ambient MS by its ability to perform surface analysis of an object exposed to some ionizing fluid in the open atmosphere. ASAP requires the application of sample to a probe and it is performed inside a closed housing. Apart from the welcome association with the acronym, ASAP would have better been termed *probe-APCI*. Nonetheless, ASAP also bears some characteristics of ADI-MS.

13.7.2 Atmospheric Pressure Solids Analysis Probe in Practice

As in APCI, the analytes addressed by ASAP may range from low to high polarity and can have molecular masses in the 100–1500 u range. Representative applications of ASAP include screening for plasticizers in food packaging [74], the analysis of low-molecular-weight synthetic polymers [72], the high-throughput identification of anabolic steroid esters in the screening of drugs [75], or the

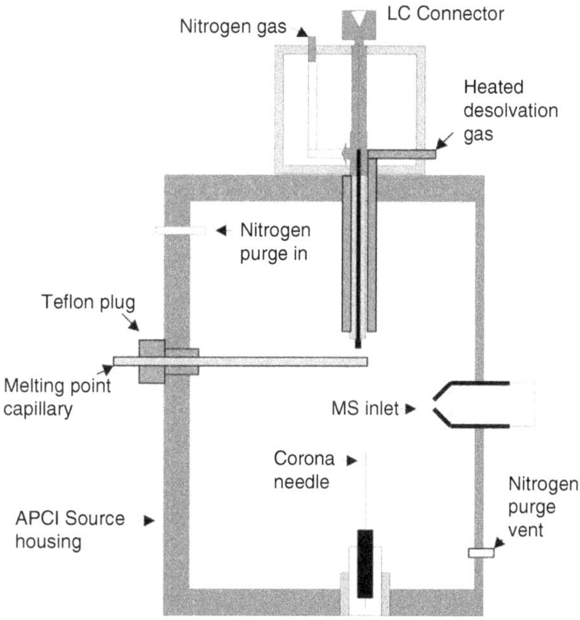

Fig. 13.23 Cross section of an atmospheric pressure solids analysis probe (ASAP) based on the standard APCI source of a Waters Q-TOF instrument (Reproduced from Ref. [70] with permission. © American Chemical Society, 2005)

analysis of nucleosides [73]. ASAP can also be used in conjunction with ion mobility-mass spectrometry as demonstrated for the detection and identification of impurities in 2-naphthalenamines [76].

One should be aware that application of sample onto the outside of a glass capillary, in particular, when provided as powder, inherently bears the risk of ion source contamination, e.g., during the process of inserting the capillary. Also, there is a tendency that dipping applies too large amounts of sample that may lead to cross contamination in subsequent runs. Therefore, care needs to be exercised to avoid these problems.

Oligomer analysis by ASAP Polystyrene of an average molecular weight of M_n = 1700 u (PS1700) was applied to the exterior of a glass capillary by dipping it into the PS powder. Positive-ion spectra in the *m/z* 50–2000 range were recorded using a Waters ASAP source mounted onto a Xevo QToF instrument. The majority of ion source parameters were set as typically the case in APCI operation (corona needle at 3.0 kV, corona discharge at 2.5 μA, nitrogen gas at 600 l min^{-1}). The temperature of the nitrogen was stepwise increased from 300 to 600 °C. The ASAP spectra showed a clear correlation between this temperature, the *m/z* range covered with PS signals, and the signal-to-noise ratio (S/N) achieved (Fig. 13.24) [72]. A minimum of 400 °C was required to form some PS ions at all, that showed up as molecular ions. Obviously, the low-polarity PS was ionized by charge transfer to form $M^{+•}$ ions. While the range covered was able to be expanded up to higher *m/z*, even the

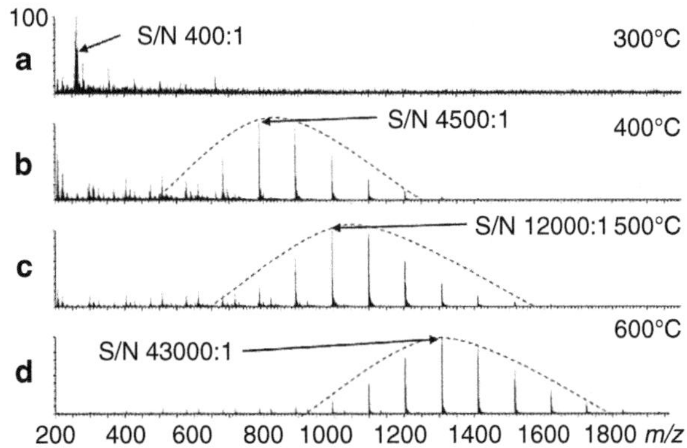

Fig. 13.24 The effect of desolvation gas temperature upon ASAP of polystyrene at (**a**) 300 °C, (**b**) 400 °C, (**c**) 500 °C, and (**d**) 600 °C (Reproduced from Ref. [72] with permission. © The Royal Society of Chemistry, 2012)

spectrum at 600 °C did not fully meet the M_n for this sample as derived from gel permeation chromatography (GPC).

13.8 Direct Analysis in Real Time

Direct analysis in real time (DART) [3], similar to ASAP in the preceding section, employs a solvent-free heated gas stream. In contrast to the aforementioned techniques, the DART gas initially carries excited noble gas atoms that have been formed in a plasma discharge. Reagent ions are then formed immediately upon interaction of these electronically excited atoms with the atmosphere. Thus, DART is related to atmospheric pressure chemical ionization (APCI) [5] and also bears some similarity to DAPCI or DAPPI.

Like DESI, DART sources are commercially available. As a powerful and highly versatile technique of ambient MS, DART has seen a vast number of applications [5, 6, 8, 9, 77–87].

13.8.1 DART Ion Source

In a DART source, a gas flow, typically helium or rarely nitrogen, is guided through a tube divided into three segments. In the first section, a corona discharge between a needle electrode and a first perforated disk electrode produces ions, electrons, and excited atoms (Fig. 13.25). The gas discharges in DART can be visibly distinguished as nitrogen emits a clear blue glare while the helium discharge shines in pale pink (Fig. 13.26).

The cold plasma passes through a further chamber where a second perforated electrode can remove cations from the gas stream that is subsequently heated and passed through a final grid electrode removing oppositely charged species. The ionizing neutral gas may either be directed towards the sampling orifice of an API

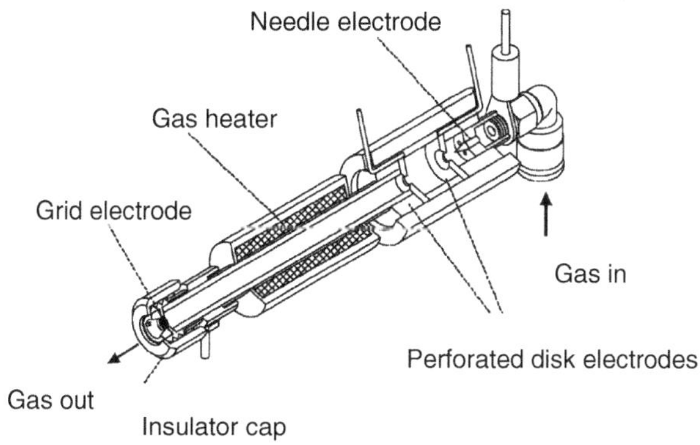

Fig. 13.25 Cutaway view of the DART source. The emanating gas effects ionization of sample independent of its state of aggregation (Reproduced from Ref. [3] with permission. © The American Chemical Society, 2005)

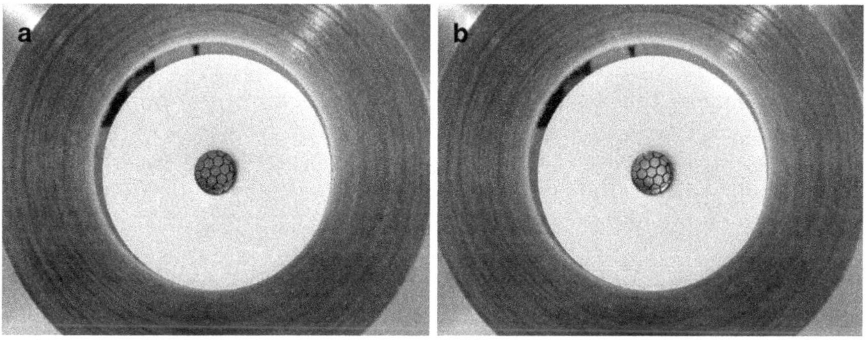

Fig. 13.26 DART discharges as seen when looking into the source. (**a**) Blue shining discharge in nitrogen, (**b**) pale pink discharge in helium. The hexagonal pattern is caused by the exit grid electrode

interface, or analogous to DESI, may hit the sample surface at an angle suitable for its reflection into the entrance of the mass spectrometer [3].

Typical operating conditions for DART use a positive discharge needle potential of 1–5 kV while the counter electrode (first perforated disk electrode) is grounded. The potentials of the second perforated electrode and the exit grid electrode are set to positive potentials for positive-ion DART and to negative potentials in the order of a hundred volts for negative-ion mode. The insulator cap protects sample and operator from any high voltage. The gas flow is adjusted to 1–3 l min^{-1} and the gas temperature may vary in the range of 50–500 °C. The DART source is adjustable over a range of angles and distances. Typically, a gap of 5–25 mm is established to insert the sample.

Type of the discharge
The DART discharge belongs to the corona-to-glow (C-G) discharge type that operates with discharge currents in the order of 2 mA at a temperature of 50–60 °C [88]. Recently, efforts have been made to provide a more efficient source for metastable atoms. A direct current *atmospheric pressure glow discharge* (APGD) sustained in helium and used in the *flowing afterglow* (FA) mode seems promising [88–90].

13.8.2 Positive Ion Formation in DART

The electrical discharge in helium produces a stream of gas containing electronically excited helium atoms (metastable atoms), ions, and electrons:

$$\text{discharge} + \text{He} \rightarrow \text{He}^* \tag{13.1}$$

The plasma gas is then heated and fully depleted of ions and electrons by passing it through electrically charged grids. When the stream exits to the open atmosphere, it may effect ionization of gases, and by direct contact also liquids and solids. The majority of the metastable helium atoms, He*, induces *Penning ionization* (Sect. 2.1.3) of nitrogen [3, 89]:

$$\text{He}^* + \text{N}_2 \rightarrow \text{He} + \text{N}_2^{+\bullet} + \text{e}^- \tag{13.2}$$

Apart from initiation by a discharge that delivers metastable helium atoms, He*, carrying 19.8 eV of energy, the pathway of reagent ion formation in DART basically follows the same route as in APCI (Sect. 7.8). Ion–molecule reactions are fast at atmospheric pressure due to high collision rates ($> 10^9\ \text{s}^{-1}$). Seemingly bimolecular reactions often are termolecular in reality, because a neutral collision partner like N_2 in Eq. 13.3 is required for immediate removal of excess energy [91–94]. Thus, the next steps lead to water molecular ions:

$$\text{N}_2^{+\bullet} + \text{N}_2 + \text{N}_{2(\text{3rdbody})} \rightarrow \text{N}_4^{+\bullet} + \text{N}_{2(\text{3rdbody})} \tag{13.3}$$

$$\text{N}_4^{+\bullet} + \text{H}_2\text{O} \rightarrow 2\text{N}_2 + \text{H}_2\text{O}^{+\bullet} \tag{13.4}$$

Then, the $H_2O^{+\bullet}$ ions quickly form cluster ions:

$$\text{H}_2\text{O}^{+\bullet} + \text{H}_2\text{O} \rightarrow \text{H}_3\text{O}^+ + \text{OH}^\bullet \tag{13.5}$$

$$\text{H}_3\text{O}^+ + n\text{H}_2\text{O} \rightarrow \left[(\text{H}_2\text{O})_\text{n} + \text{H}\right]^+ \tag{13.6}$$

Finally, the $[(H_2O)_n{+}H]^+$ ions act as reagent ions for analyte ion formation by protonation [93]:

$$M + [(H_2O)_n + H]^+ \rightarrow [M + H]^+ + nH_2O \tag{13.7}$$

Ammonium ion adducts are also observed in DART of medium polar compounds. $[M{+}NH_4]^+$ ions occur, for example, with oxygen-rich molecules, in particular in the absence of basic functional groups, e.g., polyethylene glycols, ketones, di- or triacylglycerols, and polysiloxanes:

$$M + [NH_4]^+ \rightarrow [M + NH_4]^+ \tag{13.8}$$

Ammonium ions may be delivered along with the sample, can be formed from trace amounts of ammonia in the atmosphere, or can intentionally be supplied simply by placing a vial with aqueous ammonia close to the reaction zone.

In addition to even-electron ions, DART can also yield odd-electron ions by charge transfer, i.e., DART can deliver molecular ions [95, 96]. Analyte molecular ions, $M^{+\bullet}$, can either be generated by Penning ionization with He* or more importantly by charge transfer. In the open atmosphere, the reagent ions are $N_4^{+\bullet}$, $O_2^{+\bullet}$, and NO^+:

$$N_4^{+\bullet} + M \rightarrow 2N_2 + M^{+\bullet} \tag{13.9}$$

$$O_2^{+\bullet} + M \rightarrow O_2 + M^{+\bullet} \tag{13.10}$$

$$NO^+ + M \rightarrow NO + M^{+\bullet} \tag{13.11}$$

The ratio of $M^{+\bullet}$ versus $[M{+}H]^+$ ion formation is mainly determined by analyte properties such as ionization energy, *IE*, and proton affinity, *PA* [97]. Low *IE* is going to favor $M^{+\bullet}$ ions while high *PA* promotes $[M{+}H]^+$ ion formation. Depending on the analyte, both ionic species can occur simultaneously causing the superimposition of $M^{+\bullet}$ and $[M{+}H]^+$ ion signals. Distorted isotopic patterns present a drawback for spectrum interpretation.

Helium may be replaced by argon as the DART gas in order to provide more selective or softer ionization, respectively [98, 99]. Unfortunately, argon has energetically lower metastable states of 11.55 eV ($^3P_2$) and 11.72 eV ($^3P_0$) and cannot ionize water ($IE = 12.65$ eV), causing argon-DART to have much lower sensitivity. It can be improved by a solvent make-up flow into the reaction zone, e.g., $IE_{MeOH} = 10.85$ eV. The ionization mechanism then switches from a $H_2O^{+\bullet}$-based pathway to a solvent ion-based process (replace H_2O by MeOH in Eqs. 13.4, 13.5, 13.6 and 13.7) [98, 99].

Whatever the actual process of ion formation, the high collision rates at atmospheric pressure effect immediate thermalization. As generally the case in ADI-MS, fragmentation is not really relevant in DART-MS.

13.8.3 Negative Ion Formation in DART

In negative ion mode, thermal electrons created by the reaction in Eq. 13.2 are presumed to generate mostly $O_2^{-\bullet}$ ions from air that serve as reagent ions. Of course, direct electron capture by the analyte as well as dissociative electron capture, deprotonation, or anion attachment are also feasible [92]. These $O_2^{-\bullet}$ ions form adducts by association with the analyte M:

$$O_2^{-\bullet} + M \rightarrow [M + O_2]^{-\bullet} \tag{13.12}$$

Alternatively, negative molecular ions directly formed by electron capture can attach to molecular oxygen, thereby yielding the same product:

$$M^{-\bullet} + O_2 \rightarrow [M + O_2]^{-\bullet} \tag{13.13}$$

$[M+O_2]^{-\bullet}$ may either be detected as such or may dissociate to yield radical anions:

$$[M + O_2]^{-\bullet} \rightarrow M^{-\bullet} + O_2 \tag{13.14}$$

The loss of a hydroperoxyl radical may lead to $[M–H]^-$ ions, i.e., proton abstraction, if the gas phase acidity of $[M–H]^-$ exceeds that of $HOO^\bullet$:

$$[M + O_2]^{-\bullet} \rightarrow [M - H]^- + HOO^\bullet \tag{13.15}$$

Apart from $O_2^{-\bullet}$, the atmospheric components lead to $NO_2^{-\bullet}$, $CO_3^{-\bullet}$ [100], and depending on traces of solvents also CN^-, Cl^-, OH^-, and other ions. Halogenide adduct ions can be observed when the analyte and/or a solvent are halogenated:

$$M + Hal^- \rightarrow [M + Hal]^- \tag{13.16}$$

Finally, adduct ion formation with less abundant anions such as CO_3^-, NO_2^-, or OH^- can occur.

13.8.4 ADI Methods Related to DART

There are numerous ion sources that similarly rely on Penning ionization. Some of them preceded DART by many years while the development of others may have been inspired by DART. Most of these techniques never became commercially available, and thus, sometimes are unique to a single research group. DART is the by far best established technique in the field.

Penning ionization represents only one facet of DART as it is the primary source of ionization for DART. Rather than direct Penning ionization of the analyte, in most cases reagent ions derived from atmospheric components are responsible for analyte ion generation. DART can therefore be categorized as belonging to a family

Table 13.2 Methods of ambient mass spectrometry closely related to DART

Full term	Acronym	References
Liquid surface Penning ionization	LPI	[102, 103]
Atmospheric sampling glow discharge ionization	ASGDI	[104]
Atmospheric pressure Penning ionization	APPeI	[105–107]
Plasma-assisted desorption/ionization	PADI	[108]
Dielectric barrier discharge ionization	DBDI	[109, 110]
Double cylindrical barrier discharge ionization	DC-DBDI	[111]
Atmospheric pressure glow discharge ionization	APGD	[112]
Helium atmospheric pressure glow discharge ionization	HAPGDI	[112]
Flowing afterglow atmospheric pressure glow discharge	FA-APGD	[90]
Low-temperature plasma probe	LTP	[101]
Atmospheric pressure solids analysis probe	ASAP	[70, 71, 113]
Surface-activated chemical ionization	SACI	[114, 115]
Desorption atmospheric pressure chemical ionization	DAPCI	[14, 21, 31, 101]
Desorption atmospheric pressure photoionization	DAPPI	[16]
Atmospheric pressure thermal desorption ionization	APTDI	[116]

of APCI-related ionization techniques [4]. DART and other techniques of this group have in common that they use a stream of heated gas containing ionizing species that are created in some sort of an atmospheric pressure plasma [101].

For completeness, these related techniques are compiled in Table 13.2. The multiple relationships between most of the numerous techniques mentioned here, have been visualized in a "flowergram" (Fig. 13.27) [5].

13.8.5 DART Configurations

In contrast to the gases normally contained in air, helium presents a true challenge for all types of vacuum pumps. The JEOL AccuTOF instrument that DART was originally developed for happens to possess some zig-zag ion path in the ion source optics that guides ions to the orthogonal TOF analyzer while it deflects neutrals. Thus, the use of helium was easily accepted by this instrument [3]. However, helium flow into the API interface of mass spectrometers other than the JEOL AccuTOF would cause poor if not inacceptable vacuum conditions when the DART source is in operation. To solve this problem, the so-called Vapur Interface is mounted in between the DART source and the entrance of the API interface where it serves as an additional pumping stage. A small membrane pump suffices to remove most of the helium. Furthermore, the aspirating ceramics tube improves the ion transfer from the ionization zone into the mass spectrometer (Fig. 13.28).

Initially, the DART source was configured on-axis with the sampling orifice of the API interface and objects to be analyzed were positioned tangentially to present the surface to the helium flow. Notable improvements for the analysis of single compounds and simple mixtures were made by the introduction of transmission mode DART

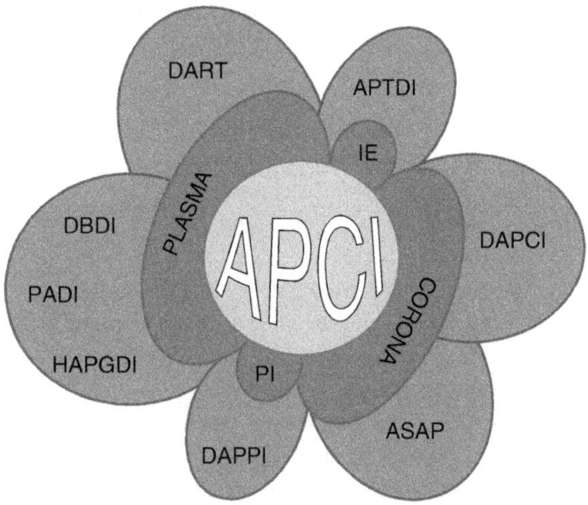

Fig. 13.27 Relationship of DART to other methods of ambient MS that basically rely on APCI-like mechanisms of ion formation. A "flowergram" illustrates the methods (*red*) where chemical ionization processes (*yellow*) are used for analyte ion formation. Reagent ion generation (*green*) is initiated by either plasma, corona discharge, ion evaporation, or photoionization (Reproduced from Ref. [5] by kind permission. © Elsevier, 2008)

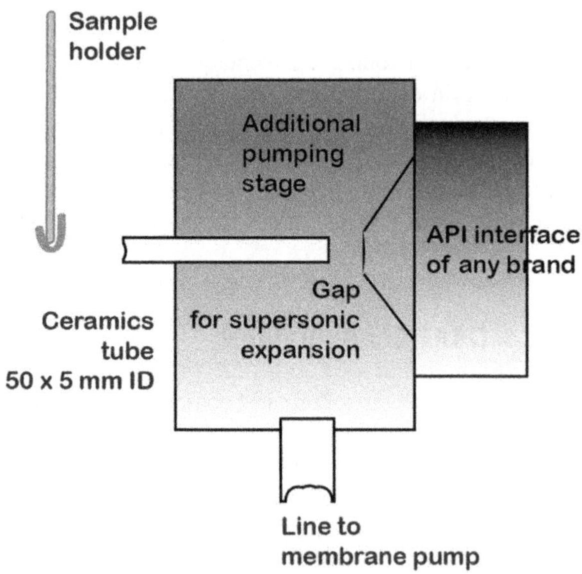

Fig. 13.28 Schematic of the Vapur Interface used to adapt the DART source to API interfaces of different instrument manufacturers. The additional pumping stage prevents compromised instrument vacuum and improves the transfer of sample ions by acting as a jet separator (Reprinted from Ref. [8] with permission. © Springer, 2013)

[117]. For transmission mode, the sample is deposited on a fine wire mesh that is then immerged into the gas stream; the mesh provides both a large surface and good transmission for the ion-carrying gas. For the DART analysis of objects, an angled configuration as used in DESI turned out to be more efficient [118]. As a consequence, DART sources can be configured in various ways to optimally meet the requirements of a variety of samples (Fig. 13.29) [8]. For routine analyses in synthetic chemistry, the Open Source, a special device for use with disposable sample cards, provides the most facile way of transmission mode DART-MS while the 45° geometry is best suited for surface mode DART (Fig. 13.30).

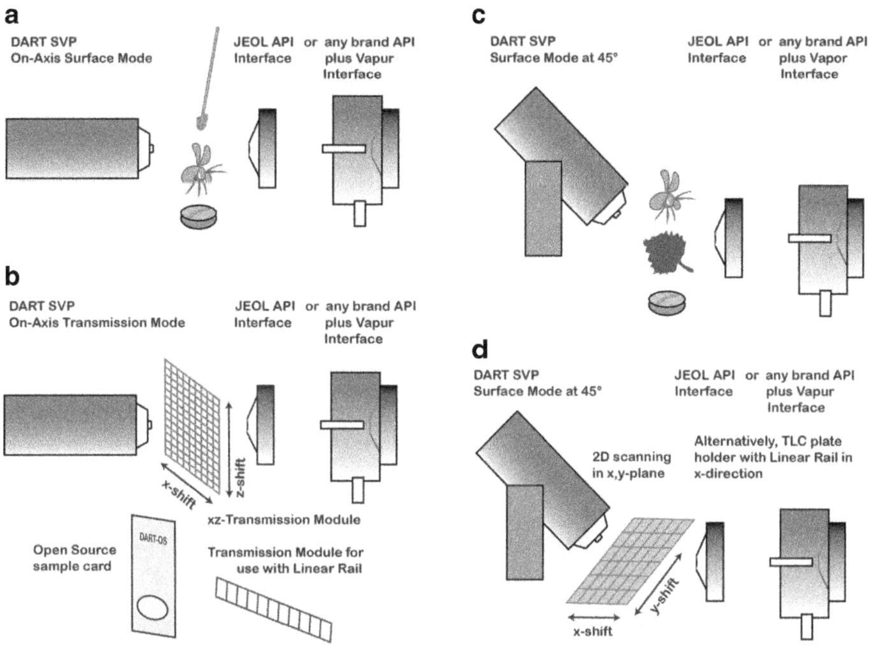

Fig. 13.29 DART configurations. (**a**) First design with axial orientation of source and orifice of the API interface, (**b**) axial orientation for transmission mode when presenting samples on a mesh, (**c**) surface mode with source at an angle for analyzing small objects, and (**d**) surface mode at an angle for automated analysis of an array of samples (Adapted from Ref. [8] with permission. © Springer, 2013)

13.8.6 Analytical Applications of DART

From the very beginning, DART has been applied to the most diverse kinds of cases [5, 6, 8, 9, 77–87]. This includes the typical safety-related and forensic usages of ambient MS like detection of explosives, warfare agents, or pharmaceuticals and drugs of abuse from cloth, banknotes, etc. [3, 92, 119], or the examination of ballpoint-pen inks on paper, e.g., signatures in cases of check fraud [120]. In the life sciences, DART serves for the rapid analysis of fatty acid methyl esters (FAMEs) from whole cells [121], for clinical studies of compounds from plasma and urine [122, 123]. DART is sensitive enough to analyze self-assembled thiol and dithioether monolayers on gold surfaces [124]. Some representative applications are depicted below to give an idea of the manifold uses of DART-MS.

Volatiles from garlic Positive-ion and negative-ion DART-MS was used for the identification of reactive sulfur-containing compounds formed from cutting different species of the genus *Allium* (garlic, onion, elephant garlic, leek, Chinese chives, and others) [125, 126]. Garlic cloves were held into the open gap between the DART source and the orifice of the API interface of a JEOL AccuTOF instrument

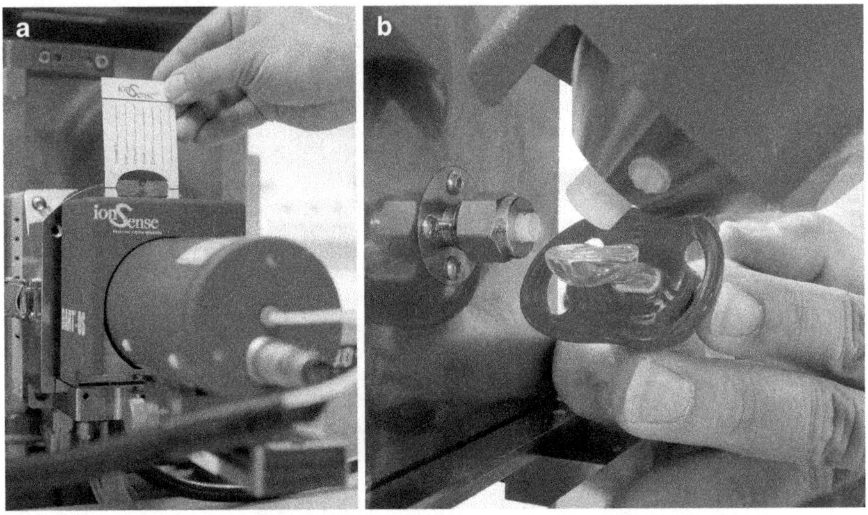

Fig. 13.30 DART configurations in use. (**a**) Open Source for transmission mode DART with disposable sample cards (corresponds to setup **b** in Fig. 13.29), (**b**) alignment at an angle of 45° for the analysis of objects placed in the gap (corresponds to setup **c** in Fig. 13.29). Both photos show the DART source attached to a Bruker instrument by means of the Vapur Interface

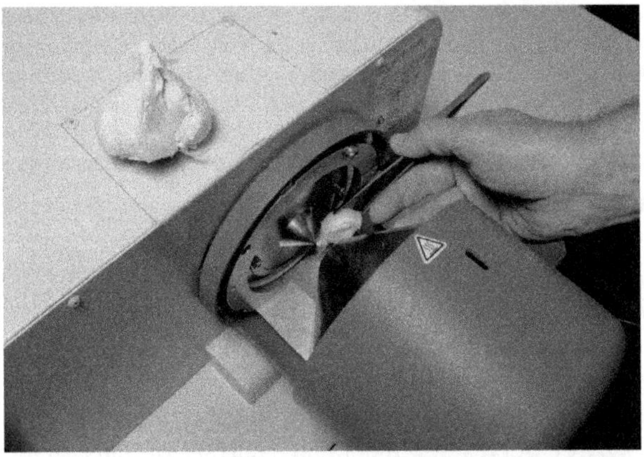

Fig. 13.31 Commercial DART source of the first generation on a JEOL AccuTOF instrument. Here it is used for the analysis of volatiles from a garlic clove [125, 126]. The sample is simply held into the open gap between the metastable atom source (*lower right part*) and the orifice of the API interface (*upper left*). Photograph by courtesy of JEOL USA

(Fig. 13.31 and mode **a** in Fig. 13.29). From cut garlic, for example, positive-ion DART showed compounds such as allicin, allyl/methyl and dimethyl thiosulfinates, diallyl trisulfane *S*-oxide, allyl alcohol, and propene. Negative-ion DART detected 2-propenesulfenic acid, 2-propenesulfinic acid, SO_2, and pyruvate. The different *Allium* species exhibited different volatile compounds.

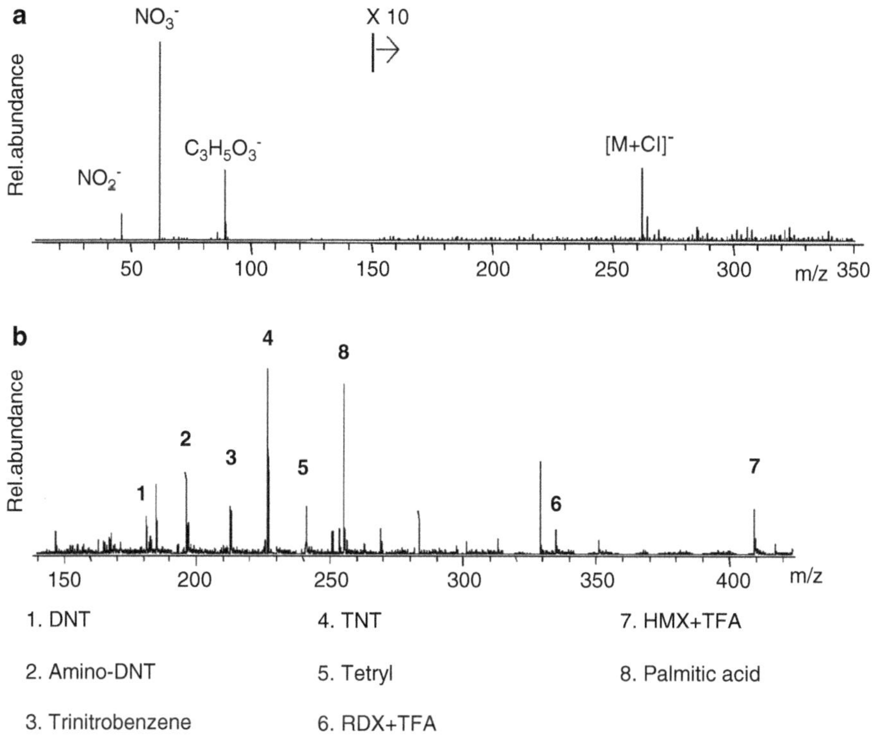

Fig. 13.32 DART spectra of explosives. Spectrum **(a)** shows nitroglycerin detected on a man's necktie 8 h after exposure to the plume from blasting at a construction site. In **(b)** a sample of contaminated pond water exhibits $[M+TFA]^-$ peaks for various explosives that are present at about 3 ppm (Reproduced from Ref. [3] with permission. © The American Chemical Society, 2005)

Negative-ion DART for explosives Still under the impression of the 2001 terrorist attack on the World Trade Center, ambient MS initially had a strong focus on the detection of explosives. Negative-ion DART is very sensitive for the analysis of explosives exhibiting extremely low but non-zero vapor pressure [92]. Nitroglycerin has been detected on a man's necktie 8 h after exposure to the plume from blasting at a construction site (Fig. 13.32a) and various explosives present at about 3 ppm in a contaminated pond water sample have been detected; placing a small open bottle with 0.1% aqueous trifluoroacetic acid (H-TFA) in proximity to the sampling zone caused them to appear as $[M+TFA]^-$ adduct peaks in the DART spectrum (Fig. 13.32b) [3].

Invading a fly's private sphere DART allows for the cuticular hydrocarbon analysis of active fruit flies *Sophophora melanogaster (Drosophila melanogaster)*. The hydrocarbon profile as measured from the exterior of female flies comprises alkenes and alkadienes in the C_{18} to C_{29} range that are detected as $[M+H]^+$ ions. The profile

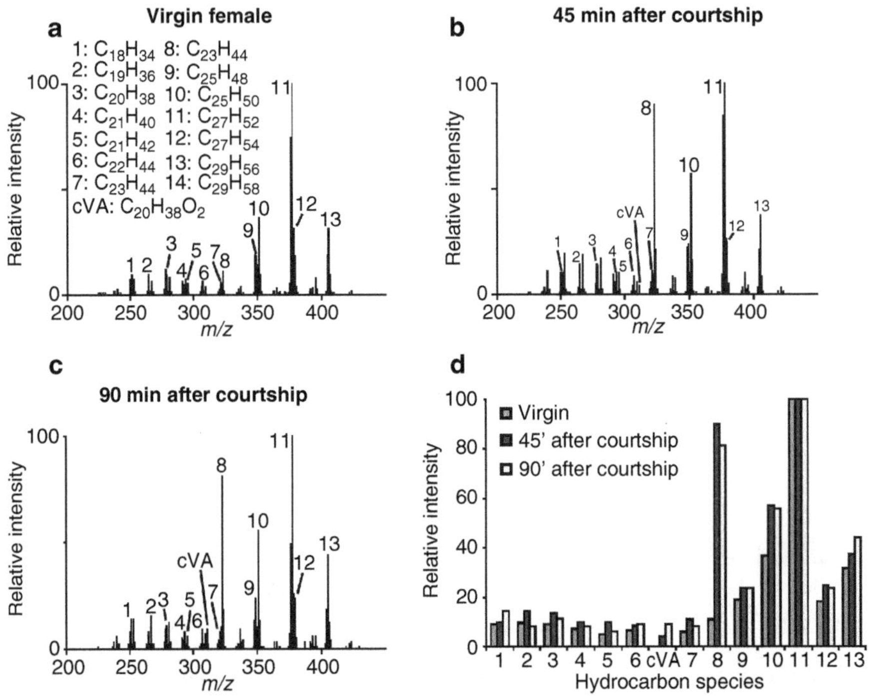

Fig. 13.33 Chemical profile changes in the same individual female fly as observed (**a**) before, (**b**) 45 min after, and (**c**) 90 min after copulation. (**d**) A histogram shows the changes in hydrocarbon concentrations, in particular, an increase in tricosene (peak 8) and pentacosene (peak 10) (Reproduced from Ref. [127] with permission. © The National Academy of Sciences of the USA, 2008)

has been found to vary depending on whether the flies are observed as virgin females, 45 min or 90 min after courtship (Fig. 13.33). There is also a difference between males and females. The advantage of DART is that the fly can be exposed to the ionizing gas stream without risk of electrical shock to both fly and researcher [127].

Silicones in household utensils and food Positive-ion DART is highly suitable for the analysis of polydimethylsiloxanes (PDMS) [128, 129], commonly known as silicone rubber. Silicone rubber is a common material of articles of daily use such as flexible silicone baking molds, watch bands, dough scrapers, pacifiers, and non-stick coatings of parchment paper, for example [130]. DART not only permits to analyze the household utensils themselves (Sect. 3.6.5) [129] but also to assess their tendency to release low-molecular-weight silicone oligomers into food during baking [129, 131, 132].

For the analysis of the household items, the DART source was mounted at an angle of 45° relative to the axis of the ceramics tube of the Vapur Interface. The entire objects were manually positioned about halfway between the helium exit and capillary entrance and directly exposed to the ionizing gas (Fig. 13.30b). For all silicone rubber items, the gas was uniformly set to 300 °C. A typical spectrum of baked goods analyzed after use of a silicone rubber baking mold is shown in Fig. 13.34. The *m/z* 200–1650 range demonstrates the relative intensities of peaks from triacylglycerols (TAGs), i.e., fat from butter, and PDMS (*right*). The series of $[M+NH_4]^+$ ions of low-mass TAGs on average exhibits the characteristic value $\Delta(m/z) = 28.0313$ due to differences by $(CH_2)_2$ units. Series of ions at higher mass with peaks of $\Delta(m/z) = 74.0185$ on average, are caused by PDMS differing by $[(CH_3)_2SiO]$ repeat units. The isotopic patterns also reveal multiple Si atoms [131]. Obviously, there is a substantial release of PDMS into the food [131, 132].

Furthermore, the distribution of peaks across the *m/z* 200–3000 range permits the use of silicone oil and grease for mass calibration in positive-ion DART-MS [128].

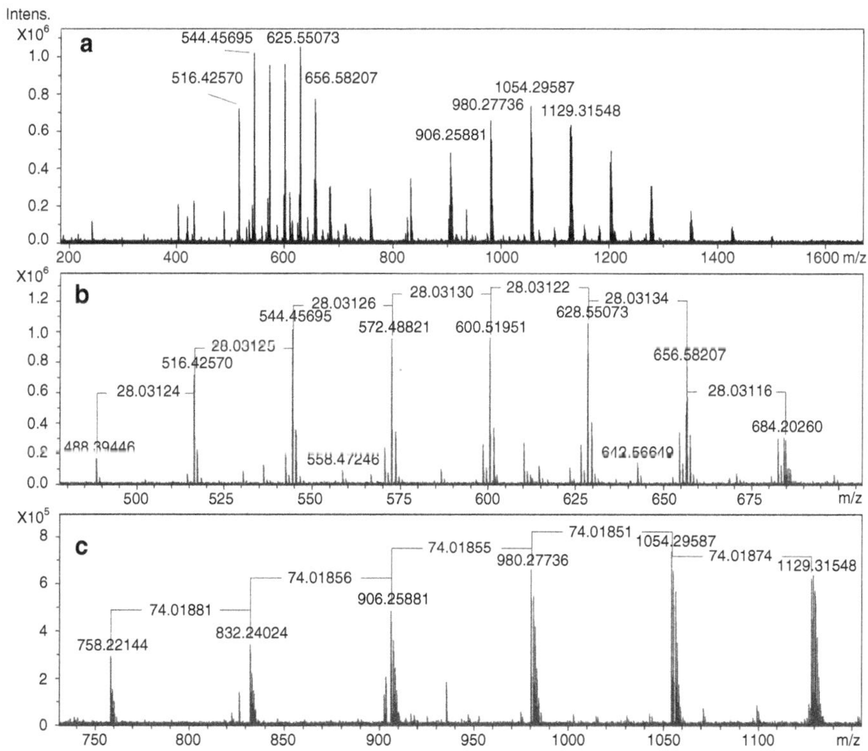

Fig. 13.34 Positive-ion DART spectra of a dough baked in a Kaiser silicone rubber baking mold. (**a**) Entire spectrum in the *m/z* 200–1650 range to show the relative intensities of peaks from TAGs (*left*) and PDMS (*right*). (**b**) Series of $[M+NH_4]^+$ ions of low-mass TAGs exhibiting the characteristic value $\Delta(m/z) = 28.0313$ on average. (**c**) Series of ions at higher mass with peaks of $\Delta(m/z) = 74.0185$ on average, owing to $[(CH_3)_2SiO]$ repeat units. The isotopic patterns also reveal multiple Si atoms (Reprinted from Ref. [131] with permission. © SAGE, 2015)

13.9 The World of Ambient Mass Spectrometry

Characteristic Feature of Ambient MS

The novel and characteristic feature of *ambient desorption/ionization* (ADI) or *ambient mass spectrometry* is that it allows instantaneous mass spectral analysis without sample preparation or sample pretreatment. Furthermore, the object to be analyzed is handled at atmospheric pressure, i.e., in a freely accessible open space in front of the atmospheric pressure interface.

Ambient MS allows for the examination of untreated samples or entire objects in the open environment while maintaining sample integrity. Ambient MS is elegant in that a sample only needs to be exposed to an ionizing fluid medium under ambient conditions.

A Family of Methods

There is no single method. Instead, the term ambient MS collects a group of techniques that all share the feature of ambient desorption/ionization. ADI-MS employs ion generation based on ESI, APCI, APPI, combinations thereof with laser desorption, and various electrical discharges to create ionizing plasmas as employed in DART.

Methods of Ambient MS

The below short table summarizes some of the more relevant ambient MS methods. They are listed in alphabetical order of their acronyms together with a key reference (Table 13.3). It should be noted, however, that only the truly simple-to-operate yet effective and rugged interfaces will survive over the years. As predicted in the previous edition of this book, DESI and DART were among the ones to persist in the long term.

Applications of Ambient MS

There is a vast range of applications for ambient MS. The major methods DESI and DART are documented in hundreds of publications each and also the numerous other methods were employed in manifold ways, sometimes to solve very specific problems. The development of ADI-MS is being pursued at a high pace.

A Word of Caution

Ambient MS methods tend to be easy to use, and in fact, can be a pleasure to use. While the range of applications is absolutely impressive, one should be aware that any of these methods only reveals what is present *on* the surface. Even there, compounds may be suppressed as others are ionized much more efficiently by the ADI method employed and under the operational conditions actually set. ADI-MS cannot reveal what is *below* the surface. Nonetheless, similar restrictions apply for any other MS method.

Table 13.3 Methods of ambient mass spectrometry

Acronym	Full term	Basic principle and key references
ASAP	Atmospheric pressure solids analysis probe	Evaporation of solids in hot gas stream and ionization by corona discharge [70]
DAPCI	Desorption atmospheric pressure chemical ionization	Sample surface exposed to APCI [21]
DAPPI	Desorption atmospheric pressure photoionization	Sample surface exposed to APPI [16]
DART	Direct analysis in real time	Sample surface exposed to ionizing noble gas stream [3]
DESI	Desorption electrospray ionization	Sample surface exposed to electrospray plume [1, 2]
DeSSI	Desorption sonic spray ionization	Sample surface exposed to sonic spray ionization plume; equal to EASI [10]
ELDI	Electrospray-assisted laser desorption ionization	LDI with post-ionization by ESI plume [55]
EASI	Easy ambient sonic-spray ionization	Sample surface exposed to sonic spray ionization plume; equal to DeSSI [42]
EESI	Extractive electrospray ionization	Sample vapor or mist admixed to electrospray plume [13, 46]
LAESI	Laser ablation electrospray ionization	IR laser ablation with postionization by ESI plume [62]
MALDESI	Matrix-assisted laser desorption electrospray ionization	Uptake of AP-MALDI plume by ESI spray and transport into API interface [60]

References

1. Takats Z, Wiseman JM, Gologan B, Cooks RG (2004) Mass Spectrometry Sampling Under Ambient Conditions with Desorption Electrospray Ionization. Science 306:471–473. doi:10.1126/science.1104404
2. Takats Z, Wiseman JM, Cooks RG (2005) Ambient Mass Spectrometry Using Desorption Electrospray Ionization (DESI): Instrumentation, Mechanisms and Applications in Forensics, Chemistry, and Biology. J Mass Spectrom 40:1261–1275. doi:10.1002/jms.922
3. Cody RB, Laramee JA, Durst HD (2005) Versatile New Ion Source for the Analysis of Materials in Open Air Under Ambient Conditions. Anal Chem 77:2297–2302. doi:10.1021/ac050989d
4. Weston DJ (2010) Ambient Ionization Mass Spectrometry: Current Understanding of Mechanistic Theory; Analytical Performance and Application Areas. Analyst 135:661–668. doi:10.1039/b925579f
5. Venter A, Nefliu M, Cooks RG (2008) Ambient Desorption Ionization Mass Spectrometry. Trends Anal Chem 27:284–290. doi:10.1016/j.trac.2008.01.010
6. Green FM, Salter TL, Stokes P, Gilmore IS, O'Connor G (2010) Ambient Mass Spectrometry: Advances and Applications in Forensics. Surf Interface Anal 42:347–357. doi:10.1002/sia.3131
7. Weston DJ, Ray AD, Bristow AWT (2011) Commentary: Challenging Convention Using Ambient Ionization and Direct Analysis Mass Spectrometric Techniques. Rapid Commun Mass Spectrom 25:821–825. doi:10.1002/rcm.4925

8. Gross JH (2014) Direct Analysis in Real Time - A Critical Review of DART-MS. Anal Bioanal Chem 406:63–80. doi:10.1007/s00216-013-7316-0
9. Hajslova J, Cajka T, Vaclavik L (2011) Challenging Applications Offered by Direct Analysis in Real Time (DART) in Food-Quality and Safety Analysis. Trends Anal Chem 30:204–218. doi:10.1016/j.trac.2010.11.001
10. Haddad R, Sparrapan R, Eberlin MN (2006) Desorption Sonic Spray Ionization for (High) Voltage-Free Ambient Mass Spectrometry. Rapid Commun Mass Spectrom 20:2901–2905. doi:10.1002/rcm.2680
11. Haddad R, Sparrapan R, Kotiaho T, Eberlin MN (2008) Easy ambient sonic-spray ionization-membrane interface Easy Ambient Sonic-Spray Ionization-Membrane Interface Mass Spectrometry for Direct Analysis of Solution Constituents. Anal Chem 80:898–903. doi:10.1021/ac701960q
12. Chen H, Zenobi R (2007) Direct Analysis of Living Objects by Extractive Electrospray Mass Ionization Spectrometry. Chimia 61:843. doi:10.2533/chimia.2007.843
13. Chen H, Yang S, Wortmann A, Zenobi R (2007) Neutral Desorption Sampling of Living Objects for Rapid Analysis by Extractive Electrospray Ionization Mass Spectrometry. Angew Chem Int Ed 46:7591–7594. doi:10.1002/anie.200702200
14. Takats Z, Cotte-Rodriguez I, Talaty N, Chen H, Cooks RG (2005) Direct, Trace Level Detection of Explosives on Ambient Surfaces by Desorption Electrospray Ionization Mass Spectrometry. Chem Commun:1950–1952. doi:10.1039/B418697D
15. Williams JP, Patel VJ, Holland R, Scrivens JH (2006) The Use of Recently Described Ionisation Techniques for the Rapid Analysis of Some Common Drugs and Samples of Biological Origin. Rapid Commun Mass Spectrom 20:1447–1456. doi:10.1002/rcm.2470
16. Haapala M, Pol J, Saarela V, Arvola V, Kotiaho T, Ketola RA, Franssila S, Kauppila TJ, Kostiainen R (2007) Desorption Atmospheric Pressure Photoionization. Anal Chem 79:7867–7872. doi:10.1021/ac071152g
17. Cooks RG, Ouyang Z, Takats Z, Wiseman JM (2006) Ambient Mass Spectrometry. Science 311:1566–1570. doi:10.1126/science.1119426
18. Wells JM, Roth MJ, Keil AD, Grossenbacher JW, Justes DR, Patterson GE, Barket DJ (2008) Implementation of DART and DESI Ionization on a Fieldable Mass Spectrometer. J Am Soc Mass Spectrom 19:1419–1424. doi:10.1016/j.jasms.2008.06.028
19. Takats Z, Wiseman JM, Gologan B, Cooks RG (2004) Electrosonic Spray Ionization. A Gentle Technique for Generating Folded Proteins and Protein Complexes in the Gas Phase and for Studying Ion-Molecule Reactions at Atmospheric Pressure. Anal Chem 76:4050–4058. doi:10.1021/ac049848m
20. Chen H, Talaty NN, Takats Z, Cooks RG (2005) Desorption Electrospray Ionization Mass Spectrometry for High-Throughput Analysis of Pharmaceutical Samples in the Ambient Environment. Anal Chem 77:6915–6927. doi:10.1021/ac050989d
21. Cotte-Rodriguez I, Takats Z, Talaty N, Chen H, Cooks RG (2005) Desorption Electrospray Ionization of Explosives on Surfaces: Sensitivity and Selectivity Enhancement by Reactive Desorption Electrospray Ionization. Anal Chem 77:6755–6764. doi:10.1021/ac050995+
22. Talaty N, Takats Z, Cooks RG (2005) Rapid in Situ Detection of Alkaloids in Plant Tissue Under Ambient Conditions Using Desorption Electrospray Ionization. Analyst 130:1624–1633. doi:10.1039/B511161G
23. Dole RB (ed) (1997) Electrospray Ionization Mass Spectrometry – Fundamentals, Instrumentation and Applications. Wiley, Chichester
24. Pramanik BN, Ganguly AK, Gross ML (eds) (2002) Applied Electrospray Mass Spectrometry. Marcel Dekker, New York
25. Denes J, Katona M, Hosszu A, Czuczy N, Takats Z (2009) Analysis of Biological Fluids by Direct Combination of Solid Phase Extraction and Desorption Electrospray Ionization Mass Spectrometry. Anal Chem 81:1669–1675. doi:10.1021/ac8024812
26. Drayß M (2005) Oberflächenanalytik mittels Desorptions Elektrospray Ionisation an einem Tripelquadrupolmassenspektrometer. Heidelberg University, Dissertation

27. Takats Z, Kobliha V, Sevcik K, Novak P, Kruppa G, Lemr K, Havlicek V (2008) Characterization of DESI-FTICR Mass Spectrometry – From ECD to Accurate Mass Tissue Analysis. J Mass Spectrom 43:196–203. doi:10.1002/jms.1285
28. Hopf C, Schlueter M, Schwarz-Selinger T, von Toussaint U, Jacob W (2008) Chemical Sputtering of Carbon Films by Simultaneous Irradiation with Argon Ions and Molecular Oxygen. New J Phys 10:093022. doi:10.1088/1367-2630/10/9/093022
29. Wiseman JM, Puolitaival SM, Takats Z, Cooks RG, Caprioli RM (2005) Mass Spectrometric Profiling of Intact Biological Tissue by Using Desorption Electrospray Ionization. Angew Chem Int Ed 44:7094–7097. doi:10.1002/anie.200502362
30. Cotte-Rodriguez I, Hernandez-Soto H, Chen H, Cooks RG (2008) In Situ Trace Detection of Peroxide Explosives by Desorption Electrospray Ionization and Desorption Atmospheric Pressure Chemical Ionization. Anal Chem 80:1512–1519. doi:10.1021/ac7020085
31. Cotte-Rodriguez I, Mulligan CC, Cooks RG (2007) Non-Proximate Detection of Small and Large Molecules by Desorption Electrospray Ionization and Desorption Atmospheric Pressure Chemical Ionization Mass Spectrometry: Instrumentation and Applications in Forensics, Chemistry, and Biology. Anal Chem 79:7069–7077. doi:10.1021/ac0707939
32. Van Berkel GJ, Ford MJ, Deibel MA (2005) Thin-Layer Chromatography and Mass Spectrometry Coupled Using Desorption Electrospray Ionization. Anal Chem 77:1207–1215. doi:10.1021/ac048217p
33. Chen H, Zheng J, Zhang X, Luo M, Wang Z, Qiao X (2007) Surface Desorption Atmospheric Pressure Chemical Ionization Mass Spectrometry for Direct Ambient Sample Analysis Without Toxic Chemical Contamination. J Mass Spectrom 42:1045–1056. doi:10.1002/jms.1235
34. Chen H, Liang H, Ding J, Lai J, Huan Y, Qiao X (2007) Rapid Differentiation of Tea Products by Surface Desorption Atmospheric Pressure Chemical Ionization Mass Spectrometry. J Agric Food Chem 55:10093–10100. doi:10.1021/jf0720234
35. Yang S, Ding J, Zheng J, Hu B, Li J, Chen H, Zhou Z, Qiao X (2009) Detection of Melamine in Milk Products by Surface Desorption Atmospheric Pressure Chemical Ionization Mass Spectrometry. Anal Chem 81:2426–2436. doi:10.1021/ac900063u
36. Luosujarvi L, Arvola V, Haapala M, Pol J, Saarela V, Franssila S, Kotiaho T, Kostiainen R, Kauppila TJ (2008) Desorption and Ionization Mechanisms in Desorption Atmospheric Pressure Photoionization. Anal Chem 80:7460–7466. doi:10.1021/ac801186x
37. Luosujarvi L, Laakkonen UM, Kostiainen R, Kotiaho T, Kauppila TJ (2009) Analysis of Street Market Confiscated Drugs by Desorption Atmospheric Pressure Photoionization and Desorption Electrospray Ionization Coupled with Mass Spectrometry. Rapid Commun Mass Spectrom 23:1401–1404. doi:10.1002/rcm.4005
38. Kauppila TJ, Arvola V, Haapala M, Pol J, Aalberg L, Saarela V, Franssila S, Kotiaho T, Kostiainen R (2008) Direct Analysis of Illicit Drugs by Desorption Atmospheric Pressure Photoionization. Rapid Commun Mass Spectrom 22:979–985. doi:10.1002/rcm.3461
39. Hirabayashi Y, Takada Y, Hirabayashi A, Sakairi M, Koizumi H (1996) Direct Coupling of Semi-Micro Liquid Chromatography and Sonic Spray Ionization Mass Spectrometry for Pesticide Analysis. Rapid Commun Mass Spectrom 10:1891–1893. doi:10.1002/(SICI)1097-0231(199612)10:15<1891::AID-RCM722>3.0.CO;2-R
40. Hiraoka K (1996) Sonic Spray Ionization Mass Spectrometry. J Mass Spectrom Soc Jpn 44:279–284. doi:10.5702/massspec.44.577
41. Hirabayashi A, Fernandez de la Mora J (1998) Charged Droplet Formation in Sonic Spray. Int J Mass Spectrom Ion Proc 175:277–282. doi:10.1016/S0168-1176(98)00129-3
42. Haddad R, Catharino RR, Marques LA, Eberlin MN (2008) Perfume Fingerprinting by Easy Ambient Sonic-Spray Ionization Mass Spectrometry: Nearly Instantaneous Typification and Counterfeit Detection. Rapid Commun Mass Spectrom 22:3662–3666. doi:10.1002/rcm.3788

43. Abdelnur PV, Eberlin LS, de Sa GF, de Souza V, Eberlin MN (2008) Single-Shot Biodiesel Analysis: Nearly Instantaneous Typification and Quality Control Solely by Ambient Mass Spectrometry. Anal Chem 80:7882–7886. doi:10.1021/ac8014005
44. Saraiva SA, Abdelnur PV, Catharino RR, Nunes G, Eberlin MN (2009) Fabric Softeners: Nearly Instantaneous Characterization and Quality Control of Cationic Surfactants by Easy Ambient Sonic-Spray Ionization Mass Spectrometry. Rapid Commun Mass Spectrom 23:357–362. doi:10.1002/rcm.3878
45. Haddad R, Milagre HMS, Catharino RR, Eberlin MN (2008) Easy Ambient Sonic-Spray Ionization Mass Spectrometry Combined with Thin-Layer Chromatography. Anal Chem 80:2744–2750. doi:10.1021/ac702216q
46. Chen H, Venter A, Cooks RG (2006) Extractive Electrospray Ionization for Direct Analysis of Undiluted Urine, Milk and Other Complex Mixtures Without Sample Preparation. Chem Commun:2042–2044. doi:10.1039/B602614A
47. Chen H, Wortmann A, Zenobi R (2007) Neutral Desorption Sampling Coupled to Extractive Electrospray Ionization Mass Spectrometry for Rapid Differentiation of Biosamples by Metabolomic Fingerprinting. J Mass Spectrom 42:1123–1135. doi:10.1002/jms.1282
48. Chang DY, Lee CC, Shiea J (2002) Detecting Large Biomolecules from High-Salt Solutions by Fused-Droplet Electrospray Ionization Mass Spectrometry. Anal Chem 74:2465–2469. doi:10.1021/ac010788j
49. Shieh IF, Lee CY, Shiea J (2005) Eliminating the Interferences from TRIS Buffer and SDS in Protein Analysis by Fused-Droplet Electrospray Ionization Mass Spectrometry. J Proteome Res 4:606–612. doi:10.1021/pr049765m
50. Chen H, Sun Y, Wortmann A, Gu H, Zenobi R (2007) Differentiation of Maturity and Quality of Fruit Using Noninvasive Extractive Electrospray Ionization Quadrupole Time-of-Flight Mass Spectrometry. Anal Chem 79:1447–1455. doi:10.1021/ac061843x
51. Chingin K, Gamez G, Chen H, Zhu L, Zenobi R (2008) Rapid Classification of Perfumes by Extractive Electrospray Ionization Mass Spectrometry (EESI-MS). Rapid Commun Mass Spectrom 22:2009–2014. doi:10.1002/rcm.3584
52. Zhu L, Gamez G, Chen H, Chingin K, Zenobi R (2009) Rapid Detection of Melamine in Untreated Milk and Wheat Gluten by Ultrasound-Assisted Extractive Electrospray Ionization Mass Spectrometry (EESI-MS). Chem Commun:559–561. doi:10.1039/B818541G
53. Chen H, Hu B, Hu Y, Huan Y, Zhou Z, Qiao X (2009) Neutral Desorption Using a Sealed Enclosure to Sample Explosives on Human Skin for Rapid Detection by EESI-MS. J Am Soc Mass Spectrom 20:719–722. doi:10.1016/j.jasms.2008.12.011
54. Quist AP, Huth-Fehre T, Sundqvist BUR (1994) Total Yield Measurements in Matrix-Assisted Laser Desorption Using a Quartz Crystal Microbalance. Rapid Commun Mass Spectrom 8:149–154. doi:10.1002/rcm.1290080204
55. Shiea J, Huang MZ, Hsu HJ, Lee CY, Yuan CH, Beech I, Sunner J (2005) Electrospray-Assisted Laser Desorption/Ionization Mass Spectrometry for Direct Ambient Analysis of Solids. Rapid Commun Mass Spectrom 19:3701–3704. doi:10.1002/rcm.2243
56. Peng IX, Shiea J, Loo RRO, Loo JA (2007) Electrospray-Assisted Laser Desorption/Ionization and Tandem Mass Spectrometry of Peptides and Proteins. Rapid Commun Mass Spectrom 21:2541–2546. doi:10.1002/rcm.3154
57. Huang MZ, Hsu HJ, Lee JY, Jeng J, Shiea J (2006) Direct Protein Detection from Biological Media Through Electrospray-Assisted Laser Desorption Ionization/Mass Spectrometry. J Proteome Res 5:1107–1116. doi:10.1021/pr050442f
58. Huang MZ, Hsu HJ, Wu CI, Lin SY, Ma YL, Cheng TL, Shiea J (2007) Characterization of the Chemical Components on the Surface of Different Solids with Electrospray-Assisted Laser Desorption Ionization Mass Spectrometry. Rapid Commun Mass Spectrom 21:1767–1775. doi:10.1002/rcm.3011
59. Lin SY, Huang MZ, Chang HC, Shiea J (2007) Using Electrospray-Assisted Laser Desorption/Ionization Mass Spectrometry to Characterize Organic Compounds Separated on Thin-Layer Chromatography Plates. Anal Chem 79:8789–8795. doi:10.1021/ac070590k

60. Sampson JS, Hawkridge AM, Muddiman DC (2006) Generation and Detection of Multiply-Charged Peptides and Proteins by Matrix-Assisted Laser Desorption Electrospray Ionization (MALDESI) Fourier Transform Ion Cyclotron Resonance Mass Spectrometry. J Am Soc Mass Spectrom 17:1712–1716. doi:10.1016/j.jasms.2006.08.003
61. Nemes P, Vertes A (2007) Laser Ablation Electrospray Ionization for Atmospheric Pressure, In Vivo, and Imaging Mass Spectrometry. Anal Chem 79:8098–8106. doi:10.1021/ac071181r
62. Nemes P, Barton AA, Li Y, Vertes A (2008) Ambient Molecular Imaging and Depth Profiling of Live Tissue by Infrared Laser Ablation Electrospray Ionization Mass Spectrometry. Anal Chem 80:4575–4582. doi:10.1021/ac8004082
63. Sripadi P, Nazarian J, Hathout Y, Hoffman EP, Vertes A (2009) In Vitro Analysis of Metabolites from the Untreated Tissue of Torpedo Californica Electric Organ by Mid-Infrared Laser Ablation Electrospray Ionization Mass Spectrometry. Metabolomics 5:263–276. doi:10.1007/s11306-008-0147-x
64. Bolt F, Cameron SJS, Karancsi T, Simon D, Schaffer R, Rickards T, Hardiman K, Burke A, Bodai Z, Perdones-Montero A, Rebec M, Balog J, Takats Z (2016) Automated High-Throughput Identification and Characterization of Clinically Important Bacteria and Fungi Using Rapid Evaporative Ionization Mass Spectrometry. Anal Chem 88:9419–9426. doi:10.1021/acs.analchem.6b01016
65. Balog J, Szaniszlo T, Schaefer KC, Denes J, Lopata A, Godorhazy L, Szalay D, Balogh L, Sasi-Szabo L, Toth M, Takats Z (2010) Identification of Biological Tissues by Rapid Evaporative Ionization Mass Spectrometry. Anal Chem 82:7343–7350. doi:10.1021/ac101283x
66. Balog J, Kumar S, Alexander J, Golf O, Huang J, Wiggins T, Abbassi-Ghadi N, Enyedi A, Kacska S, Kinross J, Hanna GB, Nicholson JK, Takats Z (2015) In Vivo Endoscopic Tissue Identification by Rapid Evaporative Ionization Mass Spectrometry (REIMS). Angew Chem Int Ed 54:11059–11062. doi:10.1002/anie.201502770
67. Strittmatter N, Rebec M, Jones EA, Golf O, Abdolrasouli A, Balog J, Behrends V, Veselkov KA, Takats Z (2014) Characterization and Identification of Clinically Relevant Microorganisms Using Rapid Evaporative Ionization Mass Spectrometry. Anal Chem 86:6555–6562. doi:10.1021/ac501075f
68. Golf O, Strittmatter N, Karancsi T, Pringle SD, Speller AVM, Mroz A, Kinross JM, Abbassi-Ghadi N, Jones EA, Takats Z (2015) Rapid Evaporative Ionization Mass Spectrometry Imaging Platform for Direct Mapping from Bulk Tissue and Bacterial Growth Media. Anal Chem 87:2527–2534. doi:10.1021/ac5046752
69. Balog J, Perenyi D, Guallar-Hoyas C, Egri A, Pringle SD, Stead S, Chevallier OP, Elliott CT, Takats Z (2016) Identification of the Species of Origin for Meat Products by Rapid Evaporative Ionization Mass Spectrometry. J Agric Food Chem 64:4793–4800. doi:10.1021/acs.jafc.6b01041
70. McEwen CN, McKay RG, Larsen BS (2005) Analysis of Solids, Liquids, and Biological Tissues Using Solids Probe Introduction at Atmospheric Pressure on Commercial LC/MS Instruments. Anal Chem 77:7826–7831. doi:10.1021/ac051470k
71. McEwen C, Gutteridge S (2007) Analysis of the Inhibition of the Ergosterol Pathway in Fungi Using the Atmospheric Solids Analysis Probe (ASAP) Method. J Am Soc Mass Spectrom 18:1274–1278. doi:10.1016/j.jasms.2007.03.032
72. Smith MJP, Cameron NR, Mosely JA (2012) Evaluating Atmospheric Pressure Solids Analysis Probe (ASAP) Mass Spectrometry for the Analysis of Low Molecular Weight Synthetic Polymers. Analyst 137:4524–4530. doi:10.1039/C2AN35556F
73. Rozenski J (2011) Analysis of Nucleosides Using the Atmospheric-Pressure Solids Analysis Probe for Ionization. Int J Mass Spectrom 304:204–208. doi:10.1016/j.ijms.2011.01.029
74. Driffield M, Bradley E, Castle L, Lloyd A, Parmar M, Speck D, Roberts D, Stead S (2015) Use of Atmospheric Pressure Solids Analysis Probe Time-of-Flight Mass Spectrometry to

Screen for Plasticisers in Gaskets Used in Contact with Foods. Rapid Commun Mass Spectrom 29:1603–1610. doi:10.1002/rcm.7255
75. Doue M, Dervilly-Pinel G, Gicquiau A, Pouponneau K, Monteau F, Le Bizec B (2014) High Throughput Identification and Quantification of Anabolic Steroid Esters by Atmospheric Solids Analysis Probe Mass Spectrometry for Efficient Screening of Drug Preparations. Anal Chem 86:5649–5655. doi:10.1021/ac501072g
76. Pan H, Lundin G (2011) Rapid Detection and Identification of Impurities in Ten 2-Naphthalenamines Using an Atmospheric Pressure Solids Analysis Probe in Conjunction with Ion Mobility Mass Spectrometry. Eur J Mass Spectrom 17:217–225. doi:10.1255/ejms.1125
77. Kusai A (2007) Fundamental and Application of the Direct Analysis in Real Time Mass Spectrometry. Bunseki 124–127
78. Saitoh K (2007) Directly Analysis for Fragrance Ingredients Using DART-TOFMS. Aroma Res 8:366–369
79. Sparkman OD, Jones PR, Curtis M (2009) Accurate mass measurements with a reflectron time-of-flight mass spectrometer and the direct analysis in real time (DART) interface for the identification of unknown compounds below masses of 500 DA. In: Li L (ed) Chemical Analysis. Wiley, Hoboken
80. Konuma K (2009) Elementary Guide to Ionization Methods for Mass Spectrometry: Introduction of the Direct Analysis in Real Time Mass Spectrometry. Bunseki 464–467
81. Chernetsova ES, Bochkov PO, Ovcharov MV, Zhokhov SS, Abramovich RA (2010) DART Mass Spectrometry: A Fast Screening of Solid Pharmaceuticals for the Presence of an Active Ingredient, As an Alternative for IR Spectroscopy. Drug Test Anal 2:292–294. doi:10.1002/dta.136
82. Kikura-Hanajiri R (2010) Simple and Rapid Screening for Target Compounds Using Direct Analysis in Real Time (DART)-MS. Food Food Ingredients Jpn 215:137–143
83. Chernetsova ES, Morlock GE (2011) Mass Spectrometric Method of Direct Sample Analysis in Real Time (DART) and Application of the Method to Pharmaceutical and Biological Analysis. Zavodskaya Laboratoriya, Diagnostika Materialov 77:10–19
84. Chernetsova ES, Morlock GE, Revelsky IA (2011) DART Mass Spectrometry and Its Applications in Chemical Analysis. Russ Chem Rev 80:235–255. doi:10.1070/RC2011v080n03ABEH004194
85. Chernetsova ES, Morlock GE (2011) Determination of Drugs and Drug-Like Compounds in Different Samples with Direct Analysis in Real Time Mass Spectrometry. Mass Spectrom Rev 30:875–883. doi:10.1002/mas.20304
86. Liao J, Liu N, Liu C (2011) Direct Analysis in Real Time Mass Spectrometry and Its Applications to Drug Analysis. Yaowu Fenxi Zazhi 31:2008–2012
87. Osuga J, Konuma K (2011) Applications of Direct Analysis in Real Time (DART) Mass Spectrometry. Yuki Gosei Kagaku Kyokaishi 69:171–175. doi:10.5059/yukigoseikyokaishi.69.171
88. Shelley JT, Wiley JS, Chan GCY, Schilling GD, Ray SJ, Hieftje GM (2009) Characterization of Direct-Current Atmospheric-Pressure Discharges Useful for Ambient Desorption/Ionization Mass Spectrometry. J Am Soc Mass Spectrom 20:837–844. doi:10.1016/j.jasms.2008.12.020
89. Andrade FJ, Shelley JT, Wetzel WC, Webb MR, Gamez G, Ray SJ, Hieftje GM (2008) Atmospheric Pressure Chemical Ionization Source. 1. Ionization of Compounds in the Gas Phase. Anal Chem 80:2646–2653. doi:10.1021/ac800156y
90. Andrade FJ, Shelley JT, Wetzel WC, Webb MR, Gamez G, Ray SJ, Hieftje GM (2008) Atmospheric Pressure Chemical Ionization Source. 2. Desorption-Ionization for the Direct Analysis of Solid Compounds. Anal Chem 80:2654–2663. doi:10.1021/ac800210s
91. Warscheid B, Hoffmann T (2001) Structural Elucidation of Monoterpene Oxidation Products by Ion Trap Fragmentation Using on-Line Atmospheric Pressure Chemical Ionization Mass

Spectrometry in the Negative Ion Mode. Rapid Commun Mass Spectrom 15:2259–2272. doi:10.1002/rcm.504

92. Song L, Dykstra AB, Yao H, Bartmess JE (2009) Ionization Mechanism of Negative Ion-Direct Analysis in Real Time: A Comparative Study with Negative Ion-Atmospheric Pressure Photoionization. J Am Soc Mass Spectrom 20:42–50. doi:10.1016/j.jasms.2008.09.016
93. Derpmann V, Albrecht S, Benter T (2012) The Role of Ion-Bound Cluster Formation in Negative Ion Mass Spectrometry. Rapid Commun Mass Spectrom 26:1923–1933. doi:10.1002/rcm.6303
94. Klee S, Derpmann V, Wissdorf W, Klopotowski S, Kersten H, Brockmann KJ, Benter T, Albrecht S, Bruins AP, Dousty F, Kauppila TJ, Kostiainen R, O'Brien R, Robb DB, Syage JA (2014) Are Clusters Important in Understanding the Mechanisms in Atmospheric Pressure Ionization? Part 1: Reagent Ion Generation and Chemical Control of Ion Populations. J Am Soc Mass Spectrom 25:1310–1321. doi:10.1007/s13361-014-0891-2
95. Cody RB (2009) Observation of Molecular Ions and Analysis of Nonpolar Compounds with the Direct Analysis in Real Time Ion Source. Anal Chem 81:1101–1107. doi:10.1021/ac8022108
96. Jorabchi K, Hanold K, Syage J (2013) Ambient Analysis by Thermal Desorption Atmospheric Pressure Photoionization. Anal Bioanal Chem 405:7011–7018. doi:10.1007/s00216-012-6536-z
97. Rummel JL, McKenna AM, Marshall AG, Eyler JR, Powell DH (2010) The Coupling of Direct Analysis in Real Time Ionization to Fourier Transform Ion Cyclotron Resonance Mass Spectrometry for Ultrahigh-Resolution Mass Analysis. Rapid Commun Mass Spectrom 24:784–790. doi:10.1002/rcm.4450
98. Dane AJ, Cody RB (2010) Selective Ionization of Melamine in Powdered Milk by Using Argon Direct Analysis in Real Time (DART) Mass Spectrometry. Analyst 135:696–699. doi:10.1039/b923561b
99. Yang H, Wan D, Song F, Liu Z, Liu S (2013) Argon Direct Analysis in Real Time Mass Spectrometry in Conjunction with Makeup Solvents: A Method for Analysis of Labile Compounds. Anal Chem 85:1305–1309. doi:10.1021/ac3026543
100. Cody RB, Dane AJ (2013) Soft Ionization of Saturated Hydrocarbons, Alcohols and Nonpolar Compounds by Negative-Ion Direct Analysis in Real-Time Mass Spectrometry. J Am Soc Mass Spectrom 24:329–334. doi:10.1007/s13361-012-0569-6
101. Harper JD, Charipar NA, Mulligan CC, Zhang X, Cooks RG, Ouyang Z (2008) Low-Temperature Plasma Probe for Ambient Desorption Ionization. Anal Chem 80:9097–9104. doi:10.1021/ac801641a
102. Tsuchiya M, Taira T (1978) A New Ionization Method for Organic Compounds. Liquid Ionization at Atmospheric Pressure Utilizing Penning Effect and Chemical Ionization. Shitsuryo Bunseki 26:333–342
103. Tsuchiya M, Taira T, Toyoura Y (1980) A New Ionization Detector for Minute Amounts of Organic Compounds in Solution. Bunseki Kagaku 29:632–637
104. McLuckey SA, Glish GL, Asano KG, Grant BC (1988) Atmospheric Sampling Glow Discharge Ionization Source for the Determination of Trace Organic Compounds in Ambient Air. Anal Chem 60:2220–2227. doi:10.1021/ac00171a012
105. Fujimaki S, Furuya H, Kambara S, Hiraoka K (2004) Development of an Atmospheric Pressure Penning Ionization Source for Gas Analysis. J Mass Spectrom Soc Jpn 52:149–153. doi:10.5702/massspec.52.149
106. Hiraoka K, Fujimaki S, Kambara S, Furuya H, Okazaki S (2004) Atmospheric-Pressure Penning Ionization Mass Spectrometry. Rapid Commun Mass Spectrom 18:2323–2330. doi:10.1002/rcm.1624
107. Furuya H, Kambara S, Nishidate K, Fujimaki S, Hashimoto Y, Suzuki S, Iwama T, Hiraoka K (2010) Quantitative Aspects of Atmospheric-Pressure Penning Ionization. J Mass Spectrom Soc Jpn 58:211–213. doi:10.5702/massspec.58.211

108. Ratcliffe LV, Rutten FJM, Barrett DA, Whitmore T, Seymour D, Greenwood C, Aranda-Gonzalvo Y, Robinson S, McCoustra M (2007) Surface Analysis Under Ambient Conditions Using Plasma-Assisted Desorption/Ionization Mass Spectrometry. Anal Chem 79:6094–6101. doi:10.1021/ac070109q
109. Na N, Zhao M, Zhang S, Yang C, Zhang X (2007) Development of a Dielectric Barrier Discharge Ion Source for Ambient Mass Spectrometry. J Am Soc Mass Spectrom 18:1859–1862. doi:10.1016/j.jasms.2007.07.027
110. Na N, Zhang C, Zhao M, Zhang S, Yang C, Fang X, Zhang X (2007) Direct Detection of Explosives on Solid Surfaces by Mass Spectrometry with an Ambient Ion Source Based on Dielectric Barrier Discharge. J Mass Spectrom 42:1079–1085. doi:10.1002/jms.1243
111. Hiraoka K, Ninomiya S, Chen LC, Iwama T, Mandal MK, Suzuki H, Ariyada O, Furuya H, Takekawa K (2011) Development of Double Cylindrical Dielectric Barrier Discharge Ion Source. Analyst 136:1210–1215. doi:10.1039/c0an00621a
112. Wetzel WC, Andrade FJ, Broekaert JAC, Hieftje GM (2006) Development of a Direct Current He Atmospheric-Pressure Glow Discharge as an Ionization Source for Elemental Mass Spectrometry Via Hydride Generation. J Anal At Spectrom 21:750–756. doi:10.1039/b607781a
113. McEwen CN, Larsen BS (2009) Ionization Mechanisms Related to Negative Ion APPI, APCI, and DART. J Am Soc Mass Spectrom 20:1518–1521. doi:10.1016/j.jasms.2009.04.010
114. Cristoni S, Bernardi LR, Biunno I, Tubaro M, Guidugli F (2003) Surface-Activated No-Discharge Atmospheric Pressure Chemical Ionization. Rapid Commun Mass Spectrom 17:1973–1981. doi:10.1002/rcm.1141
115. Cristoni S, Bernardi LR, Guidugli F, Tubaro M, Traldi P (2005) The Role of Different Phenomena in Surface-Activated Chemical Ionization (SACI) Performance. J Mass Spectrom 40:1550–1557. doi:10.1002/jms.913
116. Chen H, Ouyang Z, Cooks RG (2006) Thermal Production and Reactions of Organic Ions at Atmospheric Pressure. Angew Chem Int Ed 45:3656–3660. doi:10.1002/anie.200600660
117. Perez JJ, Harris GA, Chipuk JE, Brodbelt JS, Green MD, Hampton CY, Fernandez FM (2010) Transmission-Mode Direct Analysis in Real Time and Desorption Electrospray Ionization Mass Spectrometry of Insecticide-Treated Bednets for Malaria Control. Analyst 135:712–719. doi:10.1039/b924533b
118. Chernetsova ES, Revelsky AI, Morlock GE (2011) Some New Features of Direct Analysis in Real Time Mass Spectrometry Utilizing the Desorption at an Angle Option. Rapid Commun Mass Spectrom 25:2275–2282. doi:10.1002/rcm.5112
119. Fernandez FM, Cody RB, Green MD, Hampton CY, McGready R, Sengaloundeth S, White NJ, Newton PN (2006) Characterization of Solid Counterfeit Drug Samples by Desorption Electrospray Ionization and Direct-Analysis-in-Real-Time Coupled to Time-of-Flight Mass Spectrometry. ChemMedChem 1:702–705. doi:10.1002/cmdc.200600041
120. Jones RW, Cody RB, McClelland JF (2006) Differentiating Writing Inks Using Direct Analysis in Real Time Mass Spectrometry. J Forensic Sci 51:915–918. doi:10.1111/j.1556-4029.2006.00162.x
121. Yu S, Crawford E, Tice J, Musselman B, Wu JT (2009) Bioanalysis Without Sample Cleanup or Chromatography: The Evaluation and Initial Implementation of Direct Analysis in Real Time Ionization Mass Spectrometry for the Quantification of Drugs in Biological Matrixes. Anal Chem 81:193–202. doi:10.1021/ac801734t
122. Zhao Y, Lam M, Wu D, Mak R (2008) Quantification of Small Molecules in Plasma with Direct Analysis in Real Time Tandem Mass Spectrometry, Without Sample Preparation and Liquid Chromatographic Separation. Rapid Commun Mass Spectrom 22:3217–3224. doi:10.1002/rcm.3726
123. Jagerdeo E, Abdel-Rehim M (2009) Screening of Cocaine and Its Metabolites in Human Urine Samples by Direct Analysis in Real-Time Source Coupled to Time-of-Flight Mass

Spectrometry After Online Preconcentration Utilizing Microextraction by Packed Sorbent. J Am Soc Mass Spectrom 20:891–899. doi:10.1016/j.jasms.2009.01.010

124. Kpegba K, Spadaro T, Cody RB, Nesnas N, Olson JA (2007) Analysis of Self-Assembled Monolayers on Gold Surfaces Using Direct Analysis in Real Time Mass Spectrometry. Anal Chem 79:5479–5483. doi:10.1021/ac062276g
125. Block E, Dane AJ, Cody RB (2011) Crushing Garlic and Slicing Onions: Detection of Sulfenic Acids and Other Reactive Organosulfur Intermediates from Garlic and Other Alliums Using Direct Analysis in Real-Time Mass Spectrometry (DART-MS). Phosphorus Sulfur Silicon Rel Elem 186:1085–1093. doi:10.1080/10426507.2010.507728
126. Block E, Dane AJ, Thomas S, Cody RB (2010) Applications of Direct Analysis in Real Time Mass Spectrometry (DART-MS) in Allium Chemistry. 2-Propenesulfenic and 2-Propenesulfinic Acids, Diallyl trisulfane S-oxide, and Other Reactive Sulfur Compounds from Crushed Garlic and Other Alliums. J Agric Food Chem 58:4617–4625. doi:10.1021/jf1000106
127. Yew JY, Cody RB, Kravitz EA (2008) Cuticular Hydrocarbon Analysis of an Awake Behaving Fly Using Direct Analysis in Real-Time Time-of-Flight Mass Spectrometry. Proc Natl Acad Sci U S A 105:7135–7140. doi:10.1073/pnas.0802692105
128. Gross JH (2013) Polydimethylsiloxane-Based Wide Range Mass Calibration for Direct Analysis in Real Time Mass Spectrometry. Anal Bioanal Chem 405:8663–8668. doi:10.1007/s00216-013-7287-1
129. Gross JH (2015) Analysis of Silicones Released from Household Items and Baby Articles by Direct Analysis in Real Time-Mass Spectrometry. J Am Soc Mass Spectrom 26:511–521. doi:10.1007/s13361-014-1042-5
130. Gross JH (2015) Direct Analysis in Real Time Mass Spectrometry and Its Application for the Analysis of Polydimethylsiloxanes. Spectrosc Eur 27:6–11
131. Gross JH (2015) Polydimethylsiloxane Extraction from Silicone Rubber into Baked Goods Detected by Direct Analysis in Real Time Mass Spectrometry. Eur J Mass Spectrom 21:313–319. doi:10.1255/ejms.1333
132. Jakob A, Crawford EA, Gross JH (2016) Detection of Polydimethylsiloxanes Transferred from Silicone-Coated Parchment Paper to Baked Goods Using Direct Analysis in Real Time Mass Spectrometry. J Mass Spectrom 51:298–304. doi:10.1002/jms.3757

Hyphenated Methods

14

Learning Objectives

- Concept of chromatographic separation
- One-dimensional and two-dimensional gas chromatography
- Liquid chromatography in various pressure regimes
- Concept and technical aspects of coupling of separation methods to MS
- Basics of quantitation by MS
- Tandem MS modes for improved selectivity
- Applications of ion mobility spectrometry-mass spectrometry
- Tandem MS as a complement for chromatography coupling
- Ultrahigh resolution as a complement for chromatography coupling

The analysis of complex mixtures generally requires the combination of both separation techniques and mass spectrometry [1–3]. The first step in this direction was made by *gas chromatography-mass spectrometry* (GC-MS) coupling [4]. Soon, GC-MS became a routine method for mixture analysis [5–7]. The aim and attempt to also handle highly polar nonvolatile compounds by *liquid chromatography-mass spectrometry* (LC-MS) [8] eventually led to the development of API methods (Chap. 12) [9, 10]. The expansion of this approach to coupling of other liquid-phase separation techniques to mass spectrometry followed as *capillary zone electrophoresis-mass spectrometry* (CZE-MS) [11–15] and *supercritical fluid chromatography-mass spectrometry* (SFC-MS) [16, 17]. Regardless of the type of separation technique, it always adds an additional dimension to the analytical measurement. The hyphen used to indicate the coupling of a separation technique to mass spectrometry led to the collective term *hyphenated methods*.

Mass spectrometry itself also offers two additional "degrees of freedom". The complexity of a sample can either be resolved by high or even ultrahigh mass resolution or by employing tandem MS techniques (Chap. 9), e.g., by separating the

J.H. Gross, *Mass Spectrometry*, DOI 10.1007/978-3-319-54398-7_14

fragmentation pattern of one component from that of others in a mixture [2, 3]. In practice, the coupling of separation techniques to mass spectrometry often involves advanced MS techniques to achieve the desired level of selectivity. This altogether ensures accuracy and reliability of analytical information. (For *accuracy* and *precision* cf. Sect. 3.5.)

This chapter is about extending the range of samples that can be analyzed by mass spectrometry and about increasing the specificity of analytical information thereof. It briefly introduces the basic concepts and methodologies of the most common chromatographic techniques, handling of chromatograms, procedures for quantitation, and chromatography–mass spectrometry interfaces.

14.1 Chromatography

The term *chromatography* is derived from the Ancient Greek words for color (χρϖμα, *chroma*) and writing (γραφειν, *graphein*). Chromatography was first described about a century ago by the Russian botanist Mikhail S. Tswett as a technique for the separation of plant pigments [18].

Chromatography of any type leads to the separation of components of a mixture. The procedure relies on the equilibrium of adsorption and desorption of compounds mobilized either in the gas phase or liquid phase to and from a stationary phase [19–22].

In *gas chromatography* (GC) the mobile phase is a gas and the stationary phase is a liquid, normally presented as a thin film bound to a solid surface. This explains the original term *gas-liquid chromatography* (GLC) that was soon superseded by the shorter form *gas chromatography* (GC). In contrast to GC, the mobile phase in *liquid chromatography* (LC) is a liquid and the surface of solid particles serves as the stationary phase, i.e., the components to be separated are provided in dilute solution.

14.1.1 Chromatographic Column

Chromatographic separations are mostly performed in tubes or capillaries providing a fixed volume where the mobile phase is passed through and serving to hold the stationary phase. The tube can either be straight and several millimeters to centimeters in diameter, as in liquid chromatography, or it can be a capillary of a fraction of a millimeter in diameter that is supported on a coil, as generally the case in (capillary) gas chromatography. Such an assembly – whatever the exact form factor – represents the *chromatographic column*. The term column has been coined by the most basic setup for LC separation that is achieved by filling a vertically aligned glass pipe with silica gel or alumina and passing through the sample solution from top to bottom by virtue of gravitation. This technique is still quite common in preparative organic chemistry.

14.1.2 Equilibrium of Adsorption and Desorption

The velocity at which molecules of a compound are traveling in the mobile phase along the chromatographic column is governed by the dynamic equilibrium of adsorption to and desorption from the stationary phase.

For a compound C_i we define a *distribution coefficient* or *partition coefficient*, K_i, by the ratio of concentrations in the stationary phase, $[C_i]_{stat}$, to that in the mobile phase, $[C_i]_{mob}$:

$$K_i = \frac{[C_i]_{stat}}{[C_i]_{mob}} \tag{14.1}$$

Some compounds will adsorb more strongly to the stationary phase and thus reside for a longer time than others that only weakly interact with the stationary phase. The latter compounds move faster along the column and reach the exit earlier than those experiencing a tighter contact.

The *retention factor* k_i is used to describe the velocity of migration of a component. It is defined as the ratio of the number of molecules residing at the stationary phase, n_{stat}, to those migrating in the mobile phase, n_{mob}:

$$k_i = \frac{n_{stat}}{n_{mob}} \tag{14.2}$$

14.1.3 Dead Time and Dead Volume

Even if we assume no interaction of the pure mobile phase with the stationary phase, i.e., $k_i \approx 0$, there is a minimum time needed for the mobile phase to pass the chromatographic column. This minimum time is termed *dead time*, t_0, of a given chromatographic column. No compound can leave the system before t_0.

The dead time can either be determined by dividing the length of the column by the velocity of the mobile phase or by dividing the volume of the column by the volume flow of the mobile phase. It is important to note that this relationship refers to the free fraction of the column volume, i.e., the geometric volume minus the volume of the stationary phase inside. The volume available for filling with mobile phase is therefore called *dead volume*.

The actual dead volume of a chromatographic system is somewhat larger than the dead volume of the column alone as tubing and joints from injector to column and from column to detector also contribute to the total volume.

14.1.4 Retention Time

Depending on its individual distribution coefficient, K_i, a compound experiences stronger or weaker interaction with the stationary phase. Strong interaction means slow travel along the column because the molecules spend less time in the mobile phase. In other words, the column has greater retentiveness. The time needed for a component to pass through the column is thus termed *retention time*, t_R. The retention time is given by:

$$t_R = t_0 + t_0 \times k_i = t_0 \times (1 + k_i) \tag{14.3}$$

Vice versa, k_i can be determined from:

$$k_i = \frac{t_R - t_0}{t_0} \tag{14.4}$$

The retention time is characteristic of a compound for a given chromatographic setup. It is invariable as long as the chromatographic conditions remain unchanged. Using a longer column will increase the retention time. Increase of the volume flow of the mobile phase will reduce the retention time. Stronger interaction with the stationary phase causes an elongated retention time. Finally, the retention time is always longer than the dead time.

Chromatographic separation is thus effected by elution of individual components of a mixture at different retention times.

14.1.5 Elution and Eluate

The process of leaving the chromatographic column is termed *elution*. The fluid mixture of mobile phase (either gaseous or liquid) and separated components contained therein (either vapor or dissolved) is termed *eluate*. In preparative chromatography the eluate is collected in fractions to recover purified components. In this chapter, we deal with analytical chromatography where the eluate is either consumed by detection like in MS or discarded.

14.1.6 Separation and Chromatographic Resolution

During migration along the chromatographic column the zone occupied by a component tends to expand along the column. The extent of this longitudinal expansion, essentially smearing along the column, is determined by:

- *eddy diffusion*, *A*, caused by the different paths molecules can travel across a porous material resulting in differences in effective path length on the molecular level,

- *longitudinal diffusion*, B, of the component back and forth in the mobile phase,
- *resistance to mass transfer*, C; a collective term for any effect related to adsorption and desorption and convection during migration.

The *height equivalent of a theoretical plate* (HETP) or just *plate height*, H, can be expressed in terms of the above parameters and the velocity of the mobile phase, u, by the *van Deemter equation* [23]:

$$H = A + \frac{B}{u} + Cu \tag{14.5}$$

Van Deemter plots visualize the optimum flow of the mobile phase for a given system and help to understand which parameter is limiting in a specific situation (Fig. 14.1). The *chromatographic resolution* increases the lower the value of H as this results in the highest number of theoretical plates for a given chromatographic column.

In practice, an impression of chromatographic resolution is best obtained from the so-called *peak capacity*. The peak capacity is the number of peaks that can be fitted into a chromatogram without overlap, i.e., just separated from each other. The peak capacity roughly reflects the number of compounds that possibly can be separated by the system. It can range from several tens in quick HPLC runs to about one thousand in optimized column GC.

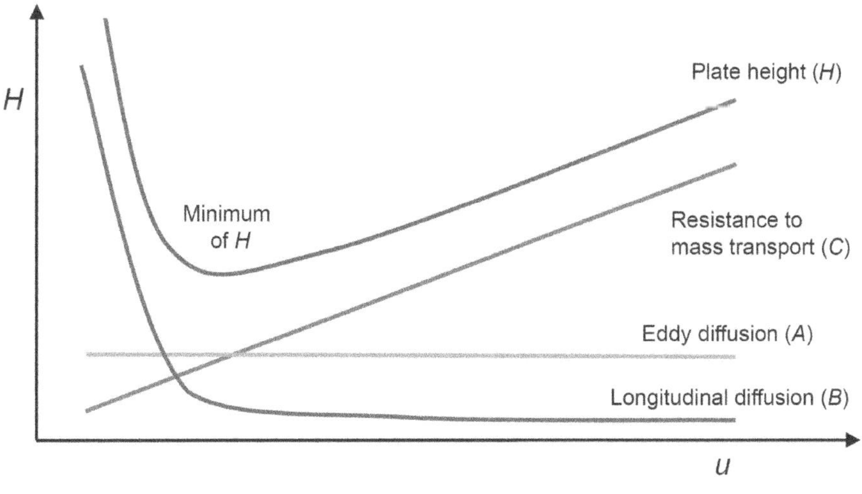

Fig. 14.1 Van Deemter plot of plate height, H, versus velocity of the mobile phase, u. The lowest value of H refers to the highest number of theoretical plates per given column length and thus marks the optimum for separation

14.1.7 Detectors

The chromatographic process effects separation of components in time. However, it does not include the means to detect whether a component is just being eluted. Even if we noticed the elution of a component there would still be no identification of this substance. With the exception of colored substances, where we may have the chance to detect the elution simply by the sudden coloration of the eluate, we need to employ some sort of *detector* to be able to judge when a colorless compound elutes.

Simple chromatographic detectors are only capable of indicating *when* a compound elutes and to provide a measure of the eluted *amount of substance* as by the relative signal intensity.

In GC, the most prominent types of detectors are *flame ionization detector* (FID), *thermal conductivity detector* (TCD), *nitrogen phosphorus detector* (NPD), and *electron capture detector* (ECD). While FID and TCD provide no or extremely low compound selectivity, NPDs only recognize nitrogen- and/or phosphorus-containing compounds and ECDs are selective for compounds with high electron affinity.

In LC, the change in UV light absorption of the eluate is normally taken as an indication of compound elution. Simple *UV detectors* rely on a single wavelength, often 254 nm, while more sophisticated *diode array detectors* (DAD) are capable of delivering a UV/Vis spectrum of the eluting component.

Mass spectrometers can serve as highly compound specific chromatographic detectors as they are capable of delivering a complete mass spectrum of every eluting compound. Occasionally, simple mass spectrometers like linear single quadrupole analyzers are referred to as *mass-selective detectors* (MSD). Here, we will certainly not follow this inappropriate habit.

More than just an inlet system
From an MS-centered view, any chromatographic system simply is another type of sample inlet, whereas from the chromatographer's point of view mass spectrometers are just detectors for their separation technique. Here, we deal with the peculiarities of those analyte-separating inlets and the associated implications for the operation of the attached mass spectrometers.

14.1.8 Chromatograms

The result of a chromatographic separation is presented as a *chromatogram* displaying the relative peak intensities versus retention time (Fig. 14.2). Ideally, all components are separated from each other and the baseline is flat. In real-world chromatography, we have to deal with overlapping peaks due to insufficient resolution, peak tailing (of polar components), baseline drift, mostly upward, e.g.,

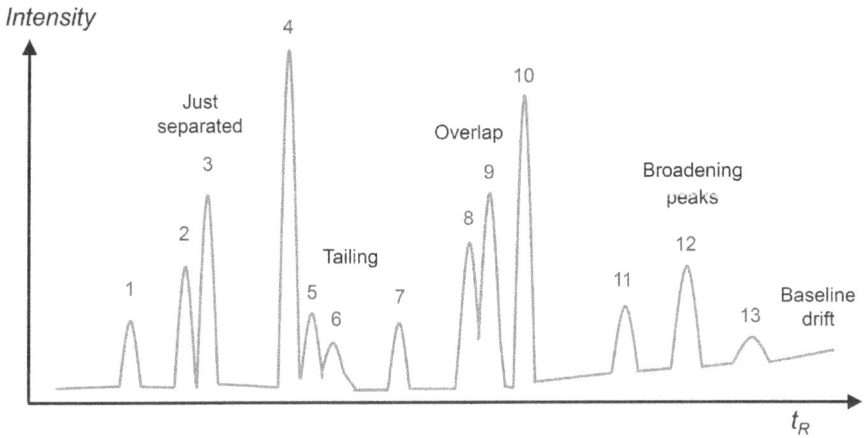

Fig. 14.2 General appearance of a chromatogram. This run shows 13 identified peaks and some frequent weaknesses like peak tailing of #6, insufficient resolution of the pair of #8, #9, and some peak broadening plus an upward baseline drift toward the end of the run

by column bleed (elution of stationary phase), and often some general peak broadening toward the end of the separation due to diffusion (cf. van Deemter plot).

14.1.9 Gas Chromatography: Practical Considerations

In *gas chromatography* (GC) the sample is evaporated and admixed to an excess of the mobile phase, i.e., an inert *carrier gas*. Normally, the sample is injected as a dilute solution in a volatile solvent. To do so, a microliter syringe is inserted into the *injector* by poking the needle through a silicone septum. The injector, essentially a hot glass tube, effects sudden evaporation and admixes the sample vapor to the carrier gas flow. Helium is frequently employed as carrier gas as it conveniently combines fast separations with perfect inertness and safety of operation. Nonetheless, the high cost of helium makes it more attractive to use nitrogen (slower separation) and hydrogen (fast separation but potentially explosive mixtures) instead.

Today, analytical GC is exclusively performed by use of *capillary columns*. Capillary columns for GC are drawn from fused silica that is transformed into a composite material by coating it with polyimide on the outside. This converts the extremely brittle quartz glass into a highly flexible material that can be wound onto a support coil (Fig. 14.3). The inner walls of the capillary are coated with a thin film of the stationary phase, mainly alkyl and aryl polysiloxanes. Typical GC capillaries are 20–60 m long, with a 0.10–0.50 mm inner diameter, and bear a film of 0.2–1.5 μm of stationary phase inside.

When the carrier gas is provided at the injector at about 1 bar, the high flow resistance of the capillary results in a gas flow in the order of 1 ml min^{-1}.

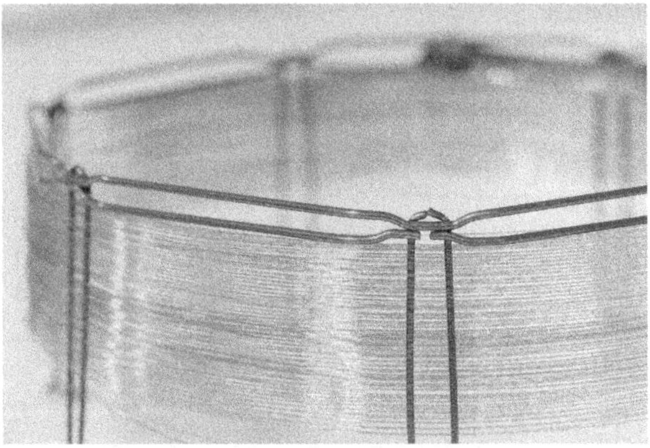

Fig. 14.3 Fused-silica capillary column for gas chromatography on a coil of about 20 cm in diameter. The golden color is caused by the outer polyimide coating of the silica capillary. While fused silica alone is extremely brittle, the composite material can easily be coiled and bent even at much smaller radius than required here

In principle, GC separations can be run at constant column temperature. However, isothermal GC separations are more time-consuming and suffer from reduced chromatographic resolution towards the end of the GC run, because elongated dwell time enhances the detrimental effect of diffusion. It is thus common to apply temperature programs that lead from low to high temperature. A gas chromatograph therefore closely resembles a convection oven wherein the column is operated under temperature control. Injector and detector are normally installed on the inside top of the housing (Fig. 14.4). As opposed to convection ovens for household use, much care is taken to achieve homogeneous temperature in the column compartment and to ensure precise and reproducible temperatures during the entire separation process. Also GC ovens reach up to at least 350 °C.

Often, the heating rate is split into a fast segment at the beginning and a slow segment covering the temperature range most efficient for the separation of the compounds of interest (Fig. 14.5). The injector and the transfer line to the detector need to be kept at higher temperature than the highest temperature of the program. Otherwise, the separated components could be condensed and thus be remixed at the column exit. Furthermore, care has to be taken that the maximum temperature specified for the actual column is not exceeded at any point of the system.

14.1.10 Comprehensive Gas Chromatography

Even though gas chromatography provides high resolution separations, this can, in some cases, be insufficient to resolve all components of complex mixtures like hydrocarbon fuels and lubricants, their combustion products, or other products of pyrolytic processes. Natural flavors and fragrances relevant for food and perfumes, aroma of spirits and wines, or coffee roasting, for example, present another field of enormous complexity.

Comprehensive gas chromatography, commonly known as GC × GC, employs a serial connection of two columns, where the first column is about 20–30 times longer than the second. The eluate of the first column is collected in an intermediate

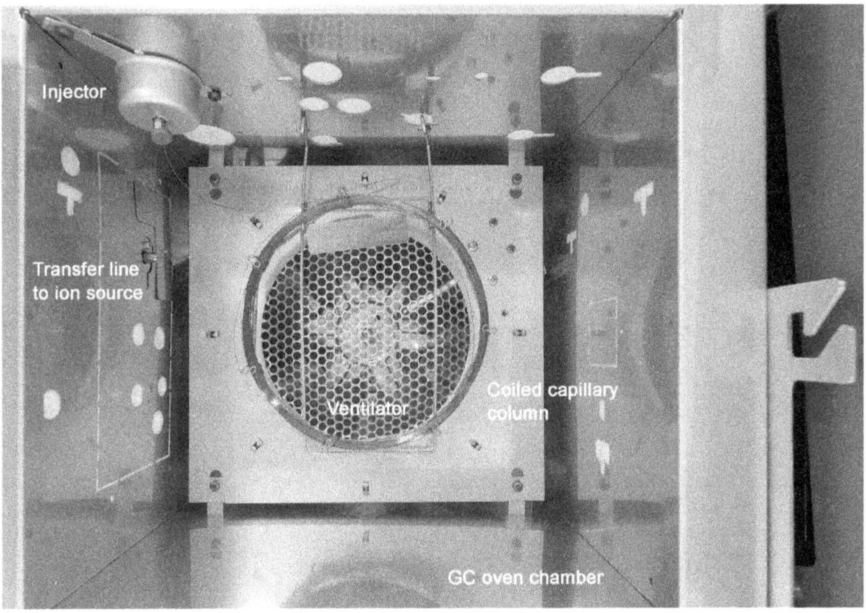

Fig. 14.4 GC oven for capillary gas chromatography with open front door. The GC column wound onto a coil is suspended to hang freely in the heated air. In this Agilent 7890B GC, the injector is on the *top left side* and the exit of the capillary to the transfer line is in the middle of the *left side lining*

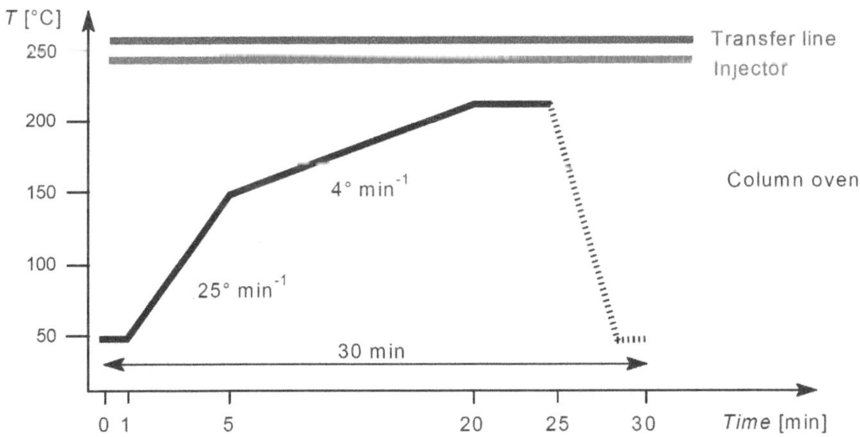

Fig. 14.5 Typical temperature program for GC operation. This program starts at 50 °C, holds that temperature for 1 min, ramps up at 25 ° C min^{-1} to 150 °C, then heats at 4 °C min^{-1}–210 °C, and holds this for 5 min before cooling down and temperature settling to get ready for the next run. Overall, this takes 30 min. Both transfer line and injector are constantly kept at about 50 °C above the highest temperature of the GC program to avoid condensation of sample

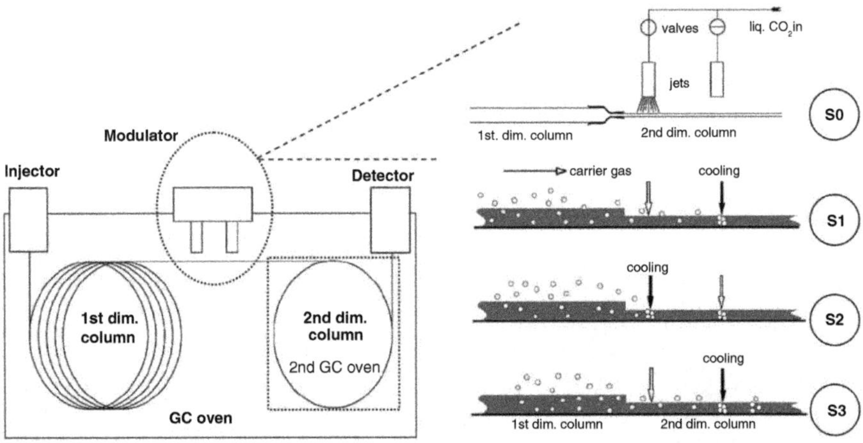

Fig. 14.6 Schematic of GC × GC instrumentation (*left*) and operation (*right*). The eluate from the first column is collected, e.g., by a dual-jet cryogenic modulator. The modulator switches from trapping to evaporation mode on two short adjacent segments at the junction of the columns (Reproduced from Ref. [24] with permission. © Elsevier, 2006)

condenser or trap [24, 25] for several seconds and then passed on in a pulsed manner to the second column (Fig. 14.6). When columns of different polarity are used, this results in an orthogonal separation, i.e., in *two-dimensional chromatography* [24–28]. Thus, co-eluting components from the first-dimension column may be separated on the second-dimension column.

GC × GC requires very fast data acquisition. Also, the amount of analytical data requires software tools capable of presenting the wealth of information. Basically, the chromatograms delivered by the high-speed second-dimension column are plotted versus the retention time of the first-dimension column (Fig. 14.7). Often, the dataset is processed further for improved visualization, e.g., for display as 2D contour plot or 3D plot. As thousands of peaks are still difficult to examine, it is common to show only zoomed-in views of the region of interest or to employ statistical tools like *principal component analysis* (PCA) to reveal common features as well as differences between samples.

14.1.11 High-Performance Liquid Chromatography

Liquid chromatography (LC) started with Tswett's work based on simple manually filled columns. The chromatographic resolution – or speed of separation at fixed resolution – can dramatically be improved by using fine and homogeneously sized particles as stationary phase [19–22]. Then, the liquid flow can only be sustained by applying high pressure in the order of 100–200 bar. This led to the development of *high-pressure liquid chromatography* (HPLC), also known as *high-performance liquid chromatography* (HPLC). HPLC was further improved when the particle size

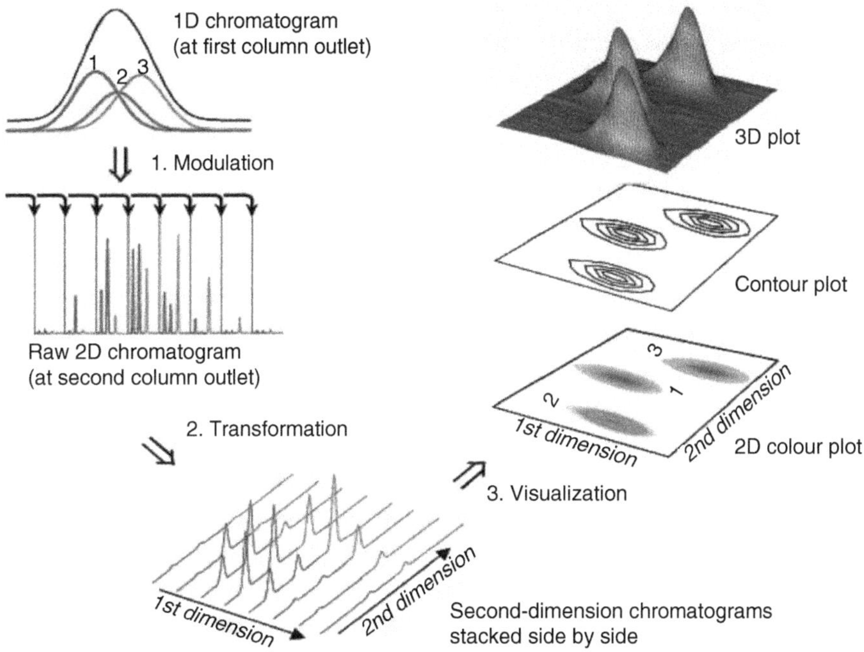

Fig. 14.7 Concept of GC × GC and data analysis. A large number of chromatograms from the second-dimension high-speed column is aligned along the retention time of the first-dimension column. Often, the data is further processed for improved visualization as contour plot or 3D plot (Reproduced from Ref. [24] with permission. © Elsevier, 2006)

could be reduced to a few micrometers causing columns to now demand pressures of up to about 1000 bar to effect flow rates of 0.5–1.0 ml min^{-1} that are useful in practice. The technique was introduced by Waters as *ultra-performance liquid chromatography* (UPLC, Fig. 14.8) and is now available from several vendors as *ultrahigh-pressure liquid chromatography* (UHPLC) [29, 30].

Most of the HPLC and UHPLC work is done on so-called *reversed phase* stationary phases. Classical LC on silica or alumina is considered as normal phases. In reversed phase chromatography the surface of the silica particles is coated with an organic layer, mostly siloxanes with various alkyl or aryl end groups. The end groups determine the interaction of the surface with the analyte molecules. Long alkyl chains, typically C_{18}, bind stronger to organic molecules of low polarity while highly polar or even ionic analytes pass by. Shorter alkyl chains like C_8 show less retentiveness to low-polarity analytes. On reversed phase columns, ionic and highly polar hydrophilic compounds may even be mobilized by pure water or water : acetonitrile = 90 : 10 (v/v). Nonpolar hydrophobic molecules require a higher fraction of organic solvent to move along the stationary phase. Overall, reversed phase chromatography leads to retention times in the order nonpolar > polar > ionic.

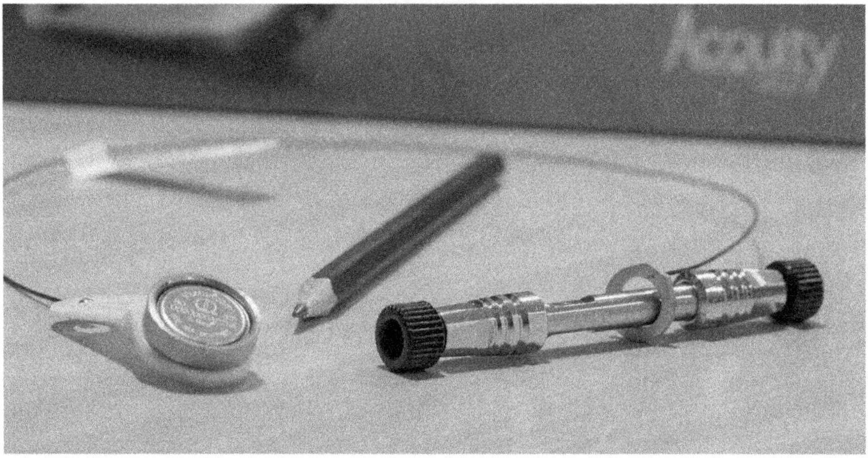

Fig. 14.8 UPLC column. The actual column (*right*), here shown with the two end caps still in place, is quite small as by comparison to the pencil. This particular column is a Waters BEH C18 reversed phase type of 50 mm length and 2.1 mm inner diameter filled with 1.7-μm-sized particles. The column is locked to a transponder (*left*) that is used to identify the column by the data system

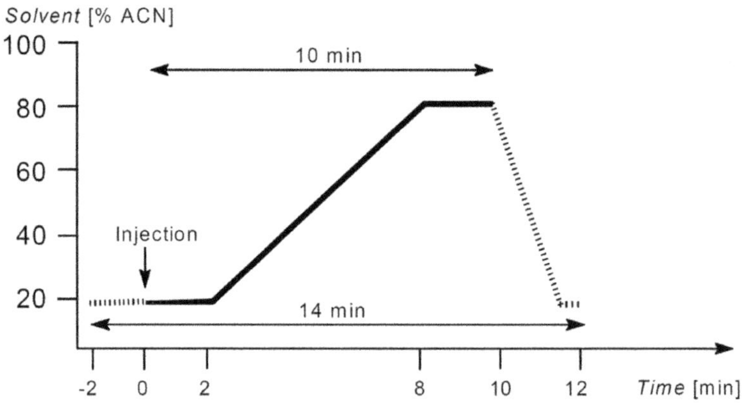

Fig. 14.9 Simple program for separation with a gradient in reversed phase UHPLC. Injection is performed after 2 min of column equilibration using a mobile phase of acetonitrile : water = 20 : 80 (v/v). After 2 min of holding this composition, the gradient leads to acetonitrile : water = 80 : 20 (v/v). Data acquisition could either stop at the end of the gradient at $t_R = 8$ min or at $t_R = 10$ min at the latest

While HPLC and UHPLC can be run at constant solvent composition, so-called *isocratic* operation, it is by far more common to employ gradually increasing concentrations of organic solvent in water to mobilize analytes of decreasing polarity. A typical *gradient* reverses the relative concentrations of two solvents (Fig. 14.9). Like the temperature program in GC, the concentration gradient in LC

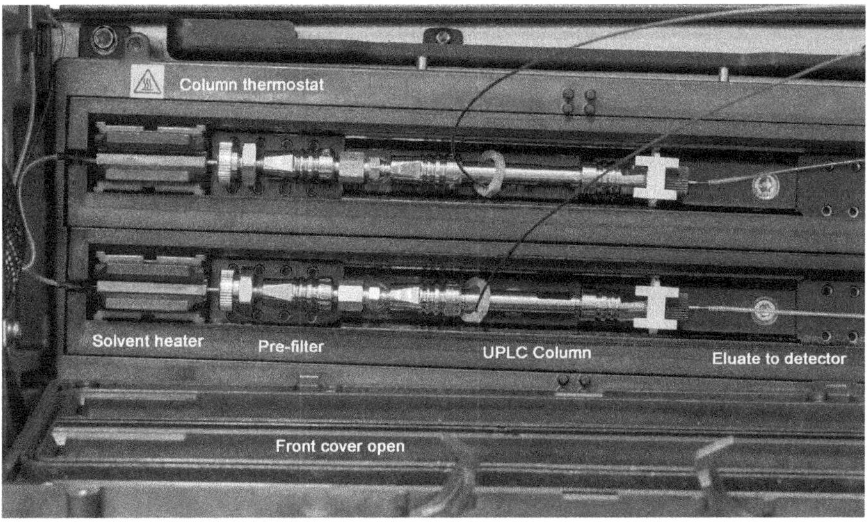

Fig. 14.10 A column thermostat of a Waters Acquity system with two UPLC columns mounted inside. The sample solution first passes a heater cartridge to ensure constant temperature equal to that of the column, then a pre-filter to prevent the column from clogging, and finally enters the UPLC column. The column compartments of the thermostat are inclined to direct solvent towards a drain in case of a leakage

serves to *i*) speed up the separation and to *ii*) preserve the level of chromatographic resolution until the end of the run.

To ensure best reproducibility, HPLC and UHPLC columns are operated at constant temperature in a thermostat (Fig. 14.10). In practice, this is most easily achieved at 30–50 °C. For practical reasons, they are run at constant flow, and thus, column pressure changes due to viscosity changes of the mobile phase.

From HPLC to UHPLC The method for transferring from conventional HPLC to UHPLC was demonstrated for the case of separating a pharmaceutical formulation containing a main product (#6) and eleven impurities (#1 – #5, #7 – #12, Fig. 14.11). The sample was analyzed in gradient mode with HPLC and UHPLC, respectively [29]. The original HPLC method used a C_{18} column of 150 × 4.6 mm with 5 μm particles at a flow rate of 1.0 ml min^{-1} that took 27 min. After transfer to UHPLC on a BEH C_{18} column of 50 × 2.1 mm with 1.7 μm particles at a flow rate of 0.6 ml min^{-1} the gradient time was shortened to 3 min. Further optimization of the UHPLC method at a flow rate of 1000 μl min^{-1} cut down the run time to 1.6 min without sacrificing resolution. In addition, the injected volume was reduced from 20 μl for HPLC to 1.4 μl for optimized UHPLC.

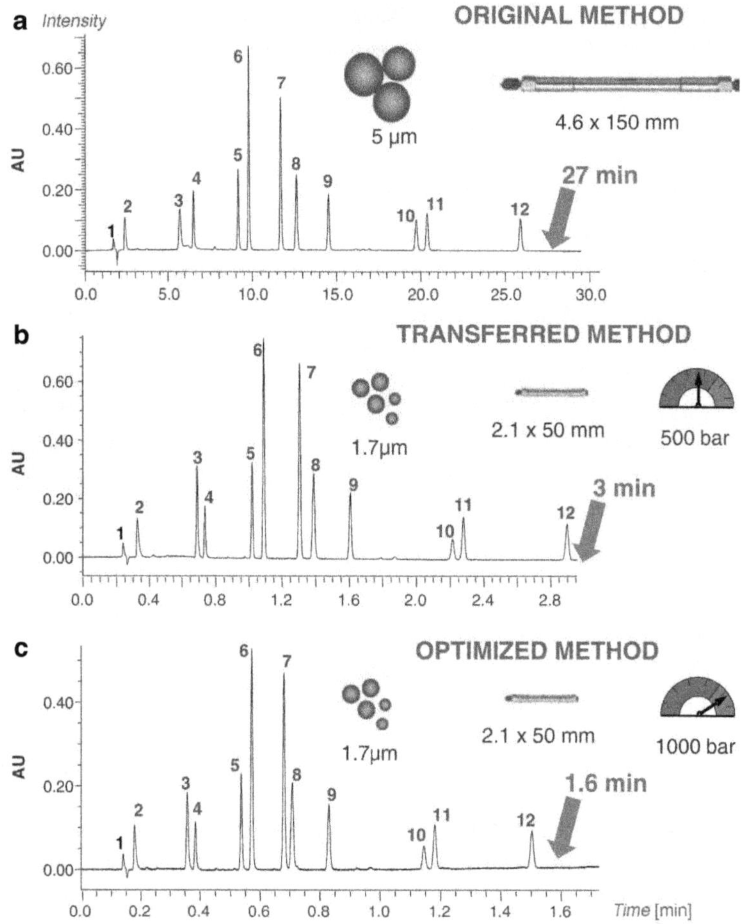

Fig. 14.11 Method transfer from conventional HPLC to UHPLC. (**a**) Original HPLC method on a C18 column of 150 × 4.6 mm lasting 27 min. (**b**) Transferred UHPLC method on BEH C18 column of 50 × 2.1 mm lasting 3 min. (**c**) Optimized UHPLC method on the same column delivering the separation in 1.6 min (Adapted from Ref. [29] with permission. © Springer, 2010)

14.2 Concept of Chromatography-Mass Spectrometry

Simple gas chromatographic detectors like the frequently employed FID deliver a chromatogram that represents the mass flow eluting from the chromatographic column. Using a mass spectrometer instead, adds a third dimension of information, i.e., the mass spectra associated to any of the eluting components (Fig. 14.12). When a mass spectrometer is employed as the chromatographic detector (also cf. Sects. 5.4 and 5.5) its output must somehow represent the chromatogram that

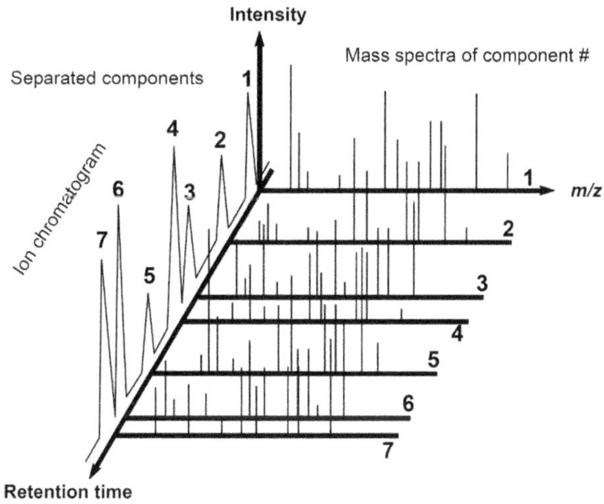

Fig. 14.12 Three dimensions of chromatography-mass spectrometry: retention time, intensity, and *m*/*z*. Each of the compounds No. 1 to No. 7 eluting from the chromatographic column is characterized by its own mass spectrum. The sum of all peak intensities of a mass spectrum at any point in retention time is used to construct the ion chromatogram

would have been obtained with other chromatographic detectors. The chromatogram as produced by the mass spectrometer is composed of a large set of consecutively acquired mass spectra. Because mass spectral chromatograms represent ionic abundances as a function of retention time, these are termed *ion chromatograms.*

14.2.1 Ion Chromatograms

Several decades ago, the *total ion current* (TIC) used to be measured by a *hardware TIC monitor* before mass analysis (nA to μA range). Today, its equivalent can be *reconstructed* or *extracted* after mass analysis [31]. Both adjectives, *reconstructed* and *extracted*, serve to illustrate that the chromatogram was obtained from a set of spectra by a computational process selecting user-defined signals to build the trace. For convenience, let us here again define some of the relevant terminology introduced in Chap. 1: The TIC represents a measure of the overall intensity of ion production as a function of time. The TIC obtained by means of *data reduction* [32], i.e., by summation of peak intensities of each mass spectrum as successively acquired during analysis, is termed *total ion chromatogram* (also abbreviated TIC). For this purpose, the sum of all ion intensities of each of the spectra is plotted as a function of time or scan number, respectively (Fig. 14.13). The term *total ion current chromatogram* (TICC) refers to a chromatogram obtained by plotting the total ion current detected in each of a series of mass spectra recorded as a function of retention times of the chromatographically separated components of a mixture (which essentially is implicated by: TIC). Unfortunately one also finds combinations such as *reconstructed total ion current* (RTIC), *reconstructed total ion current chromatogram* (RTICC), and *extracted ion chromatogram* (EIC, Table 14.1) [33].

The term *reconstructed ion chromatogram* (RIC) was and still is used by many to describe the intensity of a given *m*/*z* or *m*/*z* range plotted as a function of time or scan number. Recently, the term *extracted ion chromatogram* (EIC) has been used

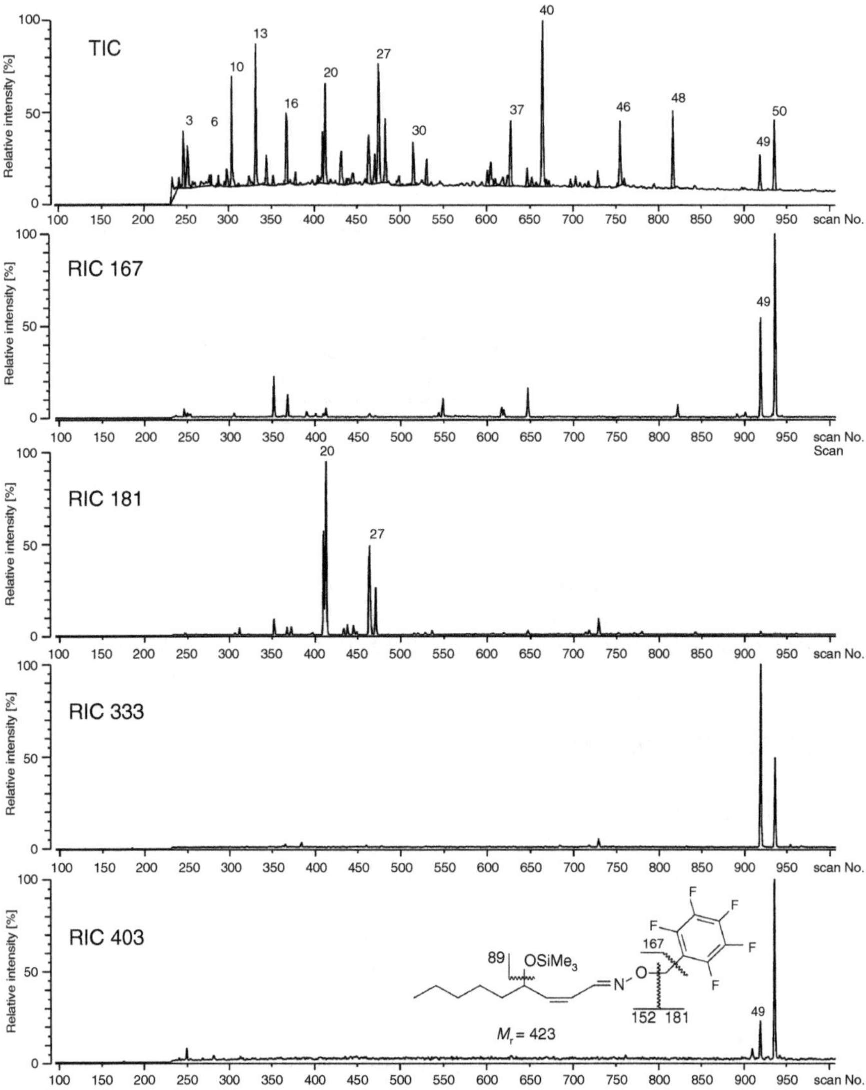

Fig. 14.13 TIC and RICs (*m*/*z* 167, 181, 333, and 403) obtained from a GC-EC-MS run of a plasma sample spiked with 4-HNE [38]. Chromatographic peaks are usually labeled using consecutive numbers to allow for their correlation to mass spectra. (The EC spectrum of the 4-HNE derivative is show in Fig. 14.14)

to describe a chromatogram created by plotting the intensity of the signal observed at a chosen *m*/*z* value or set of values in a series of mass spectra recorded as a function of retention time. Plotting RICs or EICs is especially useful to identify a target compound of known *m*/*z* from complex GC-MS or LC-MS data. In other words, the RIC allows to retrieve the retention time of the target compound. RICs

Table 14.1 Types of ion chromatograms

Acronym	Full name	Comment
TIC	Total ion chromatogram	Sum of peak intensities per spectrum vs. run time, retention time, or scan number; in practice used interchangeably. TIC is recommended here as the least complicated form
(TICC	Total ion current chromatogram)	
(RTIC	Reconstructed total ion chromatogram)	
(RTICC	Reconstructed total ion current chromatogram)	
RIC	Reconstructed ion chromatogram	Signal intensity at selected *m*/*z* vs. retention time; in practice used interchangeably
EIC	Extracted ion chromatogram	
BPC	Base peak chromatogram	Base peak intensity of each spectrum plotted vs. retention time or scan number

can also be used to elucidate the relationship of certain *m*/*z* values to different mass spectra obtained from the measurement of a single (impure) sample. Thus, RICs (EICs) often reveal valuable information on impurities accompanying the main product, e.g., remaining solvents, plasticizers, vacuum grease, or synthetic by-products (Appendix A.9).

Finally, the *base peak chromatogram* (BPC) is a chromatogram obtained by plotting the signal of the base-peak ions detected in each of a series of mass spectra recorded as a function of retention time. BPCs are particularly useful in conjunction with soft ionization methods as then the molecular mass is correlated to a chromatographic peak.

Plotting versus time or scan number
The abscissa of the TIC or RIC can either be plotted on the time scale, i.e., in units of seconds or minutes, or be labeled with scan numbers. Scan numbers are useful during data processing, while the time scale is better suited for comparison with other chromatography-mass spectrometry data.

14.2.2 Repetitive Acquisition of Mass Spectra During Elution

A widespread mode of chromatography-mass spectrometry operation is to repetitively scan the mass analyzer over the *m*/*z* range of interest during the chromatographic run [34–36]. As explained above, this generates a relationship between chromatogram and mass spectra of the eluting components. Knowledgeable handling of the TIC and suitable RICs presents the key to the effective assignment of chromatographic peaks to target compounds.

Detection of 4-hydroxynon-2-enal in plasma 4-Hydroxynon-2-enal (4-HNE) is a major aldehydic product of lipid peroxidation (LPO), its products being indicators for

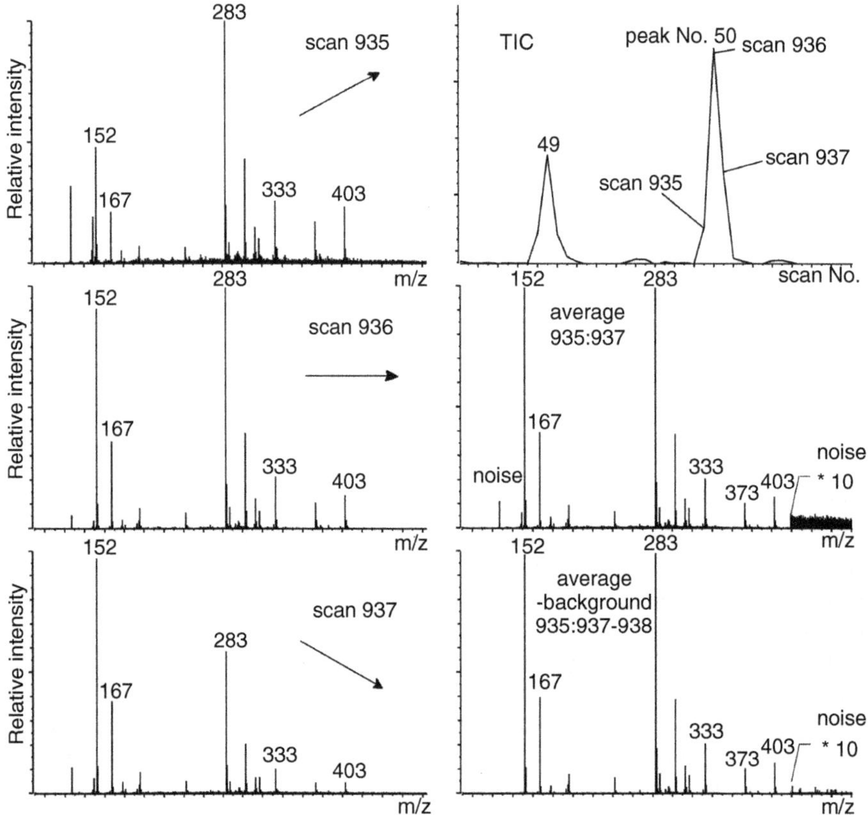

Fig. 14.14 Extraction of spectra from chromatographic peak No. 50 in the TIC of a plasma sample spiked with 4-HNE. *Left column*: single scan spectra from scans No. 935, 936, and 937 show changing relative intensities; averaging scans 935:937 levels intensity but leaves noise; background subtraction reduces noise additionally. (For explication, TIC, and RICs see preceding example and Fig. 14.13)

oxidative stress. In order to introduce LPO products as biomarkers, a GC-MS method for 4-HNE detection in clinical studies [37] was developed using a sample volume of 50 µl of plasma. For improved GC separation and subsequent mass spectral detection the aldehyde is converted into the pentafluorobenzyl-hydroxylimine and the hydroxy group is trimethylsilylated [38]. The TIC acquired in electron capture mode (EC, Sect. 7.6) exhibits 50 chromatographic peaks (Fig. 14.13). Those related to the target compounds can easily be identified from suitable RICs. The choice of potentially useful *m/z* values for RICs is made from the EC mass spectrum of the pure 4-HNE derivative (Fig. 14.14). In this case, $[M\text{–}HF]^{-\bullet}$, *m/z* 403, $[M\text{–}HOSiMe_3]^{-\bullet}$, *m/z* 333, and $[C_6F_5]^-$, *m/z* 167, are indicative, while $[CH_2C_6F_5]^-$, *m/z* 181, is not.

When the experiment is performed in the repetitive scanning mode, each point of the TIC corresponds to a full mass spectrum. The time for the acquisition of a mass spectrum has to be shorter than the time to elute a component from the chromatographic column. In capillary GC-MS, this requires scan cycle times in the order of one second. A 20-min run at one scan per second, for example, delivers a set of 1200 mass spectra. Nonetheless, the concentration of the eluting components still varies rapidly in time as compared to the time for a scan cycle. This affects the relative intensities of mass spectral peaks, i.e., high-mass ions are emphasized in an upwards mass scan at the onset of elution, but are underrepresented when elution fades out (Fig. 14.14). *Averaging* or *accumulation* of the scans contributing to a specific chromatographic peak compensates for that source of error. Additional *background subtraction* can substantially improve the signal-to-noise ratio (Sect. 1.6) of the final spectrum [35]. It is also obvious from this procedure that the number of final spectra is always lower than the actual number of scans.

Background subtraction
High-quality mass spectra suitable for interpretation and/or data base search (Sect. 5.9) are only obtained from summing/averaging plus subsequent background subtraction. Particularly for components of low concentration the value of background subtraction cannot be overestimated.

14.2.3 Selected Ion Monitoring and Targeted Analysis

The operation of mass spectrometers in the repetitive scanning mode is useful for the identification of the components of a mixture. If *quantitation* is a major issue (below), *selected ion monitoring* (SIM) is preferably employed; the term *multiple ion detection* (MID) and some others are also in use [31]. In the SIM mode, the mass analyzer is operated in a way that it alternately acquires only the ionic masses of interest, i.e., it "jumps" from one m/z to the next [39–41]. The information obtained from a SIM trace is equivalent to that from a RIC, but no mass spectra are recorded in SIM mode. Thus, the scan time spent on diagnostically useless m/z ranges or even on mere noise in the gaps between peaks is almost reduced to zero while the detector time for the ions of interest is increased by a factor of 10–100 (Fig. 14.15) [45]. An analogous improvement in detection limit is also observed.

Targeted approach
A precondition for selecting a set of m/z values to be exclusively observed during an analysis is that the *target analytes* are well defined prior to the run. In turn, the targeted approach sacrifices all data outside the selected window (s) in favor of lower detection limits for the target compounds. This explains why relevant compounds, yet unknown at the time of analysis, can be overlooked.

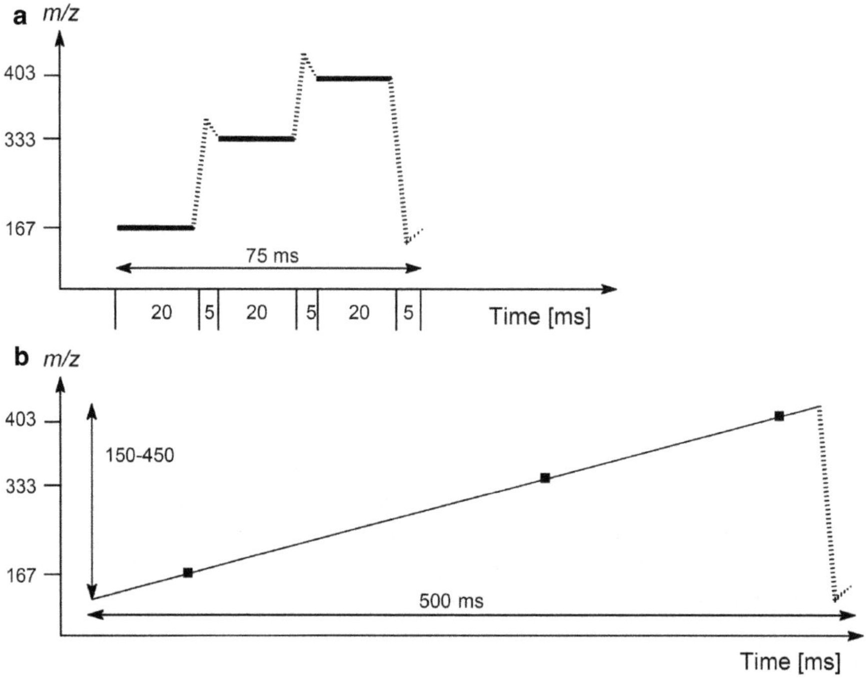

Fig. 14.15 SIM advantage over scanning mode. (**a**) Hypothetical SIM experiment to analyze 4-HNE in a plasma sample by *m*/*z* 167, 333, and 403 compared to (**b**) 500 ms-scan over the *m*/*z* 150–450 range. Only about 1.5 ms would be spent on each of the three signals during a 500 - ms-scan while 20 ms are achieved for each in a much shorter 75 ms-SIM cycle with 5 ms settling time. (Time axes not to scale.)

As the monitored *m*/*z* values are selected to best represent the target compound, SIM exhibits good selectivity that can be further increased by *high-resolution SIM* (HR-SIM) because HR-SIM almost eliminates isobaric interferences [46–49]. To ensure precise and drift-free positioning on narrow peaks, HR-SIM requires one or several *lock masses* to be employed although those are rarely explicitly mentioned in the literature [49, 50]. The role of the lock mass is to serve as internal mass reference for accurate mass measurement. (For examples cf. Sect. 14.3.)

How many ions in one run?

Normally, three to ten *m*/*z* values are monitored 20–100 ms each in one SIM cycle. Some settling time is needed for the mass analyzer after switching to the next value, e.g., 1–2 ms for pure electric scanning, 20–50 ms for a magnet scan. Due to the comparatively slow axial ion velocity in (triple) quadrupole instruments, the time to empty the quadrupole from one ionic species prior to setting it to the next has to be taken into account.

14.2.4 Retrospective and Non-targeted Analysis

The improvement of SIM mode over full spectral acquisition mode in terms of detection limits exclusively applies to scanning instruments like magnetic sector and (triple) quadrupole mass spectrometers. Quadrupole ion traps (QIT and LIT) might be operated as to deliver a SIM output. The time to achieve ion selection is, however, essentially identical to their full scan cycle time, thus canceling out the sensitivity advantage.

With any type of TOF analyzers, the SIM mode can neither be realized nor can it offer any improvement over retrieving RICs from the spectra. As many modern TOF instruments allow for both high resolution and accurate mass, this actually becomes an advantage in that the information for HR-SIM is already contained in the dataset. Thus, any RIC, even within a narrow *m/z* window, can be extracted in post-processing [51–56]. It is Therefore it is no longer necessary to restrict the analysis to a limited set of HR-SIM traces while having to discard all other information. This approach is known as *retrospective analysis*. Other comparatively fast high-resolving mass analyzers like Orbitrap and FT-ICR instruments bear the same advantage, the only difference to TOFs being somewhat slower spectral acquisition rates at, in turn, even higher resolving power and mass accuracy [54].

One can roughly compare these different instrumental concepts and their modes of operation to get an idea of where the one or the other approach will work best in terms of signal-to-noise ratio versus the number of components that are to be analyzed in one cycle (Fig. 14.16). The exact position of the lines will vary depending on the actual mass spectrometer. Also, if we were to ask instrument manufacturers, the relative positions would be shifted depending on the manufacturer's perspective.

Sometimes, compounds may only appear relevant in the aftermath of an analysis, e.g., in doping control and other forensic fields as well as in environmental analyses. Retrospective analysis offers the opportunity of investigating analytes that were not considered at the time of spectral acquisition, i.e., to retrieve *non-targeted analytes*.

Non-targeted analysis

The ability to collect as much data as possible in one run without losing neither sensitivity nor selectivity permits a *non-targeted analysis* to be performed. Even though the standard procedure may be designed to detect any one of a predefined number of compounds, the data offers the chance for re-examination to look after another set initially not considered to be relevant.

Drug residues in wastewater Drugs and their metabolites are excreted and end up in wastewater. The TIC obtained by LC-HR-TOF-MS analysis of a wastewater sample mostly showed severely overlapping chromatographic peaks (Fig. 14.17)

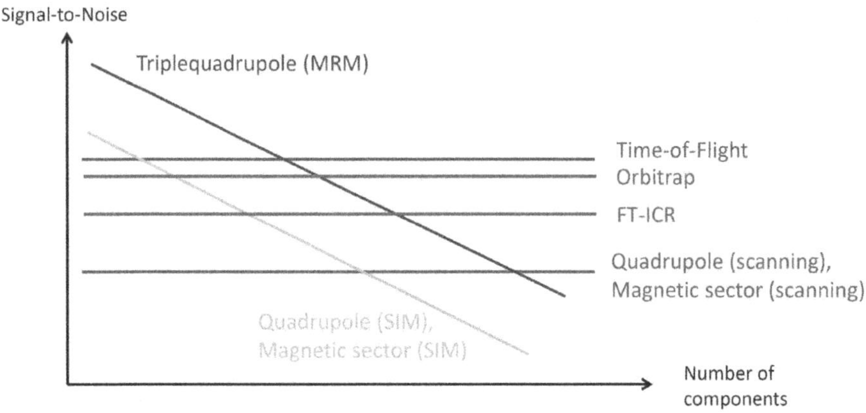

Fig. 14.16 Qualitative comparison of signal-to-noise ratios of scanning instruments, their operation in SIM or MRM modes, and nonscanning instruments versus the number of components to be analyzed per cycle

[52]. While it was impossible to detect a metabolite of the antirheumatic and antipyretic drug dipyrone from the TIC, the application of a narrow window of *m/z* 246.12 ± 0.02 characteristic of the $[M+H]^+$ ion revealed the presence of the compound. Having identified the retention time, 20.58 min, the corresponding mass spectrum could be obtained after background subtraction. It delivered a signal of the $[M+H]^+$ ion, $[C_{13}H_{16}N_3O_2]^+$ at *m/z* 246.1237, and two fragment ions, the formulas of which were also assigned by accurate mass. This demonstrates that a nontargeted analysis offers deliberate selection of target analytes during post-processing.

14.2.5 Selected Reaction Monitoring

Tandem MS adds a fourth dimension to the chromatography-MS experiment in that it allows to acquire a spectrum selectively, revealing the fragmentation of one specific ion generated of the target compound (Fig. 14.18). Like SIM, the approach of *selected reaction monitoring* (SRM, Table 14.2) requires useful ionic fragmentation pathways to be explored before their use in SRM analyses. If two or more ionic fragmentations are covered in one cycle the experiment is termed *multiple reaction monitoring* (MRM). Triple quadrupole instruments are preferred for SRM and MRM operation as they combine straightforward tandem MS operation and fast switching of *m/z* with a high linear dynamic range (10^4–10^5). (Examples of MRM and SRM are given in Sects. 14.6 and 14.8, respectively. Another procedure of four-dimensional analysis is discussed in Sects. 14.4.6.)

LC-APCI of polybrominated diphenyl ethers Hydroxylated and methoxylated polybrominated diphenyl ethers were isolated from simple organisms such as algae,

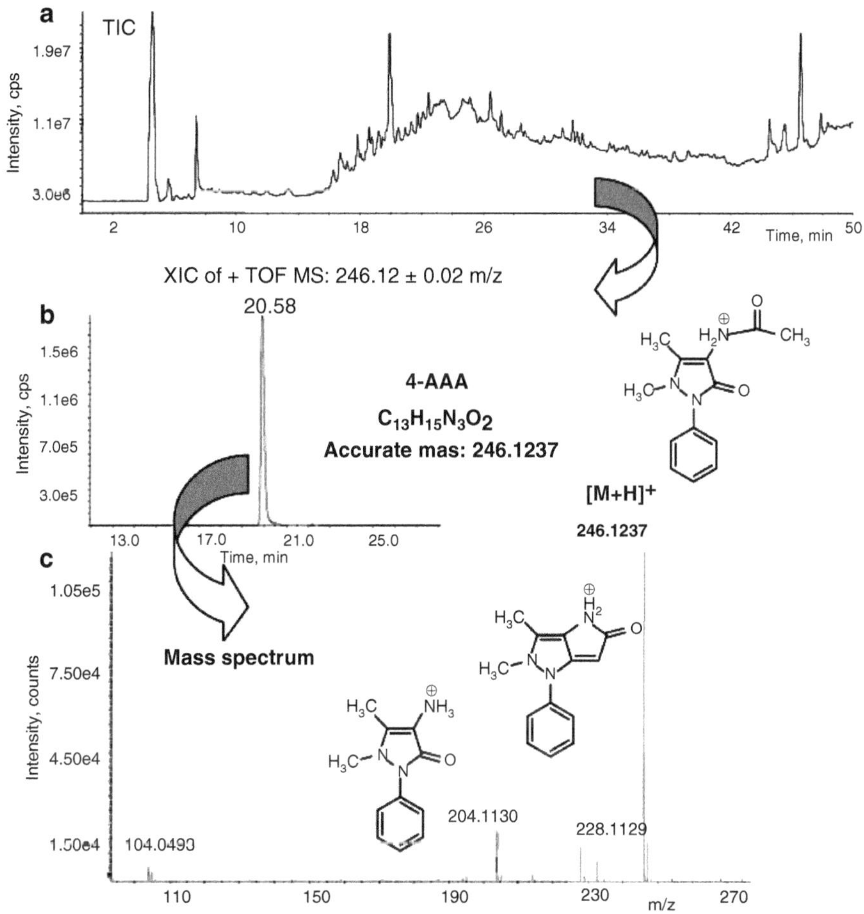

Fig. 14.17 Dipyrone metabolite in wastewater detected by LC-HR-TOF-MS. (**a**) The TIC shows severe overlap of peaks from LC analysis. (**b**) Extraction of a chromatogram at the expected *m/z* of the $[M+H]^+$ ion, *m/z* 246.12 ± 0.02, reveals the elution of the target compound, here abbreviated as 4-AAA, at 20.58 min. (**c**) Accurate mass TOF spectrum of 4-AAA as obtained after background subtraction (Adapted from Ref. [52] with permission. © American Chemical Society, 2007)

sponges, and bacteria [57]. The compounds could be separated and detected by coupling liquid chromatography to negative-ion APCI. The phenol-type compounds underwent deprotonation, and thus, formed $[M-H]^-$ ions. For higher selectivity, the compounds were not detected using full scans but by scanning for the precursor ion of their Br^- fragment ions (Fig. 14.19). As the polybrominated diphenyl ethers obviously were the only brominated compounds in these extracts, the occurrence of Br^- fragments from any of the diphenyl ether $[M-H]^-$ ions turned out to be highly characteristic for their identification. The dimethylether analogs showed a different behavior, presumably as the transient negative molecular ions

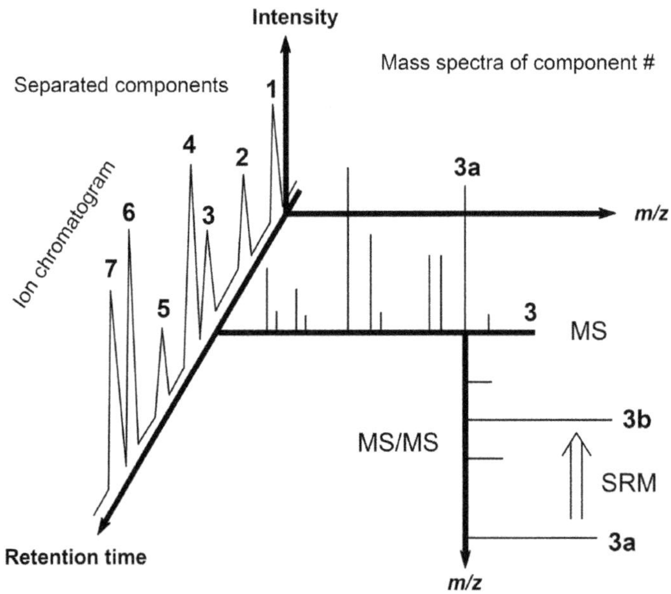

Fig. 14.18 The fourth dimension added by chromatography-tandem MS. Compound *3* has been chosen to illustrate the effect of selectively measuring the fragmentation of one precursor ion, *3a*, defined by its *m/z*. If the instrument is operated as to only detect one characteristic product ion, *3b*, the mode is termed *selected reaction monitoring* (SRM)

Table 14.2 Discontinuous modes of operation

Acronym	Full name	Comment
SIM	Selected ion monitoring	In practice used interchangeably; the term SIM is recommended.
MID	Multiple ion detection	
HR-SIM	High-resolution selected ion monitoring	To avoid isobaric interferences
SRM	Selected reaction monitoring	SIM in a tandem MS mode
MRM	Multiple reaction monitoring	More than one reaction is monitored per cycle

dissociated to yield nonetheless characteristic $[M{-}Br{+}O]^-$ and $[M{-}CH_3]^-$ ions. The bromine content resulted in clearly visible isotopic patterns.

14.3 Quantitation

Every ionization method exhibits compound-dependent ionization efficiencies (Sect. 2.3). Whether a specific compound is rather preferred or suppressed relative to another greatly depends on the ionization process employed to deliver the ions to the mass analyzer. These circumstances require a careful calibration of the

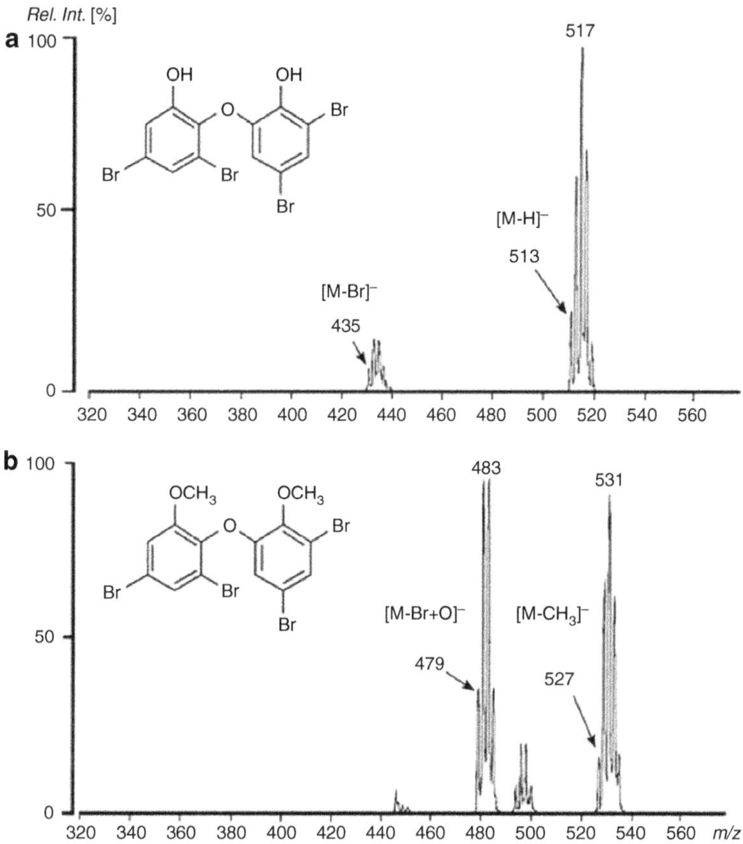

Fig. 14.19 Negative-ion Br^- precursor ion scan APCI spectra of (**a**) hydroxylated and (**b**) methoxylated tetrabromodiphenylether. The four bromine atoms are revealed by the corresponding isotopic patterns. The peak labels point at the peaks of the respective monoisotopic ions (Adapted from Ref. [57] with permission. © Springer, 2012)

instrument's response versus the sample concentration for correct *quantitation* [5, 7, 58]. While relative signal intensities are perfect for qualitative analysis, i.e., for compound characterization, some means of measuring absolute intensities would be preferred in quantitation. Basic considerations on how to approach a quantitative analysis by mass spectrometry are given below [59–62]. Readers interested in a treatment of all aspects of quantitative analysis by mass spectrometry may refer to the highly recommended book by Boyd, Basic, and Bethem [58].

14.3.1 Quantitation by External Standardization

External standardization is obtained by constructing a *calibration curve*, i.e., plotting measured intensities versus rising concentration of the target compound. Calibration curves are generally linear over a wide range of concentrations. When the concentration approaches the detection limit (Sect. 1.6) the graph deviates from linearity, either towards underestimation or towards overestimation. Underestimation can be due to losses by adsorption, overestimation may either be due to "memory" from previous injections or result from chemical background. In the regime of high concentration, saturation of the detector or of the ion source cause an upper limit (Fig. 14.20). The preparation of a calibration curve requires repeated measurements which can be very time-consuming in case of a slow chromatographic separation. In addition, drifts in instrument sensitivity, e.g., due to ion source contamination, can deteriorate the quantitation result. Depending on the instrument's dynamic range, the range of linear response is in the order of two to four orders of magnitude.

LOD versus LOQ

In practice, four or five runs at increasing concentration of the standard, preferably from well above the detection limit to close to saturation, should be run in a sequence to obtain the data for the construction of a calibration curve. Extrapolation to concentrations outside the range covered has to be strictly avoided. One should also bear in mind that the *limit of quantitation* (LOQ) of a compound is found at higher concentration than its *limit of detection* (LOD).

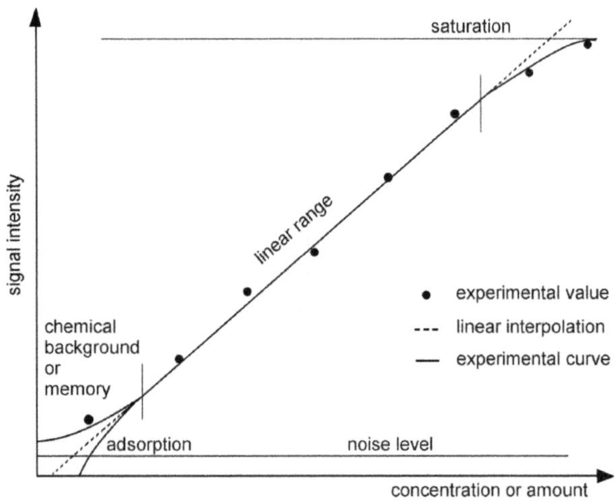

Fig. 14.20 General appearance of a calibration curve. The upper limit of the linear range is defined by saturation, the lower by memory and chemical background or adsorption. In addition, the noise level plays a role for the detection limit

14.3.2 Quantitation by Internal Standardization

Internal standardization circumvents the effects of time-variant instrument response, but does not compensate for different ionization efficiencies of analyte and standard. For internal standardization, a compound exhibiting close similarity in terms of ionization efficiency and retention time is added to the sample at a known level of concentration, e.g., an isomer or a homolog eluting closely to the analyte may serve that purpose.

It is important to add the internal standard before any clean-up procedure in order not to alter the concentration of the analyte without affecting that of the standard in the very same way. For reliable results, the relative concentration of analyte and standard should not differ by more than a factor of about ten.

14.3.3 Quantitation by Isotope Dilution

Virtually identical ionization efficiency for a pair of compounds is only given for isotopologs. As these differ from the nonlabeled target compound in mass, they can be added to the mixture at known concentration to result in a special case of internal standardization, hence the term *isotope dilution* [63]. The ratio of intensities of the peaks corresponding to target compound and labeled standard as delivered by the RICs, SIM, or MRM traces is then taken as the relative concentration of labeled internal standard and target compound. As the absolute concentration of the standard added before the analysis is known, the concentration of the analyte can reliably be calculated.

Drug metabolism A potential drug (M) and its metabolite (M') in a liver sample are quantified by LC-ESI-MS with internal standardization using trideuterated standards for each analyte (Fig. 14.21) [64]. Under these conditions it neither presents a problem that both analytes and their isotopic standards are almost co-eluting from the LC column, nor does the completely unspecific TIC play a role. If required for sensitivity reasons, this analysis could also have been performed in the SIM mode using the *m/z* values of the RICs shown.

Time windows in SIM The number of *m/z* values to be monitored in SIM is limited. Such limitations are more severe when additional lock mass peaks have to be included in case of HR-SIM. Therefore, it is commonplace to monitor different sets of SIM traces during consecutive time windows leading to a sequence of different SIM setups during a single chromatographic separation. The quantitation of halogenated dibenzo-*p*-dioxins in municipal waste incinerator fly ash at concentrations in the ppb to low-ppm range requires such a setup (Fig. 14.22) [48]. Here, a combined approach of external standardization for the $BrCl_3$-species and internal standardization for the Cl_4-species has been realized.

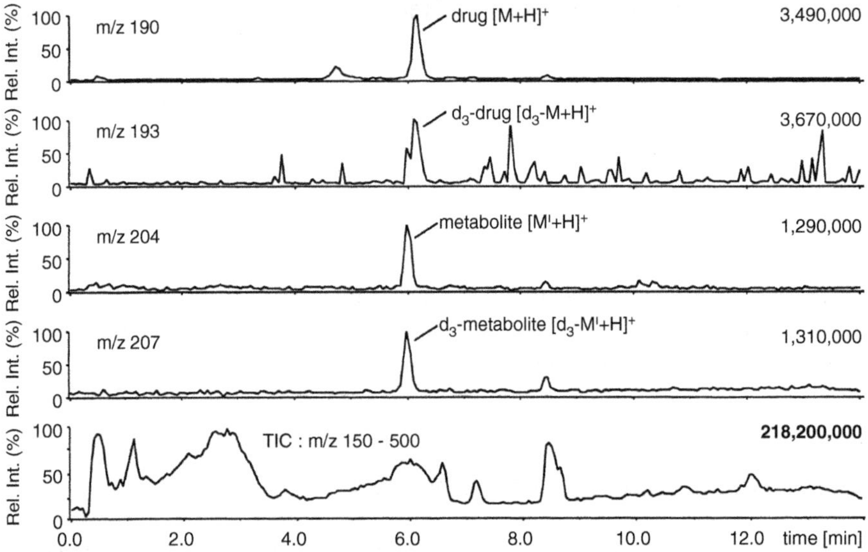

Fig. 14.21 RICs and TIC of an LC-ESI-MS quantification of a drug, $[M+H]^+$ at *m/z* 190, and its metabolite, $[M'+H]^+$ at *m/z* 204, by isotope dilution with trideuterated standards. The numbers on the top right of each trace give their absolute intensity values (Reproduced from Ref. [64] by permission. © Elsevier Science, 2001)

Getting isotopically labeled standards

According to the enormous usage of isotope dilution, ^{2}H- (D) and ^{13}C-labeled standards [65] are commercially available for a wide range of applications. Often, a methyl is exchanged for a trideuteromethyl as this safely avoids overlap with isotopic peaks of the analyte. It is also important not to select compounds with acidic hydrogens exchanged for deuterons. Other restrictions for internal standards also apply.

14.3.4 Retention Times of Isotopologs

Isotopologs exhibit somewhat different retention times in chromatography. Deuterated compounds, for example, elute from chromatographic columns at slightly shorter retention times than their nonlabeled isotopologs. Normally, the difference is less than the peak width of the corresponding chromatographic peaks, but may still be large enough to require their integration over separate time windows (Fig. 14.23).

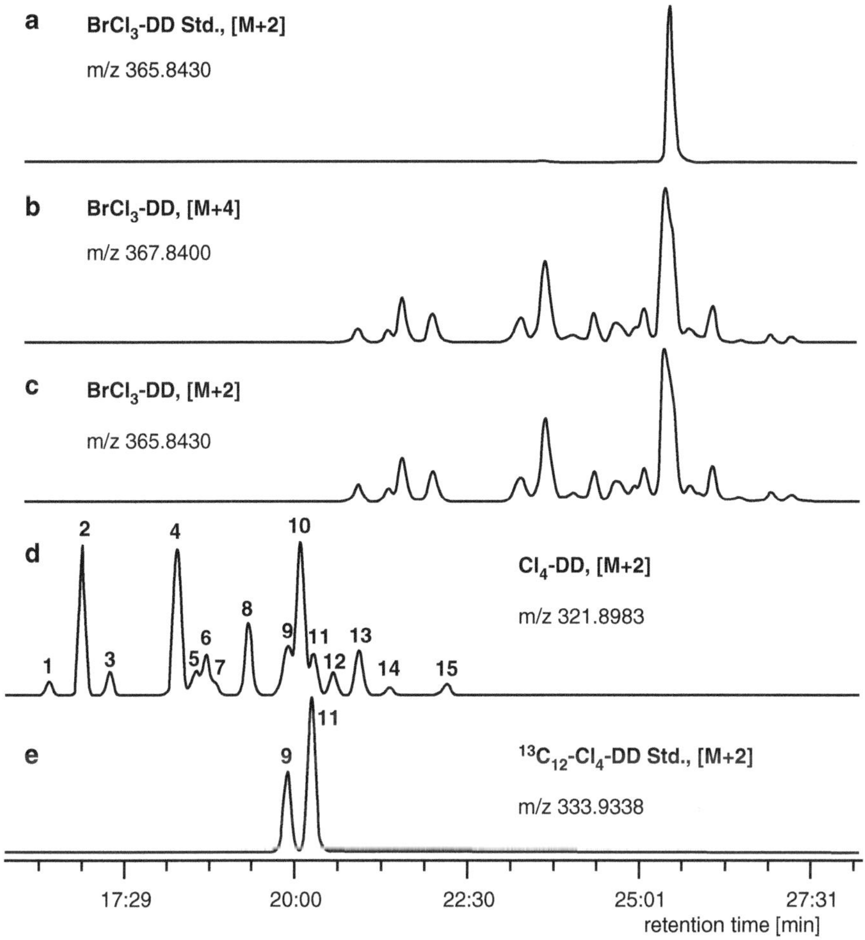

Fig. 14.22 Quantification of $BrCl_3$- and Cl_4-dibenzodioxins by HR-SIM. A $^{13}C_{12}$-labeled internal standard is added for the Cl_4-congener (Adapted from Ref. [48] by permission. © American Chemical Society, 1991)

14.4 Gas Chromatography-Mass Spectrometry

14.4.1 GC-MS Interfaces

The advent of capillary GC had a strong influence on the further development of GC-MS [66–70]. Capillary columns are operated at gas flow rates in the order of 1 ml min^{-1}, and therefore can be directly interfaced to EI or CI ion sources [71, 72]. Although the pressure inside the ion source rises due to the continuous gas load, the conditions for EI are still properly maintained. Sufficient pumping

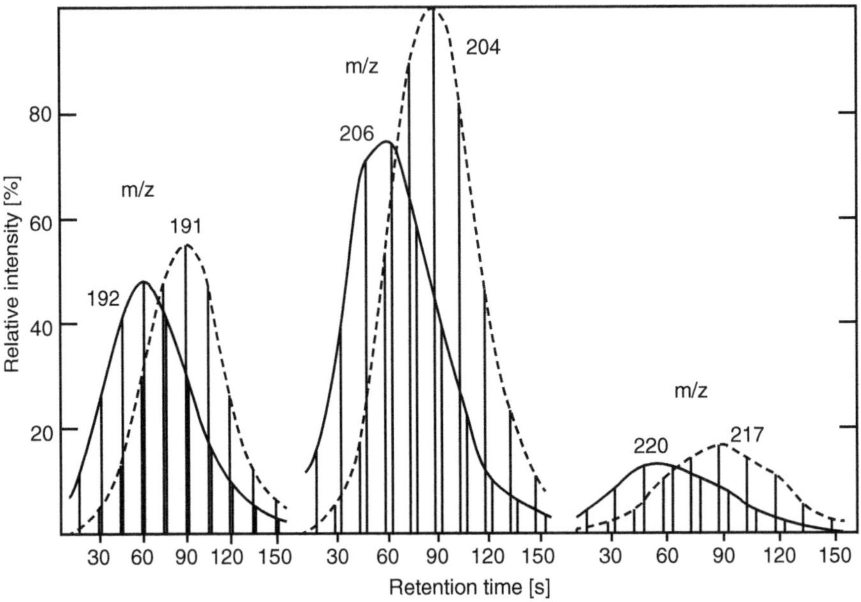

Fig. 14.23 Shorter retention times are observed for [D_7]glucose than for glucose eluting from a SE30 GC column as demonstrated for three pairs of peaks (Reproduced from Ref. [40] by permission. © American Chemical Society, 1966)

speed (≈ 200 l s^{-1}) is recommended to keep the pressure in the ion source housing below 10^{-5} mbar. Helium is the preferred carrier gas for GC-EI-MS. If CI is intended, hydrogen or methane may be used instead as these can at the same time serve as reagent gas.

To interface the GC column to the ion source the capillary column is guided by a heated glass line (Fig. 14.24). The evacuated glass line is sealed toward the atmosphere by a graphite ferrule where the GC capillary leaves the oven. Guided by the glass line the exit of the capillary column is positioned at the entrance of the ionization volume. Most EI or CI ion sources have a dedicated entrance port opposite the direct probe port for that purpose (Sect. 5.2). Thus, a modern GC-MS interface basically consists of a heated glass line bridging the distance (≈ 30 cm) between GC oven and ion source. The interface should be operated above the highest temperature employed in the actual GC separation or at the highest temperature the column can tolerate (200–350 °C). Keeping the transfer line at lower temperature causes condensation of eluting components inside the end of the column.

In contrast to sample introduction via direct probe, the components eluting from a GC capillary are quantitatively transferred into the ion source during a short time interval just sufficient to acquire about five mass spectra. Consequently, the partial pressure of the analyte is comparatively high during elution for sample amounts in the picogram range to be analyzed by capillary GC-MS.

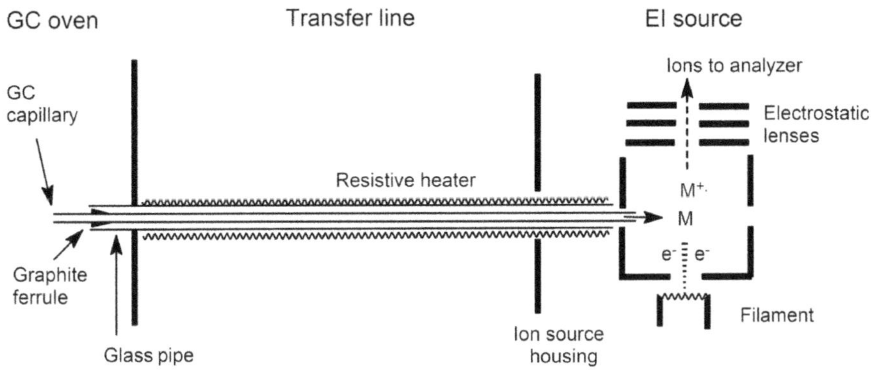

Fig. 14.24 Interfacing a capillary GC column to an EI ion source

While the market share of mass spectrometers with atmospheric pressure interface still increases, the fraction of instruments with EI sources is diminishing. It is therefore of interest to devise a means of coupling gas chromatography to APCI or APPI, for example. This can readily be accomplished by mounting the exit of the GC column into the APCI source and releasing the GC eluate into the ionization zone, which is exactly the way how ASAP is performed (Sect. 13.7) [73–75]. In recent years, GC-APCI and related techniques have found widespread application [76].

14.4.2 Volatility and Derivatization

Gas chromatography requires a certain level of volatility and thermal robustness of the analyte. Both injection block of the gas chromatograph and interface to the mass spectrometer ion source are always at high temperature even while the column oven is not. In order to adapt an analyte to these needs, *derivatization* is well established [77, 78], the most frequent derivatization procedures being silylation, acetylation, methylation, and fluoroalkylation. As derivatization transforms XH groups into $XSiR_3$, XC=OMe, XMe, or $XCOCF_3$ groups, for example, polarity of the molecules largely decreases. This causes an improved volatility even though the molecular weight increases upon derivatization. Derivatization suppresses thermal decomposition, e.g., it protects alcohols from thermal dehydration. In particular fluoroalkyl and fluoroaryl groups are extremely useful to improve detection limits in EC-MS [38, 79, 80]. There is a complete series of reviews by John Halket covering the different derivatives and their uses in mass spectrometry [81–88].

Derivatization can also introduce functional groups that induce a controlled fragmentation of the ion [89], e.g., by α-cleavage at the new functional group. This way, 3-picolinyl esters of fatty acids reveal double bond positions because the charge localizing substituent largely reduces double bond rearrangement prior to fragmentation. The alternative use of dimethyldisulfide adducts for double bond localization has already been explained in Sect. 6.5.2.

14.4.3 Column Bleed

Rising temperature of the GC column not only assists transport of less volatile components, it also causes the slow release of the liquid phase from the inner wall of the capillary. As a result of slow thermal degradation, even chemically bonded liquid phases show such *column bleed* at elevated temperature. It is a characteristic of column bleed that it continuously rises as the temperature of the GC oven is raised and it falls again upon cooling of the system. Of course, the peaks from column bleed observed in the mass spectrum depend on the liquid phase of the GC capillary in use. In case of the frequently employed methyl-phenyl-siloxane liquid phases, abundant ions at *m/z* 73, 147, 207, 281, 355, 429, etc. are observed. Within one series the peaks are aligned at $\Delta(m/z) = 74$ ($OSiMe_2$) and exhibit characteristic silicon isotopic patterns. Fortunately, column bleed is easily recognized and can be removed by careful background subtraction. Similar background ions are also obtained from *septum bleed* and silicon grease [7, 90] (Scheme 14.1).

Subtracting column bleed A portion of the TIC as obtained by GC-EI-MS of an unknown mixture on a 30-m HP-5 capillary column shows a rather small chromatographic peak at a retention time of 32.6 min (Fig. 14.25), while the chromatogram shows a rather high baseline due to continuous elution of column material. Extracting scan No. 2045 at the GC peak's apex yields a spectrum that is dominated by background ions from column bleed. This becomes obvious by averaging scans 2068 to 2082, which delivers the spectrum of column bleed alone. Averaging of all scans covering the GC peak followed by background subtraction ((2035:2052)–(2013:2020)) delivers a mass spectrum of reasonable quality, even though some background peaks are still present.

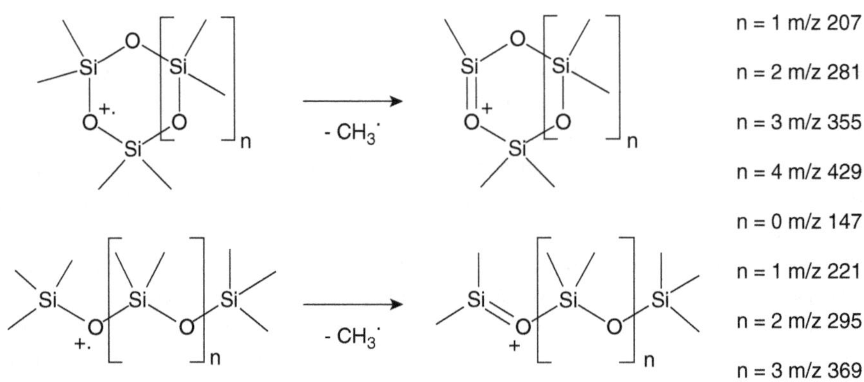

Scheme 14.1

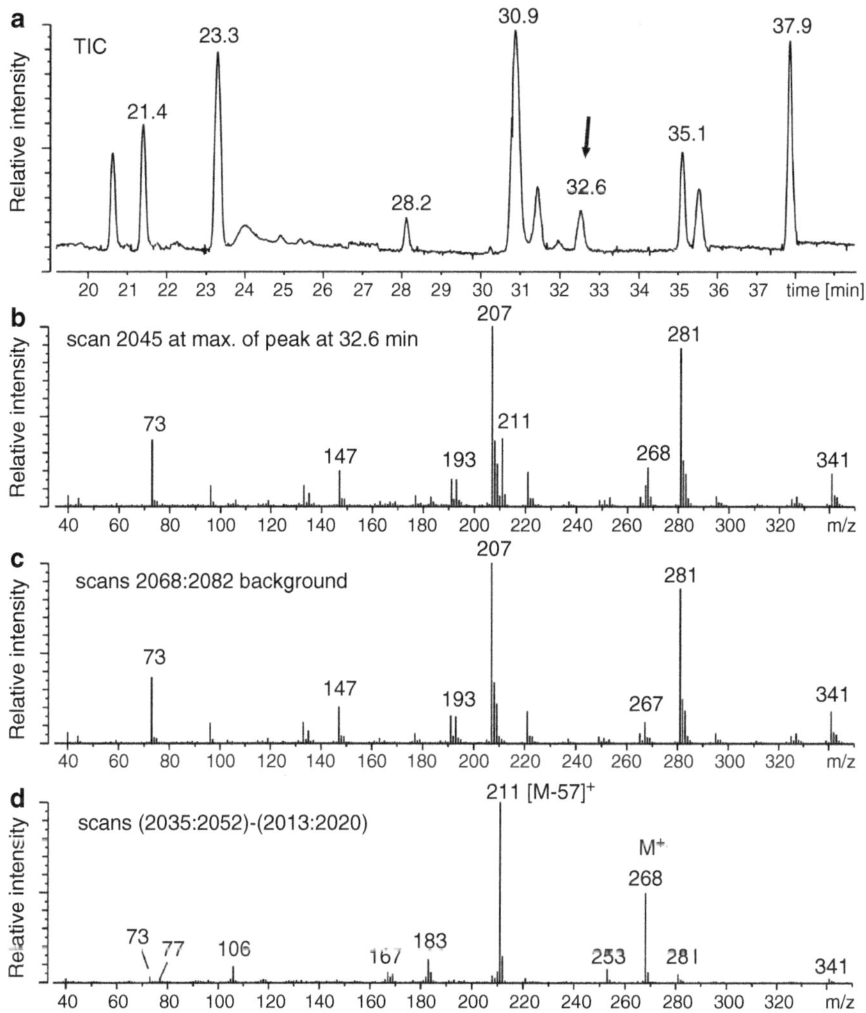

Fig. 14.25 Background subtraction to remove peaks from column bleed in GC-MS of an unknown mixture. (**a**) Partial TIC, (**b**) single scan mass spectrum from peak top at 32.6 min, (**c**) summation of scans from pure column bleed between GC peaks (cf. Scheme 14.1), and (**d**) final spectrum after averaging of scans and background subtraction

14.4.4 Fast GC-MS

When a high sample throughput is of importance, *fast GC-MS* offers a time-saving concept for mixture analysis [91–93]. The GC separation can be accelerated by replacing standard size (20–60 m × 0.25–0.53 mm i.d.) capillary columns by short narrow-bore columns (2–5 m × 50 μm i.d.) and by applying sufficient pressure

(8–10 bar) and rapid heating (50–200 °C min^{-1}). Thus, a conventional 30-min separation is compressed into a 3-min or even shorter time frame. However, in fast GC the half-life of an eluting peak is too short for use with scanning quadrupole or magnetic sector analyzers. In fast GC-MS, oaTOF analyzers (Sect. 4.2.8) are typically employed because of their ability to acquire about a hundred spectra per second. Furthermore, the high duty cycle of oaTOFs offsets the difference in sensitivity between repetitive scanning and SIM analysis. At somewhat lower rates, advanced oaTOF systems even enable accurate mass determination at good accuracy.

14.4.5 Multiplexing for Increased Throughput

Even in fast GC operation the capacity of the capillary column is not fully exploited, because gaps between loaded zones inevitably occur as the separation proceeds. Hadamard transform GC can be applied to improve the duty cycle (Sect. 4.2.10) of GC separations, i.e., the next injection onto the column is made long before all components of the preceding injection have left the column. In contrast to conventional chromatographic separation, the chromatogram then consists of several chromatograms overlapping in time. Key to mathematical deconvolution by Hadamard transform is to inject rapidly and precisely by a *multiplexing* injector according to an n-bit pseudorandom sequence (Fig. 14.26) [94, 95]. These pseudorandom injections are further divided into subsets of different concentrations, which may later serve for control of the time-shifted repetitive injections. Thus, a computer-controlled injection sequence combined with Hadamard transform of the detector output delivers the concentrations of all components at enhanced sample throughput. Using a multiplexing injector capable of up to 3000 injections per hour allowed for a 50% duty cycle of the chromatograph to be achieved.

Multiplexing means simultaneous runs

The term *multiplexing* refers to the use of one separation device for multiple samples at the same time. To achieve an improved duty cycle of the device multiplexing requires a complex mathematical deconvolution of the detector output. In contrast, *multiplexed* chromatographic systems are using one detector for multiple parallel chromatographs in a simple alternating mode (Sect. 14.4.2). Multiplexed systems use high-speed detection and are based on the assumption not to miss relevant information while the detector connects to other lines between sampling intervals.

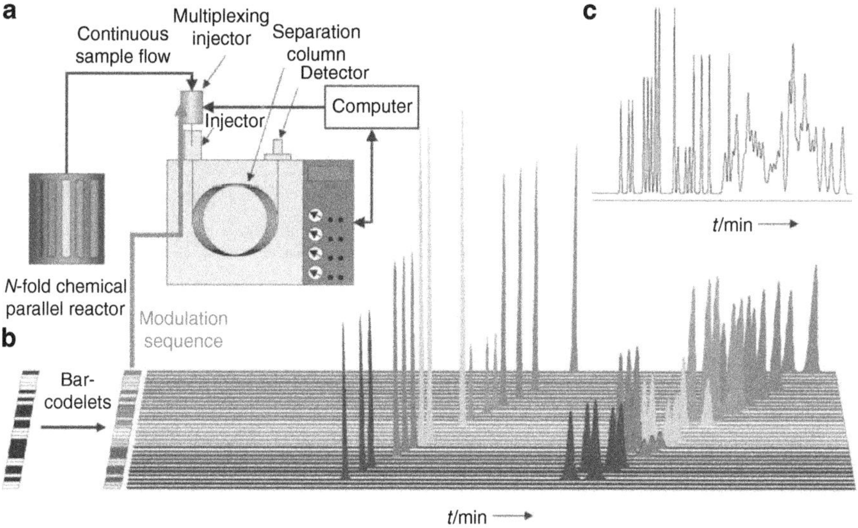

Fig. 14.26 High-throughput multiplexing gas chromatography. (**a**) Experimental setup for the analysis of the sample composition from an N-fold parallel reactor. The multiplexing injector is loading the column by short pressure pulses (1–5 ms) according to an n-bit binary pseudorandom sequence. (**b**) Temporally shifted chromatograms obtained by repetitive sample injections following the bar codelets of an n-bit sequence. (**c**) Convoluted chromatogram which is the sum of the chromatograms shown in (**b**) (Reproduced from Ref. [95] with permission. © Wiley-VCH, 2007)

14.4.6 Comprehensive Gas Chromatography-Mass Spectrometry

Like tandem MS, GC × GC adds an analytical dimension (Sect. 14.1.9). GC-MS/MS and GC × GC-MS are thus complementary in that they both provide four-dimensional analysis, either with an emphasis on separation or on enhanced-level mass analysis. The extremely high spectral acquisition rate required for GC × GC-MS does not permit GC × GC-MS/MS, however. As the mass analyzer for GC × GC-MS needs to be extremely fast, GC × GC-MS is the domain of TOF analyzers. Instruments optimized for high spectral acquisition rates are also available, like the LECO Pegasus 4D series.

Pyrolysis products from recycling of tires Pyrolysis of used tires is a promising recycling technology that yields pyrolysis liquids, carbon black, and steel [96–98]. These pyrolysis liquids are complex mixtures of organic compounds and can serve as a valuable resource similar to crude oil.

GC × GC-MS of a pyrolysis liquid was performed using a Pegasus 4D TOF analyzer and a gas chromatograph with a liquid nitrogen cryogenic modulator. A polar first column (Rxi-17SilMS, 30 m × 0.25 mm) and an apolar second column (SLB-5MS, 1.5 m × 0.1 mm) were used, i.e., different from common GC × GC conditions in reverse order of polarity [98]. A sample of 1 μl was injected at 280 °C. The GC oven program started at 35 °C and was held there for 5 min. Then, the

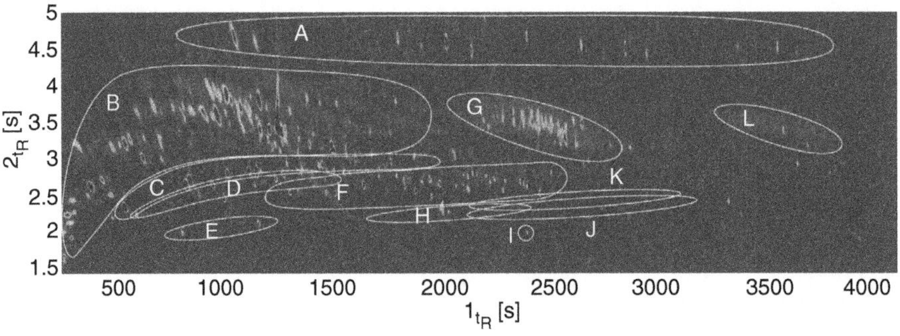

Fig. 14.27 Elution pattern of all compounds in pyrolysis liquid from tyre. The compounds are grouped as follows: *A* Alkanes, *B* cyclic hydrocarbons, *C* monocylic aromatic hydrocarbons, *D* thiophenes, *E* cycloalkanones, *F* styrenes, indanes, and indenes, *G* unidentified compounds, *H* phenoles, *I* benzothiazole, *J* benzothiophenes, *K* polycyclic aromatic hydrocarbons, and *L* unidentified compounds (Reproduced from Ref. [98] with permission. © Elsevier, 2015)

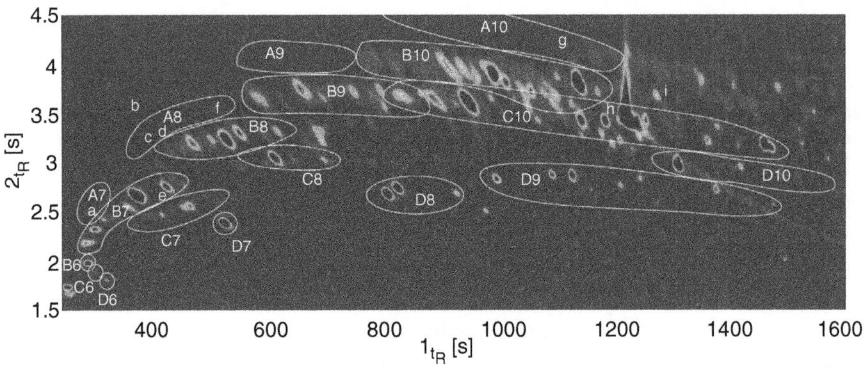

Fig. 14.28 Zoomed-in view of the elution area of hydrocarbon compounds with r + d = 1–4. The letters denote the number of r + d (A : 1, B : 2, C : 3, D : 4) and numbers denote the carbon number. The plot is based on ions of *m*/*z* 55, 67, 79, 81, 83, 91, 105, 119, 133. The positions of reference compounds are denoted by lower case letters (a: methylcyclohexane, b: octane, c: 1-octene, d: 3-octene, e: 1-methylcyclohexene, f: ethylcyclohexane, g: butylcyclohexane, h: limonene, i: *trans*-decahydronaphthalene) (Reproduced from Ref. [98] with permission. © Elsevier, 2015)

primary oven was ramped up to 300 °C at 3 °C min^{-1} and held there for another 10 min. The second dimension oven was set higher relative to the primary oven by 5 °C and the modulator higher by 40 °C.

The GC × GC-MS data can be displayed in various ways. It may reveal elution areas on the ^2t_R versus ^1t_R plane sorted by compound classes (Fig. 14.27), which, of course, requires proper selection of ions specific for each compound class of interest. Alternatively, the data can, for example, be displayed to show the elution pattern of hydrocarbons with r + d = 1–4, which is achieved by selecting ions of *m*/*z* 55, 67, 79, 81, 83, 91, 105, 119, 133 and zooming in to first-dimension retention times below 1600 s (Fig. 14.28). This demonstrates the enormous depth of analytical information contained in a single GC × GC-MS run. It also shows the need to examine the data in a selective manner, e.g., by looking at compound classes, levels of r + d, or whatever may be of interest.

14.5 Liquid Chromatography-Mass Spectrometry

Coupling of liquid chromatography (Sect. 14.1.10) to mass spectrometry has not only led to a wide variety of interfaces, it also fostered the development of new ionization methods (Sects. 7.8 and Chap. 12) [8–10, 99–102]. ESI, APCI, or APPI are suitable for LC-MS, their selection depending on sample properties like molecular mass and polarity (Sect. 12.7).

Today, LC-MS either refers to *high-pressure liquid chromatography* (HPLC) or *ultrahigh-pressure liquid chromatography* (UHPLC). For very low sample amounts, nanoLC, i.e., capillary LC, can directly be interfaced to nanoESI.

In the analytical practice, LC-MS plays a tremendous role that could be testified here by a large number of applications [8, 58, 103, 104]. However, other than proper adjustment of the interface to the liquid flow from the chromatograph the operation of LC-MS does not require dedicated techniques on the MS side. All scanning and ion monitoring techniques discussed so far in this chapter can equally well be employed for LC-MS analyses. Three examples shall highlight representative applications of LC-MS and LC-MS/MS.

Impurities in pharmaceutical preparations UV photodiode array (PDA) and ESI-TOF detection can be combined if the LC effluent is split or the PDA precedes the ESI interface. The detection methods complement each other in that their different sensitivities towards components of a mixture prevent substances from being overlooked. RICs help to differentiate a targeted compound – an unknown impurity in this case – from others and to identify eventually present isomers. Finally, accurate mass measurement helps in the identification of the unknown, the $[M+H]^+$ ion of which was assigned as $[C_{20}H_{21}N_{10}]^+$. The mass error in the order of 5 ppm was considered perfect for the oaTOF instruments of that time (Fig. 14.29) [64].

Illicit drugs in wastewater An LC-ESI-MS/MS method for the simultaneous determination of 16 illicit drugs and their metabolites in wastewater was developed [105]. Based on tandem mass spectra of the compounds, MRM experiments were set up to detect each drug by a characteristic transition (Fig. 14.30). Among others, cocaine, amphetamines, morphine, and 11-nor-9-carboxy-Δ9-tetrahydrocannabinol were found in substantial amounts in waste water treatment plants at Milan (Italy) and Lugano (Switzerland). Quantification was achieved by addition of several deuterated internal standards. Quantification ranges were found to be 0.2–1 ng l^{-1} for cocaine and 60–90 ng l^{-1} for 11-nor-9-carboxy-Δ9-THC. Illicit drugs were therefore considered ubiquitous contaminants, discharged into the environment together with pharmaceuticals presenting an environmental risk. Moreover, the

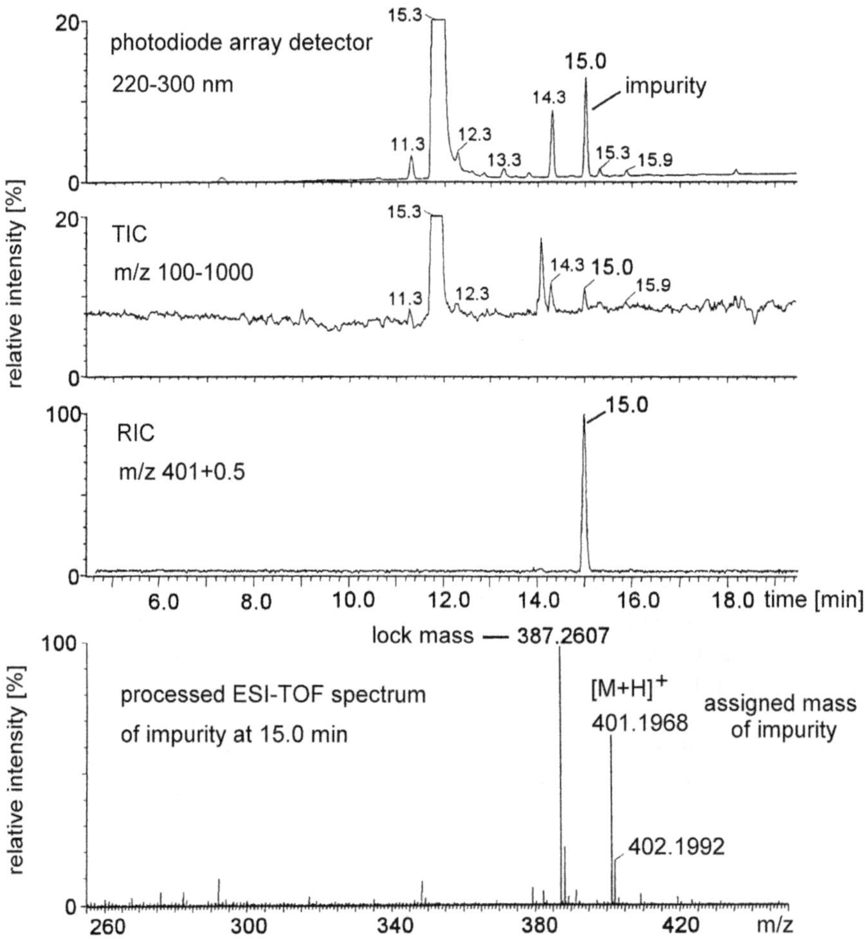

Fig. 14.29 Liquid chromatograms (*from top*) by photodiode array detection, TIC and RIC (*m/z* 401) from LC-ESI-MS, and accurate mass measurement (*bottom*) of the unknown impurity based on a one-point internal mass calibration (Adapted from Ref. [64] by permission. © Elsevier Science, 2001)

concentrations of illicit drugs in wastewater reflect their consumption by the local population.

Peptide identification from biological samples Colorectal cancer cells have been lysed and the protein fraction thereof has been subjected to 2D gel electrophoresis. A gastrointestinal-specific A33 antigen was expected in the molecular mass range of 40–45 kDa. The corresponding slice of the 2D gel was cut out and the proteins on it were subjected to tryptic digestion. Capillary column (150 × 0.2 mm C8 reversed phase) HPLC-ESI-MS of this total tryptic digest delivered a complex and mostly unresolved TIC (Fig. 14.31). A mass spectrum of a retention time span around

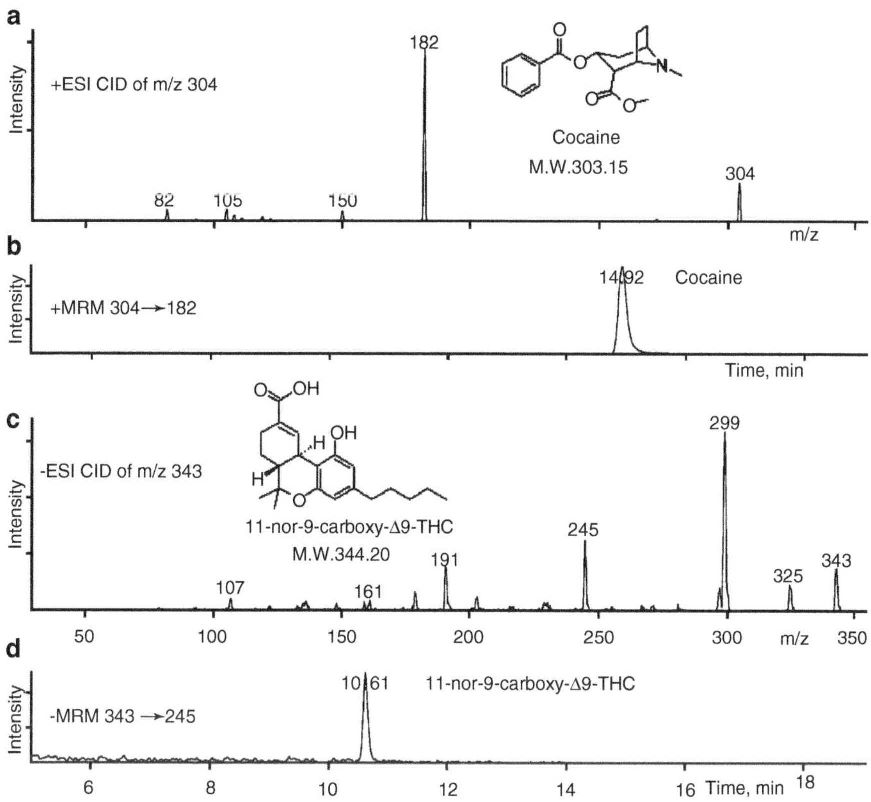

Fig. 14.30 Two examples from the analysis of illicit drugs in waste water by LC-MS/MS and MRM. (**a**) Positive-ion ESI-CID spectrum of the $[M+H]^+$ ion of cocaine and (**b**) the MRM trace derived thereof. (**c**) Negative-ion ESI-CID spectrum of the $[M+H]^-$ ion of 11-nor-9-carboxy-Δ9-THC and (**d**) the corresponding MRM trace (Adapted from Ref. [105] with permission. © American Chemical Society, 2006)

25.20 min still showed numerous peaks of protonated peptides requiring identification by mass spectrometric sequencing. One of these, an $[M+2H]^{2+}$ ion at *m/z* 1198.4, was identified as the A33 antigen peptide YNILNQEQPLAQPASGQPVSLK using SEQUEST database search.

14.6 Ion Mobility Spectrometry-Mass Spectrometry

Ion mobility spectrometry (IMS) presents an effective means of separating gaseous ions in an electric field according to their collision cross sections. From the perspective of its working principle, IMS could be regarded as gas-phase electrophoresis. As IMS is a separation method normally coupled to MS for ion detection, IMS-MS might completely be dealt with in line with GC-MS and LC-MS.

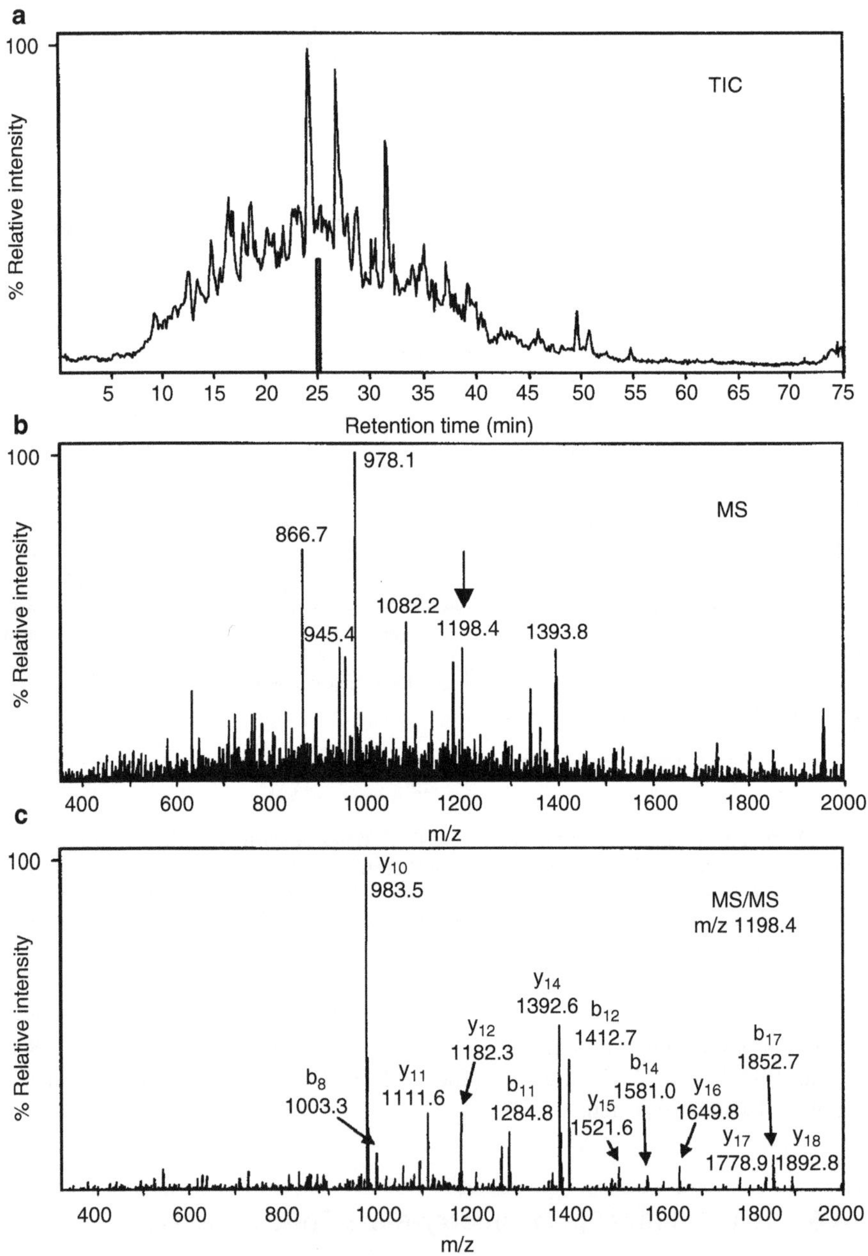

Fig. 14.31 Capillary column HPLC-ESI-MS/MS of a tryptic digest. (**a**) An unresolved TIC trace, (**b**) mass spectrum around retention time of 25.20 min, and **c**) CID spectrum of an $[M+2H]^{2+}$ ion at *m/z* 1198.4, identified as the A33 antigen peptide (Adapted from Ref. [106] with permission of publisher and author. © Wiley-VCH, Weinheim, 2000)

However, IMS is different from GC and LC in that its instrumental implementation is strongly dependent on the features of the mass analyzer attached. Accordingly, we have already discussed IMS-MS systems in the context of instrumentation (Sect. 4.10) [107, 108].

During the last decade or so, IMS-MS instrumentation has changed from custom-built to commercially available instruments. The development started with the Waters Synapt series, now available as Synapt G2-Si, In between, Agilent (Ion Mobility Q-TOF) and most recently Bruker (timsTOF) have also presented instruments in this segment and Waters also offer a second model, the Vion IMS-Q-TOF. While the Synapt G2-Si offers mass-selection in a quadrupole prior to IMS, the latter three instruments essentially have IMS-Q-TOF geometries. The Bruker timsTOF differs from the Waters Vion IMS-Q-TOF and Agilent Ion Mobility Q-TOF in that it employs the more recent technique of *trapped ion mobility spectrometry* (TIMS) [109]. This approach not only offers IMS in a compact and efficient design but also circumvents the need for an additional gas supply by employing the residual gas streaming down a modified ion funnel system for ion mobility separation. TIMS can also be adapted to FT-ICR analyzers [110].

TIMS or TIMS?
Unfortunately, the acronym TIMS is not anymore unequivocal. While TIMS once exclusively referred to *thermal ionization mass spectrometry* (Sect. 15.2), it now also serves to represent *trapped ion mobility spectrometry*. It seems as if the two communities were worlds apart.

To complement the purely instrumental approach to IMS-MS in Sect. 4.10, this section presents three selected applications. IMS-MS can be employed to:

- distinguish compound classes,
- differentiate isomers,
- separate different charge states of one molecular species,
- tell apart different gas phase conformations of otherwise identical ions [107, 111],
- separate chiral compounds when a chiral modifier is added to the inert drift gas [112, 113].

Differentiation of isomers by TIMS-MS Trapped ion mobility spectrometry-mass spectrometry (TIMS-MS) was used for the differentiation between $[M–H]^-$ ions of five isomeric hydroxylated tetrabrominated biphenyl ethers (OH-BDE) generated by negative-ion ESI [114]. TIMS provided baseline separated signals when selected binary and ternary mixtures of these compounds were injected, demonstrating ion mobility resolving power in the order of 400 (Fig. 14.32). The collision cross sections (CCS) of the isomers varied from 194.5 Å^2 to 197.2 Å^2.

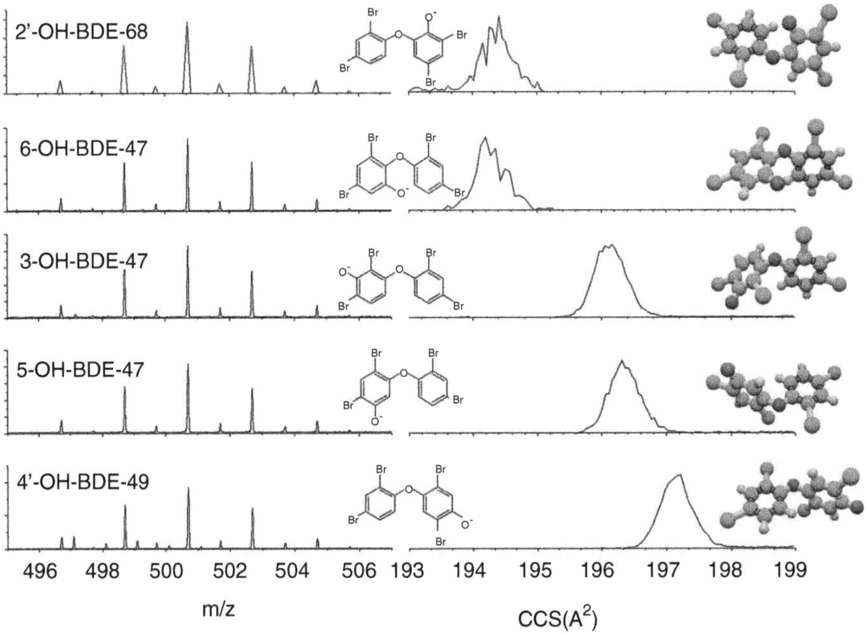

Fig. 14.32 Comparison of $[M{-}H]^-$ ions of five isomeric hydroxylated tetrabromobiphenyl ethers (OH-BDEs) by their mass spectra (*left column*), trapped ion mobility spectra (*center*), and correlation of IMS data with calculated structures (*right*) (Reproduced from Ref. [114] with permission. © Springer, 2016)

Biomolecule classification by IMS-MS Singly charged ions of biologically relevant molecular classes (96 oligonucleotides, 192 carbohydrates, 610 peptides, and 53 lipids) were generated by MALDI and subjected to IMS. Then a plot of this data, i.e., of their collision cross sections vs. *m/z* allowed for the calculation of distinct curves marking average collision cross sections vs. *m/z* distinct for each compound class. Figure 14.33 shows a plot of the MALDI-IMS-MS conformation space as obtained for a mixture of model species (roughly a dozen species for each class in the range up to 1500 u) [111]. Dashed lines correspond to regression curves for each molecular class in conformation space. There was some fragmentation of the parent ions causing the signals in the vicinity of the asterisk in the upper left corner of the diagram.

Separation of chiral compounds by IMS-MS Amino acids and other small chiral molecules can be separated by IMS-MS if a chiral modifier is admixed to the inert nitrogen drift gas (Fig. 14.34) [112]. To achieve separation of L- and D-tryptophan, (*S*)-(+)-2-butanol at a concentration as low as 10 ppm has been used as chiral modifier. The differences in drift times of the amino acid enantiomers are large enough to deliver two peaks if the mixture is subjected to chiral IMS.

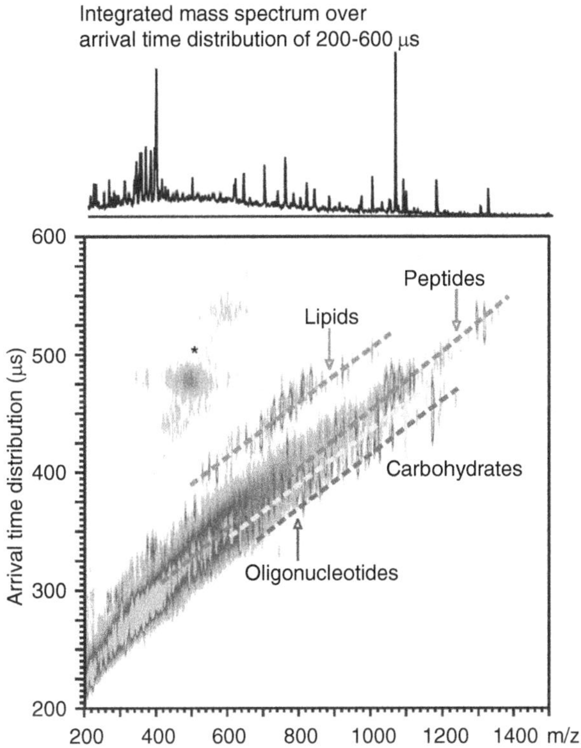

Fig. 14.33 Plot of MALDI-IMS-MS conformation space as obtained for a mixture of biomolecular model species. *Dashed lines* are for visualization purposes of where each molecular class occurs in conformation space. Signals in the vicinity of the *asterisk* arise from limited post-IM fragmentation of the parent ion species (Reproduced from Ref. [111] by permission. © Springer, 2009)

14.7 Tandem MS as a Complement to LC-MS

The principles of tandem mass spectrometry have been discussed in Chap. 9 and many different uses of tandem MS have been shown throughout this book (Table 14.3). More examples are following in this chapter showing how tandem MS offers increased selectivity [115], simplified clean-up procedures, or faster analysis as a direct result of the fourth dimension added to the analytical measurement.

Improved selectivity by tandem MS SIM is not sufficient for the LC-MS detection of 100 pg dextrometorphan (DEX) spiked into 1 ml of human plasma. The corresponding signal of the $[M+H]^+$ ion in the SIM trace at *m/z* 272 is barely detectable, whereas the SRM chromatogram obtained from the reaction $[M+H]^+ \rightarrow [M-C_8H_{15}N]^+$ shows a clean background and a signal-to-noise enhancement of more than 50-fold (Fig. 14.35) [64].

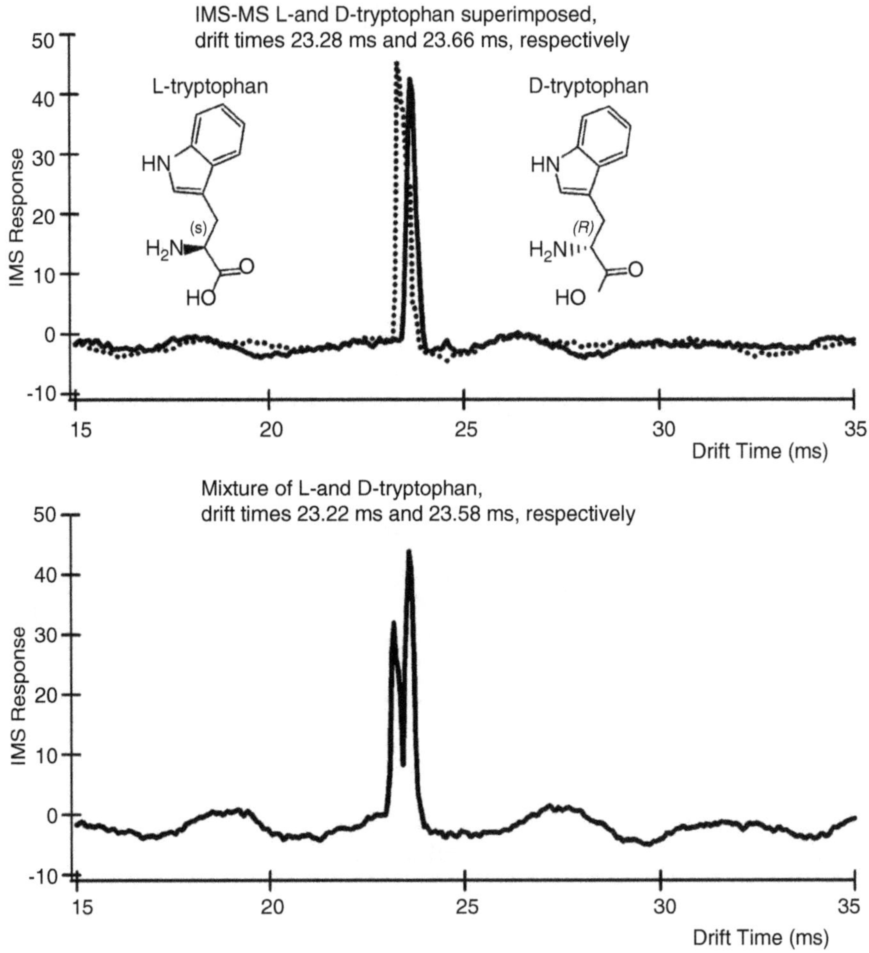

Fig. 14.34 Chiral separation of L- and D-tryptophan by IMS-MS using (*S*)-(+)-2-butanol as chiral modifier of the carrier gas (Adapted from Ref. [112] by permission. © American Chemical Society, 2006)

Suitable instruments

Triple quadrupole instruments are considered as the "gold standard" for quantification, in particular by SRM and even more so MRM. Also relevant are the high linear dynamic range, the ease of setting up SRM and MRM experiments, and the speed of switching between channels when monitoring multiple reactions. More recent QqTOF, QqLIT, and QqOrbitrap hybrids provide basically similar capabilities.

Table 14.3 Tandem MS methods and spectra referred to throughout the book

Section	Aspect of tandem MS
2.9.3	MIKES of amine molecular ions in the context of H/D isotope effects
9.3.2	CID spectrum of toluene molecular ion on a magnetic sector instrument
9.4	SID and CID of noncovalent protein complexes
9.5.1	MALDI-PSD spectrum of a peptide
9.6.5	Tandem MS with magnetic sector instruments; example: $B^2E = constant$ linked scan for caffeine quantitation using [D_3]caffeine internal standard
9.6.6	CID-FAB-MS/MS with magnetic sector instrument for peptide sequencing
9.8	Tandem MS with the quadrupole ion trap; examples: peptide sequencing by ESI-MS and LC-MS^4 to identify cyclic peptides
9.9.1	MS^4 on a QqLIT instrument for structure elucidation of a drug
9.10.1	Peptide sequencing by ESI-CID-MS/MS on LIT-Orbitrap instrument
9.10.2	Parallelized tandem MS in proteomics using a dual-LIT-Orbitrap instrument
9.11.1	Sequencing of an oligosaccharide by MALDI-SORI-FT-ICR
9.14.1	ESI-IRMPD-MS/MS of gangliosides on a FT-ICR instrument
9.14.4	ECD of doubly charged peptide ions on a FT-ICR instrument
9.15	ETD of triply protonated peptide ions on a LIT instruments
9.17	Ion–molecule reactions: in catalysis research, to elucidate peptide fragmentation, and to study short-lived species in the gas phase
11.6.3	Peptide sequencing; mechanisms and applications of MALDI-MS/MS
11.6.4	Structure elucidation of carbohydrates by PSD-MALDI-MS
11.6.7	Peptide sequencing by DIOS-TOF-MS/MS
12.3	Peptide sequencing by nanoESI-MS/MS
12.6.4	Oligonucleotide sequencing by ESI-IRMPD-FT-ICR-MS
12.6.5	Structure elucidation of a nonasaccharide by nanoESI-CID-MS/MSon a Q-TOF hybrid instrument
13.2.4	DESI-MS/MS of aspirin and of alkaloids from *Atropa belladonna* seeds

In tandem MS each stage of mass analysis provides an added step of selectivity or structural information to the analysis. Therefore, one tandem MS stage is to a certain degree equivalent to a chromatographic separation, provided the separation of isomers is not required. While chromatography separates components by their retention time, tandem MS isolates them by m/z. The next example illustrates how far MS/MS alone may go. The analysis presented in example III in Sect. 14.4, however, would have been impossible without using LC prior to MS/MS.

Tandem MS as a substitute for LC Akt is a key serine/threonine kinase controlling cellular processes such as cell survival, differentiation, proliferation, and metabolism. Three isoforms (Akt1, Akt2, and Akt3) are known in mammals. The nanoESI mass spectrum of all peptides obtained upon digestion of Akt3 with pepsin (peptic peptides) showed a large number of multiply charged ions (Fig. 14.36) [116]. The peptides were then characterized by tandem MS. The $[M+3H]^{3+}$ ions at m/z 797, for example, corresponded to a peptide of a neutral mass of 2388 u. As low-abundant peptides were difficult to identify by nanoESI-MS/MS

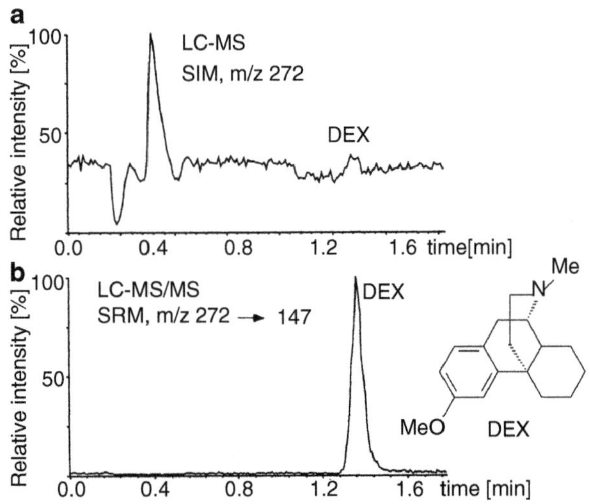

Fig. 14.35 The effect of SRM as compared to SIM in the detection of dextrometorphan. (**a**) LC-SIM and (**b**) LC-SRM (Reproduced from Ref. [64] by permission. © Elsevier Science, 2001)

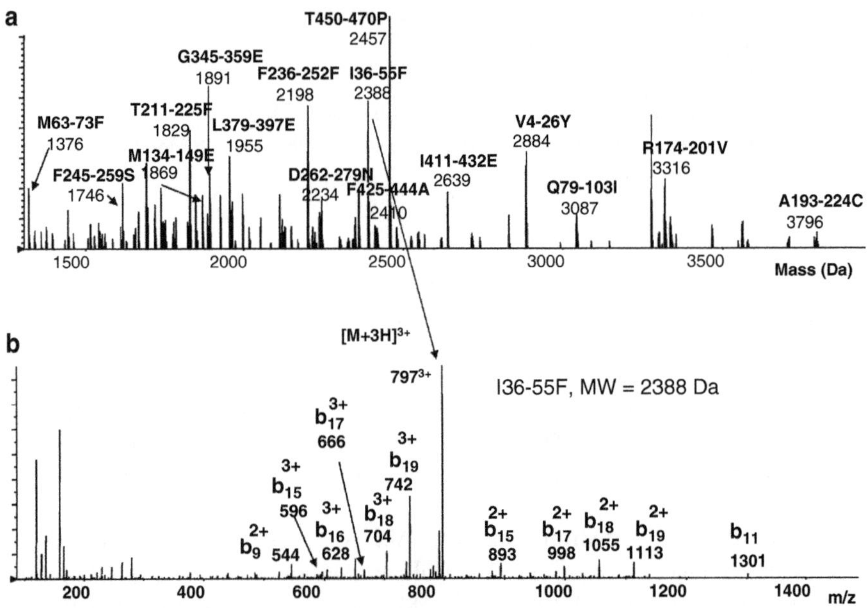

Fig. 14.36 Analysis of Akt by nanoESI-MS/MS. (**a**) Charge deconvoluted nanoESI spectrum of the complete peptic digest. (**b**) Tandem mass spectrum of the $[M+3H]^{3+}$ peptic peptide ion (I36-55F) at *m/z* 797 corresponding to a neutral peptide of 2388 u (Reproduced from Ref. [116] with permission. © John Wiley & Sons Ltd, 2009.)

alone, nanoLC/ESI-MS/MS was used in addition. Combining these approaches, a total of 24 peptide peaks were identified in both inactive and active Akt covering 70% of the amino acid sequence of Akt.

14.8 Ultrahigh-Resolution Mass Spectrometry

High and, in particular, ultrahigh resolution (Sect. 3.7) in combination with a soft ionization method such as ESI, APCI, MALDI, or FD present another way to achieve the separation of the molecular species contained in a mixture. Given a sufficient level of resolution, isobaric ions are displayed separately in the range of their common nominal mass value (Sects. 3.3 and 3.4).

The potential of ultrahigh-resolution mass spectrometry for the analysis of complex chemical mixtures is particularly illustrated by FT-ICR-MS, which currently is the definite standard. Ultrahigh resolution was applied to separate several thousand components in crude oil [117, 118], fuels [119, 120], explosion residues [121], brown coal [96], or aroma of Scotch Whisky [122]. Also, the attempts to analyze dissolved organic matter (DOM) and similar complex systems present another prominent field of application requiring the ultimate performance of FT-ICR instruments equipped with magnets of up to 15 T [123, 124].

South American crude oil In a sample of South American crude oil positive-ion ESI selectively delivers $[M+H]^+$ ions of the basic compounds, i.e., only a small fraction of the entire chemical composition. Nevertheless, the positive-ion ESI-FT-ICR mass spectrum exhibits more than 11,100 resolved peaks, of which >75% may be assigned to a unique elemental composition ($C_cH_hO_oN_nS_s$). Such a separation in mass is possible because the average mass resolution in the *m/z* 225–1000 broadband spectrum is approximately 350,000 (Fig. 14.37). This demonstrates the current upper limit for the number of chemically distinct components resolved and identified in a single step [118].

Molecular analysis of oceanic DOM *Dissolved organic matter* (DOM) substantially contributes to biomass on Earth and presents a highly complex system of mostly polar organic compounds. It requires a multi-step approach to acquire an insight into the molecular structures of DOM [124]. As a first step, reversed-phase chromatography provides bulk molecular information, but is not capable of separating individual components (Fig. 14.38). Second, the nominal mass distribution may be determined using soft ionization methods and low-resolution MS. Next, ultrahigh-resolution FT-ICR-MS separates nominally isobaric molecules, often more than a dozen per nominal mass, and delivers molecular formulas. As composition alone does still not permit the elucidation of structures, nuclear magnetic resonance (NMR) spectroscopy can be employed to reveal structural features that may, in turn, be correlated to molecular formulas.

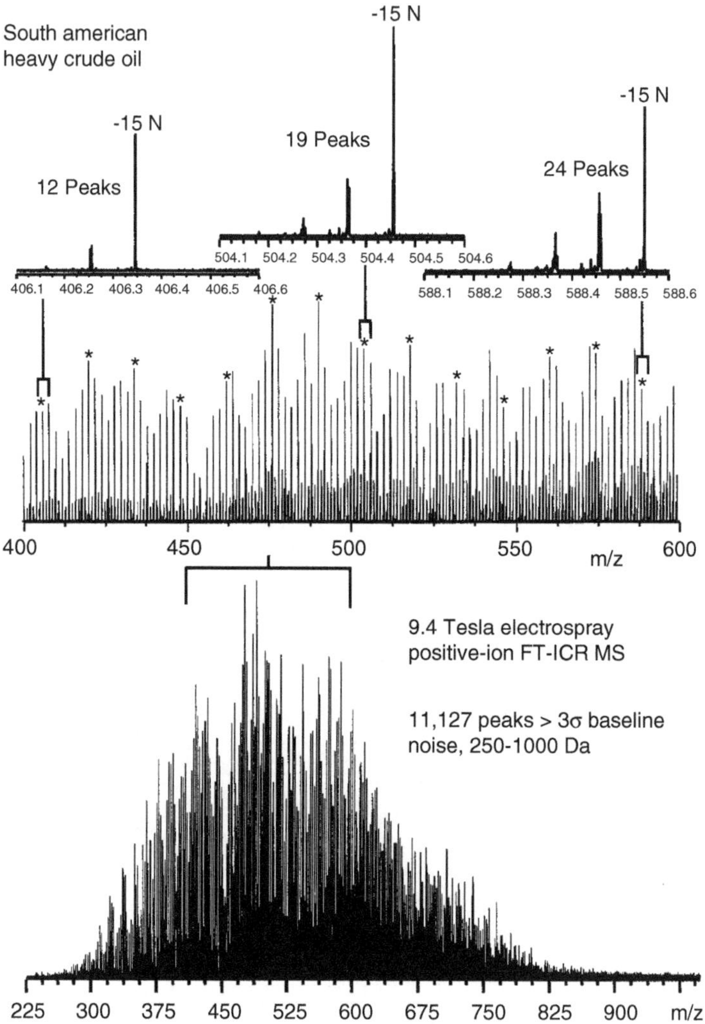

Fig. 14.37 Positive-ion ESI-FT-ICR spectrum of crude oil. The mass scale is successively expanded from the broadband spectrum to a more detailed one at three nominal mass values (Adapted from Ref. [118] by permission. © American Chemical Society, 2002.)

14.9 Summary of Hyphenated Techniques

Separation Techniques

There are numerous separation techniques available that can deal with any range of molecular mass of an analyte or its polarity, provided the analytes can either be evaporated or dissolved without decomposition. The majority of separation

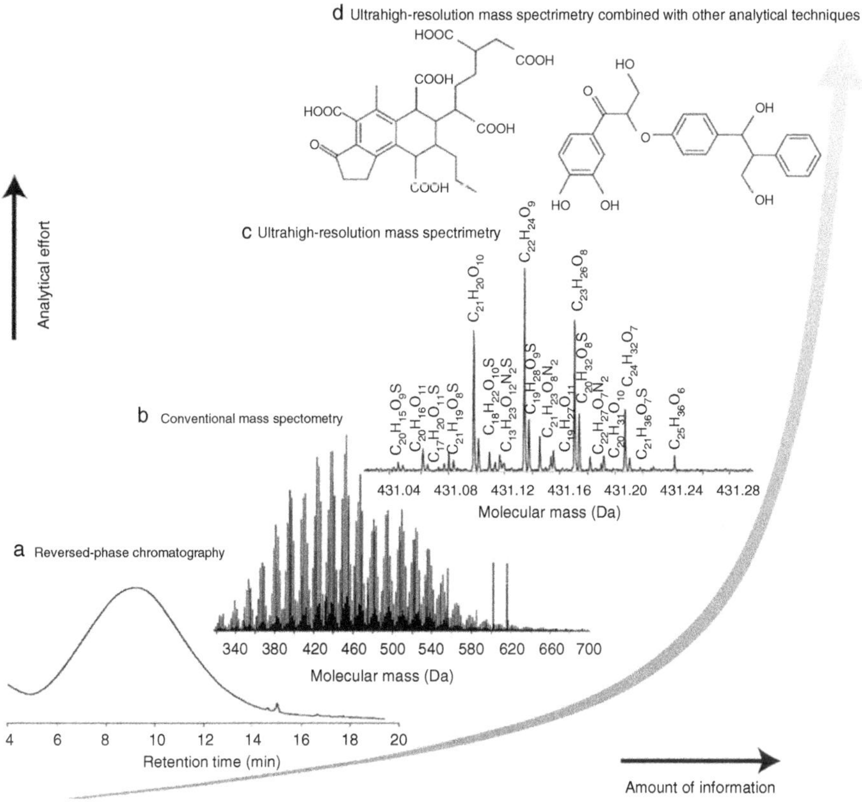

Fig. 14.38 Stepwise increasing depth of analytical information versus analytical effort in the analysis of DOM (Adapted from Ref. [124] with permission. © Springer Nature, 2009)

techniques are of chromatographic nature. A chromatographic system's ability to separate components of a mixture is expressed in terms of the height equivalent to a theoretical plate (HETP) or the number of theoretical plates. The factors influencing HETP are described by the van Deemter equation. In practice, the peak capacity of a system is more intuitive in describing its ability to resolve individual components of a mixture.

Dimensionality of an Analysis

Mass spectrometry provides a two-dimensional analysis, i.e., intensity versus *m/z*, as does chromatography, i.e., intensity versus retention time. Combining both techniques leads to three-dimensional analysis, i.e., intensity versus *m/z* versus retention time. Both tandem MS and comprehensive gas chromatography (GC × GC) add another dimension of analytical information. Thus, four-dimensional analysis can either be achieved by LC-MS/MS, GC-MS/MS, or GC × GC-MS.

Alternatives to Chromatography–Mass Spectrometry Coupling

Ion mobility spectrometry (IMS) presents a technique of separating isolated gas phase ions and can replace chromatographic separation in front of the mass spectrometer, at least to some extent. Alternatively, components of mixtures can be selected as precursor ions and analyzed by tandem MS. The tandem MS approach to mixture analysis is particularly promising in combination with soft ionization methods. In contrast to separation techniques, tandem MS cannot distinguish between isomeric precursor ions. Finally, ultrahigh-resolution MS is useful in analyzing complex mixture of related compounds.

The Method of Choice

Finding the method of choice to deliver the utmost depth of analytical information can be a tedious task as it is not easy to predict which instrumental approach will deliver the best result. Often, the techniques at hand in the particular laboratory have to be used anyway, even though others may exist. Also, different analytical approaches may be used interchangeably and experience with proven methods may counterbalance the potential of techniques used elsewhere.

References

1. Williams JD, Burinsky DJ (2001) Mass Spectrometric Analysis of Complex Mixtures Then and Now: the Impact of Linking Liquid Chromatography and Mass Spectrometry. Int J Mass Spectrom 212:111–133. doi:10.1016/S1387-3806(01)00460-2
2. McLafferty FW (2001) Tandem Mass Spectrometric Analysis of Complex Biological Mixtures. Int J Mass Spectrom 212:81–87. doi:10.1016/S1387-3806(01)00474-2
3. Kondrat RW (2001) Mixture Analysis by Mass Spectrometry: Now's the Time. Int J Mass Spectrom 212:89–95. doi:10.1016/S1387-3806(01)00516-4
4. Gohlke RS, McLafferty FW (1993) Early Gas Chromatography/Mass Spectrometry. J Am Soc Mass Spectrom 4:367–371. doi:10.1016/1044-0305(93)85001-E
5. Budde WL (2001) Analytical Mass Spectrometry. ACS/Oxford University Press, Washington, DC/Oxford
6. Sparkman OD, Penton ZE, Kitson FG (2011) Gas Chromatography and Mass Spectrometry: A Practical Guide. Academic Press, Oxford
7. Hübschmann HJ (2015) Handbook of GC-MS – Fundamentals and Applications. Wiley-VCH, Weinheim
8. Ardrey RE (2003) Liquid Chromatography-Mass Spectrometry – An Introduction. Wiley, Chichester
9. Vestal ML (1984) High-Performance Liquid Chromatography-Mass Spectrometry. Science 226:275–281. doi:10.1126/science.6385251
10. Abian J (1999) The Coupling of Gas and Liquid Chromatography with Mass Spectrometry. J Mass Spectrom 34:157–168. doi:10.1002/(SICI)1096-9888(199903)34:3<157::AID-JMS804>3.0.CO;2-4
11. Smith RD, Barinaga CJ, Udseth HR (1988) Improved Electrospray Ionization Interface for Capillary Zone Electrophoresis-Mass Spectrometry. Anal Chem 60:1948–1952. doi:10.1021/ac00169a022

12. Siethoff C, Nigge W, Linscheid M (1998) Characterization of a Capillary Zone Electrophoresis/Electrospray-Mass Spectrometry Interface. Anal Chem 70:1357–1361. doi:10.1021/ac970950b
13. Schrader W, Linscheid M (1997) Styrene Oxide DNA Adducts: In Vitro Reaction and Sensitive Detection of Modified Oligonucleotides Using Capillary Zone Electrophoresis Interfaced to Electrospray Mass Spectrometry. Arch Toxicol 71:588–595. doi:10.1007/s002040050431
14. Hsieh F, Baronas E, Muir C, Martin SA (1999) A Novel Nanospray Capillary Zone Electrophoresis/Mass Spectrometry Interface. Rapid Commun Mass Spectrom 13:67–72. doi:10.1002/(SICI)1097-0231(19990115)13:1<67::AID-RCM453>3.0.CO;2-F
15. Tanaka Y, Kishimoto Y, Otsuga K, Terabe S (1998) Strategy for Selecting Separation Solutions in Capillary Electrophoresis-Mass Spectrometry. J Chromatogr A 817:49–57. doi:10.1016/S0021-9673(98)00373-2
16. Smith RD, Felix WD, Fjeldsted JC, Lee ML (1982) Capillary Column Supercritical Fluid Chromatography Mass Spectrometry. Anal Chem 54:1883–1885. doi:10.1021/ac00248a055
17. Combs MT, Ashraf-Khorassani M, Taylor LT (1998) Packed Column Supercritical Fluid Chromatography-Mass Spectroscopy: A Review. J Chromatogr A 785:85–100. doi:10.1016/S0021-9673(97)00755-3
18. Sakodynskii KI (1972) Life and Scientific Works of Michael Tswett. J Chromatogr A 73:303–360. doi:10.1016/S0021-9673(01)91213-0
19. Ahuja S (2003) Chromatography and Separation Science. Academic Press, San Diego
20. Fanali S, Haddad PR, Poole CF, Schoenmakers P, Lloyd D (eds) (2013) Liquid Chromatography: Fundamentals and Instrumentation. Elsevier, Amsterdam
21. Fanali S, Haddad PR, Poole CF, Schoenmakers P, Lloyd D (eds) (2013) Liquid Chromatography: Applications. Elsevier, Amsterdam
22. Lundanes E, Reubsaet L, Greibrokk T (2013) Chromatography: Basic Principles, Sample Preparations and Related Methods. Wiley-VCH, Weinheim
23. van Deemter JJ, Zuiderweg FJ, Klinkenberg A (1956) Longitudinal Diffusion and Resistance to Mass Transfer as Causes of Nonideality in Chromatography. Chem Engin Sci 5:271–289. doi:10.1016/0009-2509(56)80003-1
24. Adahchour M, Beens J, Vreuls RJJ, Brinkman UAT (2006) Recent Developments in Comprehensive Two Dimensional Gas Chromatography (GC x GC) Introduction and Instrumental Set-Up. Trends Anal Chem 25:438–454. doi:10.1016/j.trac.2006.03.002
25. Adahchour M, Beens J, Vreuls RJJ, Brinkman UAT (2006) Recent Developments in Comprehensive Two-Dimensional Gas Chromatography (GC x GC). II. Modulation and Detection. Trends Anal Chem 25:540–553. doi:10.1016/j.trac.2006.04.004
26. Adahchour M, Beens J, Vreuls RJJ, Brinkman UAT (2006) Recent Developments in Comprehensive Two-Dimensional Gas Chromatography (GC x GC). III. Applications for Petrochemicals and Organohalogens. Trends Anal Chem 25:726–741. doi:10.1016/j.trac.2006.03.005
27. Adahchour M, Beens J, Vreuls RJJ, Brinkman UAT (2006) Recent Developments in Comprehensive Two-Dimensional Gas Chromatography (GC x GC). Trends Anal Chem 25:821–840. doi:10.1016/j.trac.2006.03.003
28. Adahchour M, Beens J, Brinkman UAT (2008) Recent Developments in the Application of Comprehensive Two-Dimensional Gas Chromatography. J Chromatogr A 1186:67–108. doi:10.1016/j.chroma.2008.01.002
29. Guillarme D, Ruta J, Rudaz S, Veuthey JL (2010) New Trends in Fast and High-Resolution Liquid Chromatography: A Critical Comparison of Existing Approaches. Anal Bioanal Chem 397:1069–1082. doi:10.1007/s00216-009-3305-8
30. Fekete S, Schappler J, Veuthey JL, Guillarme D (2014) Current and Future Trends in UHPLC. Trends Anal Chem 63:2–13. doi:10.1016/j.trac.2014.08.007

31. Price P (1991) Standard Definitions of Terms Relating to Mass Spectrometry. A Report from the Committee on Measurements and Standards of the Amercian Society for Mass Spectrometry. J Am Soc Mass Spectrom 2:336–348. doi:10.1016/1044-0305(91)80025-3
32. Todd JFJ (1995) Recommendations for Nomenclature and Symbolism for Mass Spectroscopy Including an Appendix of Terms Used in Vacuum Technology. Int J Mass Spectrom Ion Proc 142:211–240. doi:10.1016/0168-1176(95)93811-F
33. Murray KK, Boyd RK, Eberlin MN, Langley GJ, Li L, Naito Y (2013) Definitions of Terms Relating to Mass Spectrometry (IUPAC Recommendations 2013). Pure Appl Chem 85:1515–1609. doi: 10.1351/PAC-REC-06-04-06
34. Hites RA, Biemann K (1967) A Computer-Compatible Digital Data Acquisition System for Fast-Scanning, Single-Focusing Mass Spectrometers. Anal Chem 39:965–970. doi:10.1021/ac60252a043
35. Hites RA, Biemann K (1968) Mass Spectrometer-Computer System Particularly Suited for Gas Chromatography of Complex Mixtures. Anal Chem 40:1217–1221. doi:10.1021/ac60264a013
36. Hites RA, Biemann K (1970) Computer Evaluation of Continuously Scanned Mass Spectra of Gas Chromatographic Effluents. Anal Chem 42:855–860. doi:10.1021/ac60290a009
37. Bertholf RL (2000) Gas chromatography and mass spectrometry in clinical chemistry. In: Meyers RA (ed) Encyclopedia of Analytical Chemistry. Wiley, Chichester
38. Spies-Martin D, Sommerburg O, Langhans C-D, Leichsenring M (2002) Measurement of 4-Hydroxynonenal in Small Volume Blood Plasma Samples: Modification of a Gas Chromatographic-Mass Spectrometric Method for Clinical Settings. J Chromatogr B 774:231–239. doi:10.1016/S1570-0232(02)00242-8
39. Henneberg D (1961) Combination of Gas Chromatography and Mass Spectrometry for the Analysis of Organic Mixtures. Z Anal Chem 183:12–23. doi:10.1007/BF00478266
40. Sweeley CC, Elliot WH, Fries I, Ryhage R (1966) Mass Spectrometric Determination of Unresolved Components in Gas Chromatographic Effluents. Anal Chem 38:1549–1553. doi:10.1021/ac60243a023
41. Crosby NT, Foreman JK, Palframan JF, Sawyer R (1972) Estimation of Steam-Volatile *N*-Nitrosamines in Foods at the 136 mg/kg Level. Nature 238:342–343. doi:10.1038/238342a0
42. Brooks CJW, Middleditch BS (1972) Uses of Chloromethyldimethylsilyl Ethers As Derivatives for Combined Gas Chromatography-Mass Spectrometry of Steroids. Anal Lett 5:611–618. doi:10.1080/00032717208064338
43. Young ND, Holland JF, Gerber JN, Sweeley CC (1975) Selected Ion Monitoring for Multicomponent Analyses by Computer Control of Accelerating Voltage and Magnetic Field. Anal Chem 47:2373–2376. doi:10.1021/ac60364a032
44. Tanchotikul U, Hsieh TCY (1991) An Improved Method for Quantification of 2-Acetyl-1-pyrroline, a "Popcorn"-Like Aroma, in Aromatic Rice by High-Resolution Gas Chromatography/Mass Spectrometry/Selected Ion Monitoring. J Agric Food Chem 39:944–947. doi:10.1021/jf00005a029
45. Middleditch BS, Desiderio DM (1973) Comparison of Selective Ion Monitoring and Repetitive Scanning During Gas Chromatography-Mass Spectrometry. Anal Chem 45:806–808. doi:10.1021/ac60326a014
46. Millington DS, Buoy ME, Brooks G, Harper ME, Griffiths K (1975) Thin-Layer Chromatography and High Resolution Selected Ion Monitoring for the Analysis of C_{19} Steroids in Human Hyperplastic Prostate Tissue. Biomed Mass Spectrom 2:219–224. doi:10.1002/bms.1200020411
47. Thorne GC, Gaskell SJ, Payne PA (1984) Approaches to the Improvement of Quantitative Precision in Selected Ion Monitoring: High Resolution Applications. Biomed Mass Spectrom 11:415–420. doi:10.1002/bms.1200110810
48. Tong HY, Monson SJ, Gross ML, Huang LQ (1991) Monobromopolychlorodibenzo-*p*-dioxins and Dibenzofurans in Municipal Waste Incinerator Fly Ash. Anal Chem 63:2697–2705. doi:10.1021/ac00023a007

49. Shibata A, Yoshio H, Hayashi T, Otsuki N (1992) Determination of Phenylpyruvic Acid in Human Urine and Plasma by Gas Chromatography/Negative Ion Chemical Ionization Mass Spectrometry. Shitsuryo Bunseki 40:165–171. doi:10.5702/massspec.40.165
50. Tondeur Y, Albro PW, Hass JR, Harvan DJ, Schroeder JL (1984) Matrix Effect in Determination of 2,3,7,8-Tetrachlorodibenzodioxin by Mass Spectrometry. Anal Chem 56:1344–1347. doi:10.1021/ac00272a032
51. Cajka T, Hajslova J (2004) Gas Chromatography-High-Resolution Time-of-Flight Mass Spectrometry in Pesticide Residue Analysis: Advantages and Limitations. J Chromatogr A 1058:251–261. doi:10.1016/S0021-9673(04)01303-2
52. Hernandez F, Portoles T, Pitarch E, Lopez FJ (2007) Target and Nontarget Screening of Organic Micropollutants in Water by Solid-Phase Microextraction Combined with Gas Chromatography/High-Resolution Time-of-Flight Mass Spectrometry. Anal Chem 79:9494–9504. doi:10.1021/ac0715672
53. Portoles T, Pitarch E, Lopez FJ, Sancho JV, Hernandez F (2007) Methodical Approach for the Use of GC-TOF MS for Screening and Confirmation of Organic Pollutants in Environmental Water. J Mass Spectrom 42:1175–1185. doi:10.1002/jms.1248
54. Peters RJB, Stolker AAM, Mol JGJ, Lommen A, Lyris E, Angelis Y, Vonaparti A, Stamou M, Georgakopoulos C, Nielen MWF (2010) Screening in Veterinary Drug Analysis and Sports Doping Control Based on Full-Scan, Accurate-Mass Spectrometry. Trends Anal Chem 29:1250–1268. doi:10.1016/j.trac.2010.07.012
55. Hernandez F, Portoles T, Pitarch E, Lopez FJ (2011) Gas Chromatography Coupled to High-Resolution Time-of-Flight Mass Spectrometry to Analyze Trace-Level Organic Compounds in the Environment, Food Safety and Toxicology. Trends Anal Chem 30:388–400. doi:10.1016/j.trac.2010.11.007
56. Kang W, Zhang F, Su Y, Guo Y (2013) Application of Gas Chromatography-Quadrupole-Time-of-Flight-Mass Spectrometry for Post-Target Analysis of Volatile Compounds in *Fructus Amomi*. Eur J Mass Spectrom 19:103–110. doi:10.1255/ejms.1218
57. Kato Y, Okada S, Atobe K, Endo T, Haraguchi K (2012) Selective Determination of Mono- and Dihydroxylated Analogs of Polybrominated Diphenyl Ethers in Marine Sponges by Liquid-Chromatography Tandem Mass Spectrometry. Anal Bioanal Chem 404:197–206. doi:10.1007/s00216-012-6132-2
58. Boyd RK, Basic C, Bethem RA (2008) Trace Quantitative Analysis by Mass Spectrometry. John Wiley & Sons, Chichester
59. Busch KL (2008) Mass Spectrometry Forum: Quantitative Mass Spectrometry Part IV: Deviations from Linearity. Spectroscopy 23:18–24
60. Busch KL (2008) Mass Spectrometry Forum: Quantitative Mass Spectrometry. Part III: An Overview of Regression Analysis. Spectroscopy 23:16–20
61. Busch KL (2007) Quantitative Mass Spectrometry: Part II. Spectroscopy 22:14–19
62. Busch KL (2007) Quantitative Mass Spectrometry: Part I. Spectroscopy 22:13–19
63. Heumann KG (1986) Isotope Dilution Mass Spectrometry of Inorganic and Organic Substances. Fresenius Z Anal Chem 325:661–666. doi:10.1007/BF00470971
64. Hoke SHII, Morand KL, Greis KD, Baker TR, Harbol KL, Dobson RLM (2001) Transformations in Pharmaceutical Research and Development, Driven by Innovations in Multidimensional Mass Spectrometry-Based Technologies. Int J Mass Spectrom 212:135–196. doi:10.1016/S1387-3806(01)00499-7
65. Calder AG, Garden KE, Anderson SE, Lobley GE (1999) Quantitation of Blood and Plasma Amino Acids Using Isotope Dilution Electron Impact Gas Chromatography/Mass Spectrometry with U-^{13}C Amino Acids as Internal Standards. Rapid Commun Mass Spectrom 13:2080–2083. doi:10.1002/(SICI)1097-0231(19991115)13:21<2080::AID-RCM755>3.0.CO;2-O
66. Lindeman LP, Annis JL (1960) A Conventional Mass Spectrometer as a Detector for Gas Chromatography. Anal Chem 32:1742–1749. doi:10.1021/ac50153a011

67. Gohlke RS (1962) Time-of-Flight Mass Spectrometry: Application to Capillary-Column Gas Chromatography. Anal Chem 34:1332–1333. doi:10.1021/ac60190a002
68. McFadden WH, Teranishi R, Black DR, Day JC (1963) Use of Capillary Gas Chromatography with a Time-of-Flight Mass Spectrometer. J Food Sci 28:316–319. doi:10.1111/j.1365-2621.1963.tb00204.x
69. Dandeneau RD, Zerenner EH (1979) An Investigation of Glasses for Capillary Chromatography. J High Res Chromatogr 2:351–356. doi:10.1002/jhrc.1240020617
70. Dandeneau RD, Zerenner EH (1990) The Invention of the Fused-Silica Column: An Industrial Perspective. LC-GC 8:908–912
71. Gudzinowicz BJ, Gudzinowizc MJ, Martin HF (1977) The GC-MS Interface. In: Fundamentals of Integrated GC-MS Part III. Marcel Dekker, New York
72. McFadden WH (1979) Interfacing Chromatography and Mass Spectrometry. J Chromatogr Sci 17:2–16. doi:10.1093/chromsci/17.1.2
73. McEwen CN, McKay RG (2005) A Combination Atmospheric Pressure LC/MS:GC/MS Ion Source: Advantages of Dual AP-LC/MS:GC/MS Instrumentation. J Am Soc Mass Spectrom 16:1730–1738. doi:10.1016/j.jasms.2005.07.005
74. Schiewek R, Lorenz M, Giese R, Brockmann K, Benter T, Gaeb S, Schmitz OJ (2008) Development of a Multipurpose Ion Source for LC-MS and GC-API-MS. Anal Bioanal Chem 392:87–96. doi:10.1007/s00216-008-2255-x
75. Bristow T, Harrison M, Sims M (2010) The Application of Gas Chromatography/Atmospheric Pressure Chemical Ionisation Time-of-Flight Mass Spectrometry to Impurity Identification in Pharmaceutical Development. Rapid Commun Mass Spectrom 24:1673–1681. doi:10.1002/rcm.4557
76. Li DX, Gan L, Bronja A, Schmitz OJ (2015) Gas Chromatography Coupled to Atmospheric Pressure Ionization Mass Spectrometry (GC-API-MS): Review. Anal Chim Acta 891:43–61. doi:10.1016/j.aca.2015.08.002
77. Blau K, King GS, Halket JM (eds) (1993) Handbook of Derivatives for Chromatography. Wiley, Chichester
78. Zaikin V, Halket JM (2009) A Handbook of Derivatives for Mass Spectrometry. IM Publications, Chichester
79. Aubert C, Rontani JF (2000) Perfluoroalkyl Ketones: Novel Derivatization Products for the Sensitive Determination of Fatty Acids by Gas Chromatography/Mass Spectrometry in Electron Impact and Negative Chemical Ionization Modes. Rapid Commun Mass Spectrom 14:960–966
80. Shin HS, Jung DG (2009) Sensitive Analysis of Malondialdehyde in Human Urine by Derivatization with Pentafluorophenylhydrazine Then Headspace GC-MS. Chromatographia 70:899–903. doi:10.1365/s10337-009-1235-4
81. Halket JM, Zaikin VG (2003) Derivatization in Mass Spectrometry: 1. Silylation. Eur J Mass Spectrom 9:1–21. doi:10.1255/ejms.527
82. Zaikin VG, Halket JM (2003) Derivatization in Mass Spectrometry: 2. Acylation. Eur J Mass Spectrom 9:421–434. doi:10.1255/ejms.576
83. Halket JM, Zaikin VG (2004) Derivatization in Mass Spectrometry: 3. Alkylation (Arylation). Eur J Mass Spectrom 10:1–19. doi:10.1255/ejms.619
84. Zaikin VG, Halket JM (2004) Derivatization in Mass Spectrometry: 4. Formation of Cyclic Derivatives. Eur J Mass Spectrom 10:555–568. doi:10.1255/ejms.653
85. Halket JM, Zaikin VG (2005) Derivatization in Mass Spectrometry: 5. Specific Derivatization of Monofunctional Compounds. Eur J Mass Spectrom 11:127–160. doi:10.1255/ejms.712
86. Zaikin VG, Halket JM (2005) Derivatization in Mass Spectrometry: 6. Formation of Mixed Derivatives of Polyfunctional Compounds. Eur J Mass Spectrom 11:611–636. doi:10.1255/ejms.773

87. Halket JM, Zaikin VG (2006) Derivatization in Mass Spectrometry: 7. On-Line Derivatization/Degradation. Eur J Mass Spectrom 12:1–13. doi:10.1255/ejms.785
88. Zaikin VG, Halket JM (2006) Derivatization in Mass Spectrometry: 8. Soft Ionization Mass Spectrometry of Small Molecules. Eur J Mass Spectrom 12:79–115. doi:10.1255/ejms.798
89. Anderegg RJ (1988) Derivatization in Mass Spectrometry: Strategies for Controlling Fragmentation. Mass Spectrom Rev 7:395–424. doi:10.1002/mas.1280070403
90. Spiteller G (1982) Contaminants in Mass Spectrometry. Mass Spectrom Rev 1:29–62. doi:10.1002/mas.1280010105
91. Leclerq PA, Camers CA (1998) High-Speed GC-MS. Mass Spectrometry Reviews 17:37–49. doi:10.1002/(SICI)1098-2787(1998)17:1<37::AID-MAS2>3.0.CO;2-A
92. Prazen BJ, Bruckner CA, Synovec RE, Kowalski BR (1999) Enhanced Chemical Analysis Using Parallel Column Gas Chromatography with Single-Detector Time-of-Flight Mass Spectrometry and Chemometric Analysis. Anal Chem 71:1093–1099. doi:10.1021/ac980814m
93. Hirsch R, Ternes TA, Bobeldijk I, Weck RA (2001) Determination of Environmentally Relevant Compounds Using Fast GC/TOF-MS. Chimia 55:19–22
94. Trapp O, Weber SK, Bauch S, Hofstadt W (2007) High-Throughput Screening of Catalysts by Combining Reaction and Analysis. Angew Chem Int Ed 46:7307–7310. doi:10.1002/anie.200701326
95. Trapp O (2007) Boosting the Throughput of Separation Techniques by "Multiplexing". Angew Chem Int Ed 46(5609–5613):S5609–S5601. doi:10.1002/anie.200605128
96. Rathsack P, Wolf B, Kroll MM, Otto M (2015) Comparative Study of Graphite-Supported LDI- and ESI-FT-ICR-MS of a Pyrolysis Liquid from a German Brown Coal. Anal Chem 87:7618–7627. doi:10.1021/acs.analchem.5b00693
97. Rathsack P, Rieger A, Haseneder R, Gerlach D, Repke JU, Otto M (2014) Analysis of Pyrolysis Liquids from Scrap Tires Using Comprehensive Gas Chromatography-Mass Spectrometry and Unsupervised Learning. J Anal Appl Pyrolysis 109:234–243. doi:10.1016/j.jaap.2014.06.007
98. Rathsack P, Riedewald F, Sousa-Gallagher M (2015) Analysis of Pyrolysis Liquid Obtained from Whole Tyre Pyrolysis with Molten Zinc as the Heat Transfer Media Using Comprehensive Gas Chromatography Mass Spectrometry. J Anal Appl Pyrolysis 116:49–57. doi:10.1016/j.jaap.2015.10.007
99. Horning EC, Carroll DI, Dzidic I, Haegele KD, Horning MG, Stillwell RN (1974) Atmospheric Pressure Ionization (API) Mass Spectrometry. Solvent-Mediated Ionization of Samples Introduced in Solution and in a Liquid Chromatograph Effluent Stream. J Chromatogr Sci 12:725–729. doi:10.1093/chromsci/12.11.725
100. Blakley CR, Vestal ML (1983) Thermospray Interface for Liquid Chromatography/Mass Spectrometry. Anal Chem 55:750–754. doi:10.1021/ac00255a036
101. van der Greef J, Niessen WMA, Tjaden UR (1989) Liquid Chromatography-Mass Spectrometry. The Need for a Multidimensional Approach. J Chromatogr 474:5–19. doi:10.1016/S0021-9673(01)93898-1
102. Niessen WMA, Voyksner RD (eds) (1998) Current Practice of Liquid Chromatography-Mass Spectrometry. Elsevier, Amsterdam
103. Siuzdak G (2006) The Expanding Role of Mass Spectrometry in Biotechnology. MCC Press, San Diego
104. Ramanathan R (ed) (2009) Mass Spectrometry in Drug Metabolism and Pharmacokinetics. Wiley, Hoboken
105. Castiglioni S, Zuccato E, Crisci E, Chiabrando C, Fanelli R, Bagnati R (2006) Identification and Measurement of Illicit Drugs and Their Metabolites in Urban Wastewater by Liquid Chromatography-Tandem Mass Spectrometry. Anal Chem 78:8421–8429. doi:10.1021/ac061095b

106. Simpson RJ, Connolly LM, Eddes JS, Pereira JJ, Moritz RL, Reid GE (2000) Proteomic Analysis of the Human Colon Carcinoma Cell Line (LIM 1215): Development of a Membrane Protein Database. Electrophoresis 21:1707–1732. doi:10.1002/(SICI)1522-2683 (20000501)21:9<1707::AID-ELPS1707>3.0.CO;2-Q
107. Bohrer BC, Merenbloom SI, Koeniger SL, Hilderbrand AE, Clemmer DE (2008) Biomolecule Analysis by Ion Mobility Spectrometry. Annu Rev Anal Chem 1:293–327. doi:10.1146/annurev.anchem.1.031207.113001
108. Kanu AB, Dwivedi P, Tam M, Matz L, Hill HH Jr (2008) Ion Mobility-Mass Spectrometry. J Mass Spectrom 43:1–22. doi:10.1002/jms.1383
109. Fernandez-Lima F, Kaplan DA, Suetering J, Park MA (2016) Gas-Phase Separation Using a Trapped Ion Mobility Spectrometer. Int J Ion Mobil Spectrom 14:93–98. doi:10.1007/s12127-011-0067-8
110. Ridgeway ME, Wolff JJ, Silveira JA, Lin C, Costello CE, Park MA (2016) Gated Trapped Ion Mobility Spectrometry Coupled to Fourier Transform Ion Cyclotron Resonance Mass Spectrometry. Int J Ion Mobil Spectrom 19:77–85. doi:10.1007/s12127-016-0197-0
111. Fenn LS, Kliman M, Mahsut A, Zhao SR, McLean JA (2009) Characterizing Ion Mobility-Mass Spectrometry Conformation Space for the Analysis of Complex Biological Samples. Anal Bioanal Chem 394:235–244. doi:10.1007/s00216-009-2666-3
112. Dwivedi P, Wu C, Matz LM, Clowers BH, Seims WF, Hill HH Jr (2006) Gas-Phase Chiral Separations by Ion Mobility Spectrometry. Anal Chem 78:8200–8206. doi:10.1021/ac0608772
113. Enders JR, McLean JA (2009) Chiral and Structural Analysis of Biomolecules Using Mass Spectrometry and Ion Mobility-Mass Spectrometry. Chirality 21:e253–e264. doi:10.1002/chir.20806
114. Adams KJ, Montero D, Aga D, Fernandez-Lima F (2016) Isomer Separation of Polybrominated Diphenyl Ether Metabolites Using NanoESI-TIMS-MS. Int J Ion Mobil Spectrom 19:69–76. doi:10.1007/s12127-016-0198-z
115. Moritz T, Olsen JE (1995) Comparison Between High-Resolution Selected Ion Monitoring, Selected Reaction Monitoring, and Four-Sector Tandem Mass Spectrometry in Quantitative Analysis of Gibberellins in Milligram Amounts of Plant Tissue. Anal Chem 67:1711–1716. doi:10.1021/ac00106a010
116. Guo M, Huang BX, Kim HY (2009) Conformational Changes in Akt1 Activation Probed by Amide Hydrogen/Deuterium Exchange and Nano-Electrospray Ionization Mass Spectrometry. Rapid Commun Mass Spectrom 23:1885–1891. doi:10.1002/rcm.4085
117. Hughey CA, Hendrickson CL, Rodgers RP, Marshall AG (2001) Kendrick Mass Defect Spectrum: A Compact Visual Analysis for Ultrahigh-Resolution Broadband Mass Spectra. Anal Chem 73:4676–4681. doi:10.1021/ac010560w
118. Hughey CA, Rodgers RP, Marshall AG (2002) Resolution of 11,000 Compositionally Distinct Components in a Single Electrospray Ionization FT-ICR Mass Spectrum of Crude Oil. Anal Chem 74:4145–4149. doi:10.1021/ac020146b
119. Hsu CS, Liang Z, Campana JE (1994) Hydrocarbon Characterization by Ultrahigh Resolution Fourier Transform Ion Cyclotron Resonance Mass Spectrometry. Anal Chem 66:850–855. doi:10.1021/ac00078a015
120. Hughey CA, Hendrickson CL, Rodgers RP, Marshall AG (2001) Elemental Composition Analysis of Processed and Unprocessed Diesel Fuel by Electrospray Ionization Fourier Transform Ion Cyclotron Resonance Mass Spectrometry. Energy Fuels 15:1186–1193. doi:10.1021/ef010028b
121. Wu Z, Hendrickson CL, Rodgers RP, Marshall AG (2002) Composition of Explosives by Electrospray Ionization Fourier Transform Ion Cyclotron Resonance Mass Spectrometry. Analytical Chemistry 74:1879–1883. doi:10.1021/ac011071z
122. Kew W, Goodall I, Clarke D, Uhrin D (2017) Chemical Diversity and Complexity of Scotch Whisky As Revealed by High-Resolution Mass Spectrometry. J Am Soc Mass Spectrom 28:200–213. doi:10.1007/s13361-016-1513-y

123. Hertkorn N, Ruecker C, Meringer M, Gugisch R, Frommberger M, Perdue EM, Witt M, Schmitt-Kopplin P (2007) High-Precision Frequency Measurements: Indispensable Tools at the Core of the Molecular-Level Analysis of Complex Systems. Anal Bioanal Chem 389:1311–1327. doi:10.1007/s00216-007-1577-4
124. Dittmar T, Paeng J (2009) A Heat-Induced Molecular Signature in Marine Dissolved Organic Matter. Nat Geosci 2:175–179. doi:10.1038/ngeo440

Inorganic Mass Spectrometry 15

Learning Objectives

- Ionization of inorganic samples
- Elemental analysis by MS – special instrumentation
- Accurate isotopic compositions
- Lateral distribution of elements and mass spectral imaging
- Elemental MS for assessing biological systems
- Element speciation in organic materials and biological tissues

Mass spectrometry resulted from an endeavor to analyze gaseous ionic matter. The discovery of isotopes and the determination of their masses and relative abundances, i.e., *isotope ratios,* were a direct result of the pioneering work of Thomson, Aston, Dempster, and many others [1, 2]. Soon, the results of such measurements became the driving force for new discoveries in physics. The detection of mass defect, for example, was direct proof of the mass–energy equivalence as postulated by Einstein's special theory of relativity. It was not until the late 1940s that mass spectrometry was developed as a tool for the analysis of organic compounds, but within a decade or two, this branch flourished. In 1968, the journal *Organic Mass Spectrometry* was founded, and soon, the leap into *biomedical mass spectrometry* (also a journal title from 1974 to 1985) was taken. The majority of mass spectrometrists is now working in proteomics or metabolomics, in environmental, clinical and forensic trace analysis to name a few. Meanwhile, what became known as *inorganic mass spectrometry* [3–8] or *element mass spectrometry* has experienced equally revolutionary developments [9, 10] as its organic and biomedical counterpart – of which it could be considered a "sibling".

J.H. Gross, *Mass Spectrometry*, DOI 10.1007/978-3-319-54398-7_15

15.1 Concept and Techniques of Inorganic MS

The determination of molecular formulas via accurate mass measurements relies on isotopic masses accurate to at least 1 in 10^8 [11]. Elemental trace analysis is required for the detection of radioactive nuclides in the environment, of transition metals such as Pt in exhaust fumes from automobiles [12], and in the quality control of low-sulfur fuels for the same. All electronic devices demand for high-purity semiconductors and the properties of alloys are critically influenced by trace elements [13]. Age determinations from isotope ratios are applied in archeology, paleontology, and geology [4, 14, 15]. More recently, elemental MS and biomedical MS are jointly employed to unveil the presence and preferably location of metals in proteins or DNA as well as their lateral distribution in tissues [16–20], a field of research basically going back to seminal work by Houk in 1980 [21]. Moreover, the prominent role of metal ions in physiological processes gave rise to a new field of research: *metallomics* [22–24]. Finally, we are wittnessing a rapid expansion of imaging techniques based on former methods of element MS into the exploration of complex biological systems [25–28]. This altogether makes it mandatory to include at least a compact chapter on *inorganic mass spectrometry* in this book.

Inorganic mass spectrometry generally addresses either of the following analytical tasks:

- Determine the elemental composition of metals, alloys, rock samples, semiconductors, and other inorganic materials.
- Detect and quantify elements at low concentrations or trace levels in a sample.
- Detect and quantify trace isotopes in a sample.
- Image the lateral distribution of one or multiple elements in a sample.
- Determine the accurate mass of stable or radioactive isotopes.
- Determine the accurate isotopic composition of an element in a sample.

When accurate ratios of (stable) isotopes are to be determined, this is referred to as *isotope ratio mass spectrometry* (IR-MS; for the δ notation in IR-MS and an example of IR-MS cf. Sect. 3.1.6.) [3, 6–8]. While the techniques of inorganic MS are mainly referenced according to the ionization method in use, IR-MS describes the analytical approach. Thus, IR-MS may employ different ionization techniques, and vice versa, TIMS for example, may be employed in IR-MS (Table 15.1).

Both the reliable determination of isotope ratios and the quantitation of trace elements are generally accompanied by complete destruction of all molecular entities. Opposed to what is normally desired in organic and bio-organic mass spectrometry, ionization methods in inorganic mass spectrometry therefore use conditions which erase any molecular structure, i.e., inorganic mass spectrometry particularly employs high temperature plasmas to achieve atomization prior to ionization and mass analysis [29]. Furthermore, ion–neutral reactions need to be suppressed or their products destroyed in order to ensure isotopic patterns free from interferences with isobars [30, 31].

Table 15.1 Techniques in inorganic mass spectrometry

Acronym	Technique
IR-MS	Isotope ratio mass spectrometry
TIMS	Thermal ionization mass spectrometry
SSMS	Spark source mass spectrometry
GDMS	Glow discharge mass spectrometry
ICP-MS	Inductively coupled plasma mass spectrometry
LA-ICP-MS	Laser ablation-inductively coupled plasma mass spectrometry
SIMS	Secondary ion mass spectrometry
AMS	Accelerator mass spectrometry

It does not surprise that neither a single type of mass spectrometer nor a single method of ion generation can fulfill all of the requirements for measuring all varying sample types and compositions equally well. While accelerator mass spectrometers, for example, deliver very high abundance sensitivity and low background, they have low sample throughput and need larger amounts of sample. ICP mass spectrometers, on the other side, tend to have higher sample throughput while being more susceptible to isobaric interferences. These different types of instruments are best viewed as complementing each other in their analytical capabilities (Fig. 15.1) [32, 33].

Identification of metalloproteins The function of metalloproteins critically depends on their interaction with a metal, e.g., Cu, Zn, Fe, Mo, or metalloid such as Se or As. The living cell not only depends on its genome and proteome, but also on its metallome, i.e., the distribution of those elements among different biomolecules. It is estimated that about 30% of the proteome is made up by metalloproteins [24]. The complexity of speciation analysis demands for a combined approach of separation techniques and different methods of mass spectrometry. This is best illustrated by the metallomics toolbox that reflects the current understanding of how the metallome can be explored (Fig. 15.2) [23].

Speciation of selenium in yeast proteins The speciation of selenium incorporated in yeast proteins shows the high degree to which elemental and biomedical MS are interrelated by now. The analysis started with a tryptic digest of the water-soluble protein fraction that had been isolated by size-exclusion chromatography. Analysis of the digest by reversed-phase HPLC-*inductively coupled plasma mass spectrometry* (ICP-MS) provided identification of the selenopeptide fraction, which was then analyzed by MALDI-TOF-MS in order to select target ions for tandem MS. Finally, the sequences of the selected selenopeptides were derived from ESI-CID spectra. This combined approach using ICP-MS, MALDI-MS, and ESI-MS allowed for the first time the identification of the heat-shock protein HSP12 (M_r = 11,693 u) in which the only methionine residue was replaced by selenomethionine (Fig. 15.3) [34].

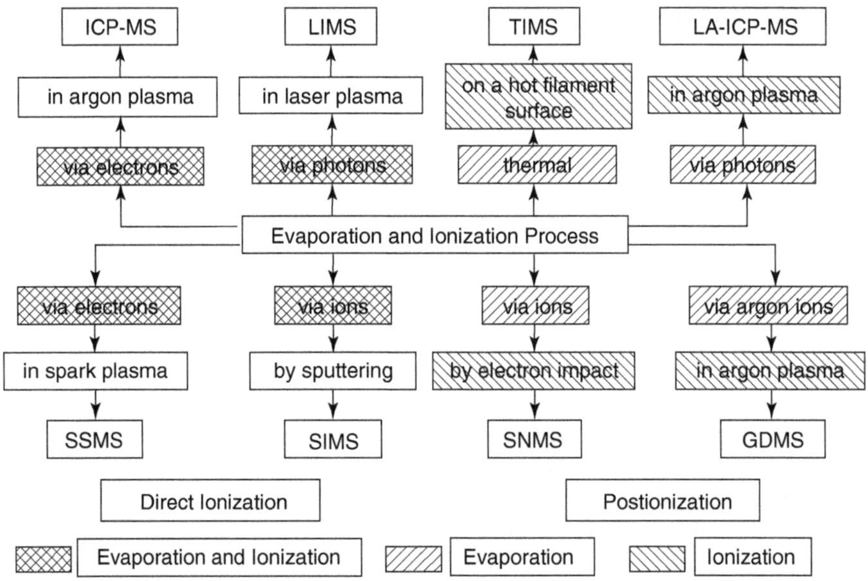

Fig. 15.1 Elemental MS techniques classified with respect to their evaporation and ionization processes (Reproduced from Ref. [32] with permission. © Elsevier Science Publishers, 2000)

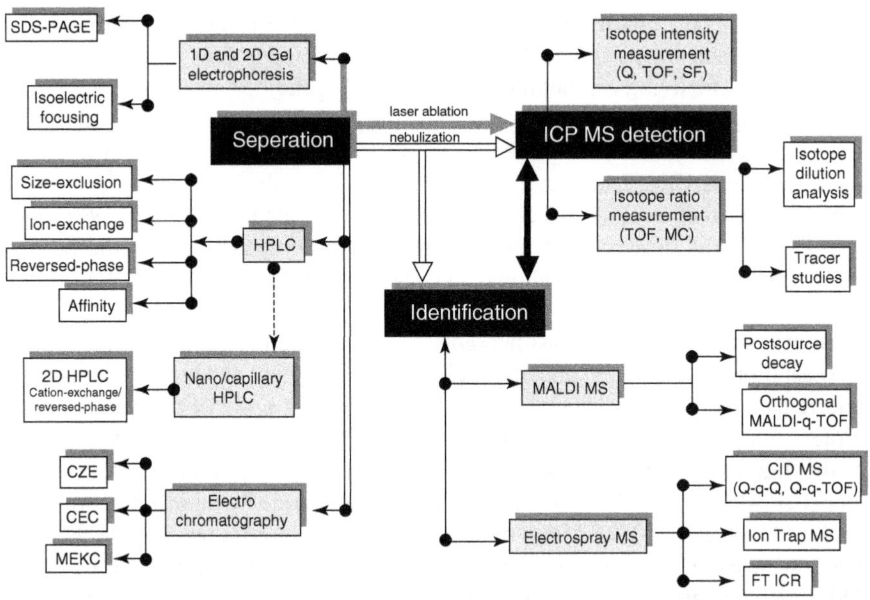

Fig. 15.2 The state-of-the art toolbox with hyphenated techniques for element speciation analysis and metallomics. The *upper right* section presents the tools of inorganic mass spectrometry (Reproduced from Ref. [23] with permission. © Wiley Periodicals Inc., 2006)

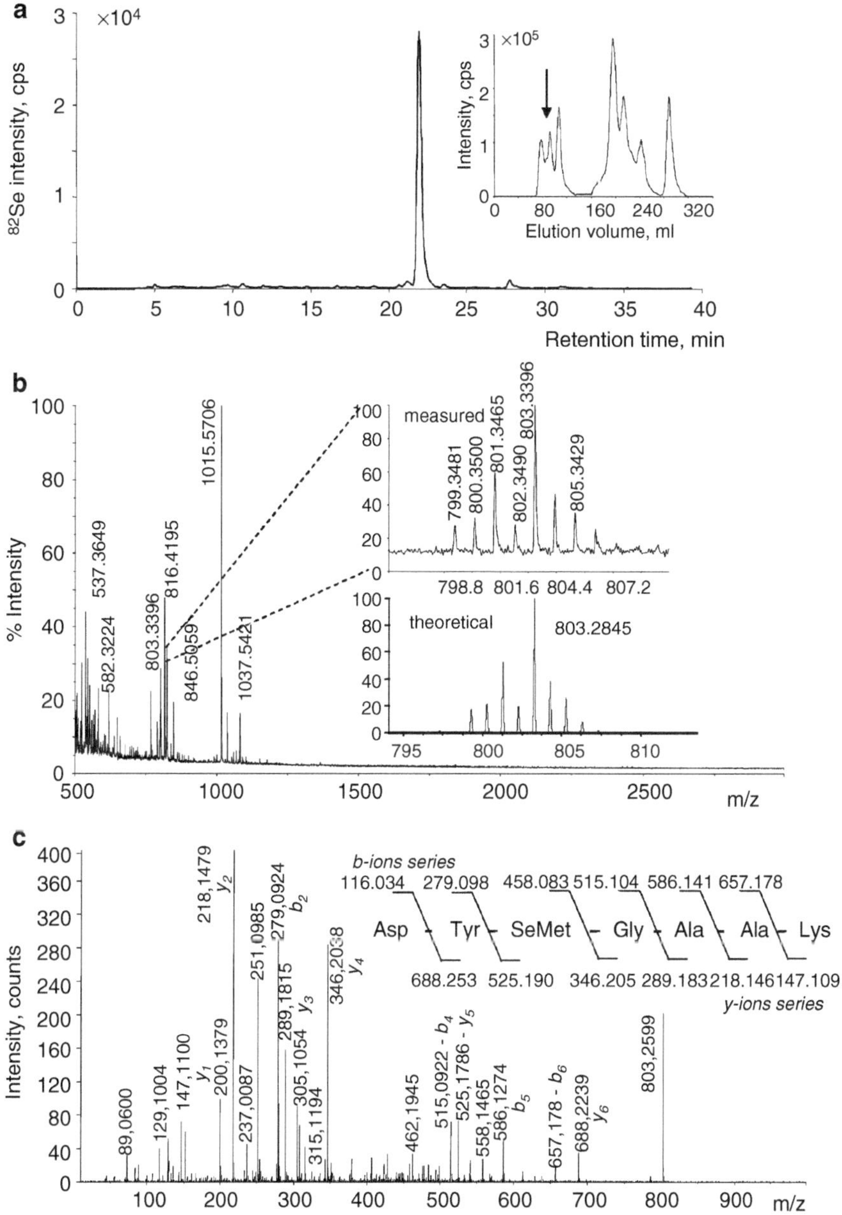

Fig. 15.3 Identification of the selenopeptide of the HSP12 protein: (**a**) Reconstructed ion chromatogram based on ^{77}Se and ^{82}Se from reversed-phase HPLC-ICP-MS of the Se-containing protein fraction (as obtained from the marked region in the size-exclusion chromatogram in the inset); (**b**) MALDI-TOF mass spectrum of the fraction producing the peak correlated to Se in part (**a**); (**c**) ESI-CID mass spectrum of the $[M+H]^+$ ion, *m/z* 803.25, of the selenopeptide (Reproduced from Ref. [34] with permission. © American Chemical Society, 2003)

15.2 Thermal Ionization Mass Spectrometry

Atomic and eventually molecular ions can be formed by *thermal ionization* (TI), also known as *surface ionization* (SI). For *thermal ionization mass spectrometry* (TI-MS), a metal salt, metal oxide, or metal is placed onto the surface of a rhenium or tungsten filament where it is heated in vacuum to 400–2300 °C. In practice, an assembly of one to three ribbon filaments in close proximity is employed for TI (Fig. 15.4). The first filament is loaded with the sample and heated to evaporate the analyte. The neutral atoms or molecules emerging thereof may then be ionized on the second filament. Electron transfer *to* the bulk metal results in positive ions while electron transfer *from* the filament yields anions. The third filament of a triple filament assembly is normally used to deliver a standard that can be analyzed alternating with the unknown under virtually identical ion source conditions. Double and triple filament assemblies have the advantage that evaporation and ionization temperature can be independently controlled. While evaporation is preferably performed at comparatively low temperature in order to obtain long-lasting signals and minor isotopic fractionation, ionization requires high temperatures for good ionization efficiency. Careful control of filament temperature [35] ensures that nanogram to microgram amounts of sample yield signals for hours because evaporation rates are in the order of picograms per second. Thoroughly chosen evaporation conditions are also vital for the reliability of the results [33]. Normally, 10–20 filament assemblies are mounted on one carousel-like sample turret in order to avoid frequent breaking of the vacuum. Once loaded and pumped to high vacuum, the instrument may be operated for days until all samples are measured.

Ion formation in TI relies on the blurring of the discrete electronic states of the neutral at high temperature. This way, the Fermi levels of adsorbed neutral and bulk metal can merge into a common band causing the charge state of the weakly surface-bound particle to be purely determined by Fermi statistics. In other words, as the electrons move freely between the adsorbed atom and the surface the atom is positive at times. Assuming ideal conditions, the degree of ionization,

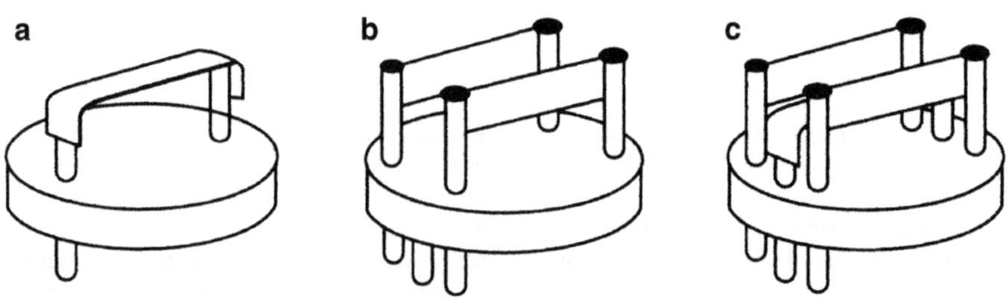

Fig. 15.4 From left (**a**) single filament, (**b**) double filament, and (**c**) triple filament assemblies for thermal ionization of metal salts and oxides (Reproduced from Ref. [3] with permission. © John Wiley & Sons Ltd., 1997)

i.e., the ratio of ions and neutrals leaving the surface, is described by the *Saha-Langmuir equation*. The degree of positive ionization α^+ is given as

$$\alpha^+ = \frac{N^+}{N^0} = \frac{g^+}{g^0} \exp\left[\frac{e(\Phi - IE)}{kT}\right] \tag{15.1}$$

$$= \frac{g^+}{g^0} \exp\left[1.16 \times 10^4 \frac{(\Phi - IE)}{T}\right] \tag{15.2}$$

where g^+/g^0 is the ratio of electronic states of the ion and the neutral, *IE* is the ionization energy of the atom or molecule to be ionized, Φ is the work function of the filament material, and T is the temperature of the ionizing filament. Best ionization efficiency is therefore obtained when metals of low *IE* are exposed to high temperature on filament materials that have large Φ. This is achieved by using filaments made of rhenium ($\Phi_{Re} = 4.98$ eV, *m.p.* = 3180 °C) or tungsten ($\Phi_W = 4.58$ eV, *m.p.* = 3410 °C; Fig. 15.5).

Vice versa, nonmetallic elements with high *IE* and metal oxides may form negative ions [36, 37]. The degree of ionization α^- is then obtained from the modified Saha-Langmuir equation

$$\alpha^- = \frac{g^-}{g^0} \exp\left[1.16 \times 10^4 \frac{(EA - \Phi)}{T}\right] \tag{15.3}$$

where *EA* is the electron affinity of the adsorbed atom.

Due to the low spatial and energetic spread of ions from TI, the method can be combined with single-focusing magnetic sector mass analyzers or quadrupoles [38]. Nonetheless, TI ion sources require dedicated instrumentation, frequently

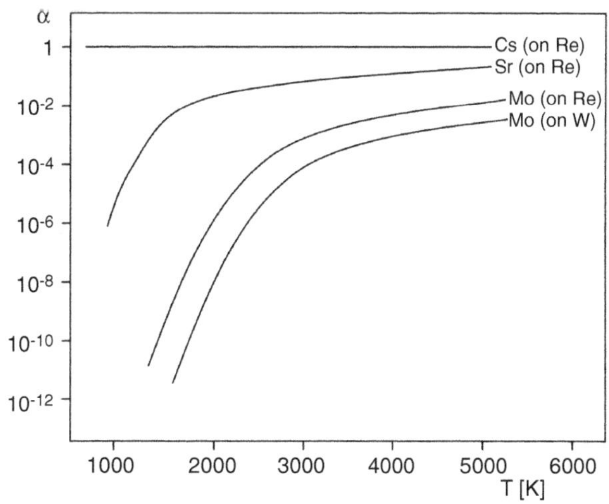

Fig. 15.5 Thermal ionization efficiency α^+ vs. filament temperature. The curves for Mo reflect the dependence of α^+ on the filament material. The advantage of the Re over the W filament follows from Eqs. 15.1–15.2 (Reproduced from Ref. [7] with permission. © John Wiley & Sons Ltd., 2008)

equipped with *multicollector* (MC) systems to insure the highest accuracy for the isotope ratios measured (Sects. 3.3.2 and 7.2 in [3]).

The favorite application of TI is *isotope ratio mass spectrometry* (IR-MS) and trace elemental analysis of metals and inorganic metal compounds. This is, however, in no way limiting the applicability of TI-MS to the elemental analysis of organic material including food. Such samples are transformed into suitable compounds by (extensive) work-up such as freeze-drying, oxidative treatment with concentrated HNO_3 or HNO_3/H_2O_2, ashing, or electrolytic deposition [39, 40]. TI of organic salts remained a rare exception [41]. TI-MS is not suitable for mixture analysis and multi-element determinations where ICP-MS is normally employed. Due to its high precision, TI-MS is important as a reference method to calibrate other techniques of isotope ratio MS, such as MC-ICP-MS that, while also requiring matrix separation, is still able to deliver higher sample throughput (Sect. 15.4). TI-MS also serves for the certification of reference materials because accuracy and precision of the method are excellent [42].

TI-MS or TIMS?

In the element MS community it is common to use the acronym TIMS without hyphen rather than the form TI-MS. The same is observed in case of other techniques employed for element MS, e.g., *secondary ion mass spectrometry* is abbreviated SIMS rather than SI-MS.

15.3 Spark Source Mass Spectrometry

The *spark source* (SS) developed by Dempster in 1935, provided the first truly multi-element and isotopic trace element method [43]. In *spark source mass spectrometry* (SS-MS), a solid sample is vaporized under vacuum by a high-voltage radiofrequency spark. The electric discharge is maintained between two pin-shaped electrodes (about 10 mm in length and 1–2 mm in diameter) in vacuum.

SS-MS is best suited for conducting samples, because the electrodes may then be directly prepared from the solid to be analyzed. Prior to insertion into the ion source, the electrodes have to be carefully cleaned, e.g., by etching, to avoid surface contamination (Sect. 5.2 in [6], Sect. 2.2 in [7]). If the sample is not itself conducting, high-purity graphite, or if neccessary silver or gold powder are used as scaffolding for the electrodes. Often, an *internal standard element* or an *isotopically enriched spike* are admixed to this powder before the finely ground analyte-containing material is added. Typically, 50 mg of powdered material, e.g., a rock sample, is mixed with the graphite powder and then compressed into electrode pins [44].

The detection limits for the elements from Rb through U generally vary between 0.001 and 0.1 ppm (equivalent to 0.001–0.1 $\mu g\ g^{-1}$). Certain elements such as Nb, Zr, Y, Sn, Sb, and Th can even be measured at the ppb ($ng\ g^{-1}$) level [45].

Trace ≠ small sample

Although an element may be detected at the ultratrace level by SS-MS, the amount of sample required is comparatively large since electrodes lasting for several hours of operation are needed. This reminds us that detection of a component present at the ppm level of concentration is not automatically equal to a tiny amount of sample.

Obviously, SS-MS is not suited for elemental analysis of small sample amounts, but SS-MS offers a high dynamic range making it very powerful for multiple element analysis including those present at trace level in alloys, ores, and similar samples. SS-MS also offers wide element coverage, an extensive concentration range and analysis of solids without dissolution.

The spark is initiated by emission of electrons from the cathode by field emission (opposite process to FI), which becomes possible due to the high local field strengths (10^8–10^9 V m^{-1}) at edges of the microscopically rough surface. The electrons are then accelerated towards the anode. There, the energy of the impinging electrons causes evaporation of the anode material (sample) that is subsequently ionized in the gas phase by electron ionization.

Proper operation of a spark source is not simple. It requires a high voltage supply of several tens of kilovolts, normally at 1 MHz radiofrequency that is generated in short pulses of variable length (20–200 μs) with a repetition frequency of 1–10^4 s^{-1} to achieve uniform ablation of both electrodes (Fig. 15.6) [44]. In order to maintain a stable ion current, the electrodes need to be carefully adjusted and dynamically re-adjusted during the measurement (0.1–0.5 mm tip to tip) [46], and special techniques such as *gliding spark source mass spectrometry* (GSS-MS) are sometimes employed for the analysis of nonconducting materials [47]. Finally, the ions emerge from the discharge with a wide kinetic energy distribution (keV range), which makes a double-focusing mass analyzer mandatory for SS-MS. To partially

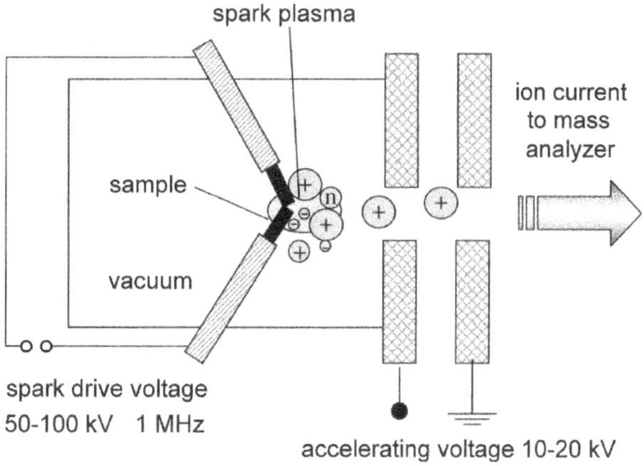

Fig. 15.6 RF spark source (Reproduced from Ref. [7] with permission. © John Wiley & Sons Ltd., 2008)

compensate for this high energy spread, accelerating voltages on the order of 20–25 kV are typical.

Opposed to all other current MS techniques, photoplate detection and subsequent densiometry on a series of exposures is still widespread in SS-MS. In practice, 15 consecutive spectra are acquired by exposing the plate streak-by-streak in a range from 0.001 to 300–2000 nCi, requiring total measurement times of about 0.5–3 h per sample. Translation of densiometric data into ion abundances is not trivial and detailed procedures have been developed for this crucial step of SS-MS analysis [43–45]. More recently, *multi-ion counting* (MIC) systems have been due to their improved sensitivity, precision, and sample throughput [45, 46]. Simultaneous detection in Mattauch-Herzog geometry SS-MS instruments using MIC is also advantageous for applications such as isotope dilution analysis of several isotopes. Furthermore, SS-MS is well suited for C, N, O determination in semiconductors, because the combination of a high vacuum source without sputter gas with a high frequency discharge allows for the analysis of samples even those of resistivities [48].

Carbon in gallium arsenide SS-MS has been used for the quantification of carbon in a gallium arsenide (GaAs) sample produced by high-pressure liquid-encapsulated Czochralski (HP-LEC) crystal growth. The carbon might originate from the graphite susceptor, the ambient gas, or be present as a trace element in both gallium and arsenic starting material. The partial SS mass spectrum shows strong signals due to $^{69}Ga^{6+}$, $^{71}Ga^{6+}$, and $^{75}As^{6+}$ in close proximity to the carbon peak at *m/z* 12 (Fig. 15.7) [49].

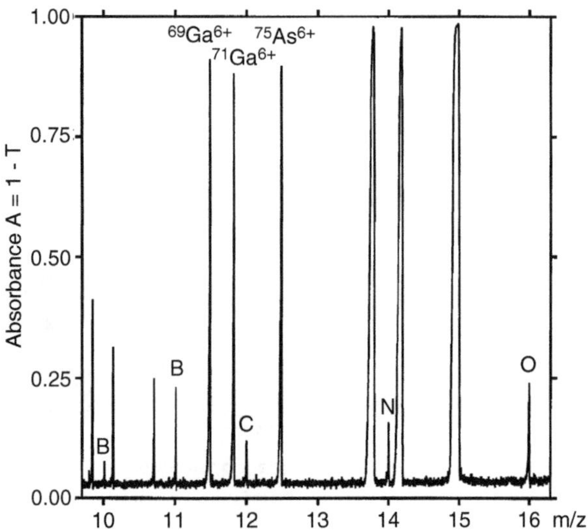

Fig. 15.7 Partial SS mass spectrum of a HP-LEC GdAs sample by photoplate detection after exposure to $Q = 3 \times 10^{-7}$ Ci Reproduced from Ref. [49] with permission. © Springer-Verlag, 1999)

15.4 Glow Discharge Mass Spectrometry

The first report of the formation of positive ions of gases from a *glow discharge* (GD) in his so-called channel ray tube was by Goldstein in 1886 [7]. Since the launch of the first commercial instrument for *glow discharge mass spectrometry* (GD-MS) in 1984, GD-MS has become sort of industry standard for the analysis of trace elements in metals and semiconductors [50, 51]. The pioneering work and much of the development of GD-MS has been done by Harrison and Marcus [52–56]. In fact, GD-MS appears as the successor to SS-MS, and at present, GD-MS is one of the most powerful solid-state analytical methods for the determination of trace impurities and depth profiling of solids. It allows direct trace element determination in solids down to concentrations as low as 1 ppb (ng g^{-1}) [32]. GD-MS is an essential technique for the quality control and characterization of high-purity metals in the electronics industry [57, 58].

The direct current (DC) glow discharge is a self-sustaining low pressure gas discharge dominated by space charges and represents a low-energy plasma making the GD ion source a compact small volume source that operates a low wattage. It is inexpensive to build and maintain, and plasma gases are modestly consumed (ml min^{-1}). Also, unlike the spark source, the GD source is inherently stable [59]. Typically, in a GD ion source [48, 51, 59–63] a discharge current of 1–5 mA is maintained through a low-pressure argon atmosphere (10^1–10^3 Pa) by applying a DC voltage of 500–2000 V across the ionization volume. The cathode is represented by the solid sample which may either be a disk (so-called *Grimm-type GD source* [59]) or a stick and an anode present as the housing and the ion source exit plate (Sect. 5.3 in [6], Sect. 7.5 in [3]).

The low-temperature Ar plasma serves as a source of primary ions, excited atoms and electrons. In the cathode dark space, a region where a large potential drop exists, the positive argon ions are accelerated towards the sample cathode and the sample material is sputtered from the cathode's surface by ion bombardment (cf. FAB, LSIMS, Chap. 10). The kinetic energies of the impinging ions are in the range of 100–500 eV [51]. Sputtered atoms and molecules depart from the surface with kinetic energies of 5–15 eV and are then ionized in the quasineutral glow discharge plasma (so-called *afterglow*). The electron density in the plasma can reach up to 10^{14} cm^{-3} [64] and their energy covers a wide distribution from thermal to energetic. Although they are by about a factor of 1000 less abundant in the plasma, metastable Ar* atoms are also effective for ionization because they carry 11.55 eV. Therefore, Penning ionization, electron ionization, and charge transfer contribute to ionize the neutrals (Fig. 15.8).

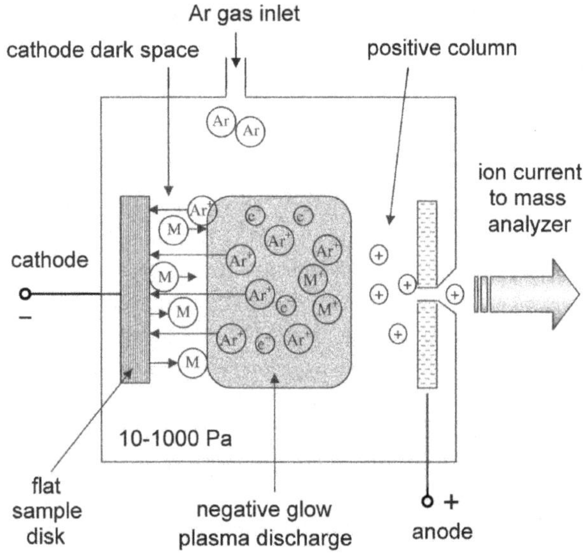

Fig. 15.8 GD ion source with disk-shaped cathode (Reproduced from Ref. [7] with permission. © John Wiley & Sons Ltd., 2008)

Shining brightly
The afterglow (or negative-glow) region shines brightly because excited atoms are emitting their characteristic visible radiation. This phenomenon not only gave rise to the method's name but also led to the construction of the neon lamp. For more applications of GDs a review by A. Bogearts is highly recommended [65].

Due to its general setup, GD has the advantage that the atomization and ionization processes are separated in space and time, resulting in only minor variations in sensitivity and a low matrix dependence. This enables the quantification of elements without the need for standards tailored to the actual type of sample matrix [48, 51].

On the downside, there are isobaric interferences such as $[XAr]^{+\bullet}$ and $[XH]^{+}$ ions that require $R > 5000$ to avoid overlap with pure atomic ions $X^{+\bullet}$ [51]. Therefore, double-focusing magnetic sector instruments present the most successful mass analyzers in GD-MS [48]. Another disadvantage of GD-MS as compared to LA-ICP-MS or SIMS (Sects. 15.4 and 15.5), for example, is the lack of spatial resolution.

Quality control of superalloy In the manufacture of aircraft engines and gas turbines superalloy is widely used due to its excellent performance, which to a great extent depends on the content of trace elements in the alloy. Critical control of the alloy's composition is therefore essential for the safe operation of such

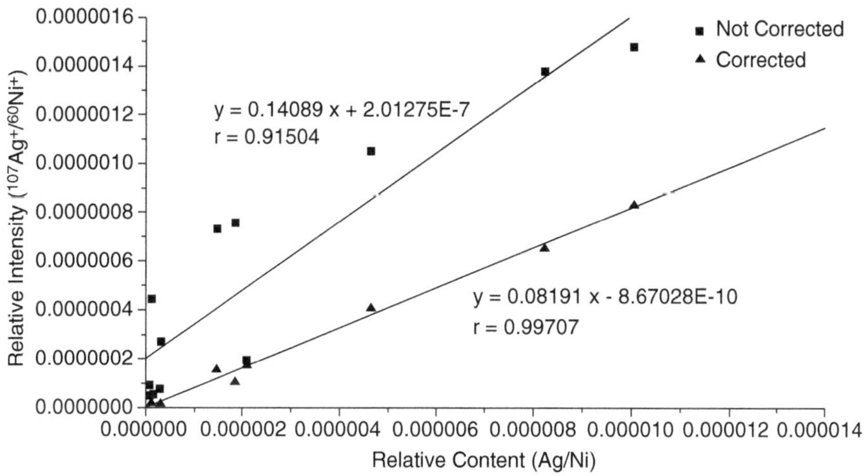

Fig. 15.9 Comparision of ^{107}Ag calibration curves in superalloy between the uncorrected results and those corrected by multivariable linear regression. The relevance of corrections when no separation by high-resolution is available is immediately apparent (Adapted from Ref. [66] with permission. © IM Publications, 2008)

engines. The obvious method to avoid isobaric interferences is to select isotopes where no interferences exist. While Tl, Pb, and Bi meet this criterion, in case of Sn only the $^{118}Sn^{+\bullet}$ ion is free of superimpositions, whereas $^{120}Sn^{+\bullet}$ has serious interferences from $^{40}Ar_3^{+\bullet}$, $^{92}Mo^{14}N_2^{+\bullet}$, and $^{120}Te^{+\bullet}$. To determine the correct content of elements in superalloy on a quadrupole GD instrument also when no suitable isotope exists, both matching the sample matrix by use of external standards and multivariable linear regression have extensively been used (Fig. 15.9) [66].

In a DC GD, nonconducting samples would rapidly cause the breakdown of the discharge due to electrostatic charging. Radiofrequency (RF) discharges circumvent this problem [54–56, 61, 67]. By applying an RF voltage at one of the two electrodes (called the *RF-electrode*), the accumulated positive charge on the sample surface will be neutralized by the negative charge accumulation during the second part of the RF-cycle thereby avoiding net charges. Typically voltages of 2 kV at an RF of 13 MHz are employed.

The atomic collision processes in the GD are sufficiently robust to break many tenaciously bonded species [59]. Nonetheless, GC-GD-TOF-MS has even been demonstrated to be capable of delivering spectra of organic molecules and elemental information [68–70].

Need to zoom in

The analytical problems of inorganic MS often require only certain selected isotopes or narrow *m/z* ranges to be measured. Multicollector systems, for example, are adjusted to simultaneously detect a few isotopes for the purpose of accurate isotope ratio determinations or to quantify a low-abundant isotope together with an isotopic standard for internal reference. Thus, the data is more often presented in tabular form or in plots of concentration versus variables such as depth of invasion, age of samples, or location on a surface. Mass spectra covering a wider range are only acquired for survey multi-element detection.

15.5 Inductively Coupled Plasma Mass Spectrometry

In *inductively coupled plasma mass spectrometry* (ICP-MS), atomization and ionization are achieved in a radiofrequency argon plasma at atmospheric pressure. Since a seminal publication in 1980 [21], ICP-MS has become one of the most frequently employed methods of elemental MS ([57, 58], Sect. 7.3 in [3], Chap. 4 in [6], Sect. 5 in [7]). The wide acceptance of ICP-MS is due to its comparatively robust, yet versatile sampling mode. An ICP not only offers high ionization efficiency for elements of low *IE*, e.g., 98% for $IE = 7$ eV, it is still applicable to nonmetals such as P and even Cl (ionization efficiency is 1% for $IE = 13$ eV).

The core of an ICP source is formed by a so-called *plasma torch*. It consists of three coaxially aligned quartz tubes that are inserted along the central axis of a water-cooled RF coil. After ignition by an electric spark discharge, the coil (typically RF of 27 MHz) feeds the plasma by coupling electric energy (1–2 kW) into the gas, because the fluctuating magnetic field causes ion motion which in turn heats up the gas and maintains a continuously flowing plasma. The outer quartz tube is about 20 mm in diameter and has its walls cooled by an argon gas flow of 12–20 l min^{-1}. The middle tube supplies another stream of argon, the so-called auxiliary gas flow of 1–2 l min^{-1} that is feeding the plasma. The sample is then introduced into the center of the toroidal plasma by an argon carrier gas flow of 1–1.5 l min^{-1}. This carrier gas passes through a nebulizer and leads to the dissipation and transfer of a liquid sample as micrometer-sized droplets (depending on the type of nebulizer), which can be vaporized, atomized, and ionized within the ICP. Typical sample consumption is in the order of 0.02–1 ml min^{-1} (Fig. 15.10).

The ICP approaches a temperature of 10,000 K in the induction zone close to the coil, in the center of which evaporation and atomization occur at about 8000 K. While the plasma flows away from the coil, excitation of the neutrals is effected at 7500 K followed by ionization in a zone well after the coil at about 6000 K (Fig. 15.10). Thereafter, recombination in the plasma's tail causes molecular interferences, which can be reduced by placing a collision cell in the ion beam, for example [30, 31, 72, 73].

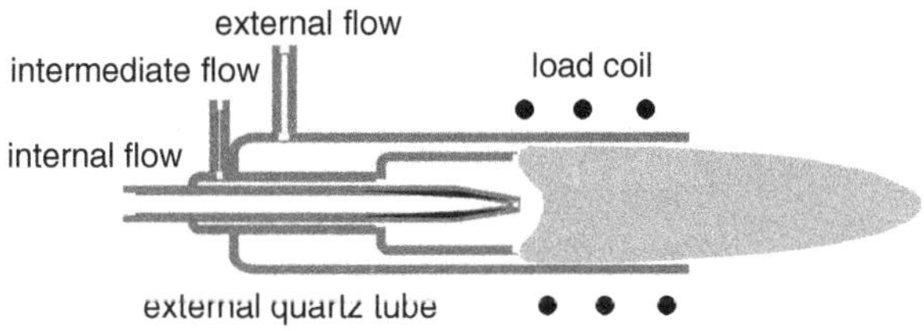

Fig. 15.10 ICP torch. Three concentric quartz tubes deliver the internal flow containing the sample, the intermediate argon flow to support the plasma, and an external flow to provide cooling to the outer wall. The temperature reaches about 10,000 K inside the coil and drops to about 6000 K at the tip of the plasma from where ions are collected at the sampling cone (Adapted from Ref. [71] with permission. © Royal Chemical Society, 2015)

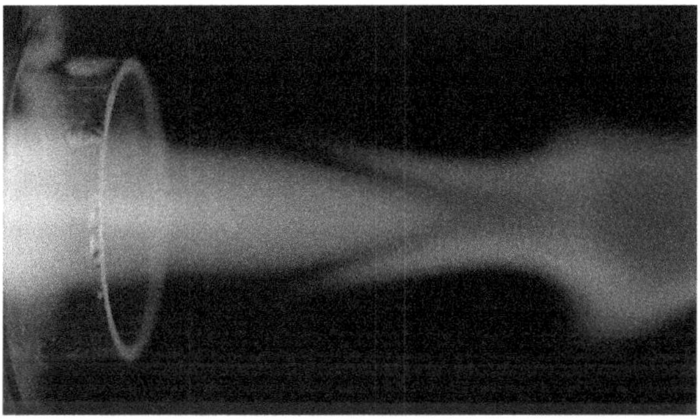

Fig. 15.11 ICP plasmas can be beautiful. This photograph shows a plasma as obtained during the analysis of yttrium (Reproduced from Ref. [74] with permission. © Royal Chemical Society, 2003)

The appearance of the plasma varies and depends on liquid and gas flow, nebulizer design, and of course, the type and concentration of the analyte. In some cases, the ICP can be extraordinarily beautiful (Fig. 15.11) [74]. Careful observation of the ICP by high-speed photography can reveal carryover of particles from laser ablation (LA) or of droplets into the ICP due to overly high liquid flow [74].

Analogous to ESI (Chap. 12), ion transfer into the mass analyzer is accomplished via a differentially pumped interface. A small portion of the plasma enters the first pumping stage through a hole in the center of the sampling cone. Water cooling of the sampling cone preserves its surface from rapid destruction due to the exposure to the hot plasma. Next, the ions are guided through the entrance of the skimmer by application of an electric potential, while most neutrals are pumped off the supersonic expansion in this region (Fig. 15.12). Analogous to early atmospheric pressure ion sources of organic MS, the first implementation of ICP-MS was attached to a quadrupole analyzer due to its acceptance of moderate vacuum conditions [21].

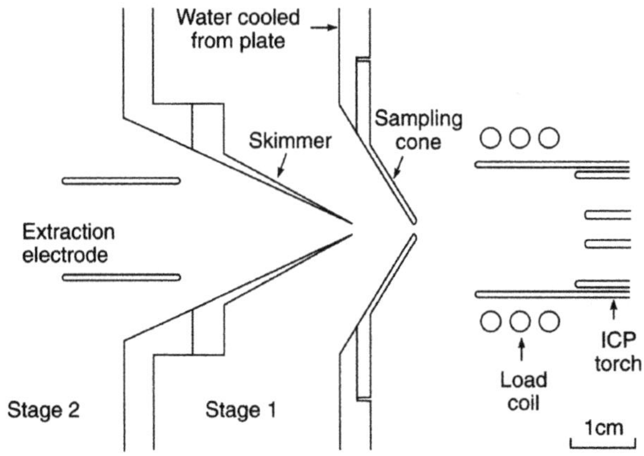

Fig. 15.12 Ion extraction interface for ICP-MS. Ions arrive from the right, a small portion is transmitted through the water-cooled sampling cone into the first pumping stage (rotary pump), the center of the free-jet expansion is then transmitted through the second skimmer cone, behind which it is guided by electric potentials through the second pumping stage (turbo pump) into the mass analyzer (Reprinted with permission from Ref. [3]. © John Wiley & Sons Ltd., 1997)

Nowadays, ICP sources are used with magnetic sector [13, 75], to an important extent time-of-flight (TOF) [76–81], and even Fourier transform ion cyclotron resonance (FT-ICR) mass analyzers [82].

The interest in high-resolution ICP instruments is driven by polyatomic interferences between the plasma gas and the matrix introduced, which are indeed limiting factors for ICP-QMS. Isobaric interferences are less problematic than it might appear on first sight, since most of the elements have more than two isotopes to select from. Anyway, none of the isobaric interferences can be resolved by the current sector or TOF mass spectrometers since they require a mass resolution above 12,000 [83].

Multicollector detection systems are an important feature of element MS instrumentation as simultaneous detection of all ions of interest provides the most accurate isotope ratios [84, 85]. The traditional approach employs multiple Faraday cups that can be adjusted along a sophisticated rail to collect a set of ions. A more recent ICP mass spectrometer allows ions along the 120-mm focal plane of a small Mattauch-Herzog geometry analyzer to be detected simultaneously. This is accomplished by use of a large direct charge semiconductor detector that provides 4800 channels covering the focal plane. Thus, 210 nuclides from ^{6}Li to ^{238}U can be monitored without scanning, i.e., at constant magnetic field [85]. The particular ICP mass spectrometer even relies on a permanent magnet and its ion optical path is complemented by a 127° electrostatic sector as pre-filter in front of the Mattauch-Herzog analyzer in order to prevent photons and neutrals from the ICP from entering the actual mass analyzer.

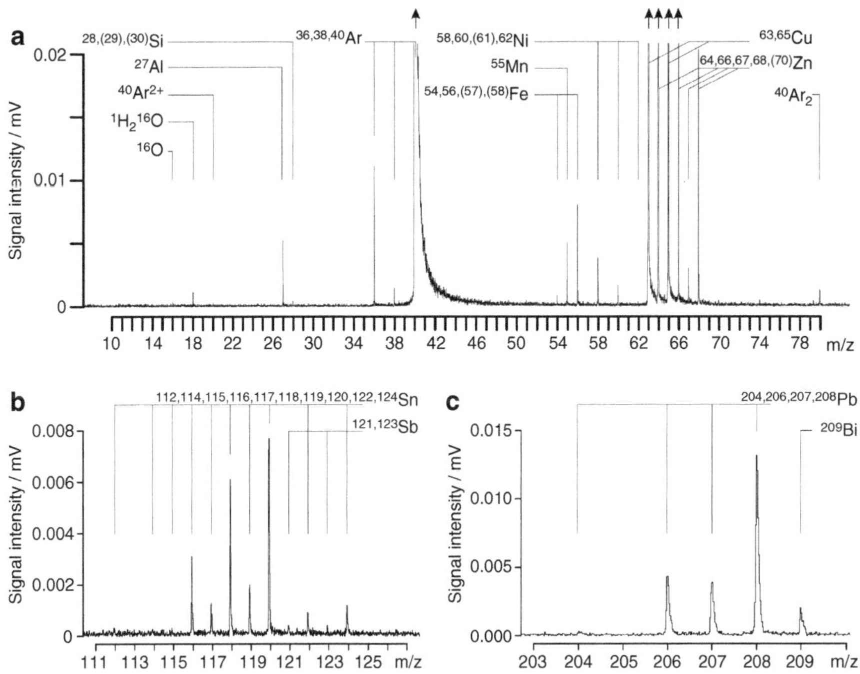

Fig. 15.13 The ICP-TOF mass spectrum of brass. The peaks due to N, O, H_2O, Ar^{2+}, Ar^+, and Ar_2^+ are present as a blank spectrum of the ICP. In range (**a**) up to *m/z* 80, Si, Mn, Fe, and Ni are detected at low levels while Cu and Zn are dominant as expected for brass. The sections (**b**) and (**c**) show overlapping signals from Sn and Sb as well as Pb and Bi, respectively (Adapted from Ref. [81] with permission. © Springer-Verlag, 2008)

Distinguished acronyms

In inorganic mass spectrometry, the type of mass analyzer occasionally becomes part of the acronym: a quadrupole leads to ICP-QMS, a magnetic sector field leads to ICP-SFMS, and use of a double-focusing analyzer may be indicated by ICP-DFMS, respectively. Thus, a time-of-flight analyzer attached to an ICP source would be referred to as ICP-TOFMS. Again, this is slightly different from the customs in organic and biomedical mass spectrometry where only TOF and FT-ICR tend to be included in the acronym and normally are separated by a hyphen from MS.

Liquid sample introduction is still the standard in ICP-MS. Consequently, the coupling of liquid chromatography or capillary electrophoresis to ICP instruments is straightforward. This way, not only the presence of an element in a sample can be detected, but also the assignment to molecular species becomes feasible. This explains the relevance of ICP-MS for the identification of non-C,H,N,O elements in proteins, i.e., for metallomics (cf. first two examples of this chapter).

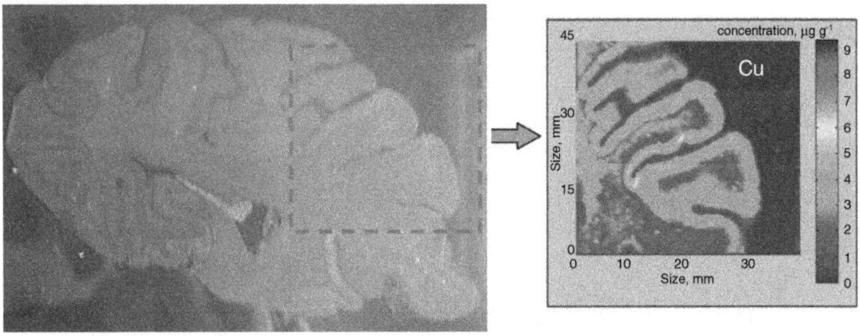

Fig. 15.14 Mass spectral imaging to unveil the quantitative distribution of Cu in tissue. The average concentration of Cu was 3–7 µg g^{-1} tissue. Light photograph of a thin tissue section of human brain (*left*) and the Cu distribution in the marked region as obtained by LA-ICP-MS (*right*) (Adapted from Ref. [18] with permission. © The Royal Society of Chemistry, 2007)

ICP-TOFMS of brass Three categories of signals are contributing to the ICP mass spectrum of brass. The background peaks due to $^{14}N^{+}$, $^{16}O^{+}$, $^{1}H_2{}^{16}O^{+\bullet}$, $^{40}Ar^{2+}$, $^{36,38,40}Ar^{+}$, and $^{40}Ar_2{}^{+}$ are contributions of the ICP background spectrum. Then, the polyisotopic elements Cu and Zn represent the main components of brass, and thus, cause strong peaks. Finally, Si, Mn, Fe, Ni, Sn, Sb, Pb, and Bi are present at low concentration (Fig. 15.13). Instead of nebulizing a solution of the alloy, in this particular case the brass has been fed into the ICP by in-torch laser ablation [81].

Need for sample preparation
ICP-MS is commonly mentioned in the context of high throughput and claimed to have no need for extensive sample preparation. In analytical practice, however, every sample needs to be treated individually; digestion prior to analysis usually takes about 2 h per sample. Furthermore, as is the case with TIMS for example, matrix separation is required for precise and accurate isotope ratio determinations. In particular, if MC-ICP-MS is going to be used as a complementary technique for TIMS, high throughput is only achieved on the expense of precision.

15.5.1 Laser Ablation ICP-MS

To further complement the sampling repertoire for ICP-MS, a gas stream, typically helium, may be employed to take up a laser-generated aerosol. This technique is known as *laser ablation* (LA) ICP-MS. Its first realization by the Hieftje group in

1996 [86] was based on the previously introduced ICP-TOF instrumentation [76–78]. LA-ICP-TOF-MS can be used for sampling from solid surfaces of bulk material, or alternatively, for imaging of element distributions. LA-ICP mass spectral imaging allows to monitor the lateral distribution of elements across a solid structure [87], to identify metals and metalloids on a 2D gel [88, 89], or to reveal element concentrations in biological tissues and similar samples (Fig. 15.14) [17, 18, 20, 89, 90].

15.6 Secondary Ion Mass Spectrometry

When a beam of (primary) ions possessing keV-energies strikes a surface, the energy transferred by the incident particles causes a collision cascade that sets several atomic layers in motion and is accompanied by complex processes of energy transfer and electronic interaction in the surface zone of the solid. It results in the emission of electrons, photons, atoms, and molecules, both of the latter either neutral or ionic, whereby the surface under bombardment experiences irreversible changes [91]. The ions that are emitted are termed *secondary ions* and the method is therefore called *secondary ion mass spectrometry* (SIMS). Nearly the same processes of sputtering and ion formation are effective in FAB and LSIMS (Chap. 10) [92], and in fact, SIMS paved the road for the development of FAB and LSIMS to analyze organic samples. Nonetheless, SIMS is not simply a precursor of FAB, but a reputable method of its own serving nicely for analyzing inorganic samples that range from rocks to alloys and semiconductors [93, 94].

The emission of secondary ions of both polarities from instrument construction materials produced as a by-product of ion source operation was first observed by Arnot [95, 96] and was developed into an analytical instrument by Herzog and Viebóck [97]. Inspired by these experiments, an early SIMS instrument was constructed in the 1960s to analyze lunar rocks from NASA's Apollo missions. Much of the breakthrough of SIMS for *i)* bulk analysis of solids, *ii)* depth profiling of thin layers, *iii)* imaging at high lateral resolution, and *iv)* monolayer analysis is also the merit of the Benninghoven group [91, 93, 98, 99].

15.6.1 Atomic SIMS

Applied to solid materials, especially semiconductors and thin films, SIMS can determine trace levels of all elements in the periodic table. Spatial microanalysis is provided by collimating the primary ion beam to about 1 μm in diameter and control of where the beam strikes the sample surface. This way, SIMS provides lateral and depth distributions of these elements within the sample. Currently, SIMS is being adapted to achieve lateral resolutions well below 100 nm. The driving force comes from the progress in microelectronics aiming at structures that approach 10 nm. Also, the depth resolution needs to come close to the atomic scale [100].

SIMS surface analysis is classified into two modes of operation, the so-called *static SIMS* and *dynamic SIMS* mode.

Static SIMS employs an extremely low sputtering rate, often with a pulsed primary ion beam, for better sensibility to the characteristics of the top monolayer and even may reveal molecular information (see below) [101]. In static SIMS, the primary ion dose is kept below 10^{12} ions s^{-1} cm^{-2}.

Dynamic SIMS uses high sputtering rates of a constant primary ion beam (10^{17} ions s^{-1} cm^{-2}) resulting in very high sensitivities to trace impurities (ppm to ppb). It delivers elemental and isotopic information as do the other methods of inorganic mass spectrometry. Magnetic sector or quadrupole mass analyzers are frequently in use for dynamic SIMS. Continuous analysis while sputtering yields information as a function of depth, called a *depth profile*.

Each impact an event of its own

A single sputtering event, i.e., penetration, lattice perturbation by impact cascades, and final particle ejection, takes less than 10^{-12} s. Interestingly, for primary ion beam densities $<10^{-6}$ A cm^{-2} (equal to 6×10^{12} ion s^{-1} cm^{-2}) no interference of processes caused by different primary ions will occur, because the maximum cross section of an impact is only in the order of 10 nm^2. In other words, each impact is independent of prior, subsequent, or nearby synchroneous hits [91, 92]. In the time domain this means that a given surface area suffers 10–100 hits min^{-1} in dynamic SIMS, but only 0.01–0.1 hits min^{-1} in static SIMS. For a monoatomic layer, observation times in the order of 1 h can thus be realized in static SIMS, i.e., the attribute *static* refers to the extended preservation of the surface.

15.6.2 Instrumentation for Atomic SIMS

The primary ions for SIMS are usually generated by either a thermal ionization source delivering Cs^+ ions or by a *duoplasmatron source*. Depending on its mode of operation, the duoplasmatron is working somewhere between electron ionization and a glow discharge. It can be used to generate a collimated beam of positive (Ar^+, O^+) as well as negative primary ions ($O_2^{-\bullet}$) [102, 103]. Positive oxygen ion bombardment increases the concentration of oxygen in the surface layer and creates M–O bonds there. Breaking these bonds during the process of bombardment and ion desorption builds up negative charge that is readily consumed by the oxygen because of its high electron affinity. Thus, more metal atoms remain positively charged. Strongly electropositive elements are therefore analyzed as positive secondary ions from oxygen bombardment for best sensitivity. Opposed to oxygen, cesium ions implanted into the sample surface reduce its work function, thereby providing more secondary electrons, which enable effective negative ion formation.

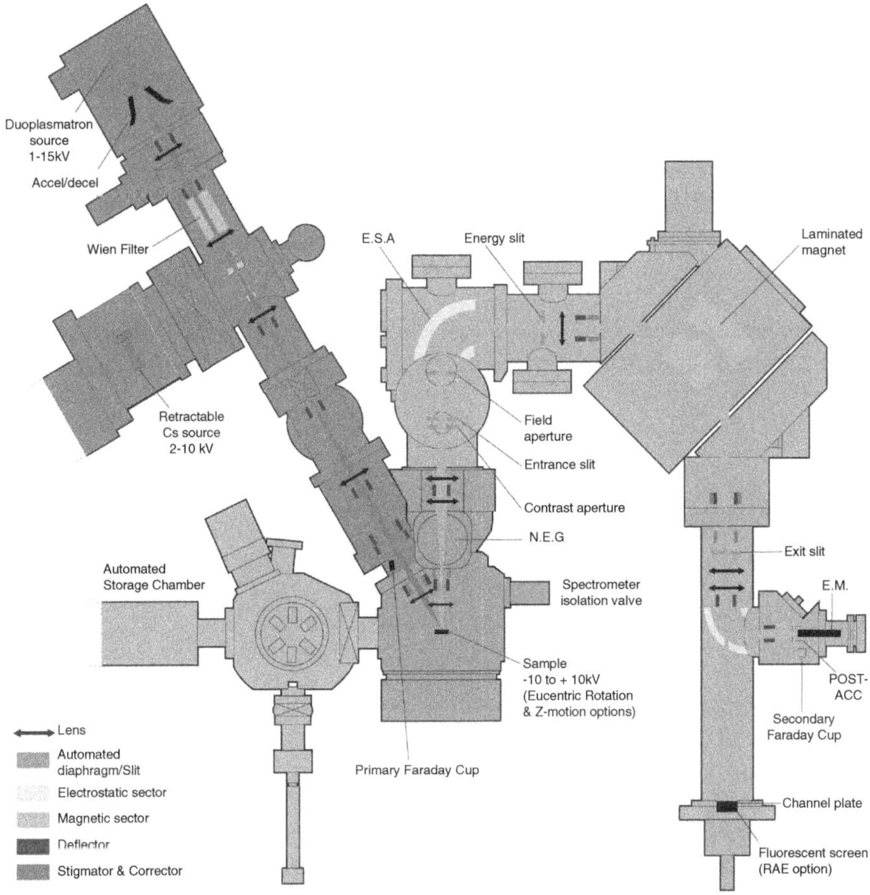

Fig. 15.15 Schematic of the CAMECA IMS 7f-Auto showing the main components of a high-resolution ion microprobe SIMS instrument. For flexibility the sample can be bombarded with either Cs^+ ions (by TI) or ions from a duoplasmatron source, which can deliver noble gas or oxygen ions. The double-focusing magnetic sector instrument of EB geometry offers high resolution and ion detection by either SEM, Faraday cup, or MCP (Reproduced from CAMECA technical literature with kind permission. © CAMECA Germany, 2016)

Consequently, semimetals and nonmetals as well as group VIII transition metals are preferably analyzed by Cs^+ bombardment as negative ions.

Another well-established class of primary ion sources are *liquid metal ion guns* (LMIG) delivering Ga^+ or In^+ ions. They offer very fine beams to achieve high lateral resolution. The Ga^+ LMIG currently provides the smallest probe size (less than 10 nm) with the highest current density (1–10 A cm^{-2}) of any ion gun. The LMIG normally consists of a field emitter tip coated with Ga from where a high electric field extracts Ga^+ ions. To ensure optimal focusing of the beam, the Ga^+ ions are accelerated by 20–60 kV (Fig. 15.15) [104].

Sputtering as a result of primary ion bombardment delivers diverse ion species ranging from monoatomic ions of various charge states to multi-atomic clusters and eventually simple molecular ions. Sputtering is generally accompanied by isotopic and chemical fractionation, i.e., the secondary ion yield is not independent of the material to be analyzed. SIMS produces spectra that are characterized by numerous interferences between different charge states of atomic ions and simple reaction products such as oxides, hydroxides, halides, etc. As with any other elemental MS technique before, high-resolution instruments provide the most effective and reliable means of dealing with superimposing isobars.

Ions generated by SIMS The positive secondary ion spectrum of a silicon surface shows peaks that can be assigned to Si^{2+}, Si^+, Si_2^+, Si_3^+, Si_4^+, etc. while the negative secondary ion spectrum yields signals corresponding to Si^-, Si_2^-, Si_3^-, and Si_4^-. In case of a two-component lattice such as a metal (M) oxide, SIMS will deliver positive ions of the type $[M_nO_{n-1}]^{x+}$ (normally $x = 1$) and negative ions of the general type $[M_{n-1}O_n]^-$. The number ratios of M and O will naturally depend on the metals' prevailing oxidation state. Accordingly, more complex systems result in additional cluster ion compositions. SIMS of salts preferably yields the cation or anion and corresponding cluster ion series as already mentioned for FD, FAB, or ESI (Chaps. 8, 10, and 12, respectively) [91, 98, 99].

15.6.3 Molecular SIMS

Static SIMS, i.e., conditions of low primary ion flux, can preserve molecular information, but this is effected at the expense of correspondingly low secondary ion yields. The combination of static SIMS conditions with scanning mass analyzers is therefore disadvantageous and the outcome of experiments with SIMS for organic molecules such as amino acids in the "pre-FAB era" was not too exciting [101]. Here again, the TOF analyzer plays to its strength as it is capable of analyzing all ions contained in a package created by a short primary ion pulse. As only few ions are lost (due to imperfect transmission) there is a more than 1000-fold gain in sensitivity when using a TOF rather than a quadrupole analyzer [105].

The first TOF-SIMS instrument [106] employed a pulsed alkali primary ion source. The primary ions were created from alkali aluminosilicate by thermionic emission, accelerated by up to 25 keV and focused onto the monomolecular sample layer on gold or silver surfaces in bursts of 5–50 ns. (This type of Cs^+ primary ion sources is still in use for LSIMS.) Useful spectra of amino acids and nucleosides [106, 107] and even peptides [108] were obtained in this way. Soon, TOF-SIMS became a major competitor of PD-MS [109–111] and the development of FAB and LSIMS led to fruitful approaches such as TOF-LSIMS [112].

Modern TOF-SIMS applications are often in the field of synthetic polymer analysis, but rarely for the determination of molecular weight distributions which is the domain of MALDI. More frequently, low-molecular-weight additives or surface modifications are analyzed as there is no interference with a matrix as

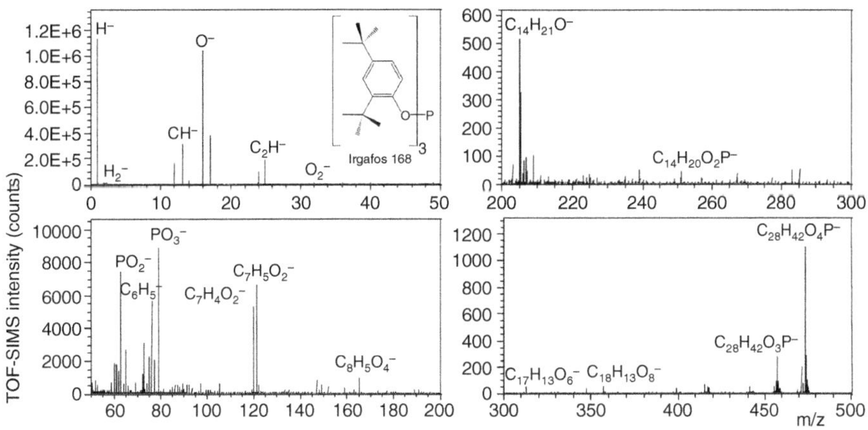

Fig. 15.16 Negative-ion TOF-SIMS analysis of Irgafos 168 on PETi. The compound undergoes significant fragmentation, and thus, no $[M–H]^-$ peak (*m/z* 645) is included. Note the tremendously decreasing ion abundances with rising *m/z*, which is also the reason for the segmented representation of the mass spectrum (Reproduced from Ref. [117] with permission. © John Wiley & Sons, Ltd., 2002)

would be the case with MALDI [113–117]. In essence, only SIMS can truly analyze the native surface.

Polymer additives by SIMS Additives are intentionally added to a polymer to stabilize or improve different polymer properties. They act as antioxidants, UV stabilizers, antistatic agents, flame retardants, etc. However, their migration towards the surface may result in blooming, thereby negatively affecting surface properties that are required for specific applications. TOF-SIMS is ideally suited to characterize surface compositions because it offers molecular information on the uppermost monolayers at high sensitivity. Here, the antioxidant Irgafos 168 (0.3 wt.%) has been analyzed on the copolymer PETi, a poly(ethylene terephthalate (60%) isophthalate (40%)) (Fig. 15.16) [117].

15.6.4 Polyatomic Primary Ion Beams

More recently, SIMS has gained enormous impetus from the introduction of heavy primary ion beams such as gold [118] or bismuth clusters [119–121] or fullerene molecular ions [27, 122–124]. Especially their combination with TOF-SIMS instrumentation has rejuvenated the whole field of SIMS. As we already know from FAB and LSIMS, and as has been veryfied also for SIMS [125], higher-mass xenon beams create a higher yield of secondary ions and are more effective for larger molecules than argon or neon, for example. Before the advent of heavy primary ion sources, the ions which could be detected by TOF-SIMS were limited to a mass range of about 300 u mainly because the primary ions where very inefficient in desorbing larger molecular species. With polyatomic primary ion beams the secondary ion emission is drastically enhanced while the surface damage is not as severe [126]. Polyatomic primary ion beams can effectively cover the range up to *m/z* 1500 at lateral resolutions in the order of 1 μm.

Experiments and molecular dynamics theory suggest that the efficient ionization of large molecular species requires the concerted action of a number of collision cascades. Atomic primary particles focus the energy deposition in a very small area but quite deep into the solid. Polyatomic primary ions, on the other side, break apart upon collision with the surface, this way creating numerous weaker impacts over a wider range [123]. The concerted action of a number of soft impacts can effect the desorption of the molecule [105]. Molecular dynamics simulations suggest that an acoustic wave is generated that essentially pushes the secondary ions off the surface. Especially fullerene ion sources ($C_{60}^{+\bullet}$ primary ions [105]) lead to energy deposition in the uppermost sample layers.

Surfactins from *Bacillus subtilis* Even with the advent of cluster ion sources, TOF-SIMS imaging favors hydrophobic molecules. Surfactins are a family of heptacyclodepsipeptides where the C-terminal carbonyl is linked with the β-hydroxy group of a fatty acid that is acylating the N-terminal function of a glutamic acid residue. The fatty acyl chain is 12–16 carbon atoms long. These compounds are secreted by the Gram-positive bacterium *Bacillus subtilis* and play an important role in the formation of dendritic patterns. Mapping of these surfactins by TOF–SIMS imaging showed that they were mainly located in the central mother colony, in a 'ring' surrounding the pattern and along the edges of the dendrites (Fig. 15.17). Surfactins with shorter chain lengths are found in the interior of the dendrites, whereas surfactins with longer fatty acyl chain lengths were found in the ring surrounding the swarm community [126].

Data handling and storage

Mass spectral imaging creates sort of a "chemical map" filled with enormous amounts of data. A standard image of 256 × 256 pixels requires 65,536 mass spectra each possessing about 10^5 data points. Therefore, effective software tools for data evaluation, representation, and eventually compression for long-term storage are necessary to deal with those gigabytes of data.

The future for SIMS seems bright and promising. From a seemingly disappearing technology at the very beginning of this millennium [27], it has stood up to deliver impressing results such as the imaging of bones, tissues, and even single cells [25, 27, 121, 123, 127, 128]. Advanced sample preparation techniques such as cryofreezing of tissues open up the new capabilities of holding these samples under low vacuum conditions for the time span of the experiment.

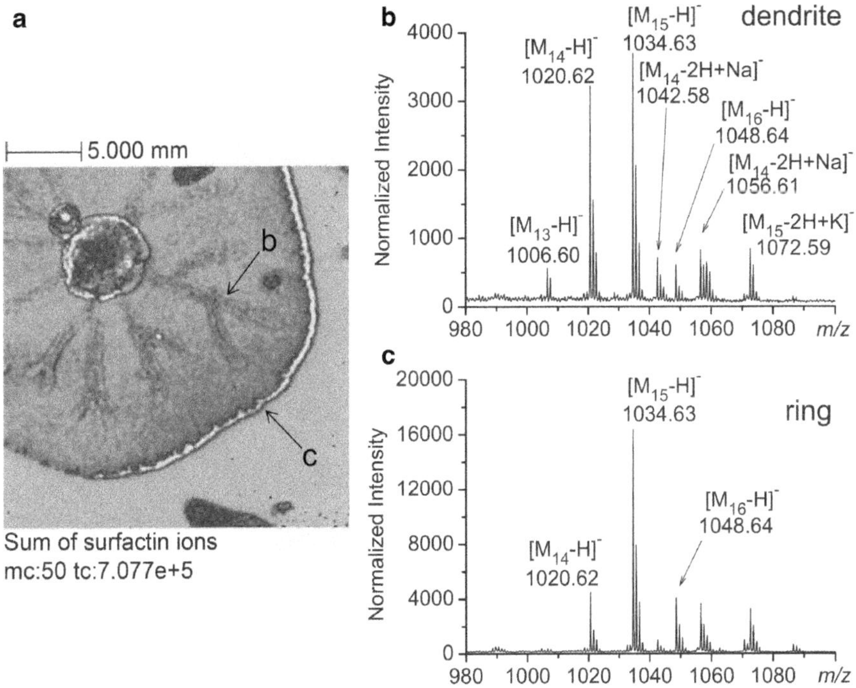

Fig. 15.17 (**a**) TOF-SIMS image of the sum of surfactin ions at the surface of a *Bacillus subtilis* swarming community. The maximal number of counts in a pixel (mc) and the total number of counts (tc) are indicated below the image. Field of view 23 × 23 mm^2, 256 × 256 pixels, pixel size 90 μm, Bi_3^+ primary ion fluence 1 × 10^9 ions cm^{-2}. (**b**) Partial mass spectrum obtained from a region of interest drawn around a dendrite. (**c**) Partial mass spectrum obtained from a region of interest drawn around the ring. M_n refers to compounds possessing an alkyl chain being n carbon atoms long (Adapted from Ref. [126] with permission. © Springer-Verlag 2009)

Recently, MALDI and SIMS imaging are seen as complementary techniques to assess complex biological systems [26]. While MALDI can deliver information on peptides, proteins, oligosaccharides, and other high-mass constituents, TOF-SIMS is the tool of choice for the analysis of lipids, unaltered surfaces, and extremely fine structures [26, 28, 104, 124, 126]. The imaging community is now also using common instrumentation such as a SIMS/ESI/MALDI quadrupole-TOF instrument [129].

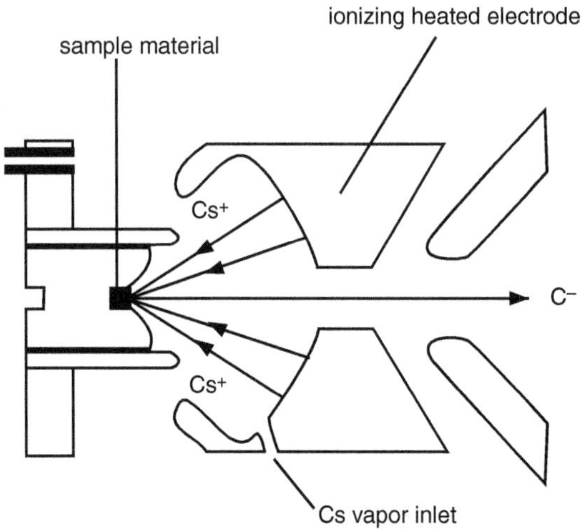

Fig. 15.18 High-intensity Cs sputter source for AMS. Cs^+ ions are created by thermal ionization of Cs vapor on a large heated tantalum anode that is placed over the sample like a dome. Secondary (analyte) ions exit through an axial aperture. Having the sample at negative high voltage accelerates the Cs^+ ions away from the anode to bombard the sample and also forces the analyte anions out of the source (Reproduced from Ref. [130] with permission. © Wiley Periodicals Inc., 2008)

15.7 Accelerator Mass Spectrometry

15.7.1 AMS Experimental Setup

The methodology of *accelerator mass spectrometry* (AMS) clearly differs from all other approaches to analyzing of atomic mass so far referred to in this book [4, 130]. While ions to be analyzed by a quadrupole analyzer are injected at kinetic energies of about 10 eV, those for a sector instrument at 5–10 keV, and those for TOFs at 15–30 keV, in AMS ions have several MeV. Another unique and key feature of the technique is that the ions experience dramatic changes in kinetic energy and charge state during the experiment.

To achieve this, the accelerator mass spectrometer consists of several stages. First, negative secondary ions of the sample are created by Cs^+ ion bombardment (Fig. 15.18). The primary step of mass analysis is conducted in a more-or-less conventional double-focusing magnetic sector unit. Mass-selected ions are then passed into a linear *Van de Graaff accelerator* or a *tandem accelerator*. These devices are frequent in nuclear physics. In a tandem accelerator, negative ions are attracted by high positive voltage, V_a, towards the high voltage terminal in the center of the vessel. An ion with z_1 elementary charges e has a charge $q = z_1e$ and by the accelerator therefore receives an additional kinetic energy of $E_a = z_1eV_a$. This ion is then passed through a so-called (charge) *stripper*. Two types of charge

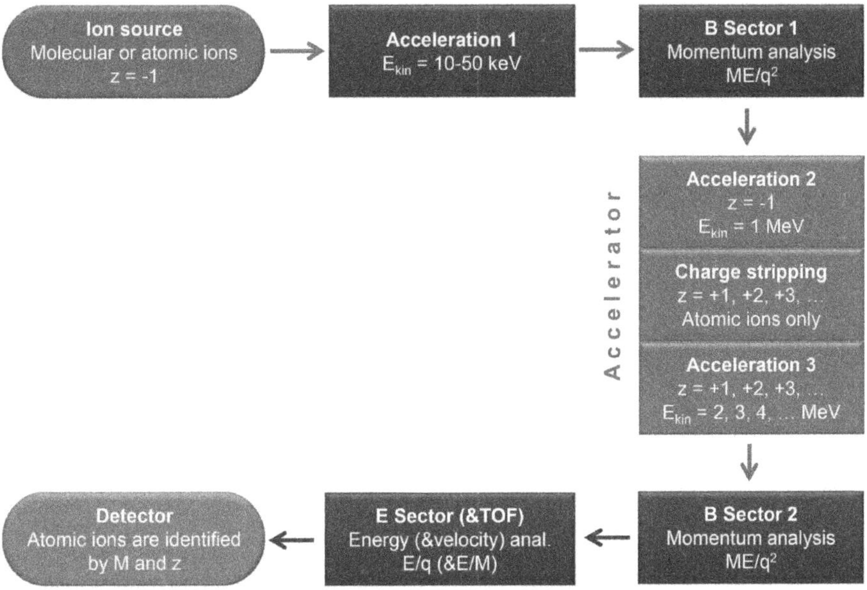

Fig. 15.19 Sequence of events and general experimental setup of AMS [4]. The instrument consists of a medium ion kinetic energy section, an ion accelerator, and a high-energy section to detect multiply charged atomic ions at highest sensitivity and specificity

stripping devices are in use: *i)* foil strippers, where the beam is shot through a thin carbon foil, and *ii)* gas strippers, essentially gas collision cells. Both serve to strip off all electrons from the anion, thereby converting it into a multiply charged positive ion, i.e., $q = -z_2e$. This extreme degree of charge inversion is the main purpose of the high collision energy – a very welcome side effect being the highly effective ion counting in the detector. The atomic cations are then pushed away from the high voltage terminal towards the exit of the accelerator on its opposite side. Due to their individual charge states the multiply charged positive ions gather different amounts of kinetic energy on the second stage of acceleration. After having passed the accelerator, the total kinetic energy received is given by $E_a = V_a \times (z_1e + z_2e)$. They are then separated according to their momentum, charge, and energy, and finally counted individually. This second unit also represents a sort of large magnetic sector instrument but it may have additional components such as a TOF analyzer for ion velocity analysis (Fig. 15.19) [4].

15.7.2 AMS Facilities

In particular, due to the accelerator, the classical AMS facility requires an area of some hundred square meters for instrumentation (Fig. 15.20). In recent years, the increasing demand for AMS measurements has led to the design of significantly smaller AMS instruments for dedicated purposes; this "miniaturization" has much

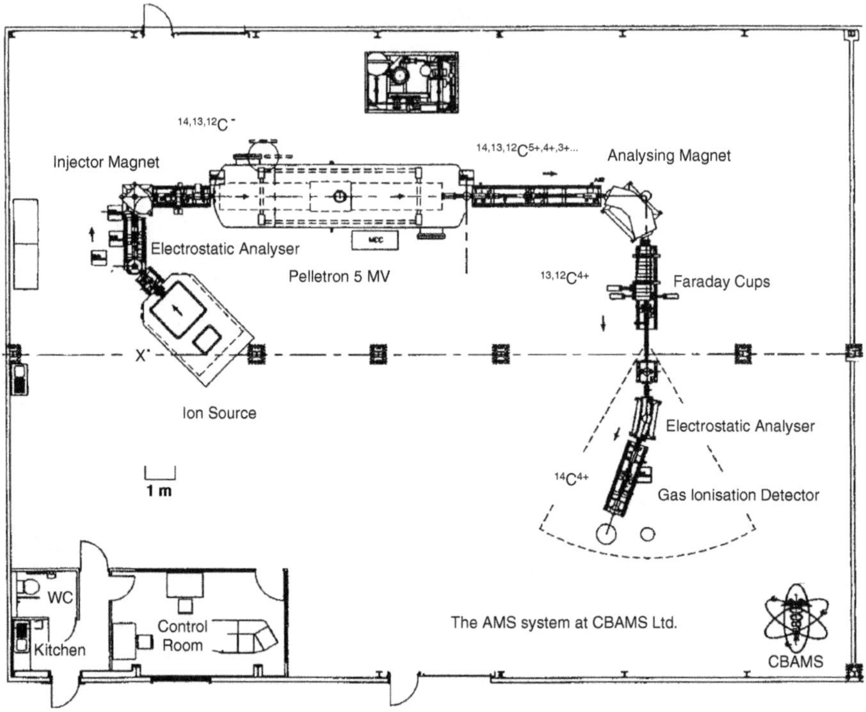

Fig. 15.20 AMS facility of CBAMS. The instrument is typical for its kind. Note the scale bar for 1 m. CBAMS, founded in 1997, is the first private company in the world to offer a fully commercial analytical service using an accelerator mass spectrometer (Reproduced from Ref. [14] with permission. © John Wiley & Sons, Ltd., 1999)

been driven by Suter in Zurich [131–133]. The concise review by Hellborg and Skog is recommended for further readings [130].

15.7.3 Applications of AMS

The great advantage of these MeV-energies is that they are able to help avoiding ambiguities in identification of atomic ions, because eventually interfering molecular species are completely destroyed at the stage of the charge stripper. Furthermore, selection of a suitable high charge state characteristic of the isotope to be analyzed allows to unequivocally identify the species. For example, the nuclei of ^{14}C, ^{26}Al, and ^{129}I are free of superimpositions from isobaric ^{14}N, ^{26}Mg, and ^{129}Xe, because the negative ions of the latter are unstable.

AMS is an extremely sensitive technique for isotopic analysis, in particular for measuring isotope ratios over an extreme dynamic range. For some elements such as carbon, isotope ratios of as low as 1 in 10^{15} can be determined. This is by a factor of 10^5 lower than by any other MS technique [4]. Moreover, about 1 mg of sample is sufficient for AMS, which is equivalent to a content of only about 10^6 atoms of the isotope of interest. Thus, AMS is ideally suited for isotope ratio measurements of low-abundant isotopes, especially those having too long half-lives for determining radioactive decay from small sample amounts such as carbon-14. In fact, carbon-14 dating led to AMS [134, 135] and is still applied in various ways [14, 130, 136]. AMS is nowadays also employed for determination of isotopes such as ^{10}B, ^{26}Al, ^{36}Cl, ^{41}Ca, ^{129}I and others including stable isotopes. The versatility of AMS has led to impressing applications in the life sciences, geosciences, archeology, and extraterrestrial research [15, 19, 130, 137–139].

AMS wins over radioactive counting To illustrate the capabilities of AMS, we compare carbon-14 determination by radioactive counting to AMS. A sample of 1 g of environmental carbon contains 6×10^{10} atoms of ^{14}C (and 1.2×10^{12} times more ^{12}C atoms). Due to the 5730 years half-life of ^{14}C, only 13 atoms will decay per minute. For a statistical precision of 0.5% as normally required in radiocarbon dating, decays from 1 g of carbon need to be counted for more than 48 h. AMS does not have to wait for the decays, it is more efficient because it uses the whole sample. A sample of 1 mg carbon, only one thousandth of the material needed for decay counting, is completely sputtered in the ion source within 1–2 h and delivers about 6×10^5 atoms, which is 1% of the total ^{14}C content, to the AMS detector system. Conventional mass spectrometers cannot be used here, because the ^{14}C ions are superimposed by atomic and molecular isobars that are by orders of magnitude more abundant. These are $^{14}N^+$ and small fragments such as $^{13}CH^+$, $^{12}CH_2^{+\bullet}$, $^{12}CD^+$, and $^7Li_2^+$. Abundance sensitivity also plays a role by limiting the ^{14}C detection due to minor overlap with stretching peak bases from ^{12}C and ^{13}C. Conventional MS is therefore limited to isotope ratios of $^{14}C/^{12}C$ of approximately 10^{-7} at best. AMS achieves $^{14}C/^{12}C$ detection down to approximately 10^{-15}.

15.8 Summary

Concept of Inorganic Mass Spectrometry

Inorganic mass spectrometry or element mass spectrometry are collective terms for the field of MS aiming at the analysis of the elemental composition of a sample, the detection of trace elements or trace isotopes, and the determination of isotope ratios.

Instrumentation

Instrumentation of inorganic MS varies widely. It ranges from dedicated instruments in stable isotope ratio analysis to highly versatile secondary ion mass spectrometers that can be adapted to deliver the bulk composition of samples – even some molecular information – or even to provide images in terms of lateral distributions of elements. Magnetic sector mass analyzers, single-focusing as well as double focusing, play an important role while quadrupole and time-to-flight instrumentation only account for a small fraction of instruments. Accelerator mass spectrometers, presumably the most exotic instruments, are a class of their own.

Ionization

Mostly, ionization conditions are harsh and simultaneously break up all molecular entities. Thus, atomic ions are delivered for elemental analysis. While some techniques only suffer from isobaric interferences of isotopes belonging to different elements, others may also be complicated by some molecular interferences. Especially plasma-based methods like GD-MS and ICP-MS are prone to formation of diatomic ions, mostly of the plasma gas, that may superimpose on atomic ions of the analyte.

Applications

In the past, the methodology has focused on metals, semiconductors, minerals, and gases. Element MS thus plays a major role in geological research, materials science, metallurgy, fabrication of electronic devices, oceanology, and climate studies, for example. Trace elemental analysis can reveal the geographical origin of a sample and isotope ratios may do the same. Also, isotope ratios can be used for determining the age of a sample, either of artwork or a prehistoric relic such as wood or bones of a dinosaur buried under sediment.

In the twenty-first century, samples of biological origin have gained relevance, especially as the combination of element MS and biomedical MS allows for the speciation, i.e., the assignment of elements to a specific molecule, typically a metal or semimetal to a certain protein.

Conclusion and Outlook

Mass spectrometry is no longer just organic, inorganic, physicochemical, biomedical, or environmental. On the contrary, mass spectrometry comprises a large number of facets and applications. The success of LA-ICP-MS, TOF-SIMS with polyatomic primary ion beams, and AMS in both the biomedical and the geological field marvelously exemplifies how a certain methodology can bridge the gap between extremes. The exploration of increasingly complex systems from cells and tissues to soils, ocean waters, and the atmosphere demands for the joint use of all techniques that enable crossing of interdisciplinary boundaries.

While working as a mass spectrometrist is necessarily correlated to a certain field of personal expertise, one should also be aware – at least to the degree of a good educational background in mass spectrometry – of the entire spectrum of this impressively versatile method – mass spectrometry, a domain of science in itself.

References

1. de Laeter JR, Kurz MD (2006) Alfred Nier and the Sector Field Mass Spectrometer. J Mass Spectrom 41:847–854. doi:10.1002/jms.1057

2. Budzikiewicz H, Grigsby RD (2006) Mass Spectrometry and Isotopes: A Century of Research and Discussion. Mass Spectrom Rev 25:146–157. doi:10.1002/mas.20061
3. Platzner IT, Habfast K, Walder AJ, Goetz APlatzner IT (eds) (1997) Modern Isotope Ratio Mass Spectrometry. Wiley, Chichester
4. Tuniz C, Bird JR, Fink D, Herzog GF (1998) Accelerator Mass Spectrometry – Ultrasensitive Analysis for Global Science. CRC Press, Boca Raton
5. Taylor HE (2000) Inductively Coupled Plasma Mass Spectroscopy. Academic Press, London
6. de Laeter JR (2001) Applications of Inorganic Mass Spectrometry. John Wiley & Sons, New York
7. Becker JS (2008) Inorganic Mass Spectrometry: Principles and Applications. John Wiley & Sons, Chichester
8. Prohaska T, Irrgeher J, Zitek A, Jakubowski N (eds) (2015) Sector Field Mass Spectrometry for Elemental and Isotopic Analysis. Royal Society of Chemistry, Cambridge
9. Douthitt CB (2008) Commercial Development of HR-ICPMS, MC-ICPMS and HR-GDMS. J Anal At Spectrom 23:685–689. doi:10.1039/B800341F
10. Hieftje GM (2008) Emergence and Impact of Alternative Sources and Mass Analyzers in Plasma Source Mass Spectrometry. J Anal At Spectrom 23:661–672. doi:10.1039/B717319A
11. de Laeter JR, De Bièvre P, Peiser HS (1992) Isotope Mass Spectrometry in Metrology. Mass Spectrom Rev 11:193–245. doi:10.1002/mas.1280110303
12. Ma R, Staton I, McLeod CW, Gomez MB, Gomez MM, Palacios MA (2001) Assessment of Airborne Platinum Contamination via ICP-Mass Spectrometric Analysis of Tree Bark. J Anal At Spectrom 16:1070–1075. doi:10.1039/B102940C
13. Stuewer D, Jakubowski N (1998) Elemental Analysis by Inductively Coupled Plasma Mass Spectrometry with Sector Field Instruments: A Progress Report. J Mass Spectrom 33:579–590. doi:10.1002/(SICI)1096-9888(199807)33:7<579::AID-JMS688>3.0.CO;2-W
14. Barker J, Garner RC (1999) Biomedical Applications of Accelerator Mass Spectrometry-Isotope Measurements at the Level of the Atom. Rapid Commun Mass Spectrom 13:285–293. doi:10.1002/(SICI)1097-0231(19990228)13:4<285::AID-RCM469>3.0.CO;2-R
15. Kutschera W (2005) Progress in Isotope Analysis at Ultra-Trace Level by AMS. Int J Mass Spectrom 242:145–160. doi:10.1016/j.ijms.2004.10.029
16. Becker JS, Zoriy M, Becker JS, Pickhardt C, Przybylski M (2004) Determination of Phosphorus and Metals in Human Brain Proteins After Isolation by Gel Electrophoresis by Laser Ablation Inductively Coupled Plasma Source Mass Spectrometry. J Anal At Spectrom 19:149–152. doi:10.1039/B311274H
17. Guenther D, Hattendorf B (2005) Solid Sample Analysis Using Laser Ablation Inductively Coupled Plasma Mass Spectrometry. Trends Anal Chem 24:255–265. doi:10.1016/j.trac.2004.11.017
18. Becker JS, Zoriy M, Becker JS, Dobrowolska J, Matusch A (2007) Laser Ablation Inductively Coupled Plasma Mass Spectrometry (LA-ICP-MS) in Elemental Imaging of Biological Tissues and in Proteomics. J Anal At Spectrom 22:736–744. doi:10.1039/B701558E
19. Cheah ELC, Koh HL (2008) Biomedical Applications of Accelerator Mass Spectrometry. Curr Anal Chem 4:102–110. doi:10.2174/157341108784587786
20. Becker JS, Matusch A, Wu B (2014) ioimaging Mass Spectrometry of Trace Elements – Recent Advance and Applications of LA-ICP-MS: A Review. Anal Chim Acta 835:1–18. doi:10.1016/j.aca.2014.04.048
21. Houk RS, Fassel VA, Flesch GD, Svec HJ, Gray AL, Taylor CE (1980) Inductively Coupled Argon Plasma as an Ion Source for Mass Spectrometric Determination of Trace Elements. Anal Chem 52:2283–2289. doi:10.1021/ac50064a012
22. Szpunar J (2004) Metallomics: A New Frontier in Analytical Chemistry. Anal Bioanal Chem 378:54–56. doi:10.1007/s00216-003-2333-z
23. Lobinski R, Schaumlöffel D, Szpunar J (2006) Mass Spectrometry in Bioinorganic Analytical Chemistry. Mass Spectrom Rev 25:255–289. doi:10.1002/mas.20069

24. Swart C, Jakubowski N (2016) Update on the Status of Metrology for Metalloproteins. J Anal At Spectrom 31:1756–1765. doi:10.1039/c6ja00181e
25. Walker AV (2008) Why Is SIMS Underused in Chemical and Biological Analysis? Challenges and Opportunities. Anal Chem 80:8865–8870. doi:10.1021/ac8013687
26. Cassiday L (2008) SIMS and MALDI: Better Together. Anal Chem 80:8860. doi:10.1021/ac8021828
27. Griffiths J (2008) Secondary Ion Mass Spectrometry. Anal Chem 80:7194–7197. doi:10.1021/ac801528u
28. McDonnell LA, Heeren RMA (2007) Imaging Mass Spectrometry. Mass Spectrom Rev 26:606–643. doi:10.1002/mas.20124
29. Adams F, Vertes A (1990) Inorganic Mass Spectrometry of Solid Samples. Fresenius J Anal Chem 337:638–647. doi:10.1007/BF00323098
30. Tanner SD, Baranov VI, Bandura DR (2002) Reaction Cells and Collision Cells for ICP-MS: a Tutorial Review. Spectrochim Acta, Part B 57B:1361–1452. doi:10.1016/S0584-8547(02)00069-1
31. Koppenaal DW, Eiden GC, Barinaga CJ (2004) Collision and Reaction Cells in Atomic Mass Spectrometry: Development, Status, and Applications. J Anal At Spectrom 19:561–570. doi:10.1039/B403510K
32. Becker JS, Dietze HJ (2000) Inorganic Mass Spectrometric Methods for Trace, Ultratrace, Isotope, and Surface Analysis. Int J Mass Spectrom 197:1–35. doi:10.1016/S1387-3806(99)00246-8
33. Richter S, Goldberg SA (2003) Improved Techniques for High Accuracy Isotope Ratio Measurements of Nuclear Materials Using Thermal Ionization Mass Spectrometry. Int J Mass Spectrom 229:181–197. doi:10.1016/S1387-3806(03)00338-5
34. Encinar JR, Ouerdane L, Buchmann W, Tortajada J, Lobinski R, Szpunar J (2003) Identification of Water-Soluble Selenium-Containing Proteins in Selenized Yeast by Size-Exclusion-Reversed-Phase HPLC-ICP-MS Followed by MALDI-TOF and Electrospray Q-TOF Mass Spectrometry. Anal Chem 75:3765–3774. doi:10.1021/ac034103m
35. Halas S, Durakiewicz T (1998) Filament Temperature Stabilizer for a Thermal Ionization Mass Spectrometer. Int J Mass Spectrom 181:167–171. doi:10.1016/S1387-3806(98)14186-6
36. Kawano H, Page FM (1983) Experimental Methods and Techniques for Negative-Ion Production by Surface Ionization. Part I. Fundamental Aspects of Surface Ionization. Int J Mass Spectrom Ion Phys 50:1–33. doi:10.1016/0020-7381(83)80001-1
37. Kawano H, Hidaka Y, Page FM (1983) Experimental Methods and Techniques for Negative-Ion Production by Surface Ionization. Part II. Instrumentation and Operation. Int J Mass Spectrom Ion Phys 50:35–75. doi:10.1016/0020-7381(83)80002-3
38. Heumann KG, Schindlmeier W, Zeininger H, Schmidt M (1985) Application of an Economical and Small Thermal Ionization Mass Spectrometer for Accurate Anion Trace Analyses. Fresenius Z Anal Chem 320:457–462. doi:10.1007/BF00479812
39. Heumann KG, Kastenmayer P, Zeininger H (1981) Lead and Thallium Trace Determination in the ppm and ppb Range in Biological Material by Mass Spectrometric Isotope Dilution Analysis. Fresenius Z Anal Chem 306:173–177. doi:10.1007/BF00482091
40. Waidmann E, Emons H, Duerbeck HW (1994) Trace Determination of Tl, Cu, Pb, Cd, and Zn in Specimens of the Limnic Environment Using Isotope Dilution Mass Spectrometry with Thermal Ionization. Fresenius J Anal Chem 350:293–297. doi:10.1007/BF00322485
41. Schade U, Stoll R, Röllgen FW (1983) Thermal Surface Ionization Mass Spectrometry of Organic Salts. Int J Mass Spectrom Ion Phys 46:337–340. doi:10.1016/0020-7381(83)80121-1
42. Moens L (1997) Applications of Mass Spectrometry in the Trace Element Analysis of Biological Materials. Fresenius J Anal Chem 359:309–316. doi:10.1007/s002160050579
43. Koppenaal DW (1990) Atomic Mass Spectrometry. Anal Chem 62:303R–324R. doi:10.1021/ac00211a015

44. Verlinden J, Gijbels R, Adams F (1986) Application of Spark-Source Mass Spectrometry in the Analysis of Semiconductor Materials. A Review. J Anal At Spectrom 1:411–419. doi:10.1039/JA9860100411
45. Jochum KP (1997) Elemental analysis by spark source mass spectrometry. In: Gill R (ed) Modern Analytical Geochemistry. Addison Wesley/Longman, Harlow
46. Jochum KP, Stoll B, Pfänder JA, Seufert M, Flanz M, Maissenbacher P, Hofmann M, Hofmann AW (2001) Progress in Multi-Ion Counting Spark-Source Mass Spectrometry (MIC-SSMS) for the Analysis of Geological Samples. Fresenius J Anal Chem 370:647–653. doi:10.1007/s002160100786
47. Saprykin AI, Becker JS, Dietze HJ (1999) Investigation of the Analytical Performance of Gliding Spark Source Mass Spectrometry (GSSMS) for the Trace Analysis of Nonconducting Materials. Fresenius J Anal Chem 364:763–767. doi:10.1007/s002160051429
48. Hoffmann V, Kasik M, Robinson PK, Venzago C (2005) Glow Discharge Mass Spectrometry. Anal Bioanal Chem 381:173–188. doi:10.1007/s00216-004-2933-2
49. Wiedemann B, Alt HC, Meyer JD, Michelmann RW, Bethge K (1999) Spark Source Mass Spectrometric Calibration of the Local Vibrational Mode Absorption of Carbon in Gallium Arsenide on Arsenic Sublattice Sites. Fresenius J Anal Chem 364:768–771. doi:10.1007/s002160051430
50. Gijbels R, Bogaerts A (1997) Recent Trends in Solid Mass Spectrometry. GDMS and Other Methods. Fresenius J Anal Chem 359:326–330. doi:10.1007/s002160050581
51. Stuewer D (1990) Glow Discharge Mass Spectrometry – A Versatile Tool for Elemental Analysis. Fresenius J Anal Chem 337:737–742. doi:10.1007/BF00322247
52. Marcus RK, King FL Jr, Harrison WW (1986) Hollow Cathode Plume as an Atomization/Ionization Source for Solids Mass Spectrometry. Anal Chem 58:972–974. doi:10.1021/ac00295a067
53. Harrison WW, Hess KR, Marcus RK, King FL (1986) Glow Discharge Mass Spectrometry. Anal Chem 58: 341A–342A, 344A, 346A, 348A, 350A, 352A. doi: 10.1021/ac00293a002
54. Duckworth DC, Marcus RK (1989) Radio Frequency Powered Glow Discharge Atomization/Ionization Source for Solids Mass Spectrometry. Anal Chem 61:1879–1886. doi:10.1021/ac00192a020
55. Marcus RK (1994) Radiofrequency Powered Glow Discharges for Emission and Mass Spectrometry: Operating Characteristics, Figures of Merit and Future Prospects. J Anal At Spectrom 9:1029–1037. doi:10.1039/JA9940901029
56. Marcus RK (1996) Radiofrequency Powered Glow Discharges: Opportunities and Challenges. Plenary Lecture. J Anal At Spectrom 11:821–828. doi:10.1039/JA9961100821
57. Jakubowski N, Prohaska T, Rottmann L, Vanhaecke F (2011) Inductively Coupled Plasma- and Glow Discharge Plasma-Sector Field Mass Spectrometry, Part I. Tutorial: Fundamentals and Instrumentation. J Anal At Spectrom 26:693–726. doi:10.1039/c0ja00161a
58. Jakubowski N, Prohaska T, Vanhaecke F, Roos PH, Lindemann T (2011) Inductively Coupled Plasma- and Glow Discharge Plasma-Sector Field Mass Spectrometry, Part II. Applications. J Anal At Spectrom 26:727–757. doi:10.1039/c0ja00007h
59. Harrison WW, Klingler JA, Ratliff PH, Mei Y, Barshick CM (1990) Glow Discharge Techniques in Analytical Chemistry. Anal Chem 62:943A–949A. doi:10.1021/ac00217a001
60. King FL, Harrison WW (1990) Glow Discharge Mass Spectrometry: an Introduction to the Technique and Its Utility. Mass Spectrom Rev 9:285–317. doi:10.1002/mas.1280090303
61. Bogaerts A, Gijbels R (1999) New Developments and Applications in GDMS. Fresenius J Anal Chem 364:367–375. doi:10.1007/s002160051352
62. Nelis T, Pallosi J (2006) Glow Discharge as a Tool for Surface and Interface Analysis. Appl Spectrosc Rev 41:227–258. doi:10.1080/05704920600620345
63. Jakubowski N, Dorka R, Steers E, Tempez A (2007) Trends in Glow Discharge Spectroscopy. J Anal At Spectrom 22:722–735. doi:10.1039/B705238N
64. Penning FM (1927) Über Ionisation durch metastabile Atome. Naturwissenschaften 15:818. doi:10.1007/BF01505431

65. Bogaerts A (1999) The Glow Discharge: an Exciting Plasma! J Anal At Spectrom 14:1375–1384. doi:10.1039/A900772E
66. Xing Y, Xiaojia L, Haizhou W (2008) Determination of Trace Elements and Correction of Mass Spectral Interferences in Superalloy Analyzed by Glow Discharge Mass Spectrometry. Eur J Mass Spectrom 14:211–218. doi:10.1255/ejms.930
67. Winchester MR, Payling R (2004) Radio-Frequency Glow Discharge Spectrometry: A Critical Review. Spectrochim Acta, Part B 59B:607–666. doi:10.1016/j.sab.2004.02.013
68. Majidi V, Moser M, Lewis C, Hang W, King FL (2000) Explicit Chemical Speciation by Microsecond Pulsed Glow Discharge Time-of-Flight Mass Spectrometry: Concurrent Acquisition of Structural, Molecular and Elemental Information. J Anal At Spectrom 15:19–25. doi:10.1039/A905477D
69. Lewis CL, Moser MA, Dale DE Jr, Hang W, Hassell C, King FL, Majidi V (2003) Time-Gated Pulsed Glow Discharge: Real-Time Chemical Speciation at the Elemental, Structural, and Molecular Level for Gas Chromatography Time-of-Flight Mass Spectrometry. Anal Chem 75:1983–1996. doi:10.1021/ac026242u
70. Fliegel D, Fuhrer K, Gonin M, Guenther D (2006) Evaluation of a Pulsed Glow Discharge Time-of-Flight Mass Spectrometer as a Detector for Gas Chromatography and the Influence of the Glow Discharge Source Parameters on the Information Volume in Chemical Speciation Analysis. Anal Bioanal Chem 386:169–179. doi:10.1007/s00216-006-0515-1
71. Nagulin KY, Akhmetshin DS, Gilmutdinov AK, Ibragimov RA (2015) Three-Dimensional Modeling and Schlieren Visualization of Pure Ar Plasma Flow in Inductively Coupled Plasma Torches. J Anal At Spectrom 30:360–367. doi:10.1039/c4ja00254g
72. Bandura DR, Baranov VI, Tanner SD (2001) Reaction Chemistry and Collisional Processes in Multipole Devices for Resolving Isobaric Interferences in ICP-MS. Fresenius J Anal Chem 370:454–470. doi:10.1007/s002160100869
73. Wilbur S (2008) A Pragmatic Approach to Managing Interferences in ICP-MS. Spectroscopy 23:18–23
74. Aeschliman DB, Bajic SJ, Baldwin DP, Houk RS (2003) High-Speed Digital Photographic Study of an Inductively Coupled Plasma During Laser Ablation: Comparison of Dried Solution Aerosols from a Microconcentric Nebulizer and Solid Particles from Laser Ablation. J Anal At Spectrom 18:1008–1014. doi:10.1039/b302546m
75. Becker JS, Dietze HJ (1999) Application of Double-Focusing Sector Field ICP Mass Spectrometry with Shielded Torch Using Different Nebulizers for Ultratrace and Precise Isotope Analysis of Long-Lived Radionuclides. J Anal At Spectrom 14:1493–1500. doi:10.1039/A901762C
76. Myers DP, Hieftje GM (1993) Preliminary Design Considerations and Characteristics of an Inductively Coupled Plasma-Time-of-Flight Mass Spectrometer. Microchem J 48:259–277. doi:10.1006/mchj.1993.1102
77. Myers DP, Li G, Yang P, Hieftje GM (1994) An Inductively Coupled Plasma-Time-of-Flight Mass Spectrometer for Elemental Analysis. Part I: Optimization and Characteristics. J Am Soc Mass Spectrom 5:1008–1016. doi:10.1016/1044-0305(94)80019-7
78. Myers DP, Mahoney PP, Li G, Hieftje GM (1995) Isotope Ratios and Abundance Sensitivity Obtained with an Inductively Coupled Plasma-Time-of-Flight Mass Spectrometer. J Am Soc Mass Spectrom 6:920–927. doi:10.1016/1044-0305(95)00484-U
79. Hieftje GM, Myers DP, Li G, Mahoney PP, Burgoyne TW, Ray SJ, Guzowski JP (1997) Toward the Next Generation of Atomic Mass Spectrometers. J Anal At Spectrom 12:287–292. doi:10.1039/A605067K
80. Westphal CS, McLean JA, Acon BW, Allen LA, Montaser A (2002) Axial Inductively Coupled Plasma Time-of-Flight Mass Spectrometry Using Direct Liquid Sample Introduction. J Anal At Spectrom 17:669–675. doi:10.1039/B200771C
81. Tanner M, Guenther D (2008) Measurement and Readout of Mass Spectra with 30 μs Time Resolution, Applied to In-Torch LA-ICP-MS. Anal Bioanal Chem 391:1211–1220. doi:10.1007/s00216-008-1869-3

82. Milgram KE, White FM, Goodner KL, Watson CH, Koppenaal DW, Barinaga CJ, Smith BH, Winefordner JD, Marshall AG, Houk RS, Eyler JR (1997) High-Resolution Inductively Coupled Plasma Fourier Transform Ion Cyclotron Resonance Mass Spectrometry. Anal Chem 69:3714–3721. doi:10.1021/ac970126n
83. Becker JS, Dietze HJ (1998) Ultratrace and Precise Isotope Analysis by Double-Focusing Sector Field Inductively Coupled Plasma Mass Spectrometry. J Anal At Spectrom 13:1057–1063. doi:10.1039/A801528G
84. Yang L (2009) Accurate and Precise Determination of Isotopic Ratios by MC-ICP-MS: A Review. Mass Spectrom Rev 28:990–1011. doi:10.1002/mas.20251
85. Ardelt D, Polatajko A, Primm O, Reijnen M (2013) Isotope Ratio Measurements with a Fully Simultaneous Mattauch-Herzog ICP-MS. Anal Bioanal Chem 405:2987–2994. doi:10.1007/s00216-012-6543-0
86. Mahoney PP, Li G, Hieftje GM (1996) Laser Ablation-Inductively Coupled Plasma Mass Spectrometry with a Time-of-Flight Mass Analyzer. J Anal At Spectrom 11:401–405. doi:10.1039/JA9961100401
87. Pisonero J, Kroslakova I, Guenther D, Latkoczy C (2006) Laser Ablation Inductively Coupled Plasma Mass Spectrometry for Direct Analysis of the Spatial Distribution of Trace Elements in Metallurgical-Grade Silicon. Anal Bioanal Chem 386:12–20. doi:10.1007/s00216-006-0658-0
88. Neilsen JL, Abildtrup A, Christensen J, Watson P, Cox A, McLeod CW (1998) Laser Ablation Inductively Coupled Plasma-Mass Spectrometry in Combination with Gel Electrophoresis: A New Strategy for Speciation of Metal Binding Serum Proteins. Spectrochim Acta, Part B 53B:339–345. doi:10.1016/S0584-8547(98)00077-9
89. Chery CC, Moens L, Cornelis R, Vanhaecke F (2006) Capabilities and Limitations of Gel Electrophoresis for Elemental Speciation: A Laboratory's Experience. Pure Appl Chem 78:91–103. doi:10.1351/pac200678010091
90. Konz I, Fernandez B, Fernandez ML, Pereiro R, Gonzalez-Iglesias H, Coca-Prados M, Sanz-Medel A (2014) Quantitative Bioimaging of Trace Elements in the Human Lens by LA-ICP-MS. Anal Bioanal Chem 406:2343–2348. doi:10.1007/s00216-014-7617-y
91. Benninghoven A (1975) Developments in Secondary Ion Mass Spectroscopy and Applications to Surface Studies. Surf Sci 53:596–625. doi:10.1016/0039-6028(75)90158-2
92. Pachuta SJ, Cooks RG (1987) Mechanisms in Molecular SIMS. Chem Rev 87:647–669. doi:10.1021/cr00079a009
93. Benninghoven A, Werner HW, Rudenauer FG (eds) (1987) Secondary Ion Mass Spectrometry: Basic Concepts, Instrumental Aspects, Applications and Trends. Wiley Interscience, New York
94. Briggs D, Brown A, Vickerman JC (1989) Handbook of Static Secondary Ion Mass Spectrometry. Wiley, Chichester
95. Arnot FL, Beckett C (1938) Formation of Negative Ions at Surfaces. Nature 141:1011–1012. doi:10.1038/1411011c0
96. Arnot FL, Milligan JC (1936) A New Process of Negative-Ion Formation. Proc R Soc A 156:538–560. doi:10.1098/rspa.1936.0166
97. Herzog RFK, Viehbock FP (1949) Ion Source for Mass-Spectrography. Phys Rev 76:855–856. doi:10.1103/PhysRev.76.855
98. Benninghoven A (1969) Mechanism of Ion Formation and Ion Emission During Sputtering. Z Phys 220:159–180. doi:10.1007/BF01394745
99. Benninghoven A (1970) Analysis of Monomolecular Surface Layers of Solids by Secondary Ion Emission. Z Phys 230:403–417. doi:10.1007/BF01394486
100. Adams F (2008) Analytical Atomic Spectrometry and Imaging: Looking Backward from 2020 to 1975. Spectrochim Acta, Part B 63B:738–745. doi:10.1016/j.sab.2008.05.001
101. Benninghoven A, Sichtermann WK (1978) Detection, Identification and Structural Investigation of Biologically Important Compounds by Secondary Ion Mass Spectrometry. Anal Chem 50:1180–1184. doi:10.1021/ac50030a043

102. Coath CD, Long JVP (1995) A High-Brightness Duoplasmatron Ion Source for Microprobe Secondary-Ion Mass Spectrometry. Rev Sci Instrum 66:1018–1023. doi:10.1063/1.1146038
103. Konarski P, Kalczuk M, Koscinski J (1992) Bakeable Duoplasmatron Ion Gun for SIMS Microanalysis. Rev Sci Instrum 63:2397–2399. doi:10.1063/1.1142941
104. Pacholski ML, Winograd N (1999) Imaging with Mass Spectrometry. Chem Rev 99:2977–3005. doi:10.1021/cr980137w
105. Weibel D, Wong S, Lockyer N, Blenkinsopp P, Hill R, Vickerman JC (2003) A C_{60} Primary Ion Beam System for Time of Flight Secondary Ion Mass Spectrometry: Its Development and Secondary Ion Yield Characteristics. Anal Chem 75:1754–1764. doi:10.1021/ac026338o
106. Chait BT, Standing KG (1981) A Time-of-Flight Mass Spectrometer for Measurement of Secondary Ion Mass Spectra. Int J Mass Spectrom Ion Phys 40:185–193. doi:10.1016/0020-7381(81)80041-1
107. Standing KG, Chait BT, Ens W, McIntosh G, Beavis R (1982) Time-of-Flight Measurements of Secondary Organic Ions Produced by 1 keV to 16 keV Primary Ions. Nucl Instrum Methods Phys Res 198:33–38. doi:10.1016/0167-5087(82)90048-5
108. Jabs HU, Assmann G, Greifendorf D, Benninghoven A (1986) High Performance Liquid Chromatography and Time-of-Flight Secondary Ion Mass Spectrometry: A New Dimension in Structural Analysis of Apolipoproteins. J Lipid Res 27:613–621
109. Ens W, Standing KG, Chait BT, Field FH (1981) Comparison of Mass Spectra Obtained with Low-Energy Ion and High-Energy ^{252}Californium Fission Fragment Bombardment. Anal Chem 53:1241–1244. doi:10.1021/ac00231a026
110. Lafortune F, Beavis R, Tang X, Standing KG, Chait BT (1987) Narrowing the Gap Between KeV and Fission Fragment Secondary Ion Yields with Nitrocellulose. Rapid Commun Mass Spectrom 1:114–116. doi:10.1002/rcm.1290010707
111. Ens W, Main DE, Standing KG, Chait BT (1988) Comparison of Relative Quasi-Molecular Ion Yields for 8-keV Ion and ^{252}Cf Fission Fragment Bombardment. Anal Chem 60:1494–1498. doi:10.1021/ac00166a004
112. Olthoff JK, Honovich JP, Cotter RJ (1987) Liquid Secondary Ion Time-of-Flight Mass Spectrometry. Anal Chem 59:999–1002. doi:10.1021/ac00134a016
113. Linton RW, Mawn MP, Belu AM, DeSimone JM, Hunt MO Jr, Menceloglu YZ, Cramer HG, Benninghoven A (1993) Time-of-Flight Secondary Ion Mass Spectrometric Analysis of Polymer Surfaces and Additives. Surf Interface Anal 20:991–999. doi:10.1002/sia.740201210
114. Galuska AA (1997) ToF-SIMS Determination of Molecular Weights from Polymeric Surfaces and Microscopic Phases. Surf Interface Anal 25:790–798. doi:10.1002/(SICI)1096-9918(199709)25:10<790::AID-SIA301>3.0.CO;2-F
115. Bullett NA, Short RD, O'Leary T, Beck AJ, Douglas CWI, Cambray-Deakin M, Fletcher IW, Roberts A, Blomfield C (2001) Direct Imaging of Plasma-Polymerized Chemical Micropatterns. Surf Interface Anal 31:1074–1076. doi:10.1002/sia.1146
116. Liu S, Weng LT, Chan CM, Li L, Ho NK, Jiang M (2001) Quantitative Surface Characterization of Poly(styrene)/Poly(4-vinyl phenol) Random and Block Copolymers by ToF-SIMS and XPS. Surf Interface Anal 31:745–753. doi:10.1002/sia.1105
117. Médard N, Poleunis C, Vanden Eynde X, Bertrand P (2002) Characterization of Additives at Polymer Surfaces by TOF-SIMS. Surf Interface Anal 34:565–569. doi:10.1002/sia.1361
118. Davies N, Weibel DE, Blenkinsopp P, Lockyer N, Hill R, Vickerman JC (2003) Development and Experimental Application of a Gold Liquid Metal Ion Source. Appl Surf Sci 203-204:223–227. doi:10.1016/S0169-4332(02)00631-1
119. Nagy G, Walker AV (2007) Enhanced Secondary Ion Emission with a Bismuth Cluster Ion Source. Int J Mass Spectrom 262:144–153. doi:10.1016/j.ijms.2006.11.003
120. Touboul D, Kollmer F, Niehuis E, Brunelle A, Laprevote O (2005) Improvement of Biological Time-of-Flight-Secondary Ion Mass Spectrometry Imaging with a Bismuth Cluster Ion Source. J Am Soc Mass Spectrom 16:1608–1618. doi:10.1016/j.jasms.2005.06.005

121. Malmberg P, Nygren H (2008) Methods for the Analysis of the Composition of Bone Tissue, with a Focus on Imaging Mass Spectrometry (TOF-SIMS). Proteomics 8:3755–3762. doi:10.1002/pmic.200800198
122. Wong SCC, Hill R, Blenkinsopp P, Lockyer NP, Weibel DE, Vickerman JC (2003) Development of a C_{60}^{+} Ion Gun for Static SIMS and Chemical Imaging. Appl Surf Sci 203-204:219–222. doi:10.1016/S0169-4332(02)00629-3
123. Fletcher JS, Lockyer NP, Vickerman JC (2006) C_{60}, Buckminsterfullerene: Its Impact on Biological ToF-SIMS Analysis. Surf Interface Anal 38:1393–1400. doi:10.1002/sia.2461
124. Mas S, Perez R, Martinez-Pinna R, Egido J, Vivanco F (2008) Cluster TOF-SIMS Imaging: A New Light for in Situ Metabolomics? Proteomics 8:3735–3745. doi:10.1002/pmic.200800115
125. Briggs D, Hearn MJ (1985) Analysis of Polymer Surfaces by SIMS. Part 5. The Effects of Primary Ion Mass and Energy on Secondary Ion Relative Intensities. Int J Mass Spectrom Ion Proc 67:47–56. doi:10.1016/0168-1176(85)83036-6
126. Brunelle A, Laprevote O (2009) Lipid Imaging with Cluster Time-of-Flight Secondary Ion Mass Spectrometry. Anal Bioanal Chem 393:31–35. doi:10.1007/s00216-008-2367-3
127. Herrmann AM, Ritz K, Nunan N, Clode PL, Pett-Ridge J, Kilburn MR, Murphy DV, O'Donnell AG, Stockdale EA (2007) Nano-Scale Secondary Ion Mass Spectrometry – A New Analytical Tool in Biogeochemistry and Soil Ecology: A Review Article. Soil Biol Biochem 39:1835–1850. doi:10.1016/j.soilbio.2007.03.011
128. Fletcher JS, Rabbani S, Henderson A, Blenkinsopp P, Thompson SP, Lockyer NP, Vickerman JC (2008) A New Dynamic in Mass Spectral Imaging of Single Biological Cells. Anal Chem 80:9058–9064. doi:10.1021/ac8015278
129. Carado A, Passarelli MK, Kozole J, Wingate JE, Winograd N, Loboda AV (2008) C_{60} Secondary Ion Mass Spectrometry with a Hybrid-Quadrupole Orthogonal Time-of-Flight Mass Spectrometer. Anal Chem 80:7921–7929. doi:10.1021/ac801712s
130. Hellborg R, Skog G (2008) Accelerator Mass Spectrometry. Mass Spectrom Rev 27:398–427. doi:10.1002/mas.20172
131. Suter M (2004) 25 Years of AMS – A Review of Recent Developments. Nucl Instr Methods Phys Res B 223-224:139–148. doi:10.1016/j.nimb.2004.04.030
132. Stocker M, Doebeli M, Grajcar M, Suter M, Synal HA, Wacker L (2005) A Universal and Competitive Compact AMS Facility. Nucl Instr Methods Phys Res B 240:483–489. doi:10.1016/j.nimb.2005.06.224
133. Wacker L, Fifield LK, Olivier S, Suter M, Synal HA (2006) Compact Accelerator Mass Spectrometry: A Powerful Tool to Measure Actinides in the Environment. Spec Publ R Soc Chem 305:11–16
134. Nelson DE, Korteling RG, Stott WR (1977) Carbon-14: Direct Detection at Natural Concentrations. Science 198:507–508. doi:10.1126/science.198.4316.507
135. Bennett CL, Beukens RP, Clover MR, Grove HE, Liebert RB, Litherland AE, Purser KH, Sondheim WE (1977) Radiocarbon Dating Using Electrostatic Accelerators: Negative Ions Provide the Key. Science 198:508–510. doi:10.1126/science.198.4316.508
136. Lappin G, Garner RC (2004) Current Perspectives of ^{14}C-Isotope Measurement in Biomedical Accelerator Mass Spectrometry. Anal Bioanal Chem 378:356–364. doi:10.1007/s00216-003-2348-5
137. Brown K, Dingley KH, Turteltaub KW (2005) Accelerator Mass Spectrometry for Biomedical Research. Methods Enzymol 402:423–443. doi:10.1016/S0076-6879(05)02014-8
138. Ikeda T (2005) Instruments for Radiation Measurement in Life Sciences. VI. Use of accelerator mass spectrometry in studies on drug metabolism and pharmacokinetics. Radioisotopes 54:15–21. doi:10.3769/radioisotopes.54.15
139. Brown K, Tompkins EM, White INH (2006) Applications of Accelerator Mass Spectrometry for Pharmacological and Toxicological Research. Mass Spectrom Rev 25:127–145. doi:10.1002/mas.20059

Appendix

A.1 Units, Physical Quantities, and Physical Constants

The *International System of Units* (SI) provides the advantage of establishing uniformity and consistency of units for physical quantities – a prerequisite for communication in science.

Table A.1 SI base units

Physical base quantity	SI unit	Symbol
Length/distance	Meter[a]	m
Mass	Kilogram[b]	kg
Time	Second	s
Electric current	Ampere	A
Thermodynamic temperature	Kelvin[c]	K
Amount of substance	Mole	mol
Luminous intensity	Candela	cd

[a]1 m = 3.2808 ft. = 39.3701 in. 1 in = 2.54 cm; 1 ft. = 0.3048 m
[b]1 kg = 2.2046 lb.; 1 lb. = 0.4536 kg
[c]T[°C] = T[K] – 273.15; T[°F] = 1.8 × T[°C] + 32

Table A.2 Derived SI units with special names

Quantity	Name	Symbol	Expression in terms of base units	Expression in terms of other SI units
Frequency	Hertz	Hz	s^{-1}	
Force	Newton	N	$m\ kg\ s^{-2}$	$J\ m^{-1}$
Pressure	Pascal[a]	Pa	$kg\ m^{-1}\ s^{-2}$	$N\ m^{-2}$
Volume	Liter	l	$10^{-3}\ m^3$	
Energy	Joule[b]	J	$m^2\ kg\ s^{-2}$	N m
Power	Watt	W	$m^2\ kg\ s^{-3}$	$J\ s^{-1}$
Electric charge	Coulomb	C	A s	
Electric potential	Volt	V	$m^2\ kg\ A^{-1}\ s^{-3}$	$W\ A^{-1}$
Magnetic flux density	Tesla	T	$kg\ A^{-1}\ s^{-2}$	

[a]1 bar = 1000 mbar = 10^5 Pa; 1 Torr = 133 Pa; 1 psi = 6895 Pa = 68.95 mbar
[b]1 cal = 4.1868 J; 1 eV = 1.60219×10^{-19} J = 96.485 kJ mol^{-1}

J.H. Gross, *Mass Spectrometry*, DOI 10.1007/978-3-319-54398-7

Table A.3 Physical constants and frequently used quantities (from NIST)

Physical constant/quantity	Symbol	Quantity
Charge of the electron	e	$1.60217648 \times 10^{-19}$ C
Mass of the electron	m_e	$9.1093822 \times 10^{-31}$ kg
Mass of the proton	m_p	$1.67262164 \times 10^{-27}$ kg
Mass of the neutron	m_n	$1.67492721 \times 10^{-27}$ kg
Unified atomic mass	u	$1.66053878 \times 10^{-27}$ kg
Speed of light in vacuum	c	2.99792458×10^{8} m s^{-1}
Planck's constant	h	$6.62607004 \times 10^{-34}$ J s or $4.13566766 \times 10^{-15}$ eV s
Avogadro's constant	N_A	$6.02214179 \times 10^{23}$ mol^{-1}
Boltzmann constant	k_B	$1.38065042 \times 10^{-23}$ J K^{-1}
Universal gas constant	R	8.314459 J mol^{-1} K^{-1}

Table A.4 SI number prefixes

a	f	p	n	μ	m	c	d	k	M	G	T
Atto	Femto	Pico	Nano	Micro	Milli	Centi	Deci	Kilo	Mega	Giga	Tera
10^{-18}	10^{-15}	10^{-12}	10^{-9}	10^{-6}	10^{-3}	10^{-2}	10^{-1}	10^{3}	10^{6}	10^{9}	10^{12}

A.2 Isotopic Composition of the Elements

Table A.5 comprises the stable elements from hydrogen to bismuth with the radioactive elements technetium and promethium omitted. Natural variations in isotopic composition of some elements such as carbon or lead do not allow for more accurate values, a fact also reflected in the accuracy of their relative atomic mass. However, exact masses of the isotopes are not affected by varying abundances. The isotopic masses listed may differ up to some 10^{-6} u in other publications.

Table A.5 Isotopic mass, isotopic composition, and relative atomic mass [u] of non-radioactive elements. © IUPAC 2001

Atomic symbol	Name	Atomic No.	Mass No.	Isotopic mass	Isotopic comp.	Relative atomic mass
H	Hydrogen	1	1	1.007825	100	1.00795
			2	2.014101	0.0115	
He	Helium	2	3	3.016029	0.000137	4.002602
			4	4.002603	100	
Li	Lithium	3	6	6.015122	8.21	6.941
			7	7.016004	100	
Be	Beryllium	4	9	9.012182	100	9.012182
B	Boron	5	10	10.012937	24.8	10.812
			11	11.009306	100	
C	Carbon	6	12	12.000000	100	12.0108
			13	13.003355	1.08	
N	Nitrogen	7	14	14.003074	100	14.00675
			15	15.000109	0.369	
O	Oxygen	8	16	15.994915	100	15.9994
			17	16.999132	0.038	
			18	17.999161	0.205	
F	Fluorine	9	19	18.998403	100	18.998403
Ne	Neon	10	20	19.992402	100	20.1798
			21	20.993847	0.30	
			22	21.991386	10.22	
Na	Sodium	11	23	22.989769	100	22.989769
Mg	Magnesium	12	24	23.985042	100	24.3051
			25	24.985837	12.66	
			26	25.982593	13.94	
Al	Aluminium	13	27	26.981538	100	26.981538
Si	Silicon	14	28	27.976927	100	28.0855
			29	28.976495	5.0778	
			30	29.973770	3.3473	
P	Phosphorus	15	31	30.973762	100	30.973762
S	Sulfur	16	32	31.972071	100	32.067
			33	32.971459	0.80	
			34	33.967867	4.52	
			36	35.967081	0.02	
Cl	Chlorine	17	35	34.968853	100	35.4528
			37	36.965903	31.96	
Ar	Argon	18	36	35.967546	0.3379	39.948
			38	37.962776	0.0635	
			40	39.962383	100	
K	Potassium	19	39	38.963706	100	39.0983
			40	39.963999	0.0125	
			41	40.961826	7.2167	

(continued)

Table A.5 (continued)

Atomic symbol	Name	Atomic No.	Mass No.	Isotopic mass	Isotopic comp.	Relative atomic mass
Ca	Calcium	20	40	39.962591	100	40.078
			42	41.958618	0.667	
			43	42.958769	0.139	
			44	43.955481	2.152	
			46	45.953693	0.004	
			48	47.952534	0.193	
Sc	Scandium	21	45	44.955910	100	44.955910
Ti	Titanium	22	46	45.952629	11.19	47.867
			47	46.951764	10.09	
			48	47.947947	100	
			49	48.947871	7.34	
			50	49.944792	7.03	
V	Vanadium	23	50	49.947163	0.250	50.9415
			51	50.943964	100	
Cr	Chromium	24	50	49.946050	5.187	51.9962
			52	51.940512	100	
			53	52.940654	11.339	
			54	53.938885	2.823	
Mn	Manganese	25	55	54.938050	100	54.938050
Fe	Iron	26	54	53.939615	6.37	55.845
			56	55.934942	100	
			57	56.935399	2.309	
			58	57.933280	0.307	
Co	Cobalt	27	59	58.933200	100	58.933200
Ni	Nickel	28	58	57.935348	100	58.6934
			60	59.930791	38.5198	
			61	60.931060	1.6744	
			62	61.928349	5.3388	
			64	63.927970	1.3596	
Cu	Copper	29	63	62.929601	100	63.546
			65	64.927794	44.57	
Zn	Zinc	30	64	63.929147	100	65.39
			66	65.926037	57.37	
			67	66.927131	8.43	
			68	67.924848	38.56	
			70	69.925325	1.27	
Ga	Gallium	31	69	68.925581	100	69.723
			71	70.924705	66.367	
Ge	Germanium	32	70	69.924250	56.44	72.61
			72	71.922076	75.91	
			73	72.923459	21.31	
			74	73.921178	100	
			76	75.921403	20.98	

(continued)

Table A.5 (continued)

Atomic symbol	Name	Atomic No.	Mass No.	Isotopic mass	Isotopic comp.	Relative atomic mass
As	Arsenic	33	75	74.921596	100	74.921596
Se	Selenium	34	74	73.922477	1.79	78.96
			76	75.919214	18.89	
			77	76.919915	15.38	
			78	77.917310	47.91	
			80	79.916522	100	
			82	81.916700	17.60	
Br	Bromine	35	79	78.918338	100	79.904
			81	80.916291	97.28	
Kr	Krypton	36	78	77.920387	0.61	83.80
			80	79.916378	4.00	
			82	81.913485	20.32	
			83	82.914136	20.16	
			84	83.911507	100	
			86	85.910610	30.35	
Rb	Rubidium	37	85	84.911789	100	85.4678
			87	86.909183	38.56	
Sr	Strontium	38	84	83.913425	0.68	87.62
			86	85.909262	11.94	
			87	86.908879	8.48	
			88	87.905614	100	
Y	Yttrium	39	89	88.905848	100	88.905848
Zr	Zirconium	40	90	89.904704	100	91.224
			91	90.905645	21.81	
			92	91.905040	33.33	
			94	93.906316	33.78	
			96	95.908276	5.44	
Nb	Niobium	41	93	92.906378	100	92.906378
Mo	Molybdenum	42	92	91.906810	61.50	95.94
			94	93.905088	38.33	
			95	94.905841	65.98	
			96	95.904679	69.13	
			97	96.906021	39.58	
			98	97.905408	100	
			100	99.907478	39.91	
Ru	Ruthenium	44	96	95.907599	17.56	101.07
			98	97.905288	5.93	
			99	98.905939	40.44	
			100	99.904229	39.94	
			101	100.905582	54.07	
			102	101.904350	100	
			104	103.905430	59.02	

(continued)

Table A.5 (continued)

Atomic symbol	Name	Atomic No.	Mass No.	Isotopic mass	Isotopic comp.	Relative atomic mass
Rh	Rhodium	45	103	102.905504	100	102.905504
Pd	Palladium	46	102	101.905608	3.73	106.42
			104	103.904036	40.76	
			105	104.905084	81.71	
			106	105.903484	100	
			108	107.903894	96.82	
			110	109.905151	42.88	
Ag	Silver	47	107	106.905094	100	107.8682
			109	108.904756	92.90	
Cd	Cadmium	48	106	105.906459	4.35	112.412
			108	107.904184	3.10	
			110	109.903006	43.47	
			111	110.904182	44.55	
			112	111.902757	83.99	
			113	112.904401	42.53	
			114	113.903358	100	
			116	115.904755	26.07	
In	Indium	49	113	112.904061	4.48	114.818
			115	114.903879	100	
Sn	Tin	50	112	111.904822	2.98	118.711
			114	113.902782	2.03	
			115	114.903346	1.04	
			116	115.901744	44.63	
			117	116.902954	23.57	
			118	117.901606	74.34	
			119	118.903309	26.37	
			120	119.902197	100	
			122	121.903440	14.21	
			124	123.905275	17.77	
Sb	Antimony	51	121	120.903818	100	121.760
			123	122.904216	74.79	
Te	Tellurium	52	120	119.904021	0.26	127.60
			122	121.903047	7.48	
			123	122.904273	2.61	
			124	123.902819	13.91	
			125	124.904425	20.75	
			126	125.903306	55.28	
			128	127.904461	93.13	
			130	129.906223	100	
I	Iodine	53	127	126.904468	100	126.904468

(continued)

Table A.5 (continued)

Atomic symbol	Name	Atomic No.	Mass No.	Isotopic mass	Isotopic comp.	Relative atomic mass
Xe	Xenon	54	124	123.905896	0.33	131.29
			126	125.904270	0.33	
			128	127.903530	7.14	
			129	128.904779	98.33	
			130	129.903508	15.17	
			131	130.905082	78.77	
			132	131.904154	100	
			134	133.905395	38.82	
			136	135.907221	32.99	
Cs	Cesium	55	133	132.905447	100	132.905447
Ba	Barium	56	130	129.906311	0.148	137.328
			132	131.905056	0.141	
			134	133.904503	3.371	
			135	134.905683	9.194	
			136	135.904570	10.954	
			137	136.905821	15.666	
			138	137.905241	100	
La	Lanthanum	57	138	137.907107	0.090	138.9055
			139	138.906348	100	
Ce	Cerium	58	136	135.907145	0.209	140.116
			138	137.905991	0.284	
			140	139.905434	100	
			142	141.909240	12.565	
Pr	Praseodymium	59	141	140.907648	100	140.907648
Nd	Neodymium	60	142	141.907719	100	144.24
			143	142.909810	44.9	
			144	143.910083	87.5	
			145	144.912569	30.5	
			146	145.913112	63.2	
			148	147.916889	21.0	
			150	149.920887	20.6	
Sm	Samarium	62	144	143.911995	11.48	150.36
			147	146.914893	56.04	
			148	147.914818	42.02	
			149	148.917180	51.66	
			150	149.917271	27.59	
			152	151.919728	100	
			154	153.922205	85.05	
Eu	Europium	63	151	150.919846	91.61	151.964
			153	152.921226	100	

(continued)

Table A.5 (continued)

Atomic symbol	Name	Atomic No.	Mass No.	Isotopic mass	Isotopic comp.	Relative atomic mass
Gd	Gadolinium	64	152	151.919788	0.81	157.25
			154	153.920862	8.78	
			155	154.922619	59.58	
			156	155.922120	82.41	
			157	156.923957	63.00	
			158	157.924101	100	
			160	159.927051	88.00	
Tb	Terbium	65	159	158.925343	100	158.925343
Dy	Dysprosium	66	156	155.924279	0.21	162.50
			158	157.924405	0.35	
			160	159.925194	8.30	
			161	160.926930	67.10	
			162	161.926795	90.53	
			163	162.928728	88.36	
			164	163.929171	100	
Ho	Holmium	67	165	164.930319	100	164.930319
Er	Erbium	68	162	161.928775	0.42	167.26
			164	163.929197	4.79	
			166	165.930290	100	
			167	166.932045	68.22	
			168	167.932368	79.69	
			170	169.935460	44.42	
Tm	Thulium	69	169	168.934211	100	168.934211
Yb	Ytterbium	70	168	167.933894	0.41	173.04
			170	169.934759	9.55	
			171	170.936322	44.86	
			172	171.936378	68.58	
			173	172.938207	50.68	
			174	173.938858	100	
			176	175.942568	40.09	
Lu	Lutetium	71	175	174.940768	100	174.967
			176	175.942682	2.66	
Hf	Hafnium	72	174	173.940040	0.46	178.49
			176	175.941402	14.99	
			177	176.943220	53.02	
			178	177.943698	77.77	
			179	178.944815	38.83	
			180	179.946549	100	
Ta	Tantalum	73	180	179.947466	0.012	180.9479
			181	180.947996	100	

(continued)

Table A.5 (continued)

Atomic symbol	Name	Atomic No.	Mass No.	Isotopic mass	Isotopic comp.	Relative atomic mass
W	Tungsten	74	180	179.946707	0.40	183.84
			182	181.948206	86.49	
			183	182.950224	46.70	
			184	183.950933	100	
			186	185.954362	93.79	
Re	Rhenium	75	185	184.952956	59.74	186.207
			187	186.955751	100	
Os	Osmium	76	184	183.952491	0.05	190.23
			186	185.953838	3.90	
			187	186.955748	4.81	
			188	187.955836	32.47	
			189	188.958145	39.60	
			190	189.958445	64.39	
			192	191.961479	100	
Ir	Iridium	77	191	190.960591	59.49	192.217
			193	192.962924	100	
Pt	Platinum	78	190	189.959931	0.041	195.078
			192	191.961035	2.311	
			194	193.962664	97.443	
			195	194.964774	100	
			196	195.964935	74.610	
			198	197.967876	21.172	
Au	Gold	79	197	196.966552	100	196.966552
Hg	Mercury	80	196	195.965815	0.50	200.59
			198	197.966752	33.39	
			199	198.968262	56.50	
			200	199.968309	77.36	
			201	200.970285	44.14	
			202	201.970626	100	
			204	203.973476	23.00	
Tl	Thallium	81	203	202.972329	41.892	204.3833
			205	204.974412	100	
Pb	Lead	82	204	203.973029	2.7	207.2
			206	205.974449	46.0	
			207	206.975881	42.2	
			208	207.976636	100	
Bi	Bismuth	83	209	208.980383	100	208.980383
Th	Thorium*	90	232	232.038050	100	232.038050
U	Uranium*	92	234	234.040946	0.0055	238.0289
			235	235.043923	0.73	
			238	238.050783	100	

A.3 Carbon Isotopic Patterns

Provided no other element contributing to M + 1 is present, reading out the P_{M+1}/P_M ratio from a mass spectrum yields the approximate number of carbon atoms, n_C, from $n_C \approx (P_{M+1}/P_M) \times 91$. If M + 1 has an intensity of 24% of that of M, for example, we can calculate the presence of $(24/100) \times 91 \approx 22$ carbons.

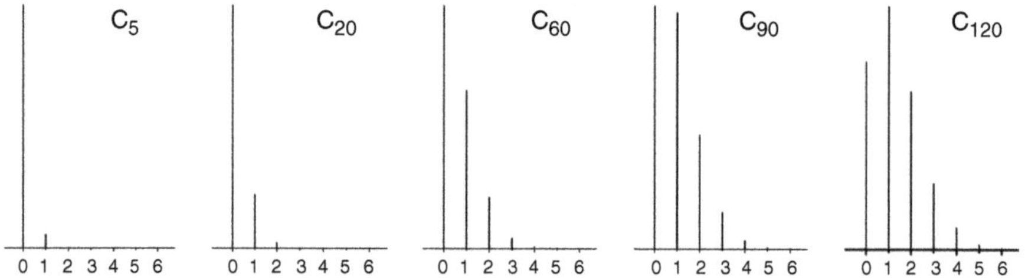

Fig. A.1 Calculated isotopic patterns for carbon. Note the steadily expanding width of the pattern as X + 2, X + 3, X + 4,... become visible. At about C_{90} the X + 1 peak reaches the same intensity as the X peak. At higher carbon number it becomes the base peak of the pattern

Table A.6 Calculated isotopic distributions for carbon

Number of carbons	X+1	X+2	X+3	X+4	X+5
1	1.1	0.00			
2	2.2	0.01			
3	3.3	0.04			
4	4.3	0.06			
5	5.4	0.10			
6	6.5	0.16			
7	7.6	0.23			
8	8.7	0.33			
9	9.7	0.42			
10	10.8	0.5			
12	13.0	0.8			
15	16.1	1.1			
20	21.6	2.2	0.1		
25	27.0	3.5	0.2		
30	32.3	5.0	0.5		
40	43.2	9.0	1.3	0.1	
50	54.1	14.5	2.5	0.2	0.1
60	65.0	20.6	4.2	0.6	0.2
90	97.2	46.8	14.9	3.5	0.6
120[a]	100.0	64.4	27.3	8.6	2.2

[a]The X peak has an intensity of 77.0% in that case

A.4 Chlorine and Bromine Isotopic Patterns

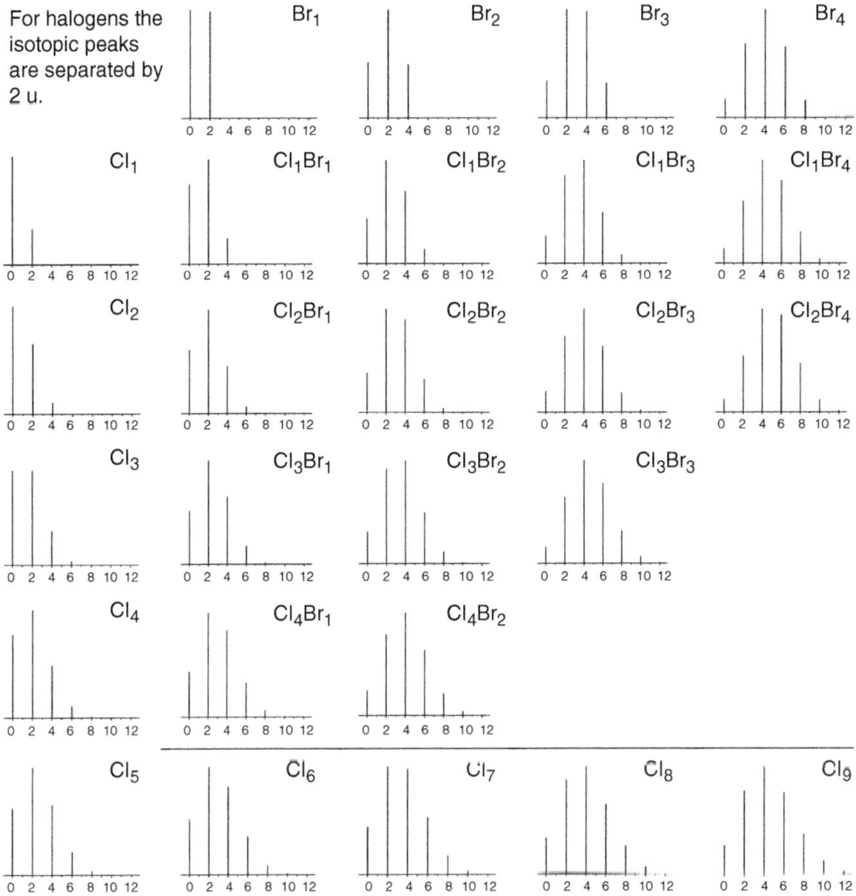

Fig. A.2 Calculated isotopic patterns for combinations of bromine and chlorine. The peak shown at zero position corresponds to the monoisotopic ion at m/z X. The isotopic peaks are then located at $m/z = \mathrm{X} + 2, 4, 6, \ldots$ The numeric value of X is given by the mass number of the monoisotopic combination, e.g., 70 u for Cl_2

A.5 Silicon and Sulfur Isotopic Patterns

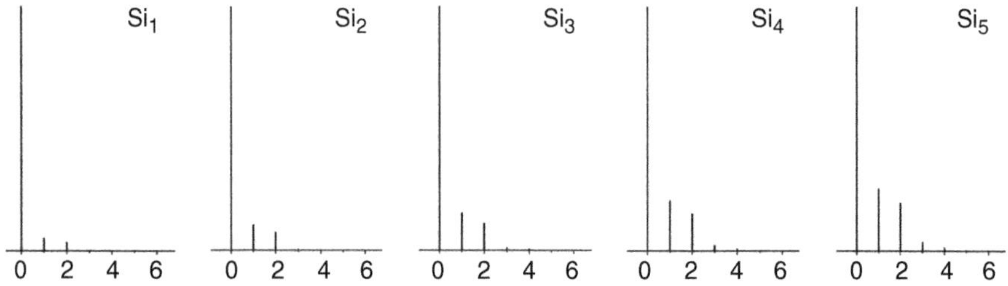

Fig. A.3 Isotopic patterns for silicon. The peak at zero position corresponds to the monoisotopic ion at *m*/*z* X. The isotopic peaks are then located at $m/z = X + 1, 2, 3, \ldots$

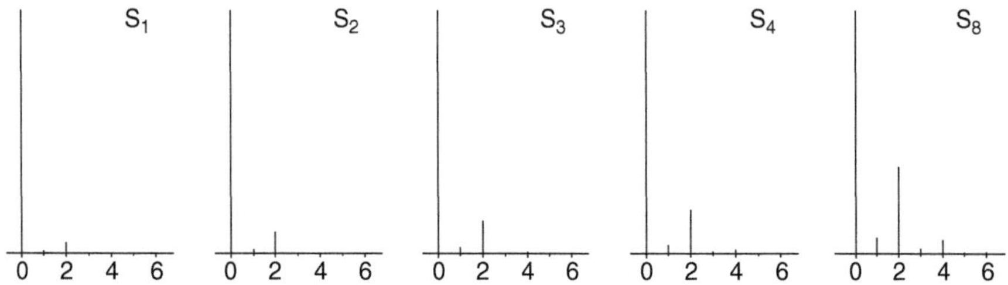

Fig. A.4 Isotopic patterns for sulfur. The peak at zero position corresponds to the monoisotopic ion at *m*/*z* X. The isotopic peaks are then located at $m/z = X + 1, 2, 3, \ldots$

A.6 Reading Isotopic Patterns

This flow chart can be used as a guideline on how to read and interpret isotopic patterns. The procedure is relevant irrespective of the ionization method employed.

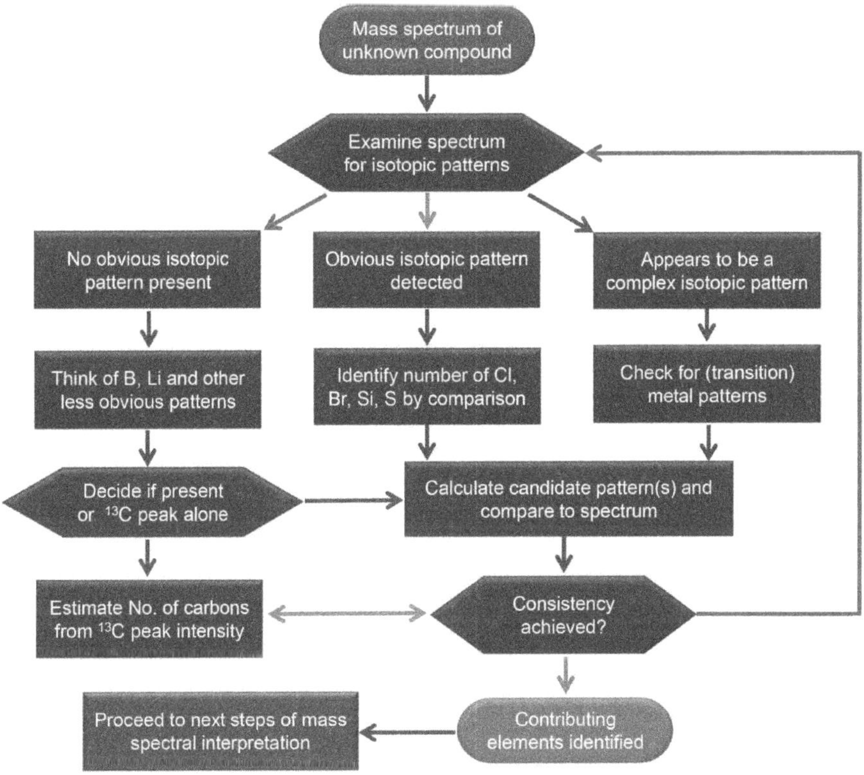

Fig. A.5 Guideline for the identification of contributing elements based on isotopic pattern analysis

A.7 Isotopologs and Accurate Mass

If isotopolog ions are resolved and sufficient mass accuracy is available, the distance between isotopic peaks can yield a new type of analytical information: the differences between isotopic masses are characteristic for certain elements.

Table A.7 Characteristic mass differences to identify the presence of elements

Pair of isotopes or modification	Δm [u]
^{6}Li vs. ^{7}Li	1.0009
^{10}B vs. ^{11}B	0.9964
^{12}C vs. ^{13}C	1.0033
^{32}S vs. ^{34}S	1.9958
^{35}Cl vs. ^{37}Cl	1.9970
^{58}Ni vs. ^{60}Ni	1.9955
^{63}Cu vs. ^{65}Cu	1.9982
^{79}Br vs. ^{81}Br	1.9980
^{191}Ir vs. ^{193}Ir	2.0023
gain or loss of H	1.0078
gain or loss of H_2	2.0156

A.8 Characteristic Ions and Losses

Care should be taken when using tables of characteristic ions and neutral losses as the values listed represent only a minor fraction of the fragmentations possible.

Table A.8 Characteristic ion series and neutral losses

Ion series	*m/z* and $[M{-}X]^+$ ions	Remarks
Carbenium ions	15, 29, 43, 57, 71, 85, 99, 113, 127, 141, ...	Any alkyl group
Acylium ions	29, 43, 57, 71, 85, 99, 113, 127, 141, 155, ...	Aliphatic aldehydes, ketones, carboxylic acids and their derivatives
Immonium ions	30, 44, 58, 72, 86, 100, 114, 128, 142, 156, ...	Aliphatic amines
Oxonium ions	31, 45, 59, 73, 87, 101, 115, 129, 143, 157, ...	Aliphatic alcohols and ethers
Sulfonium ions	47, 61, 75, 89, 103, 117, 131, 145, 159, ...	Aliphatic thiols and thioethers
From benzyl	39, 51, 65, 77, 91	Phenylalkanes
From benzoyl	51, 77, 105	Aromatic aldehydes, ketones, carboxylic acids and derivatives
	$[M{-}16]^{+\bullet}$, $[M{-}30]^+$, $[M{-}46]^{+\bullet}$	Nitroarenes
	45, 60, 73,$[M{-}17]^+$, $[M{-}45]^+$	Carboxylic acids
	59, 74, 87,$[M{-}31]^+$, $[M{-}59]^+$	Methyl carboxylates
	73, 88, 101,$[M{-}45]^+$, $[M{-}73]^+$	Ethyl carboxylates
By McL	44	McL of aldehydes
	58	McL of methyl ketones
	60	McL of carboxylic acids
	59	McL of carboxylic acid amides
	74	McL of methyl carboxylates
	88	McL of ethyl carboxylates
Halogens	$[M{-}19]^+$, $[M{-}20]^{+\bullet}$	Fluorine compounds
	35, $[M{-}35]^+$, $[M{-}36]^{+\bullet}$	Chlorine compounds (Cl pattern)
	79, $[M{-}79]^+$, $[M{-}80]^{+\bullet}$	Bromine compounds (Br pattern)
	127, $[M{-}127]^+$, $[M{-}128]^{+\bullet}$	Iodine compounds
General losses	$[M{-}1]^+$	Loss of $H^\bullet$ (strong → *α*-cleavage)
	$[M{-}2]^{+\bullet}$	Loss of H_2
	$[M{-}3]^+$	Loss of $H^\bullet$ and H_2
	$[M{-}15]^+$	Loss of methyl
	$[M{-}16]^{+\bullet}$	loss of O from nitroarenes
	$[M{-}17]^{+\bullet}[M{-}17]^+$	Loss of ammonia from amines, loss of $OH^\bullet$ from (*tert*)alcohols
	$[M{-}18]^{+\bullet}$	Loss of water from alcohols
	$[M{-}19]^+$	Loss of $F^\bullet$

(continued)

Table A.8 (continued)

Ion series	*m/z* and $[M-X]^+$ ions	Remarks
	$[M-20]^{+\bullet}$	Loss of HF
	$[M-27]^{+\bullet}$	Loss of HCN from heterocycles or HNC from aromatic amines
	$[M-28]^{+\bullet}$	Loss of CO, C_2H_4 or N_2
	$[M-29]^{+}$	Loss of $CHO^{\bullet}$ or $C_2H_5^{\bullet}$
	$[M-30]^{+\bullet}$	Loss of H_2CO from aromatic methyl ethers etc.; check for nitroarenes
	$[M-31]^{+}$	Loss of $MeO^{\bullet}$
	$[M-32]^{+\bullet}$	Loss of MeOH, O_2, (S)
	$[M-34]^{+\bullet}$	Loss of H_2S
	$[M-35/37]^{+}$	Loss of $Cl^{\bullet}$
	$[M-36/38]^{+\bullet}$	Loss of HCl
	$[M-42]^{+\bullet}$	Loss of CH_2CO or C_3H_6
	$[M-43]^{+}$	Loss of $CH_3CHO^{\bullet}$ or $C_3H_7^{\bullet}$
	$[M-44]^{+\bullet}$	Loss of CO_2
	$[M-45]^{+}$	Loss of $COOH^{\bullet}$, $EtO^{\bullet}$
	$[M-46]^{+\bullet}$	Loss of HCOOH, EtOH or NO_2
	$[M-48]^{+\bullet}$	Loss of SO from sulfoxides
	$[M-56]^{+\bullet}$	Loss of CH_3CHCO or C_4H_8
	$[M-57]^{+}$	Loss of $EtCHO^{\bullet}$ or $C_4H_9^{\bullet}$
	$[M-59]^{+}$	Loss of $COOMe^{\bullet}$ or $CH_2COOH^{\bullet}$
	$[M-64]^{+\bullet}$	loss of SO_2 from sulfolanes
	$[M-77]^{+}$	Loss of phenyl
	$[M-78]^{+}$	Loss of pyridyl
	$[M-79/81]^{+}$	Loss of $Br^{\bullet}$
	$[M-80/82]^{+\bullet}$	Loss of HBr
	$[M-91]^{+}$	Loss of benzyl or other $C_7H_7^{\bullet}$
	$[M-127]^{+}$	Loss of $I^{\bullet}$, rarely $C_{10}H_7^{\bullet}$ (naphthyl)
	$[M-128]^{+\bullet}$	Loss of HI

A.9 Common Impurities

Table A.9 Recognizing common impurities by *m*/*z*

m/*z*	Source
18, 28, 32, 40, 44	Residual air and moisture
149, 167, 279	Phthalic acid esters (plasticizers)
149, 177, 222	Diethyl phthalate (plasticizers)
73, 147, 207, 281, 355, 429	Silicon grease or GC column bleed (Si_x isotopic pattern)
27, 29, 41, 43, 55, 57, 69, 71, 83, 85, 97, 99, 109, 111, 113, 125, 127, ..., up to *m*/*z* 500	Hydrocarbons from grease or from suspensions in paraffin
32, 64, 96, 128, 160, 192, 224, 256	Sulfur (S_x isotopic pattern)
51, 69, 119, 131, 169, 181, 219, 231, 243, 281, 317, 331, ...	Background from PFK

A.10 Identification of the Molecular Ion Peak

- The molecular ion must be the ion of highest *m*/*z* in the mass spectrum (besides the corresponding isotopic peaks).
- It has to be an odd-electron ion, $M^{+\bullet}$.
- Peaks at the next lower *m*/*z* must be explainable in terms of reasonable losses, i.e., of common radicals or molecules. Signals at M–5 to M–14 and at M–21 to M–25 point towards a different origin of the presumed $M^{+\bullet}$ (Table 6.11).
- Fragment ions may not show isotopic patterns due to elements that are not present in the presumed molecular ion.
- No fragment ion may contain a larger number of atoms of any particular element than the molecular ion does.

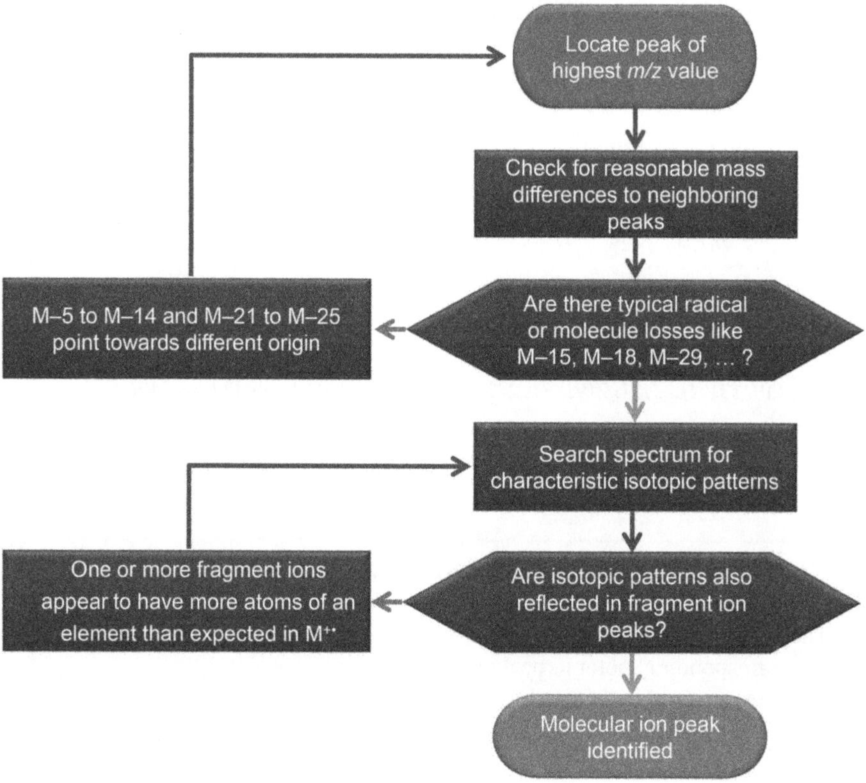

Fig. A.6 Flow chart showing decisions and criteria for the identification of the molecular ion peak

A.11 Rules for the Interpretation of Mass Spectra

- Identify the molecular ion! This is an important initial step, because it should derive the molecular composition (Sect. 6.7). If the EI spectrum does not allow for the identification of the molecular ion, soft ionization methods should be employed in addition.
- The mass differences between the presumed molecular ion and primary fragments must correspond to realistic chemical compositions (Sect. 6.7, Table 6.11).
- The calculated and experimental isotopic patterns have to agree with the molecular formula postulated (Sect. 3.2).
- The derived molecular formula must obey the nitrogen rule (Sect. 6.2.7). An odd-numbered *m/z* value of the molecular ion requires 1, 3, 5, ... nitrogen atoms to be contained, whereas an even *m/z* value belongs to 0, 2, 4, ... nitrogen atoms.
- Homolytic cleavages cause odd-numbered mass differences between fragment and molecular ion (Sect. 6.2.7). Rearrangement fragmentations cause even-

numbered mass differences. This rule toggles if odd numbers of nitrogen are contained in the neutral loss.

- In general, fragmentations obey the even-electron rule (Sect. 6.1.3). Odd-electron fragments from rearrangement fragmentations behave as if they were molecular ions of the respective smaller molecule.
- The competition of homolytic cleavages is governed by Stevenson's rule (Sect. 6.2.2). Thermodynamic stability of the pairs of products formed is decisive in selecting the preferred fragmentation route.
- Calculate r + d to check formula proposals and to derive some structural characteristics (Sect. 6.4.4).
- Write down a fragmentation scheme, thereby carefully tracking the origin of primary fragment ions and of characteristic ions used for structure assignment. From the purely analytical point of view this is very useful. However, one should keep in mind that any proposed fragmentation scheme remains a working hypothesis unless experimental confirmation is available.
- Employ additional techniques, such as measurement of accurate mass (Sect. 3.5), tandem mass spectrometry, or other spectroscopic methods to crosscheck and to refine your assignments.

A.12 Systematic Approach to Mass Spectra

- Collect background information such as origin of the sample, presumed compound class, solubility, thermal stability, or other spectroscopic information.
- Write *m*/*z* labels for all relevant peaks and calculate mass differences between prominent peaks. Do you recognize characteristic ion series or mass differences that point to common neutral losses?
- Check which ionization method was used and examine the general appearance of the mass spectrum. Is the molecular ion peak intense (as with aromatic, heterocyclic, polycyclic compounds) or weak (as with aliphatic and multifunctional compounds)? Are there typical impurities (solvent, grease, plasticizers) or background signals (residual air, column bleed in GC-MS)?
- Is accurate mass data available for some of the peaks?
- Now, follow the above rules to proceed.
- Derive information on the presence/absence of functional groups.
- Be careful when using collections of common neutral losses and *m*/*z*-to-structure relationship tables – they're never comprehensive. Even worse, one tends to get stuck on the first assumption.
- Put together the known structural features and try to assign the structure to the unknown sample. Sometimes, only partial structures of the analyte can be derived or isomers cannot be distinguished.
- Crosscheck proposed molecular structure and mass spectral data. This is also recommended between the single steps of mass spectral interpretation.

- Are there reference spectra available (at least of similar compounds) either from the literature or from mass spectral databases (Sect. 5.9)?
- Never rigidly follow this scheme! Sometimes, a step back or forth may accelerate the process or help to avoid pitfalls (Fig. A.7).

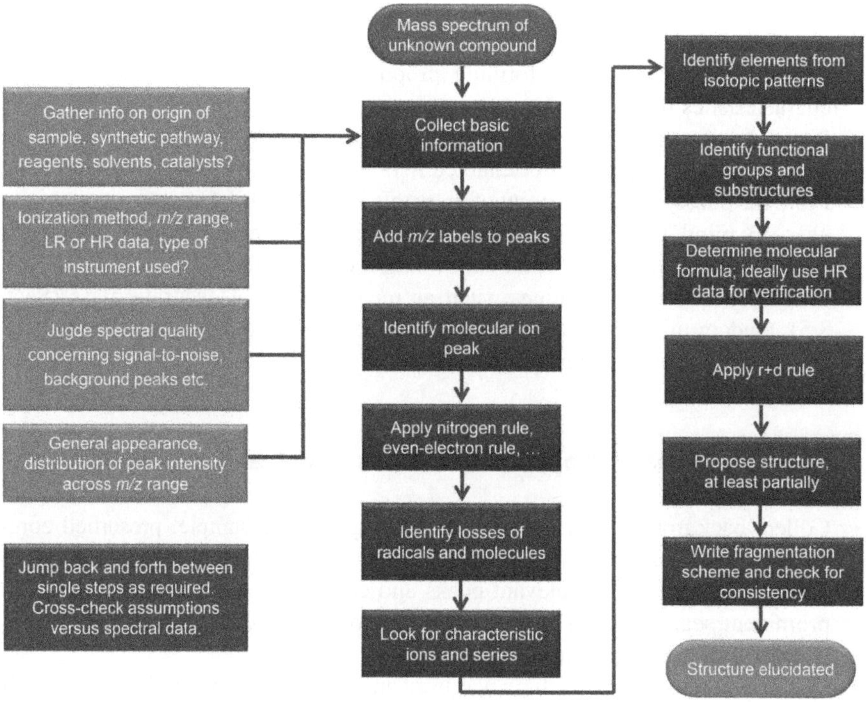

Fig. A.7 Guide to mass spectral structure elucidation

A.13 Method Selection Guide

This diagram (Fig. A.8) may help in selecting the right ionization method for analysis of a sample by MS. Often, there are several reasonable choices and it is advisable to make the best use possible of what is available at your local facility. MS results also depend on user input. Discuss your options with the MS staff at your facility.

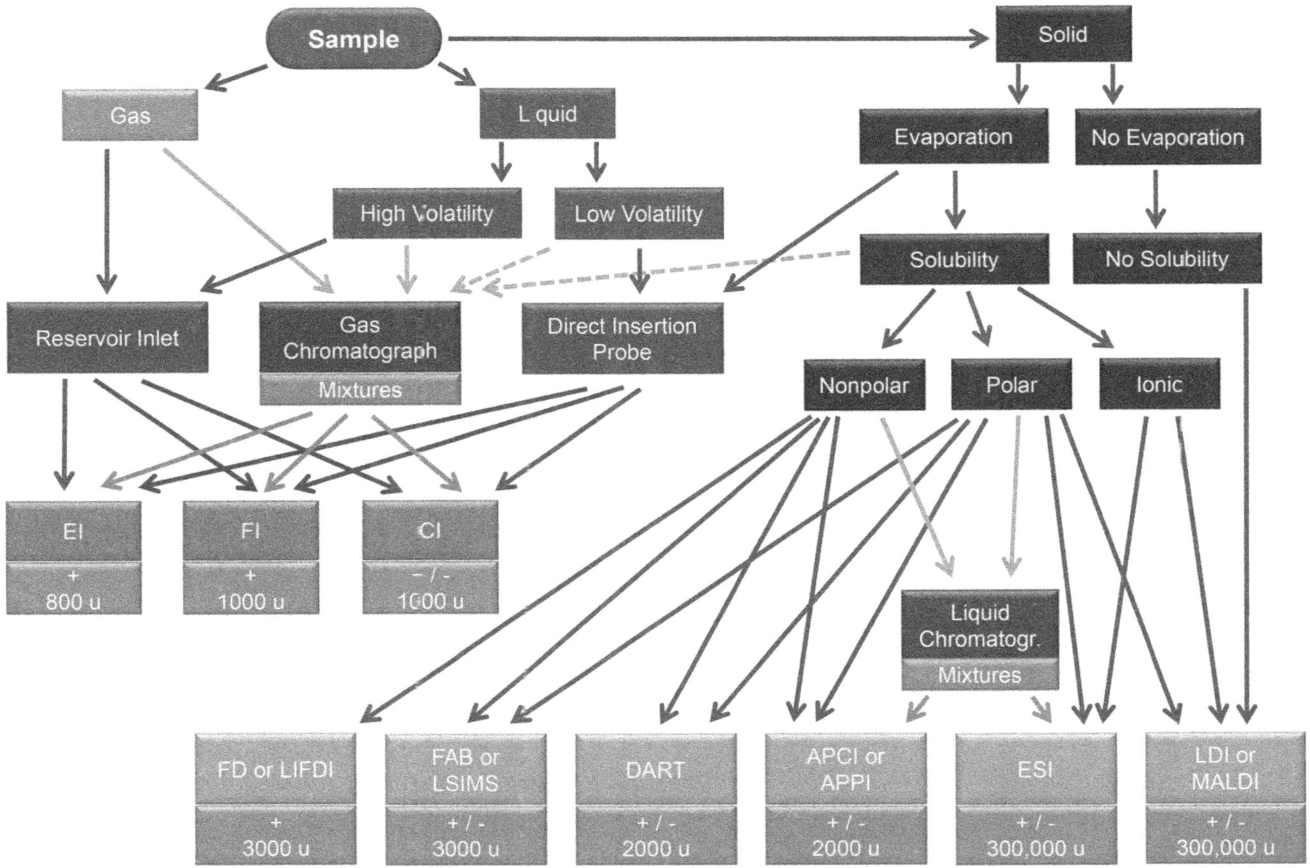

Fig. A.8 Method selection guide. Ionization methods with *bronze-colored* boxes require sample evaporation prior to ionization while methods with *orange* boxes accomplish transfer from the condensed phase along with ionization. The mass ranges are meant as guidelines and in no way define strict limits

A.14 How to Recognize Cationization

Soft ionization methods like FAB, FD, ESI, and MALDI often cause cationization by Na^+, K^+, Cs^+, and Ag^+. Especially Na^+, K^+ adducts are almost omnipresent. Other techniques like APCI and DART often yield NH_4^+ adducts in addition or competition to molecular ions and/or protonated molecules (Fig. A.9). Searching a spectrum for those characteristic $\Delta(m/z)$ values reveals the true molecular mass. It is particularly useful to identify adducts by their accurate mass differences (Table A.10).

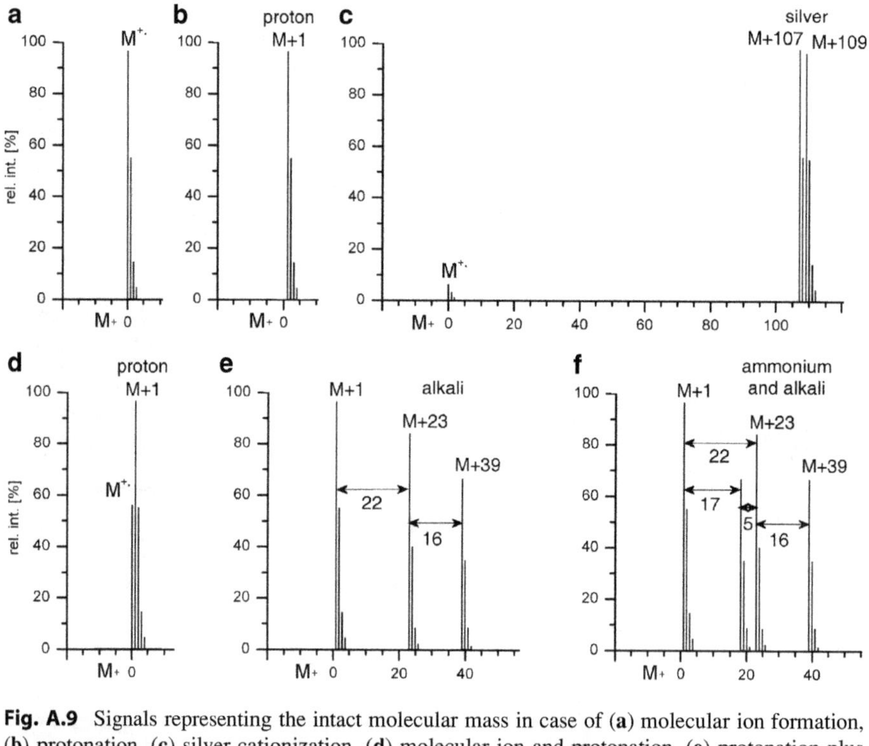

Fig. A.9 Signals representing the intact molecular mass in case of (**a**) molecular ion formation, (**b**) protonation, (**c**) silver cationization, (**d**) molecular ion and protonation, (**e**) protonation plus alkali cationization, and (**f**) protonation, ammonium plus alkali adduct formation. The relative abundances of the respective contributions are subject to wide variations. The abscissa gives the corresponding M + X nominal mass value; artificial isotopic patterns are added for more realistic appearance

Table A.10 Characteristic mass differences to identify frequent cation and anion adducts

Pair of ions	Δm [u]
$M^{+\bullet}$ vs. $^{13}C - M^{+\bullet}$	1.0033
$M^{+\bullet}$ vs. $[M + H]^+$	1.0078
$[M + H]^+$ vs. $[M + NH_4]^+$	17.0265
$[M + H]^+$ vs. $[M + Na]^+$	21.9819
$[M + H]^+$ vs. $[M + K]^+$	37.9559
$[M + Na]^+$ vs. $[M + K]^+$	15.9739
$M^{-\bullet}$ vs. $^{13}C - M^{-\bullet}$	1.0033
$[M - H]^-$ vs. $M^{-\bullet}$	1.0078
$[M - H]^-$ vs. $[M + OH]^-$	18.0106
$[M - H]^-$ vs. $[M + {}^{35}Cl]^-$	35.9767
$[M - H]^-$ vs. $[M + COOH]^-$	46.0055
$[M - H]^-$ vs. $[M + {}^{79}Br]^-$	79.9261
$[M - H]^-$ vs. $[M + CF_3COO]^-$	113.9928

A.15 Amino Acids

Table A.11 Amino acids (by order of residue mass)

Amino acid	Codes	Polarity	Charge[a]	Formula of residue	Residue nominal mass [u]	Residue accurate mass [u]
Glycine	Gly, G	nonpolar	O	C_2H_3NO	57	57.0520
Alanine	Ala, A	nonpolar	O	C_3H_5NO	71	71.0371
Serine	Ser, S	polar	O	$C_3H_5NO_2$	87	87.0320
Proline	Pro, P	nonpolar	O	C_5H_7NO	97	97.0528
Valine	Val, V	nonpolar	O	C_5H_9NO	99	99.0684
Threonine	Thr, T	polar	O	$C_4H_7NO_2$	101	101.0477
Cysteine	Cyc, C	nonpolar	O	C_2H_5NOS	103	103.0092
Leucine	Leu, L	nonpolar	O	$C_6H_{11}NO$	113	113.0841
Isoleucine	Ile, I	nonpolar	O	$C_6H_{11}NO$	113	113.0841
Asparagine	Asn, N	polar	O	$C_4H_6N_2O_2$	114	114.0429
Aspartic acid	Asp, D	polar	–	$C_4H_5NO_3$	115	115.0269
Glutamine	Gln, Q	polar	O	$C_5H_8N_2O_2$	128	128.0586
Lysine	Lys, K	polar	+	$C_6H_{12}N_2O$	128	128.0950
Glutamic acid	Glu, E	polar	–	$C_5H_7NO_3$	129	129.0426
Methionine	Met, M	nonp.	O	C_5H_9NOS	131	131.0405
Histidine	His, H	polar	(+)	$C_6H_7N_3O$	137	137.0589
Phenylalanine	Phe, F	nonpolar	O	C_9H_9NO	147	147.0684
Arginine	Arg, R	polar	+	$C_6H_{12}N_4O$	156	156.1011
Tyrosine	Tyr, Y	polar	O	$C_9H_9NO_2$	163	163.0633
Tryptophan	Trp, W	nonpolar	O	$C_{11}H_{10}N_2O$	186	186.0793

[a]Neutral amino acids are marked by O, basic AAs (+) tend to assume positive charge from protonation, acidic AAs (–) tend to be negative by dissociation of the acidic group

A.16 Nobel Prizes for Mass Spectrometry

Table A.12 Nobel laureates highly regarded in mass spectrometry

Laureate	Category and year	Prize motivation
Joseph John Thomson	Physics 1906	In recognition of the great merits of his theoretical and experimental investigations on the conduction of electricity by gases
Francis William Aston	Chemistry 1922	For his discovery, by means of his mass spectrograph, of isotopes in a large number of nonradioactive elements, and for his enunciation of the whole-number rule
Wolfgang Paul and Hans G. Dehmelt	Physics 1989	For the development of the ion trap technique
John B. Fenn jointly with Koichi Tanaka	Chemistry 2002	For their development of soft desorption ionization methods for mass spectrometric analyses of biological macromolecules

A.17 One Hundred Common Acronyms

ADC	Analog-to-digital converter
AE	Appearance energy
AMS	Accelerator mass spectrometry
APCI	Atmospheric pressure chemical ionization
API	Atmospheric pressure ionization
AP-MALDI	Atmospheric pressure matrix-assisted laser desorption/ionization
APPI	Atmospheric pressure photoionization
ASAP	Atmospheric solids analysis probe
B	Magnetic sector (as part of an instrument configuration)
CE	Capillary electrophoresis
CE	Charge exchange (equivalent to CT)
CI	Chemical ionization
CID	Collision-induced dissociation
CT	Charge transfer (formerly CE)
DART	Direct analysis in real time
DCI	Desorption (or direct) chemical ionization
DEI	Desorption (or direct) electron ionization
DE	Delayed extraction
DESI	Desorption electrospray/ionization
DIP	Direct insertion probe
E	Electrostatic sector (as part of an instrument configuration, cf. ESA)
EA	Electron affinity
EC	Electron capture
ECD	Electron capture dissociation

EDD	Electron detachment dissociation
EI	Electron ionization
ESA	Electrostatic analyzer (cf. E)
ESI	Electrospray ionization
ETD	Electron transfer dissociation
FAB	Fast-atom bombardment
FD	Field desorption
FI	Field ionization
FT-ICR	Fourier-transform ion cyclotron resonance
GB	Gas phase basicity
GC	Gas chromatography
GC-MS	Gas chromatography-mass spectrometry
GD	Glow discharge
HDX	Hydrogen–deuterium exchange
HR	High resolution
HV	High vacuum
HV	High voltage
ICP	Inductively coupled plasma
ICR	Ion cyclotron resonance
IE	Ionization energy
IMS	Ion mobility spectrometry
IR-MS	Isotope-ratio mass spectrometry
IR-MALDI	Infrared matrix-assisted laser desorption/ionization
IRMPD	Infrared multiphoton dissociation
KER	Kinetic energy release
LA	Laser ablation
LC	Liquid chromatography
LC-MS	Liquid chromatography-mass spectrometry (includes HPLC and UHPLC)
LDI	Laser desorption/ionization
LIFDI	Liquid injection field desorption/ionization
LIT	Linear quadrupole ion trap
LOD	Limit of detection
LR	Low resolution
LSIMS	Liquid secondary ion-mass spectrometry
MALDI	Matrix-assisted laser desorption/ionization
MCP	Microchannel plate
MID	Multiple ion detection
MIKES	Mass-analyzed ion kinetic energy spectroscopy
MS	Mass spectrometry (not to be used for 'mass spectrometer' or 'mass spectrum')
MS/MS	Mass spectrometry/mass spectrometry or tandem mass spectrometry
MRM	Multiple reaction monitoring
MUPI	Multiphoton ionization

nanoESI	Nano electrospray ionization
NCI	Negative-ion chemical ionization.
NICI	Negative-ion chemical ionization.
PA	Proton affinity
PCI	Positive-ion chemical ionization
PICI	Positive-ion chemical ionization
PIE	Pulsed ion extraction
PTR-MS	Proton transfer reaction-mass spectrometry
Py	Pyrolysis
Q	Linear quadrupole (as part of an instrument configuration)
q	RF-only linear quadrupole (as part of an instrument configuration)
QET	Quasi equilibrium theory
QIT	Quadrupole ion trap
RE	Recombination energy
REMPI	Resonance-enhanced multiphoton ionization
RF	Radio frequency
RIC	Reconstructed ion chromatogram
SEC	Size exclusion chromatography
SEM	Secondary electron multiplier
SIM	Selected ion monitoring
SIMS	Secondary-ion mass spectrometry
SRM	Selected reaction monitoring
SSMS	Spark source mass spectrometry
TI	Thermal ionization
TIC	Total ion chromatogram
TIMS	Thermal ionization mass spectrometry
TMP	Turbomolecular pump
TOF	Time-of-flight (analyzer)
TWIG	Traveling wave ion guide
UHR	Ultrahigh resolution
UHV	Ultrahigh vacuum
UV-MALDI	Ultraviolet matrix-assisted laser desorption/ionization.
YIKES	Well, after reading all that
ZEKE	Zero kinetic energy electron

Index

J.H. Gross, *Mass Spectrometry*, DOI 10.1007/978-3-319-54398-7

U

V